Textbook of Hearing Aid Amplification

Second Edition

A Singular Audiology Text
Jeffrey L. Danhauer, Ph.D.
Audiology Editor

Textbook of HEARING AID AMPLIFICATION

Second Edition

Edited by

Robert E. Sandlin, Ph.D.

Adjunct Professor of Audiology
San Diego State University
San Diego, California

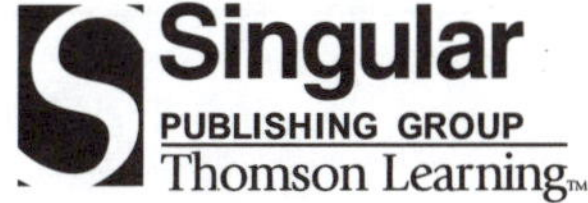

MW

Singular Publishing Group
Thomson Learning
401 West A Street, Suite 325
San Diego, California 92101-7904

Typeset in 10/12 Palatino by So Cal Graphics
Printed in Canada

Library of Congress Cataloging-in-Publication Data

The textbook of hearing aid amplification / editor, Robert E. Sandlin.— 2nd ed.
p. cm.
Rev. ed. of: handbook of hearing aid amplification. 1st ed. 1988.
Includes bibliographical references and index.
ISBN 1–56593–997–2 (softcover : alk. paper)
1. Hearing aids—Handbooks, manuals, etc. I. Sandlin, Robert E.

RF300 .H36 1999
617.8'9—dc21 99–047214

11/21/02

Contents

Preface

In 1988, the first edition of the *Handbook of Hearing Aid Amplification* (Volumes I and II) was published by Little, Brown and Company; a second printing was published by Singular Publishing Group in 1995. It was gratifying that each volume was well received in this country and abroad. There came a point in time, however, when the content was not sufficiently current to be of reasonable value to hearing health care professionals who select and fit hearing aid devices and who manage the acoustic and counseling needs of patients with hearing impairment.

When publishing a textbook dealing in part with technological advances in hearing aid design and function, it is readily evident that obsolescence is inevitable. When the first edition of the *Handbook of Hearing Aid Amplification* was released, members of our profession knew little if anything about the contributions of digital signal processing hearing instruments. Although we were aware of their potential, it was not until 1996 that wearable DSP devices became commercially available. The reader will find an excellent overview of digital signal processing hearing systems, as well as a review of DSP programming strategies in this new edition. An historical overview sets the stage for a review of technological advances over the past several decades. The principles of acoustic measurement and their clinical contributions are presented as an objective method of assessing hearing aid response. A discussion of the principles of signal processing applied to hearing aids is offered, providing the reader with an increased awareness of acoustic signals and what the hearing aid must do to amplify essential features of these signals to contribute to optimal speech discrimination. Advances in microphone technology, especially directional microphones, are reviewed, and their beneficial effect on signal-to-noise ratios is stressed. A treatise on taking earmold impressions, as well as on earmold acoustics and earmold resonances, is presented to assist the reader in gaining a better understanding of the processes involved. An overview of the principles of high-fidelity hearing instruments provides additional insights relating to some of the electroacoustic advances made in the 1990s. Attention is given to the technical and clinical aspects of sound-field audiometry. A review of hearing aid fitting methods brings fresh insights into their clinical applicability, in view of the development of more sophisticated analog and DSP devices. A current analysis of central processing disorders and hearing aid use offers additional insights into the clinical management of patient so afflicted. Assistive listening devices are reviewed, with emphasis given to the rationale for selection and use by those needing amplification assistance not provided by current hearing aids.

A discussion of the principles and application of cochlear implants contributes greatly the hearing health care professionals awareness of the assistance provided to those with profound hearing impairment who cannot benefit from more conventional amplification systems. Additionally, other advances in the selection and fitting process involving the psychological make-up of the patient with hearing impairment, ethical considerations and management practices, understanding the amplification needs of the geriatric population, and methods of assisting patient satisfaction with hearing aid amplification are reviewed. The hearing health care professional is becoming increasingly aware of the importance of understanding patient motivation in the acceptance and use of amplification systems. There is a growing sense of awareness that instrumental measurement of hearing aid performance is not an infallible indicator of user satisfaction. The value of aural rehabilitation is reviewed, with emphasis given to the need for dispensers to reassess their rehabilitative practices. Other subjectively based measurement tools for assessing hearing aid benefit contribute to our understanding of the human dynamics involved. A final chapter assesses future developments in hearing aid design, function, assessment, and user benefit.

In Volume II of the first edition, the author made the following statement: "There is a certain arrogance among those who comment about future considerations for hearing and amplification systems and those who use them. It is not that this arrogance is premeditated or intended, but rather that, in the absence of general consensus, any forecasting of that which should be becomes a very personal review and one subject to criticism." In this second edition, we have a greater ability to make statements about future advances in instrumental performance, and patient management strategies are not based solely on wishful thinking or flights of fancy, but on logical advances of existing technology.

In the new edition, the contributor's discuss a broad range of topics. To do otherwise would have been an abdication of responsibility to those who select and fit hearing aids. The successful use of amplification systems involves more than just determining the acoustic needs of the patient. It involves a level of understanding of human dynamics as they relate to the use and acceptance of hearing aids.

In the preface to Volume II of the first edition, the author stated, "Clinical approaches to the selection, fitting, and verification of hearing aid devices used by individuals with acoustic impairments often have appeared contradictory and less than absolute in meeting needs of persons who use amplification. The text is not intended to offer a resolution to all of the differences existing in decision-making processes regarding hearing aids, but rather to present ideas and clinical experiences of those professionals who deserve to be heard."

The opinion expressed then still holds today. We do not have common consensus about what needs to be addressed to determine appropriate hearing aid systems. Nonetheless, we have much more information about patient needs, and we have achieved greater advances in hearing aid technology to meet those needs. Although this textbook falls short of offering a panacea, it does offer current information that may contribute to the elimination of some uncertainties relating to the use of amplification.

As a final note, we have been fortunate to bring together a number of highly qualified individuals who have contributed their skills and clinical experiences to produce a textbook worthy of their efforts. An earnest attempt has been made to expand the content of this textbook to make it more current and clinically valuable. Conversely, we have deleted content that no longer has significant relevance to the selection and fitting of hearing aid devices. Those who contributed to the original edition have revised their chapters to bring them current with existing knowledge. There are several new authors who bring their expertise to bear on topics of interest to those who manage the hearing aid needs of the acoustically impaired. It is because of their scholarship and expertise that this textbook will be of value to the hearing health care professional.

As with most books to which a number of authors contribute, there is a certain amount of redundancy in this text. Every effort has been made to reduce needless redundancy, except where it clarifies what the author is describing and contributes to understanding the subject being discussed.

Acceptance of this book by those involved in the assessment, selection, and fitting of hearing aid amplification devices and their application to specific hearing impairments will serve as justification for the considerable effort put forth by the contributors who made it possible.

Contributors

Rose Bongiovanni, M.A., CCC-A
Private Practice
Newport Beach, California

Carl C. Crandell, Ph.D.
Department of Communication Sciences and Disorders
Institute for the Advanced Study of Communicative Processes
University of Florida
Gainesville, Florida

Laurel A. Christensen, Ph.D.
Etymotic Research
Elk Grove Village, Illinois

Inga Holube, Ph.D.
Head of Audiologic Research
Siemens Audiologishceh Technik GmbH
Erlangen, Germany

Holly Hosford-Dunn, Ph.D., CCC-A
Managing Member
Arizona Audiology Network, LLC
Tucson, Arizona

Judy L. Huch, M.S., CCC-A
President
Oro Valley Audiology, Inc.
Tucson, Arizona

Mead C. Killion, Ph.D.
President
Etymotic Research
Elk Grove Village, Illinois
Adjunct Professor of Audiology
Northwestern University
Evanston Illinois
Visiting Professor of Audiology
Rush University
Chicago, Illinois

Dawn Burton Koch, Ph.D.
Clinical Research Scientist
Advanced Bionics Corporation
Sylmar, California
Research Associate Professor
Northwestern University
Evanston, Illinois

Samuel F. Lybarger, B.S.
Retired

Edward H. Lybarger, B.A.
President
Arden Communications Group, Inc.
Meadow Lands, Pennsylvania

Robert Martin, Ph.D.
Private Practice
San Diego, California

Phillip T. McCandless, Ph.D.
Department of Communication Disorders
University of Mississippi Medical Center
Jackson, Mississippi

William McFarland, Ph.D.
Associate Professor
Department of Communicative Disorders
California State University–Long Beach
Long Beach, California

Michael J. Metz, Ph.D.
Private Practice
Audiology Associates
Irvine, California

Robert E. Novak, Ph.D.
Associate Professor
Program Director
Communication Disorders Program
University of Virginia
Charlottesville, Virginia

Mary Joe Osberger, Ph.D.
Director of Clinical Research
Advanced Bionics Corporation
Sylmar, California

Chester Z. Pirzanski, B.Sc.
Process Engineer
Starkey Labs Canada
Mississauga, Ontario
Canada

Robert E. Sandlin, Ph.D.
Adjunct Professor of Audiology
San Diego State University
San Diego, California

Joseph J. Smaldino, Ph.D.
Department of Communicative Disorders
University of Northern Iowa

Wayne J. Staab, Ph.D.
Wayne J. Staab & Associates
Phoenix, Arizona

Brad A. Stach, Ph.D.
President and Chief Executive Officer
Nova Scotia Hearing and Speech Clinic
Professor
School of Human Communication Disorders
Dalhousie University
Halifax, Nova Scotia
Canada

Robert W. Sweetow, Ph.D.
Director of Audiology
Professor of Audiology
University of California, San Francisco
San Francisco, California

Michael Valente, Ph.D.
Associate Professor of Otolaryngology
(Audiology)
Division of Adult Audiology
Washington University School of Medicine
St. Louis, Missouri

Andrew F. Valla, M.S., CCC-A
Clinical Audiologist
University of California, San Francisco
San Francisco, California

Therese M. Velde, Ph.D.
Siemens Hearing Instruments
New Jersey

Theodore H. Venema, Ph.D.
Manager of Audiology
Department of Research and Development
Unitron Industries
Kitchener, Ontario
Canada

Gary Walker, Ph.D.
National Acoustics Laboratories of Australia
Sydney, Australia

Sören E. Westermann, M.Sc.
Research Manager
Widex APS
Copenhagen, Denmark

Acknowledgments

I wish to acknowledge the support of many friends and colleagues who have contributed invaluable suggestions relative to the content and structure of this book. To those who have revised their chapters and to those who contributed new chapters, my sincere thanks.

This textbook is dedicated to students and health care professionals who seek a broader understanding of hearing aid amplification and of those who benefit from its use.

May it serve as a guide to appropriate decision making.

CHAPTER 1

A Historical Overview

SAMUEL F. LYBARGER, B.S.
EDWARD H. LYBARGER, B.A.

OUTLINE

Hearing impairment has been recognized as a handicap for many centuries. Amplification devices to ameliorate its effects date back at least several centuries, with their effectiveness increasing rapidly when electrical and electronic technologies became available. This chapter outlines some general history and gives a number of specific examples.

The authors acknowledge Dr. Kenneth W. Berger's book, *The Hearing Aid—Its Operation and Development* (1984), as one of the primary sources of historical material for this chapter. No material in the first edition was dated later than about 1987, and many important developments related to hearing aids have occured since then. Although it will be possible to mention only a limited number of these in this new edition, it is hoped that those selected will illustrate the important advances in technology and the tremendous reduction in size of today's hearing aids.

The authors received help from many sources, and particularly want to thank Elmer Carlson, Mead Killion, George Frye, Wayne Staab, and Dave Preves for their assistance. The 50th anniversary issue of *The Hearing Journal*, current issues of it and *The Hearing Review,* and our file of back issues of *Hearing Instruments* provided much help.

THE TIME FRAME

Hearing aid technology to date may be divided roughly into five main periods. The first is the acoustic era, during which devices such as horns, trumpets, and speaking tubes were utilized to amplify sound. The second is the carbon hearing aid era, during which telephone technology was adapted to hearing aid construction. The third is the vacuum tube era, which made possible greater amplification, wider response range, and reduced internal noise. The fourth era is the transistor era, and the fifth has been designated as the microelectric/digital era. Figure 1–1 illustrates these periods.

The Acoustic Era

Perhaps the first acoustic hearing aid was simply the hand cupped behind the ear. Berger (1984) noted that it has been recorded that the Roman emperor Hadrian (A.D. 117–135) used this method. There is considerable benefit from this universally available aid, which collects and reflects sound toward the pinna. Figure 1–2 shows curves of cupped-hand insertion gain. The solid curve is from de Boer (1982), who made the test on a manikin. The

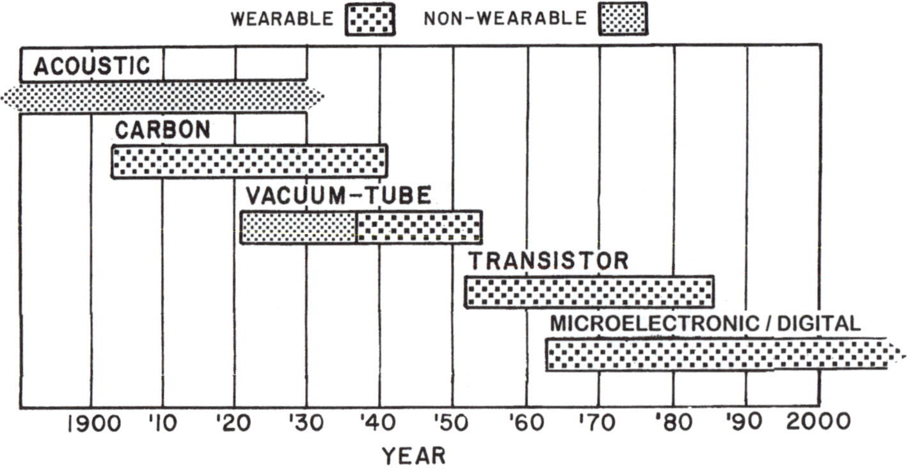

Figure 1–1. Principal hearing aid technology eras.

dotted curve was derived from data in a report by Filler, Ross, and Wiener (1945). It can be seen that there is quite useful amplification in the 1000 to 3000 Hz range.

According to Berger (1984), animal horns were used to aid hearing as early as the thirteenth century. De Boer (1982) measured the insertion gain of the horn shown in Figure 1–3 on a manikin and obtained the gain curve shown in Figure 1–4. Useful amplification is indicated between 250 and 2000 Hz.

References to man-made trumpets to aid hearing appeared in the 17th century. The idea of devices with a large opening tapering down to a small exit hole at the ear canal became well established in that century. Berger (1984) reported that the earliest illustration of a trumpet, a relatively simple funnel device, appeared in a book by Dekkers in 1673. In 1692, Nuck showed a rather complex trumpet, with a coiled section between a horn and the eartip.

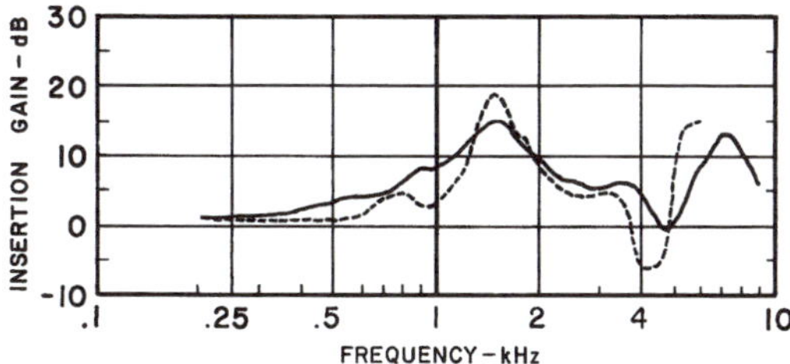

Figure 1–2. Insertion gain from a cupped hand. Solid curve from de Boer, 1982; dotted curve from Filler, Ross, and Wiener, 1945.

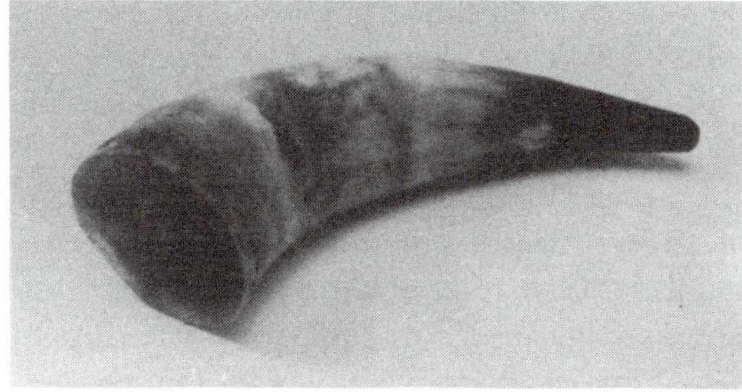

Figure 1–3. Antique animal horn. From de Boer, 1982. Reprinted with permission.

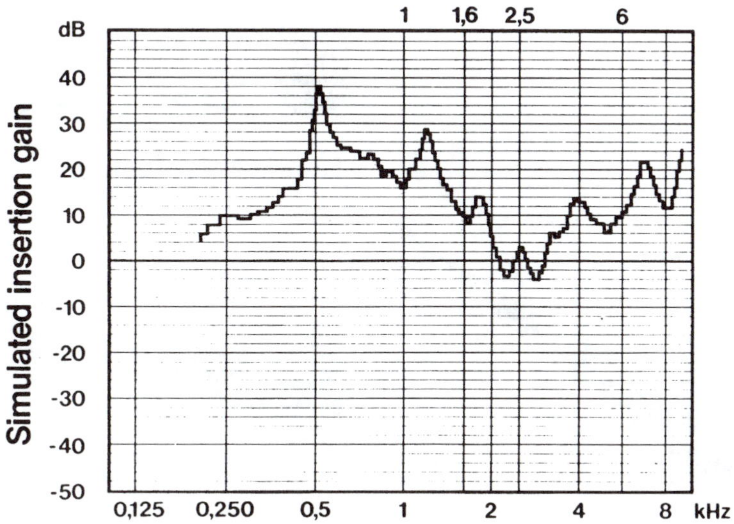

Figure 1–4. Insertion gain of animal horn. From de Boer, 1982. Reprinted with permission.

Further development of ear trumpets took place in the 1700s and particularly in the 1800s. These trumpets included, in addition to conical trumpets, "ladle" trumpets, pipe-shaped trumpets, and "dome" trumpets. The speaking tube long remained a standard item.

A "tin trumpet" illustrated in a catalog of William V. Willis & Co. (ca. 1930) was stated to be "the best known and most used of all hearing devices" (Figure 1–5). Cone diameters available ranged from 3¾ to 6 inches. Figure 1–6 shows a "London trumpet" from the same catalog. It was a folded horn to reduce length. Many other acoustic devices appeared in this catalog. One of them was called "auricles" (Figure 1–7). Not only was this a wearable acoustic device, but it was also binaural.

De Boer (1982) measured the insertion gain of several antique trumpets on a KEMAR manikin. One type is shown in Figure 1–8. The average insertion gain of four trumpets tested by de Boer is shown in Figure 1–9, along with curves for two transistor aids.

Acoustic devices are still being patented and used today (e.g., Goode, 1985). They have had the longest history by far of any form of hearing aid. Although not very acceptable cosmetically, the larger acoustic devices actually provided a great deal of gain and were of real benefit when no other means of amplification was known.

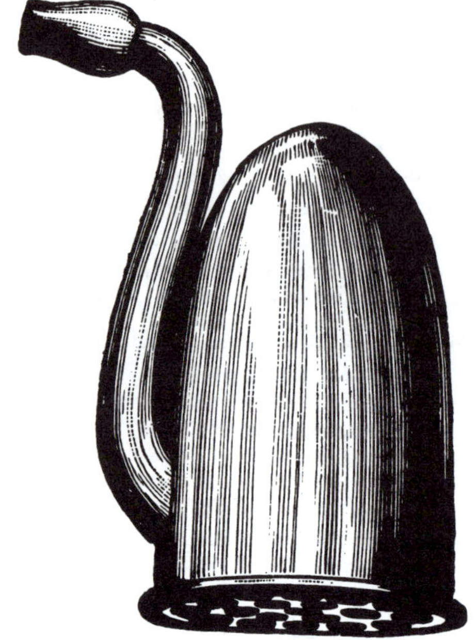

Figure 1–6. London trumpet from V. Willis & Co. catalog.

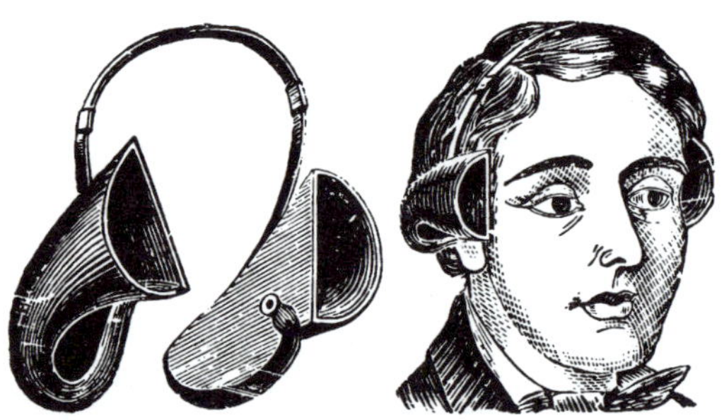

Figure 1–7. Auricles from Willis & Co. catalog.

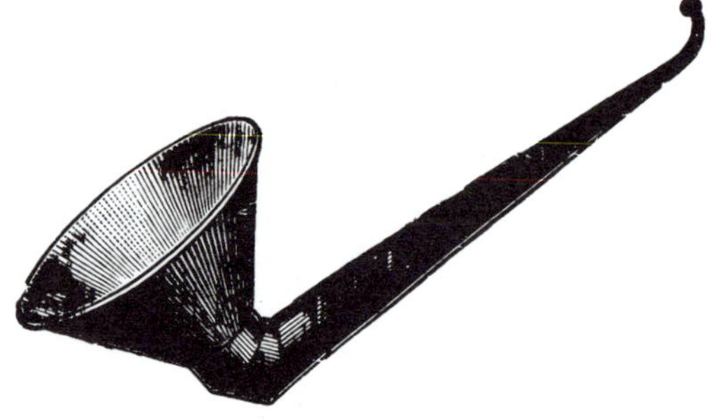

Figure 1–5. Tin trumpet from V. Willis & Co. catalog (CA. 1930).

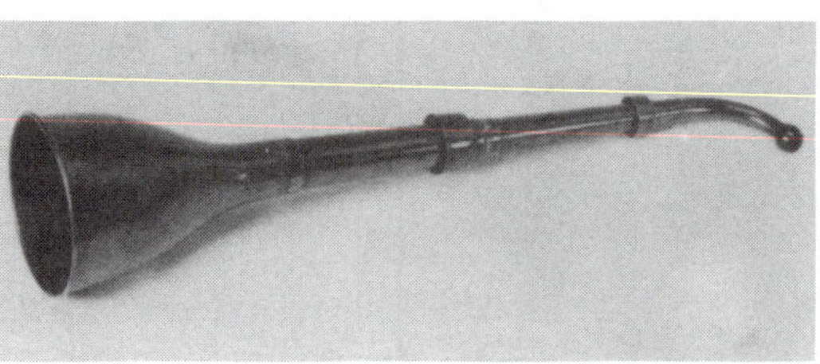

Figure 1–8. Antique trumpet. From de Boer, 1982. Reprinted with permission.

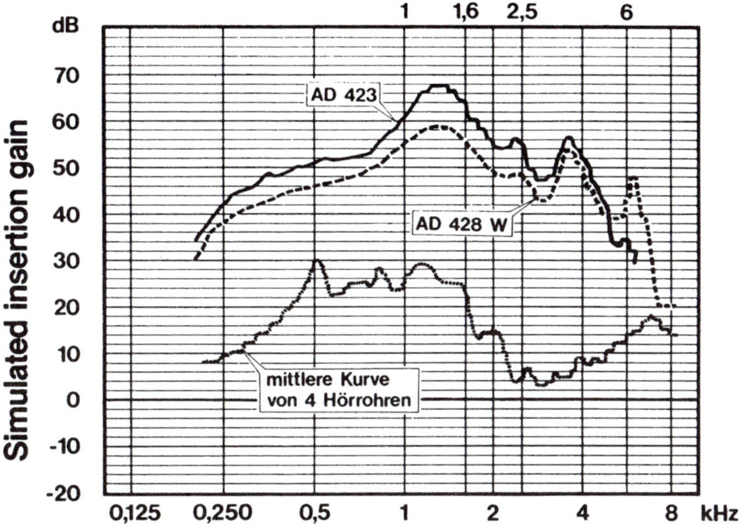

Figure 1–9. Average insertion gain of four antique trumpet (bottom curve, compaired to two transistor curves above). From de Boer, 1982. Reprinted with permission.

The Carbon Era

The telephone, invented by Alexander Graham Bell in 1876, used a magnetic microphone, which did not amplify sound. The invention of carbon transmitters by Blake and by Hughes in 1878 provided the amplification capability that made telephone technology adaptable to hearing aids.

The first practical commercially available wearable carbon hearing aid in the United States was made by Miller Reese Hutchinson in 1902, although Hutchinson had received a patent as early as 1899. His invention became the basis for "Acousticon" hearing aids. Berger (1984) gave excellent historical information on the adapation of telephone techniques to hearing aids.

Construction

The simple carbon hearing aid consisted of three elements: a sensitive carbon microphone, a magnetic receiver, and a battery, plus necessary connecting cords. An example of a simple but quite sensitive hearing aid microphone of 1930 is shown in Figure 1–10. The cover and diaphragm have been taken off to show the carbon backplate with eight pockets, each containing four highly polished 1.0 mm diameter carbon spheres (termed *globules*). With the 2¼ inch diameter by 0.015 inch thick carbon diaphragm held in place a few thousandths of an inch from the backplate by screwing on the cover, and with the microphone in a vertical position, the carbon globules rest gently against the diaphragm and the sloping sidewalls of the pockets. Vibration of the diaphragm produces relatively large variations in the microphone resistance and the battery current passing through the magnetic receiver winding is modulated correspondingly.

Instead of globules, some microphones used carbon granules similar to those used in telephone transmitters. These were held in a shallow cylindrical pocket between the diaphragm and a backplate. A washer of felt or similar material held the granules in place. The surface areas of the diaphragm (if metal) and the back electrode were often gold-plated.

Figure 1–11 shows some of the types of carbon used. In the left ring is carbon granule material, which was used in both microphones and carbon amplifiers, particularly by Western Electric. In the center ring are small highly polished carbon globules, typically 0.5 or 0.6 mm in diameter, used mainly in carbon amplifiers. In the right ring are the larger 1.0 mm polished carbon globules used in microphones such as that in Figure 1–10.

Magnetic receivers, either bipolar or monopolar, were used with carbon aids. Early receivers were of the large "watch-case" size; miniaturized receivers followed in the 1920s. An open view of a 1930 miniature receiver is shown in Figure 1–12. Three permanent magnets were used. A coil on the central soft iron core was wound to give the desired

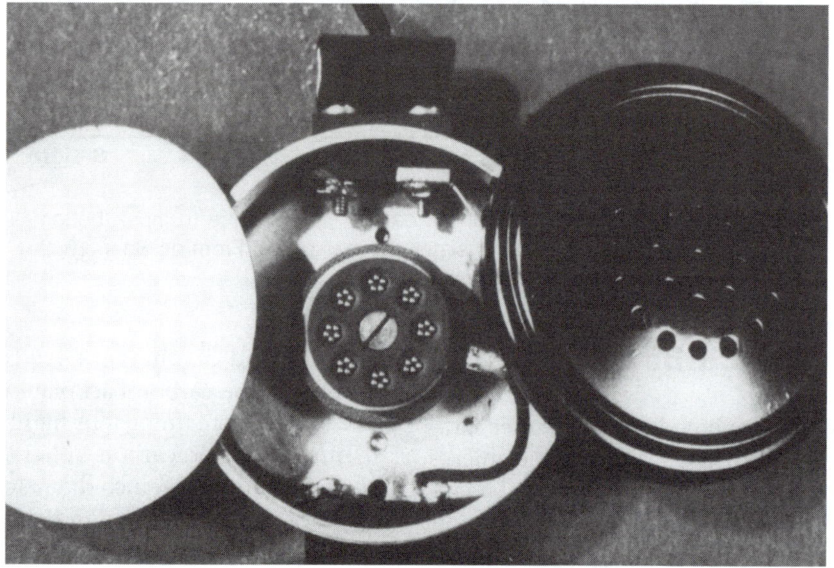

Figure 1–10. 1930 carbon microphone with cover removed.

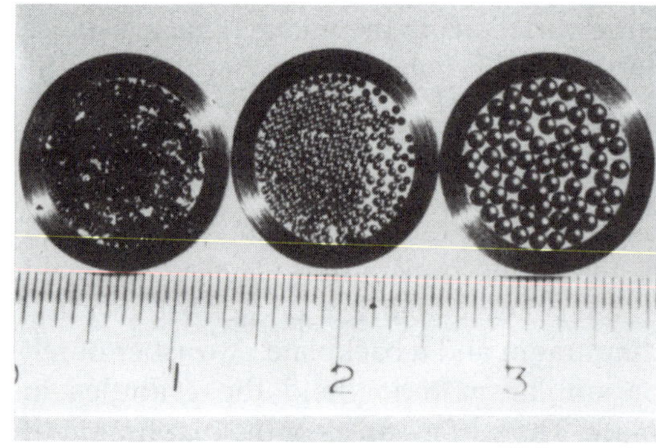

Figure 1–11. Types of carbon. Left: carbon granules. Center: 0.5 mm polished globules. Right: 1.0 mm polished globules.

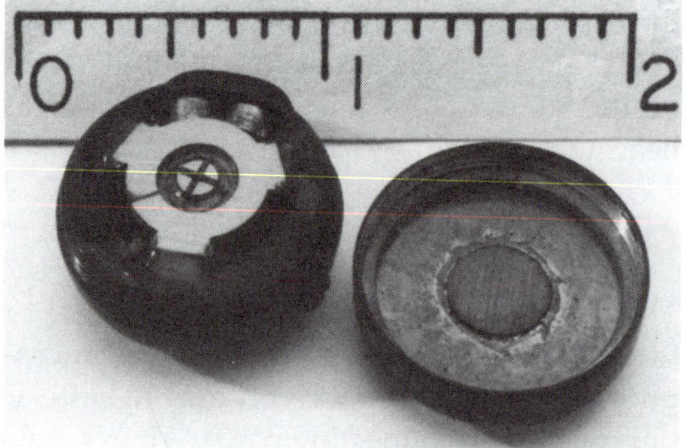

Figure 1–12. 1930 miniature magnetic receiver.

electrical impedance. The diaphragm, which has a soft iron armature attached, was clamped in the receiver cap. Accurate adjustment of the air gap was made by screwing the cap on the case to the correct position.

Batteries for carbon hearing aids were of the carbon-zinc type, mostly two or three cell. Batteries usually were custom made, with sockets to fit a particular manufacturer's hearing aids. Some hearing aids could use flashlight batteries.

The microphone shown in Figure 1–10 is of the "direct" type, with sound impinging directly on the diaphragm through holes in the cover. "Indirect" microphones had the diaphragm facing away from the talker and into a dish-shaped reflector-resonator. The sound entered the reflector through openings surrounding the basic microphone case. The indirect construction is shown in Figure 1–22. Microphone output could be increased by 5 or 10 dB by the reflector, mostly in the 1000 to 3500 Hz range.

Multiple microphones, both direct and indirect, were used in an effort to increase gain and output. Hearing aids with two microphones were extensively used.

Carbon Amplifiers

Because of the limited gain of the simple carbon hearing aid, carbon amplifiers were developed. Similar devices, called microphonic relays, had been used in telephony. An early carbon amplifier was invented by Sell (1925) for Siemens hearing aids (Figure 1–13). Carbon amplifiers, or "boosters," were used widely in the 1930s.

The principle of the carbon amplifier is simple. The vibration of the receiver diaphragm, instead of producing amplified sound in the ear canal, is used to drive another microphone, or carbon cell, that further increases the signal delivered to the receiver. In Figure 1–13, the magnetic system, receiving the energy from the microphone, causes a diaphragm (35) to vibrate. The opposite side of the diaphragm forms one electrode of a shallow cylindrical carbon cell in which there are carbon granules (41). The back of the carbon cell is formed by electrode 43.

Another type of carbon amplifier is shown in Figure 1–14. In this design, a vibrating reed carries a carbon electrode spaced a small distance from an insulating block in which there

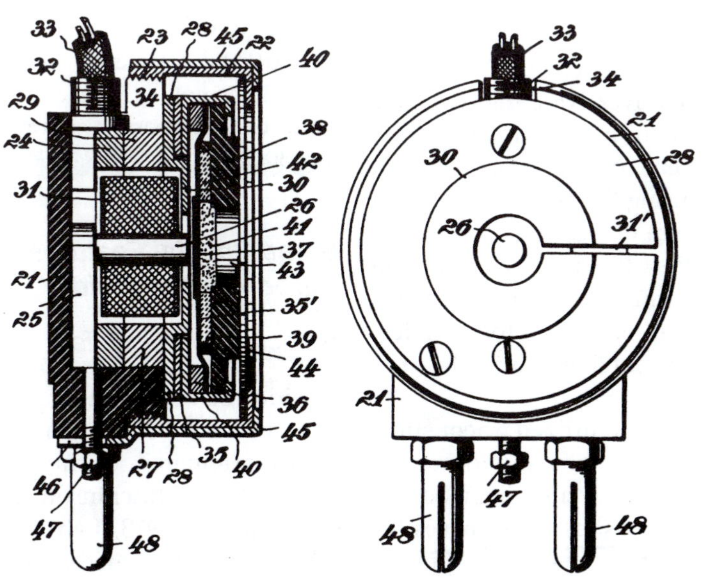

Figure 1–13. Carbon amplifier (Sell, 1925).

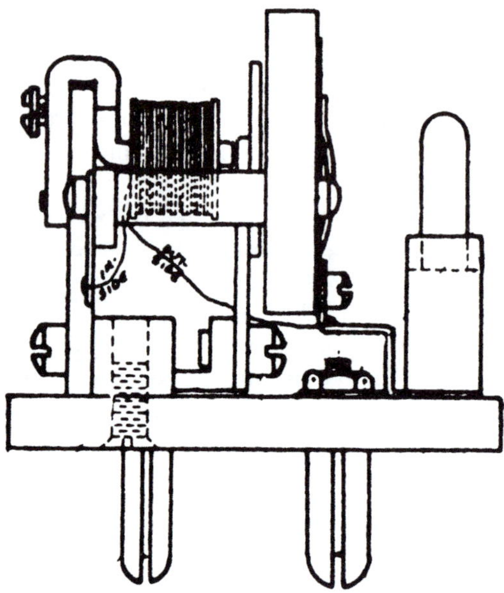

Figure 1–14. Carbon amplifier—vibrating reed type. (CA. 1934).

is a shallow cylindrical carbon cell. Carbon globules rather than granules were used in this device. A second carbon electrode closed the cell.

Figure 1–15 shows a circuit for an amplified carbon hearing aid. One battery current loop includes the microphone and the amplifier winding; a second loop includes the carbon cell and the receiver. Note the two variable resistance sections in the volume control, necessary to prevent common impedance in the loops from causing "motorboating." Even internal resistance in the batteries sometimes can cause oscillation. It is interesting to note that the motorboating problem, which has plagued hearing aid engineers for decades, was present even in amplified carbon hearing aids.

Although not standardized, acoustical measurements that gave some idea of carbon hearing aid performance were being made by 1932. Figure 1–16 shows response curves for two hearing aids as given in a 1932 engineering report. A large condenser microphone was used to measure the sound pressure level in both the field and in the coupler (see Figure 1–50), which had a volume of about 0.5 cc. The solid curve is for an amplified Western Electric Model 38-A. The dotted curve is for an unamplified Radioear Model B-7A. The dash-dot curve shows the useful increased gain when the B-7A was placed in its small carrying case.

Figure 1–17 shows the gain of the 38-A amplifier alone. Gain up to 1500 Hz averages about 12 dB; peak gain is about 26 dB. Figure 1–18 indicates 1937 gain curves for a Radioear model. This model had three available microphones, four amplifiers, one flat and three miniature air receivers, and three bone receivers.

Figure 1–18 shows the gain using a #1 microphone and a #2 miniature air receiver in combination with four different amplifiers and without any amplifier (lowest dotted curve). These tests would have been made with a coupler employing a one-half inch microphone.

Figure 1–19 shows response curves for the carbon amplifiers. The amplified gain is the response curve minus the lowest dotted curve, which was made without any amplifier in the test circuit. Gain ranged from about 8 to 17 dB in the low frequencies to about 21 to 29 dB at the peaks.

It will be noted that the high frequency cutoff of carbon hearing aids generally was below 3000 Hz.

Some Special Features of Carbon Hearing Aids

Selective Amplification

The idea that different amplification patterns were needed for different types of hearing losses originated during the carbon era. Miller Reese Hutchinson, in 1905, Hincks (England), in 1913, Lybarger, in 1938, and others patented devices to select combinations of carbon hearing aid components.

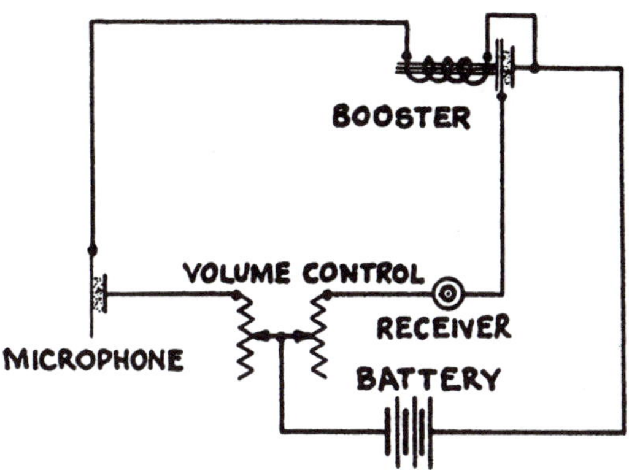

Figure 1–15. Circuit for an amplified carbon hearing aid.

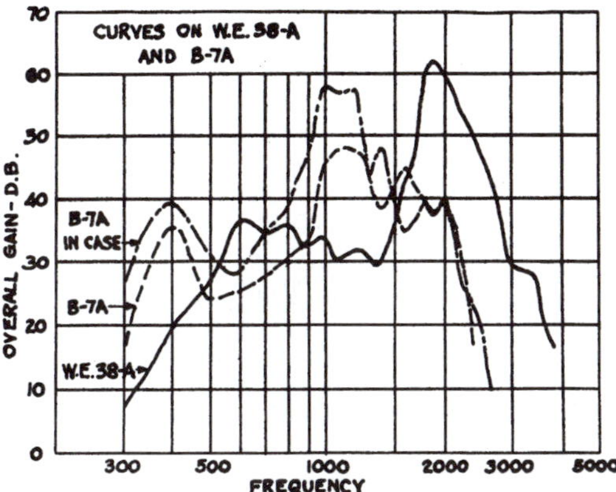

Figure 1–16. Response curves of an amplified and unamplified carbon aid.

Bone Conduction

The first wearable bone conduction hearing aid was introduced by Sonotone Corporation in 1932. The bone receiver (Lieber, 1933) had a small projecting gold-plated button attached to a vibrating strip driven by a magnetic system. It was held against the mastoid by a headband. A regular amplified carbon hearing aid was used to drive the receiver. According to an available engineering report, this early bone conduction hearing aid produced a somewhat lower sensation level on a normal ear than would be produced by direct listening in a sound field. Thus, the gain for a normal ear was negative. However, if a large air-bone gap existed, the gain could be substantial. Figure 1–20 is a graph from the report.

The pressure of the small button of the receiver against the head made it uncomfortable to wear. Also, the air gap, and thus the sensitivity, changed with static force. One later receiver (Lybarger, 1941) distributed the static force over a much larger smooth receiver face and also kept the air gap nearly constant with respect to static force.

A major improvement in bone receiver construction was made by Greibach of Sonotone, a construction that is the principal one in use today. After long patent interference litigation with Koch of Acousticon, Greibach (1939) was granted a patent on a "reaction" type bone receiver. Its magnetic air gap was

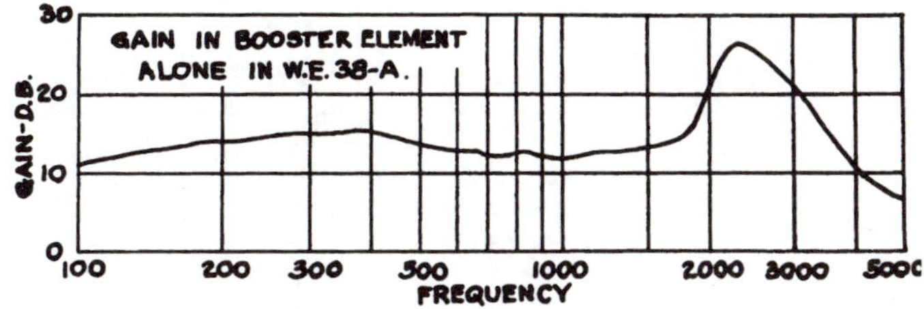

Figure 1–17. Gain of amplifier alone (Western Electric model 38-A carbon hearing aid).

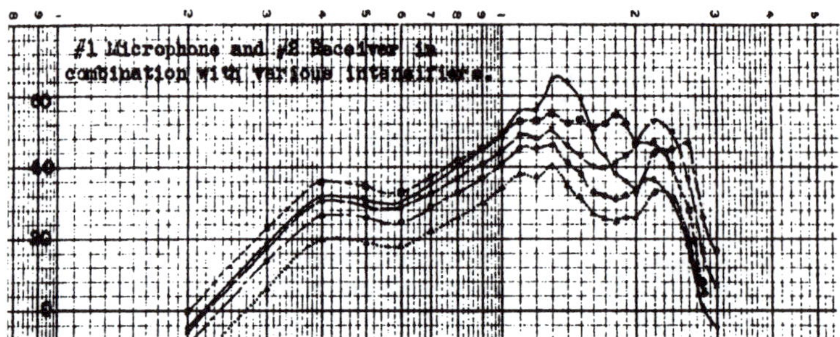

Figure 1–18. Gain curves of a Radioear carbon hearing aid model.

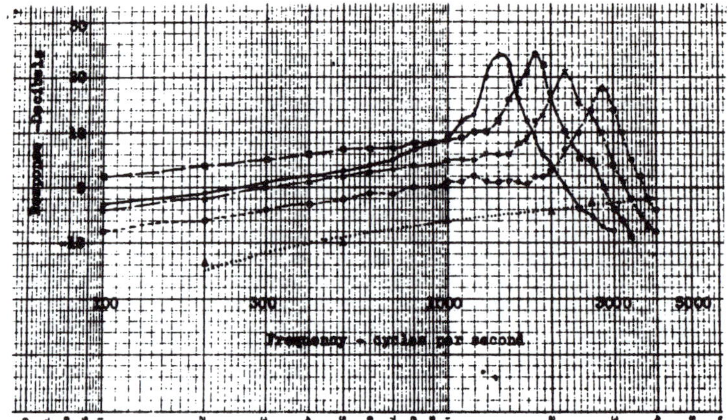

Figure 1–19. Amplifier response curves (Radioear carbon aid).

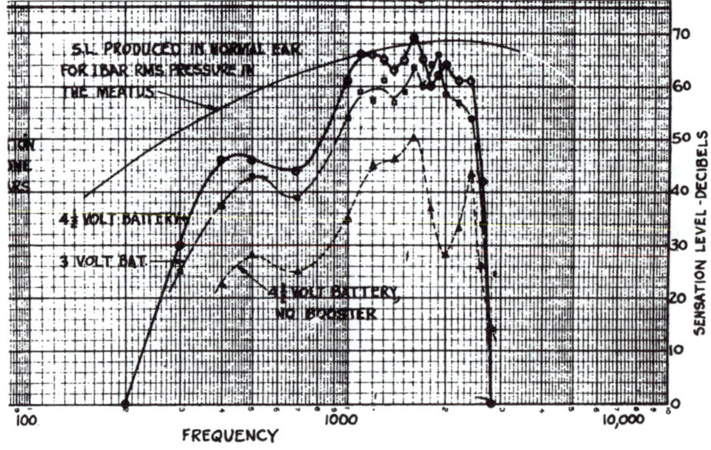

Figure 1–20. Sensation levels for normal ears with and without the first Sonotone bone conduction carbon aid (Lieber, 1933).

unaffected by external force against the case, which was completely closed. A floating mass inside the case, actually that of the magnetic driving system, was vibrated by the magnetic driving system through a spring attached to the case. The reaction force developed was transmitted to the mastoid by the case. Figure 1–21 shows a form of the device.

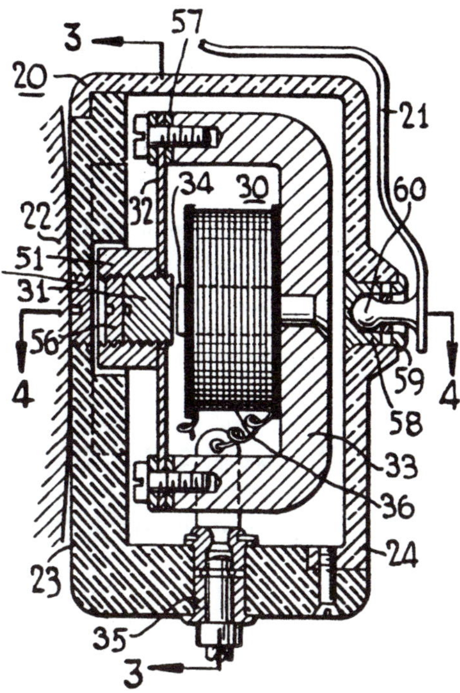

Figure 1–21. Diagram of Greibach bone vibrator.

Telephone Use

Using the telephone with a carbon hearing aid was a problem. The direct type hearing aid shown in Figure 1–10 had a raised ring on the front cover to center the telephone receivers of that day. With indirect carbon microphones, the diaphragm faced the wrong way and was inside the reflector. One solution to this problem is shown in Figure 1–22. Holes were put in the back of the microphone (now facing forward) to allow sound from the telephone receiver to enter the microphone case and reach the diaphragm. A shutter arrangement was provided to close the

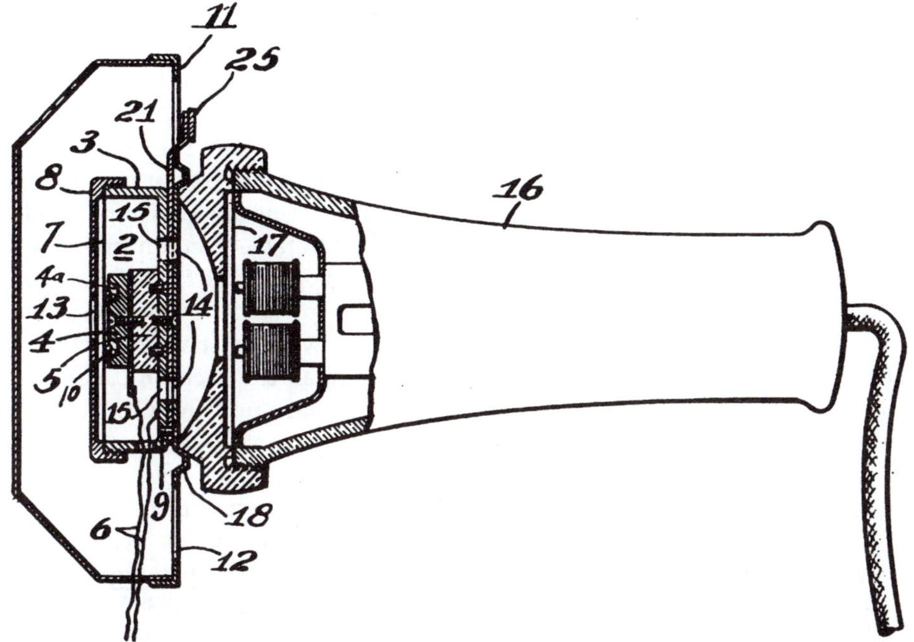

Figure 1–22. Telephone shutter device, indirect carbon microphone.

holes when the telephone was not in use to prevent a serious loss of low-frequency response.

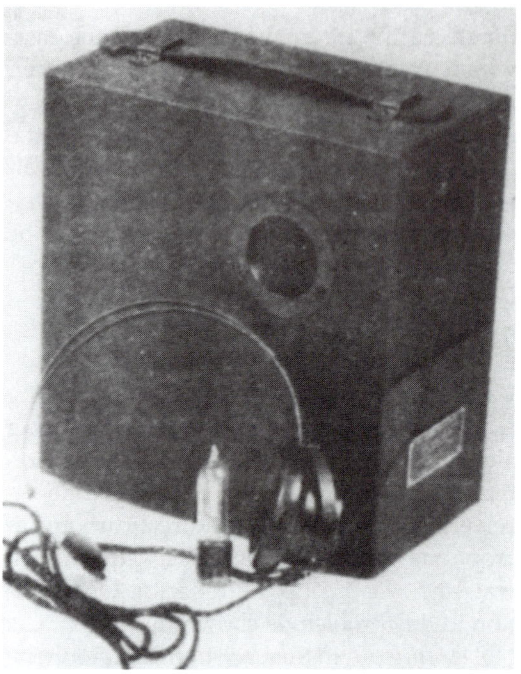

Figure 1–23. Hanson "Vactuphone" from V. Willis & Co. catalog.

Summary

During its approximately four-decade duration, the carbon era, in spite of its many limitations, contributed much to the well-being of the hearing impaired. During this era, many techniques and concepts were developed that enhanced later hearing aid technologies.

The Vacuum Tube Era

Lee DeForest invented the triode vacuum tube in 1907. It was quickly adapted to radio and telephone applications. The first hearing aid using a vacuum tube was the "Vactuphone," invented by Hanson (1920). It was made by Western Electric Company and distributed by Globe Phone Company starting in October 1921. It used a carbon microphone and one Western Electric type 215 "peanut tube" (Figure 1–23).

Patents issued to Tillyer (1923) and Kranz (1928) showed carbon microphones and vacuum tube amplifiers and were primarily concerned with adjusting the frequency response to meet the characteristics of hearing impairment. Berger (1984) mentioned several other early vacuum tube hearing aids that presumably used carbon microphones.

In 1924, a large multitube hearing aid was developed by E. A. Myers. It became available as the Radioear hearing aid in about 1925. It employed a moving coil microphone, which was superior to a carbon microphone because of its amplitude linearity and freedom from internal noise. A rubber diaphragm was used in an effort to obtain a smoother response. Figure 1–24 shows the interior of an early battery-operated Radioear (ca. 1926). Five Daven triodes were used. A six-volt storage battery supplied the filaments and the magnetizing winding of the microphone. Three large "B" batteries supplied 135 volts (V) for the plate circuits. The Myers device is further described by Lybarger (1987).

The Rochelle salts crystal microphone appeared in nonwearable vacuum tube hearing aids as early as 1936. A Tel-audio table model appeared that year. The Sonotone "Perceptron," a carryable crystal microphone vacuum tube hearing aid, was introduced in 1937.

Truly wearable vacuum tube hearing aids did not appear in the United States until 1937 and were preceded by such hearing aids in England, where initial production of small battery-operated vacuum tubes took place. The High Vacuum Valve Co., Ltd., of London (Hyvac) produced "midget" triodes, pentodes, triode-diodes, and variable-μ tubes. They ranged from $\frac{5}{8}$ to $\frac{25}{32}$ inch in diameter and from 2 inches to $2\frac{1}{2}$ inches long. Battery drains were somewhat high for wearable hearing aids. Hyvac's 1938 book of specification sheets included quite a number of hear-

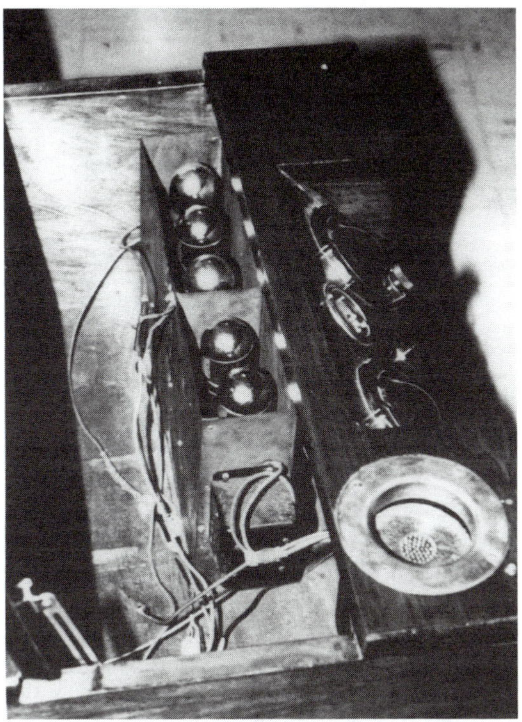

Figure 1–24. Interior of battery-operated vacuum tube Radioear that used a moving coil microphone (ca. 1926).

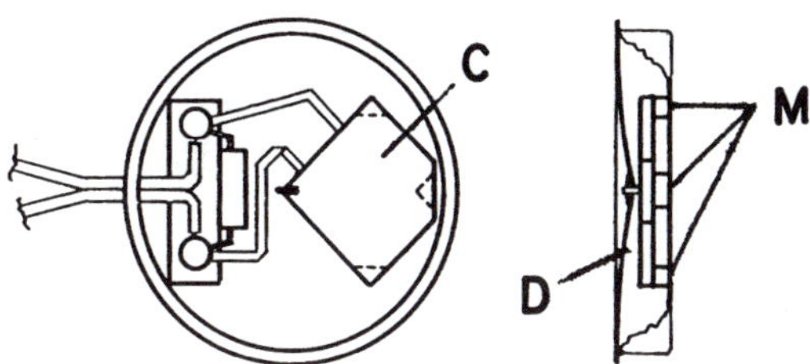

Figure 1–25. Hearing aid type crystal microphone. C: Rochelle salts crystal. M: viscous mounts. D: aluminum diaphragm.

ing aid circuit diagrams. Among them were diagrams for automatic gain control (AGC) aids, using the diode section of a triode output tube to supply the rectified voltage to control the gain of the variable-μ amplifier stages.

The bimorph Rochelle salts crystal microphone was of equal importance to small vacuum tubes in developing wearable vacuum tube hearing aids. Invented by Sawyer of Brush Development Company, this type of microphone had small size, high output, good frequency response, and high impedance well suited to work into the grid of a vacuum tube. Figure 1–25 is a diagram of a typical hearing aid crystal microphone construction. The twister type of crystal was supported on three corners by viscous pads to reduce the sharpness of the resonant peak. The thin aluminum diaphragm was fastened to the fourth corner.

Crystal receivers, notably the Brush DJ, had the advantages of light weight and wider frequency response than most magnetic receivers. However, both crystal microphones and receivers were affected by humidity and by temperatures exceeding about 110°F.

Probably the earliest wearable vacuum tube hearing aid made in the United States was Arthur Wengel's "Stanleyphone," available in 1937 and 1938 according to Watson and Tolan (1949). This hearing aid used Hyvac tubes, as did an early Telex hearing aid. It is likely that the earliest hearing aid using United States-made vacuum tubes was the Aurex, developed by Walter Huth and introduced in May of 1938. Figure 1–26 shows the interior of this hearing aid. It used four small triode tubes made by Aurex and had a large Brush crystal microphone. The case was five inches long, but thinner at the edges to fit comfortably in a pocket.

The Aurex hearing aid had low clothing rub noise, much better than the Wengel hearing aid, in which the microphone was firmly attached to the case. The favorable clothing noise condition of the Aurex was achieved by a soft rubber microphone mounting plus a lead mass attached to the microphone. Cubert of Aurex applied for a patent on this arrangement. Carlisle of Sonotone and Lybarger of Radioear filed patent applications on vibration mounts at about the same time and a patent interference case resulted. The interfer-

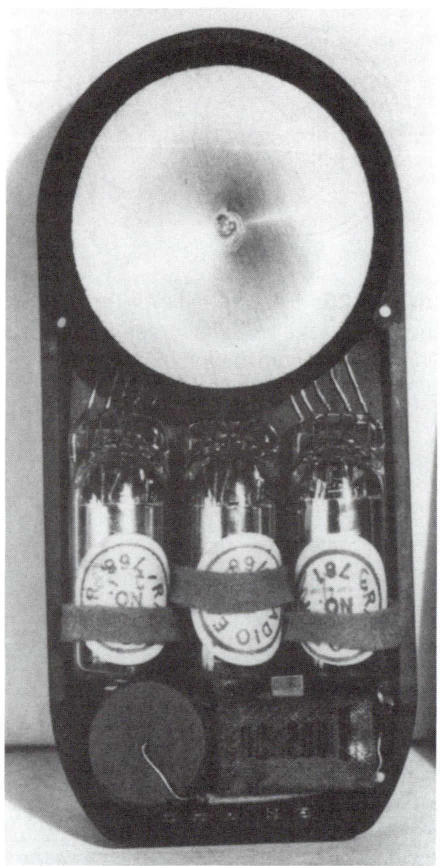

Figure 1–26. Radioear aid with first Raytheon subminiature tubes (1939).

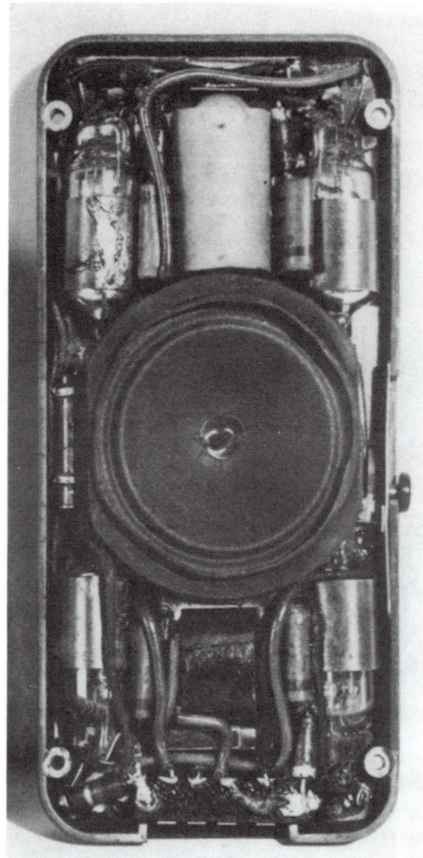

Figure 1–27. Four-triode Aurex aid (ca. 1938).

ence was won by Cubert; the others received royalty-free licenses by prior agreement.

In 1938, the Raytheon Company released its first series of subminiature pentode vacuum tubes and became the predominant supplier of hearing aid tubes. Interestingly, Raytheon's subminiature tube production (in later years for purposes other than hearing aids) continued until January of 1986.

The first Raytheon types were the CK501X voltage amplifier and the CK502X and CK503X output tubes. They were slightly over ½ inch in diameter and were 1½ inches long. Figure 1–27 is an inside view of a 1939 Radioear aid that used these early tubes. A crystal microphone and either a crystal or magnetic receiver could be used with this hearing aid.

A problem with early tubes was vibration of the filament when the tube received a tap. This microphonic effect created an objectionable ringing sound in the output. Tubes, particularly those used in the early amplifier stages, were inspected for this characteristic and rejected if the microphonics were too strong. Improved tube construction and shorter filaments of later voltage amplifier tubes eventually eliminated the problem.

By 1942, Raytheon's change to a flat tube shape (0.285 × 0.385 inch) allowed hearing aids to be made thinner. Another important development was the 0.625 V filament voltage amplifier tube. Two filaments could now be connected in series to reduce "A" battery current drain. Figure 1–28 shows the interior of a 1942 hearing aid using flat tubes. The fil-

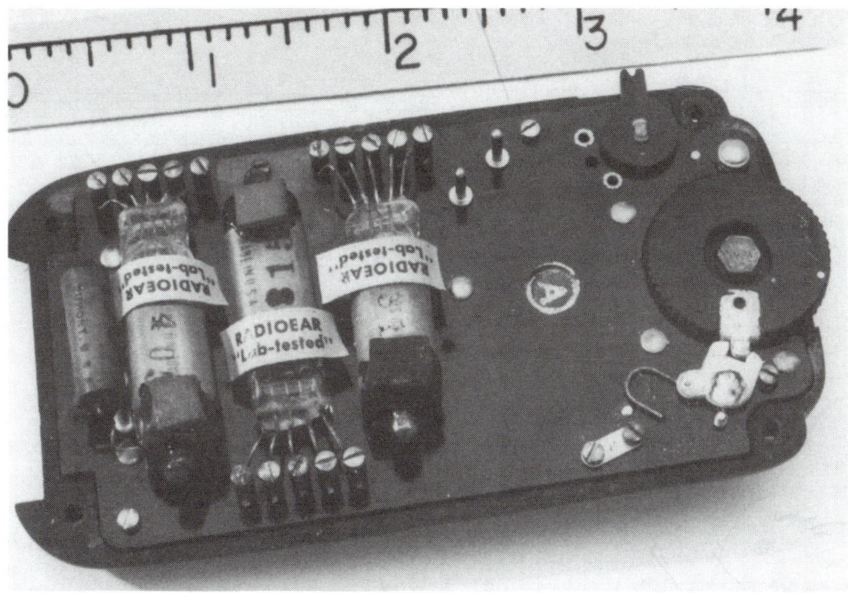

Figure 1–28. 1942 hearing aid using Raytheon flat tubes.

ament drain was 60 mA total. By 1947, filament drain for three tubes was down to 40 mA and further reductions followed. In 1949, tube size again dropped to 0.220 × 0.285 inch in section and to a shorter length.

One-piece Hearing Aids

Until 1944, vacuum tube hearing aids required large external "A" and "B" batteries. Two battery developments changed the picture. The RM-4 Ruben mercury battery, originally made by Mallory for military applications, made an excellent "A" battery. It was much smaller than a carbon-zinc battery of equal capacity and had a much flatter discharge curve. The other development was a small layer type "B" battery made by Eveready that had good capacity. Using these batteries, Beltone introduced a one-piece vacuum tube hearing aid in July 1944 that received immediate acceptance. Only one cord, from the hearing aid to the receiver, was needed. Within two or three years, most hearing aids used the one-piece construction and further reductions in size continued.

Performance

Vacuum tube hearing aids had higher gain, wider frequency range, and lower distortion than carbon hearing aids. Figure 1–29 shows full-on gain curves for some 1940 hearing aids. The solid curves are for full "A" and "B" voltages; the dashed curves are for both batteries at the end of useful life. Note that frequency response extends up to about 4000 Hz, some 1000 Hz higher than that typical of carbon hearing aids. Saturation output was typically around 120 dB SPL, but well over 130 dB in powerful hearing aids. At least one powerful hearing aid had six vacuum tubes. Extensive detail on vacuum tube hearing aids is found in Watson and Tolan (1949). Hector, Pearson, Dean, and Carlisle (1953) give information on vacuum tube hearing aid technology just prior to the introduction of transistors.

Special Features

Adjustment

Many innovations took place during the vacuum tube era. With electronic circuitry, it be-

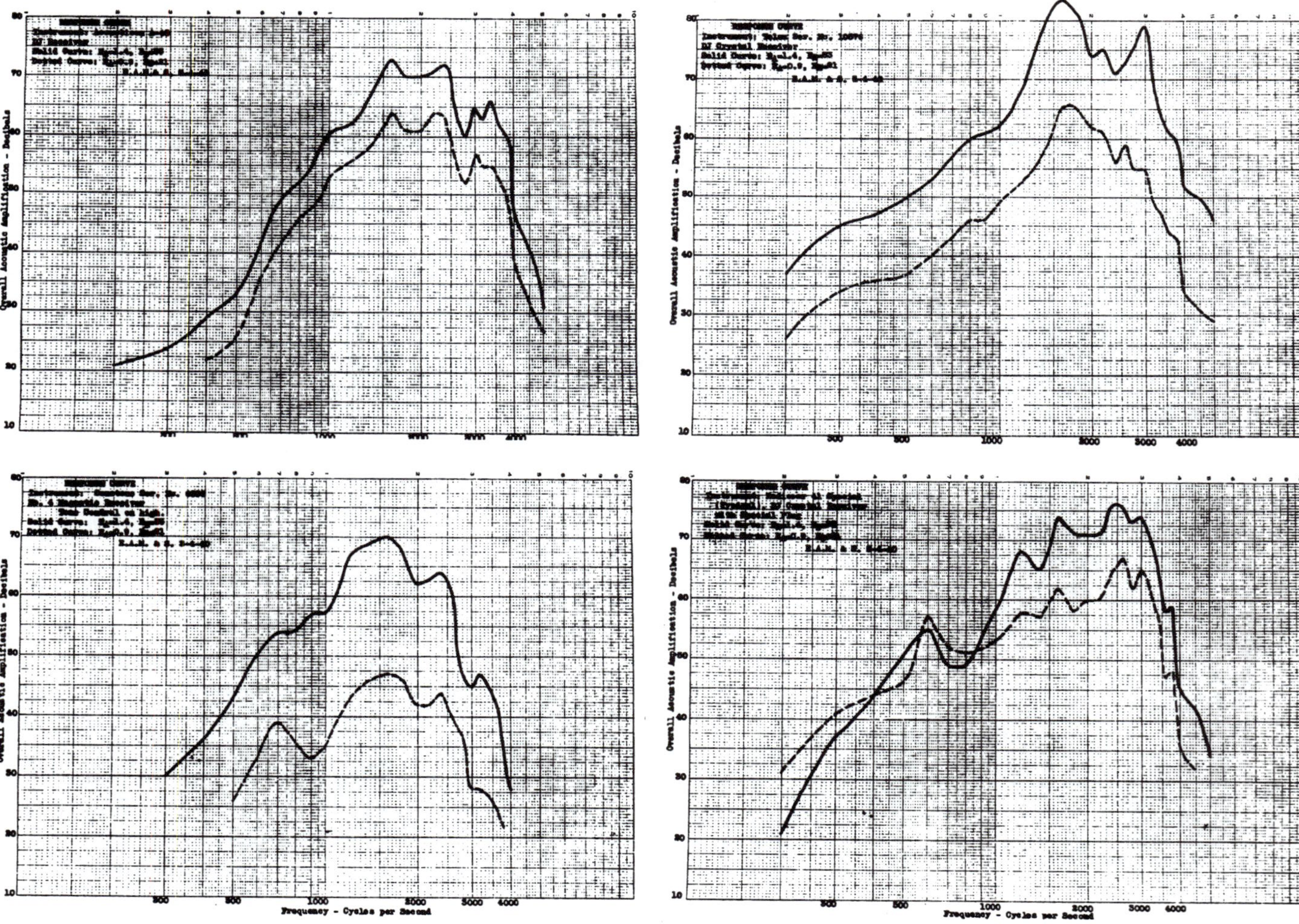

Figure 1–29. Full-on gain curves for some 1940 vacuum tube hearing aids.

came easy to cut lows or highs and to limit maximum gain and output. Thus, the flexibility of control was much greater than for carbon hearing aids.

Telephone Use

An innovation that has remained important is the telephone induction coil. In 1936, Tel-Audio introduced an AC-operated desk aid that had a large external telephone induction pickup coil, as shown in Figure 1–30. In 1946, a wearable Radioear vacuum tube aid with a built-in telephone pickup coil was introduced. Within a few years, other manufacturers adopted the idea and today nearly all moderate-to high-gain aids have built-in "telecoils."

Magnetic Microphone

Another 1946 innovation was the introduction of the magnetic microphone, primarily by one manufacturer. An input transformer was used between the microphone and the grid circuit of the first tube. The magnetic microphone had a big advantage over the crystal microphone: it was not damaged by temperature or humidity conditions normally encountered. It also turned out that the magnetic microphone was exceptionally well suited for use with transistors. Figure 1–31 shows a cross section of the 1946 Radioear magnetic microphone. Note the horizontally spaced sound entrance slots which make the microphone directional. This was probably the first hearing aid with this feature (Lybarger, 1947). The position of the telephone pickup coil can also be seen in this figure.

Earmold Venting

Grossman (1942) invented earmold venting. Its initial use was with the "button" type receivers on vacuum tube aids. Grossman had an adjustable vent opening in a short tube between the receiver and a shallow earmold. Venting, in many forms, has become a standard fitting technique when needed.

Summary

The vacuum tube era served the needs of the hearing impaired extremely well. Many tech-

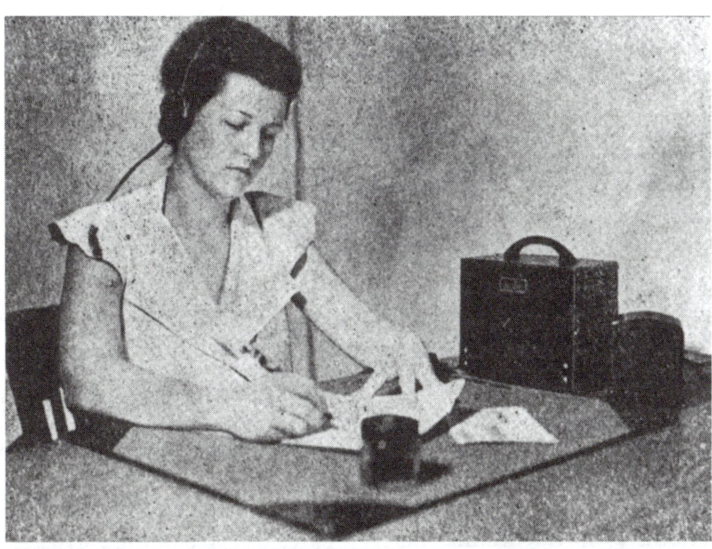

Figure 1–30. Tel-Audio desk aid with large external telephone induction pickup coil (1936).

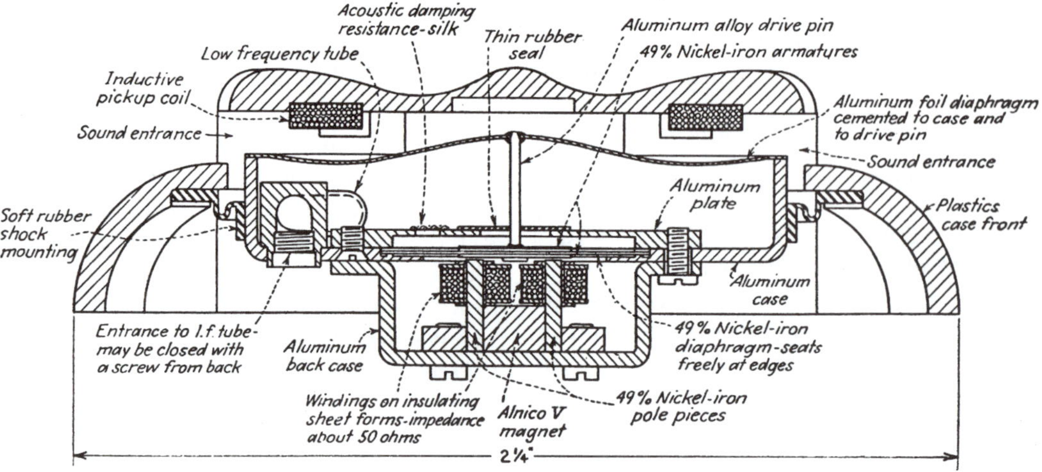

Figure 1–31. Cross section of a magnetic microphone used in a 1946 vacuum tube hearing aid.

nological advances were made. It should also be mentioned that it was during this era that the birth of audiology took place.

The Transistor Era

The transistor era started late in 1952 and produced dramatic improvements in hearing aid technology. Invented at Bell Telephone Laboratories, the transistor was first described in a 1948 article in the *Physical Review.* The first transistor was a "point-contact" type, possibly never used in hearing aids. Late in 1952, Raytheon Company released their CK718 PNP alloy junction germanium transistor for hearing aid use. The change from vacuum tubes to transistors did not significantly change acoustical performance, but did vastly reduce the cost of operation and the size of the battery supply; only a single low voltage battery was needed. There was about a 100 to 1 reduction in battery power requirements.

The input impedance of early transistor amplifiers was about 1000 ohms, much too low for the generally used crystal microphone. Three solutions were developed: a "hybrid" amplifier with two vacuum tube stages preceding a current saving output stage, a step-down transformer coupling the crystal microphone to the first transistor stage, or a magnetic microphone with impedance matching that of the transistor input stage. The latter approach became the standard method for many years.

Figure 1–32 shows a magnetic microphone all-transistor hearing aid released early in 1953. Three transistors were used. The receiver was a magnetic type with impedance suitable for direct series connection from the battery to the collector of the transistor output stage. One, two, or three RM-1 mercury batteries could be used, or, for extremely long life, a single RM-12 battery could give some 2,000 hours of operation.

Several improvements and size reductions were made in germanium transistors by Raytheon. Planar silicon transistors replaced the germanium types about 1960. In addition to providing high reliability and low noise, these also greatly reduced the number of components needed. The higher input impedance of the silicon transistors proved valuable when ceramic and electret microphones became available. Figure 1–33 compares the size of the early germanium transistor with that of a tiny discrete silicon transistor later available.

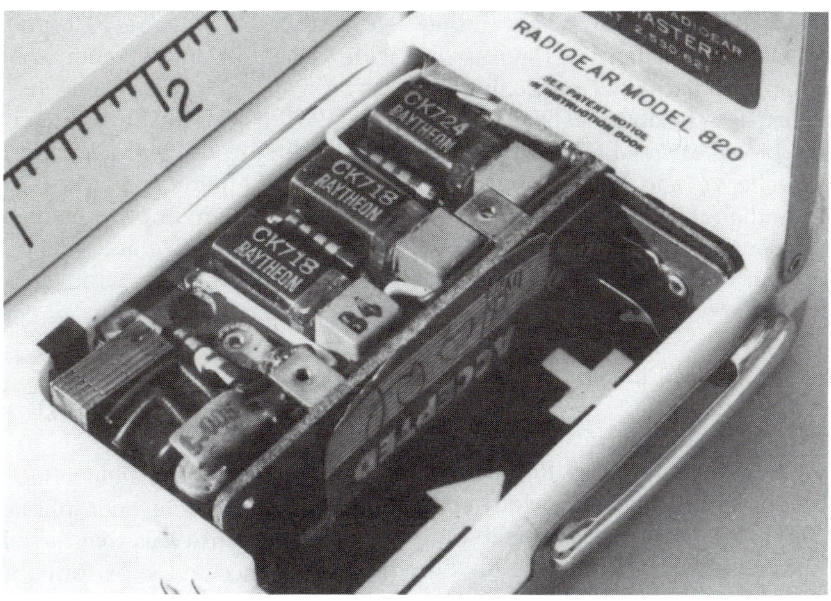

Figure 1–32. 1953 hearing aid that used three Raytheon CK718 transistors and a magnetic microphone.

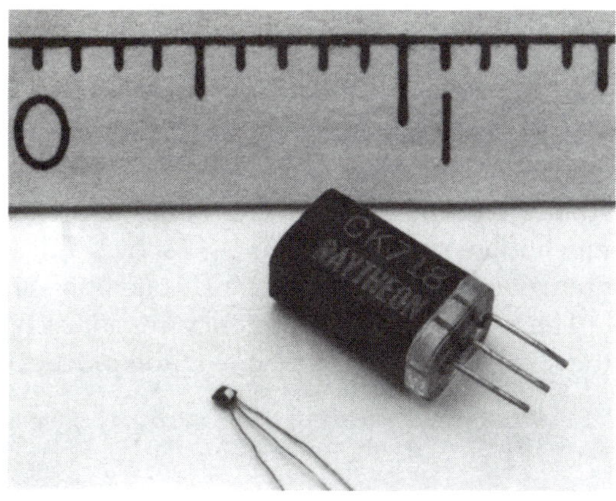

Figure 1–33. Size of Raytheon CK718 transistor compared with later Raytheon planar silicon transistor.

During 1953, miniaturized balanced-armature magnetic microphones for hearing aids appeared. One early unit was made by Shure Brothers (Bauer, 1953). It was about one inch in diameter and ⅜ inch thick. In 1953, Knowles Electronics began to produce small, rectangular shaped balanced-armature microphones. As a result of continued research and development, Knowles improved performance and reduced the size of balanced armature transducers, becoming the primary supplier to the hearing aid industry for these devices.

With increased transistor and component availability, a wide variety of transistorized body aids was produced. Size dropped as smaller microphones, batteries, and other components became available. The hearing aid industry and the hearing impaired are heavily indebted to the foresight and competence of component suppliers, who have made continued size reduction and improved acoustical performance possible.

By 1955, the size of body aids had come down significantly. That year is important, however, because it marked the beginning of ear level hearing aid development with the introduction of the eyeglass aid by Otarion. In this aid, the components were built into the two eyeglass temples and connected by wiring across the fronts. The receiver, a rectangular balanced armature unit, was in the temple opposite that containing the microphone and had a sound outlet projecting toward the ear canal. A flexible plastic tube carried the sound to an earmold. The temples of this aid were heavy and bulky and some manufacturers thought the eyeglass aid was too large to be successful. However, eyeglass aid construction improved rapidly and by 1959 constituted about 50 percent of United States hearing aid sales. In due course, it became possible to put all the components in one temple.

The eyeglass aid made practical the utilization of the CROS (Contralateral Routing of Signals) concept, originated by Harford and Barry (1965). The original concept was to put a microphone on the side of the head with the bad ear and "inject" the sound picked up there into the canal of the good ear on the other side of the head. By eliminating head shadow, excellent results were obtained for unilateral hearing losses. The eyeglass hearing aid was ideally suited for CROS, because concealed wires could be carried across the eyeglass fronts. It turned out that the frequency response characteristics resulting from the venting action of the small tubing in the open ear canal were extremely beneficial for the large number of persons with "ski-slope" type hearing loss who had previously had poor results from hearing aids. The "open canal" fitting has remained very important.

The ear level concept had many advantages. It eliminated clothing noise, put the microphone in a more favorable location near the ear, eliminated cords, and made binaural hearing with hearing aids truly significant.

The behind-the-ear (BTE) aid was an outgrowth of the eyeglass aid. As components became smaller, they could all be put into the portion of the eyeglass temple behind the pinna. When this was done, it was quite logical to remove the front portion of the eyeglass temple, leaving a BTE hearing aid. By 1959, BTE aids constituted 25% of United States hearing aid sales; by 1962 they exceeded eyeglass hearing aid sales. They remained the dominant type of aid until they were overtaken by the in-the-ear (ITE) type in 1985. A wide variety of amplification characteristics has been available in BTE aids.

In 1964, a BTE aid introduced by Zenith was the first to use an integrated circuit (IC) amplifier, the latter made by Texas Instruments. Since then, improvements in IC technology to reduce size and expand functions have made ICs very desirable for use in all forms of hearing aids.

The Microelectronic/Digital Era

The invention of the field effect transistor (FET) made possible microphone developments in the late 1960s that have had a profound influence on the performance and size of hearing aids. The frequency response advantages of a medium-size ceramic microphone over a magnetic microphone were realized in a 1967 body aid that used a separate FET with its characteristic very high input impedance.

A landmark advance took place in 1968, when a ceramic element and an FET with its associated circuitry were enclosed in a tiny metal case (Killion & Carlson, 1970). This microphone gave much smoother and wider response than magnetic microphones and was much more rugged. Figure 1–34 shows a diagram of one type of ceramic/FET microphone.

The excellent low frequency response of the ceramic/FET microphone made practical

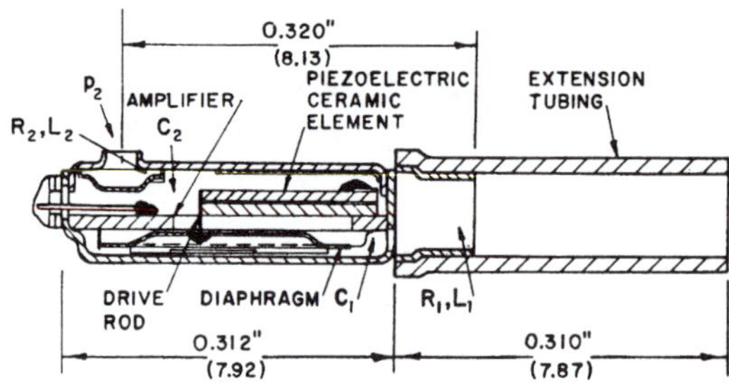

Figure 1–34. One type of Knowles ceramic/FET microphone (Courtesy of Knowles Electronics, Inc.).

the miniature directional microphone in 1969. The first of these was made in Germany using United States-made ceramic/ FET microphones and were incorporated in United States hearing aids made by Maico. Microphones made in the United States followed (Carlson & Killion, 1974). The directional microphone has remained an available feature in a number of BTE aids and in some ITE aids.

An even more dramatic development in 1971 was the very tiny electret/FET microphone (Killion & Carlson, 1974). This microphone was capable of very smooth and wide band response. A very important feature was its far lower sensitivity to mechanical vibration than either the magnetic or ceramic/FET microphones. This was of great importance in any type of aid in which the microphone and receiver were in the same small case, such as BTE, ITE, and in-the-canal aids. Figure 1–35 shows the construction of one type of electret/ FET microphone. Intensive development of this type of microphone has reduced its size significantly. Figure 1–36 shows a tiny 1986 Knowles electret/FET microphone alongside an early Knowles magnetic microphone.

To illustrate the remarkable reduction in size that has occurred in very recent years, Figure 1–37 shows a Knowles FI amplified microphone in actual size, with amplification information to its right. Figure 1–38 shows the Etymotic D-Mic, which has two ports for its directional operation and a third port for non-directional operation. The D-Mic is only ¼ inch in diameter and fits easily on an ITE faceplate.

As late as 1961, hearing aids were considered by some to be "low fidelity" devices (Harris, Haines, Kelsey, & Clark, 1961). Not

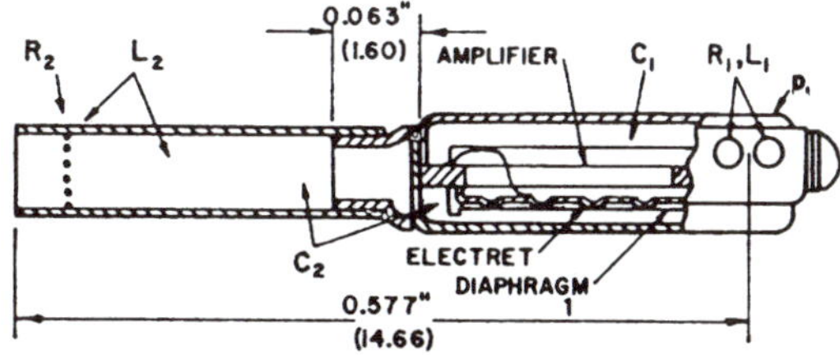

Figure 1–35. One type of Knowles electret/FET microphone (Courtesy of Knowles Electronics, Inc.)

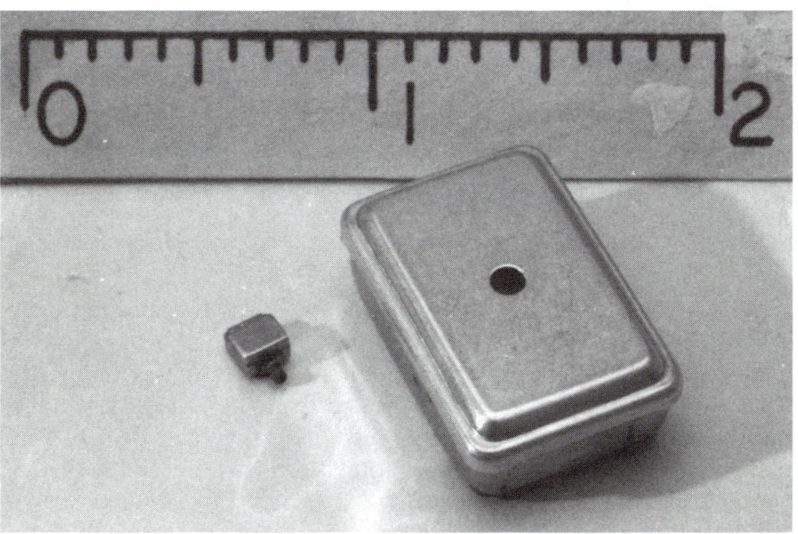

Figure 1–36. Comparison of early Knowles magnetic microphone (ca. 1953) with a tiny 1986 Knowles electret/FET microphone.

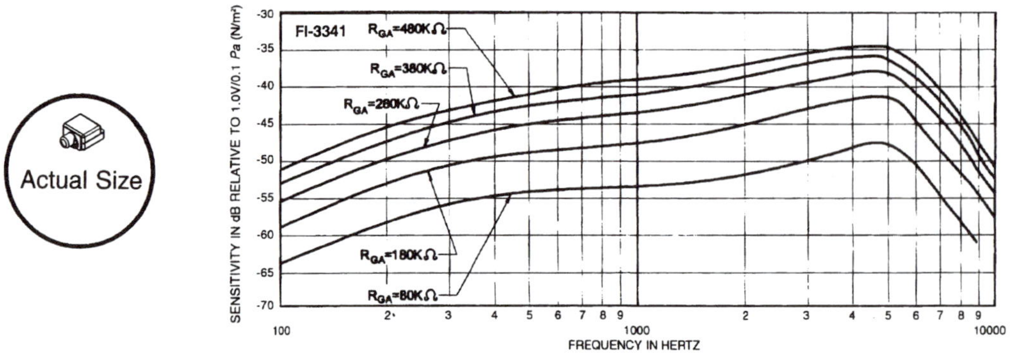

Figure 1–37. Ultra-small Knowles Electronics FI Series electret microphone with self-contained amplifier providing up to 30 dB of gain (per curves at right) 1998.

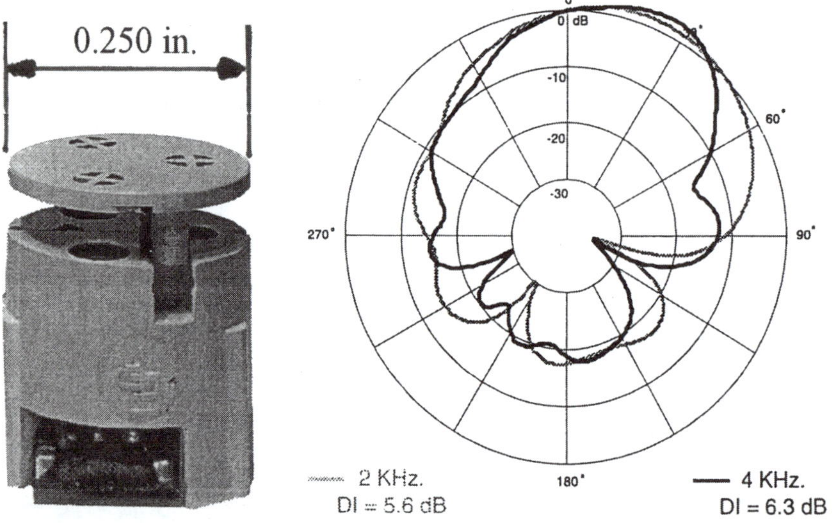

Figure 1–38. Extremely small D-MIC directional microphone with polar curves. (Courtesy of Etymotic Research)

everyone agreed with this, of course. It has been demonstrated that almost any desired degree of "high fidelity" can be achieved in hearing aids, were it to be found useful. Whereas the upper frequency limit for carbon aids was typically 3000 Hz or less and about 4000 Hz for most vacuum tube aids, major advances in receiver design and in "earmold plumbing" raised the upper limit to almost any desired useful value in the transistor era. Knowles and Killion (1978) described the performance of the BP-1817 receiver, which, when used with appropriate tubing connections, was capable of delivering good response to 9000 Hz. Killion (1981) summarized earmold options for wideband hearing aids. Many receiver designs became capable of wideband response.

The Knowles Amplified Receiver

This very small, highly efficient device, released in October 1988, has contributed tremendously to the development of very tiny hearing aids, even those that fit completely in the ear canal (CIC). By having the output-stage electronics within the receiver, space is released in the hearing aid electronics area to make the aid smaller. The use of a Class D amplifier stage reduces size and battery current and increases output power with low distortion.

The production development of the amplified receiver was accomplished by the joint efforts of Elmer Carlson (Knowles) and Mead Killion (Etymotic Research). It was designated as the Knowles EP Receiver. It is only .250 inches long, .171 inches wide, and .119 inches thick, as shown in Figure 1–39.

In order to provide room for the microelectronic Class D amplifier inside the receiver case, a new transduction mechanism arrangement is used, as shown in Figure 1–40. The smaller coil-winding space suitable for the Class D circuit provides space within the receiver housing for the amplifier. To keep battery current as low as possible for the amount of output power needed, three models of the EP receiver were made available.

The operation of the Class D amplifier is explained in detail in an article by Carlson (Carlson,1988). The concept of including the Class D amplifier in the receiver case was

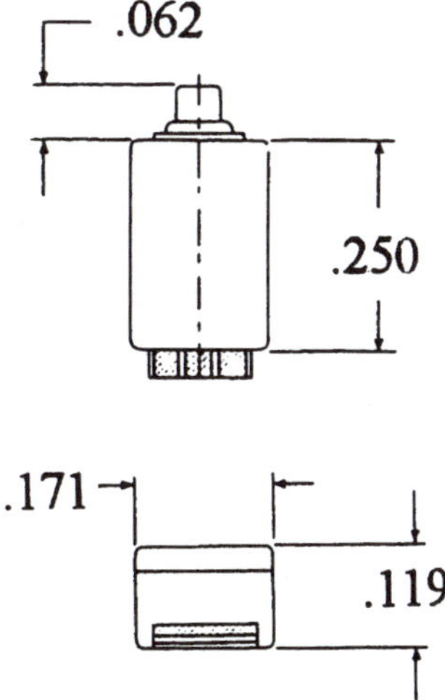

Figure 1–39. Dimensions of Knowles Electronics EP Amplified Receiver (inches).

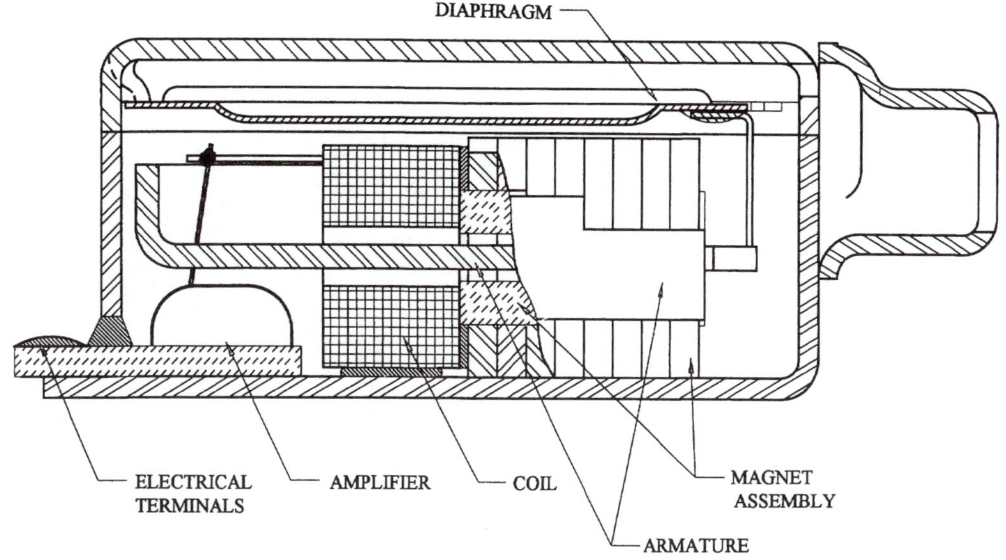

Figure 1–40. Cross section of Knowles Electronics EP Amplified Receiver, about 15 times actual size. (Courtesy of Elmer V. Carlson)

covered in patents by Killion (Killion 1983,1987).

The K-Amp

An article by Mead C. Killion entitled "An Acoustically Invisible Hearing Aid" appeared in *Hearing Instruments* magazine in October, 1988.The article was a progress report on a "K-AMP" integrated circuit amplifier then under development. Actual delivery of K-AMP amplifiers began in about 1989.

The K-AMP concept originated following Mead Killion's 1979 doctoral studies at Northwestern University (Killion,1979). It was based on the idea that high fidelity amplification for persons with hearing impairment was beneficial and could be provided.

A first consideration was that the input/output curve of a hearing aid should be modified to reduce overloading of the ear at high levels. Figure 1–41 shows a more desirable situation (Killion,1993).

A second consideration was that distortion for high level input signals should be reduced. This was achieved by the use of the Class D amplified receiver.

A third consideration was that the frequency response of a hearing aid should change with the input sound pressure level, as shown in Figure 1–42 (Killion,1993).

Other features of the K-AMP amplifier further increased its flexibility (Kruger & Kruger, 1993).

The circuitry required to achieve these desirable amplifier objectives was necessarily complex, but achieved in a remarkably small size. The size was later reduced sufficiently to fit into small in-the-canal aids. Figure 1–43 shows one type of 1998 K-AMP. It is extremely tiny, considering the complex circuitry provided, and has received wide industry acceptance.

In 1998, a programmable version of the K-AMP became available.

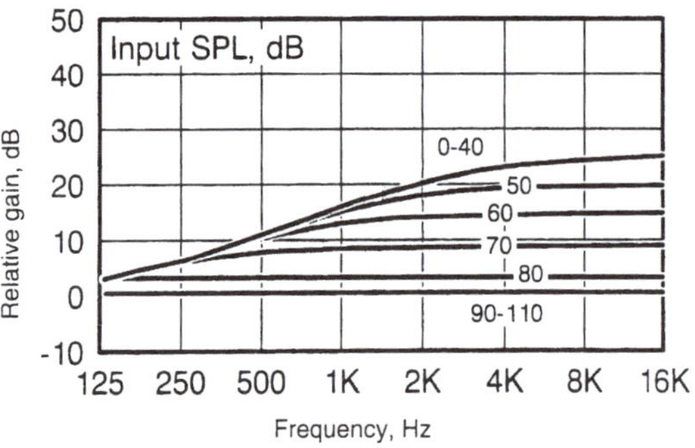

Figure 1–42. Relative gain vs. frequency for increasing input levels with K-AMP.

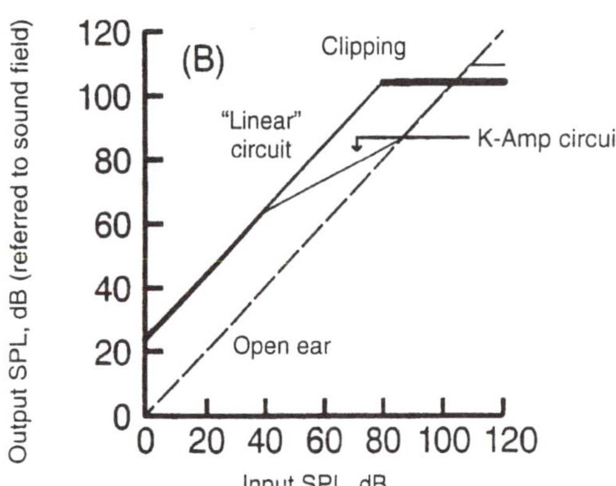

Figure 1–41. Preferred input-output characteristics for a high-fidelity hearing aid.

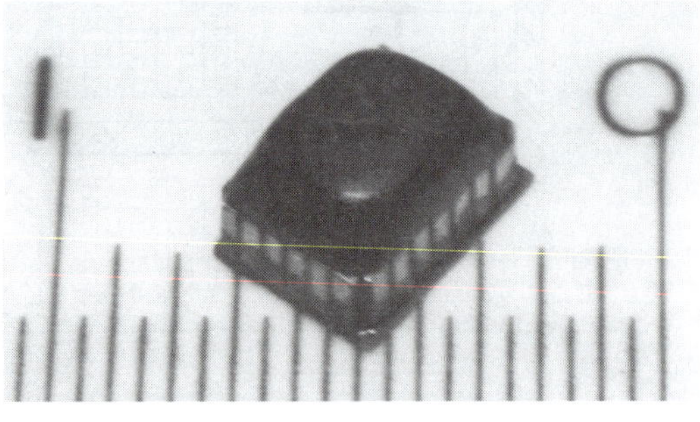

Figure 1–43. Enlarged photograph of a 1998 Etymotic Research K-AMP. Scale divisions under it are ½ millimeter apart. The complex amplifier measures only .132 × .181 × .100 inches.

Further Size Reductions

In-the-ear (ITE) aids started to appear statistically in 1961 and puttered along at a low market percentage through 1974. Early ITE aids were sometimes more out-of-the-ear than in-the-ear. However, as a result of major reductions in the size of microphones, receivers, batteries (a significant development in 1977 was the zinc-air battery, which has about double the capacity of a mercury or silver oxide battery of the same size and does not require relatively scarce materials) and other components, ITE technology took on new life and by 1975 had captured 18% of the market. A decade later, the ITE market share was approximately 65%, including the relatively new in-the-canal (ITC) instruments introduced in 1983. By 1989, ITC aids were a full 20% of the total ITE market. Further size reductions became possible in the 1990s, beginning with the Siemens XP peritympanic model which sat almost at the eardrum and required a fairly complex impressioning procedure to insure complete safety.

CIC Instruments

The development of new silicone impression materials led to more easily obtainable deep canal impressions that did not impinge on the tympanic membrane. In 1993–94, Starkey and Argosy introduced completely-in-the-canal (CIC) instruments in which the shells terminated some 5 to 7 mm beyond the second bend of the canal and the microphones sat 1 to 2 mm inside the aperture. By seating these instruments into the bony portion of the canal, it was possible to reduce significantly (and in some cases eliminate) the occlusion effect, allowing unvented instruments—almost a necessity when working with the available space in the canal.

Because of the microphone location and the smaller cavity adjacent to the eardrum, the actual performance of a CIC aid is considerably higher than indicated by a 2 cc coupler test. Preves and Leisses estimate that that the microphone inlet location could increase gain by about 7 dB and that the deep canal placement of the receiver might result in a further gain of about 6 dB compared to a full-shell ITE aid. (Preves & Leisses, 1995).

Due to relative inaccessibilty of the CIC instrument, the usual type of volume control cannot be used. Various means of handling this problem have been devised, such as a magnetic control or signals from a hand-held control.

Not all hearing losses can be fit with ITE products, and BTE instruments continue to represent almost one-fifth of all hearing aid sales. The evolution of extremely soft silicone earmolds in 1989–90 allowed the BTE style to replace most body instruments by providing a better seal within the canal to reduce the incidence of acoustic feedback.

In 1997, more than 1.8 million hearing aids were sold in the United States, with 64% of all fittings involving binaural amplification. The 1997 breakdown by style follows:

ITE (Full Shell)	37.2%
ITC	23.8%
BTE	18.8%
CIC	11.8%
Half-shell	7.2%

Programmable Hearing Aids

A programmable aid is one in which the gain, output, and frequency response can be set to meet requirements indicated by the user's audiogram, using a computer in which the output is connected to a multiple contact terminal on the hearing aid by a cable from the computer. Various fitting systems in the computer program are available.

The earliest date for the availability of programmable aids may have been 1988 (3M, Widex), followed in 1989 by Maico and in 1991 by Siemens.

The subject of digitally programmable hearing aids was extensively discussed by Staab in a review article in the *British Journal of Audiology* (Staab, 1990).

In 1992 the Hi-Pro standard interface for programmable instruments became available and is still in use.

In 1995, the first programmable CIC was introduced by Maico. Siemens introduced a programmable CIC in 1996.

The availability of programmable hearing aids has increased significantly in recent years. Many manufacturers currently utilize the "NOAH" system for programming, available through the Hearing Instrument Manufacturers Software Association (HIMSA).

Digital Hearing Aids

The earliest wearable digital hearing aid was made in experimental form in 1983 by Audiotone. It had a behind-the-ear portion that contained the analog-to-digital (A/D) converter, the digital signal processing (DSP), and the digital-to analog (D/A) converter. It was described fully in the October 1983 *Hearing Aid Journal* under the title "A Wearable Digital Hearing Aid." The authors were James Nunley, Wayne Staab, John Steadman, Perry Wechsler, and Bonnie Spencer. In addition, David Egolf and Robert Brechbiell participated in the project (Nunley, Staab et al., 1983).

The digital processing used in this device (and in most later wearable hearing aids) is described as follows:

1. The hearing aid microphone picks up airborne speech signals.
2. These analog speech signals are digitized in real time by the A/D converter.
3. The central processing unit (which is a very small computer or microprocessor) mathematically manipulates these digitized data according to programmed instructions. For example, the central processing unit may be programmed to change the frequency pattern to increase the high frequencies and reduce the low frequencies of the incoming signal. This would be a relatively simple operation. On the other hand, the ability to adapt to changing environments and to suppress noise is much more difficult.
4. The resulting output sequence is changed to analog form by the D/A converter.
5. The analog output signal is used to drive the hearing aid receiver.

Several benefits from the digital processing are mentioned in the article, including reduction of feedback, adjustment of programming to meet user requirements, improving signal-to-noise ratio, and more precise and adjustable response characteristics.

A comprehensive article by Wayne J. Staab, entitled "Digital Hearing Instruments" shows the basic circuitry in a digital hearing aid (Staab, 1987). An analog input portion precedes the digital portion, which is followed by an analog output portion, as shown in Figure 1–44.

According to the *Hearing Journal's* 50th Anniversary issue, the first digital ear level aids were introduced in 1995, by both Oticon and Widex.

An open platform digital hearing aid was introduced by Philips in 1997. In this instrument, the user can select any one of four different algorithms in the hearing aid (an algorithm is a prescribed set of well-defined rules or processes for the solution of a problem in a finite number of steps). A DSP chip developed by Philips manages all aspects of signal processing. BTE or ITE units on each ear are operated by a remote controller using infrared signals.

The hand-held remote controller turns the aid on or off, switches to telephone mode if desired, controls gain, and has push buttons that select one of the four algorithms available, as follows:

1. Single-channel broadband input and output audio gain control (AGC), maximizing fidelity.
2. Two-channel TILL (treble increases at low level) input and output AGC, emphasizing comfort.
3. Two-channel BILL (bass increases at low level) input and output AGC, emphasizing clarity.
4. Four-channel input and output AGC having independent control of performance in each channel to allow equalizing.

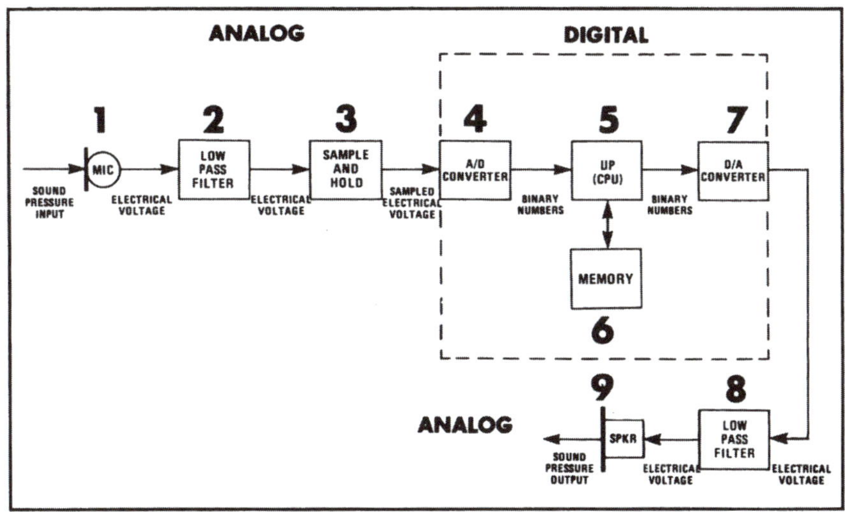

Figure 1–44. Block diagram of a digital hearing instrument. (From "Digital Hearing Instruments," Wayne J. Staab, 1987. *Hearing Instruments, 38*. Reprinted with permission.)

In a paper given at the 1998 American Auditory Society meeting, Staab reported on a study made on 14 subjects using open platform digital hearing aids. The conclusions reached were:

- Signal processing preferences by hearing aid users do change over time.
- Patients indicate a desirability to have multiple signal processing schemes at their disposal.
- Patient-preferred signal processing preferences bear little resemblance to recommendations made by audiologists.
- An "open platform" system allows multiple signal processing approaches to satisfy patient preferences.

HEARING AID MEASUREMENT

The earliest measurement tool for hearing aid testing was the human ear. Engineers and technicians tested hearing aids by listening to them or by having someone with a hearing impairment listen and report the results. An experienced listener could do much better than one might expect; some very good hearing aids were developed with this still-useful technique.

To measure any acoustical device accurately requires the measurement of sound pressure or intensity. The first accurate device for this was the Rayleigh disk (Rayleigh, 1882), a small, light disk supported by an easily twisted suspension. In a strong sound field, the disk turned an amount proportional to the sound intensity. It was used as a primary standard well into the 1930s, and possibly longer (Ballantine, 1932; Beranek, 1949; Inglis, Gray & Jenkins, 1932; Olson & Massa, 1934).

In 1917, Wente of Bell Telephone Laboratories invented the condenser microphone (Wente, 1917). This device, in improved forms, has remained the most important means of sound pressure measurement. Early condenser microphones were large and heavy. Figure 1–45 shows a large microphone that was used by the author for hearing aid measurement as early as 1932. Its diaphragm diameter was 1.687 inches and its outside diameter 3$\frac{3}{16}$ inches. It weighed 1$\frac{1}{4}$ pounds without its preamplifier.

Although the Rayleigh disk or thermophone (see Beranek, 1949) was useful for cali-

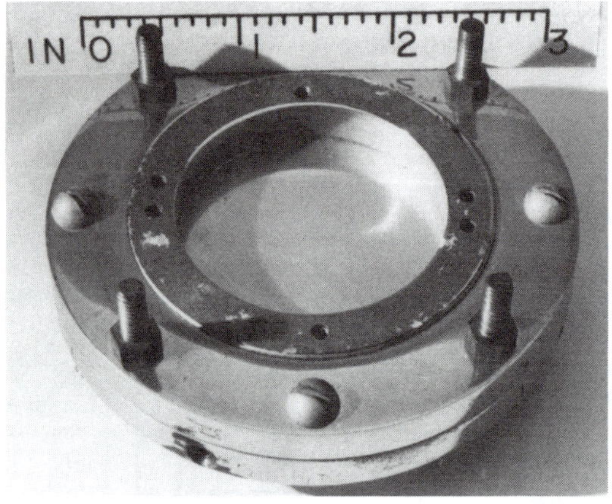

Figure 1–45. Large condenser microphone (1932).

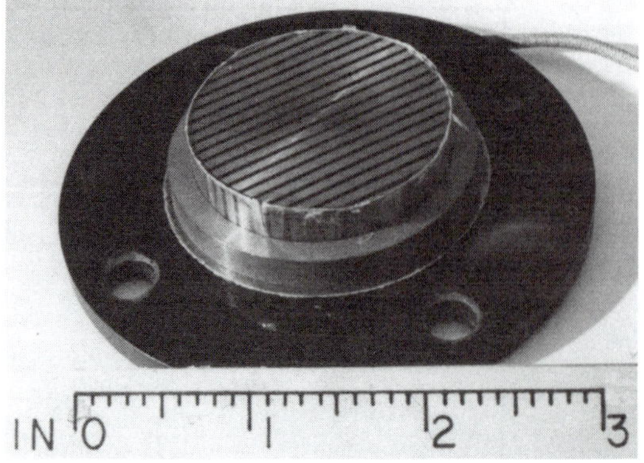

Figure 1–46. Electrostatic grille for condenser microphone calibration (1932).

bration, the electrostatic grille, or actuator, described by Ballantine (1932) was preferable. A carefully machined metal grille having alternate bars and slots was placed a small, accurately known distance from the microphone diaphragm. The open slots prevented acoustic loading of the diaphragm. The edge of the grille was insulated from the microphone by a thin mica sheet. A DC polarizing and a sine wave voltage were applied. The diaphragm was vibrated by electrostatic attraction and the equivalent sound pressure calculated. A grille used by the author in 1932 is shown in Figure 1–46. The cavity in front of the diaphragm and diffraction effects had to be taken into account to derive the free field calibration from the grille calibration (Ballantine, 1932).

Descriptions of smaller condenser microphones appeared in 1932 (Hall, 1932; Harrison & Flanders, 1932). In the 1930s, the Western Electric 640-A, predecessor of the well-known 640-AA, was developed.

Smaller companies frequently did not have funds for expensive state-of-the-art devices and had to make their own equipment. Figure 1–47 shows a 1932 half-inch diaphragm condenser microphone used by the author. It was patterned somewhat after the Hall design, but used a prestretched .0005 inch aluminum diaphragm. This microphone was

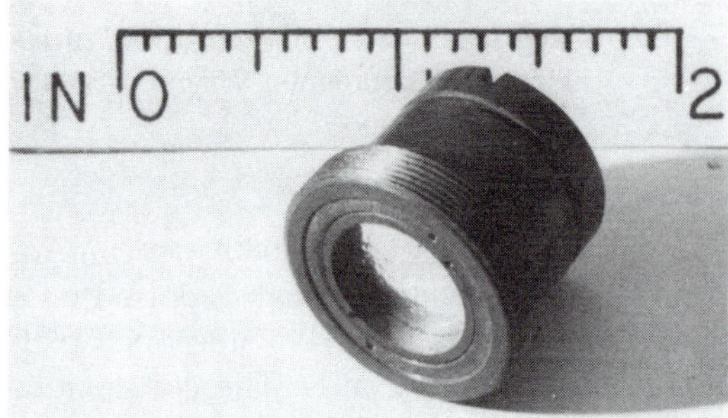

Figure 1–47. Half-inch diaphragm condenser microphone (1932).

used for both field and coupler measurements. It appears first to have been calibrated by comparison with a grille-calibrated large condenser microphone. A later (ca. 1937) in-house half-inch condenser microphone, made for coupler use, is shown in Figure 1–48. A small electrostatic grille was used to calibrate this and subsequent in-house half-inch microphones.

Cook (1940) reported on a new and precise primary method of calibrating condenser microphones, the reciprocity method. This method was further developed by DiMattia and Wiener (1946), and was fully described by Beranek (1949). It remains the basic precision method of microphone calibration.

Another device for moderately accurate primary calibration at low frequencies is the pistonphone. A pistonphone calibration at a low frequency plus an electrostatic grille frequency response curve can provide satisfactory accuracy for many purposes.

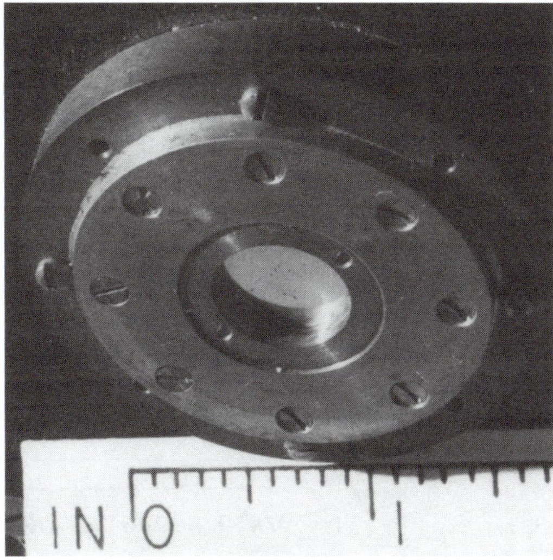

Figure 1–48. Half-inch condenser microphone used in coupler (ca. 1937).

A large step forward in sound pressure measurement was made in 1943 with the introduction of the Western Electric 640AA condenser microphone. By making the entire metal structure out of stainless steel, including the 0.00025 inch thick diaphragm, excellent stability was achieved. This microphone soon became the preferred sound pressure measurement device. An exploded view of the 640-AA from Beranek (1949) is shown in Figure 1–49. The outside diameter is 0.936 inch and the free diaphragm diameter 0.726 inch.

Some years after the introduction of the 640-AA, a series of measurement condenser microphones was developed by Bruel and Kjäer that included nominal diameters of 1 inch (Type L, similar to the 640-AA), ½ inch, ¼ inch, and ⅛ inch. In addition to the 1 inch, the ½ inch microphone is of particular interest for hearing aid measurements. It is useful for measuring input sound pressure levels and sound pressure levels in ear simulators, such as the Zwislocki coupler. It has good characteristics to at least 20 kHz.

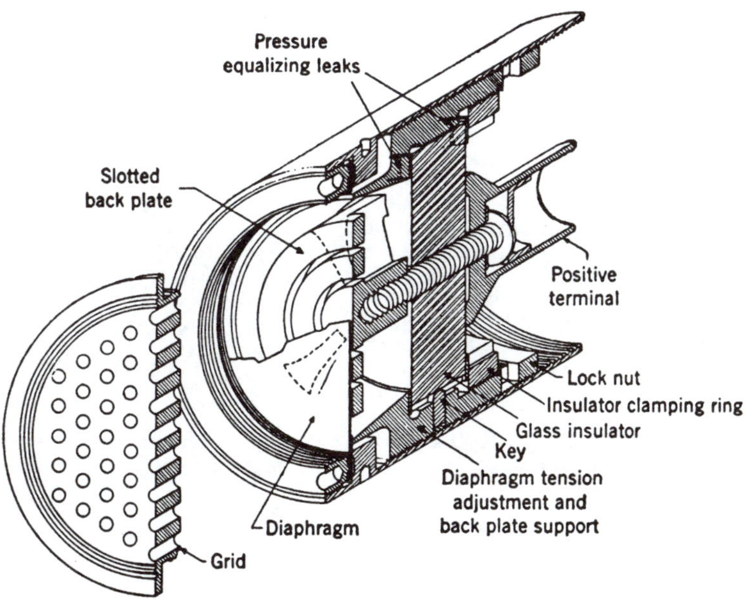

Figure 1–49. Construction of the Western Electric 640-AA condenser microphone. (From *Acoustic Measurements*, by L. L. Beranek, 1949. p. 217. Copyright 1949 John Wiley and Sons. Reprinted with permission.)

Couplers

The use of couplers for measuring earphone performance dates back at least to the 1920s. A simple coupler consists of a cylindrical cavity of chosen volume, with a calibrated condenser microphone diaphragm forming all or part of an end wall. According to Inglis and colleagues (1932), couplers had been used for some years.

The earliest coupler located in the elder author's 1932 records used a large condenser microphone. The cavity was very thin and had a volume of about 0.5 cc, as shown in Figure 1–50. The smaller volume would have given higher SPLs than a 2 cc coupler. Another coupler from the author's 1933 records used a half-inch microphone. It had a tube ¼ inch in diameter and 11/16 inch long to simulate the earmold hole and a volume of 0.5 cc beyond that.

West (1930) described an artificial ear that added an acoustic resistance element to a coupler for measuring supra-aural earphones. This was based on measurements of the impedance of real ears (West, 1929). The design had a long acoustic transmission line leading out of the coupler cavity.

About 1936, the author adapted the acoustic line idea for measuring insert earphones. A one-half inch in-house condenser microphone was used (see Figure 1–48). The coupler or "artificial ear" arrangement is shown in Figure 1–51. A tube about ⅛ inch in diameter and ¹¹⁄₁₆ inch long led from the receiver nub to a 0.75 cc cavity. A ¼ inch diameter acoustic line about 8 feet long led out of the cavity and provided about 128 acoustic ohms of resistance. Graduated amounts of yarn were placed at the far end of the line to minimize reflection. This device was used for testing both carbon and vacuum tube hearing aids until general acceptance of the 2 cc coupler.

The 2 cc coupler was first described by Romanow at a 1940 meeting of the Acoustical Society of America. Publication followed as *Bell Telephone System Monograph B-1314* and then in the *Journal of the Acoustical Society* (Romanow, 1942). Figure 1–52 shows the form of the 2 cc coupler used by Romanow. Romanow's paper has been the foundation on which hearing aid test standards have been

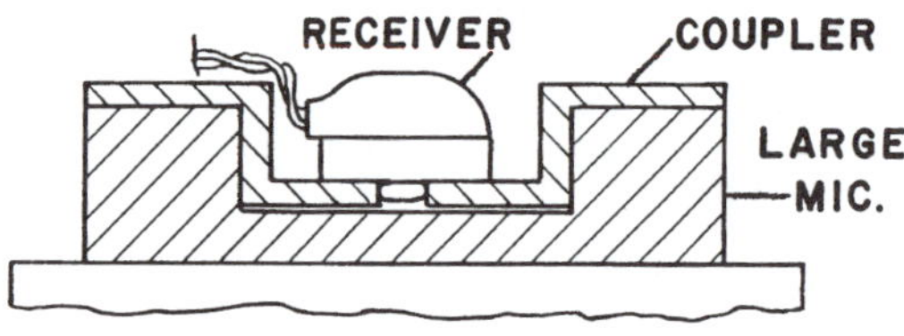

Figure 1–50. Insert earphone coupler using a large condenser micophone (1932).

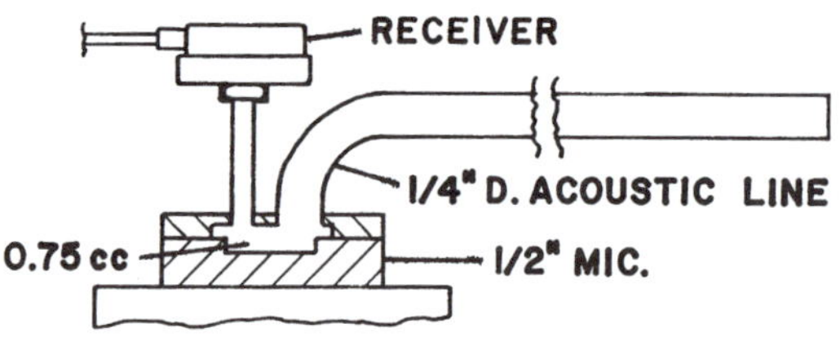

Figure 1–51. 1937 coupler with acoustic line.

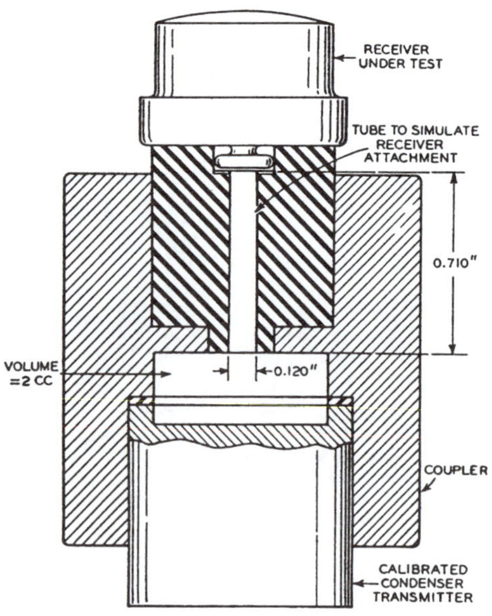

Figure 1–52. Romanow 2 cc coupler.

based. The 2 cc coupler has proved to be an accurate and reproducible device for comparing hearing aid performance. Results obtained with it can be processed to estimate insertion gain for typical average situations. It is not useful for measuring the effects of earmold venting because it lacks acoustic damping. West (1929) and Inglis and colleagues (1932) made ear impedance measurements applicable for supra-aural earphones. Zwislocki (1971) measured ear canal and eardrum impedance on human ears and invented an earlike coupler well suited for measuring insert earphones. The Zwislocki coupler, slightly modified (Sachs & Burkhard, 1972), was employed in the Knowles Electronics Manikin for Acoustic Research (KEMAR). It is shown in Figure 1–53. It has an ear canal simulating section terminated by a half-inch B&K condenser microphone. Four tuned acoustic networks are coupled to the central hole to produce the desired acoustic impedance characteristics.

The KEMAR manikin (Burkhard & Sachs, 1975) simulates the head and torso of an average human adult. It has made possible more realistic overall measurement of hearing aid performance and takes into account the acoustic effects of the body, head, pinna, and ear canal. Tests on the manikin with and without a hearing aid provide a measure of typical insertion gain.

Prior to the early 1970s, the measurement of hearing aid performance was limited to manufacturing and repair facilities due to the extent and cost of the equipment required for it. In 1973, Bruel & Kjaer (B&K) introduced a test system designed to be used in dispensers' offices, but it was quickly eclipsed in the same year by Frye Electronics' first digital hearing aid analyzer. That device featured automatic readout of amplitude and distortion, and was the forerunner of all automated in-office hearing aid test gear (Skafte, 1990). Frye and others continually have developed and further automated their systems for both the manufacturer and dispenser.

As hearing aids have been reduced further in size to fit entirely within the ear canal, yet another coupler has evolved (see Figure 1–54) to take into account the smaller volume of air through which the amplified sound passes. The HA-1 coupler may understate at-the-eardrum gain by as much as one-half (see Figure 1–55), due to its large physical volume relative to that of the unfilled canal between the tip of the hearing aid and the tympanic membrane, and the frequency-dependent impedance changes of the TM itself.

Although not yet conforming to any standard, the CIC coupler (in conjunction with correction factors built into the test gear) will provide much more accurate gain and output curves than will a standard HA-1 unit. (Frye, 1996)

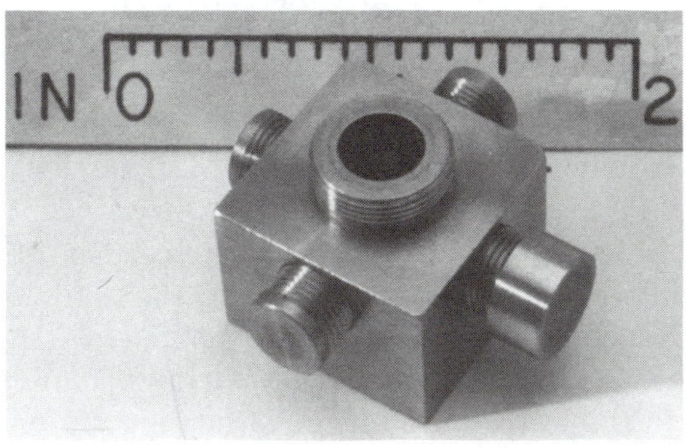

Figure 1–53. Knowles DB100 ear simulator—Zwislocki type.

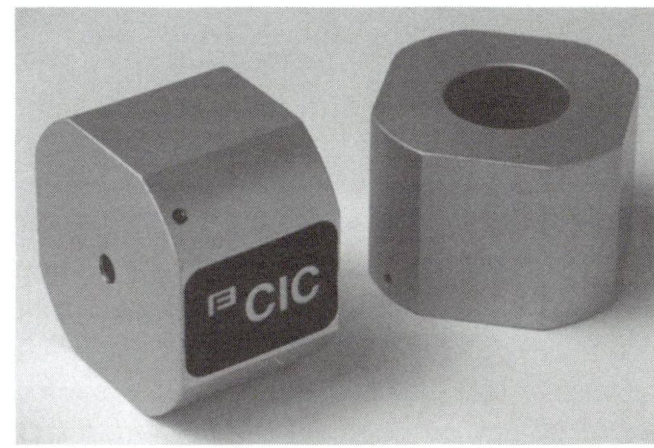

Figure 1–54. CIC coupler (Courtesy of Frye Electronics, Inc.)

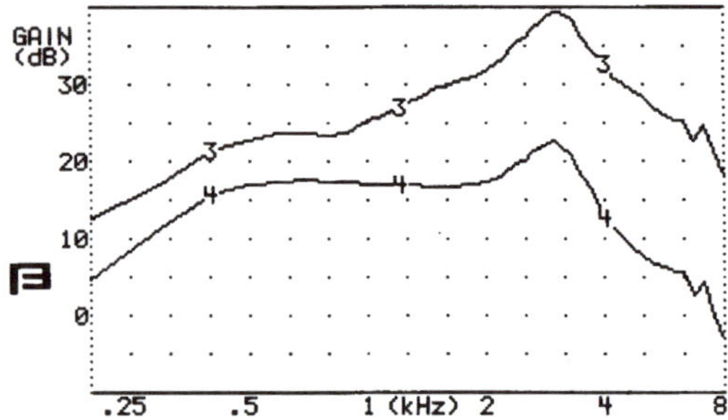

Figure 1–55. Comparison of same hearing aid measured through both CIC (Curve 3) and HA-1 (Curve 4) couplers. (Courtesy of Frye Electronics, Inc.)

Bone Conduction Couplers

A mechanical coupler for bone receivers was described by Hawley (1939). It used a vibration pickup to measure the vibration at a central point of the bone receiver face. A leather load simulated the headbone impedance. Carlisle and Pearson (1951) described a very practical strain gauge type artificial mastoid that integrated the vibration of the bone receiver surface. An IEC standard, *Publication 373,* defines a mechanical coupler that can be used for audiometer or hearing aid bone vibrator measurements.

Probe Tube Measurements

Probe tube measurement of hearing aid performance on the ear of the person being fitted, employing computerized leveling, programming, and display is becoming widespread. The concept of using a probe tube to measure sound pressure in the ear canal dates back at least to Inglis and colleagues (1932). They placed a very small probe tube coupled to a condenser microphone in the open ear canal to measure the SPL produced by a sound source. Then they derived the SPL produced by a supra-aural earphone by loudness comparison. The probe tube was calibrated by a Rayleigh disk.

Filler, Ross, and Wiener (1945) reported their historic study on the pressure distribution in the auditory canal in a progressive sound field. They used a small metal probe tube (i.d. = .025 inch) coupled to a Western Electric 640-AA microphone. A soft plastic tube (i.d. = .038 inch) was added for insertion into the ear canal to avoid possible damage. Their comprehensive study of the acoustic properties of the ear canal was published by Wiener and Ross (1946).

The first reported direct use of a probe tube for measuring hearing aid performance is believed to have been by Nichols and colleagues (1945) in *OSRD Report 4666.* A probe tube was run through the earmold to its tip, as shown in Figure 1–56 and the sound pressure in the ear canal was measured. The purpose was to compare real-ear SPLs with those measured in a 2 cc coupler to correct coupler measurements accordingly. Real-ear versus 2 cc coupler corrections measured by Nichols and colleagues for various receivers were shown in Beranek (1949).

More recently, the use of probe tubes in earmolds to measure insertion gain was descibed by Dalsgaard (1976), and has had considerable influence in stimulating the insertion gain concept.

Hearing Aid Test Standards

The paper by Romanow and work by others that started as early as 1935 or 1936 formed a basis for standardizing methods of hearing aid measurement. In 1944, under the auspices of the American Hearing Aid Association, the first United States hearing aid measurement standard, "Tentative Code for Measurement of Performance of Hearing Aids," was completed. Dr. Fred W. Kranz was chairman of the committee that developed the standard. It was later published in the *Journal of the Acoustical Society of America* (Kranz, 1945). Since that time, a number of hearing aid or related standards have been published by the American Standards Institute or its predecessors. An article on the history of hearing aid

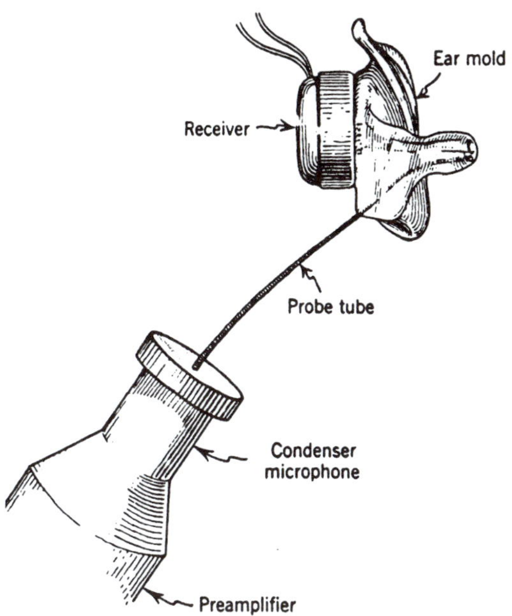

Figure 1–56. Probe tube in earmold (From Electro-acoustical Characteristics of Hearing Aids [*OSRD Report 4666*], by R. H. Nichols, R. J. Marquis, W. G. Wiklund, A. S. Filler, D. B. Feer, and P. S. Veneklasen, 1945. Copyright 1949 by Harvard University Electro-Acoustic Laboratory.)

measurement standards has been accepted for publication by the *American Journal of Audiology* in the near future. It lists ANSI standards of interest. Also, a complete series of International Electrotechnical Commission (IEC) hearing aid measurement standards have been published. Brief descriptions of ANSI and IEC standards were given by Lybarger and Olsen (1983).

Development of new hearing aid standards and updating of existing standards in the United States is being continued by working groups of ANSI Committee S3 on Bioacoustics.

REVIEW QUESTIONS

1. What acoustic aids were used prior to the introduction of electrical hearing aids?
2. What were the first electrical hearing aids?
3. When were vacuum tube aids first introduced?
4. When were magnetic microphones first used in wearable hearing aids?
5. Who invented the transistor and when?
6. What was the first ear level type hearing aid?
7. When were completely in-the-canal hearing aids introduced?
8. When did programmable hearing aids become available?
9. Who introduced wearable digital hearing aids?
10. When was the 2 cc coupler first described?

REFERENCES

Ballantine, S. (1932). Technique of microphone calibration. *Journal of the Acoustical Society of America, 25,* 319–360.

Bauer, B. B. (1953). A miniature microphone for transistorized amplifiers. *Journal of the Acoustical Society of America,* 25, 867–869.

Beranek, L. L. (1949). *Acoustic measurements.* New York: John Wiley & Sons.

Berger, K. W. (1984). *The hearing aid—Its operation and development.* Livonia, MI: National Hearing Aid Society.

Burkhard, M. D., & Sachs, R. M. (1975). Anthropometric manikin for acoustic research. *Journal of the Acoustical Society of America, 58,* 214–222.

Carlisle, R. W., & Pearson, H.A. (1951). A strain gauge type artificial mastoid. *Journal of the Acoustical Society of America, 23,* 300–302.

Carlson, E. V. (1988). An output amplifier whose time has come. *Hearing Instruments, 39,* 30–32.

Carlson, E. V., & Killion, M. C. (1974). Subminiature directional microphones. *Journal of the Acoustical Society of America, 22,* 92–96.

Cook, R. K. (1940). Absolute pressure calibration of microphones. *Journal of Research of National Business Standards, 28,* 489–503.

Cook, R. K. (1941). *Journal of the Acoustical Society of America., 12,* 415–420.

Dalsgaard, S. C., & Jensen, O. D. (1974). Measurement of insertion gain of hearing aids. *Proceedings of the Eighth ICA Congress,* London.

Dalsgaard, S. C., & Jensen, O. D. (1976). Measurement of the insertion gain of hearing aids. *Journal of Audiologic Technology, 15,* 170–183.

de Boer, B. (1982). *An investigation into the performance of antique hearing aids from the pre-electric era.* [Private publication of Mr. de Boer].

de Boer, B. (1984). Performance of hearing aids from the pre-electronic era. *Audiologic Acoustics, 23,* 34–55.

DiMattia, A. L., & Wiener, F. M. (1946). On the absolute pressure calibration of condenser microphones by the reciprocity method. *Journal of the Acoustical Society of America, 18,* 344.

Filler, A. G., Ross, D. A., & Wiener, F. M. (1945). *The pressure distribution in the auditory canal in a progressive sound field (Report No. PNR 5).* Cambridge, MA: Harvard University, Psycho-Acoustic Laboratory.

Frye Electronics, Inc. (1996). *Operator's Manual for FONIX® FP-40 Hearing Aid Analyzer.*

Goode, R. L. (1985). *Ear acoustical hearing aid.* U.S. Patent 4,556,122.

Greibach, E. H. (1939). *Bone conduction hearing device.* U.S. Patent 21,030. Filed Nov. 11, 1933; issued March 14, 1939.

Griffing, T. S., & Heide, J. (1983). Custom canal and mini in-the-ear hearing aids. *Hearing Instruments, 34,* 31–32.

Grossman, F. M. (1942). *Electrically and acoustically excited hearing aid.* U.S. Patent 2,363,175. Filed Aug. 26, 1942; issued Nov. 21, 1944.

Hall, W. M. (1932). Miniature condenser transmitter for sound field measurements. *Journal of the Acoustical Society of America, 4,* 83.

Hanson, E. G. (1920). *Telephone apparatus for the deaf.* U.S. Patent 1,343,717. Filed June 11, 1919; issued June 15, 1920.

Harford, E., & Barry, J. (1965). A rehabilitative approach to the problem of unilateral hearing impairment: Contralateral routing of signals (CROS). *Journal of Speech and Hearing Disorders, 30,* 121–138.

Harris, J. D., Haines, H. L., Kelsey, P. A., & Clack, T. D. (1961). The relation between speech intelligibility and the electroacoustic characteristics of low fidelity circuitry. *Journal of Auditory Research,* 1, 357–381.

Harrison, H. C., & Flanders, P. B. (1932). Efficient miniature condenser microphone system. *Journal of the Acoustical Society of America, 4, 51*(S).

Hawley, M. S. (1939). An artificial mastoid for audiphone measurements. *Bell Laboratories Record, 18,* 73–75.

Hector, L. G., Pearson, H. A., Dean, N. J., & Carlisle, R. W. (1953). Recent advances in hearing aids. *Journal of the Acoustical Society of America, 25,* 1189–1194.

Hincks, E. T. (1913). British Patent 10,000.

Hutchinson, M. R. (1905). U.S. Patent 789,915.

Inglis, A. H., Gray, C. H. G., & Jenkins, R. T. (1932). A voice and ear for telephone measurements. *Bell System Technical Journal,* 293–317.

Killion, M. C. (1979). *Design and evaluation of high-fidelity hearing aids.* Unpublished doctoral dissertation, Northwestern University, Evanston, IL.

Killion, M. C. (1981). Earmold options for wideband hearing aids. *Journal of Speech and Hearing Research, 46,* 10–20.

Killion, M.C. (1983). U. S. Patent 4,592,087.

Killion, M. C. (1987). U. S. Patent 4,689,819., show concept of including amplifier in receiver case.

Killion, M.C. (1993). The K-AMP hearing aid: an attempt to present high fidelity for persons with impaired hearing. *American Journal of Audiology, 2,* 52–74.

Killion, M. C., & Carlson, E. V. (1970). A wideband miniature microphone. *Journal of the Audiologic Engineering Society, 18,* 631–635.

Killion, M. C., & Carlson, E. V. (1974). A subminiature electret-condenser microphone of new design. *Journal of the Audiologic Engineering Society, 22,* 237–243.

Knowles, H. S., & Killion, M. C. (1978). Frequency characteristics of recent broad band receivers. *Journal of Audiologic Technology, 17,* 86–99.

Kranz, F. W. (1928). *Apparatus for aiding hearing.* U.S. Patent 1,679,532. Filed Oct. 10, 1921; issued August 7, 1928.

Kranz, F. W. (1945). Tentative code for measurement of performance of hearing aids. *Journal of the Acoustical Society of America, 17,* 144–150.

Kruger, B. & F. M. (1993). The K-AMP hearing aid: a summary of features and benefits. *Hearing Instruments, 44/1,* 30–35; *44/2,* 26–28

Lieber, H. (1933). U.S. Patent 1,940,533.

Lybarger, S. F. (1938). *Method and apparatus for selecting and prescribing audiophones.* U.S. Patent 2,112,560.

Lybarger, S. F. (1941). *Bone conduction receiver.* U.S. Patent 2,230,499. Filed Oct. 5, 1938; issued Feb. 4, 1941.

Lybarger, S. F. (1947, November). Development of a new hearing aid with magnetic microphone. *Electrical Manufacturing.*

Lybarger, S. F. (1987). An early auditory training system. *Journal of the Audiologic Engineering Society, 35,* 270–275.

Lybarger, S. F., & Olsen, W. O. (1983). Hearing aid measurement standards: An update and bibliography. *Hearing Journal, 36,* 19–20.

Nichols, R. H., Marquis, R. J., Wiklund, W. G., Filler, A. S., Feer, D. B., & Veneklasen, P. S. (1945). *Electro-acoustical characteristics of hearing aids* (OSRD Report 4666). Cambridge, MA: Harvard University, Electro-Acoustic Laboratory. (Library of Congress, Order No. PB 143405)

Olson, H. F., & Massa, F. (1934). *Applied acoustics.* Philadelphia: P. Blakiston's Son & Co., Inc.

Preves, D. A. & Leisses, M. E. (1995). Some questions about CIC hearing aids. *Audecibel, 44,* 10–16

Rayleigh, L. (1882). On an instrument capable of measuring the intensity of aerial vibrations. *Phil. Magazine, 14,* 186–187.

Romanow, F. F. (1942). Methods for measuring the performance of hearing aids. *Journal of the Acoustical Society of America, 13,* 294–304.

Sachs, R. M., & Burkhard, M. D. (1972). *Zwislocki coupler evaluation with insert earphones* (Report No. 20022–1). Franklin Park, IL: Knowles Electronics.

Sell, H. (1925). *Microphonic relay.* U.S. Patent 1,624,511. Filed May 6, 1925; issued April 12, 1927.

Skafte, M. D. (1990). 50 years of hearing health care. *Hearing Instruments, 4.*

Staab, W. J. (1987). Digital hearing instruments. *Hearing Instruments, 38.*

Staab, W. J. (1990). Digital/programmable hearing aids—an eye toward the future. *British Journal of Audiology, 24,* 243–256.

Tillyer, E. D. (1923). *Ear trumpet.* U.S. Patent 1,659,965. Filed May 7,1923; issued Feb. 21, 1928.

Walker, G., & Dillon, H. (1982). *Compression in hearing aids: A review and some recommendations* (NAL Report No. 90). Canberra: Australian Government Publishing Service.

Watson, L. A., & Tolan, T. (1949). *Hearing tests and hearing instruments.* Baltimore, MD: Williams & Wilkins.

Wente, E. C. (1917). A condenser transmitter as a uniformly sensitive instrument for the absolute measurement of sound intensity. *Physics Revue,* 10, 39–63.

West, W. (1929). Measurements of the acoustical impedance of human ears. *Post Office Electrical Engineering Journal, 21,* 293–300.

West, W. (1930). An artificial ear. *Post Office Electrical Engineering Journal, 22,* 260–263.

Wiener, F. M., & Ross, D. A. (1946). The pressure distribution in the auditory canal in a progressive sound field. *Journal of the Acoustical Society of America,* 18, 401–408.

Zwislocki, J. J. (1971). *An earlike coupler for earphone calibration.* (Report No. LSC-S-9). Syracuse, NY: Syracuse University, Laboratory Sensory Communication.

CHAPTER 2

Speech Perception and Hearing Aids

WILLIAM H. McFARLAND, Ph.D.

OUTLINE

A basic assumption by those who manufacture and fit hearing aids for individuals with hearing impairment is that each aid should be chosen and adjusted to maximize speech understanding for the particular person being fitted. Although there occasionally may be exceptions, this assumption is usually true. Advances in hearing aid technology over the last 10 years have improved the ability of hearing healthcare professionals to provide better hearing of speech by people with hearing impairment, especially in quiet. Patient performance in noise, however, has not reached a level that is satisfactory or equal in improvement to the increase in cost to the patient over earlier technology.

Part of the dilemma is most likely related to the diverse needs of people with hearing losses, both personal and physiological, and to the almost impossible task that hearing aids are assigned. Conversational speech sounds vary from 65–70 dB SPL for the low frequency vowels and diphthongs, while the consonants may be as much as 30 dB lower in intensity (Fletcher, 1953). Speech may be embedded in a background of noise as much as 20 to 30 dB higher. The net result must be amplified to audibility, yet many impaired ears will not have enough residual hearing to detect, let alone recognize, many of the high-frequency consonants that are processed. In ears with enough residual hearing, there still may be poor discrimination of a variety of speech cues.

Finally, there remains the possibility that the hearing aid itself may eliminate important speech sound information due to its inherent limitations, necessary adjustments by the audiologist, or limitations of advanced circuits that may enhance speech in some situations, but make speech perception worse in others.

THE ACOUSTICAL NATURE OF SPEECH

Speech sounds have a wide range of intensities. Fletcher (1953) described a range of 680 to 1 in the power of the strongest vowel /ɔ/ to the weakest consonant /θ/. This can result in a range of almost 30 dB between different sounds in the same utterance. In general, vowels and diphthongs are the most intense sounds and carry the least amount of information for recognition and understanding of ongoing speech, while the consonants are the weakest of speech sounds and yet carry the most importance for the correct understanding of speech.

The sensation level of speech is also important with regard to understanding. Figure 2–1 illustrates the performance/intensity function for listeners with normal hearing when processing monosyllabic words. Note that, to achieve 100% understanding, the words must be presented at least 25 dB above threshold for the same words (threshold being defined as the level at which 50% of the words are understood) or as much as 40 dB above speech detection level (the level at which the presence of speech is noted, but discrimination may not exist). The performance/intensity function for hearing impaired listeners with cochlear hearing loss shown in the same figure varies significantly

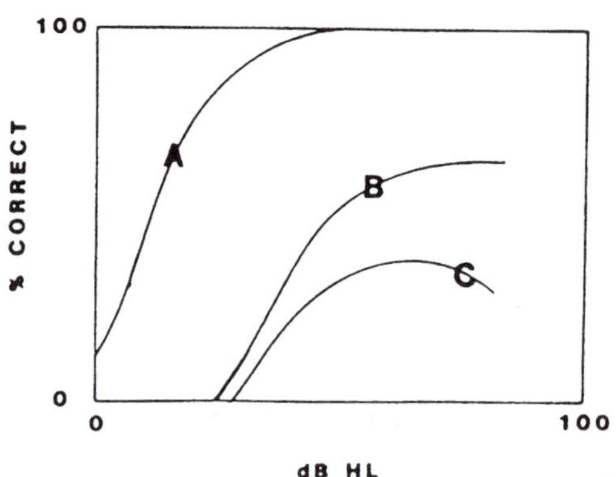

Figure 2–1. Performance-intensity functions. **A.** Normal hearing. **B.** Sensorineural hearing loss. **C.** Retrocochlear disorder. (From "Discrimination of Acoustic Signals," by W. R. Hodgson, in R. E. Sandlin [Ed.], *Handbook of Hearing Aid Amplification, Volume I*, 1988 [p. 290]. Copyright 1995 by Singular Publishing Group, Inc. Reprinted with permission.)

from patient to patient but is notably different from that for listeners with normal hearing in that:

- The range of intensities at which any speech understanding is possible is much reduced;
- Maximum understanding is often less than 100 % and in some instances may be very poor;
- Understanding may get worse as the intensity of speech increases beyond a certain level.

The intelligibility of individual speech sounds is enhanced by a complex interaction of the frequency, intensity, and temporal characteristics of each sound. In addition, speech sound spectra vary considerably from the effect of coarticulation. Amazingly, speech sounds still retain their identity, at least to listeners with normal hearing, in spite of a wide variety of speakers and adjacent speech sounds. Resonance in the vocal tract results in formant patterns that represent various positions of the tongue, lips, and oral cavity as they create vowels and diphthongs. These formants also provide some information as to the following consonant sounds (Danhauer, Osberger, & Pickett, 1973; Martin, Pickett, & Colten, 1972).

Temporal resolution is also important in speech sound recognition. Changes in duration, pausing, and syllable-rate tempo provide some assistance in understanding (Minifie, 1973). Minifie also stated that absolute prediction of intelligibility cannot be made solely on the basis of the spectral characteristics of speech sounds in relation to the configuration of the hearing loss. It is clear, however, that speech spectra are of primary importance in this process.

Figure 2–2 represents the results of a study by Hirsch, Reynolds, and Joseph in 1954. They measured the intelligibility of monosyllabic words in the Central Institute for the Deaf Auditory Test W22. These investigators examined the effect of various band-pass filter settings on speech intelligibility. The authors found that for low-pass filtering there was little loss of information with filter cutoffs as low as 1600 Hz. Performance did begin to decline below this, however, and dropped by 25% when the low-pass cutoff reached 800 Hz. High-pass filtering had little effect until 1600 Hz. Above this frequency performance began to decrease markedly. Clinical guidelines from studies such as this have led to the belief that intact hearing between the frequencies of 500 and 2000 Hz is necessary for normal speech understanding.

How hearing loss configuration degrades speech understanding, given these important speech frequencies, and how the use of hearing aids recovers this lost function is still of utmost importance to the audiologist.

HEARING LOSS CONFIGURATION AND SPEECH PERCEPTION WITH HEARING AIDS

Hodgson (1977) offered the following generalizations about speech intelligibility and hearing loss configuration:

> Persons with flat loss will probably have better discrimination than those with sloping high frequency hearing loss.
>
> Individuals with good low frequency hearing and a high frequency loss will hear vowels well and consonants poorly.
>
> There is no impressive evidence that persons with profound loss, fragmented audiograms and no measurable sensitivity over the speech range (500–2000 Hz) can learn to discriminate speech independent of visual clues.

Perhaps the most commonly used theory in calculating speech perception loss due to hearing loss or speech perception gain after amplification is the Articulation Index (Fletcher, 1929; Fletcher & Galt, 1950, Kryter, 1962a, 1962b.) The standardized version

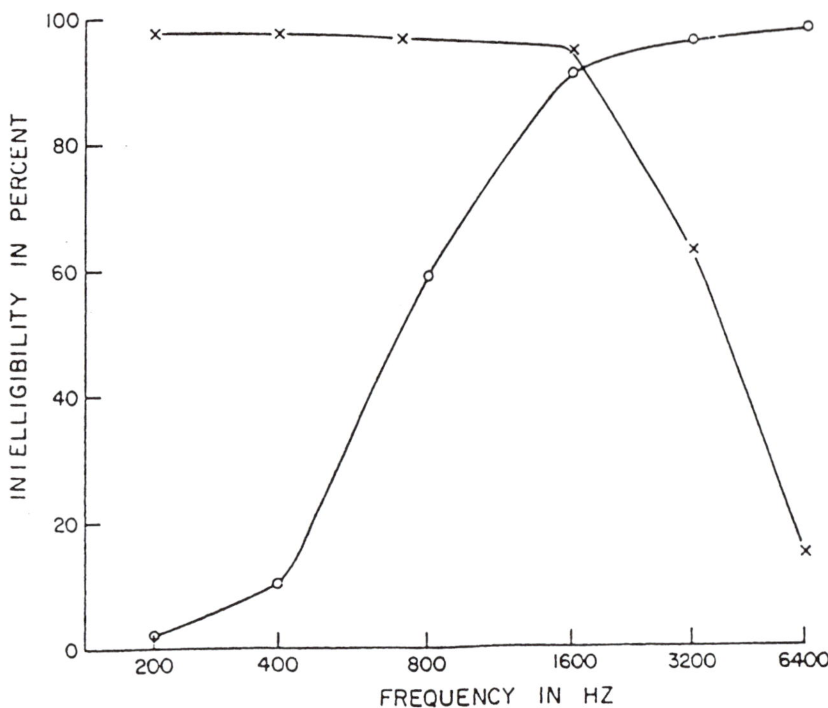

Figure 2–2. Relationship between high- and low-pass filtering and intelligibility of speech. (From "Speech Acoustics and Intelligibility," by I. Hirsch, E. Reynolds, and M. Joseph, in W. R. Hodgson [Ed.], *Hearing Aid Assessment and Use in Audiologic Habilitation,* 1955 [p. 95]. Copyright 1986 by Williams & Wilkins. Reprinted with permission.)

(ANSI S 3.5-1969) identifies the long-term speech spectrum and its overall bandwidth, divides this bandwidth into 20 narrower contiguous bands of different widths but of equal weighting with regard to the contribution toward intelligibility. The standard also incorporates the amplitude fluctuations that contribute to the understanding of speech. The important amplitudes cover a 30 dB range across the range of frequencies included in the index (200 Hz–6100 Hz). This 30 dB range is asymmetrically distributed around the rms value of the average long-term speech spectrum. The resolution of the amplitude fluctuations in each band is 1 dB. Thus, this method is more accurate if smaller increments are used in testing than the typical 5 dB increment.

Once pure-tone thresholds are known, the number of decibels of speech above threshold in each band and the weight of each band are calculated to give the total proportion of the speech spectrum that is audible. For example, if all of the spectrum is audible, the articulation index would be 1.0. If only half was audible, it would be 0.5, and so on. Clinical measures of pure-tone thresholds typically provide frequency information at only 6 to 9 points across the frequency range. Thus the use of 20 bands may be more appropriate to the researcher than the clinician. Popelco and Mason (1987) described a nine-band method that would conform better to the octave and half-octave frequencies available to the clinician. The Articulation Index focuses on hearing sensitivity across frequencies. It can give an estimate of the loss of speech intelligibility as a result of hearing loss and also help the clinician calculate the amount of gain needed across the frequency range to elevate the speech spectrum above threshold. Popelco and Mason (1987) cautioned that the Articulation Index only quantifies audibility but does not predict the actual speech recognition performance an individual might have. With complete audibility of the speech spectrum, many individuals with hearing loss still have difficulty understanding speech. This may be a result of suprathreshold auditory processing deficits inherent in the impaired auditory system, limitations of hearing aid processing, or both.

SUPRATHRESHOLD CONSIDERATIONS IN HEARING LOSS OF COCHLEAR ORIGIN

A common complaint of people with sensorineural hearing loss is: "Even with my hearing aid(s), I can hear but I can't understand." Moore (1996) stated that, for hearing losses up to 45 dB, audibility is the most important factor. But for losses greater than 45 dB, poorer discrimination of suprathreshold stimuli is also of major importance. This belief is critical when hearing aids are considered as a way of improving speech intelligibility. Take, for example, a patient who is encouraged to spend significantly more money than he or she has previously spent for advanced programmable digital technology, yet misunderstands important speech information frequently enough to cause dissatisfaction with the hearing aids. The potential for improvement may have been compromised by the poorer suprathreshold processing related to cochlear dysfunction. If there are additional processing difficulties at higher levels of the nervous system (Stach, 1995), the potential for improvement becomes even more restricted.

Hodgson (1995) reported average speech discrimination scores for normal hearers and persons with acquired sensorineural hearing losses (Table 2–1). It should be noted that these results were obtained at suprathreshold levels with amplification deemed enough to provide the best speech understanding. The results show a steady deterioration of speech understanding from 97% for borderline-normal hearing losses to 26% for severe losses (poorer than 66 dB).

A wide body of research has identified several suprathreshold processing skills that are diminished by cochlear loss.

COCHLEAR DAMAGE AND FREQUENCY SELECTIVITY

Frequency selectivity refers to the ability of the auditory system to separate or resolve the components of a complex sound (Moore, 1996). It has been demonstrated that psychophysical tuning curves obtained on animals with cochlear damage are markedly broader than those obtained from animals with normal hearing. Figure 2–3 reveals the wider tuning curve associated with sensorineural hearing loss. Broader psychophysical tuning curves have been found on humans with cochlear losses in studies that used notched-noise maskers (Dubno & Dirks, 1989; Leek & Summers, 1993; Stone, Glasberg, & Moore, 1992). These studies agree that the auditory filters in persons with cochlear loss are broader than normal and that the degree of broadening increases with increasing hearing loss (Moore, 1996).

A behavioral consequence of these broader tuning curves may result in poorer fre-

Table 2-1. Auditory discrimination scores of patients with acquired sensorineural hearing loss.

Thresholds (db re: ANSI 1969 norm)	*Age*	*Number of Ears*	*Mean Score (%)*
Normal	Under 65	175	97.31
(0–10 dB)	Over 65	5	96.40
Borderline normal	Under 65	75	97.07
(11–25 dB)	Over 65	15	94.67
Mild loss	Under 65	55	88.36
(26–45 dB)	Over 65	57	83.12
Moderate loss	Under 65	12	63.83
(46–65 dB)	Over 65	24	66.33
Severe loss	Under 65	2	26.00
(66–85 dB)	Over 65	4	26.50
Profound loss	Under 65	2	2.00
(86+ db)			

Source: From *Basic Audiologic Evaluation*, by W. R. Hodgson, 1980, Baltimore: Williams & Wilkins. Copyright 1980 by Williams & Wilkins. Reprinted with permission.

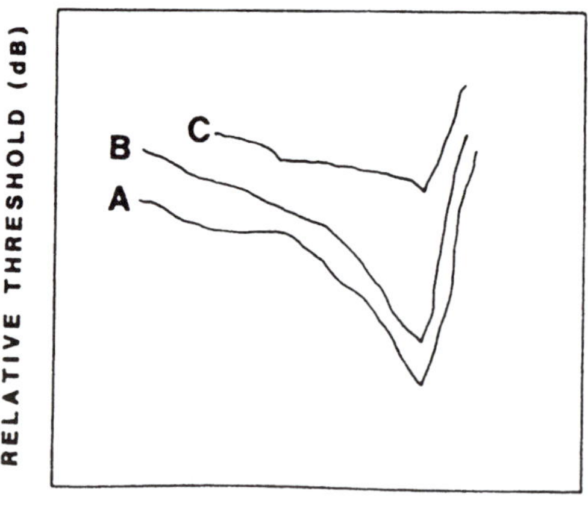

Figure 2–3. Tuning curves. **A.** Idealized tuning curve of an auditory neuron. **B.** Idealized psychophysical tuning curve. **C.** Psychophysical tuning curve of an individual with sensorineural hearing loss. (From "Discrimination of Acoustic Signals," by W. R. Hodgson in R. E. Sandlin [Ed.], *Handbook of Hearing Aid Amplification, Volume I*, 1988 [p. 284]. Copyright 1995 by Singular Publishing Group. Reprinted with permission.)

quency discrimination. Hodgson (1995) stated that difference limen for frequency (DLF) is increased on individuals with sensorineural hearing loss; that is, they require a greater change in frequency to detect a difference in pitch than do individuals with normal hearing.

Preminger and Wiley (1985) compared consonant intelligibility with psychoacoustic acoustic tuning curve data and found that sensorineural hearing loss subjects with nearly normal psychoacoustic tuning curves yielded better consonant intelligibility test results.

The upward spread of masking phenomena has been found to influence persons with high-frequency sensorineural hearing loss (Danhauer & Pickett, 1975; Scharf & Florentine, 1982). This potential interference with consonant recognition is exacerbated if hearing aids deliver excessive low-frequency amplification. Not all studies confirm the importance of spread of masking with sensorineural subjects (Hodgson, 1996). Humes (1982) cautioned that upward spread of masking may not be as much a trait of sensorineural hearing loss as the higher sound pressure level (SPL) of the stimuli used in testing subjects with sensorineural hearing loss.

Patients with sensorineural hearing loss have much greater difficulty hearing in noise than do normal listeners or persons with conductive or mixed hearing losses (Hodgson, 1995; Olsen & Tillman, 1968). Part of the difficulty may relate to the broader filtering activity of the cochlear loss and some may be related to the upward spread of masking.

COCHLEAR DAMAGE, LOUDNESS PERCEPTION, AND INTENSITY RESOLUTION

Interestingly, the point at which sounds become uncomfortably loud, or the loudness discomfort level (LDL), is about the same SPL for persons with sensorineural hearing loss as it is for others. This creates a phenomenon known as recruitment (Hodgson, 1995). Loudness recruitment and its relationship to losses of cochlear origin are well known (Fowler, 1936; Steinberg & Gardner, 1937). This abnormally rapid loudness growth is related to the fact that that absolute threshold is elevated, but the level at which sounds become uncomfortably loud is still normal. The net result is a much narrower range of loudness between what is barely heard and what is too loud. This narrowed dynamic range obviously presents a challenge when considering the use of a hearing aid. Because of recruitment, one might expect people with cochlear hearing losses to have intensity discrimination that is better than normal. People with cochlear hearing loss perform as well or better than normal if one compares them at equal sensation levels (SL); however, at equal sound pressure levels (SPL), the person with impaired hearing may be worse than normal for intensity discrimination (Moore, 1996). Moore further stated that, "in everyday life, hearing impaired people often listen at lower SL's than normally hearing people, so their intensity discrimination can be worse than normal. However, this does not appear to lead to marked problems, because it is rare in every day life for critical information to be carried by small changes in intensity."

COCHLEAR DAMAGE AND TEMPORAL RESOLUTION

There are several measures of temporal resolution, and subjects with hearing impairment perform poorly on some but not all. For example, the detection of gaps in bands of noise is more difficult for the persons with hearing impairment, as are some forms of recovery from forward masking. Again, individuals with impaired hearing are markedly worse if comparisons to normal function are made at the same SPL; they are only slightly worse if made at the same SL (Glassberg, Moore, & Bacon, 1987). For the detection of gaps in sinusoids or a series of clicks, individuals with cochlear hearing loss may actually perform a little better than normal subjects (Jesteadt, Bilger, Green, & Patterson, 1976; Moore & Glassberg, 1988).

Measures of temporal modulation transfer function (TMTF) show the amount of amplitude modulation required for the detection of the modulation, plotted as a function of the modulation rate. It has been assumed that listeners who are hearing impaired are less able to perceive high rates of modulation than are normal listeners. This may be true for individuals who have high-frequency sensorineural hearing losses (Bacon & Viemeister, 1985).

When high-frequency hearing loss is simulated through low-pass filtering in people who have normal hearing, they decline in the ability to detect high rates of modulation. Furthermore, when Bacon and Gleitmand (1992) measured TMTFs in individuals with relatively flat hearing losses, they found that, at equal SPLs, they performed similarly to individuals with normal hearing, but were better able to detect high modulation rates when they were presented at equal but low sensation levels to both groups.

Thresholds of speech sounds are also affected differentially as a function of the duration of the sound in individuals with normal hearing and those with losses of cochlear origin. Sounds of longer duration need a larger increase in amplitude than do shorter duration sounds.

Moore (1996) stated that, even though persons with cochlear hearing loss do not suffer decline in performance on some measures of temporal resolution with controlled artificial laboratory stimuli, they do in general have more difficulty than listeners with normal hearing in the unpredictable fluctuations of sounds in everyday life.

NOISE AND SPEECH PERCEPTION IN PERSONS WITH HEARING IMPAIRMENT

It is well known that individuals with hearing losses of cochlear origin have much greater difficulty in perceiving speech in a background of noise than do listeners with normal hearing or persons with conductive or mixed losses. This increased disability in noise may be due, in part, to the spread of masking described by Martin and Pickett (1970) and the abnormal widening of critical bands in pathological ears (Preves, 1995).

Plomp (1994) described a variety of research that measured the speech reception threshold for sentences (s SRT) in a background of noise. The results are expressed in signal-to-noise (S/N) ratios necessary to yield 50% understanding of the sentence material. Invariably, persons with cochlear hearing loss needed an increase in the signal relative to the noise for understanding. The necessary increase ranged from 2.5 dB for mild hearing losses to 7 dB for moderate to severe losses. An even larger increase in SNR is needed when the noise fluctuates, as with a single competing speaker. The increase in speech intensity necessary to achieve threshold in this type of competing noise can range from 9 dB to as much as 25 dB (Baer & Moore, 1994; Festen & Duqesnoy, 1983; Eisenberg, Dirks, & Bell, 1995). Figure 2–4 from Killion (1997) illustrates the increase in signal-to-noise ratio from normal required to maintain 50% intelligibility as a function of hearing loss. As is evident in the figure, persons with a 30 dB hearing loss would require a 4 dB increase in S/N ratio, while people with an 80 dB hearing loss may need as much as a 12 dB increase in S/N ratio to maintain the same 50% level of comprehension.

MODERN HEARING AIDS AND SPEECH PERCEPTION IN QUIET AND NOISE

A wide variety of signal processing strategies have been incorporated in hearing aids over the past several years. These include adaptive compression, directional microphones, multichannel compression, BILL processing, TILL processing, wide dynamic range compression, and syllabic compression. These have been incorporated in programmable and now digital hearing aids. Multimemory hearing aids allow the user access to different combinations of these processing variables designed to suit different listening situations. Although many of these features have enhanced speech understanding in quiet, they have fallen short of the mark in noise (Killion, 1997).

Compression in its various forms can limit the output of a hearing aid to a level that is safe and comfortable to the listener. With adjustments to compression threshold (CT) and compression ratio (CR), compression can also allow the listener to maintain high-

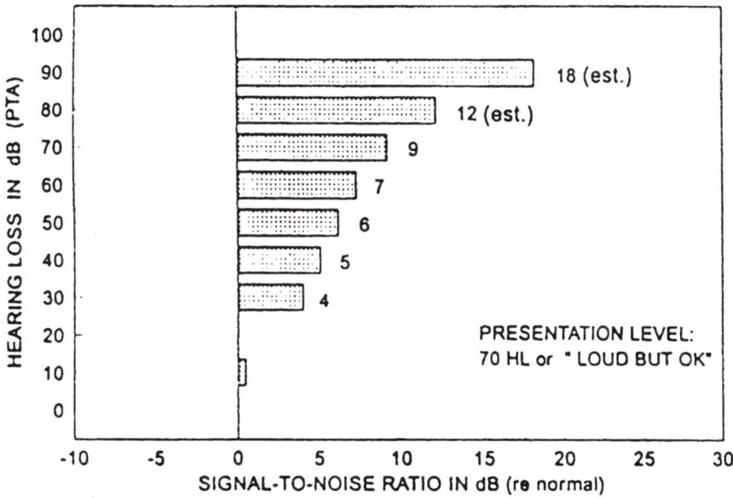

Figure 2–4. Smoothed-average SNR versus HL data. (From "Hearing Aids, Past, Present, and Future: Moving toward normal conversations in noise," by M. Killion, 1997, p. 145, *British Journal of Audiology, 31,* pp. 141-148. Copyright 1997 by Academic Press. Reprinted with permission.)

er gain for faint and mid-level sounds than he or she would be able to do with a linear instrument. Compression also reduces the need for repeated volume adjustments by the listener.

The question of whether speech perception is better through compression or linear aids is less clear. Compression applied to low-frequency amplification, as in so-called automatic signal processing (ASP) aids has produced mixed results (Moore, 1995). Studies that seem to suggest benefits may be partly due to the reduction in distortion that such aids provide for sounds at high input levels (Van Tassel & Crain, 1992).

Multiband compression has been found to provide improvement in the comprehension of speech when a wide range of levels was used (Laurence, Moore, & Glasberrg, 1983; Moore, Glasberg, & Stone, 1991; Villchur, 1973). When high-level speech is presented, however, compression does not show an improvement over linear amplification. In some studies, fast-acting compression has been found to improve speech understanding in noise as long as the number of bands was kept small (Laurence, Moore, & Glasberg, 1983; Moore, Glasberg, & Pulvinage, 1992; Moore, Glasberg, & Stone, 1991).

Moore (1995) stated that, in part, the lack of advantage for compression instruments in some studies may be related to unrealistically high gain settings chosen for the comparison linear instruments, settings that make sense theoretically for research but would not be maintained by the patient in real-life due to difficulty in tolerating loud sounds.

Multiband compression systems are intended to perform better in noise than single band systems and linear aids by allowing more gain in the high frequencies in the presence of predominately low-frequency noise. Separate CT and CR for each band should allow the audiologist to enhance speech for each person with impaired hearing. When noise exceeds the compression thresholds in the more important high-frequency bands, however, the speech signal will be reduced along with the noise and the result may be a reduction in comprehension.

The number of bands of compression that are optimal for improved speech understanding in noise is unclear, although it seems that large numbers may not be better than smaller numbers. Yund and Buckles (1995) described improvement in speech understanding in noise with increasing bands until the number of bands reached 8. Moore (1995) suggested that too many bands may reduce the spectral contrasts in speech, thus compromising understanding. Hickson and Byrne (1997) expressed concern that with single-band compression audiologists may unwittingly alter the consonant-vowel ratio and thus degrade intelligibility.

Wide dynamic range compression instruments are often sold as self-adjusting instruments. It is advantageous to have at least two bands of compression to differentially compensate for recruitment, which is usually worse in the high frequencies. Moore (1995) stated that there is little evidence that these instruments restore loudness perception to normal, and although many elderly patients appreciate the elimination of a need for a volume adjustments, a significant number of patients prefer to modify the overall gain in specific situations.

The use of directional microphones still provides the greatest improvement in speech comprehension in noise. Improvements in directional microphone design now routinely offer a 5 to 6 dB improvement in S/N ratio (Killion et al., 1998). For some hearing-impaired listeners, this can translate to as much as a 60% increase in speech discrimination performance. Directional microphones may create additional problems in some situations. Take, for example, a business executive who may hear better at a conference when the person across the table speaks, but hears much worse when persons on either side make their comments.

Assistive listening devices such as frequency modulation (FM) systems with remote microphones can provide even greater improvement in S/N ratio than directional microphones. They are seldom accepted, however, because of cosmetic considerations or because they impose additional constraints which the user may not be willing to accept.

Perhaps in the future, artificial modification of speech sounds may make them more audible in a background of noise and thus improve speech understanding. Baer, Moore, and Gatehouse (1993) demonstrated that spectral enhancement of consonant sounds does lead to the improvement of consonant recognition in noise.

DIGITAL HEARING AIDS

The emergence of digital hearing aids brings both exciting new possibilities and elimination of many constraints inherent in analog hearing aids. Most manufacturers are striving to have at least one digital hearing aid available to the public. It is estimated that by the year 2000 there will be as many as 20 different digital models to choose from (Sweetow, 1998).

In 1999, at some clinics, digital hearing aids were being sold for more than four times the cost of traditional analog hearing aids and more than twice the cost of many programmable hearing aids. Do people hear two to four times better with digital hearing aids when one considers overall hearing in a variety of situations? Do they hear 10% better? Or 20% percent better? Unfortunately, it is currently difficult to answer these questions, although some information is becoming available.

Killion (1997) stated that, once background noise (especially cocktail party noise) reaches 85 dB or greater, "the best thing any hearing aid can do is to stay out of the way" (p. 142). In his guest editorial on hearing aids and noise, Killion stressed that progress in both analog and digital hearing aid design over the past several years has led to improvement: Hearing aids no longer make hearing worse in noise, but they have yet to offer improvement in speech understanding in noise unless directional microphones or assistive listening devices (which are not unique to digital hearing instruments) are also used.

Naylor (1997) discussed technical and audiological factors related to digital hearing aids and stated that an immediate challenge was to invent good algorithms that would yield improved signal processing. Clearly, this must be the case as most signal processing schemes available in digital hearing aids are similar to those available in their predecessor analog programmable hearing aids, for example, multichannel compression; low-frequency gain reduction to reduce background noise, multiple memories, directional microphones, and so on. The speed and accuracy of these processing variables appear to be increased with digital instruments. However, it remains to be demonstrated whether there are accompanying functional improvements.

Naylor further stated that there are five perceptual deficits associated with sensorineural hearing loss:

Threshold elevation

Dynamic range/loudness distortion,

Reduced frequency selectivity,

Reduced temporal resolution, and

Reduced binaural processing

Only threshold elevation is satisfactorily corrected with digital instruments. It should be mentioned, however, that a digital hearing aid designed to restore binaural processing cues should be available shortly (Van Tassell, 1998).

Sweetow (1998) compared analog programmable to digital hearing aids, as shown in Table 2–2. The features compared include low kneepoints, multiple bands, noise reduction, and feedback control. Although the advantage appears to go to digital hearing aids in each category, it is unclear at this time whether these advantages lead to noticeable improvements in hearing. Furthermore, it is not clear whether some of the features discussed are truly advantageous. For example, a low kneepoint may be an advantage to one

Table 2–2. A comparison of a few of the capabilities of currently available analog programmable versus digital hearing aids.

Feature	*Analog Programmable*	*Digital*	*Advantage*
Low kneepoints	Down to 45 dB SPL	Down to 20 db SPL	Digital
Multiple bands	Up to 3	Up to 14	Digital
Noise reduction	Automatic Low-frequency gain Reduction based on amplitude Considerations	Automatic Low-frequency gain Reduction based on amplitude and temporal Considerations	Digital
Feedback control	Reduction in gain for Narrow-band or high Frequencies	Automatic reduction of of low-input gain and/or phase control	

Source: From "Selection Considerations for Digital Signal Processing Hearing Aids," by R. E. Sweetow, 1998, *Hearing Journal*, *51*(11), p. 35. Copyright 1998 by Lippincott, Williams & Wilkins. Reprinted with permission.

patient and a disadvantage to another or may be advantageous to one patient in a certain situation but disadvantageous to the same patient in another situation.

Valente et al. (1998) compared the comprehension of 50 subjects using the Widex SENSO digital hearing aid and the subjects' current analog hearing aids, using both objective tests of speech recognition in noise and subjective measures of subject attitude. The subjects were tested at two locations at different signal-to-noise levels. Of the 12 different stimulus conditions across the two sites, only one revealed a significant difference between the SENSO and traditional hearing aids. This was the low probability Speech Perception in Noise (SPIN) test at 50 dB signal input level at only one of the sites. Among the other test conditions, none of the Hearing In Noise Test (HINT) (Soli & Nilson, 1994) results were significantly different for the digital and analog aids or for other stimulus conditions.

There was a tendency, however, for the subjects to prefer the SENSO aids over their own hearing aids on the subjective measures. For example on the Abbreviated Profile of Hearing Aid Benefit (APHAB) subjects preferred the SENSO in the " ease of communication" and "reverberation" categories. The subjects also showed a preference for the SENSO in a questionnaire prepared by the authors.

Knebel and Bentler (1998) compared two different digital hearing aids; the Oticon Digifocus and the Widex SENSO on 20 persons with sensorineural hearing loss. Each subject was allowed to wear each hearing aid for a period of 4 weeks. An extensive battery of objective and subjective measures was used to determine each subject's performance and perceived benefit from each hearing aid. Tests included: real ear insertion gain and saturation responses, the Speech In Noise (SIN) test (Fikret-Pas, 1993), the Hearing In Noise (HINT) test (Soli & Nilsson, 1994), the City University of New York (CUNY) sentence test (Levitt & Neuman, 1990), the Categorical Rating Scale (Bakke, Neuman, & Levitt, 1995), the Abbreviated Profile of Hearing Aid Benefit (APHAB) (Cox & Alexander, 1995), the Attitudes Toward Loss of Hearing Questionnaire (ALHQ) (Saunders & Cienkowski, 1996), the Glasgow Benefit Inventory (GBI) (Robinson, Gatehouse, & Browning, 1996), and finally an exit questionnaire/interview.

Knebel and Bentler found no significant differences between the two digital hearing aids on the myriad of objective and subjective measures. There appeared to be a slight subjective preference toward the Widex SENSO but the authors caution that the preference may be largely related to nonacoustic differences (e.g., the physical characteristics of the aids: position of switches, battery doors, etc.)

The REIR results indicated that the Oticon Digifocus provided more high-frequency gain than the SENSO. Although this did not appear to translate into performance differences, it may have contributed to the increase in the "aversiveness" rating for the Digifocus on the APHAB. This may also have contributed to the slight preference for the SENSO. Oticon believes that the extra high-frequency gain is useful and suggests that it should be introduced slowly to the patient over a period of time to combat any negative reaction by the patient.

Their subjects also reported that the most benefit received from the digital hearing aids was in quiet environments and the least benefit was in noise, similar to what is reported for conventional or programmable hearing aids. Finally, the authors reported that the APHAB benefit scores were in the 20th to 30th percentiles for successful users of linear hearing aids, which may mean that the benefit provided by the digital technology alone is not noteworthy.

Valente et al. (1999) examined the performance differences of 40 subjects with hearing impairment wearing the Widex Senso C* (omnidirectional) and C9 (directional) digital hearing aids and their own analog hearing aids. The authors evaluated speech discrimination in noise with the Revised Speech Perception In Noise (R-SPIN) test (Bilger et al., 1984). Their subjects subjective preferences were also examined through the use of a questionnaire.

These investigators found that the mean performance of the SENSO C9 hearing aid with the directional microphone was significantly better than the mean performance of the of the SENSO C8 (digital with the same signal processing but with the omnidirectional microphone). The magnitude of the difference between these two hearing aids increased as S/N ratio became more difficult. Furthermore, there was not a significant difference between the SENSO C8 and their own hearing aids. This suggests that having a digital aid does not lead to better hearing in noise, but having a directional microphone does, and these are available on much less expensive analog hearing aids. The questionnaire results indicated that a strong preference for the Widex SENSO C9 in comparison to the subjects' hearing aids after wearing the C9 for 30 days.

Arlinger et al. (1998) compared speech recognition in noise with the Oticon Digifocus and 33 subjects' own hearing aids. Speech recognition was measured by determining the S/N ratio that resulted in 40% correct recognition of test words using tests of low redundancy sentences in an adaptive test procedure. In contrast to the HINT procedure, the speech level was held constant and noise levels were adaptively varied. Two different speech levels were used: 60 and 75 dB SPL. Subjective data were assessed by questionnaires, including APHAB and the Gothenburg Profile. The results revealed a small but significant difference in S/N ratio in favor of the Digifocus at 75 dB but no significant difference at 60 dB. The difference was 0.7 dB. The subjective test results revealed a preference for the Digifocus, which sounded clearer to the subjects than their own aids. In addition, subjects' perceived handicap was less while wearing the digital hearing aid.

From the above review of the research on the effectiveness of digital hearing aids, at this time, it appears that there is no clear evidence that users will hear and understand speech significantly better with digital than analog hearing aids. Although there is a subjective preference toward digital hearing aids, it may be related to comfort, a bias toward the latest technology, or other factors than hearing. Clinically, patients have remarked to this author that sound quality was more natural through digital aids or that speech seemed clearer. Although these observations may be valid, it does not necessarily hold that speech perception would be better as well.

All of the above investigators used speech perception in noise as the primary measure of speech perception. This is certainly appropriate because hearing in noise is the most important challenge for the hearing aid industry. Current digital hearing instruments that claim to reduce noise and enhance speech may eliminate important speech information when the noise is multiple-talker speech (one of the most common types of background noise). The ReSound 5000 digital hearing aids assesses the degree of modulation inherent in multitalker noise and reduces the gain in those bands with noise, proportional to the amount of noise estimated. The degree to which this strategy may improve speech understanding in a background of multitalker noise remains to be demonstrated. Even if detection algorithms work perfectly, a major weakness remains in the most common noise elimination strategy: filtering out the frequencies in the area of the noise. This generally means the reduction of an area of response important for the perception of speech. Hopefully, at some time in the future, algorithms will be developed for digital hearing aids that will allow the extraction of noise from surrounding speech but leave enough components of direct speech present to permit understanding.

CONCLUSION

Moderate, severe, and profound hearing losses of cochlear origin often have accompanying residual hearing that is markedly poorer in its ability to discriminate the frequency, intensity, and timing cues in sound—factors that are more important to the understanding of speech than the residual hearing associated with milder losses. Furthermore, the degree of residual impairment appears to be related to the degree of hearing loss: Individuals with profound hearing losses tend to have less useful residual hearing than persons with severe losses, and so on. The same individuals have significantly greater difficulty understanding speech in a background of noise than persons with normal hearing or milder hearing losses.

This reduced ability to understand speech in noise is most likely related to the poorer suprathreshold discrimination abilities of these individuals, as well as the spread-of-masking phenomenon.

It should be remembered that these deficits have been identified utilizing laboratory equipment that offers much a greater ability to reach residual hearing across the frequencies for an individual with hearing impairment than do personal hearing aids. Practical clinical realities often further reduce important sounds of speech needed for optimal understanding. Examples of these clinical realities are: (1) feedback and the unfortunate need to reduce important high-frequency gain to control it; (2) the patient's personal demand to use only the smallest cosmetically appealing hearing aid, such as a completely in the canal (CIC) hearing aid. (These small aids may not have enough gain for the hearing loss being treated); or automatic gain reductions imposed by a hearing aid either through its compression circuit or its noise reduction circuit. Although these automatic reductions in gain may improve user comport or reduce background noise, they typically also reduce some useful speech information.

New technology, especially digital technology, has improved our ability to address these limitations; however, the question remains open as to whether the purchase of these more expensive devices with their more intricate processing is wasted on individuals who cannot hear or discriminate the nuances they offer.

Successful fitting of hearing aids to persons with sensorineural hearing losses of cochlear origin is no small task. These hearing lpresent not only losses of hearing sensitivity but also deficits in the frequency, intensity, and temporal processing acuity for sounds that are audible. Advances in hearing aid technology, such as varying types of compression and multiple channels, allow more flexibility in the shaping of the frequency– gain characteristics of the instrument. Nontheless, improvements in speech comprehension in noise have been modest and remain the primary challenge of the 21st century.

REVIEW QUESTIONS

1. An Articulation Index of _____ indicates that a person should receive about half the speech information necessary for understanding.

2. The Articulation Index addresses amplitude fluctuations over a _____ dB range

3. The weakest sound of speech is: _____

4. With sensorineural hearing losses, an increase in the presentation level of speech can result in _______________ .

5. Hirsch, Reynolds, and Joseph (1954) found that speech intelligibility began to decline when low pass filters were adjusted below _____ Hz.

6. Moore (1996) stated that, for hearing losses below _____ dB, the primary reason a person does not understand is his or her threshold.

7. Persons with sensorineural hearing losses often have psychophysical tuning curves that are __________ than normal.

8. TMTF stands for ________________ .

9. A narrowed dynamic range between threshold and loudness discomfort indicates the presence of ________.

10. The most significant improvement, at this time, in hearing aid technology to reduce background noise is ________ ________________.

REFERENCES

ANSI (S3.5-1969). *American National Standard Methods for the Calculation of the Articulation Index.* New York: American National Standards Institute.

Arlington, S., Billermark, E., Oberg, M., Lunner, T., & Hellgren, J. (1998). Clinical trial of a digital hearing aid. *Scandinavian Audiology, 27,* 51–61.

Bacon, S., & Gleitman, R. (1992). Modulation detection in subjects with relatively flat hearing losses. *Journal of Speech and Hearing Research, 35,* 642–653.

Bacon, S., & Viemeister, N. (1985). Temporal modulation transfer functions in normal and hearing-impaired subjects. *Audiology, 24,* 117–134.

Baer, T., & Moore, B. (1994). Effects of spectral smearing on the intelligibility of sentences in the presence of interfering speech. *Journal of the Acoustical Society of America, 95,* 2277–2280.

Baer, T., Moore, B., & Gatehouse, S. (1993). Spectral contrast enhancement of speech in noise for listeners with sensorineural hearing impairment: Effects on intelligibility, quality and response times. *Journal of Rehabilitation Research and Development, 30,* 49–72.

Bakke, M., Neuman, A., & Levitt, H. (1995). Evaluation of a hearing aid rating procedure. Poster session presented at National Institute of Deafness and Communication Disorders/Veterans Administration conference on hearing aids, Washington, DC.

Beattie, R., Barr, T., & Roup, C. (1997). Normal and hearing impaired word recognition scores for monosyllabic words in quiet and noise. *British Journal of Audiology, 31,* 153–164.

Bilger, R., Nuetzel, J., Rabinowitz, W., & Rzeckowski, C. (1984). Standardization of a test of speech perception in noise. *Journal of Speech and Hearing Research, 27,* 32–48.

Cox, R., & Alexander, G. (1995). The abbreviated profile of hearing aid benefit. *Ear and Hearing., 16,* 176–186.

Danaher, E., Osberger, N., & Pickett, J. (1973). Discrimination of formant frequency transitions in synthetic vowels. *Journal of Speech and Hearing Research, 16,* 439–451.

Danaher, E., & Pickett, J. (1975). Some masking effects produced by low-frequency vowel formants in persons with sensorineural hearing loss. *Journal of Speech and Hearing Research, 18,* 261–271.

Dubno, J., & Dirks, D. (1989). Auditory filter characteristics and consonant recognition for hearing-impaired listeners. *Journal of the Acoustical Society of America, 85,* 1666–1675.

Eisenberg, L., Dirks, D., & Bell, T. (1995). Speech recognition in amplitude modulated noise of listeners with normal and listeners with impaired hearing. *Journal of Speech and Hearing Research, 38,* 222–233.

Fikret-Pasa, S. (1993). *The effects of compression ratio on speech intelligibility and quality.* Unpublished doctoral dissertation, Northwestern University, Evanston, IL.

Fletcher, H. (1929). *Speech and hearing.* New York: Van Nostrand.

Fletcher, H. (1953). *Speech and hearing in communication.* Princeton, NJ: Van Nostrand.

Fletcher, H., & Galt, R. (1950). The perception of speech and its relation to telephony. *Journal of the Acoustical Society of America, 22,* 89–151.

Fowler, E. (1936). A method for the early detection of otosclerosis. *Archives of Otolaryngology, 24,* 731–741.

Glasberg, B., & Moore, B. (1992). Psychoacoustic abilities of subjects with unilateral and bilateral cochlear impairments and their relationship to the ability to understand speech. *Scandinavian Audiology,* (Suppl. 32), 1–25

Glasberg, B., Moore, B., & Bacon, S. (1987) Gap detection and masking in hearing-impaired and normal hearing subjects. *Journal of the Acoustical Society of America, 81,* 1546–1556.

Hellman, R., & Meiselman C. (1990). Loudness relations for individuals and groups in normal and impaired hearing. *Journal of the Acoustical Society of America, 88,* 2596–2606.

Hickson, L., & Byrne, D. (1997). Consonant perception in quiet: Effect of increasing the consonant-vowel ratio with compression amplification. *Journal of the American Academy of Audiology, 8,* 322–332.

Hirsh, I., Reynolds, E., & Joseph, M. (1954). Intelligibility of different speech materials. *Journal of the Acoustical Society of America, 26,* 530–538.

Hodgson, W. (1995). Discrimination of acoustic signals In R. Sandlin (Ed.), *Handbook of hearing aid amplification. Volume 1: Theoretical and technical considerations* (pp. 281–297). San Diego, CA: Singular Publishing Group.

Hodgson, W. (1997) Speech acoustics and intelligibility. In W. Hodgson & P. Skinner (Eds.), *Hearing aid assessment and use in audiologic habilitation.* Baltimore: Williams and Wilkens.

Humes, L. (1982) Spectral and temporal resolution by the hearing impaired. In G. Studebaker & F. Bess (Eds.), *The Vanderbilt Hearing Aid Report. Monographs in Contemporary Audiology,* pp. 16–31, Upper Darby, PA:

Jesteadt, W., Bilger, R., Green, D., & Patterson, J. (1976). Temporal acuity in listeners with sensorineural hearing loss. *Journal of Speech and Hearing Research, 19*, 357–370.

Killion, M. (1997). Hearing aids: Past, present and future. Moving toward normal conversation in noise. *British Journal of Audiology, 31*, 141–148.

Knebel, S., & Bentler, R. (1998). Comparison of two digital hearing aids. *Ear and Hearing, 19*, 280–289.

Kryter, K. (1962a). Methods for the calculation and use of the articulation index. *Journal of the Acoustical Society of America, 34*, 1689–1697.

Kryter, K. (1962b). Validity of the articulation index. *Journal of the Acoustical Society of America, 34*, 1680–1702.

Laurence, R., Moore, B., & Glasberg, B. (1983). A comparison of behind-the-ear high fidelity linear aids and two channel compression hearing aids in the laboratory and in every-day life. *British Journal of Audiology, 17*, 31–48.

Leek, M., & Summers, V. (1993). Auditory filter shapes of normal-hearing and hearing-impaired listeners in continuous broad band noise. *Journal of the Acoustical Society of America, 94*, 3127–3137.

Levitt, H., & Neuman, A. (1990). *A sentence test*. Paper presented at the 13th annual RESNA conference. Washington, DC.

Martin, E., & Pickett, J. (1970). Sensorineural hearing loss and the upward spread of masking. *Journal of Speech and Hearing Research, 13*, 426–437.

Martin, E., Pickett, J., & Coltin, S. (1972). Discrimination in vowel formant transitions by listeners with severe sensorineural hearing loss. In G. Fant (Ed.), *Speech communication ability and profound deafness* (Paper 9). Washington, DC: A. G. Bell Association for the Deaf.

Miller, G. & Nicely P. (1955). An analysis of perceptual confusions among some English consonants. *Journal of the Acoustical Society of America, 27*, 338–352.

Minifie, F. (1973) Speech acoustics In F. Minifie, T. Hixon, & F. Williams (Eds.), *Normal aspects of speech, hearing and language* (chap. 7). Englewood Cliffs NJ: Prentice-Hall.

Moore, B. (1996). Perceptual consequences of cochlear hearing loss and their implications for the design of hearing aids. *Ear and Hearing, 17*, 133–161.

Moore, B., & Glasberg, B. (1988). Gap detection with sinusoids and noise in normal, impaired and electrically stimulated ears. *Journal of the Acoustical Society of America, 83*, 1093–1101.

Moore, B., Glasberg, B., & Stone, M. (1991) Optimization of a slow-acting automatic gain control system for use in hearing aids. *British Journal of Audiology, 25*, 171–182.

Naylor, G. (1997). Technical and audiological factors in the implementation and use of digital signal processing hearing aid. *Scandinavian Audiology, 26*, 223–229.

Olsen, W. & Tillman, T. (1968). Hearing aids and sensorineural hearing loss. *Annals of Otology, Rhinology. and Laryngology, 7*, 717–726.

Plomp, R. (1994). Noise, amplification and compression: Considerations of three issues in hearing aid design. *Ear and Hearing, 15*, 2–12.

Popelka, G., & Mason, D. (1987). Factors which affect measures of speech audibility with hearing aids. *Ear and Hearing*, 8(Suppl.), 109S–118S.

Preminger, J., & Wiley, T. (1985). Frequency selectivity and consonant intelligibility in sensorineural hearing loss. *Journal of Speech and Hearing Research, 28*, 197–206.

Preves, D. (1995). Principles of signal processing. In R. Sandlin (Ed.), *Handbook of hearing aid amplification. Volume 1: Theoretical and technical considerations* (pp. 81–120). San Diego, CA: Singular Publishing Group.

Robinson, K., Gatehouse S., & Browning, G. (1996). Measuring patient benefit for ORL surgery and therapy. *Annals of Otology, Rhinology, and Laryngology, 105*, 415–422.

Saunders, G., & Cienkowski, K. (1996). Refinement and psychoacoustic evaluation of attitudes towards loss of hearing questionnaire. *Ear and Hearing, 17*, 505–519.

Scharf, B., & Florentine, M. (1982). Psycho-acoustics of elementary sounds. In G. Studebaker & F. Bess (Eds.), *The Vanderbilt Hearing Aid Report. Monographs in Contemporary Audiology* (pp. 3–15). Upper Darby PA:

Soli, S., & Nilsson, M. (1994). Assessment of communication handicap with the HINT. *Hearing Instruments, 45*, 12–16.

Stach, B. (1995). Hearing aid amplification and central processing disorders. In R. Sandlin (Ed.), *Handbook of hearing aid amplification. Volume 2: Clinical considerations and fitting practices* (pp. 87–112). San Diego, CA: Singular Publishing Group.

Steinberg, J., & Gardner M. (1937). The dependency of hearing impairment on sound intensity. *Journal of the Acoustical Society of America, 77*, 621-627.

Stone, M., Glasberg, B., & Moore, B. (1992). Simplified measurement of impaired auditory filter shapes using the notched-noise method. *British Journal of Audiology, 26*, 329–334.

Sweetow, R. (1998). Selection considerations for digital signal processing hearing aids. *The Hearing Journal, 51*(11), 35–42.

Valente, M., Fabry, D., Potts, L., & Sandlin, R. (1998). Comparing the performance of the Widex SENSO digital hearing aid with analog hearing aids. *Journal of the American Academy of Audiology, 9*, 342–360.

Valente, M., Sweetow, R., Potts, L., & Bingea, B. (1999). Digital versus analog signal processing effect of directional microphone. *Journal of the American Academy of Audiology, 10*, 133–150.

Van Tassel, D. (1998). New DSP instrument designed to maximize binaural benefits. *The Hearing Journal, 51*(4), 40–49.

Van Tassel, D., & Crain, T. (1992). Noise reduction hearing aids: Release from masking and release from distortion. *Ear and Hearing, 13,* 114–121.

Villchur, E. (1973). Signal processing to improve speech intelligibility in perceptive deafness. *Journal of the Acoustical Society of America*, 53, 1646-1657.

Watson, T. (1964). The use of hearing aids by hearing impaired children in ordinary schools. *Volta Review, 66,* 741–744, 787.

Yund, E., & Buckles, K. (1995). Enhanced speech perception at low signal-to-noise ratios with multichannel compression hearing aids. *Journal of the Acoustical Society of America, 97,* 1224–1240.

CHAPTER 3

Hearing Aid Selection: An Overview

WAYNE J. STAAB, PH.D.

OUTLINE

A properly selected and fitted hearing aid or aids, should, at a minimum: (a) allow the wearing of hearing aids at a comfortable loudness level, (b) allow for little unnecessary overamplification of loud sounds, (c) improve communicative ability of the normal conversational speech level range, (d) provide better aided hearing than the user experiences without aid, (e) allow fit-and-modify opportunities to the hearing aid, (f) provide a means to evaluate the selection, and (g) realize that hearing aid selection is not a static event, but an ongoing process.

One of the difficulties an author faces when writing on the same topic several times, is that the content and text begin to share similarities with previous works. In other words, it becomes difficult to say the same thing many times in different ways and still make the text seem original. This was a difficulty in writing this chapter. As a result, the outline and a number of the graphs are similar to a previous work by the author (Staab, 1996).

HEARING AID CANDIDACY: AUDIOLOGICAL FACTORS

Every individual with a hearing impairment may be a potential candidate for hearing aid use. Realistically, however, emphasis should be on the *handicap* and the problems a particular loss presents and not on the degree of hearing loss as evidenced by essentially all hearing aid fitting philosophies today.

> "Hearing aids are not fitted based on the degree of hearing loss necessarily, but on the degree of hurt—and only when that hurt is great enough, whether socially, economically, financially, or psychologically, does this individual become a candidate for hearing aids."
>
> Staab, 1968

When that "hurt" occurs is individual because the realization threshold varies dramatically, often as a result of work and living conditions. Current efforts to penetrate the untapped hearing aid market attempt to educate the individual about the necessity for good hearing. We have not been successful to date. Part of the reason is that although we, as professionals, believe that hearing function is extremely important, many people who have a hearing loss do not believe that it is a big deal, especially when they can get along reasonably well without amplification.

Pathology (Type of Loss)

Conductive Loss

Often, the patient may choose to have a conductive loss corrected by medical and/or surgical intervention. When these approaches are unacceptable, due to extenuating circumstances or personal choice, good success can be generally expected with hearing aids. Because the loss of hearing is related mostly to a loss of loudness and not of speech recognition, the amplification provided by hearing aids is often sufficient to overcome the problems related to the hearing loss.

Sensorineural Loss

Hearing aids are the primary rehabilitative means for this type of hearing loss, and it is to this type that most hearing instruments today are fitted. The prognosis for success varies dramatically, depending on the location (peripheral or central nervous system), degree of loss, and expectations of the patient. Prognosis is not as good as it is for conductive losses and is generally poorer when the loss extends to the central auditory nervous system (CANS).

Degree of Loss and Hearing Aid Expectations

Hearing classification by degree of loss is somewhat arbitrary and varies among authorities. The following levels are the author's and are based on the pure-tone average of 500, 1000, and 2000 Hz (Staab, 1996, 1999). A greater number of categories are identified at the milder levels than most other authors provide, allowing the hearing health care provider to more realistically identify the decisions that are becoming increasingly important to the fitting of hearing aids. A given hearing threshold may overlap several categories.

Near Normal/Borderline (< 25 dB)

- Hearing almost everything well but may have to listen carefully in important listening situations
- Might create some problems if communication is very important
- May be more of a problem if hearing in the high frequencies (beyond those used in this average) is poor
- Hearing handicap is questionable
- Still, some believe a hearing aid is critical to their work or learning environment
- Amplification, if accepted, will seldom involve more than part-time use
- Not usual candidates for amplification

Mild Hearing Impairment (26–40 dB)

- Slight handicap for some, significant for others
- May have difficulty hearing faint or distant speech but is likely to "get along" in most situations
- Has difficulty hearing and understanding soft-spoken individuals (including women and children)
- Has difficulty understanding in a noisy environment
- Sustained attention is frequently difficult
- Speech and language are learned normally, monitored by traditional auditory feedback mechanism
- May or may not need amplification
- Most will find that HAs are too noisy unless:
  a. some type of open canal fitting is employed
  b. some unique noise suppression/cancellation approach is used
- If hearing aids are worn, they most likely are not worn constantly

Moderate Hearing Impairment (41–55 db)

- Listening is a strain, and sustained attention is difficult
- Has trouble hearing and understanding in ideal situations
- Understands conversational speech at relatively close distances without great difficulty
- Under normal conditions speech may have to be repeated often
- Has substantial difficulty understanding in noisy conditions
- Speech may show articulation problems (omissions, substitutions, and distortions of speech sounds)
- May benefit well from hearing aid use

Moderately Severe Hearing Impairment (56–70 dB)

- Understands conversational speech only if it is loud, in close proximity, or both
- Considerable difficulty expected in group or noisy situations
- Appears "not to pay attention"
- Communicates with great difficulty under all conditions
- Enough hearing is present to learn or maintain language and speech through the auditory feedback mechanism when amplification takes place
- Excellent benefit from hearing instruments can be expected; may be the most successful users of hearing aids

Severe Hearing Impairment (71–90 dB)

- May hear sound or loud voice very close to the ear
- Identifies environmental noises and may distinguish vowels but not consonants
- Seems to be "ignoring" communication
- Language and speech will not develop spontaneously in a youngster and may deteriorate significantly if the loss occurs over time, as with an adult
- Hearing aids enable them to become relatively functional for ordinary purposes of life

Profound Hearing Impairment (>91 dB)

- Does not rely on hearing as primary avenue of communication
- Speech and language must both be developed through careful and extensive training because they cannot be learned by ear alone, even with amplification
- Hearing levels in this category are often identified as being in the "deaf" range
- Hearing aids are intended to allow the user to maintain contact with environment and to allow the utilization of any auditory clues that might be presented
- Many do not utilize amplification, but rely on manual communication

Slope of Hearing Loss

The contour of the hearing threshold levels provides additional generalizations about the prognosis with amplification. Generally, flat, gradually rising, or gradually falling hearing losses respond best to amplification. As the contour of the hearing thresholds becomes steeper, is saucer-shaped, or as irregular dips and peaks occur, success with amplification becomes less. The least favorable contours for successful hearing aid use include precipitous losses (the lower in frequency the drop occurs, the less success), islands of hearing, reverse slopes, or residual hearing at the low frequencies only.

Speech Recognition

Within limits, the higher the speech recognition score, the better are the prospects for good results with amplification. When using CID W-22 word lists, scores of 90% and higher suggest probable good results; scores of 70–90% suggest mild difficulty; scores of 50–70% suggest poor results; and scores of 50% and lower are likely to result in amplification that has little success (Berger & Millin, 1971).

Dynamic Range (DR)

A person's dynamic range (DR) is ordinarily defined as the UCL (uncomfortable level) minus the SRT (Speech Reception Threshold). Individuals with wider DRs are more likely to experience success with amplification than are those having narrow DRs. Sensorineural hearing losses can have significantly reduced DRs, resulting in hearing aid circuit selections that have varying degrees and types of compression. One of the goals of a successful hearing aid fitting is to provide amplification that does not exceed the upper limit of the DR.

FACTORS INFLUENCING RECOMMENDATION AND CHOICE OF HAs

Some individuals respond much better to amplification than do others, even when their hearing losses are similar. Psychological and motivational issues are involved and are often beyond the scope or observation of the hearing aid fitter. Regardless, it is the responsibility of the dispenser to be able to judge the "hurt" caused by the loss and to counsel and fit accordingly.

Loss Related to Onset

The timing of when the hearing loss occurs can have a significant impact on successful use of hearing aids. If the loss occurs suddenly and hearing aid use is recommended closely following the incident, fewer difficulties are experienced in hearing aid use. If the hearing loss is gradual, long-standing, or if the loss is congenital, however, considerable difficulties can be expected. In these situations longer adjustment periods, along with more frequent or better counseling, are required.

General Attitude of the User

Complete acceptance depends on the motivation of the patient and also on an understanding of what constitutes successful hearing aid use.

Cost

Hearing aids are selected on the basis of cost at times. While this issue is important, it should assume importance commensurate with other considerations, such as benefit, satisfaction, and results.

Age

Hearing aids for children suggest special considerations and should be recommended by those familiar with educational and language development requirements. Prelingual (prior to speech and language development) children in particular require programs that involve a number of specialties to properly diagnose the hearing loss and to develop habilitative programs centered around appropriate amplification and educational paradigms.

Hearing aids fitted to postlingual individuals require varying treatment strategies, depending on the age of hearing loss onset, age at which hearing aids are fitted, type and degree of loss, the individual's work and recreational environments, mental capacity, and motivation of the individual. Hearing health care professionals must recognize that varying degrees of success will be achieved, and they must develop appropriate skills, based on knowledge, to counsel patients appropriately relative to prognosis. Generally, the later in life that hearing aids are recommended for a given hearing loss, the poorer are the expectations for their successful use.

Who Suggested Amplification?

Until the patient accepts the fact that he or she has a hearing loss, successful use of hearing aids will be minimal. Recommendations for amplification from the medical community are more likely to be accepted, however, than from other hearing health care providers or even from family members.

Cosmetic Considerations

Individuals are more likely to accept hearing aids if their use enhances self-image. If a person believes that the hearing loss is not significant, hearing aids that are more visible are less acceptable. A basic issue that many dispensers attempt to satisfy, then, is whether the patient will wear the type of hearing aid recommended, especially in the company of others. Patients and dispensers often take this approach, even when the most cosmetic hearing aids may not be the most appropriate. No hearing aid is acceptable unless the individual wears it, and in an attempt to mediate the decision between hearing aid acceptance and success, cosmetic considerations often become the deciding factor.

Dexterity

Manufacturers continue to reduce the size of hearing aids and their components. Some devices may include remote controls or switches or buttons under the patient's control. Some may also require decision-making. Dexterity of the potential user, therefore, must be considered when recommending hearing aids, taking into account the individual's age (young or elderly) and physical ability.

Part-Time or Full-Time Use?

The wearer will most likely determine the part-time or full-time use of hearing aids based on the listening demands and the benefit achieved when wearing them. The type and degree of hearing loss will likely have an impact, with individuals having milder losses being less likely to wear the instruments on a full-time basis.

PRESELECTION OF AMPLIFICATION: STYLE AND PLACEMENT

A variety of hearing aid types and styles are available. Often, the degree and type of hearing loss determines the style and or manner of placement of the instrument. Following are general comments relating to the different types of hearing aids based on their styles.

Completely-in-the-Canal (CIC) and Peritympanic Hearing Aids

These are the most cosmetically appealing (and smallest) of the hearing aid styles. They are intended to fit completely in the ear canal. The faceplate of the instrument should be at least flush with the opening of the ear canal, and the instrument should extend past the second bend to provide amplification advantages ordinarily associated with deep canal fittings (Staab & Finlay, 1991). These include (a) greater overall sound pressure level, especially in the high frequencies; (b) a reduction of the occlusion effect; (c) greater hearing aid headroom; (d) reduced feedback because of the lower gain/output required to fit a given loss when compared with other type hearing aid fittings; and (e) the opportunity to fit a more severe hearing loss with less gain. The degree to which these advantages are achieved depends on the way the instrument is terminated in the ear canal beyond the second bend. CIC instruments require about 5 to 10 dB less gain than in-the-canal (ITC) HAs for the same level of hearing impairment.

In-the-Canal (ITC) Hearing Aids

These instruments are between the CIC and in-the-ear (ITE) in size, and became popular during the Reagan Administration in 1983 because of his acknowledgment of hearing loss and his use of this type of instrument. Because of their size, their range of use is more limited than that of ITE instruments but greater than that of CIC aids. Even though they have less gain and output than ITE aids, the location of the microphone and slightly deeper insertion of the aid provide a smaller residual volume and, therefore, require approximately 5 dB less amplifier gain to fit a comparable hearing loss. Overall, the losses are usually less severe than for ITE instruments.

In-the-Ear (ITE) Hearing Aids

In-the-ear (ITE) aids fill the bowl of the ear. They have the greatest variety of styles, features, and range-of-loss fittings available among the custom-molded products. When selecting among the variations of ITEs (full concha, low profile, half concha, etc.), the component demands of the aid largely determine the choice.

These instruments are most successful for use with losses having pure-tone averages between 35 and 70 dB, with the upper limit primarily due to feedback limitations and the lower limit having less success because fairly good low-frequency hearing is generally present, resulting in little noticeable amplification benefit. Of the custom-molded instruments, this style lends itself best to venting, although benefit is minimized if large vents are used, which lead to increased feedback.

Behind-the-Ear (BTE) Hearing Aids

Of all styles of hearing aids, these instruments fit the widest range of hearing losses (from mild to profound) and offer the dispenser the greatest possibilities for hearing aid adjustment. Known as postauricular or over-the-ear hearing aids, they are housed in curved cases that fit neatly behind or over the ear. A custom earmold made to the shape of the ear canal is used with these aids to provide anchorage and also to direct the amplified sound into the ear. They are available in a variety of sizes, ordinarily have a telecoil switch that allows for telephone use, and many can be connected to external sound sources, such as televisions and additional assistive listening devices.

Eyeglass Hearing Aids

These are similar to BTE models in terms of range of the hearing loss fitted and the flexibility of adjustment; however, they are built into an eyeglass frame. They have been replaced largely by ITE instruments. Historical difficulties have centered around matching the optics with the hearing aid frames, temples, and hinges. Some BTE instruments have an attachment that allows the BTE instrument to be fitted to the end of eyeglass hearing aids.

Body-Worn Hearing Aids

Body-worn (pocket-worn) hearing aids have larger components, larger sized cells, and are carried in pockets or attached to clothing. An external receiver (speaker) is attached to the aid by a flexible wire cord. The receiver is attached to a custom-molded ear piece to direct sound into the ear.

These instruments are used most often with profound hearing losses or for persons who have difficulty manipulating the controls of smaller hearing aids. The separation of the microphone (on the aid) and receiver (at the earmold) allows for greater gain and output before feedback than with any other type of instrument style.

Special Function Hearing Aids

Hearing aids have been developed to manage a variety of listening conditions and demands. Some of these are variations of the noninvasive instruments described previously, while others involve invasive procedures.

Noninvasive Special Function Units/Features

CROS (Contralateral Routing of Offside Signals) Hearing Instruments

CROS hearing aids and their variations are often used by persons who have no aidable hearing in one ear but have fairly normal hearing or a slight loss of hearing in the other. The signal is picked up by a microphone located on the poor ear side and is transmitted (either via wires or by a radio frequency [RF]) signal to the better ear.

Bone-Conduction Hearing Aids

These instruments drive a vibrator that generally lies against the skull and sends a vibration rather than the auditory signal. Historically, these instruments have been reserved most often for conditions in which a chronic discharge from the ears renders fitting earmold-type hearing aids impractical. A recent offering, however, provides a distinct variation of this by transposing incoming signals into an audible ultrasound (30–40 kHz) and then directing the signal through a bone-conducted oscillator to individuals having profound hearing losses (Staab, et al., 1998).

Directional Microphone (Beam-forming) Hearing Aids

These instruments have a microphone system that allows signals from the front to be heard more easily than sounds from the rear, where much of the noise is located. These arrangements are proven to improve the signal-to-noise ratio (SNR). Some devices allow the user to switch between a regular and the directional microphone, and some have multiple microphones to provide even greater directionality.

Hearing Aid Telephone Induction

This feature, identified also as T-Switch, telecoil, T-coil, telephone pickup switch, telephone induction coil, telephone induction pickup coil among others, describes the special feature on hearing aids that use the principle of inductive coupling. The stray electromagnetic energy from a telephone is picked up by an induction coil in the hearing aid and converted into amplified sound. Because the hearing aid's microphone is not functional during this action, the only sound amplified is that directly from the telephone, without any outside interference. This inductive coupling can be used with a hearing-aid-compatible telephone and also can be used with assistive listening devices and loop systems. Essentially, the smaller the hearing aid, the less effective the induction feature and the less probable that it is a feature of the instrument.

Auditory Trainers

A limitation of hearing aids is that they tend to amplify essentially all sounds equally. Therefore, whenever the sound source is distant, distracting noises that are closer cause interference. Additionally, reverberation (echoing of sound back and forth from one surface to another) is distracting.

In these situations, the key is to place a microphone closer to the primary sound source and to deliver it to a unit worn on the user's head. Units of this type are often referred to as auditory trainers and have as their primary function the goal of reducing background noise. Some of these systems involve hard-wire connections or AM, FM, infrared, tactile, or magnetic induction transmission from the sound source to the unit worn by the person with hearing impairment. Although auditory trainers can be used in almost any environment, they are most often found in schools and places of worship.

Transposer Hearing Aids

These devices are intended to take signals that are high in frequency and shift them into the lower frequencies where the patient may have some residual hearing.

Invasive (Implantable) Special Function Aids

These instruments involve the surgical implantation of a portion of the hearing aid function into some part of the listening channel anatomy. The power supply, electronics, and input transducer (microphone) are primarily external and require some type of physical connection to the implanted feature. These implantable devices may be in the outer ear canal, attached to the tympanic membrane, or placed in the middle-ear cavity, in the cochlea, or in the bone-conduction pathway. The fact that they have not yet achieved wide-range acceptance will not deter continued efforts. Consideration of these special devices should be approached carefully and with a full knowledge of what they attempt to accomplish and of what the patient is willing to accept and expect.

Cochlear Implants

These devices convert sound to electrical impulses that are transmitted directly through a wire or wires placed inside the cochlea to stimulate the auditory nerve. Placing a cochlear implant and programming it for personal use requires a highly skilled team. These instruments have, traditionally, been limited to the postlingual deafened adult, but more recently, specialists have fit selected children with cochlear implants as well.

Middle-Ear Implants

These approaches involve affixing a magnet, piezoelectric crystal, or some other driving mechanism to the tympanic membrane or to one of the auditory ossicles. A wire or magnet powers the driving mechanism from an external power source. The degree and type of hearing losses recommended for these fittings are not yet well established.

Bone-Conduction

These units are similar to the middle-ear implants except that the driving mechanism (bone-conduction vibrator) is implanted in the skull, generally on the mastoid process. A magnet or direct attachment connects the bone-conduction vibrator to the external power source and amplification unit.

BINAURAL VERSUS MONAURAL AMPLIFICATION

The general consensus is that, unless significant contradictions exist, binaural amplification is the fitting arrangement of choice. Reasons given are that dichotic hearing (one complete aid to each ear) provides for improved (a) depth perception, (b) localization of sound, (c) utilization of the sound shadow caused by the head, (d) binaural summation to increase the apparent loudness of sound, (e) binaural loudness squelch effect (improvement in SNR when two ears are involved), (f) masking level difference (the ability to separate primary sounds from background or unwanted sounds), and (g) improved speech understanding in noise.

If nothing else, binaural amplification should be evaluated and the patient given an opportunity to experience it before decisions are made about which ear does not need amplification for a successful fitting. For some, a period of adjustment might be required before the benefits of binaural amplification can be demonstrated. Contrary to what many believe, the true advantage of binaural hearing is not that it makes the ears the same, but that it creates differences between the ears, including differences in frequency, phase, time of arrival, bandwidth, sound pressure, duration, and other acoustical and temporal differences. It is these factors that collectively provide for the advantages of binaural listening.

The impact of auditory deprivation when only a single hearing aid is recommended is an additional concern. Silman, Gelfand, and Silverman (1984) identified reduced word-recognition scores in the unaided ear following a period of asymmetrical stimulation. Poorer performance was found in 40% of the monaural hearing aids wearers.

Binaural Candidacy

Generalized criteria (Briskey, 1980) for binaural candidacy include:

1. A correctable impairment in both ears
2. Thresholds between the ears within 15 dB of each other
3. Word recognition scores within 8 to 12% of each other.

Still, it would be inappropriate to eliminate binaural amplification as a consideration if these criteria are not met, just as much as it would be inappropriate to insist on binaural amplification just because these criteria *are* met. Good judgment and understanding of the patient's needs should be the determining factors.

Monaural Candidacy

Decisions on when to fit a hearing aid monaurally are difficult and may have little to do with hard-and-fast fitting rules. In practice, these are often based on the expressed financial status of the patient or considered in those cases where the patient is uncertain about the need for hearing aids to begin with. When a decision is made to consider a monaural hearing aid, the ear to select is often the one that has (a) the widest dynamic range, (b) the best word-recognition score, and (c) ear preference, including fitting the ear that is less likely to be used most frequently on the phone.

HEARING AID SELECTION PROCEDURES

To recommend hearing aids for a given loss based on hearing performance is not yet a science, but there is consensus that some kind of hearing aid evaluation procedure is desirable. As evidence, myriad and divergent procedures have been employed since the late 1930s to select, verify, and monitor wearable amplification systems with no single procedure emerging as "the" accepted standard. The reality is that literally every approach to hearing aid selection has its satisfied users and can be considered to be successful to some degree. Still, certain directions or philosophies have emerged based on the ease of implementation and successes and failures to demonstrate measurable improvement to some ideal or optimum level. What follows is not an exhaustive attempt to describe all of the procedures, but an attempt to show the general philosophies and directions that hearing aid selection has taken, demonstrating how they seem to have been built on each other to bring us to the procedures most frequently used today. (*Significant contributions to hearing aid selection procedures can be found in McCandless, 1995, and Staab, 1996.*)

Two divergent *general philosophies* for the selection of hearing aids include (1) nonselective recommendations and (2) selective amplification.

Nonselective Recommendations for Hearing Aid Amplification

These philosophies espouse that little or no differences in amplification requirements exist among individuals with hearing impairment, and therefore, comparative evaluations or predictive measures are not necessary. The belief is that generally designed hearing aids are sufficient and that counseling about the expectations of hearing aid use is the most important contributor to successful fitting (Resnick & Becker, 1963).

The argument is made that "flat" or "high fidelity" amplification (amplification provided equally to all frequencies in the speech range), or some other standard response with the slope expressed in dB per octave (i.e., a range of slope between 0 and +6 dB/octave), along with various other recommended parameters, is the desired response for the majority of patients with hearing impairment (Davis et al., 1947; United Kingdom Medical Research Council, 1947).

Arguments against nonselective amplification fitting procedures are that they do not account for our understanding of ear physiology and the needed circuitry to manage these differences, that there is no attempt to verify the aided performance, and that use failures are related solely to the manufactured product. There seems to be currently little support for nonselective hearing aid recommendation procedures.

Selective Amplification Approach to Hearing Aid Fitting

Selective amplification refers to the belief that some unique combination of hearing aid performance characteristics provides for optimal listening for each individual's hearing loss. Some of these approaches provide for an aided *comparison* of hearing aids, while others attempt to *prescribe* (predict) aided hearing aid performance. Comparative approaches focus on the *auditory experience* (comparisons following listening experiences, ranking, retrocomparative judgements, and trial-and-error methods). They test for a quality or measured difference from a finite number of hearing aids. Prescriptive approaches, on the other hand, focus on *auditory potential*. They attempt to specify the required electroacoustic characteristics based on audiometric or psychoacoustic measurements, or both. Some procedures use a combination of the two, prescription and comparison. Regardless of how selective amplification is accomplished, a variety of procedures have been used.

Selective amplification procedures assume that (a) differences in hearing aids exist, (b) differences in amplification requirements for patients exist, and (c) that these differences are sufficient to be measured. These assumptions may be based on the following features (or a combination of them): the patient's pure-tone or speech thresholds, word-recognition scores or other aspects of speech, comfort levels, dynamic range, loudness judgments, or other features/measurements (Staab, 1996, pp. 454–455). The diagram in Figure 3–1 (adapted from McCandless, 1995) shows nicely an outline of selective amplification hearing aid selection procedures.

Comparative Hearing Aid Selection Approaches

"Traditional" (Carhart; Classical; Sound Field Comparisons) Hearing Aid Evaluation

This procedure was recommended by Carhart (1946) to be used for U.S. veterans of World War II with hearing impairment. It emphasized the ranking of hearing aids based on word-recognition performance when comparing a variety of preselected hearing aids. Based on sound-field (loudspeaker) speech presentations, the instruments were compared, and the instrument(s) that provided the greatest improvement in SRT, the best word-recognition score in quiet and noise, and the widest dynamic range were judged as being the most appropriate for the patient.

A subjective preselection of hearing aids that the evaluator thought might meet the needs of the patient were used for the evaluation. Generally, the instruments had similar electroacoustical characteristics. These instruments' performances were then *compared* to each other using speech stimuli. The instrument that provided the best improvement in aided SRT and the highest word-recognition score was considered to be optimal and was recommended.

Comparative procedures, especially those based on the Carhart principles, have been subjected to criticism for having poor reliability (Shore, Bilger, & Hirsh, 1960), including that selection of hearing aids based on SRTs and word-recognition scores do not accurately reflect nor identify the electroacoustic characteristics that are important and that single speech scores cannot help determine which of the numerous electroacoustic parameters require adjustment to improve speech intelligibility function. Speech function scores provide little or no assistance in determination of the frequency/gain adjustments required for the proper fitting of hearing aids.

In spite of the above criticisms, there have been many efforts to make the Carhart procedure more acceptable. "Improvements" have intended to shorten the evaluation time or to improve its reliability. A short list of some of the changes includes:

1. Shortening word recognition lists from 50 to 25 words, and even some 10-word lists (the latter of questionable value)
2. Making the words themselves more difficult by selecting from those having high-frequency emphasis

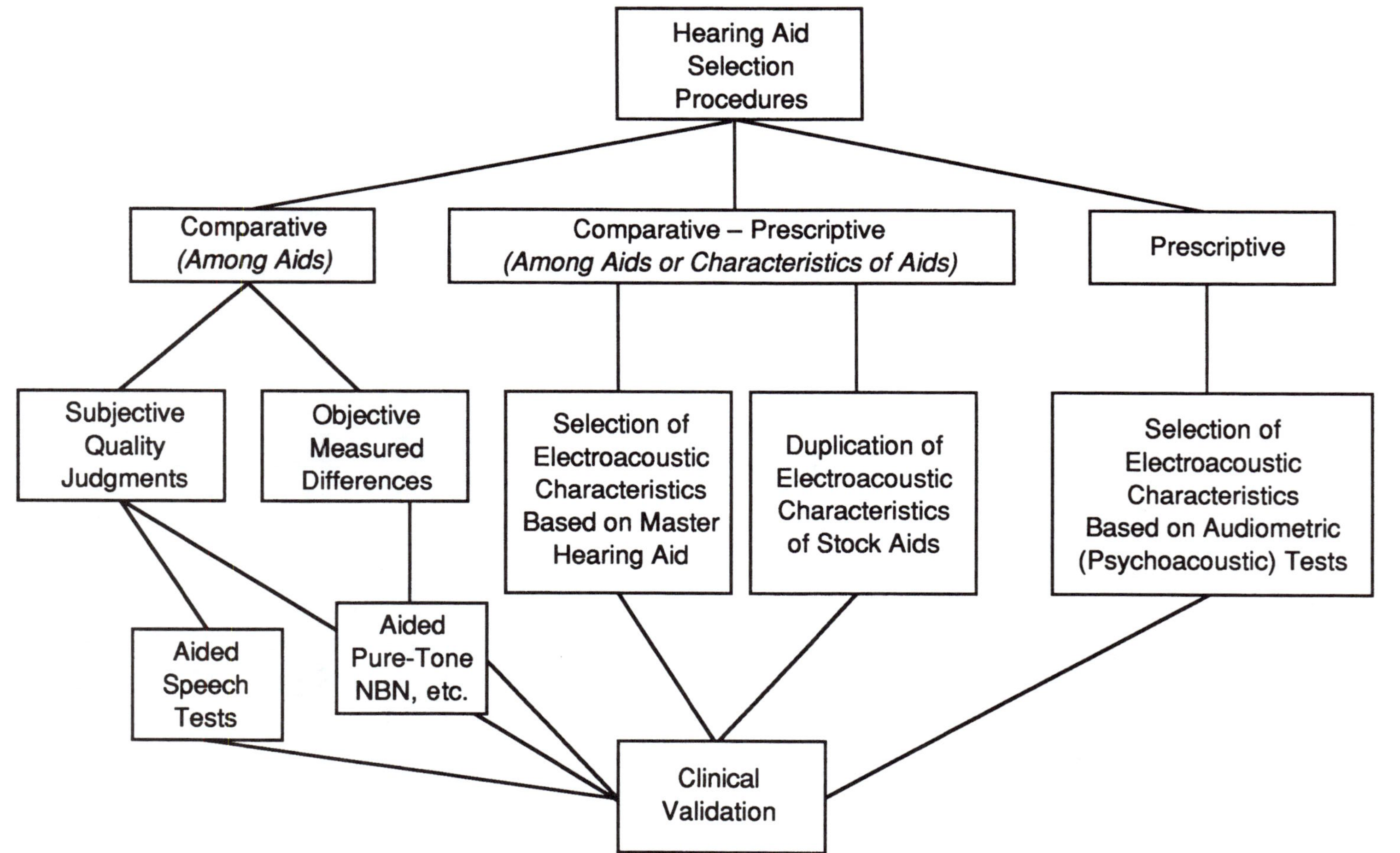

Figure 3–1. Selective amplification procedures. Diagram of comparative, comparative/prescriptive, and prescriptive hearing aid fitting procedures. (From "Hearing Aid Formulae and Their Application," by G. A. McCandless. In *Handbook of Hearing Aid Amplification,* Vol. I (p. 233), R. E. Sandlin, (Ed.), 1995, San Diego, CA: Singular Publishing Group. Copyright 1995 by Singular Publishing Group. Adapted with permission.)

3. Differentiating between "unaided" and "aided" PB Max scores by "normalizing" the presentation levels of the words. Because both unaided and aided testing were presented at a comfortable loudness level (PB Max), it was difficult to demonstrate amplification advantages when both the "unaided" and "aided" scores were approximately the same (in fact, often poorer under the aided condition). To circumvent this unacceptable approach, unaided word recognition was sometimes performed at a level of 50 dB HTL (close to 65 dB SPL) regardless of the hearing thresholds, to approximate normal conversational speech levels. This provided a more realistic example of how the patient understood under normal unaided conditions and how this then compared to the patient's performance under unaided conditions. In this way, the advantages of having sound amplified by the hearing aid could be demonstrated.

Today the Carhart procedure is considered to be too subjective, too time consuming , and is rarely used.

Comparative-Prescriptive Hearing Aid Selection Approaches

Comparative-prescriptive hearing aid techniques are often used when a hearing aid from a specific manufacturer is to be recommended. This approach, as currently practiced, is identifiable with "master hearing aid" evaluation units.

Specific electroacoustic features of hearing aids are produced from settings of a master hearing aid, and the final selection is made from a comparison of the settings using speech materials. The second, or prescriptive, step is to specify the set of optimum electroacoustic characteristics that are to be integrated in the patient's aid, duplicating the master hearing aid settings (McCandless, 1995).

Master Hearing Aid

The intent of a "master hearing aid" is to identify patient-specific information by comparison of electroacoustical changes to which the patient can respond. Presented as a practical, operational device by Lybarger in 1938, master hearing aid characteristics were expressed in sound pressure and, consequently, were often referred to as pressure-measuring instruments, SPL audiometers, suprathreshold testing devices, or hearing aid simulators. The use of master hearing aids eliminated the need for "stock" hearing aids for comparison purpose.

Early master hearing aids often were combined with an audiometer and shared a single HTL dial that expressed levels in HTL, SPL (for speech), and acoustic gain for MCL. The master hearing aid portion of the audiometer featured the ability to change the frequency response (slope), gain, output, binaural versus monaural, AGC, and sometimes other characteristics for the hearing aid(s) to be selected.

Early master hearing aids had an advantage in that they could simulate a wide range of different hearing aid characteristics. Major problems related to the fact that hearing aid performance was presented through audiometric earphones rather than through hearing aid receivers, which had poorer frequency responses and did not account for earmold coupling, and wider band microphones were used than what the hearing aid was assembled with. The result was a final hearing aid rather different from the characteristics suggested by the master hearing aid. More recent master hearing aids attempted to correct these inaccuracies by attachment of a wearable hearing aid containing actual hearing aid transducers to the master hearing aid and using the patient's own earmold. This approach functioned fairly well until the advent of custom-molded products and the use of multiple microphones and receivers to achieve specific hearing aid performance characteristics.

Master hearing aids estimate gain by determining the SPL required to provide adequate loudness of speech (MCL) for the patient. An input speech level of 60–70 dB (depending on the manufacturer of the device) is subtracted to provide a gross estimate of the gain required. The complete selection process requires also finding the combination of gain and response (or slope) that produces the best word-recognition scores. Most master hearing aids offer the option of binaural versus monaural evaluation.

Hearing aid output requirements are obtained by measuring the Threshold of Discomfort (TD), Loudness Discomfort Level (LDL), or Uncomfortable Level (UCL) for speech in SPL and limiting the hearing aid to that level. The TD is obtained while using both ears to achieve balanced output levels (identified as directly in the center of the head or equally loud in both ears). This avoids a final fitting in which the signal lateralizes to the ear where the aid has the higher output.

Master hearing aids provide frequency-response alternatives, from among which the most appropriate is selected. The hearing aid fitted eventually is expected to possess approximately the same frequency response (slope, gain per octave, rise per octave, pitch) that provided the clearest, most distinct, or most intelligible speech.

The final step is to note the "optimum" characteristics and send them to the manufacturer for inclusion in the hearing aid(s).

The Programmable Hearing Aid as a Master Hearing Aid

Programmable hearing aids currently substitute for most original-type master hearing aids and now offer true in situ circuit selection. In the past, these instruments were identified also as digitally programmable hearing aids or analog hearing aids with digital control. Today, however, they include completely digital hearing aids as well (digital chips rather than analog chips as the hearing aid memory module), as long as they are programmable, which most are.

Today's devices allow the dispenser and patient to work together to access a multitude (literally hundreds) of realistic hearing aid performance characteristics using the actual hearing aid the person will wear, attached to the ear with the exact ear coupling. In reality, these represent the first "true" master hearing aids.

Programmable hearing aids consist of two primary components: (a) a hearing aid that houses a memory module chip (analog or digital), offering numerous options in electroacoustical performance, and (b) some kind of external control to "fix" the electroacoustical performance desired within the memory module chip. The memory module replaces the conventional and even nonconventional trimmer potentiometer functions of the hearing aid while the control (sometimes referred to as an "electronic screwdriver") is most often an external microprocessor (computer) that accesses the memory locations or features within the chip. Together, they provide more varied and precise control of the hearing aid's performance than nonprogrammable devices. Once the desired electroacoustic performance is obtained, its characteristics are set and maintained within the hearing aid until such time they are reprogrammed. Some programmable hearing aids are simple and extremely portable in terms of their hardware; others are nonportable and more complex.

Most programmable hearing aids select electroacoustic performance involving both prescriptive and comparative approaches. Prescriptive application involves the use of one or any number of fitting formulae to pure-tone thresholds or to suprathreshold data (such as MCL, range of comfortable loudness, or loudness growth) and use these data to project a target gain/frequency response and other performance settings. This often is followed with a paired-comparison procedure in which the patient is allowed to subjectively make decisions about the performance of one group of settings versus another. Many of the programmable hearing aid systems allow also for some form of real-ear or functional gain measurement to verify how closely the target was met. Adjustments can then be made through the external microprocessor (programmer device).

Some programmable hearing aids offer a user-operated remote control that allows the user to select preset electroacoustic characteristics within the hearing aid for different listening environments or to adjust the gain of the instrument. Some of the remotes also allow the dispenser to program the hearing aid directly through the remote. Still other programmable devices offer the ability to store patient data and electroacoustic performance in a database management system for later use.

Programmable hearing aids lend themselves well to paired-comparison methods. These approaches emphasize the patient's judgement of "best" aided hearing. The patient is provided a number of different performance-significant configurations in a given listening environment. The patient then selects from these various configurations what he or she judges as best for that environment. Paired-comparison approaches have considerable value in that the patient participates in the decision-making process by determining "by comparison" which performance is best. Potential limitations of using this approach are that "best" may not be good in another environment and that the switching between configurations must be rapid to be meaningful.

Prescriptive Hearing Aid Selection Approaches

Prescriptive (predictive, formulae) hearing aid selection approaches are based on the assumption that optimum or desired electroacoustic characteristics can be specified prior to actual hearing aid fitting based solely on measurements of the auditory system (audiometric and/or psychoacoustic). Although derived from diverse philosophies, they have as goals the restoration of functional acuity, equal loudness, or speech spectrum to a comfortable listening level. These procedures assume that if average conversational speech is amplified to the listener's comfortable level, the fitting will result in user satisfaction by providing acceptable sound quality, clarity of speech, and comfort (McCandless, 1995). Prescriptive approaches have flourished, in part, because of the inconsistencies documented in word-recognition-based hearing aid selection procedures. Prescriptive fitting assumes, therefore, that measures other than speech stimuli will be used to specify the gain/response/output of the hearing aid. The stimuli might include pure tones or narrow band noise. Still, even though speech materials are not used, prescriptive approaches are designed to allow specific electroacoustic characteristics to be calculated that suggest optimum aided word recognition.

Prescriptive, or formulae approaches, started shortly after the advent of electronic hearing aids in 1930 (Balbi, 1935). Their popularity grew with the introduction of "objective" hearing aid selection procedures by Watson and Knudson (1940), Victoreen (1973), Byrne and Tonnison (1976), Berger (1977), and McCandless and Lyregaard (1983), and with the dissatisfaction of speech-based comparative procedures (Shore, Bilger, & Hirsh, 1960). The advent of custom-molded hearing aids solidified prescriptive fitting because audiometric data were sent to the manufacturer along with the ear impression(s) to have instruments made to fit the loss. The manufacturer applied some form of prescriptive formulae based on "average" ear needs to the audiometric data to give the instruments acceptable electroacoustic performance.

Inherent in prescriptive procedures is a verification or validation requirement to ensure that the prescriptive target has been approximated and that the fitting is appropriate and effective. The topic of validation will be discussed following the descriptions of prescriptive procedures and is discussed further in Chapter 15 by Hosford-Dunn.

Prescriptive Procedures – General Philosophies

Two general philosophies have emerged to calculate the prescribed gain/response of hearing aids to a comfortable listening level. Based on audiometric (psychacoustic) tests, one uses pure-tone threshold data, and the other uses suprathreshold data. The following section discusses the milestone procedures in chronological order, first for those based on pure-tone thresholds and then for those based on suprathreshold data.

PURE-TONE THRESHOLD-BASED PRESCRIPTIVE PROCEDURES

Considered advantages of using pure-tone threshold data are that: (a) pure tones are efficient and repeatable, (b) the gain/response can be calculated easily, and (c) thresholds can be obtained on the widest variety of patients (children, elderly, those having language and/or verbal difficulties).

Inverted Audiogram (Audiogram Fitting, Direct Mirror Fitting)

The objective is to set the frequency response of the HA to mirror the image of the hearing loss (Watson & Knudsen, 1940). Gain is recommended at each frequency that is identical to the dB loss at that frequency (to move the aided threshold to "normal" or to essentially 0 dB) (Figure 3–2). This concept is often embraced as having face validity for those new to hearing aid fitting procedures, but sufficient evidence exists to support the contention that this is not a reasonable approach. Unfortunately, it suffers from not recognizing that: (a) the patient utilizes speech at a suprathreshold rather than at a threshold level; (b) amplified speech at or near normal sensitivity levels would overpower a listener easily because the gain required confuses physical and subjective sound; (c) equal loudness contours tend to flatten at suprathreshold levels, suggesting strongly that gain requirements based on a 1:1 dB ratio between gain and HTL will lead to overamplification; (d) normal conversation speech is assumed to be 65–70 dB SPL at 1 meter, and if this input level is coupled with the gain requirements suggested, the output at 1000 Hz would be 125 to 130 dB for normal conversational speech (65 + 60 = 125; or, 70 + 60 = 130), without any consideration for reserve; (e) SPL (hearing aid output) and HTL (audiometric level) cannot be compared directly; and (f) the effects of earmold coupling and potential effects of upward spread of masking are not taken into consideration. Nevertheless, this concept serves as a reasonable starting point in understanding many of the procedures that follow.

Adjusted Audiometric Pure-Tone Data (Fractional Mirror Fitting)

A number of selection approaches have recognized the limitations of direct mirror fitting, and instead use the hearing threshold levels as a starting point for the formula, but then adjust the gain levels recommended according to some predetermined criteria (Berger, 1976a; Byrne & Dillon, 1986; Byrne & Tonnison, 1976; de Vos, 1971; Fletcher, 1952; Libby, 1986; Lybarger, 1944, 1963; McCandless & Lyregaard, 1983, 1989; Pascoe, 1975, 1990; Reddell & Calvert, 1966; Seewald & Ross, 1988). A general approach is to prescribe gain proportional to, but not equal to, the loss at each frequency. These procedures use the pure-tone thresholds, but rather than provide acoustic gain equal to the loss at each frequency, they reduce gain by approximately 10–15 dB, or some other constant value, at each frequency.

Half-Gain Rule

The "Use Gain" estimate, introduced initially by Lybarger for the Radioear Hearing Aid Company in 1944, served as the formation of the "Half Gain Rule" for which Lybarger will always be remembered. It has been modified slightly over time to reflect knowledge about the effects of amplification on the auditory system, including the significance of speech spectra, binaural amplification, and conductive losses (Lybarger, 1963). This major prescriptive for recommending "operating gain" was derived from attempts to relate the average gain required in the hearing aid to the average gain actually used for a given hearing loss. This was based on the assumption that average intensity of conversational speech was 65 dB SPL at 1m distance. Hearing aid gain was believed to be appropriate where the user's threshold was amplified into the normal speech range. The actual gain used is called the "operating" or "functional" gain. Essentially, this concept emphasizes that a rough estimate of the actual gain a person will use (require) from the hearing aid, will be one half the hearing threshold levels. The half-gain formula, as defined by Lybarger, serves as the basis for literally all hearing aid fitting formulae based on pure-tone thresholds and is also the foundation for most MCL-based procedures. The use gain formula as described by Lybarger for a monaural fit is:

Use, Operating, or Functional Gain (Actual gain person will use) $= \frac{A}{2} + \frac{(A-B)}{4}$

Where: A = Average air/conduction threshold (.5, 1, and 2 kHz)
B = Average bone/conduction threshold (.5, 1, and 2 kHz)

$\frac{(A-B)}{4} =$ Correction factor for an air-bone gap

For maximum gain, a 15 dB reserve is added to the operational gain, and a –10 dB correction was recommended for a binaural fit.

In this formula, an average 50 dB monaural hearing loss, having no air-bone gap, would require an operating gain of 25 dB and a maximum gain of 45 dB (reserve added).

Figure 3–3 illustrates how the half-gain rule relates to restoring average conversational speech (considered to be 55 dB HL or 65 dB

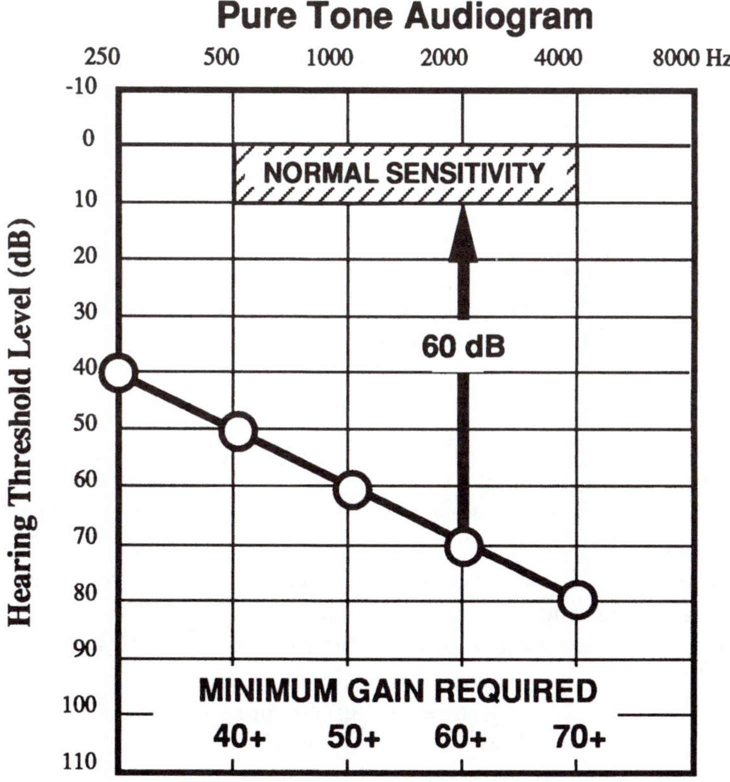

Figure 3–2. Inverted audiogram concept: A 50 dB pure-tone threshold at 500 Hz would require 40 dB gain from the hearing aid at 500 Hz to restore the pure-tone thresholds to the "normal sensitivity" range; 60 dB of hearing aid gain would be required to overcome the 70 dB pure-tone loss at 2000 Hz, and so forth. This is essentially a direct mirror fitting of the audiogram.

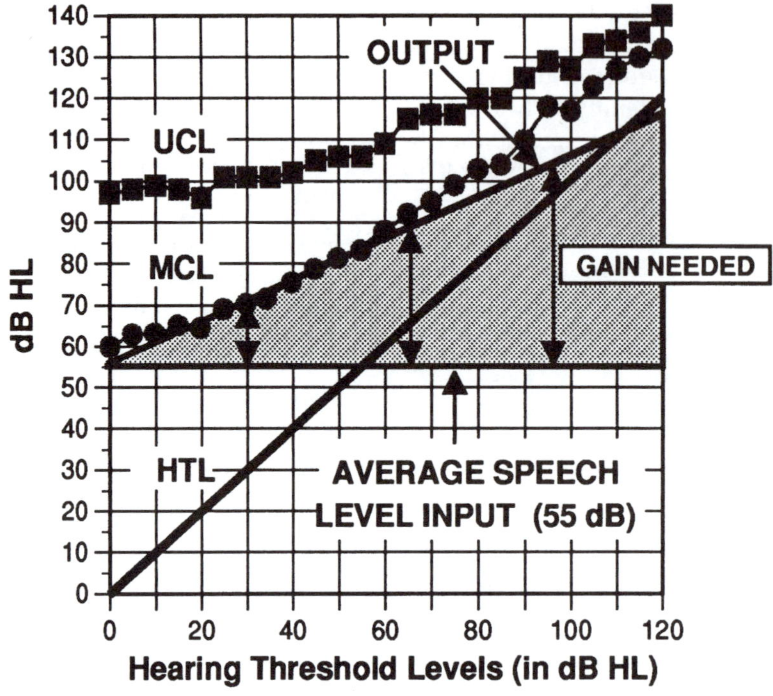

Figure 3–3. Comparison of average MCL and UCL (LDL; TD) levels as they relate to varying levels of hearing loss (in HTL). This supports the half-gain rule for losses up to at least 60 dB, intending to raise a 55 dB SPL input level of speech to the MCL. (From data in "Clinical Measurements of the Auditory Dynamic Range and Their Relation to Formulas for Hearing Aid Gain," by D. P. Pascoe. In *Presbyacousis and Other Age Related Aspects,* Proceedings of the 14th Danavox Symposium, 1990.)

SPL, when presented in the sound field) to MCL, at least up to hearing threshold levels of about 60 dB. When losses are greater than 60 dB, slightly greater gain is required as the loss becomes more severe. These trends can be identified in various hearing aid selection formulae and support clinical practice procedures that select initial frequency/gain characteristics on the half-gain rule. The threshold-based fitting formulae that follow are not necessarily presented in their order of publication, but in a systematic way to move from those easiest to understand to those that are more complex.

Lybarger (1944) also introduced other adjustments to the half-gain rule that attempted to take into consideration the impact of the long-term average speech spectrum, in other words, frequency shaping. His 1944 patent application for the Radioear Company was the first to suggest the use of audiometric HTL multiplied by a frequency-dependent factor. The formula multiplied thresholds by a factor between 0.3 and 0.7, depending on the expected contribution for different frequencies. High frequencies generally were given more importance than were low frequencies. He later introduced the Radioear "one-fourth slope rule," which split the frequency range into two bands with 1000 Hz serving as the dividing line (Lybarger, 1955). Based on the pure-tone thresholds, a slope was recommended for the low band and also for the high band. Gain recommendations from the recommended slope were adjusted on the basis of one fourth of the departure from a flat audiogarm. Also introduced were corrections for body baffle, another first.

An equally important contribution by Lybarger (1955) was the recognition of the impact of saturation output on successful hearing aid use. The Radioear one-fourth rule for output provided for the selection of the saturation output *before* the selection of gain. This rule related the average saturation output to the average air-conduction thresholds and air-bone gap, and provided a look-up to facilitate ease of use. The reason it was called the one-fourth rule was because the recommended saturation output increased one fourth as fast as the hearing loss for a given AC−BC difference. (The one-fourth gain and one-fourth output rules might not be readily available to many readers, but a description, along with the formula and the look-up tables, can be found in Staab, 1996, pp. 464–468).

Slide Rule Formulae

The mid-1970s produced a number of manufacturer-specific formulae presented with a form of slide rule in which the HTL thresholds for the different frequencies were entered and recommended gain for each frequency was displayed gain (Maico, 1974; Zenith, 1975; and others).

De Vos (1971)

Although actual measurement of the MCL and tolerance measurements for pure tones is the preferred method to present sound at or near the patient's MCL, a formula can be used to calculate target insertion frequency/gain requirements based on pure-tone data only.

$$\frac{\text{HL 500} - 6\text{ dB}}{2} \quad \frac{\text{HL 1000}}{2} \quad \frac{\text{HL 2000} + 5\text{ dB}}{2}$$

Berger (1976a)

This formula is based on an assumption that the amount of gain required should amplify sounds to average speech spectrum levels, that low-frequency amplification should be reduced slightly to keep it from degrading hearing, that amplification should be provided at those frequencies only where some residual amplification remained, that speech sounds above 4000 Hz are relatively unimportant to intelligibility, and that excessive gain and output should be avoided because they reduce intelligibility.

The formula is based on applying the half-gain rule to thresholds obtained under earphones. These threshold values are divided (or multiplied) by numbers that reflect the importance of speech at those frequencies. Correction factors are also available for conductive and mixed losses, monaural versus binaural, as well as for hearing aid microphone pickup locations (BTE, ITE, ITC, body-worn).

Major contributions of the Berger formula were that it provided a test sequence to validate the fitting, that the formula provided "*target*" (operating gains) at each frequency against which to compare aided performance in a sound field, and that it included *both* gain and output calculations.

Frequency (Hz)	Operational Gain or Insertion Gain	Reserve
500	0.30 × HTL*	+10
1000	0.63 × HTL	+10
2000	0.67 × HTL	+10
3000	0.59 × HTL	+10
4000	0.53 × HTL	+10

* × 0.50 for a > 50 dB HTL

The top portion of Figure 3–4 diagrams the most recent calculations of the Berger formula for hearing aid prescription, and the bottom portion illustrates the plotting or setting of the operational or "target" gain based on this prescription. The actual operational gains for the different frequencies are expressed in terms of "*functional gain*" (how much gain actually occurs), and verified via sound-field threshold measurements using narrow band stimuli.

Berger Formula

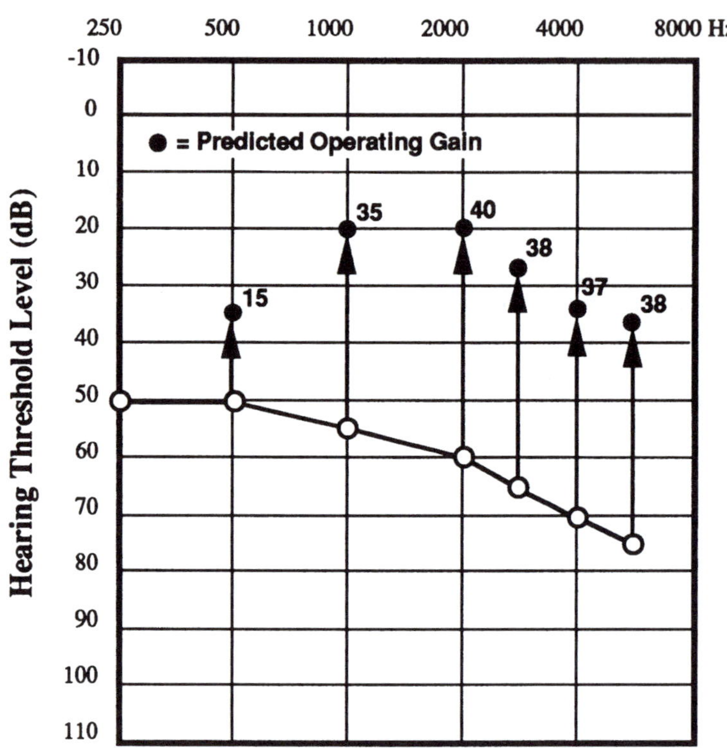

WORKSHEET

	.25	.5	1	2	3	4	6k Hz
HTL	50	50	55	60	65	70	75
X by	–	0.30*	0.63	0.67	0.59	0.53	0.50
Operating Gain		15	35	40	38	37	38
Reserve Gain		10	10	10	10	10	10
Maximum Gain		25	45	50	48	47	48

* 0.50 for a 50 dB HTL

Figure 3–4. Diagram concept of the Berger formula for hearing aid prescription. The predicted operating gains are the "target" or "insertion gains" to be achieved as measured with functional gain or microphone-probe real-ear measurements.

Recommended saturation outputs are based on sound-field pulsed tone UCLs at 125, 250, 500, 1000, 2000, 3000, and 4000 Hz in SPL. The recommended saturation outputs are as follows (Berger, 1977):

125 Hz = No higher than 250 Hz

250 Hz = 6 dB lower than 500 Hz

500 Hz = UCL + 8 dB or 110 dB, whichever is lower

1000 Hz = UCL + 4 dB

2000 Hz = UCL + 6 dB

3000 Hz = UCL + 5 dB

4000 Hz = UCL + 6 dB

POGO (1983)

POGO is an acronym for Prescription of Gain and Output (McCandless & Lyregaard, 1983). This formula provides a fairly straightforward approach to defining the insertion gain and output required across the frequency range for a closed earmold system. It was derived by evaluating other formulae and integrating insertion gain data from successful hearing aid users. Hearing thresholds are obtained under earphones, with the goal to amplify speech to MCL. POGO follows the half-gain rule closely. For example, the *gain* portion of the formula is

Frequency (Hz)	Insertion Gain	Reserve
250	½ HTL – 10	+10
500	½ HTL – 5	+10
1000	½ HTL	+10
2000	½ HTL	+10
3000	½ HTL	+10
4000	½ HTL	+10

Because of upward spread of masking possibly leading to lower word recognition in noise, the gain at 250 and 500 Hz is reduced from the half-gain rule by –10 and –5 dB respectively. A reserve gain of 10 dB is added to the calculated score with the final total score used in selecting hearing aids from the 2 cc coupler data provided by manufacturers. Insertion gain at 6000 Hz appears to have been dropped in more recent descriptions of the formula (McCandless, 1995).

Peak hearing aid *output* in SPL, not to be exceeded with an aid, is calculated from the average UCL (in HTL) for 500, 1000, and 2000 Hz. Taking into consideration that 2 cc coupler measurements are made in dB SPL, a 4-dB correction factor is added to this value. Additional correction factors are applied for earmold modifications, such as vents or horns.

$$\frac{\text{UCL@500 Hz} + \text{UCL@1000 Hz} + \text{UCL@2000 Hz}}{3} + 4$$

To determine how closely the aided performance is to the prescribed performance, verification by either (a) real-ear probe-tube microphone measurements or (b) sound-field functional gain measurements are recommended (McCandless, 1988).

NAL; NAL(R) (1976, 1986)

This formula, based on pure-tone theshold data, is an acronym for National Acoustics Laboratory (of Australia). It was based originally on approximating the half-gain rule, but included a low-frequency correction to minimize the effects of background noise (Byrne & Tonnison, 1976). In reality, the formula was 4.6 dB real ear gain rather than 5.0 dB for each 10 dB hearing loss. The formula was modified later to NAL (R) or NAL Revised (Byrne & Dillon, 1986) because it was deemed not to meet the goal of amplifying all frequency bands of speech to the 60 phon equal loudness contour target.

In NAL (R) the thresholds are multiplied by 0.31 at each frequency and are combined with a one third slope rate to control for excessive gain in the high frequencies for steeply sloping hearing losses. Speech spectrum corrections are factored in for each frequency and a gain constant having a value of 0.05 times the summed HTL at 500, 1000, and 2000 Hz is applied also.

Frequency	Insertion Gain	Sp. Spectrum Correction	+ Constant
250 Hz	HTL × 0.31	–17	+X
500	HTL × 0.31	–8	+X
750	HTL × 0.31	–3	+X
1000	HTL × 0.31	+1	+X
1500	HTL × 0.31	+1	+X
2000	HTL × 0.31	–1	+X
3000	HTL × 0.31	–2	+X
4000	HTL × 0.31	–2	+X
6000	HTL × 0.31	–2	+X

How closely the hearing aid meets the target gain is measured best by probe-tube microphone systems. Functional gain measured could be used also but is not recommended (Byrne & Dillon, 1986). Byrne and Dillon recommend a formula for deriving 2 cc coupler gain, but it is beyond the scope of this chapter. No clear formula was identified for output selection.

Libby One-Third Gain Rule (1986)

This formula was based on an assumption that the gain in mild-to-moderate hearing losses more closely approximates a one-third gain rule as a target insertion gain. Libby (1986) suggested that mild hearing losses used little amplification in real-life situations. For hearing losses greater than moderate, he suggested a two-thirds gain rule. Corrections were applied to the lower frequencies to prevent excessive amplification and to eliminate the possible upward spread of masking.

Frequency (Hz)	Insertion Gain
250	⅓ HTL – 5
500	⅓ HTL – 3
1000	⅓ HTL
2000	⅓ HTL
3000	⅓ HTL
4000	⅓ HTL

Articulation-Index-Based Predictive/Comparative Measurements

Articulation-Index-Based Hearing Aid Performance Measurement Approaches

Hearing health care practitioners have constantly sought good predictors of how well hearing aids function on humans, with little success. Such efforts included traditional speech discrimination testing (Shore, Bilger, & Hirsh, 1960). For this, and other reasons to be identified in the text that follows, Articulation Index (AI) procedures have been proposed as a means to help differentiate among the effects of different hearing aid electroacoustic performance characteristics. Additionally, they may allow accurate *estimates* of hearing aid performance on a given individual (Pavlovic, 1989; Studebaker & Wark, 1980). It is for this latter reason that they are included in this section of the chapter. Articulation Index procedures are available also to compare the performance of hearing aids fitted.

The theory on which this index is based postulates that speech intelligibility is uniquely related to a quantity termed "Articulation Index." The Articulation Index (AI) can be computed from the intensities of speech and competing noise reaching the ear of the listener for any specified, normal-hearing speaker-listener pair. The earliest report of Articulation Index (AI) use can be traced to Collard (1930). Its use with implications to hearing aids, however, is traced better to work by Beranek (1947), Fletcher (1952), French and Steinberg (1947), and Kryter (1962a, 1962b). The American National Standard (ANSI S3.5-1969) for AI is based largely on work by Kryter.

The AI has been modified over the years in a number of ways. It has been changed for simplicity by reducing the number of band contributions (to 15 from 20) and the long-term average levels have been reevaluated in each band to produce a speech dynamic range of 30 rather than 36 dB (Beranek, 1947), to correct for upward spread of masking, calculation from octave and one third octave band analysis, and to make an allowance for loudness discomfort levels (Kryter, 1962a, 1962b); and to develop an optimum amplification curve (Fletcher, 1952). The primary purpose of the AI by these authors was to explain and predict the impact of hearing loss on speech intelligibility in quiet and in noise for electronic communication systems. Later authors used the AI to predict the patient's aided intelligibility with hearing aids (Bergenstoff, 1990; Berger, 1992; Briskey, Greenbaum, & Sinclair, 1966; Fabry & Van Tasell, 1990; Humes, 1986, 1991; Korabic, 1993; Mueller & Killion, 1990; Pavlovic, 1987, 1988; Rankovic, 1991).

What is the AI? It is a number having a range from 0.00 to 1.00. The number represents the overall fractional part of the total speech signal available to a listener relative to the total speech signal. When a signal is presented, the AI represents the portion of the *entire* speech signal that can still be *heard* (not understood), in spite of the hearing loss. A number of 1.00 indicates that all the speech signal is audible to the listener. A value of 0.00 means that none of the speech signal is audible. The AI attempts to *predict*, based on the speech that is audible, rather than *measure* the intelligibility of speech. Table 3–1 shows the relationship that exists among the AI and speech intelligibility (ANSI, 1969). Because the AI is used to determine the amount of speech information that is *available* to the listener, the term *Audibility Index* rather than *Articulation Index* was recommended to be used for hearing aid use (Killion, Mueller, Pavlovic, & Humes, 1993), possibly based on the argument for the term "weighted audibility index (WAI)" which was already in use by Studebaker (1991).

Calculation of the AI is made by dividing the frequency range into equal intelligibility bands and then determining each band's contribution by the dynamic range of speech that is available to the listener in that band. French and Steinberg (1947), for example, identified that if a 5% contribution was expected from each band, then the hearing range would have 20 bands. The theory holds that the intelligibility of the band is determined by the audibility of that band. The contribution to intelligibility of each band depends at least on the following issues: (1) the number of bands, (2) the type of speech material, (3) the speaker, (4) the level at which measurements are made, (5) the noise level, and (6) the type of hearing impairment. The number of bands varies among procedures, with reports ranging from 4 to 21. Table 3–2 shows 20-band contributions from three different sources for three different types of speech signals.

Why use the AI? It is attractive as an outcome measurement of hearing aid performance because it (a) provides a clear visual illustration of the effects of threshold (unaided

Table 3–1. Comparison of Articulation Index and speech intelligibility.

Articulation Index	*Speech Intelligibility*
1.00	100%
0.80	99%
0.60	98%
0.40	93%
0.20	50%
0.10	18%
0.05	8%

AI	*% Sentence Understood*	*Speech Intelligibility*
0.40–1.00	95–100	Excellent
0.20–0.40	80–95	Acceptable
0.10–0.20	30–80	Poor
0.00–0.10	0–30	None

Table 3–2. Twenty frequency bands of equal contribution (5%) to speech intelligibility.

Band No.	Frequency Limits (in Hz) ANSI S3.5-1969	Frequency Limits (in Hz) French & Steinberg (1947)	Frequency Limits (in Hz) Studebaker et al. (1987)
1	200–330	250–375	150–300
2	330–430	375–505	300–355
3	430–560	505–645	355–408
4	560–700	645–795	408–458
5	700–840	795–955	458–515
6	840–1000	955–1130	515–592
7	1000–1150	1130–1315	592–697
8	1150–1310	1315–1515	697–824
9	1310–1480	1515–1720	824–990
10	1480–1660	1720–1930	990–1189
11	1660–1830	1930–2140	1189–1407
12	1830–2020	2140–2355	1407–1641
13	2020–2240	2355–2600	1641–1915
14	2240–2500	2600–2900	1915–2234
15	2500–2820	2900–3255	2234–2568
16	2820–3200	3255–3680	2568–2951
17	3200–3650	3680–4200	2951–3390
18	3650–4250	4200–4860	3390–4213
19	4250–5050	4860–5720	4213–5361
20	5050–6100	5720–7000	5361–8000

and aided) on speech, (b) allows for a comparison of different hearing aids' speech intelligibility contribution without the need for speech testing, (c) provides graphical suggestions on how to adjust the hearing aid to maximize the AI, and (d) can be used with other indexes of user satisfaction. There are caveats: (a) a high score does not necessarily suggest the "best" hearing aid, and (b) there is an inverse relationship between accuracy and ease of use. To facilitate the understanding of the concept and use of the AI for hearing aid use, the following "walk-through" procedure, adapted from Pavlovic (1987) is used. This is followed with a more simplified method for calculating the AI by Mueller and Killion (1990).

AI Modification (Pavlovic, 1987, 1988)

This approach is an attempt to illustrate how the primary parameters and procedures for use in speech intelligibility predictions are derived. The author has found this useful in describing AI basics as used to measure hearing aid outcome performance. Other AI approaches, although somewhat different, can be understood by reference to the series of illustrations that follow in Figures 3–5A through 3–5G.

Concept 1: Speech spectrum dynamic range (SSDR). The range and frequency distribution of the important speech spectrum dynamic range is identified as the white

Articulation Index Basics

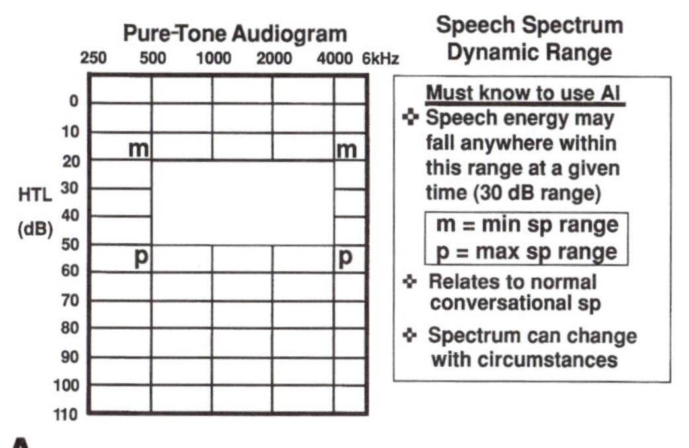

A

AI Calculation

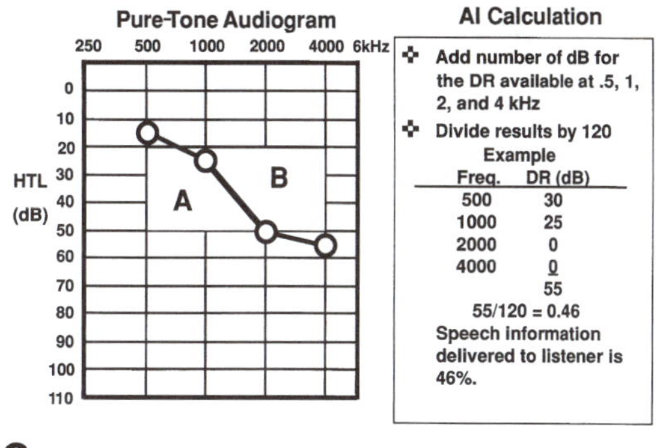

C

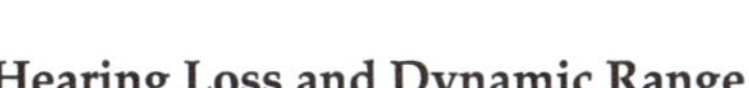

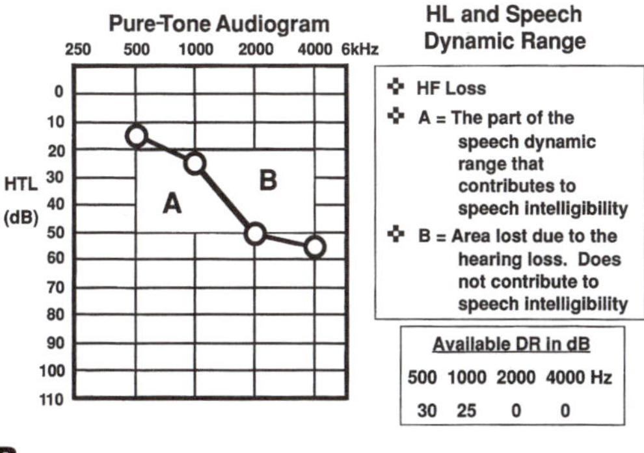

B

Hearing Aid Improvement

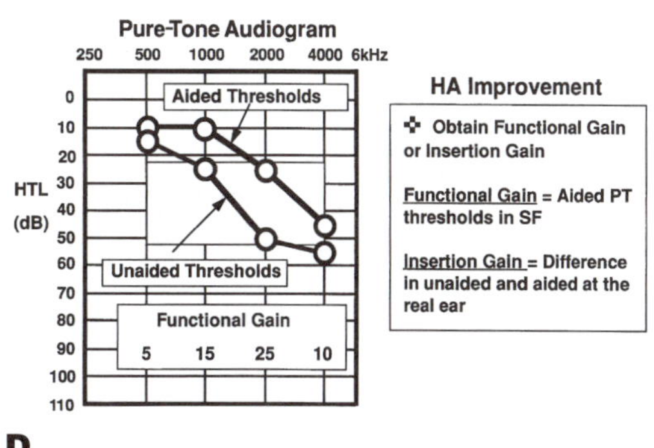

D

Figure 3–5. **A** through **G** are an attempt to explain the basics of the Articulation Index (AI) as modified for use in hearing aid evaluation. Note that other approaches will be somewhat different but also can be understood by referring to these series of figures. This figure identifies the range of frequency distribution of the important speech spectrum dynamic range. (From "AI Predictions of Speech Intelligibility in Hearing Aid Selection," by C. V. Pavlovic. *Asha, 30*, 1988. Copyright 1988 American Speech and Hearing Association. Reprinted with permission.) **A.** Defining the available dynamic range (DR) in dB by comparing the audiogram to the speech spectrum dynamic range of 30 dB as expressed in HTL on an audiogram. **B.** The relationship of hearing loss to the DR. Area "A" represents the audible hearing remaining and "B" represents lost audibility caused by the loss. The DR for this loss that remains (at the frequencies tested) is identified in the lower right box. **C.** AI calculation using the available DR information in dB. The total is divided by 120 (arrived at because four frequencies, each having a range of 30 dB, is 120). The unaided AI is 0.46, meaning that 46% of the speech information is being delivered to the listener (difference between the unaided and aided thresholds at the different frequencies). **D.** Plotting of hearing aid improvement, whether by functional gain (FG) or insertion gain (IG). The block at the bottom lists the functional gain improvements for the frequencies considered. The effect is to modify the speech spectra, rather than thresholds, by moving it downward on the audiogram by the amount of FG or IG. *(continued)*

FG or IG Effect on Speech Spectra

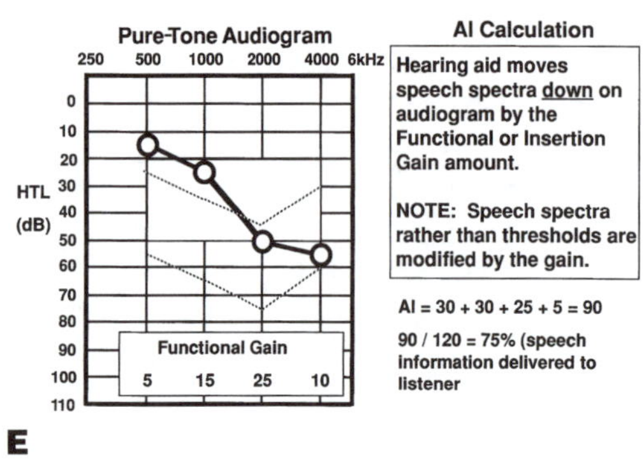

AI to Compare Hearing Aids

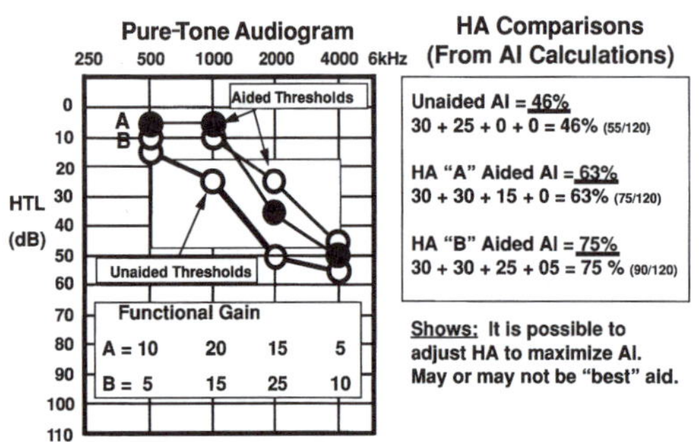

Potential AI Problem With UCL

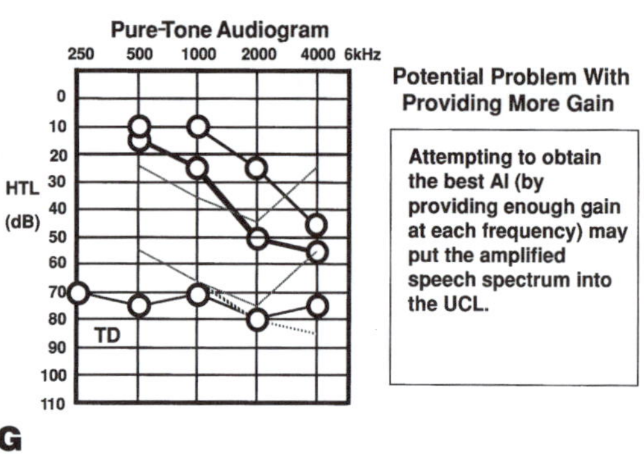

Figure 3–5. *(continued)* **E.** This illustrates a calculated AI, now calculated with hearing aid use. The functional gain improvements from **D** move the speech spectra down to the functional gain values recorded. The new DR values for the frequencies being evaluated are now 30, 30, 25, and 5 dB for the frequencies of 500, 1000, 2000, and 4000 Hz respectively. The aided is now 0.75, indicating that 75% of the speech information is delivered to the listener as compared to the unaided AI of 46% in **C. F.** The AI can be used to compare different hearing aids. This suggests also that hearing aids can be adjusted to maximize the AI. Even if maximized, however, there is no evidence to suggest that the higher AI will provide the "best" hearing aid. What it means is that more speech information is available for the patient to use. **G.** In some cases, too high an AI can infringe on the patient's UCL. Care should be exercised so that continued attempts at gain improvement at a given frequency do not shift the speech spectrum too far downward to impinge on the UCL.

area on the audiogram (Figure 3–5A). Normal conversational speech is considered to have a dynamic range of 30 dB (20 to 50 dB on the audiogram), with "m" representing the minimal level for this range and "p" representing the maximum level of this range. For hearing aid use, this example considers the frequency range to be from 500 through 4000 Hz. It is understood that (a) speech energy may fall anywhere within this range at a given time, (b) this range relates to normal conversational speech, and (c) the spectrum can change with circumstances.

Concept 2: Relating hearing loss to the speech spectrum dynamic range. Figure 3–5B defines the available dynamic range. The portion marked "A" shows what remains of hearing in the speech dynamic range to audibility (and assumed intelligibility). The area marked "B" shows the audibility lost in the SSDR as a result of the hearing loss. This does not contribute to audibility or intelligibility. The small box in the lower right hand corner indicates the available DR in dB. At 500 Hz, the entire DR exists. At 1000 Hz, only 25 dB of the 30 dB DR is available as a result of the hearing loss. At 2000 and 4000 Hz, the hearing loss has resulted in no speech spectrum information being audible.

Concept 3: AI calculation. Calculation of the AI is made by using the available DR information in dB (Figure 3–5c). The summed total of the available DR is divided by 120. (The divisor, 120, is arrived at by taking the DR of 30 dB at 500, 1000, 2000, and 4000 Hz and totaling them). The unaided AI, in this example, is 0.46 (DR of 55 divided by the total DR available of 120), meaning that 46% of the speech information is delivered to the listener.

Concept 4: Plot of hearing aid improvement. Functional gain (aided pure-tone thresholds in sound field) or insertion gain (difference in unaided and aided performance at the real ear) is superimposed onto the same audiogram (Figure 3–5D). The "Functional Gain" block at the bottom of the audiogram is merely a numeric description of what was plotted.

Concept 5: Hearing aid improvement effect on the speech spectrum. The effect of functional or insertion gain on the speech spectrum is illustrated in Figure 3-5E. The effect is that it moves the speech spectrum *downward* on the audiogram in an amount equal to the functional or insertion gain improvement. It is important to understand that hearing aid improvement does not change the person's thresholds but places the speech spectrum in a range more readily heard by the listener. Just as an AI could be calculated for the unaided performance, it can be calculated for the aided performance. In this case the functional or insertion gain has moved the speech spectrum downward, resulting in new dynamic ranges for the various frequencies of 30 dB at 500 Hz, 30 dB at 1000 Hz, 25 dB at 2000 Hz, and 5 dB at 4000 Hz. The aided AI is now 0.75, meaning that 75% of speech information is delivered to the listener. As before, the available DR at the frequencies identified is totaled and divided by 120.

Concept 6: Hearing aid comparisons and suggestions for improvement. Figure 3–5F illustrates how two different hearing aid performances can be compared when using the AI (there is no limit on how many can be compared). From this example, one can see that hearing aid "B" provides a higher AI than does Hearing aid "A". This can be attributed directly to the functional or insertion gain improvement of "B" over "A". Such a comparison can be extremely useful in providing a clear visual illustration of possible methods of hearing aid adjustment to maximize AI.

Concept 7: The AI and UCL. The aided spectrum should fall between threshold and UCL. Care must be exercised, however, when attempting to obtain the highest AI score by providing additional gain at certain frequencies, especially the highs (Figure 3–5G). Too much gain may put the amplified speech spectrum into the UCL, rendering the hearing aid inappropriate as a hearing loss solution.

Generally, the AI approach provides useful information about the *relative* benefits of a number of hearing aids for an individual, even though the AI may not predict the actual speech recognition performance. Still, many believe that for a given individual, the hearing aid having the highest AI will also provide the highest speech intelligibility. Because the instrument having the highest AI may not suggest the "best" hearing aid, it is wise to use the AI with other indexes of user satisfaction: quality, patient reactions, speech recognition scores, and so forth. An AI of 1.0 does not mean the auditory system is functioning normally. Lastly, the application of the AI to nonlinear circuits is not clear.

Fletcher (1952)

Fletcher's modification of the AI used the audiogram and a formula to develop an optimum amplification curve. This involved complex calculations and was based on data developed in the Harvard Report (Davis, et al., 1947). Conductive and sensorineural components of the hearing loss were factored into the formula, and "proficiency factors" attempted to account for the reduced speech intelligibility of those having a sensorineural hearing loss. For sensorineural hearing losses, the optimum amplification curve tended to be a slightly rising-with-frequency amplification curve, while for conductive losses the optimum amplification curve was a mirror image of the audiogram (resulting in a downward sloping curve for a rising audiogram).

ANSI Standard S3.5-1969

The American National Standards Institute (ANSI) method for calculating the AI is based on work by Kryter. Developed to optimize telecommunications systems, it contains the equal contribution to speech intelligibility of 20 individual frequency bands. The standard contains useful tables showing these contributions. While the AI is intended to be an objective method to evaluate the social hearing handicap (or conversely, the benefit of amplification with hearing aids), the ANSI standard method of calculation is impractical and too time consuming for hearing aid use. As a result, modifications to the AI have been proposed to predict the patient's aided intelligibility with hearing aids (Briskey, Greenbaum, & Sinclair, 1966; Humes, 1986, 1991; Mueller & Killion, 1990; Pavlovic, 1991). These modifications differ primarily in (a) the number of bands, (b) the weightings assigned to each band, and (c) the type of speech stimuli.

"Count the Dots" (Mueller & Killion, 1990)

This simple and visual example of a method to calculate the AI follows the principles outlined in the "AI Modification" by Pavlovic (1988) discussed earlier in this chapter. It is based on taking the speech spectrum dynamic range and plotting it on the audiogram in HTL. One hundred dots are distributed unevenly throughout the 30 dB speech dynamic range on the audiogram, with each dot corresponding with the importance of speech at that frequency (Figure 3–6). Each dot contributes equally to speech intelligibility, assuming that speech is presented at 50 dB HTL (roughly 70 dB SPL). From this template, one can see that the high frequencies contribute most to speech understanding. To calculate the AI, count the number of dots that exceed threshold and divide that number by 100. If the threshold falls on top of a dot, or if one half or more falls below the threshold, the dot is counted. The result is an AI somewhere between 0.00 and 1.00. As an example, an AI of 0.5 means that 50% of the acoustic information contributing to speech intelligibility is available to the listener and can be used when speech is at normal conversational levels. Other "count the dot" procedures have been proposed but vary somewhat from that described here (Humes, 1991; Pavlovic, 1991).

Threshold Data to a Range of Loudness Comfort Levels

DSL (1988) and DSL [i/o] (1994)

The Desired Sensational Level (DSL) approach was developed originally for linear circuit

Count the Dots AI

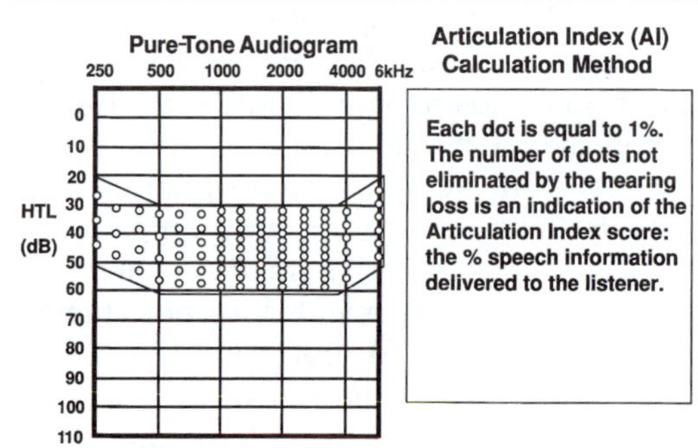

Figure 3–6. "Count the Dots" Articulation Index calculation method. An explanation of its use is provided in the box and in the text. (From "An Easy Method for Calculating the Articulation Index," by H. G. Mueller & M. Killion, 1990, *Hearing Journal, 43*, p. 15.. Copyright 1990 by *The Hearing Journal.* Adapted with permission.)

hearing aid selection, fitting, and verification of hearing aids with preverbal children (Seewald & Ross, 1988; Seewald et al., 1985). The procedure addresses three major areas: (a) the selection and fitting of hearing aids to children when based on limited information, (b) the recognition that the acoustic properties of young children's ears are substantially different than adults', and (c) the fact that amplification to learn speech and language must allow children to hear not only the speech of others, but to hear themselves as well for self-monitoring of their own speech.

A major feature of the DSL is the ability to use limited data (i.e., a single frequency threshold) and through computer software that has stored in it a wide range of information for infant and young children's ears, to calculate (a) the desired sensation levels (DSLs) for amplified speech, (b) target REAR (real ear aided response) and RESR (real ear saturation response) values, and (c) target aided sound field thresholds (Seewald, 1994).

Similar to many other procedures, the goal is to select hearing aid frequency/gain characteristics that place as much as possible of the long-term speech spectrum into the amplified range. Hearing thresholds are measured preferably via insert earphones in SPL, or converted to SPL, and compared to the long-term speech spectrum information stored in the computer database. The computer software calculates the amount of gain required to place the speech spectrum at the desired sensation levels for amplified speech. The desired real ear output levels are estimated because UCL data is seldom obtainable in children.

Once the hearing aid and its coupling that meet the calculated requirements have been selected, aided performance is verified using real ear measurements (although functional gain could be used as well). Measurements are obtained within the ear canal, with the patient serving as his or her own reference, regardless of age. As such, gain is in situ, as opposed to insertion gain. In situ gain measurements allow RECD (real ear to coupler differences) to account for the individual's ear and hearing aid coupling acoustics. Because these measurements define the differences between the real ear and coupler, electroacoustic response shaping can be performed in the hearing aid test box with accurate predictions of how the hearing aid will perform on the individual (Seewald, 1994). Figure 3–7 shows a block diagram of the general structure and options (inputs and outputs) comprising the DSL method for hearing aid fitting in infants and children (Seewald, 1995). Figure 3–8A illustrates the electroacoustic information derived for a given threshold (dB HL), and Figure 3–8B shows the information plotted on a DSL SPL-P-GRAM.

The DSL has been proposed more recently for adults as well, and a modification suggestion has been offered also for evaluating nonlinear (specifically wide dynamic range compression), as well as linear hearing aids. With this latter modification, identified as the DSL [i/o] (Coenelisse, Seewald, & Jamieson, 1994), the fitting procedure has become a common method for predicting and verifying hearing aid performance.

DSL [i/o] (1994)

The DSL (i/o) uses not only the information that is commonly available when hearing aids are selected (i.e., pure-tone thresholds), but additional measurements (LDL, RECD) are encouraged and should be used if available. If not, appropriate estimates are used.

The goal is to prescribe nonlinear hearing aids by specifying the desired output characteristics of the device for a *range of input levels*. This is similar to other fitting protocols that call for making recommendations for soft, normal, and loud speech, rather than to reach MCL for normal speech only (as did most earlier formulae). The expanded use of automatic gain control (AGC) hearing aids to fit the dynamic range of sounds heard by a normal hearing listener into the residual auditory area of a hearing aid wearer has fostered this interest.

When used to predict performance for a wide dynamic range compression aid, the DSL (i/o) selects compression characteristics relative to the user's perceived growth of loudness. At low input levels (soft speech),

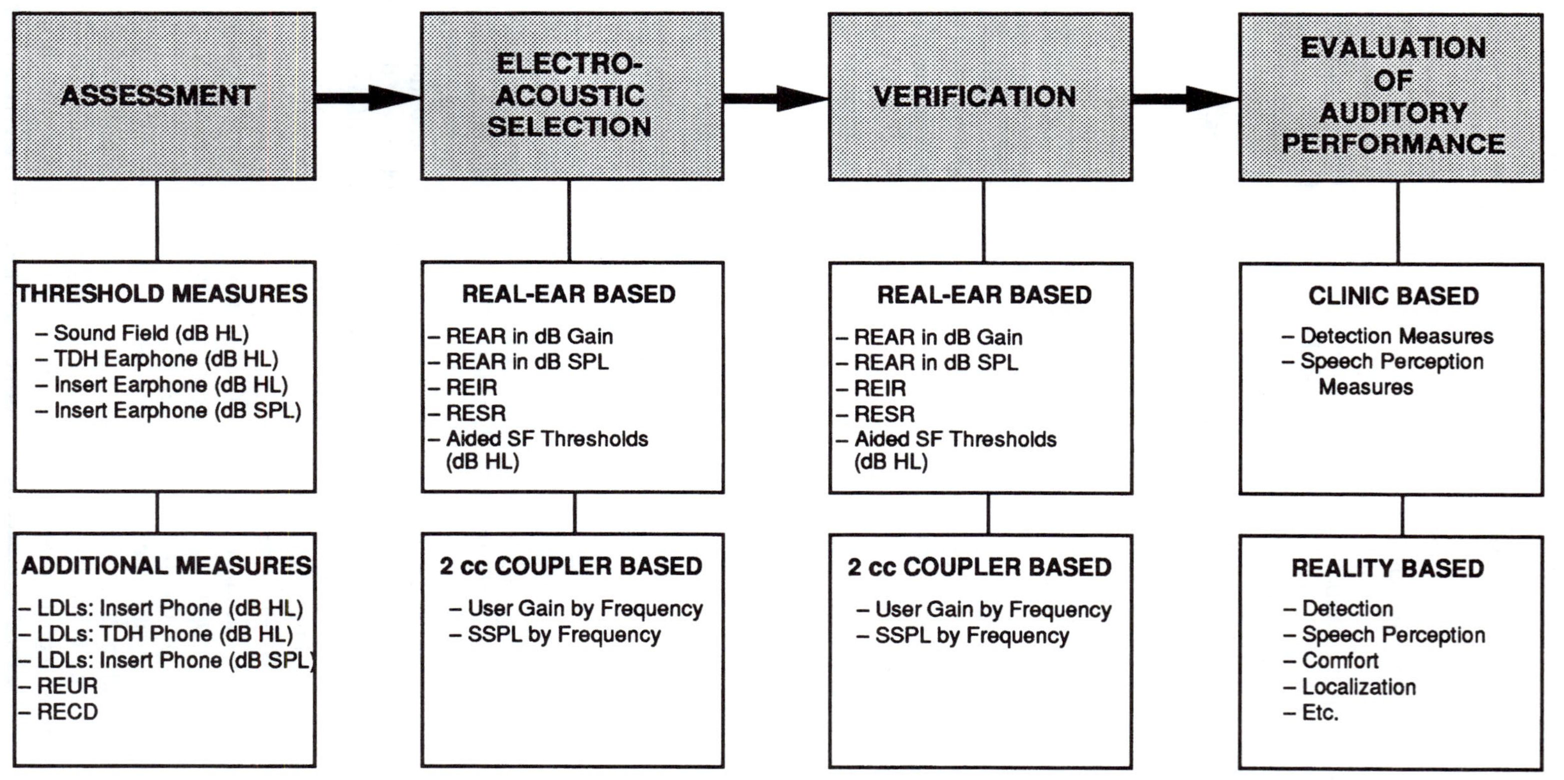

Figure 3–7. Block diagram of the general structure and options (inputs and outputs) compromising the DSL method for hearing aid fitting. (Adapted from "The Desired Sensation Level (DSL) Method for Hearing Aid Fitting in Infants and Children, by R. C. Seewald, 1995. *Phonak Focus, News/Ideas/High Technology/Acoustics,* No. 20.)

a	FREQUENCY (Hz)					
	250	500	1000	2000	4000	6000
Threshold (dB HL)	55	60	65	70	75	75
MAP (dB SPL)	73	73	75	85	90	93
DSLs (dB)	14	19	21	20	15	8
Amplified LTASS (dB SPL)	87	92	96	105	105	101
REAR (dB Gain)	24	28	39	54	63	59
RESR (dB SPL)	106	115	117	122	122	120
REIR (dB Gain)	23	26	37	42	48	52
Aided Thresholds (dB HL)	32	34	28	28	27	23

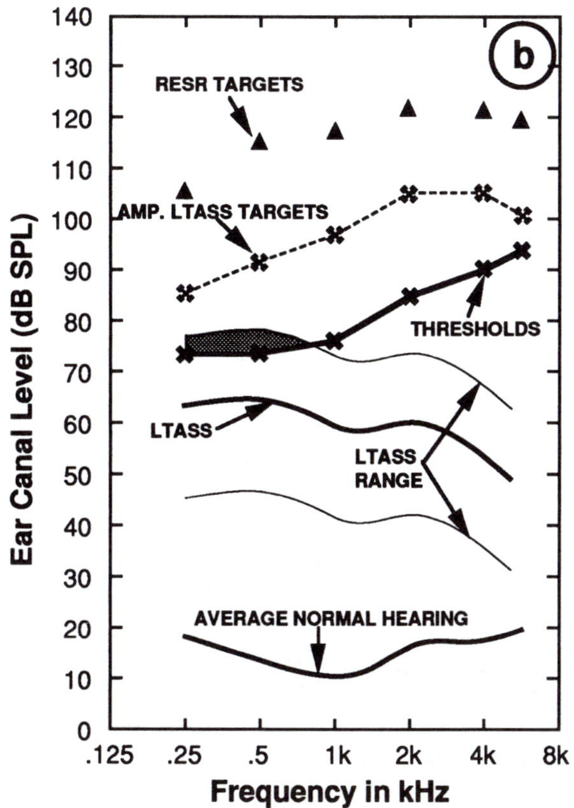

Figure 3–8. Real-ear electroacoustic results derived for the loss on the top line of **A**, using the DSL method, and by entering the threshold values only into the computer program. Seven calculations (in **A**) are made. Unaided information is recorded in SPL (ear canal level) on a DSL SPL-0-GRAM (**B**). Thresholds are shown, along with average normal hearing sensitivity, the long-term average speech spectrum (LTASS), the associated LTASS range of approximately 30 dB, the amplified LTASS targets (DSLs), and the RESR targets. The shaded area in the unamplified speech spectrum area is all that is audible to the hearing loss plotted on the top line of **A**. These values are calculated and plotted by the computer program, based on the pure-tone thresholds. The theoretical end result of a hearing aid fitting for this loss would amplify the speech spectrum to levels above the thresholds and not exceed the RESR targets. (Adapted from "The Desired Sensation Level (DSL) Method for Hearing Aid Fitting in Infants and Children, by R. C. Seewald, 1995. *Phonak Focus, News/Ideas/High Technology/Acoustics*, No. 20.)

more gain is applied to the input signal than recommended for a linear gain device; at high input levels (loud speech), but below the output limiting point, less gain is recommended than for a linear gain device. For normal conversational input level speech, the two are reasonably similar. The primary difference between the DSL (i/o) and DSL formulae (or for other formulae that are based on linear hearing aid circuit design) is that the DSL (i/o) produces *several* input-level-dependent *targets*, whereas more conventional approaches provide a *single target* only, regardless of the input signal level.

FIG6 (1995)

Designed for the fitting of nonlinear hearing aids that have wide dynamic range compression (WDRC), this computer-based fitting procedure is based on average loudness data that relates equal-loudness and threshold curves on data from several published studies (Gitles & Tillman Niquette, 1995; Killion, 1995).

Audiometric thresholds are entered into the computer program, and three fitting target insertion gain curves are calculated automatically: (1) low-level sounds at 40 dB SPL, (2) moderate-level sounds at 65 dB SPL, and (3) high-level sounds at 95 dB SPL. Three target gain curves were chosen because available knowledge of loudness growth data indicated that patients having sensorineural hearing loss typically required less gain for intense sounds and more gain for soft sounds. The use, therefore, of a single target gain was thought to be inappropriate. Although loudness growth function testing would be ideal, the ability to obtain these data was not always possible or practical. Therefore, FIG6 is based on the belief that targets based on average loudness growth data (for soft, medium, and loud input levels), provide a good first approximation of need. Killion (personal communication) recommended the use of FIG6 and WDRC hearing aids for individuals having hearing losses between 20 and 70 dB HL, although individuals having more severe losses and even those having poor word-recognition scores have been fitted successfully. FIG6 software also calculates insertion gain targets (REIG) and 2 cc coupler response targets for CIC, ITC, ITE, and BTE instruments. The 2 cc coupler targets are designed to be used in combination with a manufacturer's published electroacoustic performances or matrices. Figure 3–9 illustrates the target insertion gain curves for WDRC hearing aids having level-dependent frequency response, as compared with the NAL (R) target curves, for the audiogram at the top.

Summary of Threshold-Based Prescriptive Procedures

Linear-based formulae may have differences as great as 20 dB at certain frequencies (Figure 3-10), even when adjusted for volume control (different presentation sensation levels). There is no reason to expect that nonlinear formulae will be any different, especially for normal conversational speech input levels. Still, the linear-based formulae described (and others that have not been described in this chapter) have made and continue to make important contributions to the fitting of hearing aids. Specifically, the identification of target insertion gains and the practice of frequency/gain modifications based on verification approaches have become important mainstays in any hearing aid selection procedure. Additionally, formulae based on nonlinear hearing aids continue to follow essentially the "half-gain" rule for target insertion gains for normal conversational speech.

PRESCRIPTIVE PROCEDURES BASED ON SUPRATHRESHOLD MEASURES OF LOUDNESS JUDGMENTS

Suprathreshold prescriptive advocates believe that it is not correct to assume the MCL and UCL levels for a subject based on thresh-

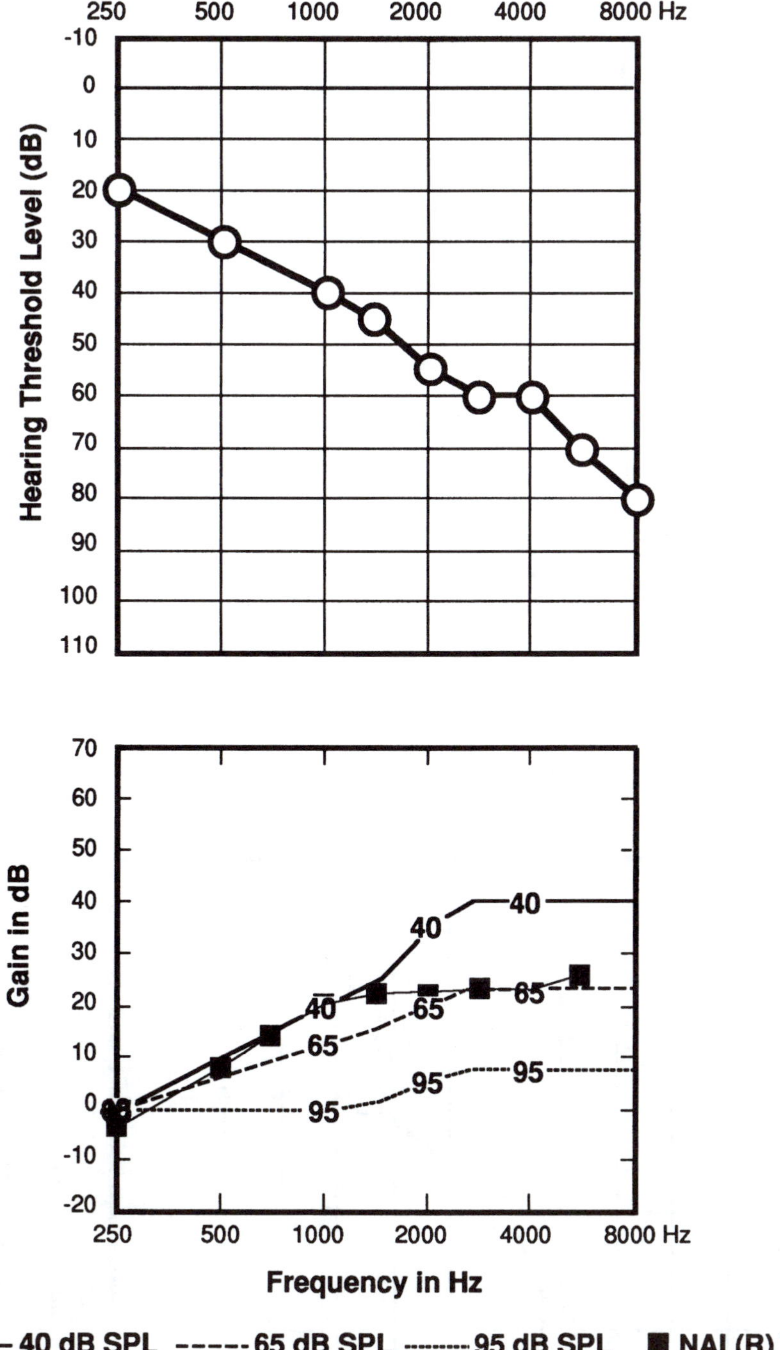

Figure 3–9. FIG6 target insertion gain curves for WDRC hearing aids with level-dependent frequency response, as compared with the NAL-R target curves, for the hearing loss illustrated on the top half of the graph. (From "FIG 6 in ten." by T. C. Gitles and P. Tillman Niquette, 1995, *The Hearing Review,* Nov/Dec, p.30. Copyright 1995 by *Hearing Review*. Adapted with permission.)

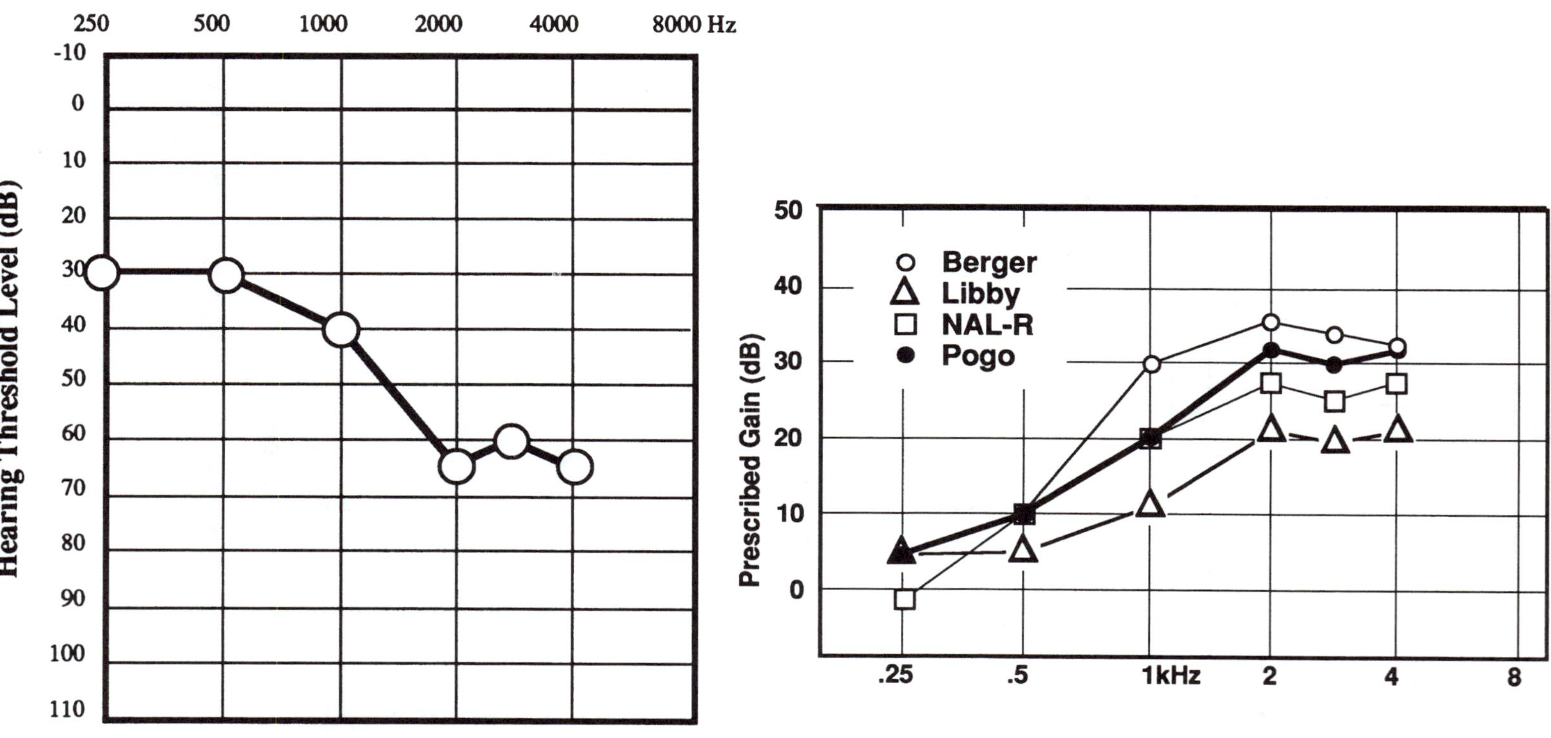

Figure 3–10. Audiogram of a moderate hearing loss (left graph) subjected to four different, common hearing aid fitting formulae, showing the differences in prescribed insertion gains. (From "Overview and Rationale of Threshold-Based Hearing Aid Selection Procedures," by G. A. McCandless. In: *Strategies for Selecting and Verifying Hearing Aid Fittings*, M. Valente, Ed. (p. 15), 1994, New York: Thieme Medical Publishers, Inc. Copyright 1994 by Thieme Medical Publishers. Adapted with permission.

old data (Humes & Halling, 1994; Kamm, Dirks, & Mickey, 1978). Suprathreshold approaches attempt to place the spectrum of normal conversational speech at the MCL or preferred listening range of the patient. The belief is that amplification must be comfortable to listen to or it will not be accepted by the patient. Although even many of the threshold-based advocates would agree with these statements, suprathreshold procedures have not been used as widely primarily because of (a) a "belief" that they take about twice as long as threshold-based procedures to perform; (b) manufacturers of custom-molded hearing aids request primarily pure-tone threshold data, and custom-molded products constitute approximately 80% of all hearing aids sold in the United States; (c) it was believed that obtaining suprathreshold MCL data is more difficult on children and on subjects who have diminished intellectual capacity; and (d) test-retest variability was thought to be greater for MCL than for threshold.

Compelling arguments in support of extended use of suprathreshold-based procedures have been given by Humes and Halling (1994):

1. Because the rationales for both suprathreshold and threshold procedures are identical (amplify speech to MCL), an understanding of one will enhance our understanding of the other.
2. The hearing aid fitting process is undergoing radical changes related to (a) the use of programmable instruments, analog and digital, and (b) the use of real-ear probe microphone systems to validate fitting targets. If a goal is to provide amplification of speech at MCL, this can be confirmed.
3. Current threshold-based procedures were not developed for nonlinear hearing aid amplifiers that allow the speech spectrum to fit within the dynamic range, and therefore, verification requires speech spectra to be measured at a number of different levels, all suprathreshold.

Suprathreshold loudness judgement measures have included the MCL primarily. Some MCL judgments are measured directly, while others are estimated or made indirectly.

Direct MCL Judgments

These procedures measure MCL directly at different frequencies and provide gain to match the MCL curve. When speech is used as a stimulus to obtain MCL, the level of normal conversational speech is subtracted from the measured MCL to calculate the gain required. (This latter procedure was identified earlier in this chapter when using Master Hearing Aids). Regardless of how it is done, the objective is to provide the user with hearing aid gain characteristics that allow speech, when amplified, to be at the user's MCL.

Watson and Knudsen (1940)

One of the first descriptions to determine the frequency response of a hearing aid, this procedure was designed to amplify speech to MCL. Gain is plotted as a mirror image of an equal loudness contour (MCL). Loudness matching occurred across octave frequencies from 125 to 8000 Hz, referenced to MCL at 1000 Hz (Figure 3–11). The text is not clear as to why a 20 dB difference exists between the MCL and the recommended gain.

Kee MCL Approach (1972)

Kee outlined a procedure that converted pure-tone thresholds to SPL so that they could be related more specifically to the hearing aid performance. All measurements were made under earphones. He also identified a procedure to evaluate the range of comfortable listening levels to allow the MCL to be identified more precisely. The procedure follows and is referenced to Figure 3–12.

1. Pure-tone hearing thresholds are measured and plotted using the HTL numbers on the right side of the graph, ensuring that the threshold is placed on the curved

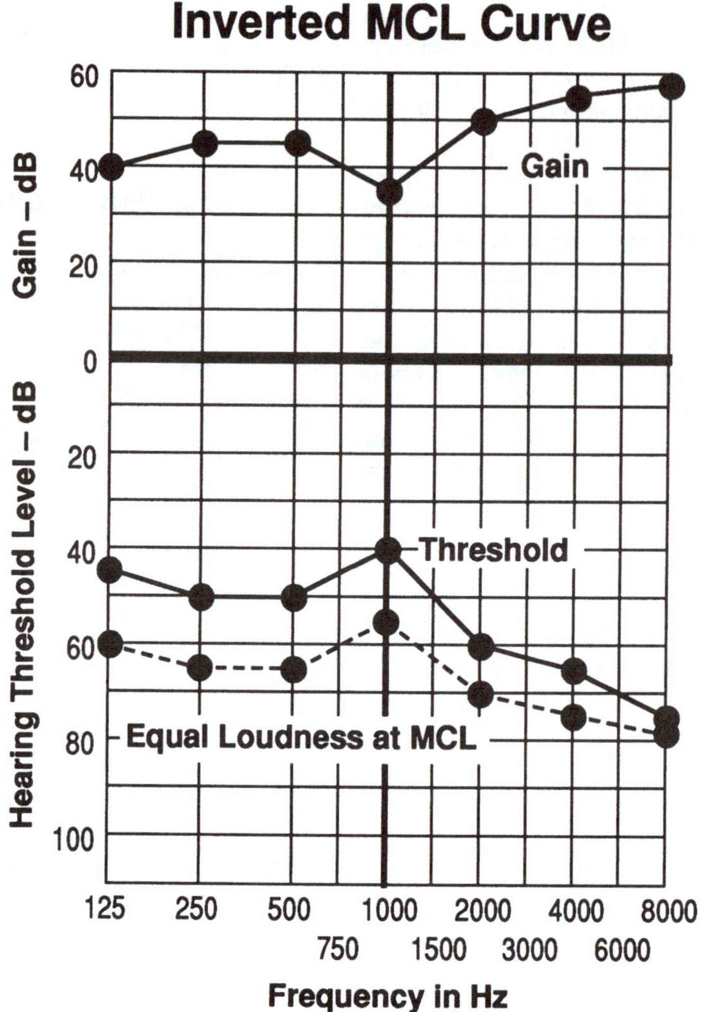

Figure 3–11. Watson and Knudsen method for hearing aid response selection based on direct MCL judgements. The gain or response curve is a mirror image of an equal loudness contour at MCL. (From "Selective Amplification—A Review and Evaluation," by S. F. Lybarger, 1978. *Ear and Hearing, 3,* 258–266. Copyright 1978 by Ear and Hearing. Adapted with permission.)

line or its corresponding relative position to the curved line. For example, a pure-tone threshold of 25 dB at 500 Hz should be placed at the midpoint between the 20 and 30 dB curves as referenced from the right. When viewed using numbers on the left (SPL) side of the graph, that threshold is read to be 35 dB SPL. This allows the determination of how much sound pressure is required at each frequency to detect the test tone.

2. A bracketing of the comfort range is determined at 500, 1000, 2000, and 3000 Hz, using pulsed pure tones. Three comfort levels are determined: too loud, comfortable, and too soft. Too loud is a little too loud to be comfortable; too soft is too low to be comfortable and is usually about 5 dB be-

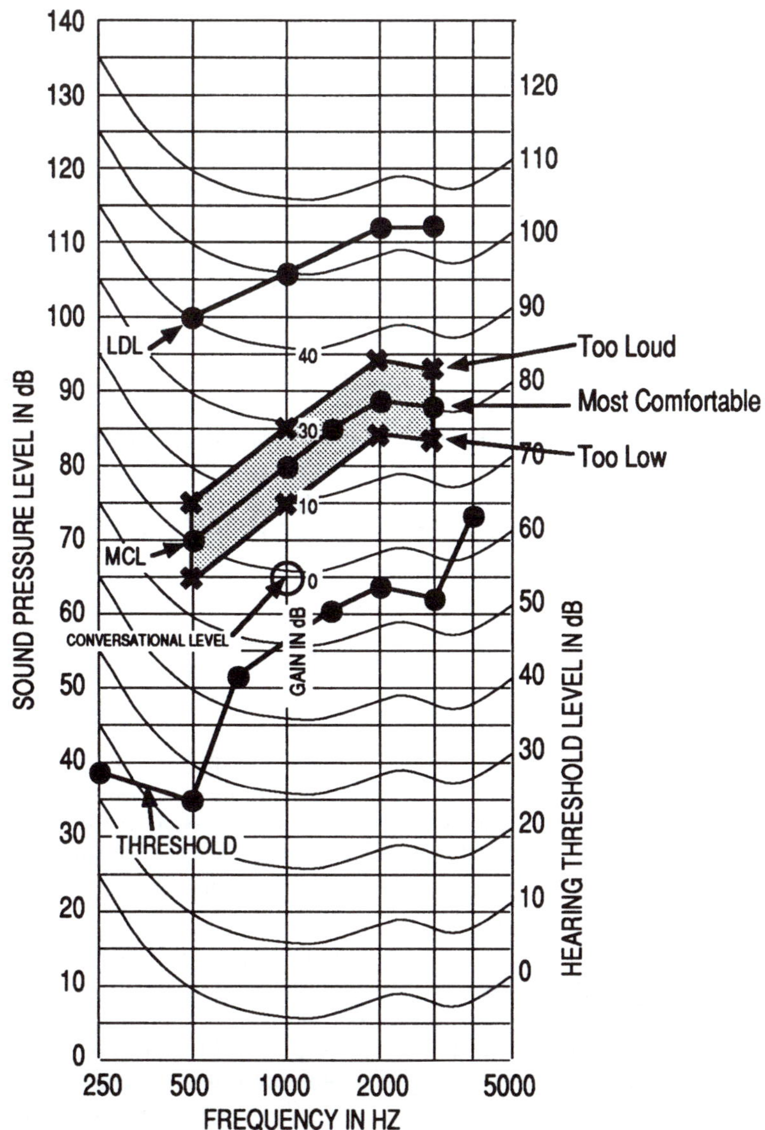

Figure 3–12. Estimated hearing aid gain for various frequencies using direct MCL judgments (after Kee, 1992). HTL data are converted to SPL and related to equal loudness contours.

low the MCL; and comfortable is usually about 5 dB below the too loud and 5 dB above the too soft.

3. The gain required is the difference between the MCL and 65 dB SPL (considered to be normal conversational speech level) at each frequency.

Shapiro MCL Approach (1975; 1976)

Using MCL measures to determine the required hearing aid gain, the recommended procedures for calculation are:

1. Obtain pure-tone threshold.

2. Measure MCLs and UCLs for pulsed narrow band noise at 500, 1000, 2000, 3000, and 4000 Hz. MCL was defined as the level 5 dB below the lowest intensity level described as being "too loud" two of three times. Using these data, Shapiro determined the ear to be aided as the one having the largest dynamic range and highest UCL. He specified that the SPL for a hearing aid should not exceed the average UCL in sound pressure for NBN.
3. The desired use gain for each frequency was calculated by subtracting 60 dB (customary input SPL for measuring hearing aid gain) from the MCLs at each frequency, except at 500 Hz where gain is to be 10 dB less than at 1000 Hz. If 250 Hz is used, 15 dB is subtracted from the gain prescribed at 1000 Hz, assuming that less gain is required at the lower frequencies.
4. A constant 10 dB is added to a final gain calculation for reserve.

The basis for this procedure was Shapiro's report that a line bisecting a patient's pure-tone threshold and UCL occurred at about the MCL for the frequencies of 2000 and 4000 Hz. At the lower frequencies the MCL occurred at higher levels than midpoint, however.

CID MCL Approach (1982, 1988)

As with other procedures, the Central Institute for the Deaf (CID) approach reported by Skinner et al. (1982) assumes that average conversational speech should be amplified close to the listener's MCL. Where it differs, however, is that it advocates amplifying the long-term average speech level (root mean square overall level of 65 dB SPL), to MCL. An understanding of the "perceived speech spectrum" that amplification is intended to reach is necessary in order to use the procedure. Although the procedure utilizes both threshold and suprathreshold measurements, the concentration on a variable MCL target results in its description in this section of the chapter.

The CID method authors believe that a single contour used to represent MCL is too arbitrary and that a graphical representation of the speech range and of average speech levels is helpful (Figure 3–13). With data plotted in SPL, the shaded speech range (having energy varying in sound pressure displayed over approximately a 30 dB range from "B" to "C") and a line approximating average speech levels (the level at which 50% of the speech energy falls below and above, line "A") are plotted. The lower level of the speech range eliminates only 1% of speech energy (1st percentile), while in the upper level of the speech range 90% of the speech energy should be detected (representing the 90th percentile). Average normal hearing thresholds are plotted at the bottom of the graph for reference. The fact that the MCL (Line "A") varies with frequency is important. It was believed that meeting the different MCL targets in specific frequency regions would provide maximum discrimination ability because they reflected the listener's loudness growth.

Use of this procedure is complicated and requires computer capability. Because a complete presentation is beyond the scope of this chapter, serious readers should explore this approach in more detail and are referred to the original articles. Still, some of the basic philosophy can be grasped with a limited explanation.

1. *The listener's auditory area is determined.* MCL and LDL (loudness discomfort level) are obtained by use of earphone-delivered, pulsed, pure-tone thresholds from 250 to 6000 Hz. These thresholds are later adjusted to reflect an unobstructed sound field environment, a more normal listening condition of speech in everyday life.
2. *The desired functional gain is determined.* The left panel of Figure 3–14 shows a sample auditory area for a patient relative to the contour of average speech levels (unaided speech) in HTL obtained in a sound field. It can be seen that the unaided speech contour is heard (above threshold) only at 250 Hz and is far below the MCL range. The right panel of Figure 3–14 indicates the functional gain required to amplify speech to the MCL range. The differences of approximation to MCL (dotted line) re-

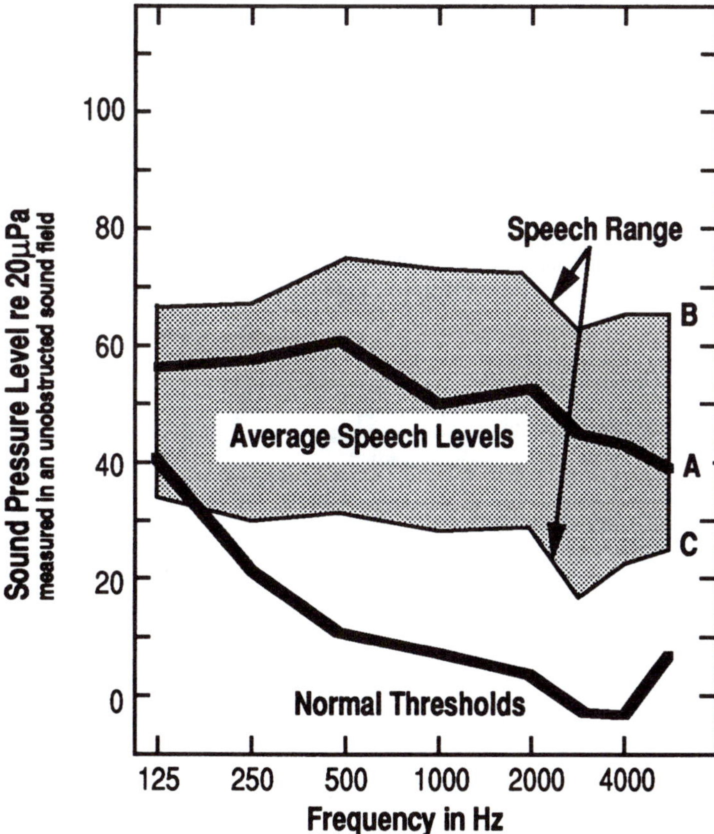

Figure 3–13. Graphic representation of hearing aid fitting target range. Speech range (shaded area) and average speech levels (50th percentile solid line) are plotted in SPL, relative to normal hearing thresholds (lower line). This shows the approximate 30 dB range of normal speech and also the level at which 50% of the speech energy falls below and above. This understanding forms an important basis for understanding the CID MCL approach to hearing aid fitting. (From "Measurements to Determine the Optimal Placement of Speech Energy Within the Listener's Auditory Area: A Basis for Selecting Amplification Characteristics," by M. W. Skinner, D. P. Pascoe, J. D. Miller, and G. R. Popelka. *The Vanderbilt Hearing-Aid Report* (p. 162), G. A. Studebaker and F. H. Bess (Eds.), 1982. Upper Darby, PA: Monographs in Contemporary Audiology. Copyright 1982 by Monographs in Contemporary Audiology. Adapted with permission.)

flect an attempt to establish *loudness* relations similar to those received by normal hearing listeners. At 250 Hz, for example, amplification is reduced to a level that brings speech to the midpoint between threshold and MCL. This is an attempt to reduce amplified low-frequency background noise. A subsequent modification (Skinner, 1988) advocates amplifying speech to halfway between threshold and MCL for 250 and 6000 Hz; 500 Hz to MCL; 1000 and 2000 Hz to 90% of the range between threshold

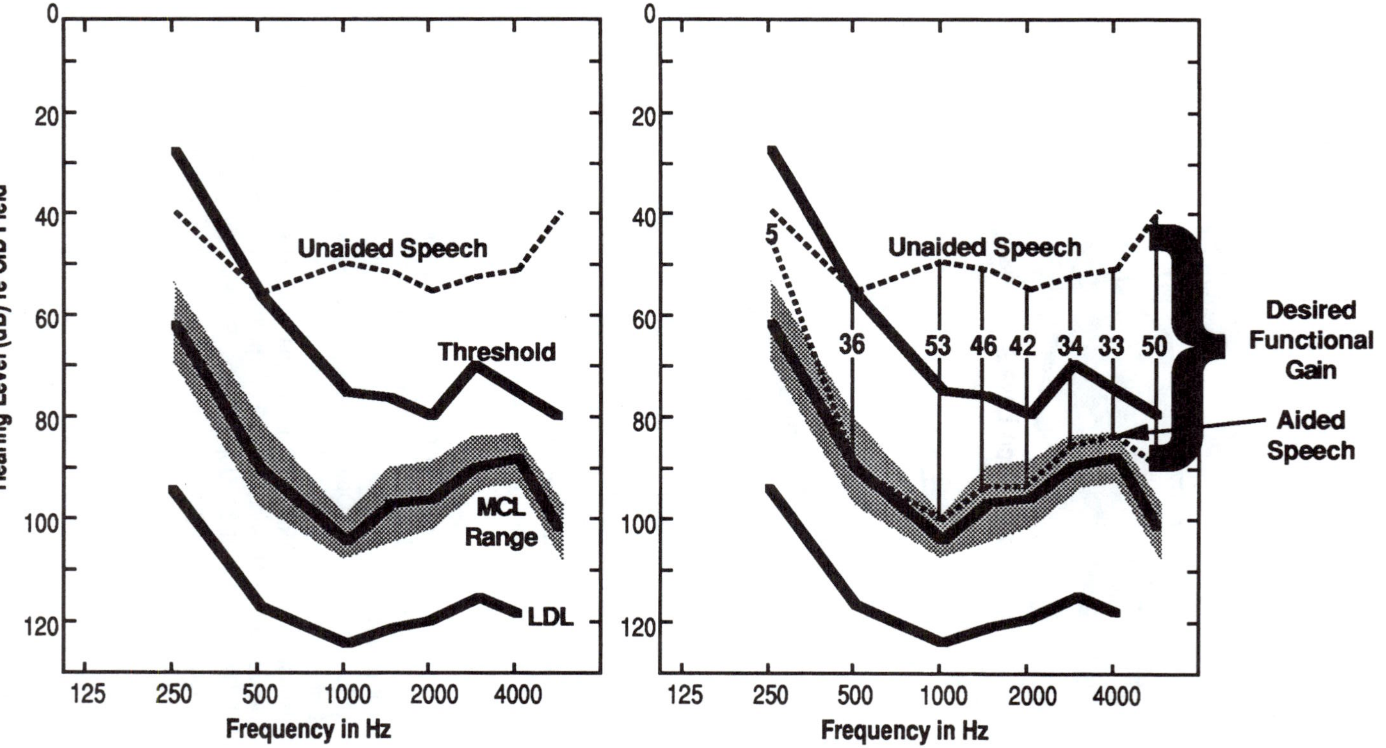

Figure 3–14. CID MCL method to determination of desired functional gain. The left panel shows a listener's auditory area in HTL (previous graph interpolated to relate the data to the audiogram). Only at 250 Hz is the unaided speech contour heard. To amplify speech in the region of the MCL range, the functional gain denoted by the numbers on the vertical lines on the right-hand panel are required. See text for additional explanation. (Adapted with permission from "Measurements to Determine the Optimal Placement of Speech Energy Within the Listener's Auditory Area: A Basis for Selecting Amplification," by M. W. Skinner, D. P. Pascoe, J. D. Miller, and G. R. Popelka, 1982, p. 162. In *The Vanderbilt Hearing-Aid Report*, G. A. Studebaker and F. H. Bess, Eds. Upper Darby, PA: Monographs in Contemporary Audiology. Copyright 1982 Monographs in Contemporary Audiology.)

and MCL; and 2000 and 4000 to 80% of the range between threshold and MCL.

3. *The target desired functional gain and actual functional gain are then compared.* Hearing aids are selected that will provide approximately the desired functional gain and output when coupled with an appropriate earmold. The patient adjusts the gain to running speech presented at 65 dB SPL to achieve maximum clarity and comfort. At this volume control setting, the actual functional gain is measured and recorded (Figure 3–15A). The measured functional gain is plotted against the target functional

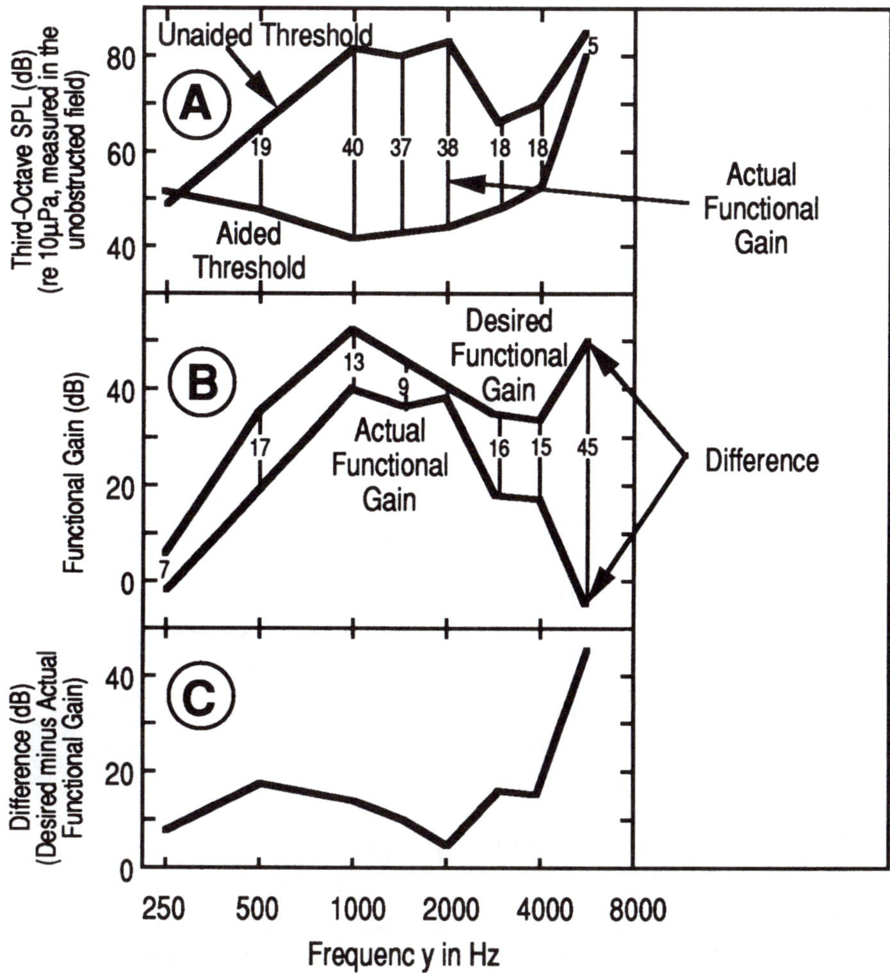

Figure 3–15. CID MCL procedure comparing the actual functional gain **(A)**, compared to the desired functional gain **(B)**, and the amount by which the patient's aid does not provide the desired functional gain **(C)**. (Adapted with permission from "Measurements to Determine the Optimal Placement of Speech Energy Within the Listener's Auditory Area: A Basis for Selecting Amplification," by M. W. Skinner, D. P. Pascoe, J. D. Miller, and G. R. Popelka, 1982, p. 162. In *The Vanderbilt Hearing-Aid Report*, G. A. Studebaker and F. H. Bess, Eds. Upper Darby, PA: Monographs in Contemporary Audiology. Copyright 1982 Monographs in Contemporary Audiology.)

gain established in Figure 3–15B, showing the differences. The amount by which the patient's aid does not provide the desired functional gain is shown in Figure 3–15C.

4. *An unobstructed-field to hearing-aid-microphone transfer function is obtained.* This provides for differences between the level at the microphone in the hearing aid test box and that at the microphone port of the aid when worn on the head. This transfer function (difference) is added to the patient's unaided thresholds, MCLs, and LDLs, and is done best by computer.
5. The difference between the *actual* coupler gain of the hearing (as measured with tubing on an artificial ear) and the desired coupler gain is added to the *desired* coupler gain.
6. *The output selection goal is to limit this level to just below the patient's LDL contour.* This can be determined more accurately by expressing the patient's LDL with reference to the output of the hearing aid. Subtract the functional gain from the unaided threshold, MCL, and LDL values. These new values represent the "aided" levels at the microphone of the hearing aid. Criteria for selecting the desired output include:
   a. If the LDL is 18 dB or greater above the average MCL range at a given frequency, select 15 dB above MCL as the maximum output. This is to allow linear amplification of the upper 15 dB of the 30 dB speech energy range, but limits higher levels that may cause fatigue.
   b. When insufficient range exists between MCL and LDL to allow this level of maximum output, a compromise can be made. One should usually limit the output to 3 dB below LDL, regardless of the range. This adjustment to the hearing aid can be performed in the test box so that the output closest to LDL is 3 dB below in the 2 cc coupler test if the maximum output is adjusted properly by presenting narrow and broad bands of noise at intensity levels likely to occur fairly often in everyday life (80–90 dB SPL). The output is appropriately adjusted if the patient reports these to be loud but acceptable. If, however, the sounds become distorted before becoming too loud, the output could be raised or compression amplification should be considered.

Indirect MCL Judgments

Indirect MCL hearing aid selection procedures also posit that hearing aids should amplify speech to the MCL. Rather than measure the MCL directly, however, the MCL is *estimated*, based primarily on (a) a value above the hearing thresholds (Seiler, 1971) or (b) some value between the hearing thresholds and the LDLs, for example, a level that bisects the dynamic range (Balbi, 1935; Bragg, 1977; Cox, 1983, 1985, 1988; Wallenfels, 1967).

Balbi Bisection Approach (1935)

Patented in 1935, this approach measured both the threshold and LDL in SPL and bisected them. The assumption was made that bisecting the range of these values would approximate the MCL and provide the shape of the amplification curve. Gain was determined as the dB SPL required to reach MCL at each frequency.

Wallenfels Bisection Approach (1967)

This procedure advocated measuring thresholds and plotting them in SPL. The procedure is outlined as follows and is illustrated in Figure 3–16:

1. Obtain the pure-tone audiogram and plot the data in SPL on a sound pressure graph.
2. Obtain the UCL using narrow bands of noise (or other stimuli) and plot these in SPL.
3. Plot the optimum listening level. This is identified as the midpoint on a line plotted between the threshold of sensitivity and the threshold of discomfort at 1000 and 4000 Hz. The bisected line connecting these two points should extend below 1000 Hz. If the audiogram indicates a precipitous loss, the drawn line continues

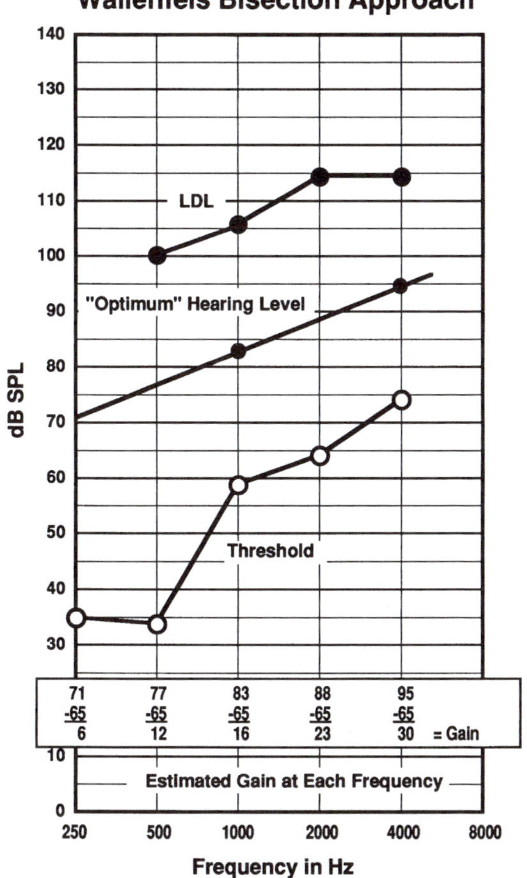

Figure 3–16. Wallenfels bisection approach to determine the estimated hearing aid gain. The pure-tone audiogram is plotted in SPL, along with the LDL. The optimal listening level is plotted as a line that bisects the thresholds of discomfort (LDL) and sensitivity at 1000 and 4000 Hz, with 65 dB (normal conversational speech) subtracted to determine the gain at each frequency. (Adapted with permission from *Hearing Aids on Prescription*, by H. G. Wallenfels, 1967, Springfield, IL: Charles C. Thomas. Copyright 1967 by Charles C. Thomas.)

downward below 1000 Hz with the same slope. If the slope between 1000 and 4000 Hz is less than 8 dB per octave, however, the recommended curve below 1000 Hz should have a slope between 8 and 10 dB per octave. The intent was to stay closer to the threshold curve if the dynamic range was narrow.

4. Subtract 65 dB (normal conversational speech level at each of the frequencies) from the "optimum" hearing levels at the various frequencies to determine the gain at each frequency. This assumption was recognized not to be accurate, and accommodations could be made to more accurately reflect the actual inputs of speech at the different frequencies.

Based on measuring hearing aid performances as worn, Wallenfels believed that the optimal hearing level was comparable to the MCL. This was based on his finding that the optimum (predicted) level and the actual (measured) listening levels were the same when patients were satisfied with their hearing aids but were not the same when they were dissatisfied with their hearing aids.

Seiler (1971)

This formula is notable because it was one of the first that considered the differences between hearing results obtained under earphones from those obtained in a sound field and also the differences resulting from aided in situ measurements. It considered transfer functions for MCL, ear resonance, the contribution of different frequencies speech recognition, the amount of gain required by the hearing aid, and differences between conductive and sensorineural loss gain requirements: it also suggested tests to help determine if possible modifications should be made in the earmold, receiver, tubing, and so forth. MCL values were estimated because it was felt that pure-tone MCLs were too difficult to obtain, and although not a straight bisection approach, it fits this category best because it estimates the MCL. The calculation for gain by frequency is as follows:

$$\text{Gain} = (TH_{HTL} + MCL_c + ER_{dB}) \times \text{Discrim\%} + 1/2\,(\text{Gain})$$

Where:

TH_{HTL} = Threshold in HTL (at .5, 1, 2, 3, and 4 kHz)

MCL_c = Calculated MCL by adding 15 dB to each pure-tone threshold

DR_{dB} = Ear resonance values for those frequencies (based on Weiner and Ross, 1946)

$Discrim_{\%}$ = Weighted speech discrimination contributions for those frequencies (Fowler and Sabine, 1947). Weighting for speech discrimination contribution is as follows: 512 Hz = 15%; 1024 Hz = 25%; 2048 Hz = 30%; 2896 Hz = 25%; and 4096 Hz = 5%, for a total of 100% (Rounded to appropriate frequencies)

Gain = Add 15 dB to the HTL thresholds at .5, 1, 2, 3, and 4 kHz to arrive at a generalized MCL value for each frequency. Sum these values and multiply them by 10% to provide a gain figure. This value is then multiplied by .5 (the half-gain rule) to arrive at the half gain figure used in the formula (Figure 3–17).

Seiler believed that completely conductive hearing losses required slight modifications in circuitry, which required a little more gain. Evaluation of the fitting included the use of cold-running speech in quiet and noise (varying levels of the latter), checking volume-control reserve when the aid is used at MCL, and word-recognition testing at MCL. Results from these tests were used for potential modifications to the fitting (earmold, receiver, tubing, etc.).

Bragg Bisection Approach (1977)

Bragg's procedure defined a desired listening level (DLL) between "too soft to hear" and "too loud to bear." The DLL, determined to be the amplification target, was obtained using a speech-shaped 70 dB overall input signal. Special "hearing aid selector" charts served as the medium for data transfer with the average normal DLL represented as 60, 61, 58, 54, and 46 dB SPLs at octave frequencies from 250 through 4000 Hz. The patient's dynamic range was bisected, and the target gain was established as halfway between threshold and LDL from 1000 to 8000 Hz, and one third between threshold and LDL at 250 and 500 Hz. If LDL was not obtainable, the level of the stapedius reflex serves as a substitute. Two different "hearing aid selector" charts were available on which the thresholds and LDL values were plotted. One chart was in HTL and the other in SPL, with see-through overlays that allowed easy comparison between the two reference levels.

The selection process goals of Bragg's approach to select and/or adjust hearing aids that best meet the following two criteria:

1. a saturation output from 250 through 4000 Hz that approaches at each frequency, but does not exceed the LDL or the acoustic reflex, and
2. gain at each frequency sufficient to raise average speech to the DDL, plus a reasonable reserve (between 5–15 dB) depending on the type of aid and the degree of conductive involvement (one fourth the conductive loss). The reserve gain can be added to each frequency when selecting the hearing aid or accounted for by setting the hearing aid volume control 5 to 15 dB below the maximum gain when adjusting the aid.

MSUv3 (1983, 1985, 1988)

This procedure, developed and modified by Cox (1983, 1985, 1988) at Memphis State University (MSU, but now renamed the University of Memphis), bisects the listener's dynamic range and establishes the target gain to where the speech spectrum (a 70 dB SPL raised voice level) is amplified halfway between threshold and the measured or calculated ULCL (upper limit of comfortable loudness). One modification to the procedure was a provision preventing the target level for amplified speech at any frequency from being higher than ULCL −15 dB. This was added to manage the narrowed listening range (less than 30 dB) between SPHL and ULCL that occurs with high-frequency losses. A second provision allows the prescriptive procedure to be used based on threshold measures only, if needed.

This fitting procedure prescribes gain and saturation output for BTE and ITE hearing aids. It calls for obtaining hearing thresholds at several frequencies in SPL (HSPL) and loudness perception measurements of the up-

Seiler Formula Calculations (1971)

Frequency in Hz	500	1000	2000	3000	4000
Threshold (example)	45	45	60	70	80
+For MCL	15	15	15	15	15
+ER dB	6	8	13	19	16
Sub Total	66	68	88	104	111
X Discrim. %	.15	.25	.30	.25	.05
Sub Total	9.90	17.00	26.40	26.00	5.55
+1/2 Gain	18.75	18.75	18.75	18.75	18.75
Response	**28.65**	**35.75**	**45.15**	**44.75**	**24.30**

MCL Th + 15 dB	
500 Hz	60
1000 Hz	60
2000 Hz	75
3000 Hz	85
4000 Hz	95
Total	375
X10%	
Gain	37.5
1/2 Gain	**18.75**

Figure 3–17. Seiler indirect MCL hearing aid gain selection formula based on pure-tone thresholds. The formula considers, MCL, the ear resonance, the contribution of different frequencies to speech recognition, and the amount of gain required by the hearing aid. See text for explanation. (Adapted with permission from "A Formula for Fitting Hearing Aids," by J. A. Seiler, 1971, p. 19. *The Hearing Dealer*. Copyright 1971 by The Hearing Dealer.)

per limit of comfortable loudness (ULCL, also in SPL) for one third octave noise bands or warble tones. The formula is designed to prescribe hearing aid gain and output based on (a) sound-field thresholds only, (b) earphone thresholds, (c) sound-field thresholds and ULCLs, or (d) any of the previous, singly or in combination with each other. Hearing aid selection is done best by computer, although hand calculations or a look-up table approach can be used (Table 3–3), using the equations from Table 3–4.

Table 3–3. MSUv3 equations to calculate hearing instrument prescription. (Numbers in parentheses refer to columns in Table 3-4)

Gain for OTE Instrument

(a) Supra-aural earphone pretest:

Gain (HA-1) = ½ ULCL + ½SPHL − (1) − (2) + (5) + (6) *

or

Gain (HA-1) = ULCL − 15 −(1) − (2) + (5) + (6) **

(b) Insert earphone pretest:

Gain HA-2) = ½ ULCL + ½ SPHL − (1) − (2) *

or

Gain (HA-2) = ULCL − 15 - (1) − (2) **

* Gain option 1

** Gain option 2

Use gain option giving lower (smaller) value

Gain for ITE Instrument

Gain = [OTE gain (HA−1)] − (3)

SSPL90 for OTE Instrument

(a) Supra-aural earphone pretest:

SSPL90 = ULCL − 5 + (4) + (5) + (6)

(b) Insert earphone pretest:

SSPL90 = ULCL − 5 + (4)

SSPL90 for ITE Instrument

SSPL90 = ULCL − 5 + (4) + (5) + (6)

Aided Sound Field Threshold (ASFT) Goals (ITE and OTE)

ASFT goal = (1) − ½ ULCL + ½ SPHL (for gain option 1)

or

ASFT goal = (1) + 15 − ULCL + SPHL (for gain option 2)

Estimation of Unaided Sound Field Threshold (USFT) from SPHL

(a) Supra-aural earphone pretest:

USFT = SPHL + (5) + (7)

(b) Insert earphone pretest:

USFT = SPHL + (6) + (7)

Insertion Gain (IG)

IG = USFT − ASFT goal

Estimation of SPHL from USFT

(a) Supra-aural earphone:

SPHL = USFT − (7) − (5)

(b) Insert earphone:

SPHL = USFT − (7) + (6)

Table 3–4. Values (dB) used in the equations of Table 3–3.

Freq (kHz)	(1) Speech Spectrum	(2) OTE Head Baffle	(3) ITE re: OTE Input	(4) 1% Peak re: Long Term RMS	(5) Eardrum re: 6 cc Coupler	(6) 2 cc Coupler re: Eardrum	(7) FF re: Eardrum
0.25	60.0	0.5	1.0	17	–7.8	–4.0	–1.3
0.5	62.0	1.0	1.0	20	1.6	–4.0	–1.8
0.8	56.5	0.75	1.5	22	2.4	–4.0	–3.0
1.0	55.0	0.0	1.0	23	2.8	–5.0	–2.5
1.6	52.0	1.0	1.0	24	4.0	–7.5	–6.5
2.5	48.0	2.0	4.5	25	7.1	–9.5	–16.5
4.0	46.0	3.0	6.0	28	5.1	–12.0	–14.0
6.3	45.5	0.0	3.0	28	3.0	–14.0	–6.5

The prescription can include (a) coupler gain at use volume control setting, (b) the saturation output of the hearing aid, (c) aided sound-field threshold targets, and (d) insertion gain at each test frequency. Use, and not full-on gain values are not provided by the prescription. Cox recommended that full-on gain be 10 to 15 dB greater than use gain at each frequency.

Saturation output is prescribed at a level considered to be high enough to avoid significant clipping of the speech signal under all likely listening conditions (12 dB added to the ULCL to account for speech peaks) and when adjusted to the highest level likely to be chosen by the patient. Because the method does not measure specifically the patient's tolerance for amplified sound (it is *predicted* based on measured or calculated ULCL, which is lower than the LDL), tolerance to loud, amplified sounds should be discussed with the patient in follow-up interviews and adjusted accordingly.

Cox suggested that ULCLs can be *predicted* from SPHL data rather than measured directly. Equations for this estimation for supra-aural or insert earphones are shown in Table 3–5. The same equations can be used for one-third-octave band and warble-tone stimuli. There is some inaccuracy in this prediction in the order of 7–8 dB. Still, it has the advantage of use for patients incapable of making loudness judgements. Cox (1988) commented that the highest level likely to be chosen by a patient for amplified speech remains somewhat lower than the contour of ULCLs determined with narrowband noise or warble-tone stimuli. This level is now estimated at ULCL −5 dB plus some other correction factor. A more complete explanation of the procedure can be found in Cox (1988).

MCL Prescriptive Procedures: Summary

Bisection techniques have been questioned at times because, although they might bisect the dynamic range visually, they may not bisect the dynamic range in loudness perception. This concern is based on the recognition that loudness grows more rapidly at lower sensation levels than at higher sensation levels for both normal and impaired ears. Additionally, if the assumption of the fitting protocol is that the speech level at all frequencies is 65 dB SPL (or some other fixed value), bisection procedures tend to under amplify high-frequency gain in high frequency losses. Long-term average speech spectra show high frequencies to have significantly less energy than low frequencies.

Table 3–5. Regression equations for estimation of ULCL (dB SPL) from SPHL (dB SPL) for supra-aural or insert earphone.

ULCL (250)	=	.37 (SPHL)	+	85
ULCL (500)	=	.25 (SPHL)	+	83
ULCL (800)	=	.45 (SPHL)	+	73
ULCL (1000)	=	.44 (SPHL)	+	71
ULCL (1600)	=	.41 (SPHL)	+	69
ULCL (2500)	=	.37 (SPHL)	+	69
ULCL (4000)	=	.39 (SPHL)	+	68
ULCL (6300)	=	.39 (SPHL)	+	68

When *comparing MCL prescriptive procedures*, whether direct or indirect, differences are generally greater for a rising-with-frequency sensorineural loss and for milder losses across all audiometric configurations. This was identified in a comparison among seven direct and indirect MCL methods compared by Humes and Halling (1994). The greatest differences among methods in their target gain recommendations appear in the average overall gain and low-frequency slope. Little difference was observed in the high-frequency slope gain target recommendations. For their overall comparison, Humes and Halling concluded that no data clearly supported the superiority of one MCL prescriptive method over another relative to the frequency of successful fittings or in the magnitude of success achieved in individual cases. They did suggest, however, that both MCL *and* threshold-based methods contribute appropriately to the hearing aid fitting process. As an example, Humes and Hackett (1990) suggested that an initial hearing aid adjustment might be made to maximize listening *comfort* (i.e., near MCL) or *sound quality*. This could be followed, if necessary, by adjusting the frequency/gain response of the hearing aid gradually to match more closely the response designed to maximize speech recognition.

PRESCRIPTIVE SELECTION PROCEDURES BASED ON A RANGE OF COMFORTABLE LOUDNESS

These procedures identify a range of comfortable loudness and then use this range in different ways to set goals for hearing aid amplification.

Otometry (1963)

This hearing aid selection approach is the precursor on which loudness scaling hearing aid selection procedures are based. Essentially all hearing aid selection procedures based on the concept of loudness growth have utilized certain concepts from otometry, directly or indirectly. The procedure is fairly involved but merits significant consideration.

Introduced by Victoreen (1963), it was based on the principle of determining a range of comfortable loudness and then of providing aided performance to return the hearing to a given equal loudness contour at 72 dB SPL. This procedure also provided a basis for hearing aid candidacy in that if the measured ear deviates from the normal flat 72 dB most comfortable loudness pressure curve (MCLP) by more than 6 dB, the ear should be considered for prosthetic correction.

The term "otometry" (a "physical" science rather than a "behavioral" science) was coined by Victoreen to reflect the concept of fitting to loudness judgements. A basic tenet of the procedure was that 2 cc coupler data (used to measure hearing aid performance characteristics) did not relate to real ear performance, nor to the audiogram in HTL. Victoreen advocated that all measurement procedures be made in sound pressure, including threshold and all loudness judgment data. Otometry was an attempt to return to the scientific method of expression, measurement, and numerical notation and to move away from the behavioral approach, the behavioral approach having found its way into audiometric measurement but not considered appropriate for hearing aid selection. Otometry was an attempt to determine how much hearing function is "left," not how much has been "lost," as does audiometry. A damped wavetrain signal was used as the stimulus because it was considered to be scientifically explainable, was truly measurable, made free-field measurements feasible and practical because the signal reduced standing waves and reflection problems, and was able to substitute for speech. The damped wavetrain signal has been described as a pure-tone burst having a constant number of cycles regardless of the frequency of the signal. Its characteristics decay rapidly or fade out, much like speech, instead of coming to an abrupt end.

Otometry did not, in itself, describe how to prescribe a hearing instrument. The principles did, however, explain how an ear functions with hearing aids (Victoreen, 1973). As such, the procedure may function best today as a measure of the "outcome" performance of the fitting. (The author has experienced that, as a predictor of the amplification required, otometry tends to suggest heavily on high-frequency electroacoustic response characteristics.) Still, when the principles are applied in conjunction with a *"measured laboratory standard hearing instrument fitted with a custom-made earmold,"* a prescription for a hearing aid for a given ear may be obtained using a substitution method (Hartenstein, 1978; Melen, 1978). When used as a prescriptive procedure for hearing aid amplification, Figure 3–18A through 3–18F illustrates the graphing and relationships of the measures required. The fitting steps that follow explain the fitting approach:

1. Measure the *unaided* free-field most comfortable loudness pressures (MCLP), identified also as the central loudness pressure locus (CLPL), for each ear separately (occlude contralateral ear if necessary). Seat the patient 28 inches at zero-degree axis with the free-field speaker. MCLP is defined as the bracketed midpoint of loudness sensation between "loud" and "soft," words printed on a card and pointed to by the patient. Using this procedure and stimulus, most individuals have a "comfortable" loudness range of about ±4 dB. The data are plotted on an otometric chart in SPL from 250 to 6000 Hz (Figure 3–18C). If the measured ear departs from the normal flat 72 dB MCLP curve significantly (usually in excess of 6 dB), that ear is considered a candidate for a hearing aid. The dotted line in Figure 3–18C represents the 72 dB MCLP curve and serves as an overall target.
2. The *aided* free-field MCLP is measured for each ear separately (Figure 3–18D), with the contralateral ear occluded, if necessary. This measurement is made with a "laboratory test aid" (a similar, standard hearing aid whose parameters can be modified as necessary by the manufacturer to fulfill the prescriptive measurements) with the actual earmold coupling. The gain control of the aid is adjusted (referenced) to MCLP for a 72 dB damped wavetrain signal at 1000 Hz. Signals at other frequencies are then presented and plotted for their most comfortable range and most comfortable loudness but with the volume control maintained at the referenced setting. In Figures 3–18D and 3–18E the target of 72 dB SPL has been modified arbitrarily at the low frequencies and is represented by the solid line. The slight adjustment calls for less gain to compensate for the potential upward spread of masking, the relative predominance of low-frequency sounds in the environment, and the relative lesser importance of low-frequency sounds for speech intelligibility. Identified as a solid line in Figure 3–18E as the "overall prosthetic objective," it rolls off at a rate of 3 dB/octave for each 10 dB of in-use gain at 1000 Hz. This makes the roll-off variable, which, for the example shown, is +6 dB at 500 Hz, and +10 dB at 250 Hz.
3. A prescription (or preselection) is tabulated by a direct substitution method. This is obtained by taking the aided measured values on the laboratory aid at the "in-use" gain setting (Figure 3–18F) and cal-

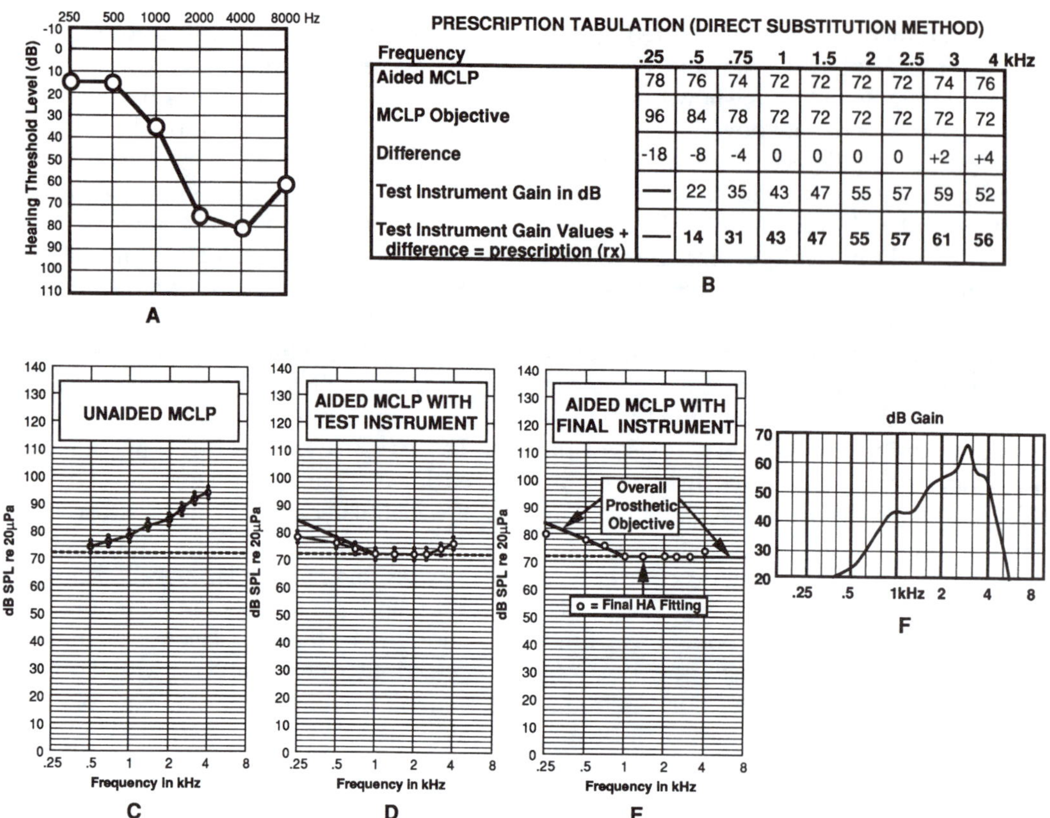

PRESCRIPTION TABULATION (DIRECT SUBSTITUTION METHOD)

Frequency	.25	.5	.75	1	1.5	2	2.5	3	4 kHz
Aided MCLP	78	76	74	72	72	72	72	74	76
MCLP Objective	96	84	78	72	72	72	72	72	72
Difference	-18	-8	-4	0	0	0	0	+2	+4
Test Instrument Gain in dB	—	22	35	43	47	55	57	59	52
Test Instrument Gain Values + difference = prescription (rx)	—	14	31	43	47	55	57	61	56

Figure 3–18. Graphing and the relationships involved in otometry as described by Victoreen (1963), using a direct substitution method. For the audiogram identified in **A**, the unaided most comfortable loudness pressures (MCLP) are identified and plotted in SPL **(C)** using a damped wavetrain signal. Normal unaided ear MCLP values are at 72 dB across the frequency spectrum (dashed line). MCLPs are then obtained from a "laboratory aid" **(D)** after the gain control is adjusted to a comfortable level matching a 72 dB damped wavetrain signal output at 1000 Hz. This is identified as the "in-use" gain setting. Other frequencies are then matched in loudness to this level, and their SPL values are recorded. The actual differences in gain required to reach these levels at different frequencies are identified as the "difference" in **B.** To obtain these values, the "laboratory aid" is measured into a 2 cc coupler with the volume control at its reference setting. The "in-use" gain at 1000 Hz is the SPL output measured gain for this patient is 44 dB at 1000 Hz. The prescription (or preselection) can be tabulated by a direct substitution method. This is obtained by taking aided measured values on the laboratory hearing aid **(F)** at the "in-use" gain setting and recording the differences between these gains and the difference values required to reach the prosthetic objective. These deviations from the prosthetic objective in measured MCLP are appropriately added or subtracted from the 2 cc coupler frequency response of the instrument, and a prescription is written (bottom line of **B**). The hearing aid prescriptive gain is the test instrument gain values plus the difference. See text for additional explanation.

culating the difference between these gains and the differences values needed to reach the prosthetic objective. These difference values are added or subtracted appropriately from the 2 cc coupler frequency response of the hearing aid, and a prescription is written (bottom line of Figure 3–18B). The hearing aid's prescribed gain is the test instrument gain values plus or minus the differences.

4. The aided MCLP values of the patient's actual hearing aid are plotted against the MCLP objective (solid line on Figure 3–18E). The final aided MCLP is to be within ±2 dB of the predicted curve.
5. Tolerance of the fitted aid is measured separately for each ear with the contralateral ear occluded if necessary. If TD is reached before the limits of the test equipment, the input sound pressure plus the gain of the aid may be used to specify the maximum tolerable pressure at that frequency.
6. To show if "stereophonic perception" has been achieved, aided binaural MCLPs are performed.

Pascoe (1975, 1978)

Proposed as a simple and less time-consuming hearing aid selection procedure, this approach was based on the acceptance of certain premises, namely:

1. The frequency response of a hearing aid must be known or defined in terms of functional gain.
2. Those changes in frequency responses that reestablish the proper balance between the low- and high-frequency components of speech (two-humped configuration in the aided perceived speech spectrum) result in improved speech reception.
3. A wider bandwidth is correlated positively with improved discrimination. Both ends of the speech spectrum must be retained to produce a pleasant, normal-sounding signal.
4. Amplification must be adjusted, when needed, to variations in the dynamic range of hearing, including compression.
5. Hearing aids can be manufactured that meet these needs.

The procedure for hearing aid selection is shown in Figure 3–19:

1. Define the dynamic range of loudness monaurally. Use pulsed one-third octave bands of noise presented at zero-degree incidence in the sound field, in SPL. Occlude the other ear.
2. The listener selects from a 5-point scale one of the following: 1 = very soft, 2 = soft but clear, 3 = just right, 4 = a little loud but OK, and 5 = too loud, uncomfortable. Three or four trains of pulses are presented, somewhat randomly, at various levels, either ascending or descending sequences. The patient assigns a scale value following each pulse train. Three scale values are obtained for each of five signal levels of eight noise bands. This number is sufficient to provide the basic information needed to select a hearing aid. At a minimum, exploration of 500, 1000, and 2000 Hz should be defined fully. While sound-field signals are preferred, earphone SPL corrections can be converted to sound field SPL levels using the suggested corrections that follow (values are to be subtracted from the earphone SPL values).

Frequency:	**250**	**500**	**1000**	**1500**	**2000**	**3000**	**4000**	**6000 Hz**
Phone – SF	−3	0	0	−2	−6	−12	−13	−9 dB

3. Define the "desired signal levels." Input levels should be reasonable facsimiles of the speech spectrum at or near normal conversational levels. If an overall input speech level of 65 dB and a 20 dB dynamic range for speech are desired, the input levels that follow are thought to approximate the 20% and 80% levels of speech as reported by Dunn and White (1940).

Frequency:	**250**	**500**	**1000**	**1500**	**2000**	**3000**	**4000**	**6000 Hz**
Maximum	68	71	60	61	62	55	54	50 dB SPL
Mean	58	61	50	51	52	45	44	40 dB SPL
Minimum	48	51	40	41	42	35	34	30 dB SPL

(One-third octave band levels)

4. Derive the functional gain of the hearing aid by frequency (functional response) required to amplify the above input levels to the patient's MCL.
5. Minimum input levels should reach the listener's thresholds, but maximum input levels should not produce discomfort. If not, consider compression amplification.

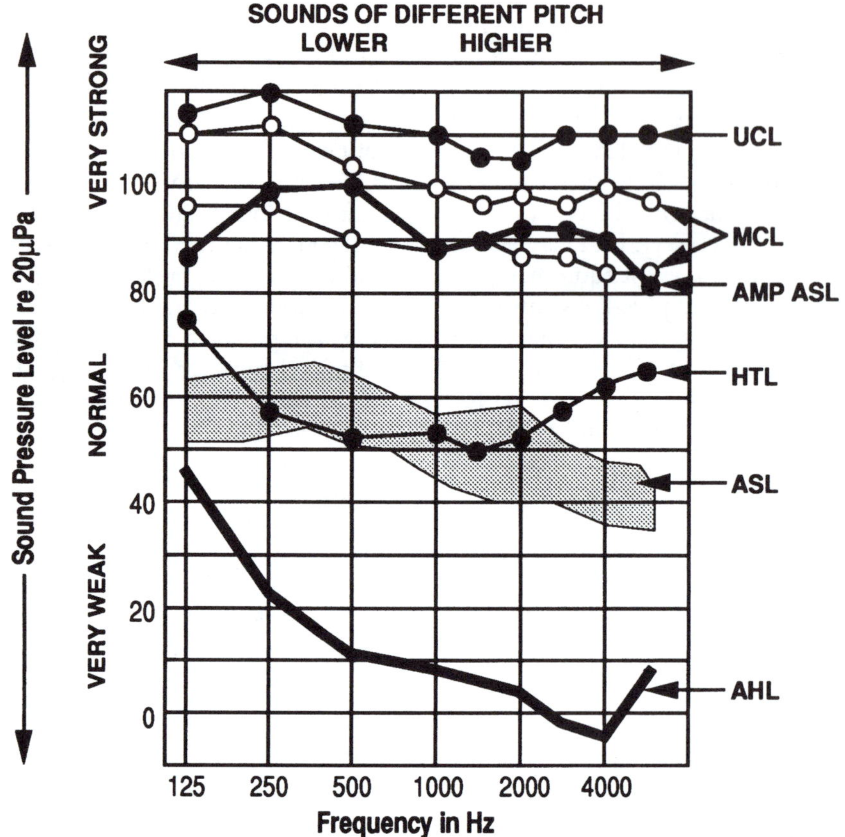

Figure 3–19. Pascoe hearing aid selection procedure and patient explanation information display shown in SPL. The goal is to have the aided performance fall within the most comfortable zone of average speech levels.

6. Saturation output levels should be just below the discomfort levels. If not, consider compression amplification.
7. Use a "test aid" to describe the hearing aid coupler gain by frequency (frequency response). The "test aid" should approximate the characteristics of the projected coupler requirements, aid type, and earmold coupling. Obtain aided thresholds at each noise band and mask the contralateral ear, if needed. Calculate the functional gain (unaided minus aided) for each frequency band. These functional gains are then compared to the hearing aid 2cc coupler gains and functional versus coupler corrections are calculated.
8. Specify the entire set of hearing aid requirements, including the style, ear fitted, gain and output characteristics, inherent noise level, and the need for and type of compression or other form of output limiting.
9. Test the fitting with Step 7 using the "desired signal levels" of Step 3. If departures from the required goals are deemed significant, electrical or acoustical adjustments can be made. Although acceptable variances are difficult to specify, the goal is to have the sensations produced by the peaks of high and low bands of speech to be within the most comfortable zone. The frequencies of 1000 to 1500 Hz should be heard and described as being "softer."

Results of this fitting procedure can be displayed in SPL (Figure 3–19) or, following translation, on an audiogram in HTL.

Loudness Growth in Octave Bands (1989)

Based on measurements of loudness sensation (Pluvinage & Benson, 1988; Pluvinage, 1989) and introduced by the ReSound Company, the LGOB measures the growth of loudness as a function of frequency, with the dynamic range of an individual's hearing impairment calculated from the data.

One-half octave bands of noise are presented, and the patient is asked to make loudness judgements based on the following categories: (0) Cannot Hear—CH, (1) Very Soft—VS, (2) Soft—S, (3) Comfortable—C, (4) Loud—L, (5) Very Loud—VL, and (6) Too Loud—TL. The noise bands are presented at each of the octave frequency midpoints from 250 to 4000 Hz. Loudness growth is plotted for each band using intensity-versus-loudness sensation, and the equal loudness contours are then displayed. Presentations of noise levels and bands are randomized and automatically presented by a programmed computer. The patient operates a hand-held selector from which the comfort level is selected for each presentation sequence, which consists of groups of three half-second bursts separated by half-second intervals of silence. The data obtained is used to determine the sound processing required to fit a patient's dynamic range of hearing. The fitting algorithm is proprietary.

The test is divided into two sections:

1. Data is collected to determine the limits of the dynamic range (VS and VL). Determining these levels eliminates them from the test sequence to shorten the test time.
2. The remaining dynamic range (minus the VS and VL presentation levels) is presented with intensity steps ranging from 6 dB (normal dynamic range) to 2 dB (very narrow dynamic range). The difference between a normal and abnormal loudness growth curves is illustrated in Figure 3–20 for a single frequency, whereas Figure 3–21 shows the loudness growth across

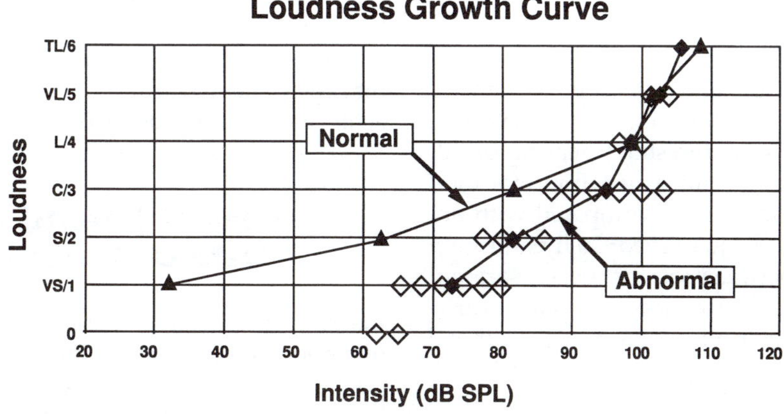

Figure 3–20. Normal and abnormal (rapid) loudness growth curve comparisons. The clear diamonds indicate individual responses, and the solid diamonds represent the average intensity level for all presentations eliciting the same loudness selection. A loudness growth curve is obtained by connecting the solid diamonds. (After Pluvinage, 1989, *Hearing Instruments, 39*, 3).

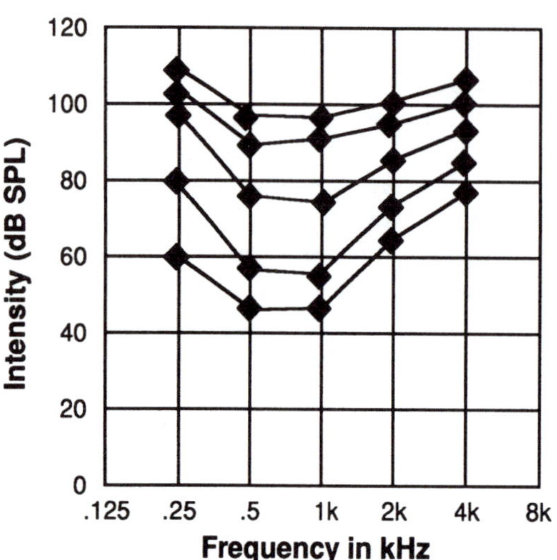

Figure 3–21. Equal loudness contours for a high-frequency hearing loss. The patient's high-frequency hearing shows a decrease in the dynamic range (spacing between the curves) for the higher frequencies.

frequencies (equal loudness contours) for a patient having a high-frequency hearing loss. Notice the decrease in the dynamic range for the higher frequencies in the latter illustration.

The LGOB test, and other loudness growth tests, provide important information about the patient's suprathreshold hearing profile. The degree of recruitment (abnormal loudness growth increase as compared with normal listeners) is quantified easily and helps distinguish between conductive, sensorineural, and mixed hearing losses. From a hearing aid fitting prescriptive, loudness growth patterns suggest sound processing options to best compensate for a particular hearing loss.

INTEGRATED HEARING AID SELECTION PROCEDURE

With the differences in recommended hearing aid selection procedures for linear versus nonlinear amplification circuits that have risen in the past few years, the emergence of new programmable hearing aids, and the expanded need for "outcome" measures to qualify the hearing aid fitting, hearing health care professionals face new challenges. Could all of these objectives be accomplished in a single fitting protocol? To this end, a group of practitioners developed the IHAFF (Independent Hearing Aid Fitting Forum) in 1994. This protocol is considered to be an ongoing process and may be somewhat different by the time this text is published.

IHAFF, a group of hearing health care professionals, developed a protocol to respond to the challenges. The protocol involves three components:

1. Prefitting data collection of hearing thresholds, but with an emphasis on suprathreshold loudness-based measures,
2. Amplification selection software, and
3. Fitting and verification of benefit.

The goal of the fitting procedure is to restore normal loudness appreciation of amplified speech cues that are audible for soft input levels, are comfortable (for normal speech levels), and are not uncomfortable or distorted for intense sounds. It is assumed that if a hearing aid restores the normal loudness perception sensations over a wide bandwidth that the patient will have an opportunity to achieve maximum speech intelligibility.

Phase I (Prefitting Data Collection)

Insert earphone measurements are recommended to provide a common reference point to hearing aid measurements (especially when the insertion depth is carefully matched between the insert earphone and the hearing aid earpiece).

1. Pure-tone thresholds are measured from 250 to 8000 Hz.
2. Loudness growth information is used to calculate the appropriate amplifier charac-

teristics necessary to restore normal loudness perception. These are measured using pulsed warble tones or narrow bands of noise loudness judgements (for seven levels ranging from very soft to uncomfortable) at a minimum of two frequencies. These data are then converted to SPL (HA-1, 2 cc coupler measures). A median taken from four ascents for each loudness judgement is used (Figure 3–22). Loudness judgements can be administered manually or by computer. A practice run from very soft to loud, followed by three ascending data collection runs for each judgement level presentation are made. The patient's loudness contour is calculated from the median value for each category.

3. An index of communicative handicap is obtained to assess the patient's needs and expectations from amplification and to es-

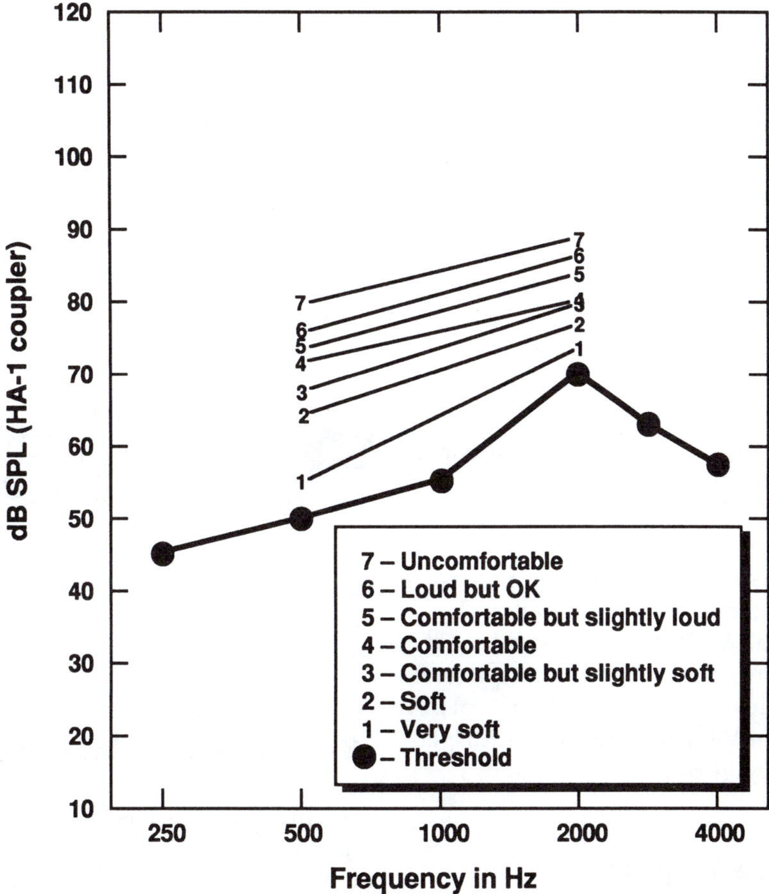

Figure 3–22. Threshold audiogram with loudness contour judgments at 500 and 2000 Hz. (After Van Vliet, 1995, p. 30. *Hearing Instruments*, March). Instructions for the loudness test: "The purpose of this test is to find your judgments of the loudness of different sounds. You will hear that increase and decrease in volume. You must make a judgment about how loud the sounds are. Pretend you are listening to the radio at that volume. How loud would it be? After each sound, tell me which of these categories best describes the loudness. Keep in mind that an uncomfortably loud sound is louder than you would ever choose on your radio no matter what mood you are in."

tablish a baseline for comparison to aided conditions. The APHAB (Abbreviated Profile of Hearing Aid Benefit), described by Cox and Alexander (1995) is used.

Phase II (Hearing Aid Selection)

This phase involves having casual, normal, and loud vocal effort speech levels targeted to fit appropriately within the individual's seven categories of loudness. After the results of the loudness perception test are entered, input/output curves derived from these data define the gain, slope, and output of the desired hearing aid. The location of the hearing aid microphone pickup, loudness summation, and other factors are considered in the equation. The program displays two input/output graphs at frequencies chosen by the dispenser, which show target values for the three speech input levels. The gain, compression ratio, compression threshold, and limiting levels of known circuits are entered by the dispenser. The practitioner then matches the resultant calculated input/output curves for a match with the target values. The process can be performed manually, but is best left to computer application. A computer program to assist in this selection process is VIOLA (Visualization of Input/Output Locator Algorithm). VIOLA assists in making the determinations as to which circuit parameters will achieve the amplification goals. A graphic of the VIOLA input/output display is shown in Figure 3–23.

Phase III (Fitting and Validation)

This phase can involve: (1) 2 cc coupler measures, (2) aided sound-field measures, (3) probe microphone assessment, and (4) a follow-up validation using APHAB.

1. The 2 cc coupler measurements allow the hearing aid to be preset to meet the specifications prescribed in Phase II. Setting the correct saturation output to ensure that distortion measures are lower than 10% at 90 dB SPL input should receive special attention.
2. Aided measures of speech and sound are recommended as follows: conversational speech (65 dB SPL) is to be perceived at a loudness ratings of 3, 4, 5; low-level input sounds should fall in the 20–30 HTL range; and high-level speech (85 dB SPL) should be perceived at a loudness rating of 6.
3. Probe microphone measures of real ear aided response (REAR) should show no excessive irregularities (peaks). The bandwidth should be as wide as practical for the user. Real ear saturation response (RESR) to a swept warble-tone or smoothed pure-tone stimulus at 90 dB SPL is obtained to verify that a loudness discomfort rating of 7 is not reached at any frequency.

COMBINED THRESHOLD AND SPEECH-IN-NOISE APPROACH

At least one fitting procedure utilizes threshold-based measurements in a different way and a suprathreshold measure other than MCL.

The "Benefit" Method (1992)

This procedure is based on two beliefs: (a) that it is best to use the hearing aid user as his or her own standard when fitting hearing aids, rather than using an average value based on pure-tone audiometry (as do pure-tone based fitting formulae), and (b) that understanding in noise is critical to successful hearing aid fitting, and it is not possible to predict word-recognition scores in noise from scores in quiet (Svard & Spens, 1992; Svard & Ahlner, 1994). The "benefit" method takes both these issues into consideration.

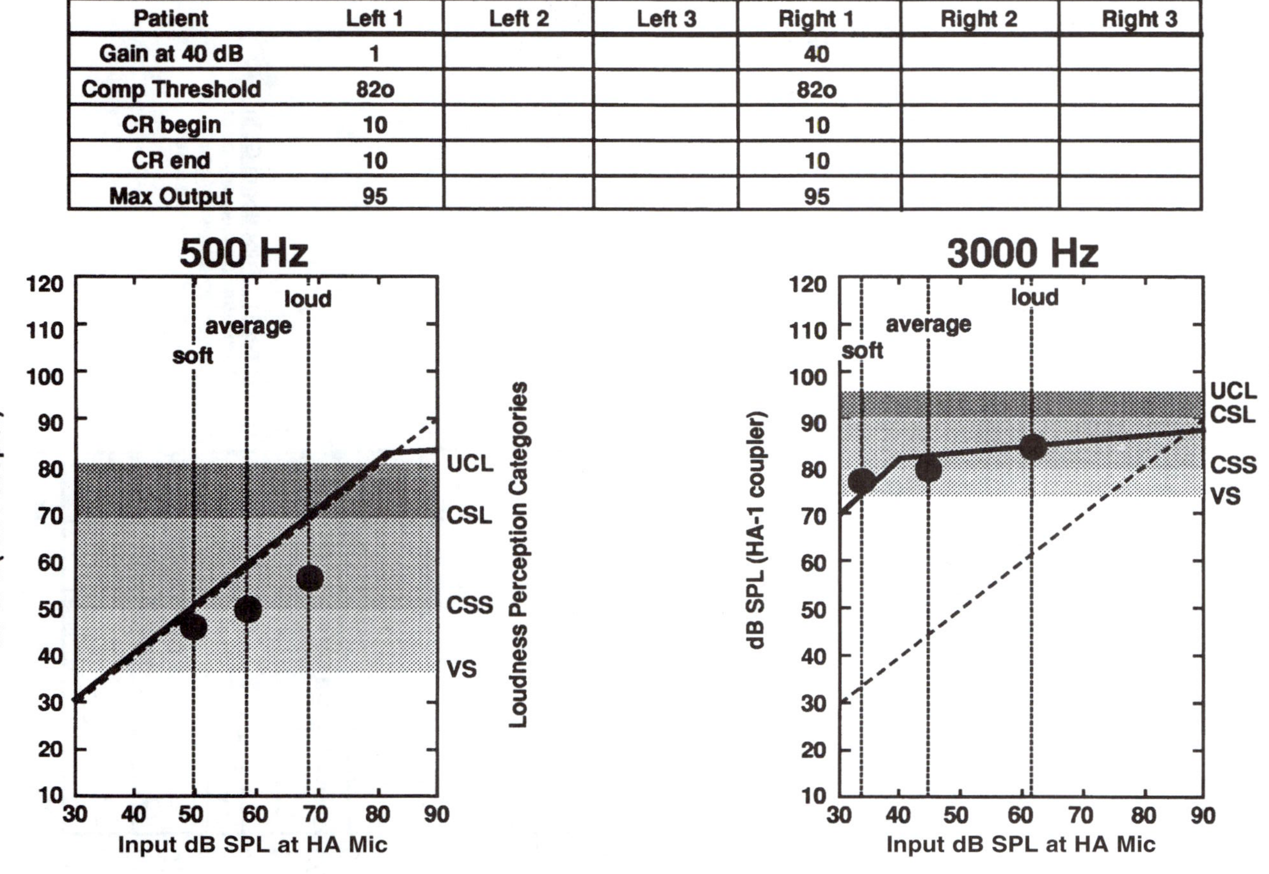

Patient	Left 1	Left 2	Left 3	Right 1	Right 2	Right 3
Gain at 40 dB	1			40		
Comp Threshold	82o			82o		
CR begin	10			10		
CR end	10			10		
Max Output	95			95		

Figure 3–23. Viola input/output display. This shows the hearing loss and loudness judgments for an individual with a mild hearing loss at 500 Hz and a severe loss at 3000 Hz. The calculated "targets" (●) for the 500 Hz band are at less than unity gain, so no gain was selected for the 500 Hz band. A linear response up to a knee of 82 dB was selected for the 3000 Hz band. The output compression hearing aid selected has a 10:1 compression ratio and is limited at 95 dB SSPL90 output. (Modified from "A Comprehensive Hearing Aid Fitting Protocol, Progress Report, by IHAFF, April, 1994.)

The patient is surrounded by four loudspeakers that create a homogeneous *noise* field that simulates the patient's difficult listening conditions. A separate loudspeaker presents the desired *signal* at a 45° angle to the patient. Test stimuli consist of damped wavetrain signals and phonetically balanced (PB) words. A "standard" against which to test the benefit of amplification is included. The test is performed as follows:

1. Measure *unaided word recognition* to assess the patient's everyday listening problem. PB words are presented by the signal loudspeaker at 75 dB SPL (S/N + 10 dB). This test also provides some indication as to the prognosis for amplification when several people are speaking at the same time.
2. Measure *unaided thresholds* using a damped wavetrain (after Victoreen, 1963), attached to a Békésy audiometer, in speech-shaped noise. Thresholds are obtained at 1000, 2000, 3000, and 4000 Hz. These thresholds are compared with the "normal" thresholds from a reference group. The difference between the two thresholds is the *minimum* gain necessary to detect signals of a normal speech level (Figure 3–24). A computer program calculates which frequencies must be amplified.
3. The hearing aid is adjusted to the *minimum* gain and step 2 is repeated, except that the signals are now *aided*. These results show the extent to which amplification can be used by the patient. The hearing aid is adjusted to reach the "reference group normal threshold," and an addition of 10 dB reserve gain is recommended. This step identifies the *optimum gain*.
4. An *aided* word-recognition score in speech noise is performed with the aid that provides the best signal detection threshold. The difference between the scores of steps

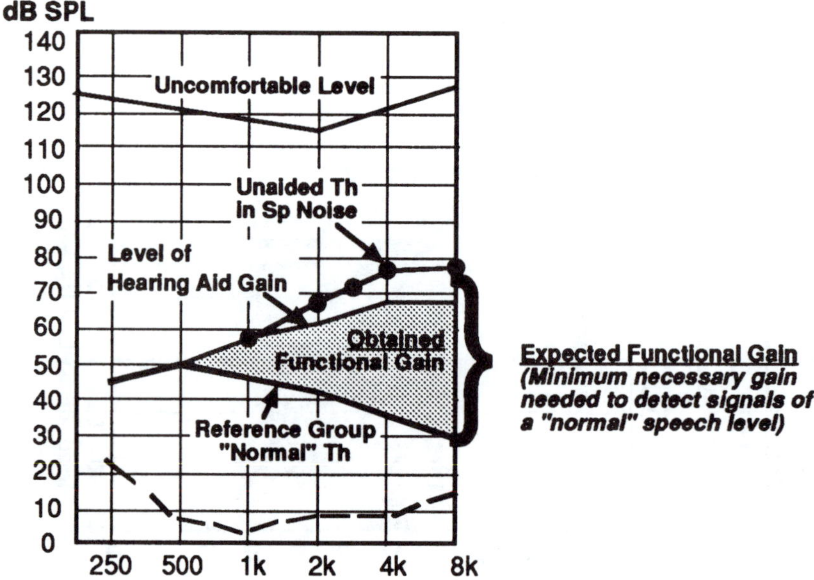

Figure 3–24. "Benefit" method graphical explanation showing the minimum necessary gain needed by the patient to obtain a "normal" threshold in noise. See text for explanation. (Adapted from "The 'Benefit Method' in the Fitting of Hearing Aids," by I. Svärd and B. H. Ahlner, 1994, *Bulletin of the American Auditory Society, 19,* 10–11, 16. Copyright 1994 by American Auditory Society.)

1 and 4 is a measure of the benefit of the chosen hearing aid. The extent to which the patient's hearing aid(s) can improve speech perception in noise is shown by the word-recognition score. This verifies the potential benefit of the prescribed hearing aid and its settings.

MAXIMUM OUTPUT SELECTION

A successful hearing aid fitting requires that the saturation output of a hearing aid be set just below the LDL. When not set appropriately, users reject a significant number of hearing aids because of loudness discomfort. An inappropriate setting may also cause the user to reduce the volume control setting to less than optimum, or restrict hearing aid use to quieter environments to avoid high level inputs that might cause the LDL to be exceeded. If set too low, the dynamic range of the hearing aid will be restricted unnecessarily, leading to distortions (Hawkins, 1984b). Additional generalized comments about the saturation output from Mueller and Bright (1994) include the following:

1. It is suggested that the optimal saturation output be slightly below the LDL but as high as possible to prevent limiting the amplified dynamic range.
2. Some individuals may show an increase in LDL of 6 to 8 dB following repeated LDL measurement sessions. As a result, it may be necessary to add an additional 3 dB to account for this variable.
3. Hearing aids that provide very low distortion may be able to use a slightly higher saturation output.
4. Binaural hearing aid fittings are treated as two separate monaural fittings. Loudness discomfort does not seem to have a summation effect.

While a number of the prescriptive hearing aid formulae detailed previously predict or prescribe the gain/frequency characteristics of amplification, they offer suggestions also on the selection of the maximum output of the hearing aid (Berger, 1976b; Bragg, 1977; Cornelisse, Seewald, & Jamieson, 1994; Cox, 1988; Lybarger, 1957; McCandless and Lyregaard, 1983.) A significant number of other formulae, however, do not specifically prescribe maximum output levels for each patient. If one of the major goals of hearing aid selection is to provide amplification that does not make ordinary sounds uncomfortable to the user, then such a recommendation should not be ignored. Because appropriate selection of the saturation output of the hearing aid is so important, this section expands on methods and ideas relative to saturation output selection, even when not related to the formulae. (In this chapter, Threshold of Discomfort (TD), Loudness Discomfort Level (LDL), and Uncomfortable Loudness Level (UCL) are used synonymously.)

Output Prediction from Pure-Tone Thresholds

These procedures attempt to *predict* the LDL (rather than measure it) from pure-tone thresholds and are helpful when it is not feasible to obtain LDL levels (for nonverbal patients, those having language problems or an inability to respond, etc.) There is, however, a nonlinear relationship between hearing levels and the LDL, and the individual variability is rather large, on the order of 20 dB across frequencies (Dillon, Chew, & Deans, 1984; Kamm et al., 1978; McCandless & Miller, 1972). Up to about a 40–50 dB hearing loss, average LDLs for patients having a cochlear loss are similar to having normal hearing. Above this loss level, the differences can be rather substantial. It is partly for these reasons that many practitioners believe the LDL should be measured directly for each individual, when possible. A method for predicting the saturation output from pure tones as has been discussed previously in this chapter (DSL).

The use of a regression equation to determine the best prediction of the LDL from pure tones was calculated by Cox (1985). The calculation was:

LDL = 100 + 1/4 Hearing Loss

Output Selection from Suprathreshold Estimates

Saturation output has been recommended based on suprathreshold measurements. Two methods for such estimation have been detailed earlier in this chapter (Cox, 1983; Skinner et al., 1982).

Output Selection from LDLs Using Stimuli Other Than Pure Tones

Direct measurements and indirect estimations of LDL have been made using a variety of stimuli. These have included, in addition to pure tones, narrow bands of noise; speech, in the forms of continuous discourse, sentences, spondees, nonsense syllables, filtered speech, and others; and warble tones.

Why use speech stimuli rather than some other type stimuli that provide frequency-specific information about the LDL? Speech is favored by some because it represents what the patient listens to and it also provides information about loudness summation. Practitioners who favor stimuli that provide frequency-specific information appreciate the fact that they allow for direct comparisons to the output curve selected.

How do the LDLs obtained using the various stimuli compare? A number of studies have investigated this topic (Beattie & Boyd, 1986; Bentler, 1993; Bentler & Pavlovic, 1989; Dirks & Kamm, 1976; Filion & Margolis, 1992; Hawkins, 1980). The following is a brief review of these studies.

- The studies tend to agree that consistency of the LDLs obtained with the different stimuli are fairly good, but as the spectrum of the signal type narrows, the LDLs are somewhat higher in the low frequencies (up to 10 dB differences between pure tones and wide band signals; Hawkins, 1980).
- Between pure tones and spondees, Dirks and Kamm (1976) found no significant differences for a group of individuals with hearing impairment.
- Between pure tones and multitone (speech-like) stimuli, Bentler and Pavlovic (1989) found multitone LDLs to be lower among both individuals with normal hearing and those with hearing impairment.
- Different kinds of environmental stimuli and annoyance judgements also resulted in LDL inconsistencies (Bentler, 1993).
- Intensities exceeding the clinical LDL were seldom judged to be uncomfortable in the real world (Filion & Margolis, 1992).
- Prescription of saturation output using six common formulae resulted in prescribed outputs differing by as much as 8 dB, but when a single individual was tested with all six formulae, differences as great as 25 dB were noted (Hawkins et al., 1992).
- Major variables that affect the LDL, and thus the saturation output selection, are the instructions to the patient, type of stimulus, and the stimulus delivery system.

Based on the results of these studies, it might be suggested that a variety of stimuli may be desirable in measuring the LDL for saturation output selection. In essence, any of the stimuli should provide reasonably good clinical LDL measurements, with the understanding that verification and modification, if necessary, are requisite to postselection.

Issues and Test Protocol for Saturation Output Selection

A number of issues arise relative to the determination of saturation output selection:

1. Should saturation output selection be made by direct measurement or by prediction of LDL? Whenever possible, a direct measurement of LDL is preferred rather than predicting it from pure-tone data. Because saturation output of a hearing aid can vary significantly as a function of frequency, more frequency-specific signals can provide important information relative to

its selection. This is especially true if the goal is to maximize the dynamic range across frequency.

2. What are appropriate instructions to give the patient for LDL determination? LDL varies as a function of the instructions given (Beattie, et al., 1980). As such, Hawkins et al. (1984, p. 163) suggested the following instructions:

> We need to do a test that will help me decide where to set the amplifier on your hearing aid. We want to set it so that sounds do not get so loud that they are uncomfortable. If we set it too high, sounds could get too loud for you, and you may not want to wear the hearing aid.
>
> You will hear some tones, and after each one I want you to tell me which of the loudness categories on this sheet (Figure 3–25) best describes the sound to you. So after each tone, tell me if it was "Comfortable," or "Comfortable, But Slightly Loud," "Loud, But OK," or Uncomfortably Loud."
>
> I will be zeroing in on this "Uncomfortably Loud" category, because that's where we want the hearing aid to stop. We want to keep the sound down in this region [point to the three comfortable categories] and not let the sound get up into here [point to the top three categories]. So for each tone, tell me which category it falls into. Understand?

LEVELS OF LOUDNESS

Painfully Loud
Extremely Uncomfortable
Uncomfortably Loud
Loud, But O.K.
Comfortable, But Slightly Loud
Comfortable
Comfortable, But Slightly Soft
Soft
Very Soft

Figure 3–25. Loudness category descriptions for LDL measurements. (After Hawkins, 1984, Selection of a critical electroacoustic characteristic: SSPL90. *Hearing Instruments, 35*, 28–32.)

3. What is a suggested procedure for LDL determination? The modified Hughson-Westlake technique for threshold determination (Carhart & Jerger, 1959) can be used effectively. LDL is obtained using an ascending approach. When a multichannel hearing aid is to be recommended, consider obtaining LDLs to pure tones at 500, 1000, 1500, 2000, 3000 Hz. If a single channel hearing aid is to be fitted, and if knowledge of the peak output of the hearing aid to be fitted is known, it may be sufficient to test LDL at that frequency only (Mueller & Bright, 1994).

   Starting at MCL, increase the intensity in 5 dB increments until the patient indicates the sound is "Uncomfortably Loud." At this response, drop the intensity level 10 dB and raise it in 5 dB increments until the "Uncomfortably Loud" level has been indicated on two of three ascends.

4. Convert data to 2 cc coupler SPL values. This is required to select the appropriate saturation output of the hearing aid.

   - For pure tones the conversion values from Table 3–6 can be used.
   - If speech was the stimulus, add 20 dB to the HTL value to derive the SPL equivalent.
   - If insert earphones were used there is no need for *average* correction factors because *precise* corrections can be made. For this use, an initial calibration for the audiometer and insert earphone combination is made, but not then for each patient. The insert receiver is placed in the 2 cc coupler, and the audiometer output is measured at the dial setting obtained for LDL. For example, if the audiometer dial reading is 80 dB and the measured 2 cc coupler reading is 85 dB, the conversion would be +5 dB. Such a procedure is appropriate

Table 3–6. Conversion values from dB HL to dB SPL in a 2 cc coupler.

Frequency (Hz)	*TDH-39*	*TDH-49 and 50*
250	20.7	21.7
500	9.9	11.9
750	7.3	7.8
1000	5.5	6.0
1500	2.5	3.5
2000	5.2	7.2
3000	5.7	5.2
4000	-0.5	0.5
6000	-0.2	-2.2

Source: From "Corrections and Transformations Relevant to Hearing Aid Selection," by D. Hawkins, 1992. In *Probe Microphone Measurements: Hearing Aid Selection and Assessment*, H. G. Mueller, D. Hawkins, and J. Northern, Eds. San Diego, CA: Singular Publishing. Copyright 1992 by Singular Publishing Group. Reprinted with permission.

for children because the residual volume between the tip of the earpiece and the eardrum is smaller than in adults. With children, the 2 cc to real-ear output difference can be greater by as much as 15 dB or more (Feign, et al., 1989).

Test Protocol for Saturation Output Verification

Mueller and Bright (1994) suggested the procedure that follows. They believe that verification is simplified if (a) careful measurements are taken during the selection procedure, and/or (b) the hearing aid has an output control that has a wide range of adjustment. Both behavioral testing and probe microphone measurements are used.

1. With pure tones:
   - Instructions: same as for saturation output selection.
   - Test at 500, 1000, 1500, 2000, and 3000 Hz.
   - Position patient 1 m in front of the loudspeaker. Calibrate the sound delivery system to determine the dial setting that corresponds to a 90 dB SPL output for each frequency.
   - Set the volume control 5 dB above the use gain or prescriptive target gain if a new user (to account for potential higher use gain in some situations).
   - Present pure tones at 90 dB SPL for the various frequencies. Determine LDL using the modified Hughson-Westlake procedure. If the saturation output of the hearing aid is set correctly, the patient will respond to "Loud, but OK." If too loud, adjust the hearing aid in any means available to reduce the output (output control, AGC knee, AGC compression ratio, etc.).
2. With probe-microphone equipment:
   - Confirm the above results with a RESR (real ear saturation response) measurement. It should correspond with target RESR.
3. Finally, expose the patient to loud sounds that are similar to those expected in the real world. At no time should the patient comment that any of the sounds are uncomfortably loud.

The following are potential correction factors for this procedure:

1. Some patients may show an increase in LDL of 6 to 8 dB following repeated LDL measurement sessions (Morgan & Dirks, 1974). As such, it may be necessary to add an additional 3 dB to account for this variable (Cox, 1981; Hawkins, 1984b; Libby, 1985).
2. A slightly higher saturation output may be used for hearing aids with low distor-

tion than is recommended by this procedure (Fortune, Preves, & Woodruff, 1991).

3. Because loudness discomfort does not seem to have a summation effect, binaural hearing aid fittings are treated as two separated monaural fittings (Mueller & Bright, 1994).

SUMMARY OF PRESCRIPTIVE HEARING AID SELECTION METHODS

A basic goal of hearing aid prescriptive formulae is to provide at least generalized or specific frequency target gains for the hearing aid(s) to be fitted. Some formulae provide additional targets for saturation output. Reasons hearing aid fitting formulae have been advocated include (Staab, 1996):

- They provide a degree of objectivity in the hearing aid selection process.
- They provide a first approximation of need and put the hearing health care provider in the proper ball park to start the fitting.
- They provide a means to verify the hearing aid fitting target by functional gain measures.
- A formula helps determine what modifications should be made to the hearing aid to more closely approximate targets.
- A formula provides a means to discuss objective data with the patient.

On the other hand, attempts at "objective" methods to determine amplified hearing aid performance via formulae have had their critics. Arguments suggesting care when applying formulae include (Staab, 1996):

- Target gains based on pure-tone thresholds are influenced by the developer's belief in the significance of different frequency bands to intelligibility.
- Essentially all procedures have been developed for linear amplifier hearing aids.
- Hearing aid formulae based on average data seem to degrade their usefulness when applied to a given individual.
- Most have been developed based on 2 cc coupler measurements.
- Almost all formulae have been derived from data obtained from sensorineural losses, occluding earmolds, and do not account for loudness growth changes.
- Most have not taken into consideration the differences in hearing aid style or gain requirements for varying degrees of hearing loss and some do not consider the UCL and subsequent saturation output requirements for the instrument.

Based on the combined pros and cons related to hearing aid fitting formulae, certain trends appear to be emerging:

- Meeting the targets of a hearing aid fitting formula are considered as a "first approximation of need" rather than as providing the final target.
- A real concern is the inability to substantiate that meeting a target provides even appropriate amplification.
- Hearing aid formulae based on average data seem to degrade their usefulness when applied to a given patient.
- Meeting the "target" is compounded by the inability of the electronics of the instrument to meet the requested target values, even with programmable systems.
- An inherent limitation of most prescriptive approaches (threshold or suprathreshold) is that they were developed to predict the *average* gain required when the input to the hearing aid is *average* conversational speech presented in a quiet, nonreverberant environment at a distance of approximately 3 feet. When input signal levels are less than this average level, the amount of gain prescribed results in under-amplification. Likewise, when the input signal levels are greater than this average conversational level, over-amplification occurs.
- Threshold testing in 5 dB increments (±5 dB variability) and the effects of ambient noise suggest that formulae based on threshold data would be expected to have at least the same variability.

- On the other hand, for some patients, threshold data may be the only information available upon which to base gain, frequency response, and output projections.
- The introduction and widespread utilization of new hearing aid options (varying compression configurations, multibands, fitting placement, etc.) require that fitting formulae will need to be modified. Some of this has been presented already in the forms of FIG6, DSL [i/o], and the IHAFF.
- Studies have not demonstrated clear advantages of one type of fitting approach over the others.

Reasons why a given formula is used by a dispenser include:

- Ease of use
- Familiarity with the procedure
- It is the procedure suggested and used by manufacturers for their own circuit selection with custom-molded hearing instruments

INTEGRATED HEARING MANAGEMENT SOFTWARE

NOAH

Early in 1993, a group of hearing aid manufacturers agreed to establish a joint development group called the Hearing Instrument Manufacturers' Software Association (HIMSA).

Their mission was twofold:

1. to design a standard for integrated hearing care software and
2. to develop an industry-wide software standard for fitting programmable hearing aids.

The NOAH software system, introduced in 1994, is the result of this cooperative effort. It is a common platform (Figure 3–26) that allows an office computer to link information from hearing aid fitting programs from different manufacturers, hearing-related test equipment (NOAH-compatible audiometers and real-ear test equipment), and office management software (i.e., Software and Systems "HearWare," Hearing Centers Network "PC/MacHear," and the Starkey "Pro-Hear").

As a pictorial-icon-driven system, a NOAH session can consist of seven application (or fewer, as desired) program modules. These consist of (right side of Figure 3–27):

1. The Client/Patient Module creates a patient record when the dispenser patient information is entered into the database in this module.
2. The Audiometric Test Module allows the dispenser to enter audiometric test data manually or to transfer it directly from an audiometer connected to the computer.
3. The Hearing Aid Selection Module allows the dispenser to choose and start up one of the manufacturer hearing aid selection modules for computer-assisted fitting of *conventional* hearing aids. These modules contain the proprietary software of those hearing aid manufacturers who are NOAH licensees and provide their product information, fitting recommendations, and fitting guidelines.
4. The Hearing Aid Fitting Programming Module allows the dispenser to utilize computer-based programming for fitting virtually all *programmable* hearing aids for NOAH licensed subscribers. It takes the proprietary fitting software from manufacturers, all using different technologies, and makes them available in a single software package. A cord supplied by the manufacturer couples the programmable hearing aid to the programming device (HI-PRO interface programmer), which in turn is coupled by cable to the computer.
5. The Real Ear Module allows the dispenser to transfer real-ear measurement data and use them in the hearing aid selection, fitting, or verification process. Real-ear equipment has been connected to the computer and linked to NOAH's software platform. This allows for accessing, storing, and retrieving insertion gain test data.

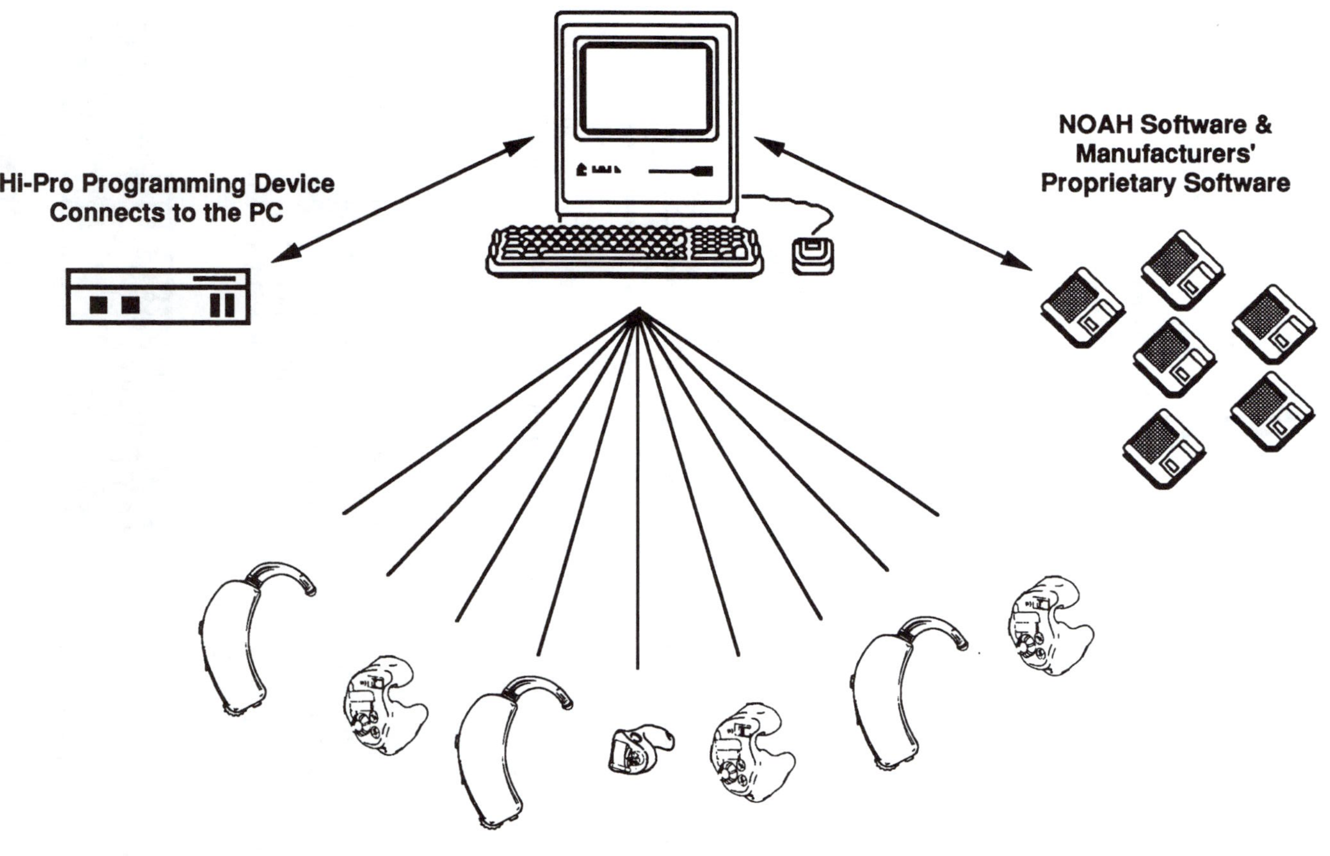

Figure 3–26. NOAH hearing care system overview.

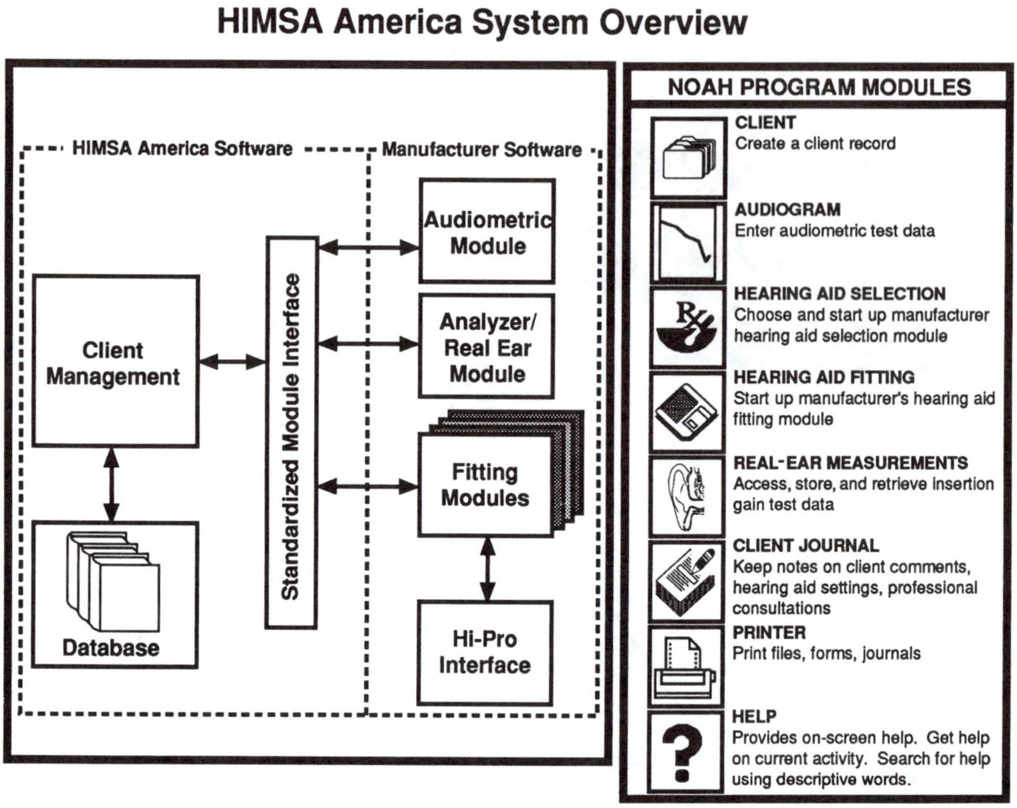

Figure 3–27. HIMSA America system overview. The left side shows the NOAH hearing care system overview and identifies HIMSA software as opposed to that required by the manufacturer. The right side shows the NOAH pictorial-icon-driven applications managed by the dispenser in his or her office.

6. The Journal Module allows the dispenser to add notes on fittings, hearing aid settings, troubleshooting activities, patient feedback, and professional consultations into a client journal.
7. The Printer Module allows the dispenser to print files, forms, or journals.

The NOAH system encourages patient interaction by providing graphs and data on a screen that help inform and educate patients about their hearing, hearing aids, and their hearing aid purchase options. NOAH can store and retrieve data within a given software module or transfer data from one software module to another automatically. It has application to a single office or can be used across multiple offices in different locations to create an extensive hearing care network. Additional hearing aid fitting systems, office management software, or the connection of test equipment can be added to at any time, provided that it is NOAH licensed.

NONCONVENTIONAL APPROACHES TO HEARING AID SELECTION

Acoustic Impedance Measures in Hearing Aid Fitting

This method has been suggested to select certain parameters of the hearing aid, especially for patients who are nonverbal or uncooperative (Horning, 1975; McCandless & Miller, 1972; McCandless, 1975; Rainville, 1976; Snow & McCandless, 1976; Tonisson, 1975).

Acoustic Reflex Thresholds (ART)

An attempt to relate acoustic reflex thresholds (ART) to loudness discomfort level (LDL) for nonverbal individuals determined these measures to be about equal at 95-100 dB SPL for both normal and cochlear losses when tested at specific frequencies (McCandless & Miller, 1972). When speech was used, however, LDLs were found to be about 5 to 10 dB higher than the ART for hearing losses greater than 75 to 80 dB HL. Their recommendation for cochlear losses up to 75 dB HL was to set the saturation output for hearing aids at about 100 dB SPL or at a level at which sounds first become uncomfortable. Snow and McCandless (1976) recommended that the saturation output of hearing aids be set to conversational speech or noise such that constant middle-ear muscle contraction would not occur. Horning (1975) and Rainville (1976) also documented the close relationship between LDL and the ART and recommended the application of these to hearing aid fitting. They recommended the use of average ARTs at 500, 1000, and 2000 Hz to specify the saturation output of hearing aids.

Other studies question the close relationship between the ART and LDL. Woodford and Holmes (1977) reported LDLs lower in intensity than the ART for the majority of children having severe to profound hearing losses. Other studies (Berger, 1976b; Denenberg & Altshuler, 1976; Rappaport & Tait, 1976) identified the ART as being much closer to the MCL than to the LDL. Keith (1976) reported the ART for speech to be related to MCL for speech and the pure-tone ART related to the LDL for speech. Preves and Orton (1978) found the ART to always be above the MCL and the LDL consistently higher than ART for pure tones and speech-spectrum noise. They concluded that for both types of stimuli, individual variability was considerable and that the ART is unreliable as an indicator of either MCL or UCL. The large variability was felt to be due to variations in stimulus type and presentation format.

Impedance Measures to Determine Real-Ear Gain

These have been used to measure the differences between the aided and unaided reflex thresholds (Tonisson, 1975). In a different application, McCandless (1975) used impedance measures to adjust the gain of hearing aids. With the hearing aid on the head and turned on, the reflex was measured in the opposite ear (speech input at 65 dB SPL). The hearing aid gain was set to just below the level of the acoustic reflex. Impedance measures to test for the most appropriate aided hearing aid frequency response have used the acoustic reflex in the unaided ear and then compared the acoustic reflex for different hearing aids (Snow & McCandless, 1976).

Synthetic Sentences

Reported by Jerger and Hayes (1976), this method uses synthetic sentences and speech competition in varying "message-to-competition ratios" (MCR). (An example of a synthetic sentence is "women view men with green paper should.")

The goals of the technique are to (a) determine the most suitable hearing aid arrangement, (b) define differences among hearing aids in real life listening conditions, (c) provide information on realistic expectations of aid use for patient counseling, and (d) make accountable rehabilitative recommendations to patients. Synthetic sentences are presented at 60 dB SPL at 0° incidence. The competing message is presented directly behind the patient, and its intensity is varied such that the message-to-competition ratio varies from +20 to –20 dB. Unaided, aided, and then again unaided scores are obtained. The patient's unaided and aided scores at each MCR are plotted graphically relative to the performance of normal listeners measured under the same conditions.

ABR

Use of auditory brainstem response (ABR), or brainstem auditory evoked response (BAER) use has been suggested as a technique to prescribe hearing aids, especially for obtaining information about performance in young children where behavioral techniques may be of limited value (Clarke-Cox & Metz, 1980; Mokotoff & Krebs, 1976). ABR is an attempt at the use of objective data to prescribe hearing aid performance characteristics.

ABR results are displayed as seven scalp-positive waves that occur within the first 10 ms following short acoustic clicks (primarily) and/or tone bursts from approximately 1000 to 5000 Hz (Figure 3–28). The seven waves resulting from the test are designated by Roman numerals. Wave V typically is considered the most stable to evaluate in ABR testing. To evaluate a hearing aid's performance, the ear(s) are fitted with the hearing aid(s), and ABR data are obtained in a sound field. An alternative is for the earphone to be suspended above the hearing aid microphone. The following methods have been used to select hearing aid amplification characteristics:

1. Wave V latency is noted in microseconds with the intensity level of the stimulus reduced in 10 dB steps. Preselected hearing aids are ranked, with the hearing aid giving the shortest latency as number one. Additionally, a hearing aid or setting that produces an ABR at the lowest intensity level could be ranked number one (Clarke-Cox & Metz, 1980). Evaluating several hearing aids having different response characteristics could provide information that would indicate which aid produced the "best" ABRs. Clark-Cox and Metz reported that the hearing aid resulting in the shortest Wave V latency also provided the best speech intelligibility score.
2. Hearing aid "benefit" was evaluated by adjusting the gain of a hearing aid until a recognizable wave form is evident. Benefit is identified by evaluating the difference

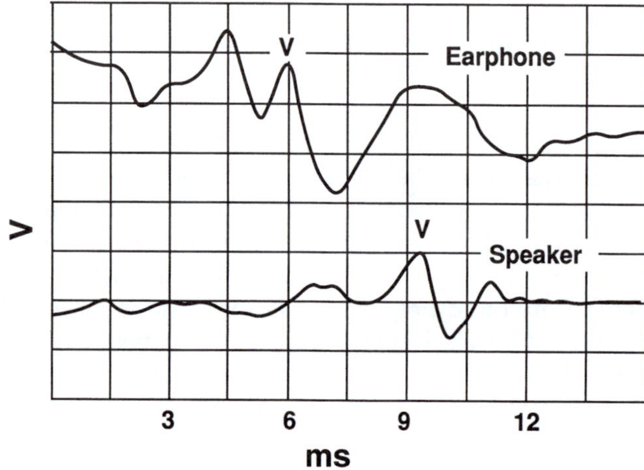

Figure 3–28. Typical auditory brainstem-evoked traces for clicks obtained from the same subject with earphones and free-field speaker at about the same intensity level for the clicks. The objective, scalp-positive waves that result from the presentation of these stimuli have been suggested for use with infants and young children to assist in the selection of hearing aids (Clarke-Cox and Metz, 1980).

between the unaided and aided ABR thresholds (Kileny, 1982; Mahoney, 1985).

3. Gain, output, and compression characteristics of a hearing aid were evaluated using ABR. These characteristics were adjusted until the aided ABR latencies closely approximated normal latency values (Hecox, 1983).

ABR results are suggested to be more accurate with some hearing loss configurations than with others. For example, Clarke-Cox and Metz (1980) found fairly clearcut results from precipitous losses but poorer results from sloping configurations. Concern had been expressed with the use of ABR because of procedural problems inherent with ABR. Seitz and Kisiel (1990) demonstrated that the abrupt click stimuli can produce ringing in the hearing aid. The use of longer duration tone bursts can create even greater artifacts (Kileny, 1982), and compression hearing aids may respond too slowly to be reflected in ABRs to click stimuli (Gorga et al., 1987).

Implications of ABR studies with respect to hearing aids suggest that it could be used with infants and young children for hearing aid selection, but serious questions remain about its effectiveness to provide an accurate picture of the hearing aid's performance. Weber (1994) acknowledged that ABR is in limited clinical use for hearing aid selection because of the procedural problems involved and concerns about the validity of the techniques.

HEARING AID VALIDATION

Determining the appropriateness and effectiveness of the hearing aid fitting continues as one of the most challenging projects of the hearing aid selection process. Verbal statements of success by the patient, while extremely important, fail to survive the "litmus test" required of third-party payers. As a result, a number of verification techniques have been advanced, and although none has emerged as the "standard," aided threshold measures or insertion gain testing appear to be extremely desirable, at least to assure that the prescriptive criteria have been met. Other measures that rely on patient self-assessment are covered elsewhere in this text.

Functional Gain and Insertion Gain

The essential difference between these two measurements, which produce essentially the same results (McCandless, 1982), is that functional gain is a psychoacoustic or behavioral measurement, whereas insertion gain is an electroacoustic term. Figure 3–29 illustrates the plotting of functional gain and insertion gain.

Functional (Use) Gain

This is the dB difference between unaided and aided thresholds. Functional gain is measured generally in a sound-field environment using warble tones at different frequencies, speech, or narrow bands of noise (Figure 3–30).

Insertion Gain

This is the dB difference between the sound pressure measured at or near the tympanic membrane, without and with the hearing aid in place. Insertion gain is used also to show the prescribed "target" gain for a particular hearing loss (Figure 3–30).

Functional and insertion gain are used in the hearing aid selection and evaluation process by identifying the prefitting calculations (targets) of the desired gain and then verifying the fitting by measuring how closely the target gains are approximated while wearing the hearing aids.

Measured functional gain or measured insertion gain is also referred to as real-ear gain (as differentiated from 2 cc coupler measurements).

Speech Audiometry

The Carhart procedure (1946) and subsequent modifications of it by others are notable examples of hearing aid verification

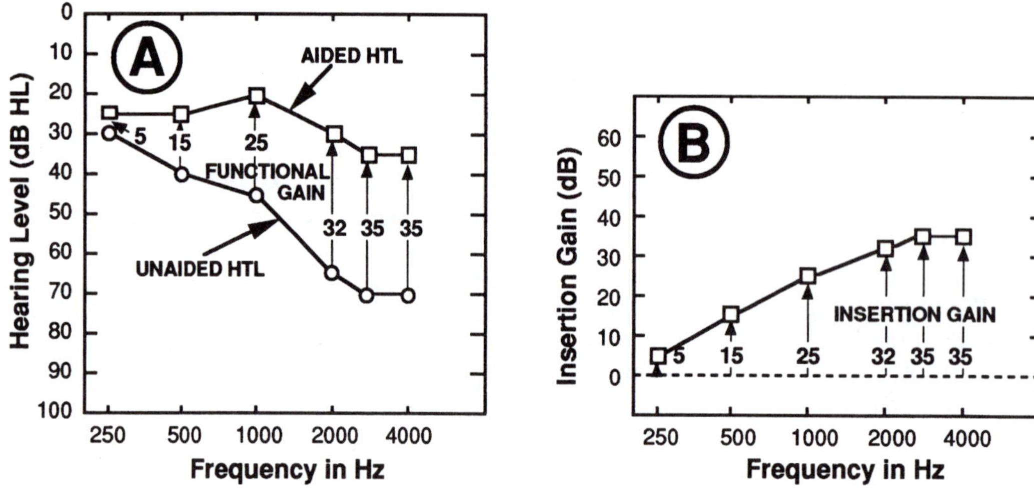

Figure 3–29. This figure shows the relationship between functional gain **(A)** and insertion gain **(B)** and how each is measured and plotted. (Adapted from "Overview and Rationale of Threshold-Based Hearing Aaid Selection Procedures," by G. McCandless, 1994, p. 7. In *Strategies for Selecting and Verifying Hearing Aid Fittings*, M. Valente, Ed. New York: Thieme Medical Publishers.)

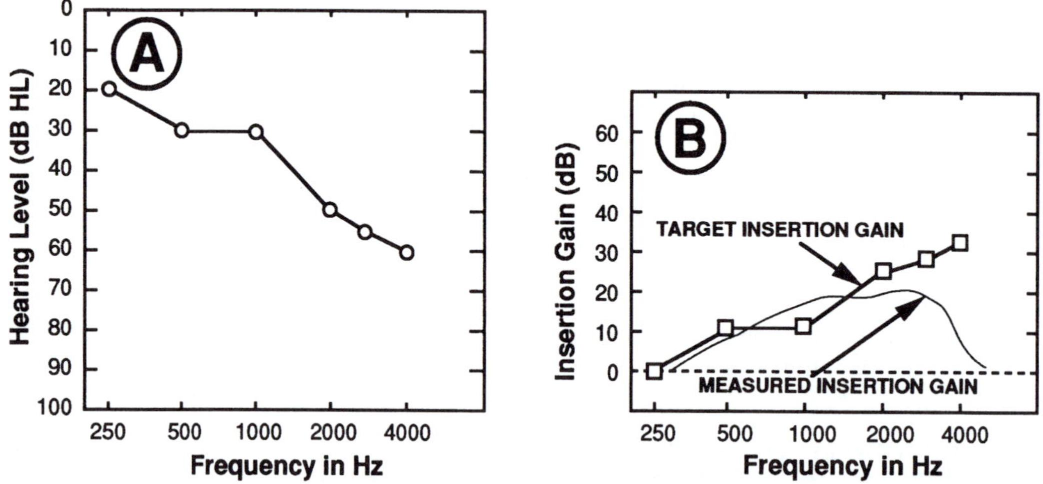

Figure 3–30. Audiogram (A) and target insertion gain calculated from the prescriptive formula POGO (B). The measured insertion gain (B) shows too much gain in the mid-frequencies and insufficient gain in the high frequencies. (Adapted from "Overview and Rationale of Threshold-Based Hearing Aid Selection Procedures," by G. McCandless, 1994, p. 7. In *Strategies for Selecting and Verifying Hearing Aid Fittings,* M. Valente, Ed. New York: Thieme Medical Publishers.)

procedures that have employed speech stimuli for verification (aided) measures. These procedures included mostly unaided-versus-aided (functional gain) measures of SRT and word-recognition scores. Word-recognition scores have been criticized widely since a report by Shore, Bilger, and Hirsch (1960) was published. Concerns evolved around the unreliability and the validity of speech stimuli. It was felt that with its wide array of uncontrollable variables, it was not a reliable predictor or evaluator of hearing aid performance. These concerns led, in large part, to the movement toward predictive procedures based on pure-tone thresholds and other stimuli.

Sound Field Pure Tones

One such procedure, advanced by Goldberg (1986), does not require language or the ability to recognize words. Instead, it plots results to steady-state sinusoidal signals presented in a calibrated, pure-tone sound field. The procedure is based on plotting three "most important" areas of hearing in SPL based on normal hearing equal loudness contours,

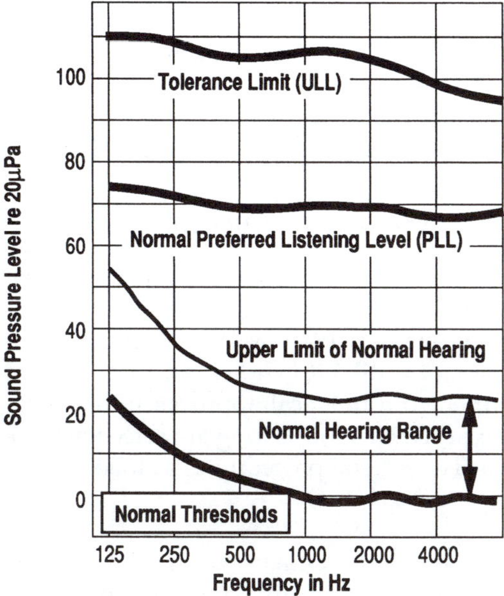

Figure 3–31. Detailed 90° sound-field audiometric chart showing the important features of normal hearing, including the normal range of threshold sensitivity, the preferred listening level for average normals (PLL), and the uncomfortable listening level (ULL). The range of normal hearing sensitivity is shown as 25 dB. (Adapted from "Psychoacoustic Aided Hearing Instruments," by H. Goldberg, 1986. *Hearing Instruments, 37*, 17, 19, 51.)

which serve as "targets" (Figure 3–31) at 250, 500, 1000, and 3000 Hz. These targets include:

1. Threshold of hearing: This target is derived from normal equal loudness contour curves for minimum audible field (MAF) and corrected for a 90° incidence presentation. The range of normal hearing sensitivity is plotted as being 25 dB.
2. Preferred listening level (PLL) for average normal ears: An acceptable aided PLL is considered to be within ±4 dB from the recommended 70 dB equal loudness contour curve (similar to that of otometry).
3. Uncomfortable listening level (UCLL): This target is derived from the 110 dB phon and corrected for a 90° incidence presentation. For the unaided and aided UCLL, speech noise is used because it should register the lowest unacceptable response and because it has great accuracy, ease of use, and repeatability.

The goal of the final aided hearing measurements is to meet or closely approximate these three basic frequency contour curves. Graphs illustrating the unaided and aided pure-tone sound-field audiogram are shown in Figure 3–32.

To overcome concerns about the possibility of standing waves resulting from the use of pure tones in a sound field, a concentrated sound field is used. The equipment uses a distance of 9 inches from the two loudspeaker projections to each ear. According to Goldberg, this allows for up to 2 inches of patient head movement when centered between the loudspeakers with a maximum error of 2 dB. Related testing in speech, room, and street noise is recommended as well, with the examiner having the ability to mix these with the sinusoidal tones to further determine the degree of difficulty in noise. For the unaided audiogram plotted on the lower curve of Figure 3–32, the upper target PLL is exceeded and would require reduction. These data can also be plotted in HTL, using correction factors based on work by Shaw (1974) and Killion (1978).

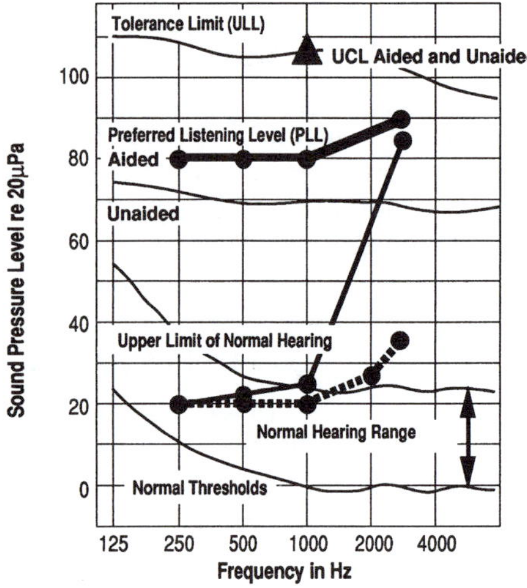

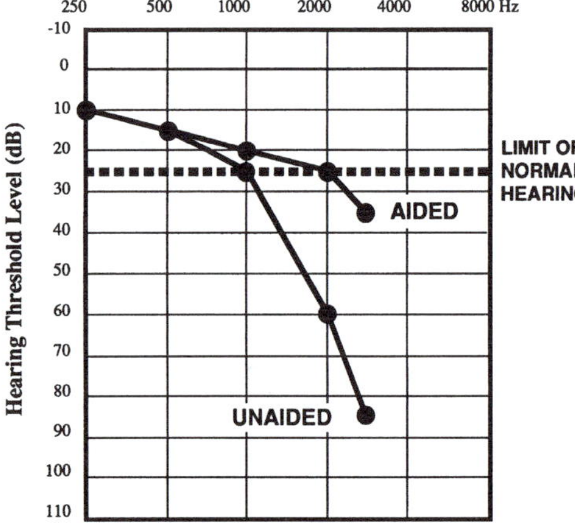

Figure 3–32. Goals of the final aided hearing aid measurements for Goldberg's (1986) sound-field pure tones. Unaided and aided pure-tone sound-field audiograms are displayed for the hearing loss shown in the lower graph. The final aided measurements, with the aid worne at the PLL, should closely approach the three basic curves at their designated intensity levels. An acceptable aided PLL is considered to be within ±4 dB from the recommended normal 70 dB equal loudness contour curve. This fitting shows that the aided response exceeds the acceptable variability and would require reduction.

Probe Microphone Measurements/Calculations

Systems that utilize probe microphones measure the amount by which a hearing aid changes the SPL in the external ear canal relative to the unaided condition. This "real-ear" approach allows the hearing aid and its associated coupling performance to be measured rapidly and objectively near the eardrum while hearing aids are actually worn (in situ). A voluntary response from the patient is not required. Essentially, probe-microphone measurements allow verification of fitting formulae, help in determining if the hearing aids meet the patient's acoustic needs, and provide an accurate display of what is occurring at the eardrum.

Probe microphone data can be used to help select, evaluate, and fit hearing aids. Although not a method of fitting hearing aids per se, these measurements allow for evaluating whether prescriptive gain targets have been achieved when hearing aids are worn. For the most part, they are used to measure the results of prescriptive fitting approaches, particularly if the prescriptive approach is based on frequency-specific gain. In general, the reliability of various probe microphone systems is relatively good, with some discrepancy at higher frequencies. For an excellent review of the use of the probe microphone with hearing aids, the reader is referred to Mueller, Hawkins, and Northern (1992).

Probe Microphone Concept

The use of probe microphones within the ear canal for measurement purposes was reported as early as 1946 by Wiener and Ross. It was not until 1981, however, that Harford presented a practical approach to use these measurements for hearing aid selection/benefit. The general procedure is as follows (Figure 3–33):

1. The natural resonance of the ear is measured near the eardrum using a probe microphone with the ear canal unoccluded (open).
2. The measurement is repeated with the probe microphone in the same position but now with hearing aid in position as worn.

Measurements and Calculations Made

Following preparation of both the equipment and the patient (calibration and appropriate

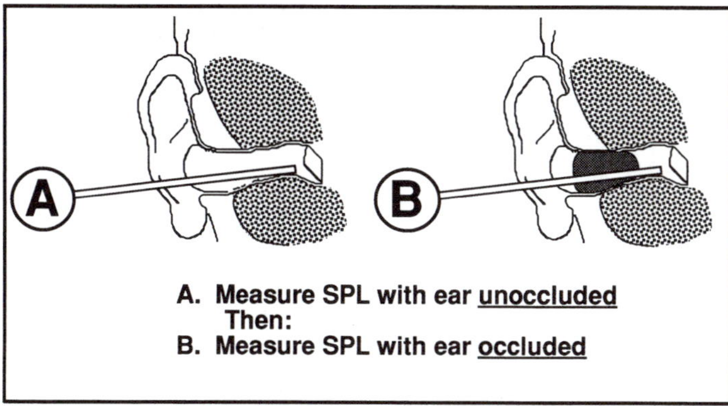

Figure 3–33. Real ear probe microphone measurement concept. In **A**, the natural resonance of the ear is measured near the tympanic membrane by a probe microphone with the canal unoccluded, and then **B**, the measurements of amplification from the hearing aid can be measured with the ear canal occluded in whatever fashion the hearing aid is worn.

positioning), a series of measurements are made to help validate the hearing aid fitting process targets.

Real Ear Unaided Response (REUR). This is generally the first measurement obtained and represents the *unaided* resonance characteristics of the open ear canal and the diffraction effects of the head, pinna, and concha (Figure 3–34). Collectively, these provide an "ear resonance." The average adult ear resonance (REUR) demonstrates a primary peak around 2700 Hz of about 17 dB and a secondary peak of about 12–14 dB in the 4000 to 5000 Hz region.

The REUR has been used in at least three ways for hearing aid validation and selection:

1. as a reference value to help calculate the hearing aid insertion gain (IG), which is used to validate prescriptive gain formulae targets);
2. when ordering custom-molded hearing aids to help determine the most appropriate 2 cc coupler response; and
3. to select a hearing aid real-ear frequency response that follows the same pattern as the REUR (this last approach is not consistent with selective amplifications prescriptive approaches and requires substantiation).

Real Ear Aided Response (REAR). This measurement normally follows the REUR and represents the *aided* ear measurement. It includes the total response of the hearing aid system, *including* the REUR and is identified also as the *in-situ response*, or the *in-situ gain*. The measurement is similar to those obtained using a 2 cc coupler, except that the patient's own ear is used as the "load" resistance rather than the 2 cc coupler.

REAR is used most commonly to calculate the *insertion gain* and in some equipment may not be displayed routinely, even though it is used in the calculation. A visual display of REAR is useful, however, to evaluate other aspects of hearing aid performance, such as directional microphone performance, trouble-shooting wearer complaints relating to feedback or unpleasant sound quality, or other types of signal processing applications.

Real Ear Occluded Response (REOR). This is the response of the ear with the hearing aid in place but not turned on. It provides an estimate of the *insertion loss* created by placing a

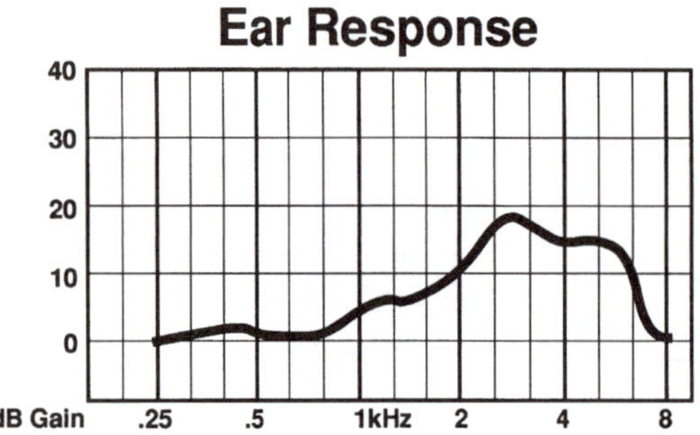

Figure 3–34. REUR (real ear unaided response). Ear response that represents primarily the resonance characteristics of the open ear canal but also the diffraction effects of the head, pinna, and concha.

hearing aid, its associated coupling, or both into the ear. Although this measurement is normally not obtained, REOR can provide an indication about the effectiveness of a vent or if feedback is being caused by the coupling.

The relationships between REUR, REAR, and REOR are illustrated in Figure 3–35.

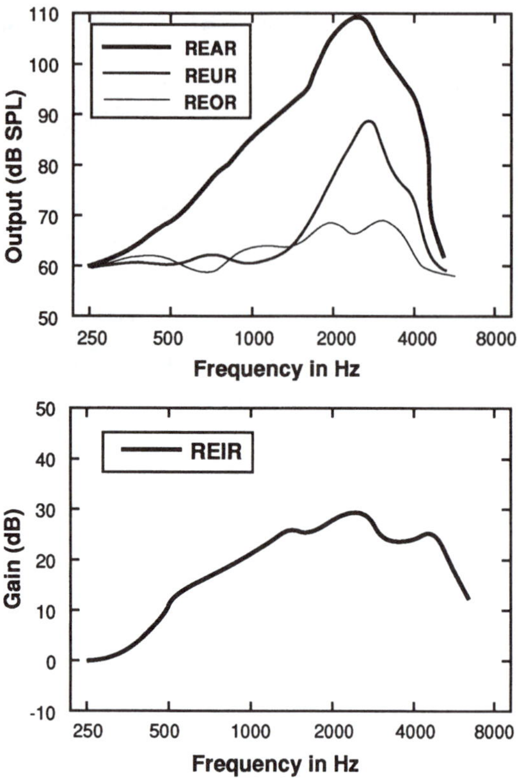

Figure 3–35. REUR, REAR, and REOR. Upper panel: Illustration of the real ear unoccluded response (REUR), the real ear occluded response (REOR), and the real ear aided response (REAR). The lower panel shows the resulting real ear insertion response (REIR) for the measurements shown in the left panel. (Adapted with permission from "Terminology and Procedures," by H. G. Mueller, 1992. In *Probe Microphone Measurements: Hearing Aid Selection and Assessment* (p. 12), H. G. Mueller, D. Hawkins, and J. Northern, Eds. San Diego, CA: Singular Publishing Group. Copyright 1992 by Singular Publishing Group.

Real Ear Insertion Response (REIR). This is a *calculation* and not actually a measurement. It is the REAR minus the REUR in dB (Figure 3–36). REIR represents the *functional gain* provided by the hearing aid and its associated coupling when worn. When the functional gain is identified at *a specific frequency*, it is referred to as the Real-Ear Insertion Gain (REIG), or Insertion Gain (IG) for short. The REUR must be subtracted because it represented the natural "gain" present prior to the hearing aid fitting.

REIR, as an electroacoustic calculation, approximates the behavioral measurement of functional gain (Dillon & Murray, 1987). Because of this feature, REIG can be used to replace functional gain targets in formulae (even in those formulae developed prior to the use of probe-microphone measurements). The importance of insertion response (gain across frequencies) is that it agrees much more closely with subjective measures of hearing aid performance than do traditional 2 cc coupler measurements.

REIR is used primarily to verify frequency-specific target gains suggested by the various formulae. Realistically, calculation of REIR without a target is meaningless. What makes REIR appealing is that almost all probe microphone test systems can calculate and display prescriptive target insertion gains if pure-tone thresholds are entered. The target gains and REIR are often used in patient

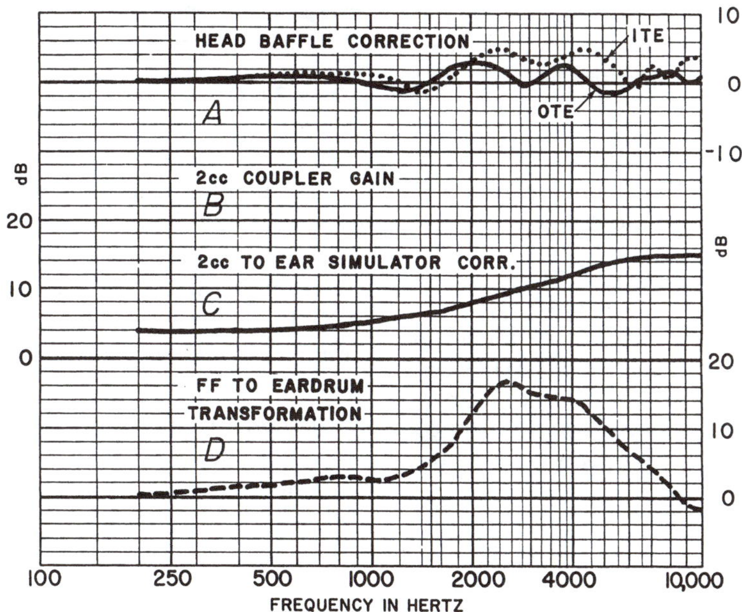

Figure 3–36. Transfer functions used to estimate insertion gain from 2 cc coupler data. (Lybarger, 1985).

counseling to visualize the success of the fitting. Care should be taken, however, because it is rare for target insertion gains to be achieved at all frequencies.

Real Ear Saturation Response (RESR). This is a measurement of the aided ear at saturation and is considered the real-ear counterpart to the saturation output measurements of the hearing aid obtained in a 2 cc coupler. This measurement seems to be especially important for the selection of hearing aid saturation outputs for those who are not able to give qualified subjective judgments of loudness discomfort levels (i.e., young children and/or nonresponsive patients).

Real Ear Coupler Difference (RECD). This is the dB difference between the output of a hearing aid measured in the real ear versus that measured in a 2 cc coupler at the same settings. This value combines the use of probe microphone measurements with a prescriptive formula to arrive at a desired 2 cc coupler gain as an *individual* personal correction factor (Punch et al., 1990). This is not the same as correcting the 2 cc coupler response to derive the desired real-ear response because it includes the REUR for a *particular* person and then corrects for differences in the frequency response in the 2 cc coupler versus that in the patient's ear. It allows for individualized target coupler gains to be specified as measured in 2 cc coupler. It would appear that such a calculation would allow prescriptive targets to be more closely approximated than are achieved currently by using average correction values.

Just Able to Follow Speech

Conversational speech is presented at 0° azimuth at a normal constant level (i.e., 65 dB SPL), along with some type of continuous competing noise from 180°. The noise is increased in 5 dB increments (2.5 might be better) until the patient can no longer follow the conversation from the front. The level of noise where this occurs is recorded. Various hearing aids, hearing aid settings, and coupling methods are presented, and the test is repeated with each alteration. The hearing aid combination of choice is often that which provides the highest noise level before speech can no longer be followed.

Insertion Gain Estimated From 2 cc Coupler Gain

Insertion gain frequency response on real ears or ear simulators (i.e., KEMAR) has been estimated from 2 cc coupler frequency response data (Burkhard, 1978; Frye, 1982; Killion & Monser, 1980; Longwell & Johnson, 1980; Lybarger, 1978; McCandless & Lyregaard, 1983). These correction factors allow approximation to any hearing aid measured according to ANSI S3. 22-1987.

Correction values can be practical if the following precautions are taken (Staab & Lybarger, 1994):

1. The correction value used must be for the type of hearing aid used and must account for the microphone pickup location.
2. The physical connection from the aid to the reference plane of the coupler or ear simulator must be identical acoustically with that of the aid when worn.
3. Corrections are applicable to closed coupler and occluded earmold conditions on a 2 cc coupler. Venting effect corrections are to be applied after the estimated insertion gain is determined.
4. All corrections are average. Large variations may exist.

In addition to the above, Lybarger (1985) has identified the different components required to estimate insertion gain from coupler data (Figure 3–36). These include:

1. Head baffle
2. 2 cc coupler response
3. 2 cc coupler-to-eardrum corrections
4. Free field-to-eardrum transformations

Estimated 2 cc coupler-to-insertion gain corrections for various types of hearing aids, by different investigators, are provided in Table 3–7.

SUMMARY

There is no doubt that each of the hearing aid selection procedures has met with some success. Hearing aid dispensers have to decide on the advantages and limitations of the system(s) they use. In the final analysis, matching a prescriptive target gain does not assure that a successful fitting has been achieved: More is involved than the electroacoustical end result, or even that speech has been made loud enough to hear. Effective patient management, necessary counseling, validation procedures, and the realization that a hearing aid fitting is an ongoing, not static, event are vital aspects of the hearing health care professional's responsibilities.

REFERENCES

American National Standards Specification of Hearing Aid Characteristics. (August, 1995). ANSI S3.22-1997, revision of ANSI S3.22-1987; 2nd draft, not approved by ANSI. New York: American National Standards Institute.

American National Standards method for the calculation of the articulation index. (1969). ANSI S3.5-1969. New York: American National Standards Institute.

Balbi, C. M. R. (1935). Adjusted sound amplification. U.S. Patent No. 2,003,875.

Beattie, R. C., & Boyd, R. L. (1986). Relationship between pure tone and speech loudness discomfort levels among hearing-impaired subjects. *Journal of Speech and Hearing Disorders, 51*, 120–124.

Beattie, R. C., Svihovec, D. A., Carmen, R. E., et al. (1980). Loudness discomfort level for speech: Comparison of two instructional sets for saturation sound pressure level selection. *Ear and Hearing*, 1, 197–205.

Bentler, R. (1993). Relationship of perceived quality dimensions to threshold of discomfort. (Abstract). *Audiology Today, 5*, 40–41.

Bentler, R., & Pavlovic, C. (1989). Comparison of discomfort levels obtained with pure tones and multitone complexes. *Journal of the Acoustical Society of America, 86*, 126–132.

Barenek, L. L. (1947). The design of speech communication systems. *Proceedings from the Institute Radio Engineers, 35*, 880–890.

Bergenstoff, H. (1990). Presbycusis and the articulation index. *Hearing Instruments, 41*(9), 18–19.

Table 3–7. Estimated 2 cc coupler to insertion gain corrections.[a]

Frequency	BTE[b] (CALC)	ITE-1[c] (CALC)	ITE-2[d] L&T ('86)	ITE-3[e] B&B ('87)	ITC[f] (CALC)
200	3.8	3.6	4.8	2.5	3.6
300	3.4	3.2	3.5	2.4	3.7
400	3.7	3.7	3.3	2.2	3.6
500	3.6	4.0	2.7	2.0	2.3
600	3.3	4.1	2.2	1.5	2.2
700	2.8	3.8	1.9	1.5	3.2
800	2.5	3.7	2.0	1.6	2.3
900	2.5	3.8	2.8	2.2	3.4
1000	2.7	4.2	2.8	1.6	5.1
1200	2.5	3.7	2.6	2.3	0.8
1400	1.4	1.1	3.2	2.7	-0.8
1600	2.2	0.7	3.4	2.0	-1.0
1800	1.5	0.4	1.8	0.8	-2.3
2000	-0.5	-0.6	1.5	-1.2	-2.4
2200	-2.8	-1.8	0.6	-2.7	-2.2
2400	-4.7	-2.4	-1.8	-4.6	-2.6
2600	-5.8	-2.4	-3.7	-5.7	-2.3
2800	-5.8	-2.1	-3.4	-5.6	-1.7
3000	-5.0	4.6	-1.2	-4.3	-1.8
3200	-3.5	-1.0	-0.9	-2.6	-2.4
3400	-1.7	-0.4	2.4	-1.0	-2.2
3600	-0.5	0.5	3.5	0.5	-1.0
3800	0.3	1.3	4.5	1.8	-0.3
4000	0.5	2.5	6.7	2.8	0.6
4500	0.3	5.2	10.0	5.1	5.1
5000	1.8	6.9	8.6	6.7	6.1
5500	4.0	7.7	10.2	10.3	7.8
6000	6.5	7.6	12.6	11.6	7.3
6500	9.6	8.5	15.3	14.8	8.9
7000	11.5	13.3	18.2	19.7	11.0
7500			16.7	17.2	
8000	15.1	14.1	15.2	16.8	
9000	15.7	19.5			
10000	17.4	20.6			

a Add values to 2 cc curves to obtain estimated insertion gain
b BTE = Calculated correction (Lybarger, 1985; Lybarger & Teder, 1986)
c ITE-1 = Calculated correction (Lybarger, 1985; Lybarger & Teder, 1986)
d ITE-2 = S3-48 Round Robin. One aid, six labs, on KEMAR (Lybarger & Teder, 1986)
e ITE-3 = Ten different ITEs on KEMAR (Burnett & Beck, 1987)
f ITC = Calculated (Lybarger, 1985; Lybarger & Teder, 1986)

Berger, K. W. (1976a). Prescription of hearing aids: A rationale. *Journal of American Auditory Society, 2,* 71–78.

Berger, K. W. (1976b). The use of uncomfortable loudness level in hearing aid fitting. *Maico Audiological Library Series, 15,* 2.

Berger, K. W. (1977). *Prescription of hearing aids: A rationale*. Columbus, OH: Kent State University.

Berger, K. W. (1992, October-November-December). Utilization of the articulation index for hearing aid selection. *Audecibel*, pp. 26–27.

Berger, K. W., & Millin, J. (1971). Hearing aids. In D. Rose (Ed.), *Audiological assessment* (pp. 471–517). Englewood Cliffs, NJ: Prentice-Hall.

Bragg, V. C. (1977). Toward a more objective hearing aid fitting procedure. *Hearing Instruments, 28*(9), 6–9.

Briskey, R. J., Greenbaum, W. H., & Sinclair, J. C. (1966). Frequency response index for audio systems. *Journal of the Audio Engineering Society, 14*, 368, 370.

Burkhard, M. D. (1978). Maniken measurements. Itasca, IL: Knowles Electronics.

Byrne, D., & Dillon, H. (1986). The National Acoustics Laboratories' (NAL) new procedure for selecting the gain and frequency response of a hearing aid. *Ear and Hearing, 7*, 257–265.

Byrne, D., & Tonisson, W. (1976). Selecting the gain of hearing aids for persons with sensorineural hearing impairments. *Scandinavian Audiology, 5*, 51–59.

Carhart, R. (1946). Selection of hearing aids. *Archives of Otolaryngology, 44*, 1–18.

Carhart, R., & Jerger, J. (1959). Preferred method for clinical determination of pure tone thresholds. *Journal of Speech and Hearing Disorders, 24*, 330–345.

Clarke-Cox, L., & Metz, D. A. (1980). ABER in the prescription of hearing aids, *Hearing Instruments, 31*, 12–15, 55.

Collard, J. (1930). Calculation of a telephone circuit from the circuit constants. *Electronic Communication, 8*, 141–163.

Cornelisse, L. E., Seewald, R. C., & Jamieson, D. G. (1994). Wide-dynamic-range compression hearing aids: The DSL [i/o] approach. *The Hearing Journal, 47*(10), 23–26.

Cox, R. M. (1981). Using LDLs to establish hearing aid limiting levels. *Hearing Instruments, 5*, 6–20.

Cox, R. M. (1983). Using WLCL measures to find frequency/gain and SSPL90. *Hearing Instruments, 7*, 17–21, 39.

Cox, R. M. (1985). A structured approach to hearing aid selection. *Ear and Hearing, 6*, 226–239.

Cox, R. M. (1988). The MSU hearing instrument prescription procedure. *Hearing Instruments, 39*, 6, 8, 10.

Cox, R. M., & Alexander, G. C. (1995). The abbreviated profile of hearing aid benefit (APHAB). *Ear and Hearing, 16*, 176–186.

Davis, H., Stevens, S. S, Nichols, R. H., Jr., Hudgins, C. V., Marquis, R. J., Peterson, G. E., & Ross, D. A. (1947). *Hearing aids, An experimental study of design objectives* Cambridge, MA: Harvard University Press.

Denenberg, L., & Altschuler, M. (1976). The clinical relationship between acoustic reflexes and loudness perception. *Journal of the American Audiological Society, 2*, 79–82.

Dillon, H., Chew, R., & Deans, M. (1984). Loudness discomfort level measurements and their implications for the design and fitting of hearing aids. *Australian Journal of Audiology, 6*, 73–79.

Dillon, H., & Murray, N. (1987). Accuracy of twelve methods of estimating the real ear gain of hearing aids. *Ear and Hearing, 8*, 2–11.

Dirks, D., & Kamm, C. (1976). Psychometric functions for loudness discomfort and most comfortable loudness level. *Journal of Speech and Hearing Disorders, 19*, 613–627.

de Vos, A. W. (1971). The possibilities and limitations of the fitting of hearing aids. *Scandinavian Audiology, 1*(Suppl. 1), 21–31.

Dunn, H. K., & White, S. D. (1940). Statistical measurements on conversational speech. *Journal of the Acoustical Society of America, 11*, 278–288.

Fabry, D. A., & Van Tasell, D. J. (1990). Evaluation of an articulation-index based model for predicting the effects of adaptive frequency response hearing aids. *Journal of Speech and Hearing Research, 33*, 676–689.

Feighin, J., Kopun, J., Stelmachowic, P., & Gorga, M. (1989). Probe-tube microphone measures of ear-canal sound pressure levels in infants and children. *Ear and Hearing, 10*, 254–258.

Filion, P. R., & Margolis, R. H. (1992). Comparison of clinical and real-life judgments of loudness discomfort. *Journal of the American Academy of Audiology, 3*, 193–199.

Fletcher, H. (1952). The perception of speech sounds by deafened persons. *Journal of the Acoustical Society of America, 24*, 490–497.

Fortune, T., Preves, D., & Woofruff, B. (1991). Saturation-induced distortion and its effects on aided LDL. *Hearing Instruments, 42*, 37–42.

Fowler, E. P., & Sabine, P. E. (1947). *American Medical Association Council on Physical Medicine.*

French, N. R., & Steinberg, J. C. (1947). Factors concerning the intelligibility of speech sounds. *Journal of the Acoustical Society of America, 19*, 90–119.

Frye, G. J. (1982). "In-situ" and "etymotic" hearing aid testing. *Hearing Instruments, 33*, 32–36.

Gitles, T. C., & Tillman Niquette, P. (1995, Nov/Dec). FIG6 in ten. *The Hearing Review, 28*, 30.

Goldberg, H. (1986). Psychoacoustic aided hearing measurements, *Hearing Instruments, 37*(6), 17, 19, 51.

Gorga, M. P., Beauchaine, K. A., & Reiland, J. K. (1987). Comparison of onset and steady-state responses of hearing aids: Implications for use of the auditory brainstem response in the selection of hearing aids. *Journal of Speech and Hearing Research, 30*, 130–136.

Harford, E. (1981). A new clinical technique for verification of hearing aid response. *Archives of Otolaryngology, 107*, 463.

Hartenstein, R. W. (1978). *Clinical use of otometry in hearing aid dispensing*. Munster, IN: The Hammond Clinic, Department of Otolaryngology.

Hawkins, D. B. (1980). The effect of signal type on the loudness discomfort level. *Ear and Hearing, 1*, 38–41.

Hawkins, D. B. (1984). Selection of a critical electroacoustic characteristic: SSPL90. *Hearing Instruments, 35*, 28–32.

Hawkins, D., Ball, T., Beasley, H., et al. (1992). A comparison of SSPL90 selection procedures. *Journal of the American Academy of Audiology, 3*, 46–50.

Hecox, K. (1983). Role of auditory brainstem response in the selection of hearing aids. *Ear and Hearing, 4*, 51–55.

Horning, J. (1975). Tympanometry and hearing aid selection. *Hearing Aid Journal, 28*(6), 8.

Humes, L. E. (1986). An evaluation of several rationales for selecting hearing aid gain. *Journal of Speech and Hearing Disorders, 51*, 272–281.

Humes, L. E. (1991). Understanding the speech-understanding problems of the hearing impaired. *Journal of the American Academy of Audiology, 2*, 59–69.

Humes, L. E., & Hackett, T. (1990). Comparison of frequency response and aided speech-recognition performance obtained for hearing aids selected by three different prescriptive methods. *Journal of the American Academy of Audiology, 1*, 101–108.

Humes, L. E., & Halling, D. C. (1994). Overview, rationale, and comparison of suprathreshold-based gain prescriptive methods. In M. Valente (Ed.), *Strategies for selecting and verifying hearing aid fittings* (pp. 19–37). New York: Thieme Medical Publishers.

IHAFF (Independent Hearing Aid Fitting Forum). (1994). A comprehensive hearing aid fitting protocol, progress report. New York, NY: Author.

Jerger, J., & Hayes, D. (1976). Hearing aid evaluation. *Archives of Otolaryngology, 102*, 214–225.

Kamm, C., Dirks, D. D., & Mickey, M. R. (1978). Effect of sensorineural hearing loss on loudness discomfort level and most comfortable loudness judgements. *Journal of Speech and Hearing Research, 21*, 688–691.

Kee, W. R. (1972, Winter). Use of pure tone measurement in hearing aid fittings. *Audecibel*, pp. 9–15.

Keith, R. (1976, November). *An acoustic reflex technique of establishing hearing aid settings*. Paper presented at the American Speech and Hearing Association Convention, Houston, TX.

Kileny, P. R. (1982). Auditory brainstem responses as indicators of hearing aid performance. *Annals of Otolaryngology, 91*, 61–64.

Killion, M. C. (1978). Revised estimate of minimum audible pressure: where is the missing 6 dB? *Journal of the Acoustical Society of America, 63*, 1501.

Killion, M. C., & Monser, E. L. (1980). CORFIG: Coupler response for flat insertion gain. In G. A. Studebaker & I. Hochberg (Eds.), *Acoustical factors affecting hearing aid response* (pp. 149–168). Baltimore: University Park Press.

Killion, M. C., Mueller, G., Pavlovic, C. V., & Humes, L. (1993). A is for audibility. *The Hearing Journal, 46*(4), 29.

Korabic, E. W. (1993). Easy as 1-2-3: Using an electronic spreadsheet to calculate AIs. *Hearing Instruments, 44*, 28–29.

Kryter, K. D. (1962a). Validation of the articulation index. *Journal of the Acoustical Society of America, 34*, 1968–1702.

Kryter, K. D. (1962b). Methods for the calculation and use of the articulation index. *Journal of the Acoustical Society of America, 34*, 1689–1697.

Libby, E. R. (1985). The LDL to SSPL90 conversion dilemma. *Hearing Instruments, 36*, 15–16, 68.

Libby, E. R. (1986). The 1/3-2/3 insertion gain hearing aid selection guide. *Hearing Instruments, 3*, 27–28.

Longwell, T. F., & Johnson, J. H. (1980). Estimating hearing aid insertion gain from coupler gain. *Hearing Instruments, 31*, 20–22, 30.

Lybarger, S. F. (1938). U. S. Patent No. 2, 112, 569.

Lybarger, S. F. (1944). U. S. Patent Application SN543-278.

Lybarger, S. F. (1955). An historical overview. In R. Sandlin, (Ed.), *Handbook of hearing aid amplification* (vol. 1, pp. 1–29). San Diego, CA: Singular Publishing Group.

Lybarger, S. F. (1957). Radioear basic fitting procedure (condensed form for clinical use). (Original written June 14, 1955, Revised July 10, 1957.) Cannonsburg, PA: Radioear Corporation.

Lybarger, S. F. (1963). Simplified fitting system for hearing aids. *Radioear Specifications and Fitting Information Manual*. Cannonsburg, PA: Radioear Corporation.

Lybarger, S. F. (1978). Selective amplification–a review and evaluation. *Journal of the American Audiology Society, 3*, 258–266.

Lybarger, S. F. (1985). Relationship between coupler measurements of hearing aids, as required by the Food and Drug Administration (FDA) labeling regulations and the performance of an aid under actual use conditions. American Auditory Society Carhart Memorial Lecture, Atlanta, GA. *Corti's Organ, 10*, No. 3.

McCandless, G. A. (1975, June). Special consideration in evaluating children and the aging for hearing aids. *Proceedings of the Lexington Hearing Aid Conference*. Lexington, NY: Lexington School for the Deaf.

McCandless, G. A. (1995). Hearing aid formulae and their application. In R. Sandlin (Ed.), *Handbook of hearing aid amplification* (Vol. 1, pp. 221–238). San Diego, CA: Singular Pulishing Group.

McCandless, G. A. (1982). In-the-ear canal acoustic measures. In G. A. Studebaker & F. H. Bess (Eds.), *The Vanderbilt Hearing-Aid Report* (pp. 170–173). Upper Darby, PA: Monographs in Contemporary Audiology.

McCandless, G. A., & Lyregaard, P. E. (1983). Prescription of gain/output (POGO) for hearing aids. *Hearing Instruments, 34*, 16–21.

McCandless, G. A., & Miller, D. L. (1972). Loudness discomfort and hearing aids. *Hearing Aid Journal, 25*(8), 7.

Mahoney, T. M. (1985). Auditory brainstem response hearing aid application. In J. T. Jacobson (Ed.), *The auditory brainstem response* (pp. 349–370). San Diego, CA: College-Hill Press.

Melen, L. A. (1978). Application of otometric principles in binaural hearing aid fittings. Project 76-12 of the Guthrie Foundation for Medical Research, Sayre, PA.

Mokotoff, B., & Krebs, D. F. (1976, November). *Brainstem auditory-evoked responses with amplification.* Paper presented at the 92nd meeting of the Acoustical Society of America, San Diego, CA.

Morgan, D.. E., & Dirks, D. D. (1974). Loudness discomfort level under earphone and in the free field: The effects of calibration methods. *Journal of the Acoustical Society of America, 56*, 172–178.

Mueller, H. G., & Bright, K. E. (1994). Selection and verification of maximum output. In M. Valente (Ed.), *Strategies for selecting and verifying hearing aid fitting* (pp. 38–63). New York: Thieme Medical Publishers.

Mueller, H. G., Hawkins, D. B., & Northern, J. L. (1992). *Probe microphone measurements: Hearing aid selection and assessment*. San Diego, CA: Singular Publishing Group.

Mueller, H. G., & Killion, M. (1990). An easy method for calculating the articulation index. *Hearing Journal, 43*, 14–17.

Pascoe, D. (1975). Frequency responses of hearing aid selection. *Hearing Instruments, 29*, 12–16, 36.

Pascoe, D. P. (1990). Clinical measurements of the auditory dynamic range and their relation to formulas for hearing aid gain. In *Presbyacousis and Other Age Related Aspects* (pp. 129–147), *14th Danavox Symposium*. Denmark: Jensen.

Pavlovic, C. V. (1987, August). Derivation of primary parameters and procedures for use in speech intelligibility predictions. *Journal of the Acoustical Society of America, 82*, 2.

Pavlovic, C. V. (1988). Articulation index predictions of speech intelligibility in hearing aid selection. *Asha, 30*, 63–65.

Pavlovic, C. V. (1989). Speech spectrum considerations and speech intelligibility predictions in hearing aid evaluations. *Journal of Speech and Hearing Disorders, 54*, 3–8.

Pavlovic, C. (1991). Speech recognition and five articulation indexes. *Hearing Instruments, 42*, 20–24.

Pluvinage, V. (1989). Clinical measurement of loudness growth. *Hearing Instruments, 39*, 3.

Pluvinage, V., & Benson, D. (1988). New dimensions in diagnostics and fitting. *Hearing Instruments, 39*(8), 28–30.

Preves, D. A. & Orton, J. F. (1978). Use of acoustic impedance measures in hearing aid fitting. *Hearing Instruments, 29*, 22–24, 34–35.

Punch, J., Chi, C., & Patterson, J. (1990). A recommended protocol for prescription use of target gain rules. *Hearing Instruments, 41*, 12–19.

Rainville, M. (1976). Impedance measurements in evaluation of hearing aid performance. *Hearing Instruments, 27*(11), 39.

Rappaport, B., & Tait, C. (1976). Acoustic reflex threshold measurement in hearing aid selection. *Archives of Otolaryngology, 102*, 129–132.

Rankovic, C. M. (1991). An application of the articulation index to hearing aid fitting. *Journal of Speech and Hearing Research, 34*, 391–402.

Reddell, R. C., & Calvert, D. R. (1966). Selecting a hearing aid by interpreting audiologic data. *Journal of Auditory Research, 6*, 445–452.

Resnick, D., & Becker, M. (1963). Hearing aid evaluation—a new approach. *Asha, 5*, 695–699.

Seewald, R. C. (1994). Fitting children with the DSL method. *The Hearing Journal, 47*(9), 10, 48–51.

Seewald, R. C. (1995). The desired sensation level (DSL) method for hearing aid fitting in infants and children. *Phonak Focus, News/Ideas/High Technology/Acoustics*, No. 20.

Seewald, R. C., Ross, M. (1988). Amplification for young hearing-impaired children. In M. Pollack, (Ed.), *Amplification for the hearing impaired* (3rd ed., pp. 213–267), Orlando, FL: Grune & Stratton.

Seewald, R. C., Ross, M., & Spiro, M. K. (1985). Selecting amplification characteristics for young hearing-impaired children. *Ear and Hearing, 6*, 48–53.

Seiler, J. A. (1971, March). A formula for fitting hearing aids. *The Hearing Dealer*, pp. 18–19, 30.

Seitz, M. R., & Kisiel, D. L. (1990). Hearing aid assessment and the auditory brainstem response. In R. Sandlin (Ed.), *Handbook of hearing aid amplification. Vol. II: Clinical considerations and fitting practices* (pp. 203–223). Boston: College-Hill Press.

Shapiro, I. (1975). Prediction of most comfortable loudness levels in hearing aid evaluation. *Journal of Speech and Hearing Disorders, 40*, 434–438.

Shapiro, I. (1976). Hearing aid fitting by prescription. *Audiology, 15*, 163–173.

Shaw, E. A. G. (1974). Transformation of sound pressure level from free field to the eardrum in a horizontal plane. *Journal of the Acoustical Society of America, 56*, 1848.

Shore, I., Bilger, R., & Hirsch, I. (1960). Hearing aid evaluation: Reliability of repeated measurements. *Journal of Speech and Hearing Research, 25*, 152–170.

Silman, S., Gelfand, S. A., & Silverman, C. A. (1984). Late-onset auditory deprivation: Effects of monaural versus binaural hearing aids. *Journal of the Acoustical Society of America, 76*, 1357–1362.

Skinner, M. W. (1988). *Hearing aid evaluation*. Englewood Cliffs, NJ: Prentice-Hall.

Skinner, M. W., Pascoe, D. P., Miller, J. D., & Popelka, G. R. (1982). Measurements to determine the optimal placement of speech energy within the listener's auditory area: A basis for selecting amplification characteristics. In G. A. Studebaker & F. H., Bess (Eds.), *The Vanderbilt Hearing-Aid Report* (pp. 161–169). Upper Darby, PA: Monographs in Contemporary Audiology.

Snow, T., & McCandless, G. (1976). The use of impedance measures in hearing aid selection. *Hearing Aid Journal, 29*, 3, 32.

Staab, W. J. (1968, May). *Monaural vs. binaural hearing aid recommendations*. North Dakota Hearing Aid Dealers, Bismark, ND.

Staab, W. J. (1996). Selecting amplification systems. In R. Sandlin (Ed.), *Hearing instrument science and fitting practices* (2nd ed., pp. 431–595). Livonia, MI: National Institute for Hearing Instruments Studies.

Staab, W. J. (1999). *Hearing aids: A user's guide* (pp. 30–31). Phoenix, AZ: Wayne J. Staab.

Staab, W. J., & Finlay, B. (1991). A fitting rationale for deep canal hearing instruments. *Hearing Instruments, 42*(6), 8–10, 50.

Staab, W. J., & Lybarger, S. F. (1994). Characteristics and use of hearing aids. In J. Katz (Ed.), *Handbook of clinical audiology* (4th ed., pp. 657–722). Baltimore: Williams & Wilkins.

Staab, W. J., Palashek, T., Nunley, J., Green, R., A., Dojan, R., Taylor, C., & Katz, R. (1998). Audible ultrasound for profound losses. *Hearing Review, 5*(2), 28–36.

Studebaker, G. A. (1991). Measures of intelligibility and quality. In G. Studebaker, F. Bess, & L. Beck (Eds.), *The Vanderbilt Hearing-Aid Report II* (pp. 185–195). Parkton, MD: York Press.

Studebaker, G. A., & Wark, D. J. (1980, November). *Factors affecting the intelligibility of hearing aid processed speech*. Paper presented at the Annual Convention of the American Speech-Language-Hearing Association, Detroit, MI.

Svärd, I. & Ahlner, B. H. (1994). The "benefit method" in the fitting of hearing aids. *Bulletin of the American Auditory Society, 19*, 10–11, 16.

Svärd, I. & Spens, K. E. (1992, August/September). *A new approach to hearing aid selection*. Paper presented at the XXI International Conference on Audiology, Morioka, Japan.

Tonisson, W. (1975). Measuring in-the-ear gain of hearing aids by the acoustic reflex method. *Journal of Speech and Hearing Research, 18*, 17–30.

United Kingdom Medical Research Council. (1947). *Medical Research Council Special Report No. 261. Hearing aids and audiometers*. London: His Majesty's Stationery Office.

Victoreen, J. A. (1963). *Hearing enhancement*. Springfield, IL: Charles C. Thomas.

Victoreen, J. A. (1973). *Basic principles of otometry*. Springfield, IL: Charles C. Thomas.

Wallenfels, H. G. (1967). *Hearing aids on prescription*. Springfield, IL: Charles C. Thomas.

Watson, N. A., & Knudsen, V. O. (1940). Selective amplifications in hearing aids. *Journal of the Acoustical Society of America, 11*, 406–419.

Weber, B. A. (1994). Auditory brainstem response: threshold estimation and auditory screening. In J. Katz, (Ed.), *Handbook of clinical audiology* (4th ed., pp. 375–386). Baltimore: Williams & Wilkins.

Weiner, F., & Ross, D. (1946). The pressure distribution in the auditory canal and progressive sound field. *Journal of the Acoustical Society of America, 18*, 401–408.

Woodford, C. M., & Holmes, D. W. (1977). Relationship between loudness discomfort level and acoustic reflex threshold in a clinical population. *Audiology and Hearing Education, 2*, 9–10, 12.

Zenith, S. E. A. (1975). *Guide to hearing instrument selection*. Chicago, IL: Zenith Hearing Instrument Corp.

CHAPTER 4

Earmold Acoustics and Technology

CHESTER Z. PIRZANSKI, B.Sc.

OUTLINE

The advent of the button-type receiver for hearing aids resulted in the invention and fabrication of the earmold. The first earmold, made over seventy years ago, was of a galvanized rubber and did not look and perform as modern earmolds do. After years of research, the options in earmold styles and materials were broadened greatly in the effort to enhance earmold comfort and acoustic seal, as well as cosmetic appearance. Successive advancements in electroacoustics resulted in the development of the damping system, horn tubes, and acoustically tuned earmolds. Constant progress also has been observed in the quality and variety of ear impression materials and procedures. The most recent addition of the digital signal processing technology made earmolds and behind-the-ear (BTE) hearing instruments an attractive option in providing a better quality of live for the hard of hearing people.

The physical fit of an earmold in the patient's ear is one of the most intriguing issues in hearing aid fittings. If a hearing instrument fitting is successfully completed, anything can be said to justify the success: years of experience, a new impression or earmold material, or the most recent development in earmold design. If the fitting fails, there are many questions but few good answers.

Field consultants commonly emphasize that there is not one impression-taking technique nor material that would guarantee a success in hearing instrument fittings. The daily practice seems to support this opinion; with most hearing instruments being successfully fitted, a number of earmolds always require a remake. This, however, does not mean that all existing options in impression taking and earmold manufacturing are equally good.

This chapter will guide the hearing health care professional through a variety of ear impression taking techniques, the selection of earmold style and material, and earmold acoustic options. Selected aspects of the manufacturing process also will be discussed. This review will begin with a look at the relationship between the human ear anatomy and the earmold fit in the ear.

THE HUMAN EAR AND THE EARMOLD

The Ear

The human external ear consists of the pinna, ear canal, and eardrum. The canal has two bends, with the eardrum located beyond the second bend. Anatomically, the section between the ear's first and second bend is made up of moderately sensitive cartilaginous tissue. This tissue is soft and forgiving and often lined with earwax produced by wax glands situated deeper in the canal. Fortunately for earmold fittings, the cartilaginous portion can be stretched by the earmold body and still remain within comfort limits. The ear canal cartilaginous tissue also is subject to shifting resulting from jaw movements. The jaw's downward movement commonly stretches the anterior (front) ear wall and increases the ear canal diameter.

Beyond the canal's second anatomical bend, the cartilage thins and eventually disappears, and the ear wall becomes more rigid. The underlying tissue of the ear canal bony section, which is quite thin, has no subcutaneous layer, is highly vascular, and is quite sensitive (Staab, 1994). An earmold that presses against the canal bony tissue creates enough pressure to make the mold difficult to tolerate. Although this tolerance to pressure varies among individuals, the feeling of discomfort is common.

The Earmold

An earmold is an individually fabricated ear insert that channels the sound reproduced by the hearing aid receiver to the eardrum. In most fittings and configurations, the earmold must:

- couple the hearing aid to the ear,
- retain the behind-the-ear hearing aid on the outer ear,
- provide satisfactory acoustic seal to prevent acoustic feedback,
- acoustically modify the gain, frequency response and output of the hearing aid,
- be comfortable to wear for an extended period of time, and
- be aesthetically acceptable to the client (Mynders, 1996).

To meet these requirements, the earmold must be crafted skillfully from an ear impression that properly reflects the anatomical structures of patient's ear. Figure 4–1 shows an earmold fitted in the human ear. Certain sections of the earmold body are designed to perform one or more functions. These functions include providing sufficient acoustic seal, adequate in-ear retention, necessary comfort, proper sound direction, and ease of insertion.

Acoustic Seal

In most earmolds, the acoustic seal occurs between the ear canal aperture and the canal second bend. The seal area does not need to be tight or long but does need to be comfortably snug and accurate. If the seal is inadequate, the hearing aid may produce external acoustic feedback. External feedback occurs when the amplified signal escapes from the ear canal, reaches the microphone, and causes the amplifier to oscillate. The earwax and moisture collected in the canal enhance the efficiency of the seal and help prevent feedback. For high-powered hearing instruments, which require a better seal, the snugger fit still must be achieved within the cartilage. If the

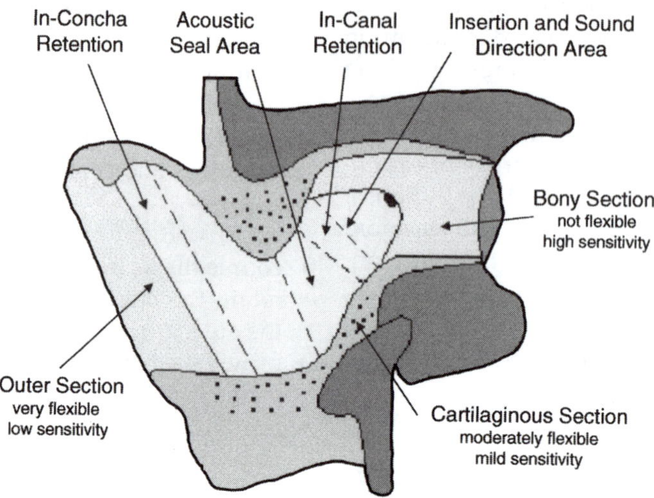

Figure 4–1. To fit securely, comfortably, and be feedback free the earmold must conform properly to the ear anatomical structures. (From *Otoplastics: Recommendations & Modifications* paper presented at the Canadian Association of Speech and Language Pathologists and Audiologists by C. Pirzanski. May 1997. Toronto, ON.)

seal area is extended into the bony portion of the canal, the earmold is often uncomfortable.

Earmold Retention

The efficiency of earmold retention depends on natural prominences present in the ear concha and canal. Retention for full concha earmolds occurs at the area of the helix, tragus, and antitragus. Retention for canal molds is found in the ear canal, commonly at the ear's second bend where the canal flares past the ear aperture. The bulge marked in Figure 4–1 is the most common retention area for canal molds. When the earmold is fitted, the bulge holds it securely in the canal. The size of the bulging area must be carefully balanced. If it is too large, the mold's insertion, removal, and comfort can be problematic. If excessively trimmed, the retention area can be ineffective.

Earmold Comfort

To be comfortable, an earmold should fit snugly in the canal cartilaginous tissue and make no contact with the bony portion of the ear. The snug fit is defined by several factors, including impression-taking technique and material, and in-lab impression trimming and coating. Comfort at the ear bony portion is achieved through in-lab impression trimming.

Earmold Sound Direction

The sound bore on the earmold should be directed towards the eardrum. This can be achieved easily in ears that have straight or moderately crooked canals. In ears that have sharp bends, the sound direction may be compromised to some extent with the earmold's insertion.

Earmold Insertion

Earmold insertion is defined in the manufacturing process through skillful trimming of the helix and canal portion of the impression. An earmold that cannot be easily inserted is most likely made from an inadequately trimmed ear impression.

EAR IMPRESSION MATERIALS

There are two types of impression materials currently in use for impression taking: silicone and ethyl methacrylate. Ethyl methacrylate also is known as acrylic material, traditional material, or liquid and powder material. Impression materials differ in their physical properties. From the dispenser's point of view, the material's after-mix viscosity, contraction ratio, and stress relaxation are the most critical variables in the process of producing a satisfactory impression. Other parameters to consider include the mixing ratio, setting time, type of cure (addition or condensation), after-cure hardness (shore value), and effectiveness of the release agent.

Viscosity

Viscosity of impression material is defined as a measure of the consistency of the material before polymerization. In technical terminology, viscous means having a thick or sticky consistency. Although the consistency of currently available impression materials significantly varies from one material to another, manufacturers generally do not provide a description of viscosity. Figure 4–2 provides research-established variances in viscosity of ear impression materials (Pirzanski, 1997a). Silicones being injected with impression guns have the lowest, type A, viscosity. Putty and putty, 1:1 mixture silicones formulated for deep canal impressions, are slightly more viscous with a type B viscosity. Other putty and putty silicones have a moderate, type C viscosity. The majority of putty with paste catalyst and putty with catalyst drops silicones are considered to be quite viscous, referred to as viscosity type D. However, some of these silicones may have a lighter consistency, typical for group C. Ethyl methacrylate (powder and liquid) material exhibits a type C viscosity.

Impression materials of type C and D viscosity are considered standard and have been used to take ear impressions for custom earmolds for decades; ethyl methacrylate from the 1940s and silicones from the 1960s.

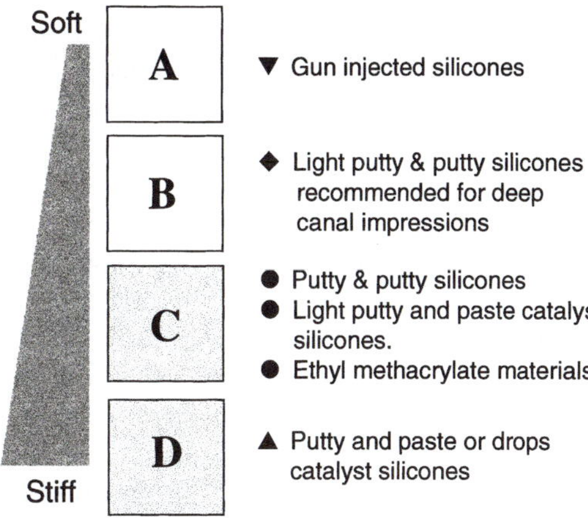

Figure 4–2. The after-mix viscosity of impression materials varies. Gun-injected silicones (viscosity type A) have a lighter consistency than syringed impression materials (B, C, and D). Standard viscosity impression materials (type C and D) appear to be the most suitable for any type of hearing instrument and hearing loss. (From "Anatomically accurate ear impressions" by C. Pirzanski, 1999, *Audecibel*, p. 11, Copyright 1999 by International Hearing Society. Reprinted with permission.)

Extra light and light impression materials, possessing viscosity type A and B, were developed in the early 1990s for the deeper impression required for peritympanic and completely-in-the-canal (CIC) instruments. The development of these materials resulted from research conducted by Termeer (1994), who claimed that discomfort in hearing aid fittings resulted from the ear tissue overstretching caused by impression material and recommended the use of extra light silicones to remedy this problem. In-field hearing aid fitting results and further research proved the idea false. Termeer (1999) is no longer supporting the use of light silicones, even for deep canal impressions. Instead, he recommends standard viscosity materials (possessing a type C viscosity in our classification scheme). Unfortunately, many manufacturers and industry consultants are still recommending light silicones. Because the cartridge gun system is very convenient, light materials are still being used to take impressions even for earmolds being made for high-powered hearing aids. If the patient's ear tissue is stiff, the fitting may go well, however, if the ear tissue is soft, the fitting may be problematic.

Figure 4–3 shows an ear impression taken with a light silicone inserted into a bisected investment cast as a negative of another impression taken from the same ear but with a standard viscosity material. The impression in the investment is obviously loose. This loose fit can lead to insecure earmold fit, feedback, unclear/intermittent sound conduction, and even discomfort. Note that the ear wall stretching occurs in the ear canal, between its first and second bend, which is cartilaginous tissue. Little stretching is evident beyond the second bend, which is the bony tissue. Interestingly, there is no evidence of stretching in the concha.

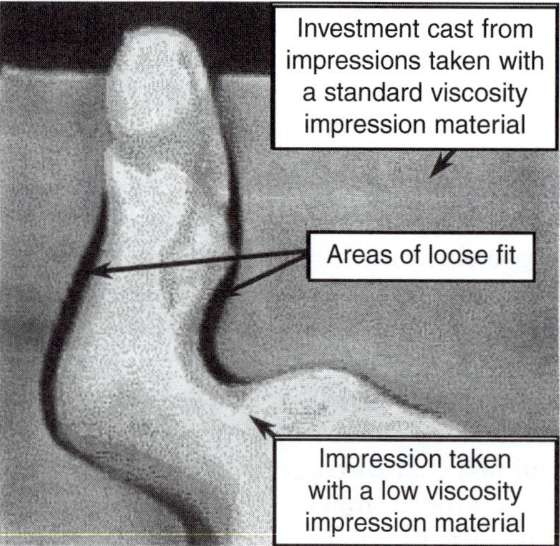

Figure 4–3. The magnitude of the ear canal tissue stretching depends on the viscosity of the impression material. The use of a low viscosity material may result in an earmold that is loose, uncomfortable, and feeds back. (From "Anatomically accurate ear impressions" by C. Pirzanski, 1999, *Audecibel*, p.10, Copyright 1999 by International Hearing Society. Reprinted with permission.)

When assessing impression material viscosity, do not rely on its color or brand name. Manufacturers of impression materials sell their product in a variety of shades to distributors. This means that a yellow silicone being sold under one brand name may be of much lighter or heavier viscosity than another yellow silicone being sold under another brand name.

Impression Dimensional Stability

The stability of a finished impression is defined by several parameters, such as tensile strength, stress relaxation, and contraction ratio.

Tensile Strength

Tensile strength relates to how much pull can be extorted on the final impression before it tears. Silicones have adequate elongation, but too much catalyst in some products can make the finished impression more vulnerable to tearing or breakage during the manufacturing process. Silicone material age and storage, as well as latex in rubber gloves, if worn while mixing the material, may affect its curing time. A silicone material that is contaminated or old may refuse to cure.

Stress Relaxation

Stress relaxation describes the viscoelastic nature of the cured material. A finished ear impression must not change shape as a result of its removal from the patient's ear, during shipping, or in-lab processing. Ethyl methacrylate impressions have inferior stress relaxation and are susceptible to heat. Excessive heat (e.g., a hot summer day) can cause the impression to melt down and distort. Due to limited stability, it is recommended to glue ethyl methacrylate impressions to the liner of the shipping box. If not secured, the impression may rest on its canal or helix against the shipping box and endure enough stress to permanently alter its shape. Some ethyl methacrylate impressions can distort even when properly secured. Figure 4–4 provides illustrations of left and right impressions sent in the same mailing box. Impression A has held it shape satisfactorily, impression B arrived to the lab severely distorted. The canal portion shifted and bent forward, and the canal aperture area sagged. If impression distortion is obvious, a new impression is requested by the earmold lab. However, slight impression distortion may be unnoticed.

Contraction Ratio

This parameter relates to the material shrinkage with time. Silicone impression materials typically shrink 0.1% to 0.7% in seven days. In ethyl methacrylate impressions, the magnitude of volume shrinkage is approximately 3% for the same period of time (Nolan and Combe, 1989). Shrinkage of 3% or below is acceptable in terms of the resulting earmold dimensional accuracy and quality of fit. Interestingly, Agnew (1986) established that, by adding more liquid (and changing the recommended mixing ratio), the volume shrinkage of ethyl methacrylate impressions exceeded 20%. The practice of adding an extra amount of liquid is incorrectly employed by some hearing health care professionals to retard the polymerization process, in order to make syringing easier or to minimize the stretching of the ear tissue.

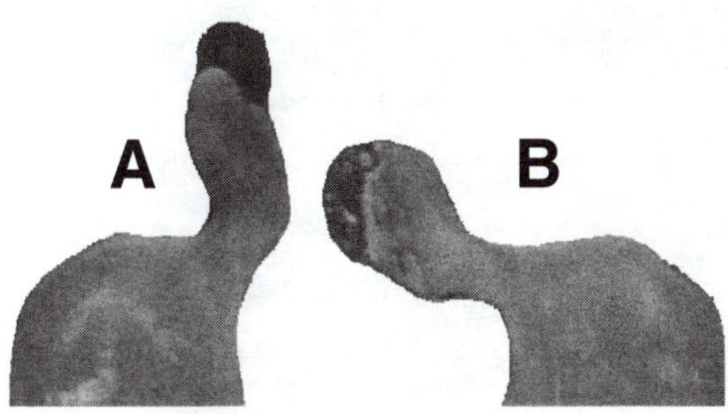

Figure 4–4. Shape distortion of ethyl methacrylate impressions can result in improper earmold fit. The left impression arrived to the lab in good condition, the other severely distorted. Long-canal, top-heavy impressions are most likely to disfigure. Impressions made from silicone materials will not distort.

Ethyl methacrylate is still the material of choice for many professionals. Even with some shrinkage and distortion occurring, properly mixed ethyl methacrylate material can examine better the potential of the ear tissues to stretch than silicones formulated for deep canal impressions. However, the use of a dimensionally stable, standard viscosity silicone is still the surest way to insure that the impression transfers to a satisfactory earmold. There are not, in the author's experience, impression materials that are too viscous (thick) to take ear impressions for the majority of patients.

Shore Value

The shore value refers to the material after-cure hardness. The lower the value, the softer the finished impression. There is no direct relationship between the impression softness and the ease of its extraction from the patient's ear, which relates more to the material release agent than to its actual softness. In addition, the shore value does not define the flow characteristics of the material before hardening, so it cannot be used to estimate the material after-mix consistency. For example, some silicones of 50 shore hardness have a much lighter after-mix viscosity than some silicones of 30 shore hardness. The shore value of ear impression materials is practically irrelevant to the hearing health care professional.

IMPRESSION TAKING TECHNIQUES

Impression-taking methods and techniques can be divided into four categories:

1. Methods of delivering the impression material into the ear,
2. Techniques for taking standard and deep canal impressions,
3. Techniques of impression-taking that require the use of two or more silicone materials, and
4. Techniques of affecting the impression shape through mandibular and head movements while the material sets in the ear.

Methods of Delivering Impression Material Into the Ear

In the hand-packing method, impression material is packed into the patient's ear by hand. In the syringe method, the material is dispensed from either an impression syringe or a cartridge impression gun. The gun can be electrically or manually operated.

Hand-packed Impression

Figure 4–5 shows several impressions. Impression A was hand-packed and impression B was syringed. To demonstrate clearly the differences between these two impressions, a bisected investment cast from the syringed impression B was used to photograph both impressions. The hand-packed impression is of inferior accuracy compared to the syringed impression. The fit of the hand-packed impression is satisfactory at the concha, but highly inaccurate in the canal area. The impression is generally loose, has a short canal, and fails to reflect the ear's second bend. The resulting earmold most likely would have a loose fit and would direct sound into the ear canal wall rather than into the actual canal.

Impression Syringe

There are several types and models of impression syringes. The most recommended are syringes that are easy to load, self-cleaning, offer a good grip, and require minimum pressure to operate. A properly designed syringe may require up to four times lower pressure to dispense the same impression material than that required for a bottom line product. Shown in Figure 4–6 are the universal syringe introduced by Microsonic and the double piston impression syringe developed

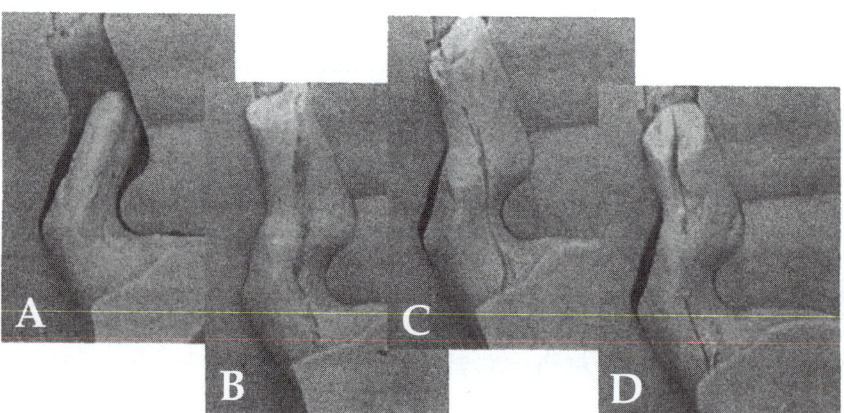

Figure 4–5. Impression-taking tools and technique affect ear impression accuracy. Impressions shown are: hand-packed (A), open jaw (B), closed jaw (C), and chewing (D). (From "Anatomically accurate ear impressions" by C. Pirzanski, 1999, *Audecibel*, p.9, Copyright 1999 by International Hearing Society. Reprinted with permission.)

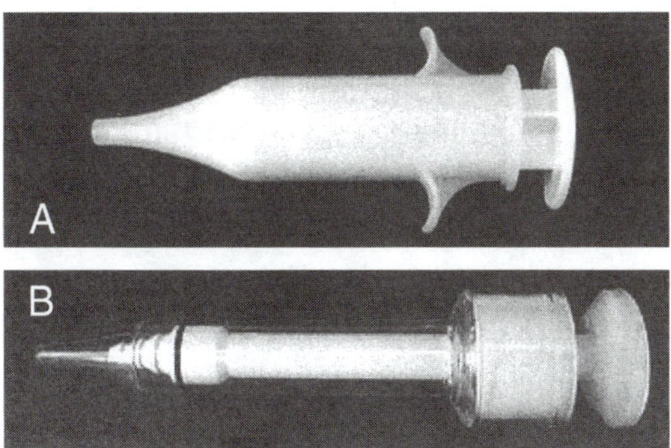

Figure 4–6. The universal impression syringe from Microsonic (A) and double piston impression syringe from Dreve (B) are premium products. (Photo courtesy of Microsonic and Dreve.)

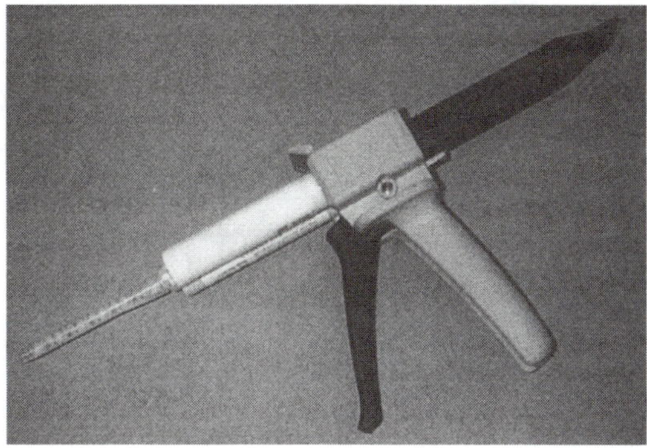

Figure 4–7. Cartridge ear impression material injector (gun). This type of injector can dispense only low viscosity (light) impression materials.

by Dreve. Both of these syringes are premium products, which require minimum pressure to operate.

Cartridge Impression Gun

Cartridge impression guns have been introduced as a tool to dispense very light silicone materials for deep canal impressions. Figure 4–7 provides an example of such an impression gun. Impression guns have gained significant popularity, because they are convenient to use, offer a mess free work environment, reduce material waste, and save time. Gun dispensed silicones polymerize within 2 to 3 minutes. Air bubbles and voids in impressions, which are common pitfalls, can be avoided by keeping the mixing tip at the margin of the mixture (as opposed to embedded in or leading in the syringe technique).

Techniques for Taking Standard and Deep Canal Impressions

Standard Canal Length Impression

An ear impression that reflects the ear canal structure 2 mm past the second canal bend is considered the standard and most satisfactory for earmold manufacturing.

All ear impressions should be taken with an oto-block inserted past the canal second bend. The use of the block helps to replicate the shape of the ear canal and, most importantly, the flexibility of the ear cartilage. When impression material is injected, the material flows up against the block, spreads, and stretches the cartilaginous canal tissue out toward the ear aperture. The canal opens up and its increased diameter is captured on the impression. This process is critical to build a comfortable and feedback-free earmold. With a shallow block position, the ear tissue stretching may be inadequate.

The magnitude of the cartilage stretching related to the oto-block position can be compared to two rulers having equal flexibility but different lengths. If the same force is used to bend the rulers, the longer ruler will flex more than the short one. A similar effect is observed in impression taking. Impression material of a given viscosity will stretch the ear tissue more with a deeply inserted oto-block, and less with a shallowly inserted block, as shown in Figure 4–8. An earmold made from a long canal impression (Figure 4–8A) trimmed to line X will have a better acoustic seal and comfort than when made from a short canal impression (Figure 4–8B).

An impression that reflects the ear in the more expanded state is more desirable for

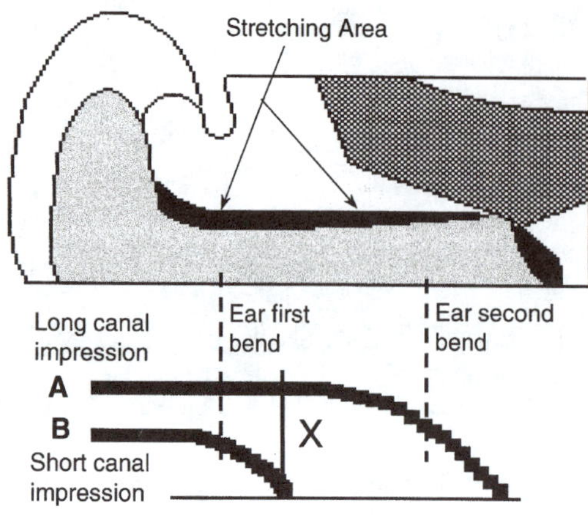

Figure 4–8. A deep insertion of the oto-block allows for more adequate ear tissue stretching than a shallow insertion. An earmold made from a long canal impression (A), trimmed to line X, will have a better acoustic seal and comfort than when made from a short canal impression (B). (From "Open wide" by A. Scott, 1998, *Advance*, p.15, Copyright 1998 by Merion Publications Inc. Reprinted with permission.)

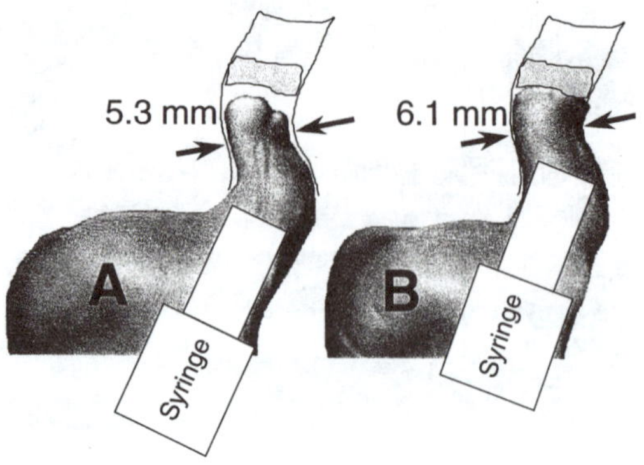

Figure 4–9. Impression material injected into the ear must flow against the oto-block, spread, and stretch the ear wall to prevent feedback in earmolds. The syringe for impression A was inserted shallowly in the ear canal. Impression B was properly taken. (From "Hearing Aids Selection," 1999, in press. Copyright by National Institute for Hearing Instrument Studies. Reprinted with permission.)

any type of earmold, including mild and moderate gain hearing instruments. Maye (1997) found that hearing instruments manufactured from long canal impressions had five to eight times fewer remakes due to feedback, loose fit, and even tight fit than instruments built from short canal impressions. For a dispenser who fits two new hearing aids every day, this translates into one remake every month or one remake every second day. The difference is considerable.

To take advantage of the proper oto-block position, the nozzle of the syringe or gun mixing tip has to be adequately inserted into the canal. When taking impression A in Figure 4–9 the syringe was shallowly inserted in the ear. Because the material did not come into contact with the oto-block, the ear tissue did not stretch, and the diameter on the impression at the seal area is smaller than on impression B, which was properly taken. The failure in taking a satisfactory ear impression is evidenced commonly by the oto-block dangling on the thread from the impression. On a properly taken impression, the block is firmly imbedded in the impression material.

The oto-block should not be removed from the finished impression before it is sent to the earmold lab. In many cases, the position of the block is helpful in assessing the actual ear canal direction past the ear second bend. Removing the oto-block may result in an incorrect sound bore position.

Deep Canal Impression

A deep canal impression is defined as an ear imprint that shows the ear canal structures at least 4 mm past the second ear bend. Figure 4–10 shows three ear impressions: a standard canal length (A), a deep canal impression (B), and an impression that shows the complete ear canal imprint (C), including the imprint of the eardrum.

Taking deep canal impressions is not common in earmolds. However, in cases of a severe occlusion effect, taking a deep canal impression may be necessary. Certification currently is required for taking such impressions.

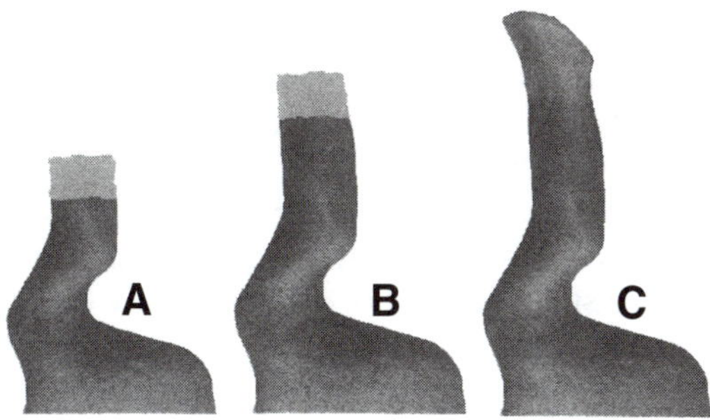

Figure 4–10. Impressions taken with varying canal lengths: **A.** Standard impression. **B.** Deep canal impression. **C.** Full canal length impression, with the imprint of the eardrum.

Prior to taking a deep canal impression, the dispenser should examine the ear canal carefully, paying special attention to the location of the canal second bend and the diameter of the canal after the bend. Depending on the findings, an oto-block of proper size should be selected. The employment of an oto-block is necessary to prevent contact between the injected material and the eardrum.

Inject the impression material carefully, constantly looking into the ear canal to see the material coming back out from the canal. Sealing the ear opening with the nozzle of the syringe or the gun's mixing tip, or using excessive force in injection, can lead to the material passing the oto-block and reaching the eardrum. If such a contact occurs, extraction of the impression from the ear can be painful to the patient. This is due to the vacuum effect that occurs when the finished impression is being pulled out from the ear. The pulling on the impression may painfully stretch the eardrum until the seal between the ear wall and impression breaks and air flows into the canal. The presence of the oto-block greatly minimizes the vacuum effect and facilitates impression extraction.

When the impression material has cured, ask the patient to open and close their mouth several times. Next, press gently the pinna away from the impression, turn the impression's helix portion forward, or lift the lower portion of the mold up. All of this will break the seal between the impression and ear wall. Bring the impression straight out from the ear while holding the thread. Re-examine the ear carefully for ear tissue soreness, slight bleeding or other potential problems.

Techniques That Require the Use of Two or More Impression Materials

The majority of ear impressions are taken by filling the patient's ear with one kind of impression material. Historically, however, other impression-taking techniques, such as the multilayer and multimedia techniques, have been developed.

Multilayer Technique

The development of this technique was driven by the need to produce earmolds with enhanced acoustic seal. A snug earmold fit typically is realized by applying a thicker coating on the impression prior to earmold manufacturing. Earmolds manufactured in such a way have a better seal but can be less comfortable. To remedy this problem, Fifield (1980) proposed taking the ear impression in several stages using impression materials possessing different viscosity, and testing the effectiveness of the seal.

Prior to impression taking, an oto-block with a vinyl tubing threaded through and glued to the block is inserted into the ear. This tubing is used at a later stage to test the seal of the impression. A heavy-bodied impression material is syringed first into the ear. When it has cured, the impression is removed from the ear and a thin coating of a medium viscosity silicone is applied to its surface. The impression then is returned in the ear before the material has begun to set. Gentle pressure is applied for a short time to the outside of the impression to assist the material to "flow." When the coating has set, the impression is removed and carefully returned to the ear. This procedure is important because it breaks the seal between the impression and ear. If it is not carried out, most impressions will stick to the ear firmly enough to demonstrate an effective air-tight seal. Next, an air pump and manometer (part of an acoustic impedance meter, or tympanometer) are attached to the tubing protruding from the impression. The pressure is increased slowly to a maximum of +200 daPa. The patient is encouraged to open and close his or her jaw, to ensure that leakage does not occur during these movements. If the pressure decreases during the test, the impression requires a build-up with another layer of the soft silicone. It is quite possible to repeat the build-up procedure a number of times, until a satisfactory seal is achieved. Figure 4–11 illustrates an impression taken with the multilayer technique. Note the tube coming out from the impression. Taking one multilayer impression may take about one hour for a professional already experienced in this procedure.

Time pressure and the fact that air-tight-seal earmolds are not required in most hearing aid fittings (Macrae, 1990) caused this technique not to gain any significant popularity.

Multimedia Technique

The multimedia technique was introduced to North America by Staab and Martin (1995). The method was developed to improve both the comfort and acoustic seal in earmolds and custom hearing aid fittings. The technique requires the use of two silicones of an addition type of cure (as opposed to condensation cure) so they can merge appropriately. First, a small amount of a low viscosity (light) silicone is dispensed deeply into the ear to fill the space around the canal's second bend. Next, standard viscosity silicone is syringed in to the remaining space of the canal and concha. The light silicone is employed to ensure the comfort at the bony portion, whereas the standard silicone is used to enhance the seal in the cartilaginous tissue.

In-field earmold fitting results did not confirm the superiority of the multimedia technique over other techniques. In fact, it was established that multimedia impressions could be of inferior quality compared to one-part impressions. A one-part impression and a multimedia impression are shown in Figure 4–12. The one-part impression was taken with a light silicone (viscosity type A). The same light silicone was used to fill the medial end of the subject's ear canal for the multimedia impression. The impression was completed with a standard viscosity silicone (viscosity type C). As marked, it is the one-part impression, not the multimedia impression,

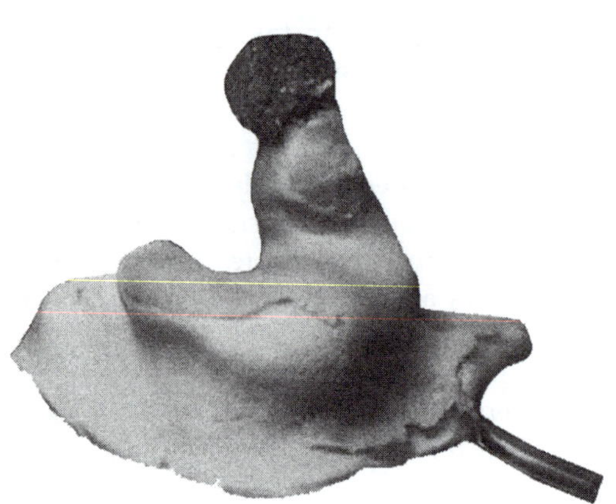

Figure 4–11. Multilayer ear impression. Note the air pressure test tube protruding from the impression the antitragus area.

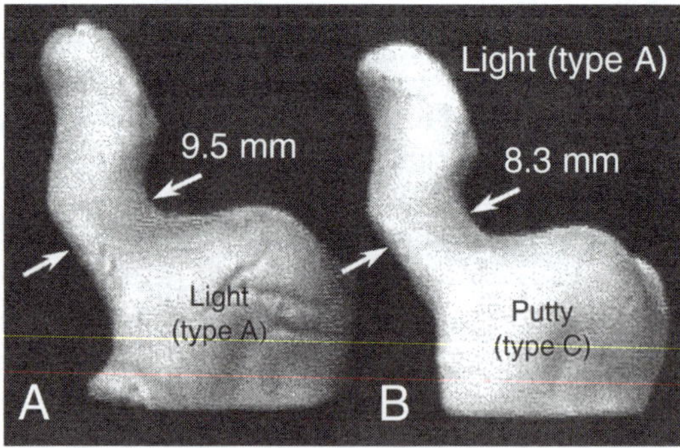

Figure 4–12. The one-part impression (A) is 1.2 mm wider at the acoustic seal area than the multimedia impression (B). (From "Hearing Aids Selection," by 1999, in press. Copyright by National Institute for Hearing Instrument studies. Reprinted with permission.)

that has the diameter of the canal at the seal area larger. The explanation of this phenomenon is simple. In both cases, the injection of the light silicone stretched the soft canal tissue somewhat. The tissue then began to relax. For the one-part impression, however, the filling in the concha resisted such relaxation. The light silicone is fast curing, therefore, it set before the tissue relaxed. This did not occur for the multimedia impression. Before the standard viscosity material was ready for injection, the canal tissue had relaxed, pushing some of the light silicone toward the concha, where it set.

Techniques of Affecting Impression Shape Through Mandibular and Head Movements

In many instances, the patient's jaw and head movements can modify the impression size and shape, if such movements occur while the material is setting in the ear. Variances in impression dimensions can be incurred through encouraging the patient to:

1. stay still or be naturally relaxed,
2. move his/her jaw from side to side, and up and down, or vigorously chew, or
3. gently bite on a mouth prop inserted at the corner of the jaw.

The first technique is called the closed-jaw technique, the last is the open-jaw technique (Pirzanski, 1996).

Impressions B, C and D in Figure 4–5 were taken with various jaw positions from the same subject's ear. Impression B was taken with the jaw wide open, impression C with the jaw closed, and impression D while the subject chewed. A gap at the anterior (front) ear wall between the investment and the closed, as well as chewing, impression is apparent. Such a gap is quite typical and usually extends from the first to second ear bend. Anatomically, it is the articulation area where the jaw movements stretch the ear tissue. The open-jaw impression has the canal 1mm wider than that obtained in the chewing impression.

Earmolds made from chewing impressions may feed back even before the patient opens his or her mouth. As illustrated, the chewing impression (D) has the diameter of the canal at the seal area smaller than the closed-jaw impression (C), which means that a "chewing" earmold will leak acoustically even with the patient's jaw closed.

Earmolds made from the closed-jaw impression may lack proper acoustic seal and retention when the jaw opens. If the mold is pushed back frequently into the ear by the patient in an attempt to achieve a more secure fit and/or to stop feedback, it will irritate the ear and commonly, but incorrectly, be reported as tight.

The jaw's downward movement can cause the instrument's sound to cut off. It is believed that this results from the earmold displacement and the receiver bore facing the ear wall. Although this may happen in some fittings, the cutting off effect commonly has another reason. With the ear canal widening, resulting from mandibular movement, the volume of air inside the canal increases, so that the receiver must move a larger volume of air than previously required. Because the level of hearing aid amplification has not changed, the sound pressure in the ear canal is considerably lower and the instrument's loudness is reduced (Pirzanski, 1997). If the reduction is greater than 5 dB, the patient will complain that jaw movements make the sound cut off.

Oliviera (1997) established that the effects of jaw movements on the ear canal wall were present in most subjects, and were commonly asymmetrical and non-linear, as per Figure 4–13. This explains why, in binaural fittings, the fitting of an earmold on one side can be more challenging than fitting the other side.

Mouth Prop

To take an open-jaw impression, the hearing health care professional should insert a mouth prop at the corner of the patient's

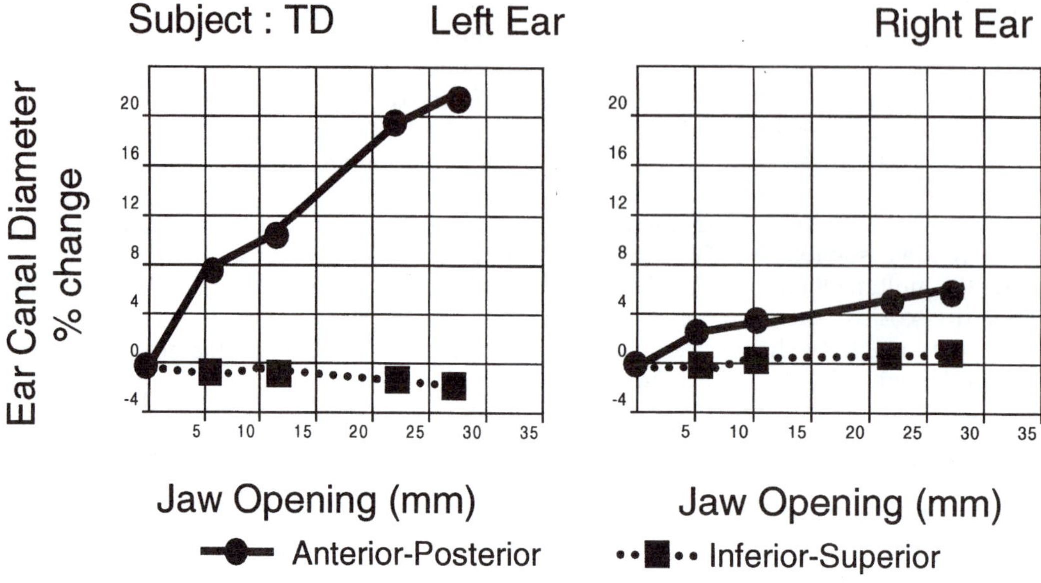

Figure 4–13. Mandibular movements are asymmetrical and non-linear, and they commonly widen one ear canal more than the other. (From *"The Human ear Canal"* by B. Ballachanda, 1995, p. 88. San Diego, CA: Singular Publishing Group, Inc. Copyright 1995 by Singular Publishing Group Inc. Adapted with permission.)

mouth, on the side that the impression will be made (see Figure 4–14). The prop must be inserted prior to injecting the impression material. Its use is recommended to prevent accidental mouth closing. Pirzanski (1998b) observed that the placement of a prop at the side of the mouth subsequently prevented acoustic feedback with chewing. Chewing on food widens the ear canal in the inferior direction and leads to feedback. The presence of the prop forces the condile of the jaw downward and stretches the ear tissue. The canal on an ear impression taken with a mouth prop may be up to 1.5 mm wider in the superior-inferior direction than on a closed-jaw impression taken from the same ear (Kieper and Berger, 1999).

Another option is to insert the mouth prop between the front teeth. This position allows for taking two ear impressions at the same time, which is not possible with the prop's side position. However, this frontal prop's position may lead to acoustic feedback when the patient is chewing food and is not recommended particularly for earmold remakes and for earmolds made for high-powered hearing aids.

Earmold labs have taken polarized positions on the use of the mouth prop. With a growing number of manufacturers that strongly support taking open-jaw impressions, there are still labs that are against it. This polarization results from different approaches to in-lab ear impression processing. The open-jaw technique is the most advanced technique and, as such, requires advanced impression trimming, particularly the impression's canal portion. An earmold made from an open-jaw impression commonly is wider at the ear canal cartilaginous area. When the patient closes his or her mouth, this creates pressure at the ear anterior wall and the earmold is shifted slightly into a posterior position. The ear cartilage between the ear canal first and second bend is forgiving enough to accommodate this shifting and the increased pressure against the canal walls. On the other hand, the ear tissue at and past the canal second bend is more sensitive and firm. This tissue will not toler-

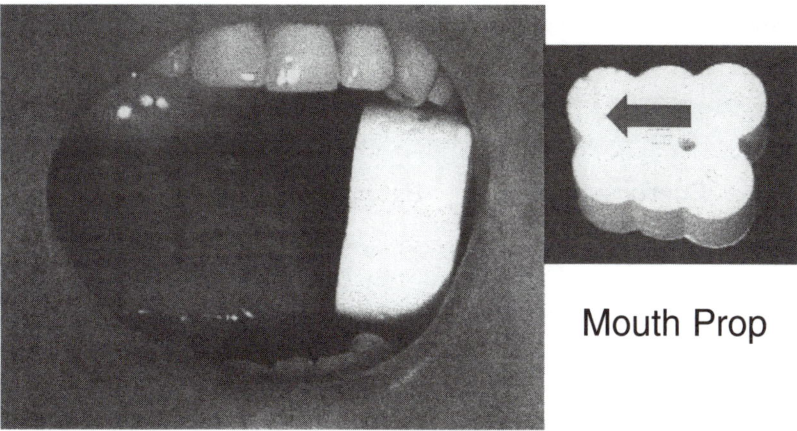

Figure 4–14. Prior to taking an open-jaw impression, insert a prop at the corner of the patient's mouth. The narrow part of the prop goes in first. (From "Techniques for successful CIC fittings" by R. Martin and C. Pirzanski, 1998, *The Hearing Journal*, p. 72 Copyright 1998 by Lippincott Williams & Wilkins. Reprinted with permission.)

ate pressure from the shifted earmold and discomfort often results. To prevent this, the ear impression must be trimmed skillfully by the earmold lab technician.

There are many advantages to taking open-jaw impressions. Earmolds made from such impressions have a better definition of fitting in the ear, more secure fit, less feedback, and commonly are reported to be more comfortable. Fishbein (1998) claimed that he succeeded with the most challenging hearing instrument fittings if an open-jaw impression was taken. Kieper and Berger (1999) determined better attenuation in earmolds made from open-jaw impressions. Jean (1999) reported that in her clinical experience open-jaw impressions effectively reduced the occurrence of the occlusion effect and feedback with hearing aids. Chasin, Pirzanski, Hayes and Mueller (1997) found that custom hearing aids manufactured from open-jaw impressions attenuated noise more effectively and performed better in noisy environments.

Ear Impression Evaluation

An ear impression, before being sent to the earmold lab, must be critically evaluated. The canal portion on the impression should be long enough to reflect the ear canal two bends in full. In addition, the impression should be free from underfilled areas. The size of the concha and canal portion should be considered while selecting the style and acoustic options of the earmold. Figure 4–15 shows an ear impression in satisfactory condition and how it relates to the anatomy of the ear and the earmold fitting. Note the parallel structure of the ear canal.

EARMOLD ACOUSTICS

The acoustic effects of earmolds are an essential part of earmold design and hearing aid fitting practices.

Insertion Loss

In an open ear canal, due to the shape of the external ear, the incoming acoustic signal will resonate around 2.7 kHz. This resonance boosts the mid-frequency range of about 10 to 15 dB, as shown in Figure 4–16. Because this natural sound amplification is present in our ears since birth, we normally are not aware of this phenomenon.

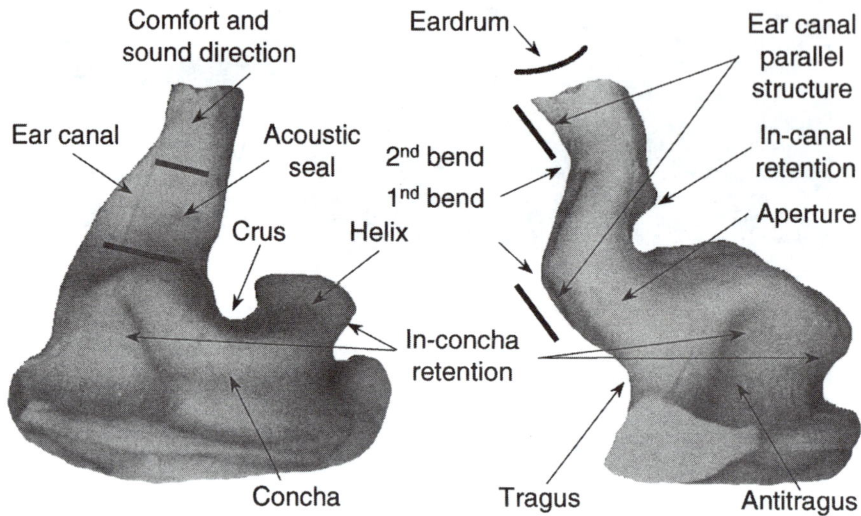

Figure 4–15. An ear impression is an anatomically correct reproduction of the patient's ear. Right ear impression shown. Note the parallel structure of the ear canal. (From "The anatomy of a perfect ear impression" by C. Pirzanski, 1998, *The Hearing Review, 51*(12), p. 22 Copyright 1998 by Fladmark Publishing Company. Reprinted with permission.)

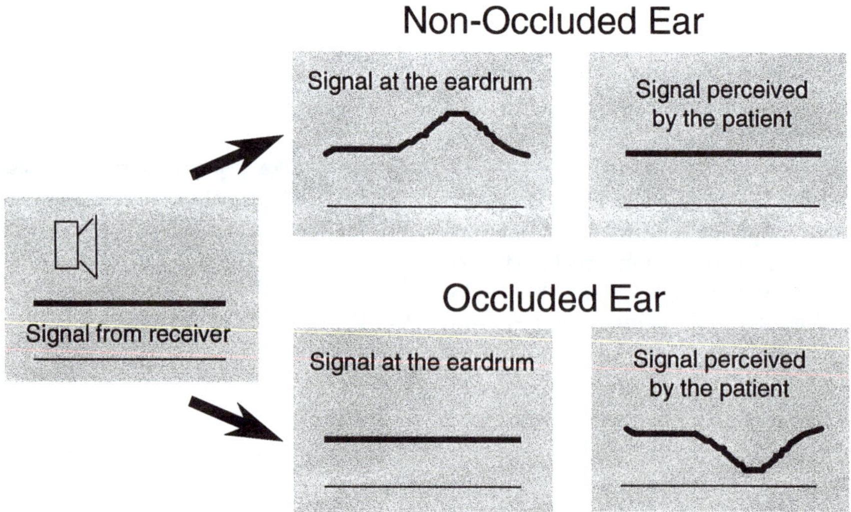

Figure 4–16. Insertion loss results from the insertion of an earmold into the patient's ear.

When an earmold is inserted in the ear, this resonance will not occur. Therefore, the acoustic signal arriving through the earmold at the eardrum will be deprived of the mid-frequency boost. This is called the insertion loss. As a result of the insertion loss, the individual will lack the information that the boosted signal would normally carry. Insertion loss can be compensated to some extent through the hearing aid response design and the earmold design.

Sound Transmission Line

The sound transmission line for a BTE hearing instrument, see Figure 4–17, includes the receiver tubing, earhook, earmold tube and, in some fittings, the medial end of the earmold canal. The receiver tubing encased in the BTE is about 5 to 8 mm long and has an internal diameter (ID) of 1 mm wide. The sound bore of the earhook is typically 20 to 30 mm long and 1.2 to 1.8 mm wide. The earmold tubing is usually 40 to 45 mm long and 1.93 mm wide. The entire transmission line is approximately 75 mm long.

Earmold tubes act like organ pipes when driven by a receiver and resonate at their preferred frequencies. In hearing aid fittings, the transmission line is closed at the receiver and opened in the ear canal. The acoustic impedance of the ear canal and the eardrum is relatively low compared to the impedance of the earmold tube. This impedance mismatch will create a ¼ wave resonance in the earmold tube with additional resonances at odd-number intervals of the fundamental frequency. These resonances can be observed in the hearing aid response as three resonant peaks at approximately 1100, 3300, and 5500 Hz (Walker, 1979). These peaks are undesirable because they degrade sound quality, introduce transients, and allow the output to exceed the listener's loudness discomfort level.

Acoustic Dampers

The effect of resonance is present in most BTE hearing aid fittings and is best dealt through damping. Damping causes acoustic resistance to the passing sound and smooths the frequency response in the mid-frequency range (1-4 kHz). This allows the user to increase the volume control setting with less probability of feedback and achieve greater useable gain and output. In addition, the reduction of the first resonant peak at 1kHz will improve word recognition in noise (Valente, Valente, Potts, & Lybarger, 1996).

Figure 4–18 shows the earmold transmission line with the three standing waves. The position of the damper in the earmold tube is critical for effective reduction of the resonant

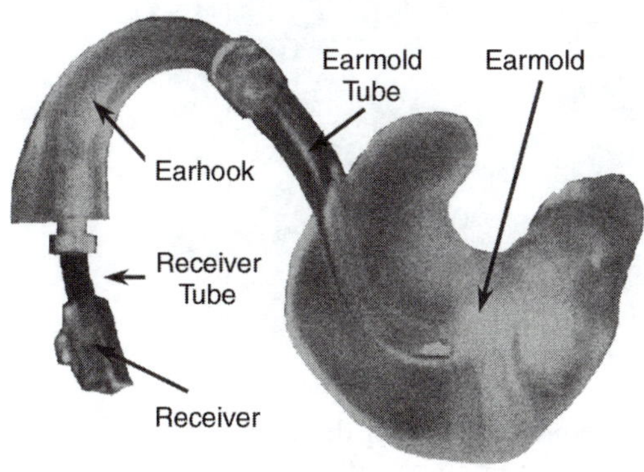

Figure 4–17. Components of the earmold sound transmission line.

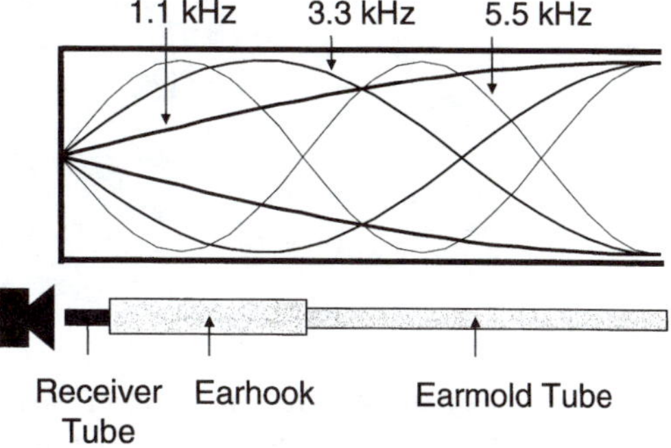

Figure 4–18. Acoustic resonance in the earmold sound transmission line.

peaks. A damper inserted into the earhook on the receiver side, position A, will not reduce the resonant peaks because, at this point, there is no air particle vibration related to the resonance. Maximum damping effect will be achieved if the damper is inserted at the end of the earmold tube, position C, where the air particles vibrate most. Such a placement, however, is impractical because moisture, cerumen, and debris would easily clog the mesh of the damper. To avoid this, acoustic dampers are being inserted at the end of the earhook, point B. At this position, a fairly good attenuation of the first and second resonant peaks still can be achieved, as provided in Figure 4–19. The frequency of the third peak is too high to be reduced effectively by damping.

To reduce the resonant peaks and achieve a smooth and gently rising hearing aid response, several types of damping materials have been developed. Knowles acoustic dampers are probably the most convenient damping system. These dampers are made in a metal housing with a color-coded mesh screen at one end. There are six Knowles dampers available: 680 (white), 1000 (brown), 1500 (green), 2200 (red), 3300 (orange), and 4700 ohm (yellow). The higher the damper value, the stronger the effect of attenuation. However, too much damping may have an adverse effect on the efficiency of the transmission line and result in increased battery drain. Other damping materials such as lamb's wool, sintered steel pellets, and the star damper are not commonly used now.

When dealing with resonant peaks in earmolds, consider that the resonance is formed in the earmold tube and is not related to the quality of the receiver. The same receiver used for an ITE hearing aid has a much smoother response than when used in a BTE

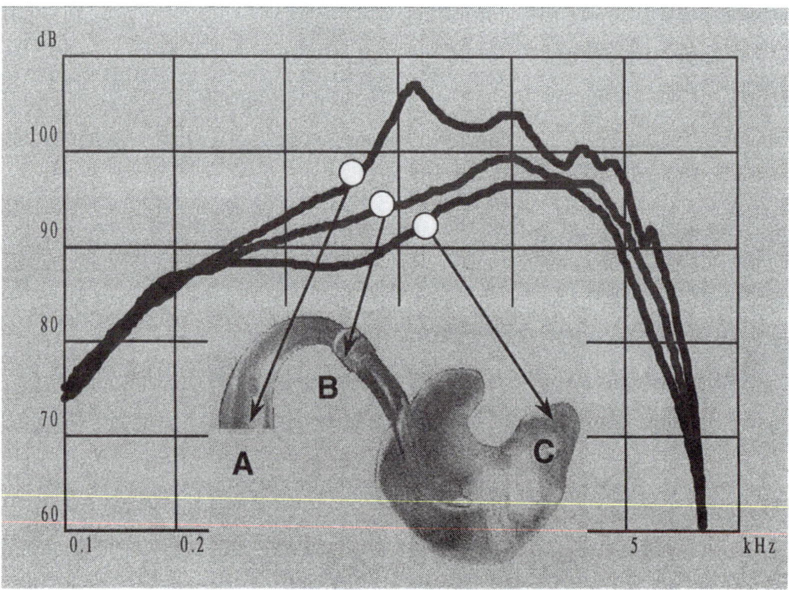

Figure 4–19. The effect of earmold damping depends on the damper's position. The most recommended is inserting the damper at the earhook end, position B. (From *Hearing Instrument Science & Fitting Practices* (p. 399) by R. Sandlin, 1996. Copyright 1996 by National Institute for Hearing Instrument Studies. Adapted with permission.)

system, as shown in Figure 4–20. Note that, due to the resonance in the earmold tube, the BTE response curve rises faster in the low frequencies than does the ITE response.

The Horn Effect

It is known from musical acoustics that the "belling" of a tube will enhance a high-frequency signal passing through the tube. The reverse is also true in that the narrowing of the end of a tube will reduce the high-frequency components.

By using a horn tube in earmolds, a significant increase in the high-frequency response can be obtained. The modern small receiver is a high impedance source. This means that it generates high sound pressure, which can move only a small volume of air. The eardrum is a moderate impedance load. A low impedance load responds to low pressures, but requires large air volume movements. An impedance "transformer" is required to transfer the energy from the receiver to the ear efficiently. A horn bore is such a transformer. It works as follows: The high pressure from the receiver moves a small volume of air in the small diameter of the tube. This in turn, moves a larger volume of air in the next larger bore of the tube and the pressure drops accordingly, and so on progressively until the conditions required by the eardrum are met. The improvement in frequencies around 6000 Hz is about 10-12 dB and depends on the ratio of the diameter of the tube at the receiver and the diameter of the bore at the earmold canal end. The bore does not need to be circular to produce the horn effect.

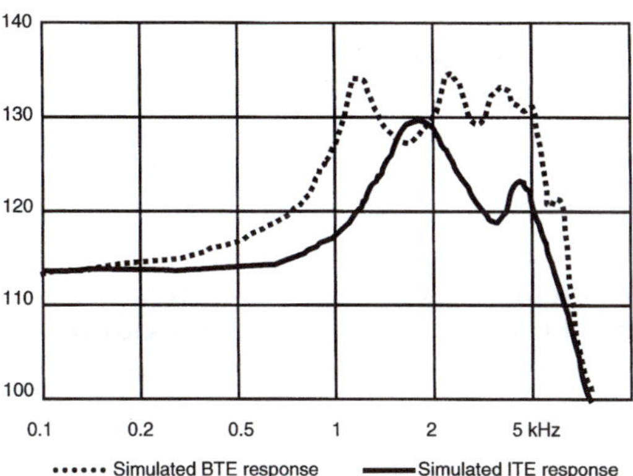

Figure 4–20. The acoustic response of the same receiver used in a custom in-the-ear (ITE) and behind-the-ear (BTE) hearing aid fitting will vary significantly. Responses of a broad band Knowles BK receiver are shown. Simulated Real Ear for BTE: 8 mm × 1 mm inside diameter (ID) + 28 mm × 1.5 mm ID + 18 mm × 3 mm ID tubing + Zwislocki coupler. Simulated Real Ear for ITE: 10 mm × 1 mm ID tubing + Zwislocki coupler. (From *Knowles data manual*. Adapted with permission.)

A very useful aspect of the horn's response is that there is a boost in signal at 2.7 kHz that will compensate somewhat for insertion loss. This helps to achieve a more natural sound. This does not happen in a 2 mm tube. In a conventional mold, an increase in the gain causes the peak areas to amplify beyond the discomfort level, causing the wearer to turn the aid down or suffer.

There are several acoustic options that provide impedance transformation and offer the boost in the high-frequency range. At the end of the 1970s Killion (1980) developed a family of earmolds that were acoustically tuned for certain acoustic effects. This series of options incorporated venting, damping, and horn tubes. The earmolds were characterized by two or three sizes of tubing cemented together and dampers precisely positioned in that tubing. The system used numbers and letters to designate the different style of earmolds. The numbers referred to the frequency involved, whereas a letter or letters referred to the effect. A final number referred to decibels. For example: 6B10 meant a 10 dB boost at 6 kHz, compared to the level of amplification at 1 kHz. This system of acoustically tuned earmolds offered significant acoustic advantages but turned out to be impractical. There was accumulation of moisture in the tubing, cosmetic objections, the difficulty of joining tubings with accurate dimensioning, and the difficulaty of replacing the tubing assembly. To overcome these disadvantages, Libby (1980) developed a one-piece earmold tube with varying diameter. This smooth tube of internal stepped-bore construction, commonly known as Libby Horn Tube, is available in 3 mm and 4 mm sizes, and is used quite frequently for high frequency hearing losses. Due to the varying diameter of the tube, the acoustic damper, typically 1500 ohms, is placed in the earhook.

Other acoustic options that boost the high-frequency range include a belled canal and horn bore. These constructions are drilled in the canal portion of the earmold. To be effective, however, the depth of the bore must to be 17 mm (Killion, 1980). This means that a belled canal that is 1 to 2 mm deep will have no acoustic effect on the hearing aid response and rather should be regarded as a cerumen trap.

The employment of the Libby Horn tube in pediatric and small ear canal fittings must be carefully considered. The 3 mm and 4 mm Libby tubes have outer diameters of approximately 4.5 mm and 5.5 mm, respectively. If the diameter of the earmold medial end is smaller than 6 mm, the Libby tube should not be requested. In hard earmolds, the plastic around the tube will be thin and may chip and hurt the ear tissue. In soft molds, the tube can stretch the mold material and make the earmold uncomfortably tight.

Interestingly, small ears may not require the use of the horned tube at all. As was already mentioned, acoustic resonance occurs as a result of the tube/ear-canal impedance mismatch. In small ears, the impedance of the ear canal and eardrum may be close to the impedance of the tube, so the hearing aid response may be satisfactorily smooth.

Venting

A vent is a channel drilled in the body of the earmold that connects the lateral surface of the mold with the medial end of the canal. Acoustically, there are several purposes of venting:

1. To reduce the sensation of plugged ears, commonly known as the occlusion effect,
2. To reduce the low frequency component in the hearing aid response, and
3. To prevent moisture condensation in earmold that would adversely affect the hearing aid performance.

Venting in earmolds can be drilled in parallel, external, or diagonal configurations, as shown in Figure 4–21. Parallel venting (A) is the most commonly recommended. It reduces the low-frequency component without altering the high-frequency response. The larger the vent bore, the more the low frequencies are reduced. External venting (B) is used for patients possessing small ear canals where accommodating two bores within the earmold canal is not feasible. The disadvantage

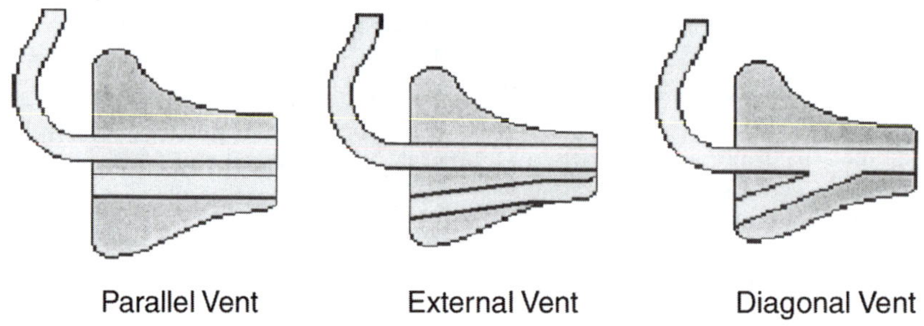

Figure 4–21. Venting configurations: **A.** Parallel. **B.** External. **C.** Diagonal. Acoustically, the parallel type of venting is recommended.

of this type of venting is that the external portion of the vent can be clogged by ear wax and moisture. Diagonal venting (C) is another option for ears with small canals. The vent begins at the earmold lateral surface and than intersects the sound bore between the end of the tubing and the end of the mold. Diagonal venting is not recommended because of its adverse effect on the high-frequency area. Figure 4–22 provides guidelines for vent selection in relation to the patient's hearing loss.

The presence of the vent increases sound leakage and feedback often results. To maintain the benefits of venting and, at the same time, to effectively prevent feedback, earmold labs developed three venting systems that allow for reversible vent modifications. Each system consists of five plastic plugs having a bore, and a zero-vent plug. The size of the bore varies. In the Select-A-Vent (S.A.V.) system, the diameter of the bore is 0.8 mm to 4.0 mm (.031 to .06 inch), in the Mini S.A.V. it is 0.5 mm to 1.9 mm (.020 to .075 inch) and in the Positive Venting Valve (P.V.V.) system the bore is 0.5 mm to 3.2 mm (.020 to .125 inch) (Microsonic, 1998).

The selection of the plugging system should be based on two factors: the patient's hearing loss and the size of the ear. Because moderate, severe, and profound hearing losses pose a higher risk of feedback, a smaller venting system, such as Mini S.A.V., is recommended for such losses. This system also is useful for patients possessing narrow ear canals that provide limited space for the ventilation channel.

Hearing loss in the range 250Hz to 1kHz	Earmold vent size [mm]				
	Non-Occluding	4-2	2-1	1-0.5	No Vent
Normal	●				
Mild		●			
Moderate			●		
Severe				●	●
Profound					●

Figure 4–22. Guidelines for earmold vent size selection.

EARMOLD MATERIALS

Earmolds can be made from a variety of hard and soft materials. The selection of these materials as well as the range of their flexibility grows constantly. The most commonly offered earmold materials include:

LUCITE - This hard acrylic material is most commonly used in earmold manufacturing. It is available in clear, translucent tint, opaque beige and brown, and any pastel color.

ULTRA-VIOLET RESIN - This is a hard photo-polymerization plastic possessing excellent hypoallergenic properties. Recommended for deep canal fittings. Available in blue and red, and other colors as described for hard acrylic.

POLYETHYLENE - This is a semi-hard waxy material recommended for extreme allergies. Earmolds made of polyethylene will float in water.

SOFT ACRYLIC - This is a semi-soft plastic, which can be used either to make earmolds or just the flexible canal portion of a Lucite earmold. The material will harden with time and absorb earwax.

SOFT ULTRA-VIOLET - This is a soft, clear, one-part photo polymerization resin recommended for deep canal fittings or for soft canals on hard body earmolds. Considered to be more hypoallergenic than soft acrylic.

SILICONE - Medical grade silicones have gained significant popularity as earmold materials due to their extreme softness and hypoallergenic properties. The softness, however, precludes the use of silicone for the Receiver and Non-Occluding earmolds. Silicone molds come in a variety of colors. With the addition of a special filler, silicone molds can be made to float.

POLYVINYL CHLORIDE - This soft thermoplastic material, also known as vinyl or PVC, is used commonly to make flexible earmolds. It is firmer than silicone, thus giving the patient freedom to insert the mold.

When considering earmold material, several categories of concern arise: power level requirements, patient manual dexterity, comfort, allergic conditions, and personal preferences.

Physical Properties of Earmold Materials

The earmold manufacturing process, for most molding materials, is based on polymerization. In its nonpolymerized condition the liquid plastic consists of monomer molecules which compound during reaction to long chains of polymers. Single monomer molecules have a greater distance to each other in liquid condition than the polymer in cured condition. The transition from noncured to cured condition causes contraction in the earmold body. The linear contraction is approximately 2% for acrylic, 1.7% for ultraviolet resin, and 0.4% for silicone. Vinyl earmolds, which are formed by injection of melted hot PVC into a gypsum casting, contract about 2.5% within 24 hours after molding. Soft acrylic earmolds shrink during and after casting up to 2% (Combe & Nolan, 1989a).

The softness of a given material is described as the shore value. Earmolds made of a soft acrylic and soft ultra-violet material have 40 to 50 shore hardness, vinyl earmolds have 30 to 50, and silicone earmolds have 25 to 55, depending on the material and manufacturer. Once again, the lower the shore value, the more flexible the material. Rigid materials have 90 shore hardness. Soft earmolds, particularly made of silicone, are more difficult for in-office modifications and require special modification tools.

Acoustic Seal

One of the most common questions asked by hearing health care professionals is whether soft earmolds provide better seal and comfort than hard earmolds. Few research studies have attempted to answer the question.

In a study of sixteen subjects, (Macrea, 1990) used one ear impression to make four earmolds for each subject. The molds were made of acrylic, vinyl, silicone, and polyethylene. In total, 64 earmolds were manufactured. The accuracy of earmold seal was tested with the same method as in Fifield's research (1980): Static air pressure was applied to the ear canal through a tube running through the earmold. If sustained pressure was measured for five seconds, the seal was considered satisfactory. If the pressure decreased, the seal was inadequate. This study failed to prove that soft earmolds seal better than hard earmolds. In fact, if the hard earmold leaked, all of the remaining three soft earmolds made for a given subject leaked as well.

Pirzanski and Maye (1999) studied remakes of earmolds manufactured from all kinds of soft and hard materials. A total of 2731 earmolds (1413 hard-body and 1318 soft-body) were investigated. The authors found that soft earmolds were prescribed more frequently for severe hearing losses and had a higher rate of remakes, as shown in Figure 4–23. They concluded that soft earmolds do not offer any obvious advantages in hearing aid fittings. These results also are consistent with my observations on earmold fittings: If a hard-body earmold does not seal the ear properly, the seal of a soft earmold, in most cases, will not be better.

Acoustic seal in earmolds depends on more factors than the softness of the mold material. It encompasses the flexibility, sensitivity, and shape of the patient's ear. It also depends on the impression material viscosity and impression-taking technique. Finally, it is

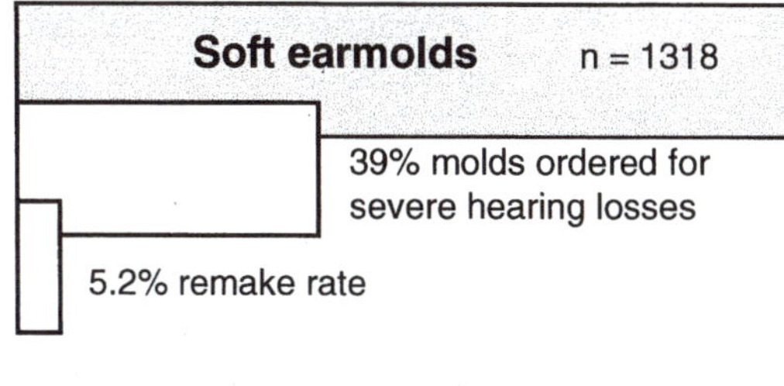

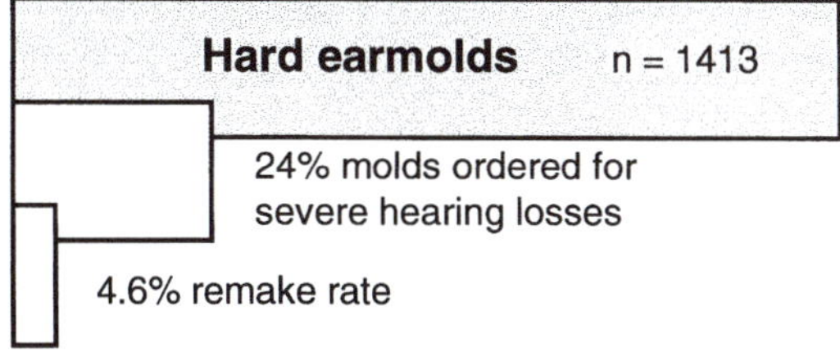

Figure 4–23. Soft earmolds do not provide superior acoustic seal and comfort compared to hard earmolds, as it is commonly claimed. With a higher usage for severe hearing losses, soft earmolds also have a higher rate of remakes due to fitting problems.

determined by impression trimming, coating, and the earmold manufacturing process. Because so many factors are involved, a successful earmold fitting cannot be credited just to the softness of the material.

In practice, the effectiveness of earmold seal is controlled through the thickness of impression coating, commonly made of wax. Macrae (1990) wondered whether there was a better method of improving earmold acoustic seal than through waxing. In a series of experiments conducted on a varying number of subjects, he compared the effectiveness of seal in earmolds made from waxed impressions with non-waxed multilayer impressions. The research results are provided in Figure 4–24. Two impressions from each subject's ear were made. The first was taken with a soft impression material, the other as a multilayer impression with the primary impression made of a heavy-bodied silicone. Four wax coatings of varying thickness were used

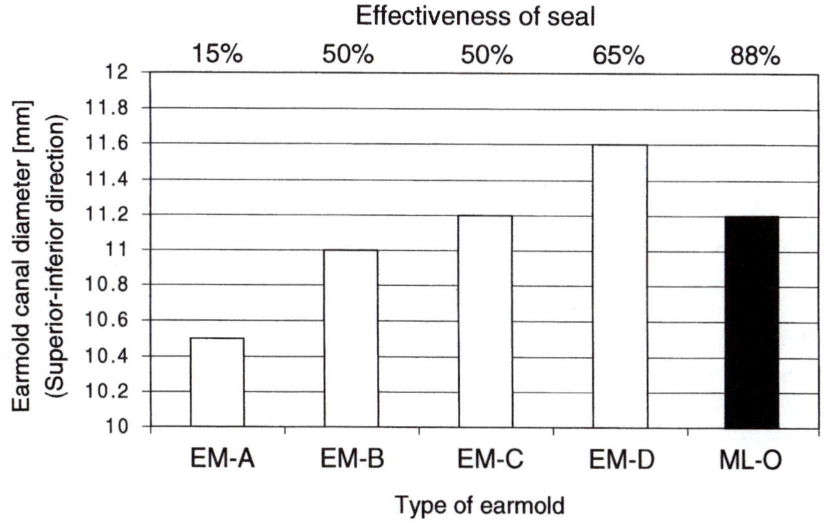

Figure 4–24. Comparison of static seal provided by earmolds manufactured under five different conditions. Earmolds EM-A, EM-B, EM-C, and EM-D were made from waxed impressions taken with a soft impression material. The thickness of the wax varied: A < B < C < D. Earmolds ML-O, which provided the most effective seal, were made from non-waxed multilayer impressions. (Data from "Static Pressure Seal of Earmolds," by J. Macrae, 1990, *Journal of Rehabilitation Research and Development, vol.* Adapted with permission.)

to make four earmolds from the first impression, one earmold for each coating condition. Earmolds EM-A were made from the thinnest impression coating A, whereas earmolds EM-D were made from the thickest coating D. Multilayer impressions were not coated prior to making earmolds ML-O. All earmolds were made of a medical grade silicone and had a vinyl tubing for the static air pressure test.

With the increase in the wax thickness, from coating A to D, a more effective seal was measured. With the thickest coating D, 65% of earmolds EM-D provided effective seal. Interestingly, earmolds ML-O had the best sealing properties, reaching 88%. This was achieved despite the fact that these earmolds had the diameter of their canals 0.4 mm smaller than EM-D earmolds. It also is worth noticing that earmolds EM-C, which had, on average, the same diameter of the canals as earmolds ML-O, provided a much less effective seal, just 50%. The superb sealing in earmolds ML-O resulted from their excellent anatomical accuracy.

The ear canal tissue is soft, but this softness is not a rubber-like flexibility. Certain areas of the cartilage appear to be more forgiving than other areas. Earmolds EM-D made from heavily coated impressions taken with a soft material did not correspond properly with the anatomical structures of subjects' ears. They overstretched the ear tissue in some areas but did not stretch the tissue enough in other areas. This resulted in a poor seal and air leakage. The most efficient seal in earmolds ML-O was achieved due to the employment of the multilayer technique. Although multilayer impressions stretched the ear tissue significantly more, the stretching reflected the natural ear tissue forgiveness. The fit of the resulting earmolds was snug but, anatomically, most accurate. Earmolds ML-O also were most likely to be more comfortable than molds EM-C and EM-D.

Does this mean that hearing health care professionals should utilize more frequently the multilayer technique and earmold labs should minimize the thickness of impression coating? If taking a multilayer impression required 10-15 minutes, such a strategy would be recommended. Unfortunately, as indicated before, the procedure requires an hour, which makes the technique impractical.

The results of Macrea's study, however, strongly support my experience that there are no impression materials and techniques that can produce a too-tight ear impression. To achieve the best results in earmold fittings, standard viscosity impression materials (as opposed to light viscosity impression materials) and the open-jaw technique should be utilized more commonly.

Comfort

Theoretically, earmolds made from soft materials should be more comfortable than those made from hard materials. Practically, the softness of the mold material is quite irrelevant. Most human ears appear to be softer than earmold materials. If so, it is the ear tissue that must conform to the earmold, not the earmold to the ear. Results in custom hearing aid fittings fully support this opinion. The majority of shells for custom instruments are manufactured from either a hard acrylic or hard ultraviolet resin. A study conducted by Maye (1997) found that, with a proper impression-taking technique and competent manufacturing, not more than 0.7% of custom in-the-ear hearing aids required a remake due to discomfort, including high gain instruments. These results would not be so good if soft materials were as critical for comfort as it is commonly claimed.

It is a little-known fact that discomfort in earmold fittings more commonly results from a loose fit than from a too tight fit. Even soft earmolds that require frequent pushing into the ear may cause ear tissue soreness. The resulting inflammation is commonly, but incorrectly, interpreted by the hearing health care professional as an indication of a tight fit.

Allergic Conditions

Hard and soft materials used to manufacture earmolds are biocompatible, so they generally do not cause irritation or sensitization to the skin in the ear. However, some patients can exhibit high sensitivity to traces of certain chemicals, particularly those found in acrylic resins, and develop soreness of the ear tissue. For such patients, the use of a hypoallergenic, rigid or soft, material is recommended.

To determine which hypoallergenic material will prove most effective for a given patient, the dispenser may administer a skin patch test in which small samples of earmold materials, provided by the earmold lab, are taped to the patient's arm or neck. The adverse reaction can range from dry itchy skin with a slight inflammation to a painful edema of the pinna, cheek, or neck area (Valente et al, 1996). The sample that does not result in an adverse reaction should be used for the earmold manufacturing.

Patients with allergies to earmold materials usually have a history of allergies to other chemical agents. If the patient appears "allergic" just to the earmold, the irritation most likely has another cause. This situation is quite evident in binaural fittings in which one earmold fits comfortably, but the other, according to the hearing health care professional, requires a remake due to an "allergic" reaction. In such fittings the ear inflammation is obviously caused by the earmold poor fit. Ear inflammation can develop due to a difficulty in the instrument insertion, earmold tightness, and surface roughness, as well as to constant tissue coverage, increased humidity in the ear canal, or lack of proper hygiene.

Temporary earmolds can be made from trimmed ear impressions if the impression material is recommended for such a use. Some impression materials contain DBTD (dibutystanbumdilauart), which is an oto-toxic component. Rykowski, Bredberg and Alsterborg (1991) found that, if a DBTD contaminated impression mold stayed in an animal's ear for one week, it often led to severe inflammation in the middle ear and even damage to hair cells.

Patient's Manual Dexterity and Personal Preferences

Hard earmold materials are recommended for patients having problems with manual dexterity and for patients whose ear canals are soft, collapsed, or have sharp anatomical bends. Such patients will find hard earmolds easier to insert into the ear. Some typical cases of difficulty in earmold insertion are discussed in the troubleshooting section of this chapter.

First-time hearing aid users typically will accept a recommendation regarding the earmold material given by the hearing health care professional. Some experienced users, however, may request that the earmold be made from a material of their preference. If the history of the patient does not indicate any difficulty in earmold fitting in the past, or if the earmold is being remade due to poor cosmetics, following the patient's specification is a good practice. If the remake is due to difficulty in insertion, feedback, a loose fit, or discomfort, the accuracy of the patient's request should be reconsidered carefully.

Soft earmold materials are recommended for children and for noise reduction plugs, because the flexible material reduces the risk of injury with blows to the head.

EARMOLD STYLE

The majority of earmold labs offer earmolds in the following configurations:

STANDARD - This earmold provides maximum in-concha retention. It is useful for profound hearing losses in which the secure fit of the instrument and the mold is most needed.

STANDARD with HELIX LOCK - The addition of the helix curl is used to improve the mold retention for ears that lack satisfactory in-concha retention.

SHELL - This earmold fills the concha like a standard mold but is slightly shelled out for better appearance.

SKELETON and SEMI-SKELETON - These earmolds have material removed from the center portion of the concha to enhance cosmetic appearance, while still providing enhanced in-ear retention. Easy to modify to other styles, such as Canal and Canal-Lock

HALF-SHELL - This earmold is essentially a shell mold with the helix and cymba area removed. Recommended for ears possessing adequate retention in the tragus/antitragus and the canal area.

CANAL - This earmold is made only from the canal portion of the impression. In some fittings, the mold may require a long canal. Recommended only for patients whose ear canals provide adequate in-canal retention.

CANAL-LOCK - This model offers improved in-concha retention in cases in which the in-canal retention is insufficient. The lock also facilitates the mold insertion and removal for patients with impaired manual dexterity.

NON-OCCLUDING - These earmolds are recommended for patients with a high-frequency hearing loss or patients complaining of occlusion. There are several styles of non-occluding molds.

RECEIVER - This earmold is designed for a body-type hearing aid that has an external button-type receiver. The receiver is snapped in a metal or plastic ring imbedded in the mold. The size of the ring will vary, depending on the type of the receiver.

All earmolds, as illustrated in Figures 4-25 and 4-26, are provided with an earmold tubing, except the Receiver style. The tubing is approximately 60 mm (2 3/8 inch) long and must be trimmed at the time the hearing aid is fitted. Tubes have regular, medium, or heavy (thick) walls. Heavy wall tubes are recommended for severe and profound hearing losses because they reduce sound radiation through the tube wall and prevent acoustic feedback. For patients having problems with moisture condensing in the earmold tube, tubes called dry-wall ought to be ordered.

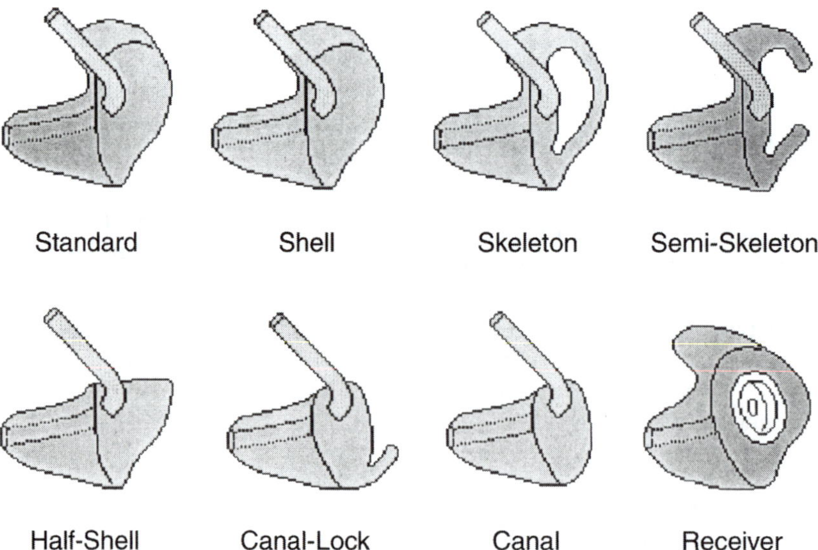

Figure 4–25. Earmold style selection.

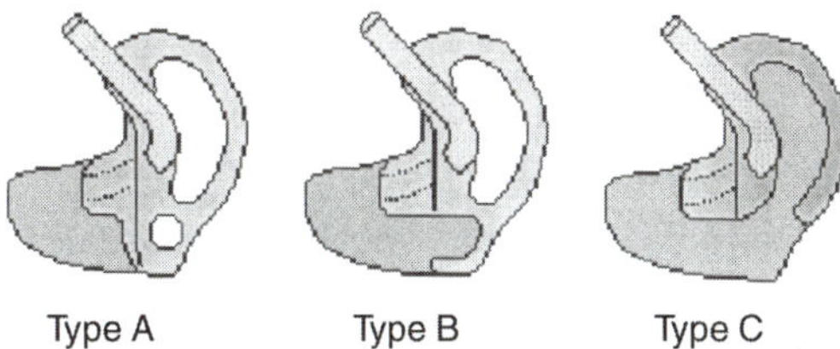

Figure 4–26. Non-occluding earmolds. Earmold type C is known commonly as the Jansen non-occluding earmold.

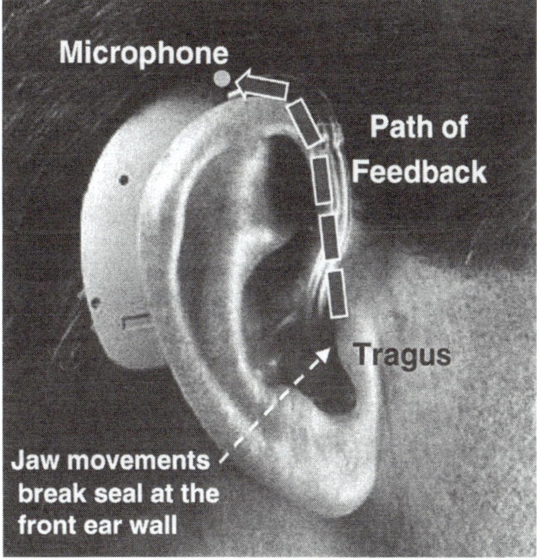

Figure 4–27. Acoustic seal in most earmold fittings breaks at the anterior (front) ear wall, allowing for non-controllable sound leakage and feedback. The impression-taking technique, viscosity of impression material, and the manufacturing process appear to be more critical for feedback prevention than the earmold style and material.

The criteria for earmold style selection are similar to those for earmold material selection. The evaluation should include the severity and type of the patient's hearing loss, anatomical properties of the ear, the patient's dexterity, personal preferences, and difficulty with any previous hearing instrument fitting.

Acoustic Seal

Earmolds made as the Canal, Canal-Lock, and Half-Shell style are prescribed commonly for mild hearing losses. Earmolds made as Skeleton or Semi-skeleton, with more material at the concha, are recommended for moderate hearing losses. For severe-to-profound losses, earmolds in the Shell or Standard style are ordered. Because it is regarded that full concha earmolds provide a better acoustic seal, these division lines for earmold selection are observed by most hearing health care professionals. Are these guidelines correct?

In most earmold fittings, the acoustic seal area is in the ear canal, between its first and second bend. Because jaw movements break the seal at the front ear wall (compare with Figure 4–5 C, D), the path of feedback most likely will be as shown in Figure 4–27: along the front ear wall, above the tragus, and then directly to the microphone of the hearing aid hanging over the ear. The path of feedback for loosely fitting earmolds (compare with Figure 4–3) will be exactly the same. The sound will always choose the shortest path from the ear canal toward the microphone. In this regard, the size of the earmold at the concha does not appear to be critical for enhancing the seal of the earmold.

Retention

Earmolds are connected with BTE hearing aids through an earmold tube and earhook. Although the tube is flexible, it still can create some pressure on the earmold that will try to pull the mold out of the ear. As the result of the pulling, a Canal earmold fitted in an ear with inadequate retention can be loosen by mandibular movements and feedback. Figure 4–28 shows two Canal style earmolds; earmold A provides adequate in-canal retention, earmold B does not. To fit securely, earmold B must be manufactured as a Shell or Skeleton earmold that provides in-concha retention.

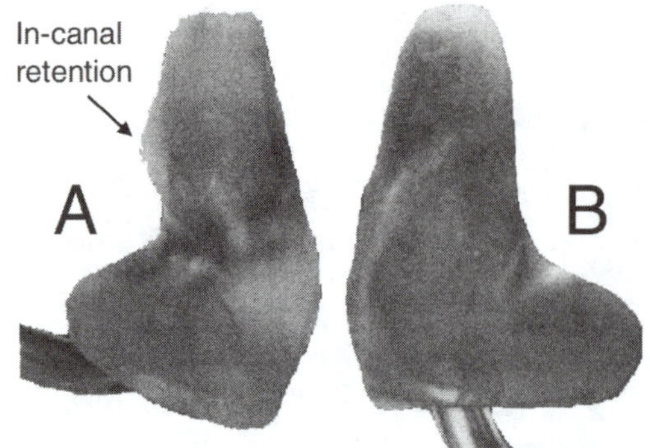

Figure 4–28. Sufficient in-canal retention is critical for fitting Canal style earmolds. Earmold A has adequate in-canal retention, earmold B does not.

Mandibular movements not only widen the ear canal but also, in some patients, change the angle between the ear canal and concha. As a result, a hard-body full-concha mold can be forced out of the ear. Such a problem can be remedied in two ways: If the ear canal provides good in-canal retention, a silicone Canal mold should be ordered. Otherwise, order a silicone Skeleton mold. The flexible concha ring of the mold will accommodate movements of the ear tissue while still securing the mold's fit in the ear.

Insufficient seal in earmolds and acoustic feedback also may result from incompetent manufacturing. Earmolds made from thinly waxed ear impressions, after buffing and shining, will be smaller than the actual ear impression and fit loosely in the ear. On the other hand, heavy impression coating can make the canal portion of the earmold longer than the patient's ear canal if the impression is not properly trimmed. Excessive impression trimming, however, may yield an earmold with poor retention. In addition, a skeleton earmold with the concha ring styled too much can be loosen easily by mandibular movements. Most of these fitting problems will not occur with Shell or Standard style earmolds. These earmolds provide maximum in-concha retention and are less likely to feed back, even when loose. That is why full-concha molds often are credited for better seal. Recent research conducted by Pirzanski, Chasin, Klenk, Maye and Purdy (1999) found that properly manufactured Canal earmolds had equal, sometimes even better, sealing properties than Standard earmolds made from the same material for the same subject.

EARMOLD FITTING AND TROUBLESHOOTING

Most earmolds have satisfactory fit and acoustic seal if manufactured from long canal impressions, taken with a standard viscosity silicone (viscosity type C or D), and with a mouth prop inserted in the patient's jaw. Some, for a variety of reasons, do not. Typical problems encountered during earmold fitting include earmold insertion, acoustic feedback, discomfort, and the sensation of plugged ears.

Earmold Insertion

Before the patient can experience any benefit from hearing aid use, the earmold must be inserted and fit comfortably in the ear.

Hand Rotation

Most patients, if not properly advised, will unintentionally rotate the hand holding the earmold while bringing it to ear level. Therefore, they will attempt to insert the earmold with its helix, or upper bowl, positioned backwards across the ear. To avoid this, the patient should be advised to bring the earmold to the ear without any rotation.

Soft Material

Insertion of an earmold made from a soft material can pose difficulty for patients possessing ears with a sharp first bend. In such ears, the flexible earmold canal can bend backwards, across the canal entrance. The sharper the ear bend or the softer the earmold material, the more challenging the insertion can be. Shortening the earmold canal is recommended. Generally, for such patients, a rigid body earmold should be considered.

Long Canal

Very few human ears have straight ear canals. Most ears have moderately to severely sharp bends. If in addition to these bends the ear tissue is firm, an earmold with a long canal can be difficult to insert. Because the acoustic seal area on an earmold occurs just past the canal aperture, the tip of the earmold canal can be shortened or tapered without encountering feedback problems. A lubricant can be used to facilitate earmold insertion.

Bottleneck Ear Canal

A constriction at the ear canal entrance can make earmold insertion painful when the wide portion on the earmold canal is forced through the narrow ear opening. To ease insertion, the bulging area on the canal should be tapered and the canal shortened. The tapering should not affect the bottleneck area, which provides acoustic seal.

Wide or Extended Helix

Some earmolds may have the helix area wide and/or extended toward the ear canal. Due to difficulty in insertion, such earmolds can be worn improperly with the helix sticking over the ear. This may lead to acoustic feedback and discomfort. Because the helix area provides retention only, the length and width of the helix can be greatly reduced without increasing the risk of feedback.

Acoustic Feedback

Most hearing instruments perform well acoustically when turned on. However, some instruments may produce acoustic feedback before the required level of amplification is reached. It is important to determine the nature of feedback properly. Feedback can be internal, due to a component failure, or external, due to the earmold loose fit, presence of a vent, or jaw movement. In the case of internal feedback, a certified technician should repair the hearing instrument. In the case of external feedback, the vent in the earmold should be plugged temporarily. If this stops the whistling, the no-vent plug can be replaced with a variable vent plug often provided with the mold. The selected vent insert should provide adequate ear ventilation without feedback. When fitting severe hearing losses, a permanent vent plugging may be necessary.

Reducing the vent size is an effective method of feedback elimination if the earmold fits snugly enough in the ear. In many fittings, however, feedback occurs due to a loose fit that allows for uncontrolled sound leakage. To reduce leakage and stop feedback, a plastic tubing of appropriate size and thickness can be pulled over the earmold canal and cemented to it. Figure 4–29 shows a Canal-Lock earmold with a seal/retention ring and several tubings in varying sizes and thickness. Such tubings can be ordered from earmold labs. The use of the tubing is the fastest and most convenient method in feed-

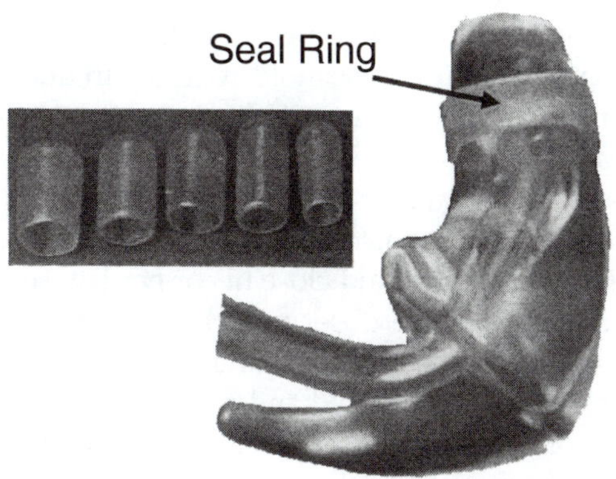

Figure 4–29. A seal ring made of a flexible tubing reduces loose fit and prevents acoustic feedback in earmolds. Tubings of varying diameters and wall thickness are available from earmold labs.

back elimination. Another solution is to apply a soft coat to the earmold canal at the seal area. If the feedback results from the patient's jaw movements, such a coating (or tubing) often is ineffective. In such cases, an earmold remake from an open-jaw impression may be necessary.

Discomfort

As a result of the earmold rubbing against the ear wall while being inserted, the ear canal can swell and, after several days, make insertion painful or not possible. If the ear is slightly irritated, the dispenser should shorten or taper the earmold canal until easy insertion is achieved. If the swelling is substantial, modification should be postponed until the irritation recedes.

An easy-to-insert earmold will not necessarily be comfortable to wear for an extended period of time. To insure thorough comfort, encourage the patient to turn his or her head, to chew, and to open his or her mouth very wide. Should this identify any problems, modify the earmold accordingly. In a case of discomfort deep in the canal, check the ear for any hard wax deposit or a growth hidden at or after the canal's second bend.

If an initially comfortable earmold begins to irritate the ear after some time, assume that the earmold has become loose. If the patient concedes that the earmold requires frequent pushing in to improve its fit or to stop feedback, this may be the case. Apply a soft coat or make a seal ring to achieve a snugger fit.

If an irritation is reported at the helix, have the patient open and close his or her jaw several times while observing the earmold. In some patients, mandibular movements are able to rotate the mold and cause abrasion in the pinna. Modify the helix area accordingly.

A soreness and itching in the ear is not necessarily an allergic reaction to the earmold material. Check the patient's history or ask questions to find out if the patient is allergic to any chemical agents. If the patient has a history of allergies, consider a remake from a hypoallergenic clear ultra-violet material or clear silicone. If not, consider difficulty in earmold insertion or its general tightness as the most likely cause of the irritation.

Sensation of Plugged Ears

This may be caused by a variety of reasons. For a first-time user who has not heard his or her own voice for a long time, echoing sounds of speaking, breathing, chewing, or walking can be quite annoying. This is called the occlusion effect. Encourage the patient to wear the hearing instrument for several days and the unpleasant sensation should diminish and eventually disappear. If you are dealing with an experienced user, increasing the vent size and/or shortening the canal is recommended.

In earmolds without vents, or with the vent blocked by earwax, air pressure in the ear can build up and be annoying. In addition, complaints of too much low-frequency energy can relate to electroacoustic characteristics of the hearing instrument (Sweetow and Valla, 1997). To eliminate the hearing aid amplification as the reason, turn the instrument off and verify the effect by asking the patient. The feeling of pressure also may come from physical discomfort resulting from the earmold pressing on the ear wall at or after the ear's second bend.

All of these issues should be considered before the hearing health care professional decides on an earmold modification, remake, or hearing aid response adjustment.

SUMMARY

As has been discussed, many problems in earmold fittings, such as feedback, insecure fit, discomfort, occlusion, and sound fading, are avoidable, provided the ear impression is properly taken.

A high quality ear impression has the canal portion extended past the ear canal second anatomical bend and has no underfilled areas. It is recommended to take ear impressions with a standard viscosity impression material and the patient's jaw wide open. Open-jaw impressions can and should be taken for all earmolds. Such impressions have a larger diameter of the ear canal area, so the resulting earmold has enhanced acoustic seal, comfort, and retention. Because this technique is new, some hearing health care professionals may approach this advice with apprehension. In such cases, it is advisable to begin taking open-jaw impressions for earmold remakes. This will allow the time necessary for learning the technique. An appreciation of its benefits can be obtained over time. Similar advice is extended to professionals who use gun-injected silicones and would consider the employment of a standard viscosity silicone material. Standard viscosity materials better reflect the ear's natural flexibility and even further enhance the definition of the earmold fit and seal. Practicing the use of such silicones when taking impressions for earmold remakes is a wonderful way to gain confidence. Once confident, the viscous silicone can be used with all patients for all hearing aids.

An anatomically accurate ear impression is subject to trimming and coating at the earmold lab. These processes are essential in ensuring the earmold satisfactory acoustic seal, comfort, easy insertion, and sufficient retention. Earmolds manufactured as "replicas" of ear impressions generally require a greater number of modifications and remakes due to fitting problems than earmolds made from properly prepared ear impressions.

The selection of earmold style and material should be considered based on anatomical properties of the patient's ear captured on the impression. For ears that provide insufficient in-canal retention, a Shell or Skeleton earmold should be ordered. Flexible earmolds may provide better comfort but not necessarily better seal, if a poor ear impression is taken. The size of the vent should be adequate for the patient's hearing loss. Larger vents are required for mild and high-frequency hearing losses.

Although the electroacoustic characteristics of modern hearing aids have improved greatly over recent years, acoustic resonance occurring in the earmold tube can deteriorate the quality of sound delivered to the ear significantly. An acoustic damper will smooth the hearing aid audio response, reduce the risk of feedback, and benefit the patient with better sound.

REVIEW QUESTIONS

1. The human ear canal observed in the transverse view commonly has:
   a. One sharp bend.
   b. A number of bends that depends on how old the patient is.
   c. Two bends that give the canal a shape similar to the letter "S".
   d. Thick hair close to the eardrum.
   e. b and d.

2. The cartilaginous tissue of the ear canal commonly is:
   a. Quite flexible.
   b. Moderately sensitive.
   c. Lined with ear wax.
   d. Changing with jaw movements.
   e. All of the above.

3. The following is/are true:
   a. The hand-packed impression-taking technique is superior to taking impressions with a syringe or gun.
   b. The use of a mouth prop is recommended to prevent accidental jaw closing while the material cures in the ear.
   c. A hearing aid has a better acoustic seal if the impression is taken with a low viscosity (runny) impression material.
   d. The shorter the canal portion of the impression, the better the instrument's retention.
   e. The oto-block should be removed from the impression before the impression is forwarded to the otoplastic lab.

4. Insertion of the oto-block past the ear's second bend is necessary to:
   a. Imprint the first and second canal bend on the impression.

b. Eliminate voids and air pockets on the impression.
c. Prevent excessive bleeding while removing the impression from ear.
d. b and c.
e. None of the above.

5. To be appreciated by the user, an earmold must have:
a. Sufficient acoustic seal.
b. Adequate in-ear retention.
c. Proper sound direction.
d. Comfortable fit for extended use.
e. All of the above.

6. An earmold manufactured from an open-jaw impression commonly:
a. Has a small vent.
b. Has better seal, retention, and comfort than an instrument built from a closed jaw or chewing impression.
c. Is more difficult to modify.
d. Is rejected by the user.
e. Has a long, crooked canal.

7. An earmold manufactured from an impression taken with a low viscosity (runny) impression material may:
a. Be loose.
b. Feedback.
c. Be uncomfortable.
d. Work out of the ear.
e. All of the above.

8. Silicone ear impression materials, compared to acrylic (liquid and powder) materials, have:
a. Better shape stability.
b. Equal quality.
c. Inferior stress relaxation.
d. Less shrinkage.
e. a and d.

9. The Shore value of an impression material refers to the material's:
a. After cure hardness.
b. Color.
c. Flow characteristics.
d. Stress relaxation.
e. None of the above.

10. The acoustic seal area in most earmolds occurs:
a. At the helix.
b. At the concha.
c. Between the ear canal anatomical first and second bend.
d. Past the second bend.
e. All over the earmold.

11. Insertion loss results from:
a. The disruption of the ear's natural resonance properties.
b. The patient's aging.
c. Lack of proper venting.
d. Earmold style.
e. Inadequate hearing aid amplification.

12. The following is/are true:
a. The behind-the-ear sound transmission line includes: the battery, amplifier, earmold tube, and the eardrum.
b. An increase in high-frequency amplification can be achieved through the use of the Libby horn tube.
c. Diagonal vent is the preferred style of venting as it increases amplification in the high frequency area.
d. Large vents are required for severe and profound hearing losses
e. The inside diameter of the earmold tube is typically 1 millimeter

13. The use of an acoustic damper is recommended to:
a. Reduce low frequency amplification.
b. Reduce high frequency amplification.
c. Keep the earmold tube clean from earwax.
d. Reduce resonant peaks on hearing aid response.
e. Reduce the size of vent.

14. The following is/are true:
a. Silicone earmold materials typically have 90 Shore hardness.
b. Shrinkage in earmold materials typically exceeds 5%.
c. Earmolds made of vinyl better prevent acoustic feedback than molds made of silicone.

d. All of the above.
e. None of the above.

15. Ear inflammation can be caused by:
a. Loose or tight hearing aid fit.
b. Allergy to earmold material.
c. Difficulty in earmold insertion.
d. All of the above.
e. b and c.

REFERENCES

Agnew, J. (1986). Ear impression stability. *Hearing Instruments, 37*(12), 10–11.

Chasin M., Pirzanski C., Hayes D., & Mueller G. (1997). The real ear occluded gain as a clinical predictor, *The Hearing Review, 4*(4), 22–26.

Fifield, D. (1980). A new ear impression technique to prevent acoustic feedback with high-powered hearing aids. *Volta Review, 82*(1), 33–39.

Fishbein, H. (1997). Thank you, thank you, thank you, Chester Z. Pirzanski! *The Hearing Journal, 50*(4), 65.

Jean, A. (1999, March). *Patient focus and case studies.* Paper presented at the Canadian University Symposium, Mississauga, ON, Canada.

Kieper, R., & Berger, E. (1999). The effect on the real-ear attenuation of using a bite block while making a custom earmold. Indianapolis, IN: AERO Company.

Killion, M. C. (1980). Problems in the application of broadband hearing aid earphones. In G. A. Studebaker & J. Hochberg (Eds.), *Acoustical factors affecting hearing aid performance* (pp. 219–264). Baltimore: University Park Press.

Libby, E. R. (1980). Smooth wideband hearing aid responses—The new frontier. *Hearing Instruments, 30*(10):12-13, 15, 18, 43.

Macrae, J. (1990). Static pressure seal of earmolds, *Journal of Rehabilitation Research and Development, 27*(4), 397–410.

Maye V. (1997). Field return analysis by account. Internal study, Canada: Starkey Labs.

Microsonic. (1998). *Custom earmold manual* (6th ed.), Ambridge, PA . Author:

Mynders, J. (1996). Acoustic couplers. In R. Sandlin (Ed.), *Hearing Instrument Science and Fitting Practices* (pp. 351–429). Livonia, MI: National Institute for Hearing Instrument Studies.

Nolan, M., & Combe, C. (1989). In vitro considerations in the production of dimensionally accurate earmolds. I. The ear impression. *Scandinavian Audiology, 19,* 35–41.

Oliveira, R. (1997). The dynamic ear canal. In B. B. Ballachanda (Ed.), *The human ear canal* (pp. 83–111). San Diego, CA: Singular Publishing Group, Inc.

Pirzanski C. (1996). An alternative impression-taking technique: The open-jaw impression. *The Hearing Journal, 49*(11), 30, 32, 34, 35.

Pirzanski, C. (1997a). Critical factors in taking an anatomically accurate impression. *The Hearing Journal, 50*(10), 41, 44, 46–48.

Pirzanski, C. (1997b). Why is the sound intermittent? *The Hearing Review, 4*(6), 28–30, 72.

Pirzanski, C., (1998, November). *CICs: Insertion, retention, comfort and feedback control.* Paper presented at the Annual Convention of the American Speech-Language-Hearing Association, San Antonio, TX.

Pirzanski, C., Chasin, M., Klenk, M., Maye, V., & Purdy, J. (1999). Acoustic seal variables in custom earmolds. Unpublished manuscript.

Pirzanski, C., & Maye, V. (1999). *Variances in the remake rate of earmolds made of hard and soft materials.* Internal study. Canada: Starkey Labs.

Rykowski, S., Bredberg, G., & Alsterborg, E. (1991). Fitting of hearing aids. *Audionytt,* 1–2.

Staab, W. (1994). Taking impressions for deep canal hearing aid fittings. *The Hearing Journal, 47*(11), 19–28.

Staab, W., & Martin, R. (1995). Mixed-media impressions: A two-layer approach to taking ear impression. *The Hearing Journal, 48*(5), 3, 24, 27

Sweetow, R., & Valla, A. (1997). Effects of electroacoustic parameters on amplification in CIC hearing instruments. *The Hearing Review, 5*(9), 8, 12, 16, 18, 22.

Termeer, P. (1994). *Ear canal expansion using different ear impression materials.* Unpublished report. Eindhoven, The Netherlands: Philips Hearing Instruments.

Walker, G. (1979). Earphone termination and the response of behind-the-ear hearing aids. *British Journal of Audiology, 13,* 41–46

Valente M. (1996). Options: Earhooks, tubing, and earmolds. In M. Valente, M. Valente, G. Potts, & S. Lybarger, (Eds.), *Hearing aids: Standards, options, and limitations* (pp 252–327). New York: Thieme Medical Publishers, Inc.

CHAPTER 5

Principles of High-Fidelity Hearing Aid Amplification

MEAD C. KILLION, PH.D.
LAUREL A. CHRISTENSEN, PH.D.

OUTLINE

The 20th century has seen the emergenc of many technologies related to the amplification of sound for the listener with hearing impairment. These technologies have ranged from a turn-of-the-century, nonelectric ear trumpet to the fully digital hearing aid of the 1990s. To determine if recent hearing aid technologies (e.g., wide dynamic range compression and digital signal processing) provide more benefit to the listener than older technologies, Bentler and Duve (1997) examined hearing aid processing strategies over the last 50 years, as well as an ear trumpet from the turn of the century. The specific technologies evaluated included (1) an 1800's ear trumpet or speaking tube, (2) a linear hearing aid from the 1930s with peak clipping to limit output (body aid), (3) a hearing aid using wide dynamic range compression only in the high frequencies (K-amp™), (4) a two-channel wide dynamic range compression hearing aid (ReSound™), (5) a digital signal processing (DSP) hearing aid from Oticon (Digifocus™), and (6) a DSP hearing aid from Widex (Senso™). Speech recognition was assessed in quiet and in noise at multiple presentation levels. Figure 5–1 shows the speech recognition results in quiet at two presentation levels (58 and 78 dB SPL). The modern technologies, K-amp, ReSound, and the two DSP hearing aids, performed essentially equally at the two levels. In addition, the performance levels were high for these modern technologies with average scores ranging from 76 to 83% for both presentation levels using the CUNY Sentence Test (Levitt & Neuman, 1990). The older technologies, linear processing with peak clipping (body aid) and the speaking tube, did not perform as well. The nonelectric speaking tube did not provide enough gain for the low input level (58 dB SPL), and the linear hearing aid, which distorted due to peak clipping at the 78 dB SPL input level, showed reduced performance at that level.

The good performance of modern instruments comes from the fact that they have eliminated the major deficits of older designs: distortion, very narrow bandwidth, and peaks in the response. From the standpoint of word-recognition scores, it is unlikely that any further improvement can be obtained with further improvements in fidelity.

From the standpoint of sound quality, however, further improvement is possible. The requirements for optimal high fidelity are discussed below. Analog hearing aids can now meet all of these requirements, but none of today's digital hearing aids do, mostly because of a limited dynamic range (effectively 13 to 14 bits equivalent in a 16 to 18 bit high-fidelity world) and limited bandwidth (7–8 kHz in a 16 kHz world). As digital aids continue to improve, such requirements will no doubt be met.

There is one problem that cannot be solved with further increases in fidelity: the difficulty of hearing in noise. Hearing aid users typically

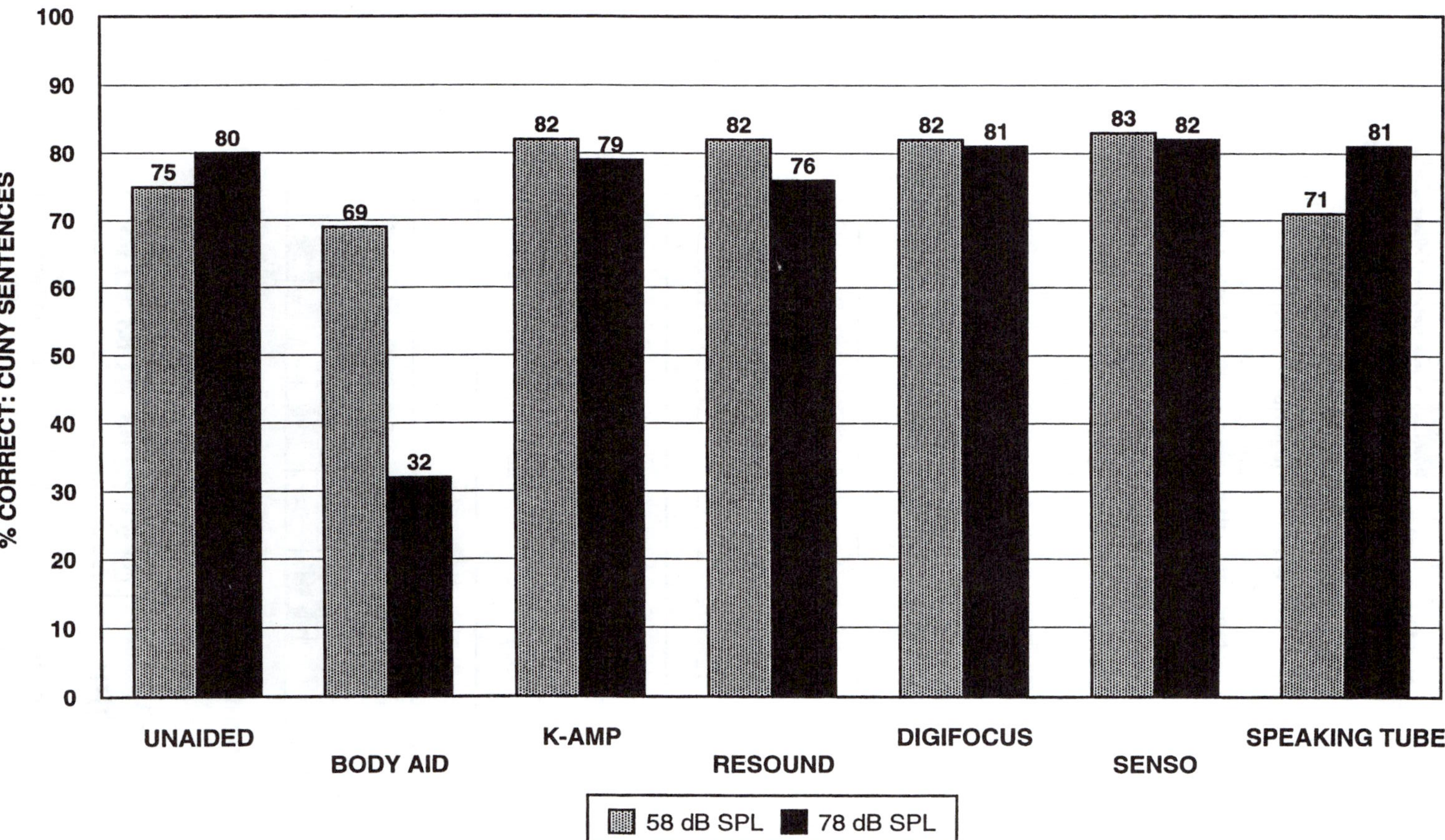

Figure 5–1. Average speech recognition scores in quiet at 58 and 78 dB SPL for the technologies evaluated in the Bentler and Duve (1997) study. (Data are from *Progression of hearing aid benefit over the twentieth century*, by R. A. Bentler and M. R. Duve, 1997, poster presented at the American Academy of Audiology Convention, Ft. Lauderdale, FL. Used with permission.)

have a 5 dB deficit in their ability to hear in noise (Killion, 1997b). Bentler and Duve (1997) tested 20 study participants with each hearing aid described above in noise at four signal-to-noise ratios (SNRs) and four presentation levels (from 55 dBSPL to 95 dB SPL). The results for the 0 dB SNR are shown in Figure 5–2. No technology provided much assistance at 0 dB SNR, although individuals with normal hearing can typically understand 30% or more of the words. Solutions to the SNR problem involve increasing the SNR directly. Methods for achieving this goal are discussed below.

THE BASIC REASONING

What Is High Fidelity?

Our first problem is to define a high-fidelity hearing aid. An object that reproduces high-fidelity sound should be acoustically and, more important, subjectively transparent. That is, listeners should receive the same auditory sensation with the high-fidelity system interposed between them and the original source of sound as they would receive listening directly to the sound.

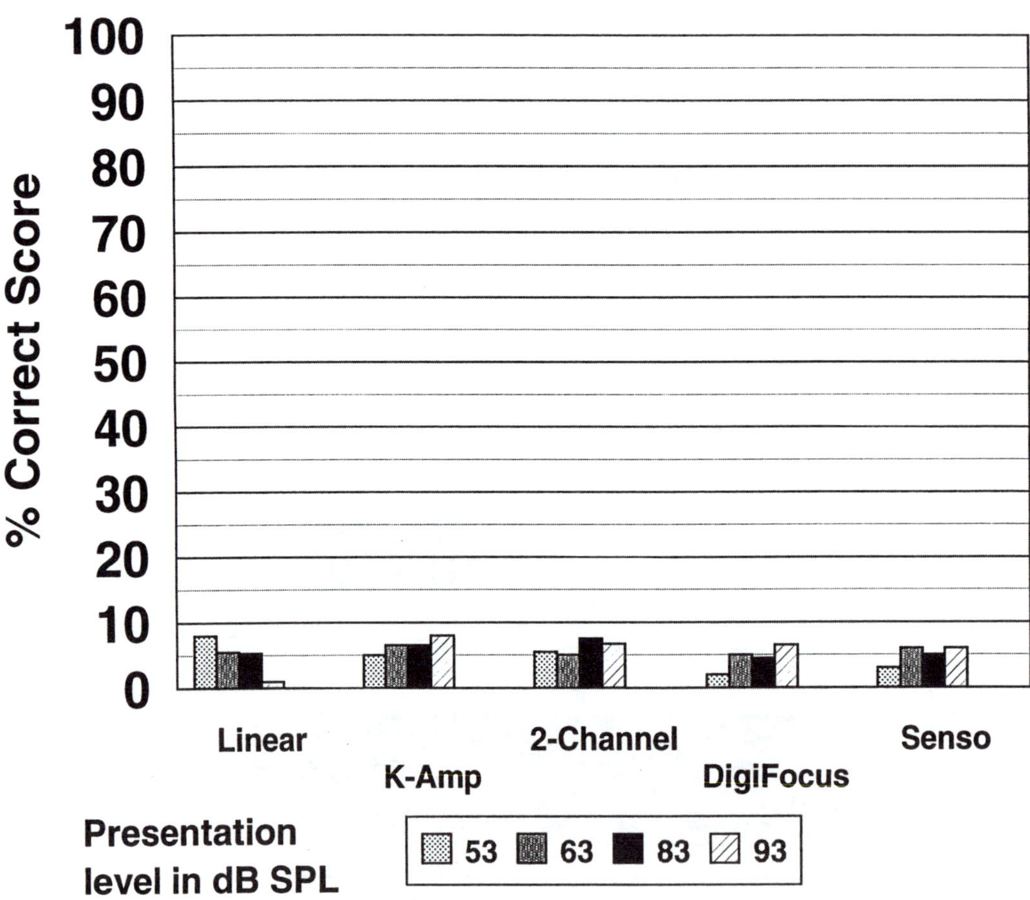

Figure 5–2. Average speech recognition scores in noise for the technologies evaluated in the Bentler and Duve (1997) study. This figure shows the results for 0 dB SNR at four presentation levels. (Data are from *Progression of hearing aid benefit over the twentieth century*, by R. A. Bentler and M. R. Duve, 1997, poster presented at the American Academy of Audiology Convention, Ft. Lauderdale, FL. Used with permission.)

Interestingly enough, if it weren't for the complications of the hearing impairment that creates the need for the hearing aid in the first place, a hearing aid worn on the head would stand a better chance of providing perfect fidelity than any other means of sound reproduction. Near-perfect subjective fidelity is difficult to achieve with recorded sound. Loudspeaker reproduction is heavily influenced by the acoustics of the listening room: Neither the directional cues nor the frequency spectrum experienced in a live concert-hall performance are preserved accurately. Headphone listening to proper binaural recordings offers the best theoretical approach, but because of the lack of head-motion cues to source localization, most listeners experience, for example, the orchestra playing in the middle of their heads. Because the hearing aid is worn in "real time," all head-motion cues to sound localization are preserved. Because the hearing aid is worn in real space, all directional cues can be preserved as well.

But hearing impairment is what creates the need for a hearing aid in the first place, and it must be accommodated. Barfod (1972) stated the goal well: "One could say that the ideal hearing prosthesis was an instrument which gave the wearer the same perception of external stimuli as a normal hearing person would have." The signal processing required to achieve this result in the regions of hearing loss may not be known or even possible, but Barfod's definition immediately suggests a direct application of the "If it ain't broke don't fix it" principle: The hearing aid should do absolutely nothing (i.e., be acoustically transparent) for sounds that fall within a region of normal hearing. In particular, this principle implies that the hearing aid should provide no amplification within a region of normal hearing.

This "don't-amplify-where-there's-no-loss" principle is well understood in the frequency domain. We know better than to use a closed earmold for individuals who have normal low-frequency hearing, for example, because they would inevitably object to the sound quality, partly because the imperfections in the hearing aid are interposed between them and the natural low-frequency sounds that they can hear quite well without the hearing aid. In addition, the closed-mold "occlusion effect" will make one's own voice sound abnormal.

This same principle has been more recently applied in the amplitude domain. Amplification is certainly necessary for quiet and moderately loud sounds. There is substantial evidence, however, that many individuals with mild or moderate hearing impairement, have normal hearing for high-level sounds. Following our don't-amplify-where-there's-no-loss principle, we conclude that whenever a person has normal or near-normal hearing for high-level sounds, the hearing aid should do absolutely nothing: It should be so acoustically transparent that it subjectively disappears. This idea was subject to much more debate in 1988 than it is today, now that wide-dynamic range compression (WDRC) circuits are common.

The term "unity acoustic gain" or simply "unity gain" (i.e., 0 dB gain) is used to describe the condition in which the hearing aid provides neither amplification nor attenuation of the incoming sound. For quiet sounds, however, a practical hearing aid must provide enough gain to make those sounds audible to an individual with a hearing loss. The amplification compensates for the loss of sensitivity to low-level sounds, or the loss of sensitivity that is measured in a threshold audiogram.

If the hearing loss for low-level sounds is frequency dependent, as in the case of what is commonly called a "sloping hearing loss," more low-level amplification may be required at some frequencies than at others. This requirement, in combination with the requirement for unity acoustic gain at some or all frequencies for high-level sounds, implies that the frequency response of the hearing aid must depend on the sound level. A WDRC circuit meets this requirement. The WDRC circuitry required to provide the variable gain and variable frequency response amplification dictated by the reasoning of the previous paragraphs should operate as unobtrusively as possible.

A Brief History of High-Fidelity Hearing Aids

A unity-gain high-fidelity sound reproduction system (as judged by listeners with normal hearing) is the sensible starting point for a high-fidelity hearing aid design, with appropriate signal processing (e.g., level-dependent gain and frequency response) added to compensate for the hearing loss. The quest for this type of high-fidelity hearing aid began in the late 1970s with the design of hearing-aid-sized microphones that were used in recording and broadcast studios. In 1979, Killion (1979a) demonstrated that hearing aids could be assembled with both objective frequency response accuracy and subjective fidelity ratings comparable to those of highly regarded loudspeaker systems. Hearing-aid earphones are now used in the ER-4 series of 16 kHz bandwidth high-fidelity earphones, which have won high praise from audiophile reviewers.

By the end of the 1970s, only two things were missing from hearing aids: a low-distortion power amplifier small enough and with a low enough battery drain to be practical for use in the smaller hearing aids and a broadcast-quality input amplifier that could handle loud voices and live orchestra concerts without distortion. Both amplifiers became a reality in tiny integrated circuit chips introduced in the late 1980s. The power amplifier is the Class-D chip developed by Etymotic Research for Knowles Electronics. The Class D amplifier will produce 110 to 115 dB maximum undistorted output, yet its internal amplifier idles at about 0.17 mA, a small fraction of the idling current of a typical hearing-aid power amplifier. The broadcast quality input amplifier was developed by Etymotic Research with the help of a $500,000 grant from the National Institute on Aging. This K-Amp™ input amplifier chip amplifies only quiet sounds (Killion, 1993). To this end, an automatic circuit operates an electronic volume control to make quiet sounds audible and a tone control to provide treble boost for quiet sounds. Loud sounds that present a problem for most hearing-aid wearers (e.g., dishes clattering, paper crunching, wind howling, people shouting) pass through without amplification just as if the hearing aid was not there. Amplification for loud sounds is available to the user if he or she chooses to use it, but it is generally not required.

Who Are the Beneficiaries?

High-fidelity hearing aids are not for everyone. There are individuals whose hearing impairment is so great that even amplified speech is not clear, especially in the presence of competing noise. Similarly, individuals with no useful high-frequency hearing will derive little benefit from wide frequency range sound reproduction (Hogan & Turner, 1998; Rankovic, 1991; Skinner, 1980). Their use may be troublesome to others because of the high-frequency feedback squeals that hearing aid users cannot hear. (One of the successful uses of low-pass filter earhooks has been high-power hearing aids and closed earmolds, for individuals with profound loss and a "corner audiogram," to eliminate the unheard-squeal problem.) Individuals with the most common hearing impairment (a mild sensorineural hearing loss that appears to be restricted to a loss of sensitivity for low-level sounds, with normal hearing for high-level sounds) are the primary beneficiaries of high-fidelity hearing aids.

The psychoacoustic and physiological evidence showing that many individuals with hearing impairment have essentially normal hearing for high-level sounds has been available for some time. Punch (1978) found no statistical difference between hearing aid sound-quality judgments obtained from 10 subjects with normal hearing and 10 subjects with sensorineural hearing loss, even though some subjects had moderate-to-severe losses at high frequencies. The subjects with sensorineural hearing loss studied by Lindblad (1982) were as good at detecting nonlinear distortion in high-level material as normal subjects were. Some of Toole's (1986) listeners had mild-to-moderate high-frequency hearing losses and still exhibited excellent relibility in their fidelity ratings of high-fidelity loudspeakers.

Steinberg and Gardner discussed such individuals in 1937, when they observed that many of those with impaired hearing had essentially normal hearing for high-intensity sounds, but a loss of normal sensitivity for low-intensity sounds. This phenomenon is commonly referred to as loudness recruitment. Figure 5–3 (Scharf, 1978) illustrates this phenomenon for a "typical listener with a 40 dB hearing loss due to a cochlear impairment."

A substantial amount of evidence has accumulated since the Steinberg and Gardner study to indicate that many (but not all) individuals with mild-to-moderate cochlear impairments may have essentially normal high-level hearing. In addition to pure-tone loudness per-

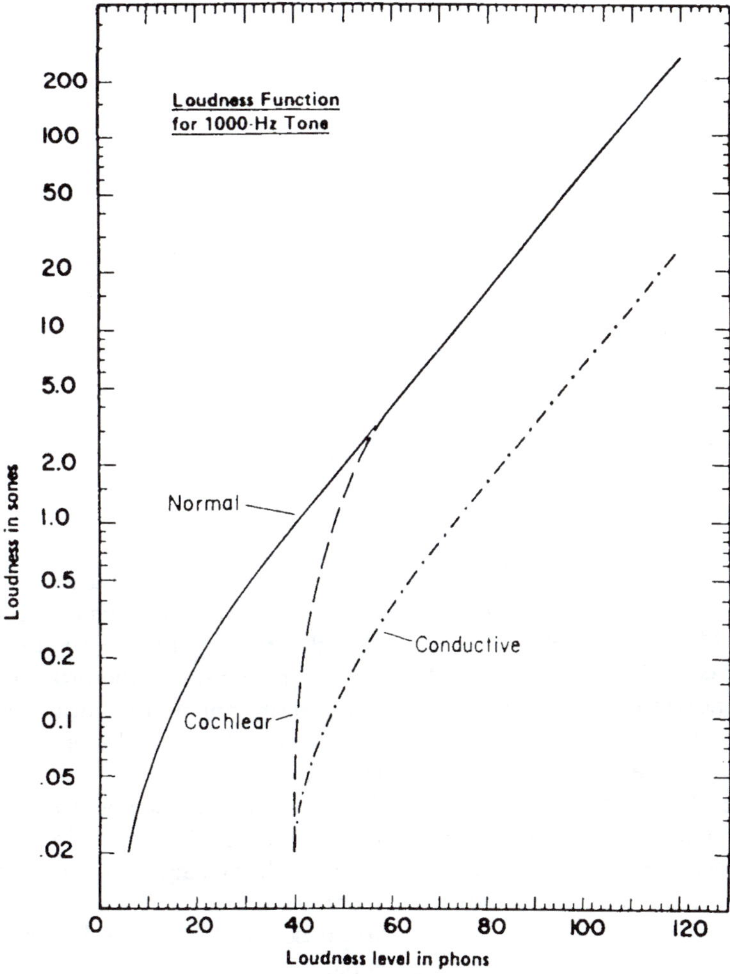

Figure 5–3. Loudness of a 1000 Hz tone as a function of loudness level for a normal listener, a typical listener with a cochlear impairment (and recruitment), and the typical listener with a conductive impairment. (From "A model of loudness. A summation applied to impaired ears," by B. Scharf, 1978, *Journal of the Acoustical Society of America, 40*, 71–78. Reprinted with permission.)

ception, the following attributes of hearing have been found to be within normal limits at sufficiently high-intensity levels, even in the presence of mild-to-moderate cochlear impairment:

1. Frequency selectivity as determined from the "Fletcher Critical Band" that can be inferred from tone-in-noise masking experiments (Jerger, Tillman, & Peterson, 1960; Palva, Goodman, & Hirsh, 1953)
2. Frequency selectivity as determined from psychophysical tuning curves (McGee, 1978)
3. Frequency discrimination (dF) (Gengel, 1973)
4. Loudness summation for complex sounds (with cochlear impairment below 50 dB) (Scharf and Hellman, 1966)
5. Loudness discrimination (dlI) (Scharf, 1978)
6. Localization abilities (see the summary given by Scharf, 1978)

In addition to the psychophysical data, recent evidence indicates that the high-level electrical potentials in the cochlea can be normal in some cases of mild cochlear impairment. The whole-nerve action potential recorded in laboratory animals (Wang & Dallos, 1972) or recorded from the ear canal in humans (Berlin & Gondra, 1976) is often normal. Indeed, both the wave form and latency of the entire auditory brainstem-evoked response may appear entirely normal at high levels in some individuals. Similarly, data obtained on laboratory animals with drug-induced outer hair cell damage (Dallos et al., 1977) indicate that it is possible to have normal bandwidth for both the psychophysical tuning curve and the classical single-unit tuning curve obtained from fibers of the auditory nerve.

A discussion of the physiology of hearing impairment is beyond the scope of this chapter, but the function of the outer hair cells may be to improve the low-level sensitivity of the ear, while the primary function of audition appears to rest on the inner hair cells. Postmortem hair-cell counts on patients with hearing impairment who had good speech recognition in noise typically show hair-cell loss restricted to outer hair cells. Thus, the loss of outer hair cells may permit normal or near-normal hearing for high-level sounds as long as most of the inner hair cells function properly.

Adaptation and Good Counseling

Even today, any observant dispenser realizes that the most important factor in a successful hearing aid fitting may have nothing to do with the aid's electroacoustic characteristics. Given appropriate counseling and an established trust between the individual with hearing impairment and the dispenser, any hearing aid that makes previously unheard sounds audible can provide a successful fitting. The old advice, "wear it a few weeks and you'll get used to it," is as true—and as useful—today as ever.

The process of "getting used to it" can be so successful that a change in the hearing aid creates a problem. Anyone servicing hearing aids is familiar with complaints that may result from restoring the frequency response of a damaged hearing aid to its original configuration, and from the use of "loaner" hearing aids during an extended repair period (Goldberg, 1965). Even when the general frequency responses of the original and loaner aid appear similar, it is not uncommon for a user to complain initially of difficulty understanding speech only to find that after a 2- or 3-week period, the loaner seems much better than the repaired original aid.

Even when change is ostensibly an improvement, it may not be welcome. Smoothing the response (i.e., by adding damping to the earmold tubing) for a long-time hearing aid wearer can result in a negative evaluation. Similarly, a low-distortion hearing aid may not sound loud enough to a user accustomed to hearing the severe distortion products that accompanied overload in an old peak-clipping hearing aid. The extraordinary ability of humans to adapt to even badly degraded sensory inputs has been a merciful boon to many hearing aid wearers but can cause unmerciful trouble to the conscientious dispenser. The success of hearing aids decades ago, when the best that could be done in terms of sound quality, intelligibility, and convenience was poor indeed, attests to the ability of the central nervous system to adapt.

High-fidelity hearing aids as described in this chapter are available today to the hearing aid user. Although these devices have been available for 10 years, how these aids differ from traditional linear amplification is still often misunderstood. In the next section, the design guidelines for high-fidelity amplification will be reviewed. We feel this review is important to understand the capability of high-fidelity amplification and the limitations of hearing aids that do not meet these desired design guidelines.

DESIGN GUIDELINES FOR HIGH-FIDELITY HEARING AIDS

In this section, we provide engineering guidelines for the design of hearing aids that can be reasonably expected to be judged as high fidelity by those with mild or moderate hearing impairment.

Frequency Response Guidelines

Recall that, at high levels, the hearing aid should deliver the same sound pressure to the listener's eardrum—at all frequencies and for all angles of incidence of the original sound—that he or she would receive without the hearing aid interposed. This requires consideration of the relationship between the sound pressure in a sound field and that found at the normal unaided eardrum.

Nature provides each of us with a natural hearing aid in the form of external-ear resonances and "horn" action, which combine to produce substantially greater eardrum sound-pressure levels than those present in an oncoming sound field. At the roughly 2.7 kHz resonance frequency of the outer ear, the gain amounts to 15 to 20 dB (Wiener & Ross, 1946).

The pressure at the microphone inlet of a head-worn hearing aid, on the other hand, will generally be only about 5 dB greater than that in the sound field, depending somewhat on the exact location of the microphone (Kuhn & Burnett, 1977; Madaffari, 1974). Thus, the hearing aid must provide some 10 to 15 dB of acoustic gain in the 2.7 kHz frequency area to compensate for the gain provided by the external ear before it was blocked by the plastic earmold. In contrast, little compensation is required at low frequencies where the eardrum pressure and the pressure available to the hearing aid microphone are essentially the same.

Insertion gain is the ratio of eardrum pressure produced by a hearing aid to the eardrum pressure produced without the hearing aid (Dalsgaard & Jensen, 1974). Expressed in dB, the insertion gain of a hearing aid is the difference between aided and unaided eardrum sound-pressure levels. At high levels, the hearing aid should have 0 dB insertion gain at all frequencies (a flat insertion gain frequency response).

Coupler Response for Flat Insertion Gain

For engineering purposes, the required frequency response tailoring is best defined in terms of the coupler response of the hearing aid. In addition to the factors discussed above (loss of external-ear resonance effects and hearing aid microphone location), the *CO*upler *R*esponse for a *F*lat *I*nsertion *G*ain (CORFIG) curve will be influenced by the choice of couplers, the selection of reference sound-field conditions, and differences among individuals in terms of their external ear resonances, eardrum impedances, and so forth.

A great deal of simplification is provided if we ignore individual differences and choose a manikin of average anthropometric dimensions and a coupler ("occluded-ear simulator") that approximates the acoustic impedance of an average ear. The KEMAR manikin (Burkhard & Sachs, 1975) meets the first requirement, while the modified Zwislocki (1970) coupler meets the second requirement up to 7 or 8 kHz (Sachs & Burkhard, 1972). Unpublished experiments comparing eardrum-pressure response on real ears to the response measured in the Zwislocki coupler were conducted at Etymotic Research during the development of the ER-4 16 kHz bandwidth high-fidelity earphone. These experiments indicated that the Zwislocki coupler provides a reasonably good representation of the ear in the 8 to 16 kHz region.

Figure 5–4 shows the Zwislocki-coupler CORFIG curves from Killion and Monser (1980) for three microphone locations and three sound-field reference conditions, based on measurements with a KEMAR manikin. The inset drawings illustrate the three different locations for the microphone inlet, for OTE (behind the ear), ITE (in the ear), and CIC (completely in canal) hearing aids. The curves for the ITE aid were obtained for a microphone inlet approximately flush with the plane of the pinna because at the time the data were obtained, most ITE aids filled the entire concha. (Throughout this chapter, we will use the term OTE to mean a behind-the-ear case in which the microphone is located over, and not behind, the ear.)

The Role of the Pinna

As illustrated in Figure 5–4, the exact shape of the CORFIG curve generally depends on the direction from which the sound is coming. The effect of the pinna flange, for example, is to increase eardrum pressure by a few dB at high frequencies for sounds arriving from the front and to reduce substantially the eardrum pressure for high-frequency sounds arriving from the rear "due to interference between the direct wave and a scattered wave from the edge of the pinna flange" (Shaw, 1974). For microphone locations outside the pinna, such as the BTE, forward-looking-inlet location discussed above, little of this directional dependence is contained in the sound available to the microphone. This loss was graphically illustrated in the data of Berland and Nielsen (1969), who compared the sound pressure available to microphones located behind, over, and in the ear for sound fields at six angles of incidence.

Even when the microphone is in an ITE hearing aid, the presence of the earmold filling the concha substantially reduces the effectiveness of the pinna. Only when the microphone inlet is located directly in front of the blocked ear-canal entrance, as with a CIC construction, are the directional effects preserved in their entirety.

With regard to auditory localization, it is clear than any of the microphone locations used in binaural, head-worn hearing aids will preserve the basic interaural time and intensity difference so important to binaural localization (Licklider, 1949) and the changes in interaural phase and intensity caused by head motion that are so important to the externalization of the sound (Wallach, 1940). What is not so clear is the relative importance of the pinna and concha to everyday localization, auditory spatial perception, and the binaural squelching of noise and reverberation.

Informal experiments (such as taping the pinna tightly to the side of the head) have provided some evidence that the pinna and concha provide relatively weak cues to localization, compared to those provided by head movement and interaural time and intensity differences. Such a conclusion is consistent with anecdotal evidence indicating that many individuals who need artificial pinnae wear them only on social occasions, that is, primarily for cosmetic reasons.

Reference Sound-Field Condition

As Figure 5–4 indicates, it is impossible to design a conventional ITE or BTE aid that will have a perfectly flat frequency response for the user (i.e., an insertion gain that is frequency independent) at all angles of incidence. The

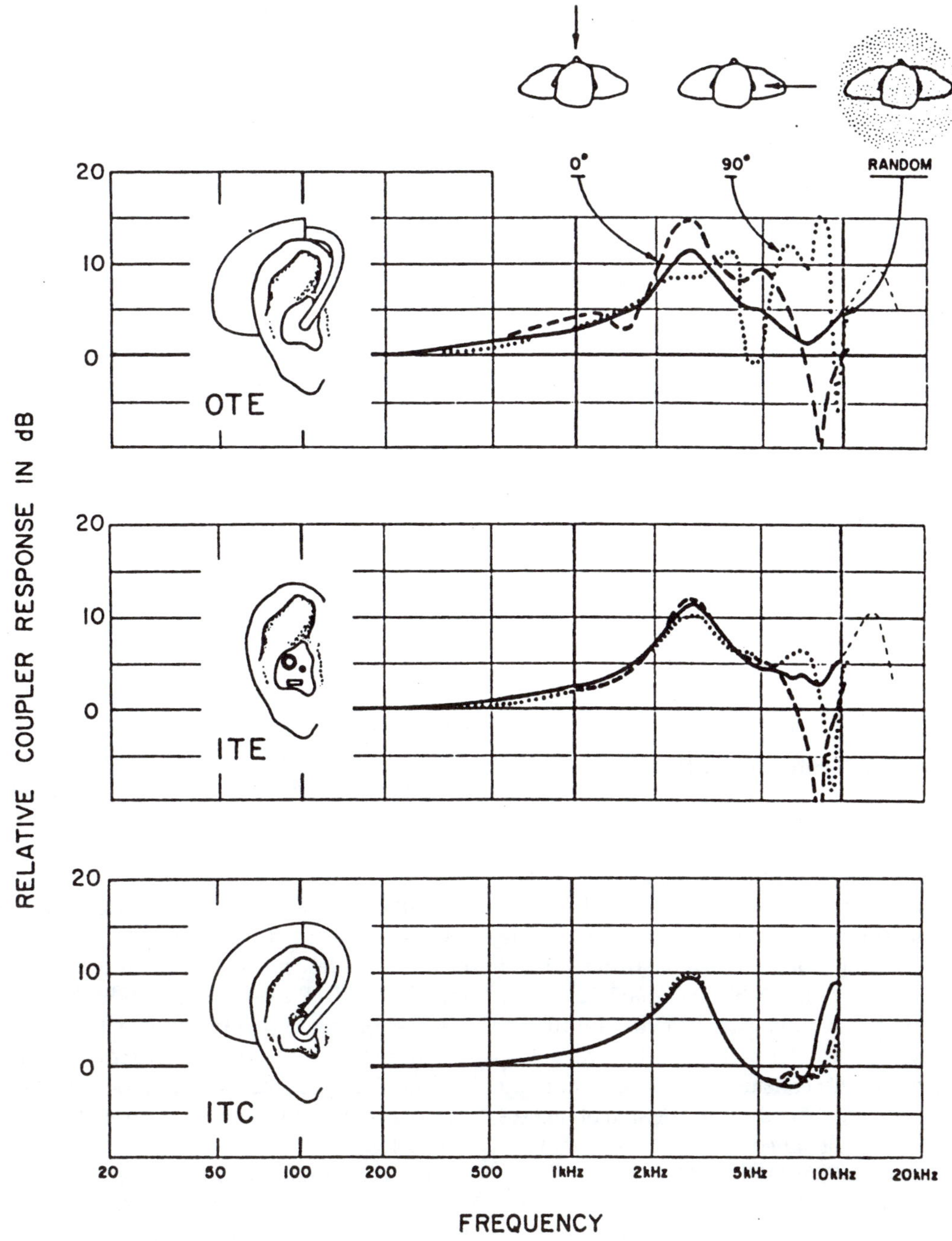

Figure 5–4. Required Zwislocki coupler response to produce flat insertion gain (CORFIG) for OTE, ITE, and CIC hearing aids under three sound field conditions. Note that only the CIC CORFIG is essentially independent of where the sound is coming from. (From *Acoustical Factors Affecting Hearing and Performance* by M. C. Killion and E. L. Munser, 1980, Baltimore, MD: Park Press. Copyright 1980. Reprinted with permission.)

acoustical effects of the unencumbered outer ear are not duplicated in either of the microphone configurations. Where speech discrimination in face-to-face (near-field condition) listening situations is the only consideration, the appropriate reference condition might be a 0°-incidence sound wave.

Where sound quality is the dominant criterion, other considerations apply. In home and concert listening, the reflected energy substantially exceeds the energy arriving directly from the sound source (Olson, 1967). Under those circumstances, the appropriate design compromise for a high-fidelity hearing aid would appear to be a flat insertion gain for random-incidence sound. This conclusion is consistent with the results of the psychoacoustic experiments reported by Schulein (1975).

The CIC aid requires no compromise between conflicting frequency response requirements because the coupler response that provides a flat insertion gain response for 0°-incidence sound provides a flat insertion gain response for all angles (and thus, trivially, for random-incidence sound as shown in Figure 5–4).

Bandwidth Requirements

After considering the available information on (a) hearing sensitivity and frequency limits of hearing for typical listeners, (b) measurements of the discomfort level of sound, (c) measurements of room noise in a wide variety of locations, and (d) measurements of the frequency limits in the maximum and minimum levels of speech, orchestral music, and various instruments of the orchestra, Fletcher (1942) concluded that "substantially complete fidelity in the transmission of orchestral music is obtained by use of a system having a volume range of 65 dB and a frequency range from 60 to 8000 cycles per second." Olson (1957) concluded that "the reproduction of orchestral music with perfect fidelity requires a frequency range of 40 to 14,000 cycles and a volume range of 70 dB." Both judgments were based on similar data, primarily those of Snow (1931), and the differences reflected the level of fidelity required. Snow's listeners gave a judged quality rating slightly in excess of 90% to a system in which the frequency range extended from 60 Hz to 8000 Hz, compared to unrestricted range reproduction. With a 40 Hz to 14,000 Hz range, the quality rating was close to 100%. Tests reported by Muraoka, Iwahara, and Yamada (1981) on the audio bandwidth requirements for unlimited digital recordings indicated that only with a 14 kHz cutoff frequency (but not with a 16, 18, or 20 kHz cutoff) could any of their listeners reliably detect the bandwidth restriction.

A frequency response extending from 60 Hz to 8000 Hz thus appears to be a reasonable goal for a high-fidelity hearing aid. This was confirmed in fidelity rating experiments undertaken by Killion in which three panels of listening judges (25 "man-on-the-street" listeners, 5 "golden ear" listeners, and 6 trained listeners) each rated a pair of experimental OTE aids with 8 kHz bandwidth as being comparable in fidelity to a pair of good studio monitor loudspeakers with 20 kHz bandwidth. (Figure 5–5, shows their frequency response curves, labled OTE and MS, respectively. The irregularity in the frequency response of the loudspeakers was apparently judged to be as important a defect as the 8 kHz bandwidth limitation of the BTE aids.) The 8-kHz-bandwidth hearing aids were rated *much* higher in fidelity than a pair of "Popular headPhones" (Koss PRO-4AA) in which exaggerated bass and treble response has been widely noted. The good fidelity ratings for the BTE aids held up under four different selections of program material, as shown in Figure 5–6, including a piano trio selection chosen because the drummer's brush-on-cymbal sound provided substantial energy above 10 kHz.

From these data, it appears reasonable to conclude that restricting the bandwidth of a hearing aid to 8 kHz, or perhaps a bit less, is not likely to be an important limitation to high-fidelity sound reproduction as judged by the hearing aid wearer. Of course, there is no harm in approaching perfection, and a 16 kHz bandwidth is also practical as demonstrated by the experimental ITE aids whose fidelity ratings are also shown in Figure 5–6.

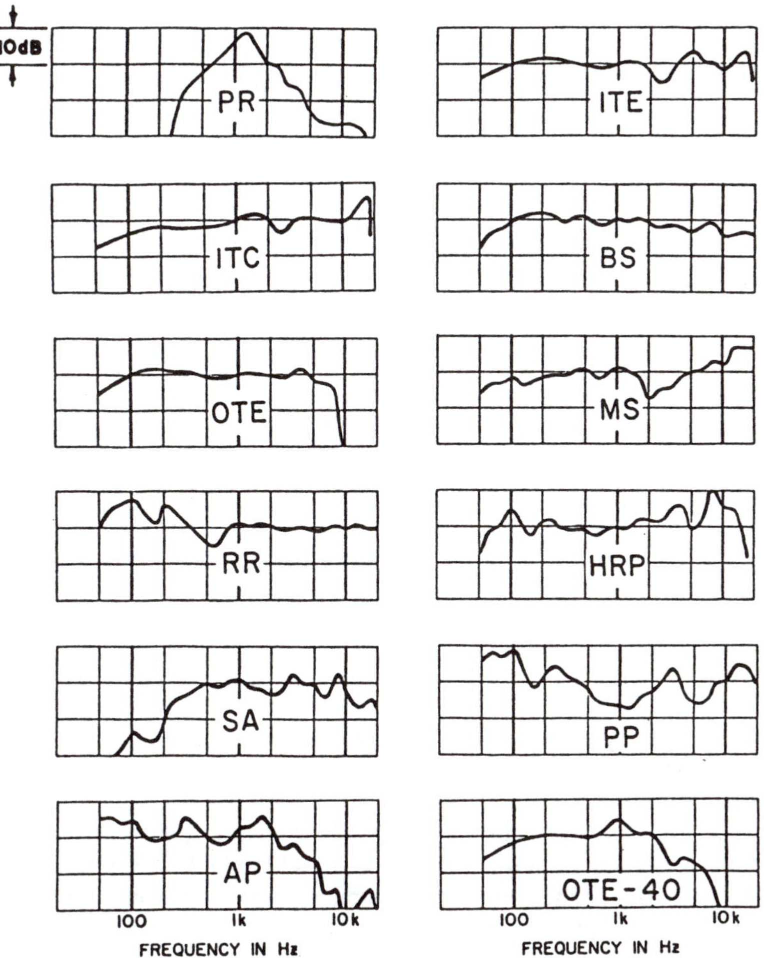

Figure 5–5. Fidelity ratings obtained with different program materials for experimental ITE hearing aids; experimental OTE hearing aids; Electro Voice Sentry V Studio Monitor Speakers (MS); Koss PRO-4AA Popular Choice Phones (PP); Simulated Speech Audiometer with TDH-39 earphones (SA); K-MART special $69.95 "High Fidelity" Discount Stereo (DS); GE $4.95 Pocket Radio in overload (PR).

Even when high-level hearing is not completely normal, informal experiments conducted by Gudmundsen and Killion, using a high-fidelity loudspeaker playing a piano trio recording, indicated that 12 of 14 hearing aid wearers could hear the difference between a 16 kHz bandwidth and the 4 to 5 kHz bandwidth typical of many aids. For these tests, the participants removed their hearing aids and the level was set for 85 dB SPL, which is typical of nightclubs. Of the 12 participants who could tell the difference, 2 preferred the narrower bandwidth. The 10 who preferred the wideband sound placed a dollar value of $20 to $10,000 on the wider bandwidth, with a median value of $100.

Response Smoothness

The question of how irregular the frequency response may be before it has a noticeable effect on fidelity has not been as well studied as the effect of restricting the frequency range.

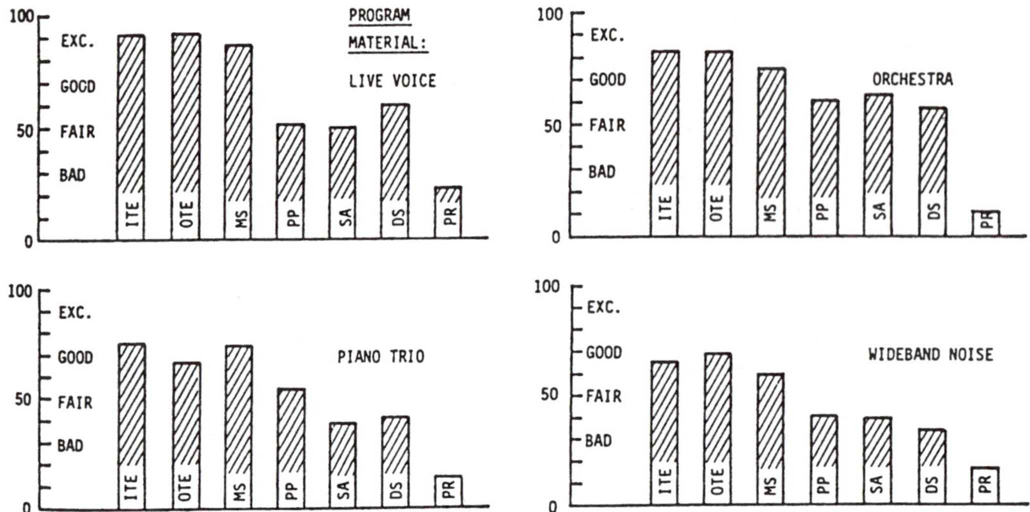

Figure 5–6. Comparison between average subjective fidelity (similarity) ratings and calculated 25-band accuracy scores for 12 systems rated on three identical program selections (orchestra, piano trio, male voice). Fidelity ratings obtained for a +3 dB shift in level as the only difference between the comparison and the reference are plotted as open symbols.

Bucklein (1962) studied the effect of, among other things, 10 and 20 dB peaks and dips at 3.2 kHz in an otherwise flat-response transmission system. The peaks and dips used appeared fairly sharp, with an apparent 3 dB bandwidth of roughly 10% of the center frequency. He found that 100% of his observers could detect both the 10 and 20 dB peak, but less than half could detect the 20 dB dip; only 10% could recognize the 10 dB dip. Flanagan (1957), in a study of the difference limen for formant amplitude, found that a change of 3 dB in the amplitude of the second formant can be detected approximately 50% of the time.

Toole (1981, 1984, 1986) published the findings from 10 years of investigation into high-fidelity loudspeakers (and high fidelity in general). He observed (personal communication) that the loudspeakers that receive the highest fidelity ratings exhibit frequency responses lying within a ±1.5 dB tolerance from 100 Hz to 1 kHz, widening to about ±3 dB between 1 and 2 kHz, and then +1.5/−3 dB from 2 kHz to 10 kHz.

From all these results, it seems reasonable to infer that a response irregularity in a high-fidelity system of approximately 3 dB can be detected under appropriate conditions when the source material is speech but is not likely to be objectionable. Even much larger response irregularities have been found to be minimally objectionable (Dillon & Macrae, 1984) or even preferable (Cox & Gilmore, 1986) under some experimental conditions.

Accuracy Scores

Is there a way to reliably estimate directly from the frequency response curve what the fidelity rating would be if an extensive (and expensive) listening test was performed? With some limitations, the answer appears to be yes. A procedure based on loudness calculations was adopted some time ago by Consumers Union (CU) for rating the frequency response accuracy of high-fidelity loudspeakers (*Consumer Reports*, 1977). With this procedure, the loudspeakers are driven with a wideband "pink" noise (equal energy in each one-third-octave band) at an overall level adjusted to produce a calculated loudness (Stevens, 1972) of 88 sones, equivalent to a level of 90 PLdB "Perceived Loudness" in the 110 to 14,000 Hz frequency range. In each of the 21 one-third-octave bands in that range, the loudness in sones corresponding to the total sound power output of the loudspeaker in that band is calculated and compared to the sones calculated for a theoretically perfect loudspeaker producing exactly 74 dB SPL in that band. (A 74 dB SPL in each of those 21 bands produces a calculated loudness of 88 sones.) A percentage accuracy is then calculated from the deviations from perfection, averaged over the 21 bands. For purposes of the accuracy calculations, the individual band deviations from perfection are obtained by subtracting the ratio of measured to ideal sones from 1.0 (perfection), and then subtracting the absolute value of that difference from 1.0. Thus, a measured power equivalent to either .5 or 1.5 times the ideal loudness would produce a 50% accuracy score for that band. For example, a loudspeaker with a perfectly flat "power response" everywhere except for a 7 dB drop-off (half loudness) in the 125-Hz band would have a calculated accuracy score of (50 + 20 × 100)/21 = 98%. For our purposes, the accuracy score described above will be called the "21-band accuracy score" to distinguish it from a "25-band accuracy score" discussed below.

The 21-band accuracy scores obtained at that time by Consumers Union on 16 models of low-priced ($100 to $200 per pair) high-fidelity loudspeakers ranged between 63% and 93%, with a median value of 80%. Listening tests were said to have borne out the utility of the accuracy scores, although CU stated that "experience has taught us that a group of listeners won't readily agree on which of two speakers is more accurate when the speakers' scores differ by eight points or less" (*Consumers Reports*, 1977).

The general utility of the accuracy score as an indication of the fidelity rating to be expected from a sound system that has no defects other than frequency response inaccuracies (i.e., which doesn't buzz, crackle, or otherwise audibly distort) was confirmed in listening test experiments (Killion, 1979a). Figure 5–7

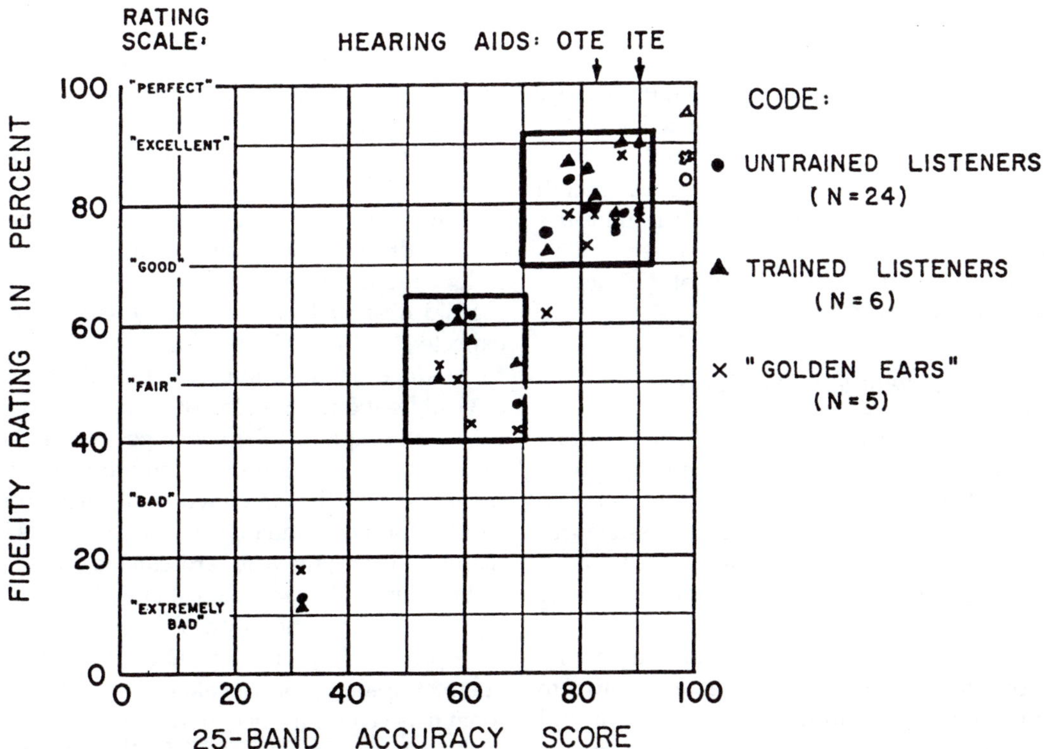

Figure 5–7. Frequency responses of sound systems used in complete listening tests and compared to calculated accuracy scores in Figure 5–6.

shows a comparison between fidelity rating and calculated 25-band accuracy score (the four one-third-octave bands below 125 Hz were added to the calculations) for a variety of loudspeakers, earphones, and hearing aids that were all rated on the same three selections of program material: orchestra, piano trio, and live voice.

A more detailed look at some examples is useful. The frequency response of six of the tested sound systems is shown in Figure 5–5. The insertion gain frequency response of the ITE aids shows a one-half-octave dip of about 4 dB at 2.7 kHz (due to insufficient compensation for the loss of external-ear resonance "hearing aid"), and a broad peak of about 3 dB at 5 kHz. This resulted in a calculated 21-band accuracy score of 91% and an average fidelity rating (for those three program selections) of 82%. The experimental CIC aids had a dip in their insertion gain response of only 3 dB at 2.7 kHz and a smooth boost of 2 dB at about 1.5 kHz. This resulted in a calculated accuracy score of 92% and an average fidelity rating (same program materials) of 86%. The studio monitor loudspeakers had a dip of 8 dB in their listening-room response at 2 kHz (the crossover frequency between the woofer and horn tweeter), with a calculated accuracy score of 83% and a fidelity rating of 80%. Finally, the BTE aids had an extremely smooth frequency response, with an 8 kHz high-frequency cutoff as their only real defect. This resulted in an accuracy score of 82% and a fidelity rating of 79%.

Individual Variation in Ears

If a separate hearing aid were to be designed for each user, it would presumably be possible to take into account individual eccentricities in external-ear ("ear canal") resonances and eardrum impedances. To be economically practical, however, a high-fidelity hearing aid design must be based on average data. Under those circumstances, individual variations in outer-ear resonance and eardrum impedance may cause the (insertion) gain and the (insertion gain) frequency response of a hearing aid to deviate substantially from the design average in a given individual.

An estimate of the individual differences in outer-ear resonance was provided in the data of Filler, Ross, and Wiener (1945). In that report, individual sound-field-to-eardrum pressure curves for 12 male and 2 female subjects were given, which can be compared to the overall average curves for the same subjects shown by Wiener and Ross (1946). The standard deviation of the individual curves (from the average curve) ranged from 1 to 2 dB below 1800 Hz up to 4 to 7 dB in the 5 to 8 kHz region with peaks at 2.1 and 3.3 kHz. The peak deviations occurred mostly because individual external-ear resonance frequencies were lower or higher than average. No individual eardrum-pressure-level curve deviated more than 7.5 dB from the average curve below 5 kHz, but the majority deviated by at least 5 dB at some frequency below 5 kHz.

As part of a study leading to a validation of the modified Zwislocki coupler, Sachs and Burkhard (1972) reported the probe-tube-microphone measurement of the sound pressures developed in 11 ears (6 male and 5 female subjects) by subminiature hearing-aid earphones. The standard deviation of the level of pressure that developed ranged from approximately 1 dB at 1 kHz to 5 dB in the 6 to 8 kHz range. Greater pressure levels were developed in female ears (by 3–5 dB at the higher frequencies).

While the variations in outer-ear resonance and eardrum impedance are only partially independent variables, it is clear that no hearing aid designed for the average ear can be expected, in the majority of individual cases, to produce an insertion gain that does not have at least one deviation of perhaps 7 dB at the worst frequency. Some perspective can be obtained from Killion's listening-test experiment in which the "large red ears" were substituted for the "standard ears" on the KEMAR manikin. Using the standard ears as the perfect reference, the large ears obtained an average fidelity rating of only 81%. (Perspective is also provided by noting that relocating a "perfect" pair of loudspeakers in a listening room may change the one-third-octave response at the listening position sufficiently to reduce a 21-band accuracy rating from 100% to 85 to 90% area.)

The subjective importance of such response inaccuracies to a long-term hearing-aid wearer has not been studied, although it is known that even larger deviations in unaided frequency response can occur due to the accumulation of ear wax in the canal in which the onset is so gradual that changes often go unnoticed until the canal becomes almost completely blocked. In most cases, it thus seems reasonable to assume that satisfactory adaptation to a slightly inaccurate insertion gain frequency response will make it unnecessary to provide modification for individual eccentricities.

There are now data on the question of individual differences. Palmer (1991) studied the importance of having the hearing aid match the individual ear's response using subjects who had normal ear-canal resonances (REUR, real-ear unaided response) and normal eardrum impedance (RECD, real-ear-coupler difference); normal REUR and abnormal RECD; and abnormal REUR and normal RECD. Each subject judged quality and intelligibility while listening to a frequency response that matched the ear-canal resonance (REUR) only, matched the eardrum impedance (RECD) only, matched both, or matched KEMAR's REUR and RECD. She found that people who were different from average, but not too different, preferred the tailored response to their own ear. People who had substantially deviant REUR or RECD preferred the average (KEMAR-based) response. The individuals with dramatically collapsed canals, for example, preferred the average response.

All things considered, a reasonable goal for the smoothness of the frequency response of a high-fidelity hearing aid would thus appear to be an accuracy score of 80% as measured on the KEMAR manikin. Such a hearing aid would have a calculated accuracy score equal to or better than half the $100–$200-per-pair loudspeakers tested in 1977 by Consumers Union. A more stringent goal would be a 21-band accuracy score equal to the median (89%) of the expensive ($600–$1,000 per pair) "state of the art" loudspeakers tested in 1978 by Consumers Reports. In either case, the response accuracy goal would presumably apply only to the idealized "average" hearing-aid wearer.

Amplitude Response Requirements

Although the distinctions are somewhat arbitrary, we generally think of the dynamic range of a sound system (between its maximum undistorted output levels and its noise levels), its nonlinear distortion (harmonic and intermodulation), and any automatic gain control (AGC) functions as taking place in the amplitude or intensity domain. Some amplitude-domain performance requirements imposed on a high-fidelity hearing aid are discussed below.

Peak Output Levels

There is no easy answer to the question of what the maximum undistorted output of a wearable unity-gain sound reproduction system should be. If the peak outputs of rock music played at a discotheque are to be reproduced, a 130 dB SPL capability may be required (R.W. Peters, personal communication). A similar capability would be required to reproduce the peak levels produced by some aircraft and industrial noise sources. As summarized by Miller (1974), however, such levels are hazardous to the hearing mechanism.

Speech and Everyday Sounds

In everyday conversational settings, the highest levels at the hearing aid microphone will normally be generated by the user's own speech. The data of Dunn and Farnsworth (1939) indicate that the overall speech levels measured at the talker's ear were about equal to the levels 30 cm in front of his or her lips. Thus, the Dunn and White (1940) data on instantaneous peak levels in speech measured at 30 cm may be used directly. For normal conversational speech, instantaneous speech peaks of 90 to 95 dB SPL occur with some regularity (in 1 to 5% of one-eighth-second intervals). (Due to the head-shadow effect, the high frequencies will be attenuated somewhat, but since the majority of the peak energy lies below 1000 Hz, this will have little effect on the overall peak levels.) Unless the conversation becomes agitated, therefore, the instantaneous peak levels at the microphone will be 90 to 95 dB SPL, a range that has often been used as the goal for the level of minimum undistorted input in hearing-aid design. If the conversation becomes agitated, a shout or forceful expletive can easily produce 100 to 105 dB instantaneous peak SPL at the microphone of the speaker's own hearing aid. The first author, a far-from-professional singer, can still sing a high "A" that has produced a 112 dB instantaneous peak SPL at the microphone of a head-worn hearing aid that was wired to an oscilliscope.

Other commonly encountered sounds, such as the clack of a typewriter key or a finger snap at arm's length, can also produce a 100 to 110 dB instantaneous peak SPL. A spoon dropped onto a plate can produce a 110 to 115 dB instantaneous peak SPL.

Live Music

In live performances of classical music, Marsh (1975) reported that in a good main-floor seat in Chicago's Orchestra Hall, "a fully scored orchestral passage in a Mendelssohn symphony reaches approximately 95 dB on a decibel meter." Marsh reported that approximately the same levels are reached during a similar passage in the front benches at outdoor amphitheaters such as Grant Park, or at the edge of the Ravinia stage. The typical instantaneous peak factor for an orchestral passage of this sort is 5 to 10 dB, indicating instantaneous peaks of 100 to 105 dB SPL at these three Chicago-area locations. Similarly, for a typical listening position in a large music hall, Olson (1967) reported the instantaneous peak sound pressure level as 100 dB SPL.

During the last 5 years, one of the authors has regularly carried a sound level meter (SLM) to concerts. The Chicago Symphony Orchestra has produced a peak SLM reading of 104 dB on the A scale during a Mahler symphony, measured in a seventh-row, center balcony seat. (At the other extreme, the quietest piano passage in Strauss's Burlesque for Piano and Orchestra in D Minor was 35 dBA. The same 35 dBA level was measured on a solo viola in Elgin and Payne Symphony No. 3. Rapid SLM reading changes of 40 to 50 dB are not uncommon.

Surprisingly high decibel levels are even encountered at audiological parties where bands are playing. Levels of 95 dB are common. At the 1999 opening night party of the American Academy of Audiology Convention, held on the beach, the levels in the dance area ranged from 108 to 112 dBA. At a Chicago blues bar, levels of 110 to 114 dBA are not uncommon.

All things considered, an undistorted input capability of 115 dB instantaneous peak SPL—referred to the sound field—appears to be a reasonable minimum requirement for a high-fidelity hearing aid intended for use at live concerts.

What is also needed for our present purposes, however, is information on the peak output levels required of the hearing aid earphone. This requires consideration not only of the frequency distribution of peak levels in music but also consideration of the increased eardrum pressure levels normally produced by external-ear resonances.

The frequency distribution of the maximum instantaneous peak levels for a 75-piece orchestra was given by Fletcher (1931) and is shown in Figure 5–8. Several more recent measurements have indicated that the high-frequency peak levels do not fall off as fast as Fletcher's curve indicated (and indeed Fletcher himself intentionally excluded the cymbals; an instrument whose inclusion would have brought the 10 kHz level back up near the level at 250 Hz). It is sometimes argued, therefore, that a no-compromise system would allow no drop in the high-frequency peak capability.

Because occasional high-frequency overload is generally found to be less annoying than a constant hiss, however, a 75 µs, high-frequency preemphasis (a 6 dB per octave upward slope above a 2.1 kHz corner frequency) remains the standard in FM broadcasting. Similarly, current AES standards on prerecorded tape and phonograph records call for a preemphasis ranging from 75 to 150 µs. The effect of the preemphasis, which is corrected in playback, is to improve the signal-to-noise ratio of recorded material at the expense of a reduced high-frequency overload capability.

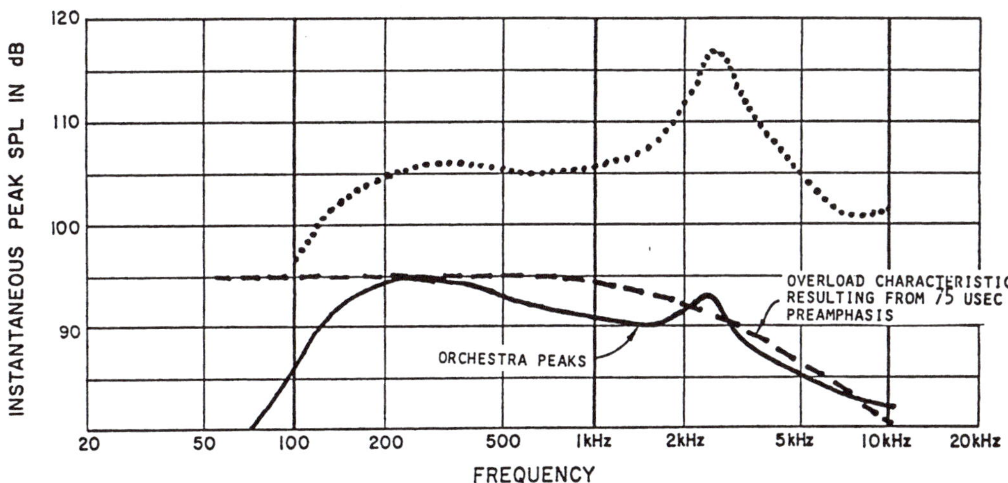

Figure 5–8. Maximum peaks produced in half-octave bands by large orchestra, referred to audience area (solid line). Instantaneous peak (of sine wave) eardrum pressure capabilities required of hearing aid to reproduce large orchestra (dotted line). (Note: Orchestra peaks correspond to instantaneous wideband peaks of 105 dB SPL or peak readings of 95 dB SPL on sound level meter set to "C, Fast.")

Not surprisingly, the frequency dependence of the instantaneous peak-pressure requirements is not much different when it is based on the Fletcher curve or on the assumption of a 75 microsecond preemphasis. This comparison is shown in Figure 5–8.

In terms of system requirements, approximately 10 dB of "headroom" is required in any half-octave band over the instantaneous peak levels shown in Figure 5–8. This comes about because the presence of energy in other frequency bands can, when added to that present in a given band, produce instantaneous peaks greater (by approximately 10 dB in the case of half-octave bands) than the peak that would be produced by the in-band energy acting alone. The measured instantaneous peak overload capability of a system at a given frequency (measured as the instantaneous peak of a sinewave signal just before clipping) must therefore exceed the half-octave-band instantaneous peak measurements of music by approximately 10 dB.

The output requirements for a hearing aid must also take into account the increase in eardrum pressure produced by outer-ear resonances. On a random-incidence basis (as in a concert hall where sounds are arriving from all directions), this increase amounts to approximately 15 dB at 2700 Hz (Shaw, 1976). When combined with the considerations of the previous paragraph, this means that a hearing aid that is to provide unity gain for high-level sounds must be capable of producing an instantaneous peak eardrum pressure level at 2700 Hz that is 25 dB greater than the peak level shown in Figure 5-8, or a maximum of 117 dB SPL at 2700 Hz. The dotted curve in Figure 5–8 shows the estimated instantaneous peak (sine-wave) output requirements for a high-fidelity hearing aid operating at unity insertion gain for high-level signals. Fortunately, even a 127 dB eardrum pressure peak corresponds to only 112 dB SPL in a 2cc coupler at 3 kHz because of the normal 15 dB RECD at 3 kHz. This output is easily reached with Class B or Class D receivers.

Input Noise Level

The input noise level of a high-fidelity hearing aid should be less than that of the ambient noise levels likely to be encountered by a user. The A-weighted noise level during a quiet listening period in a theater or auditorium may drop to 32 dB (Fletcher, 1942; Olson, 1967) and sometimes lower (author's observation). Residential noise levels are generally higher. Seacord (1940) measured noise levels in a large number of residential rooms and found an average level of 43 dB A-weighted; 90% of the levels fell between 33 and 52 dB(A). Seacord's data (1940) have found common acceptance, although it is generally believed that the greater use of forced-air heating and air-conditioning systems has acted to increase average levels since his data were obtained.

Macrae and Dillon (1986) determined the maximum hearing aid equivalent input noise levels acceptable to their subjects. A hearing aid in which input noise just met their one-third-octave limits at each frequency would have an overall A-weighted equivalent input noise of 38 dB SPL.

The input noise level in a modern hearing aid is determined almost entirely by the microphone noise level. Currently available subminiature microphones have typical A-weighted noise levels equivalent to a 26 dB SPL ambient noise level; a few are 2 to 3 dB quieter. Even in a quiet auditorium, therefore, the microphone noise level would add less than 1 dB to the apparent A-weighted ambient level. The aided threshold determined by typical microphone noise levels is within a few dB of normal threshold and can be better than normal with special design (Killion, 1976a). The internal noise of the hearing aid should thus present no impediment to a high-fidelity design.

Distortion

We will use the term distortion to mean nonlinear distortion, in the restricted sense of a distortion that results in the generation of new frequencies appearing in the output but not present in the input stimulus. An example of nonlinear distortion would be the overload of an amplifier so that clipping occurs. Common measures of nonlinear distortion are total harmonic distortion and intermodulation distortion, both of which measure the relative strength of the new frequencies created by the nonlinearity when sine-wave signals of one or more frequencies are presented to the input.

In a study of the amounts of distortion tolerable in a high-fidelity system, Olson (1957) found that total harmonic distortion levels of approximately 1% were just detectable and that total harmonic distortion levels below 3% were not considered objectionable in a system with an 8 kHz upper cutoff frequency. Two systems were tested, one using a single-ended triode amplifier and another using a single-ended triode amplifier and one using a single-ended pentode amplifier. In both cases, the distortion increased with increasing output, and the distortion percentages represented the total harmonic distortion of sine waves with an output level equal to the peak levels of the music used as program material.

Nonlinearities in the system that occur near the upper cutoff frequency are difficult to examine using harmonic distortion measures because the harmonic distortion products (at 2f1, 3f1, etc.) may lie above the cutoff frequency. High-frequency distortion can be easily detected, however, by applying two high-frequency sine waves to a system and measuring the system output at the difference frequency This has been called the "CCIF method" for measuring intermodulation distortion and is described more completely in the references below.

Tests made by the British postal service and reported by Moir (1958) indicated that CCIF intermodulation distortion on speech and music "is not detectable when the quadratic or cubic difference tones are . . . below one percent." Termin and Pettit (1952) reported that CCIF intermodulation distortion becomes objectionable at a value of 3 to 4% when the difference frequency lies in the 400 to 5000 Hz range.

Tests employing "golden ears" have produced similar results, as summarized by Milner (1977) and Davis (1978). Intermodulation distortion levels below 2% are generally inaudible on musical material, and even gross distortion levels (6 to 12%) are sometimes inaudible. In general, the barely audible distortion levels for musical material are at least

10 times greater than the barely audible pure-tone distortion levels.

One complication that arises in attempting to apply these results to hearing aids is the necessity of translating the results into ear-drum-pressure or coupler-pressure levels. Although eardrum pressure and sound field pressure are roughly equal below 1000 Hz, the combined effect of head diffraction and external-ear resonance results in a 10 to 20 dB boost in eardrum pressure levels in the 2000 to 5000 Hz region (Wiener & Ross, 1946). One consequence of the treble boost provided by the head and outer ear is that the ear is able to detect lower levels of harmonic distortion when the harmonics fall in the 2000 to 5000 Hz region. In addition, small head movements may place one ear in a "null" position for the fundamental tone in the listening room, which can result in incredibly low detection levels for pure tone distortion in real rooms.

A further complication is the level-dependence of the ear's sensitivity to distortion. At low sound pressure levels, the level of any harmonic or intermodulation distortion products may lie below the normal threshold of hearing. At high levels, the increased upward spread of masking (Wegel & Lane, 1924) and the distortion of the ear itself may mask externally generated distortion products. Thus no single-number distortion specification will apply at all listening levels.

The tests reported by Olson (1957) were carried out in a small listening room at a level of "about 70 dB." Assuming that this level was close to the 75 dB levels reported by Olson for other similar listening tests, it corresponds to instantaneous peak levels of approximately 85 dB SPL. This is only slightly greater than the 70 to 80 dB SPL that a study of the masking literature indicates is the region in which the ear should be most sensitive to distortion. Thus, the values for detectable and tolerable distortion obtained by Olson and others reasonably can be applied as a requirement for a high-fidelity hearing aid only for output levels in the range between about 50 and 90 dB SPL (measured at the eardrum or in an ear simulator). Below 50 dB and above 90 dB, a less stringent requirement is clearly in order, and a relaxation to perhaps 10% at 30 dB and 110 dB eardrum SPL appears reasonable.

The last problem in attempting to arrive at reasonable distortion specifications is probably the most important one. Unless the precise distortion mechanism (peak clipping, center clipping, curved transfer characteristic, etc.) is understood, no single distortion measurement can provide reliable information as to how clean the sound will be to a human listener. Thus, 1% of "soft peak clipping" (as employed in the determinations discussed above) may be inaudible, but 1% of center clipping distortion may be intolerable!

Similar difficulties are encountered in attempting to study the effect of distortion on speech discrimination. Thus, Peters and Burkhard (1968) found that the 40% total harmonic distortion produced by one system had negligible effect on speech discrimination, whereas another system in which the total harmonic distortion measured only 20% resulted in a loss of 40 percentage units in speech discrimination score.

In light of the available information, a reasonable initial goal for a high-fidelity hearing aid with an 8000 Hz bandwidth would appear to be a maximum total harmonic distortion or CCIF intermodulation distortion of 2% for output levels between 50 and 90 dB eardrum SPL (assuming the distortion mechanism is a simple one), with a smooth relaxation to 10% between 30 and 110 dB SPL. Figure 5–9 illustrates such a requirement. Listening tests should be employed as a final check.

Automatic Gain Control Characteristics

Recall that a unity-gain sound reproduction system is desired for high-level sounds, coupled with sufficient gain for (desirable) low-level sounds to make them audible to the hearing-aid user.

The low-level gain required of a high-fidelity hearing aid can be readily estimated. Although a gain numerically equal to the user's hearing loss would be required to restore his

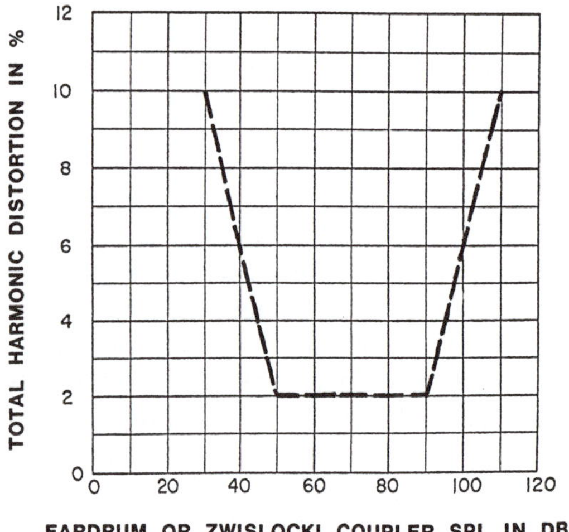

Figure 5–9. Estimated maximum hearing-aid distortion that will be inaudible on speech or music.

or her threshold down to audiometric zero levels, such a large amount of gain is commonly found to be unacceptable (Lybarger, 1944; Martin, 1973).

Under most circumstances, the masking produced by the background noise levels commonly encountered in residences, offices, and other locations render even those with unusually acute hearing incapable of detecting sounds that are less than 15 to 30 dB above commonly accepted audiometric zero levels. Based on the average room noise and spectra data of Seacord (1940) and Hoth (1941), Killion and Studebaker (1978) estimated that the masking effect of typical residential room noise produces a nearly uniform 23 dB "hearing loss" across the 250 to 4000 Hz speech frequencies. (Other investigators have made similar estimates. Thus, Olson (1957) calculated a 20 to 22 dB loss using slightly different assumptions.) Gain more than what is required to make background noises audible will be "empty gain," that makes everything louder but does not improve the detection of quiet sounds. Thus, a maximum gain sufficient to improve the aided threshold to the 15 or 20 dB hearing level generally has been found appropriate.

The input level at which the gain should be reduced to unity can also be estimated. Examination of clinical data and the literature on recruitment indicates that recruitment is typically complete (loudness sensation is essentially normal) for sounds corresponding to a hearing level of 80 dB or greater. More recently, Barfod (1978) has shown that in some cases a nearly linear relationship exists between the degree of hearing loss and the hearing level at which recruitment is complete. For Barfod's subjects, all of whom had steeply sloping high-frequency losses with nearly normal low-frequency hearing, all hearing losses below 50 dB HL were accompanied by complete recruitment above 75 dB HL. By way of illustration, Figures 5–10A and 5–10B show two hypothetical hearing losses with their corresponding areas of presumably normal hearing, based on Barfod's loudness data,

As a practical example, assume a user has a 45 dB HL cochlear impairment with complete recruitment for sounds above 80 dB HL. By our assumptions, he requires a maximum gain of 30 dB (45 minus 15) for sounds at 15 to 20 dB HL, and unity gain for sounds at 80 dB HL and above. (For speech sounds, 80 dB HL corresponds to a 95 dB SPL in a 0°-incidence sound field, or 100 dB SPL under headphones. For pure tones, 80 dB HL corresponds to approximately 80 to 90 dB SPL in the sound field in the frequency range important for speech perception.)

Optimum Amplitude Input-Output Characteristics

To avoid constant adjustments of the volume control, an Automatic Gain Control (AGC) system is required. To introduce the minimum degradation in perceived sound quality, the operation of the AGC system must be unobtrusive. Compression amplification has found wide acceptance in the broadcast and recording industry for such purposes (Blesser & Ives, 1972). As originally defined at Bell Telephone Laboratories (Mathes & Wright, 1934), compression amplification meant what is now sometimes called logarithmic compression (to distinguish it from some of the misuses of the term), that is, a constant ratio between the logarithms of the input and output signal

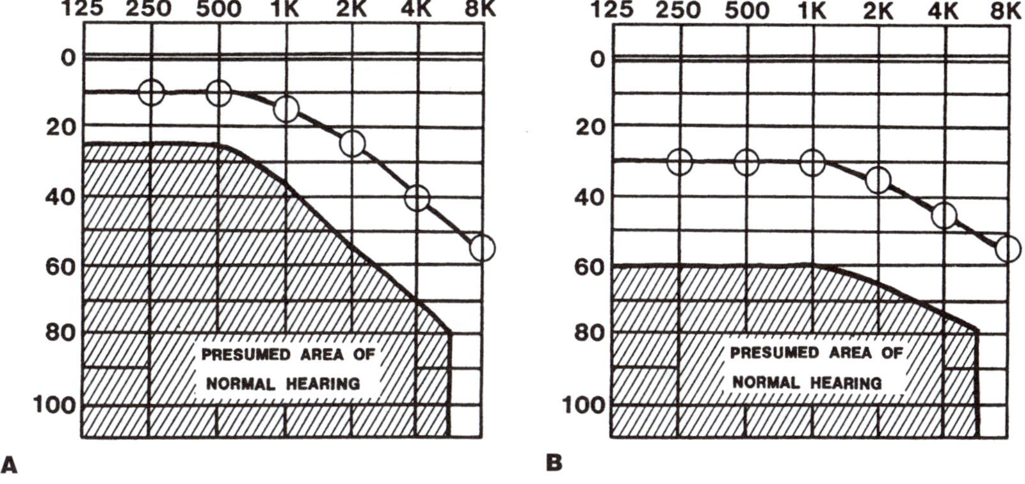

Figure 5–10. Threshold audiograms for two hypothetical subjects, with areas of presumed normal hearing based on Barfod's (1978) data.

amplitudes. When input and output levels are expressed in dB, for example, a compression ratio of 2:1 corresponds to a 5 dB increase in output level for each 10 dB increase in input level.

The idea of applying compression amplification to hearing aids is not new, dating back at least to Steinberg and Gardner (1937). Wide dynamic range compression amplification was apparently first reduced to commercial practice in wearable hearing-aid designs by Goldberg (1960, 1966).

Figure 5–11 illustrates input-output characteristic (Killion, 1979b) for a hearing aid intended to meet the requirements of the example discussed above. There are four stages of amplification illustrated in Figure 5–11: a low-level, constant-gain stage; a mid-level, constant-compression ratio (2:1) stage; a high-level, unity-gain stage; and a very high-level, compression-limiting stage.

The final compression-limiting stage requires further comment. Fast-acting, low-distortion compression limiting applied to the microphone output for sounds above roughly 100 dB hearing levels (equal to 110–115 dB SPL) was originally planned to prevent audible distortion or bias shifts in the amplifier associated with overload. Output limiting was not expected to be needed to prevent discomfort if the hearing aid was set for unity gain for loud sounds. In practice, the K-AMP circuit has never had its output limiting circuit activated, and complaints of excessive loudness have been almost nonexistent.

Note that the input-output characteristic illustrated in Figure 5–11 is quite different from any of the three other types that were commonly employed in hearing aids at the time the first edition of this chapter was written and shown for comparison in Figure 5–12: Ouput limiting (peak clipping or low-distortion compression limiting), AVC (automatic volume control), or wide dynamic range compression. Properly adjusted, output limiting can prevent amplified sounds from ever becoming too loud, but linear amplification combined with output limiting often makes a large proportion of sounds almost too loud. An automatic volume control can insure that all sounds are amplified to the most comfortable listening level, but the resulting restriction of the dynamic range lends a sameness to all sounds that is highly unnatural. Wide dynamic range compression comes closest to the "ideal" characteristic of Figure 5–11 but continues to perform signal processing even for loud sounds, when the hearing aid should be simply "getting out of the way" of the wearer's presumed normal hearing.

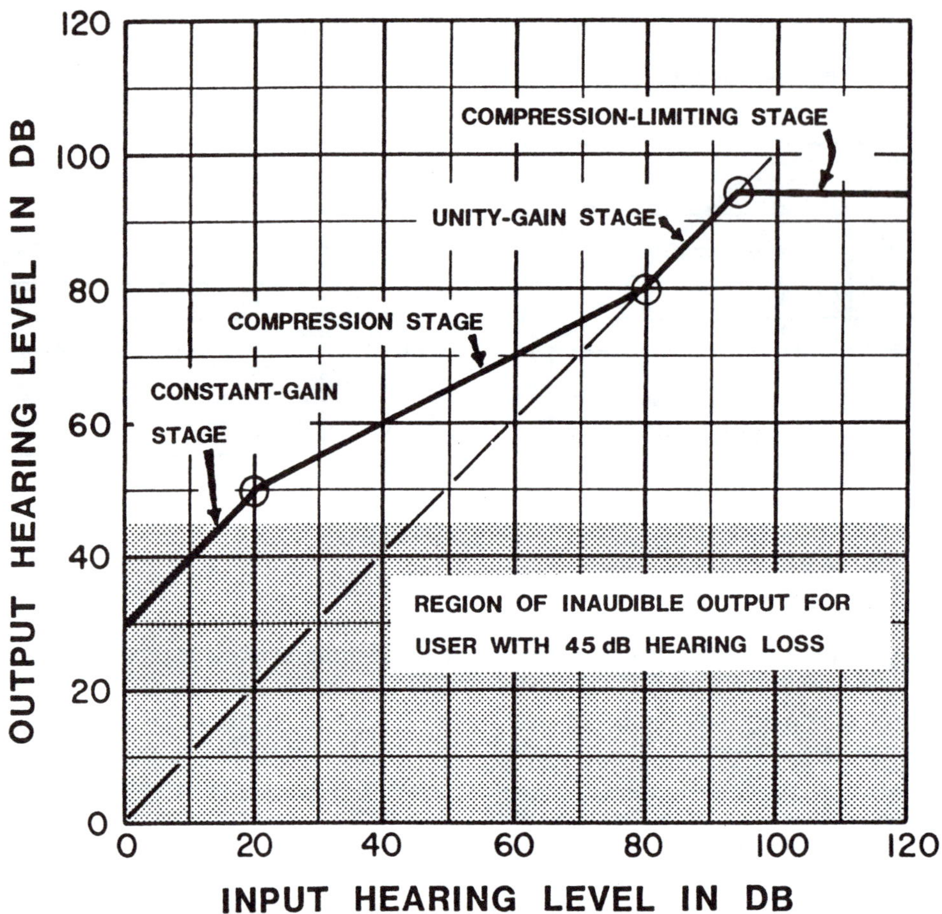

Figure 5–11. Presumed ideal hearing aid input-output characteristics for listener with 45 dB hearing loss and complete recruitment above 80 dB HL.

Level Dependent Frequency Response

Few threshold audiograms are flat. A greater loss at the higher frequencies is commonly found in those with hearing loss. For low-level sounds, a high-frequency emphasis in the hearing aid's frequency response is required to make the entire range of quiet speech sounds audible without overamplifying the low frequency sounds. For high-levels sounds, on the other hand, unity gain (and thus a flat frequency response) is required.

This need for a level-dependent frequency response can be met in several ways. The technique most often described in the literature is the use of multiple-channel compression amplification, with the compression ratio in each channel chosen to compensate for the degree of hearing loss in that frequency band (Villchur, 1973).

A simpler method that is adequate in the case of mild-to-moderate hearing impairments is to use a single-channel amplifier with a suitable capacitor in series with the gain-determining element. As an illustration of what can be accomplished with relative ease in a practical hearing aid amplifier, Figure 5–13 shows the level-dependent frequency response characteristic of the K-AMP (Killion, 1979b). A greater high-frequency emphasis at

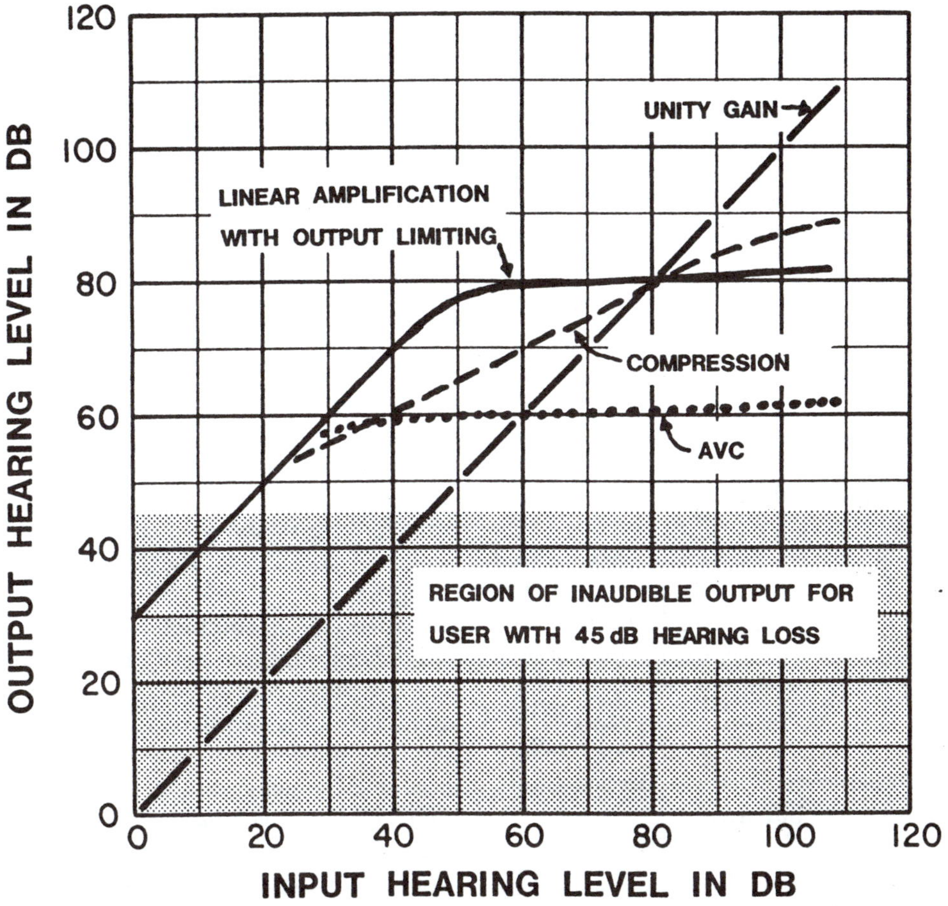

OUTPUT HEARING LEVEL IN DB

INPUT HEARING LEVEL IN DB

UNITY GAIN

LINEAR AMPLIFICATION WITH OUTPUT LIMITING

COMPRESSION

AVC

REGION OF INAUDIBLE OUTPUT FOR USER WITH 45 dB HEARING LOSS

Figure 5–12. Input-output characteristics for three conventional approaches to dynamic range reduction in hearing aids.

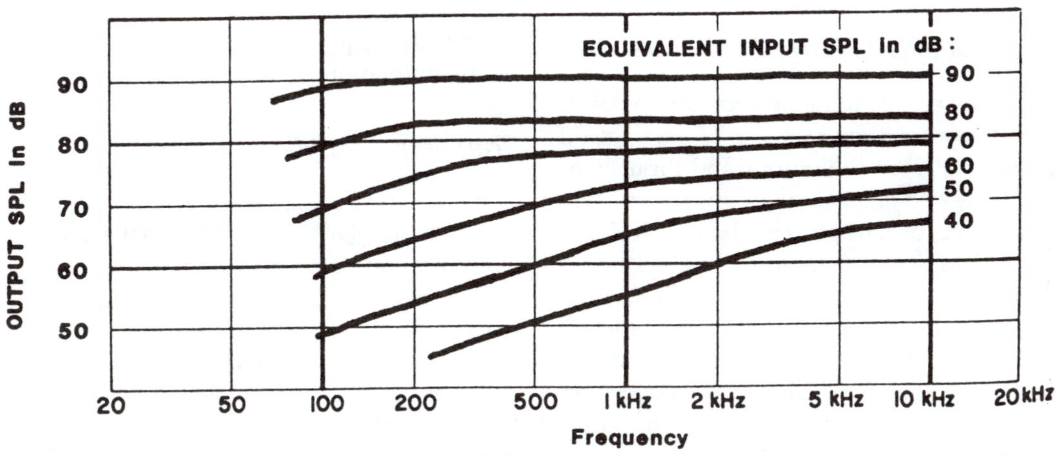

Figure 5–13. Relative amplifier frequency response versus input level in "speech mode" (compression ratio set for 2:1) of first author's experimental amplifier.

low levels would be required to meet the needs of the hypothetical individual whose audiogram was shown in Figure 5–10, but that also should be practical.

The need for a level-dependent frequency response has been discussed by Barfod (1976), Goldberg (1960, 1972), Skinner (1976, 1980), and Villchur (1973, 1978). Whatever the optimum characteristic, properly executed compression amplification should, in the ideal, not significantly degrade the fidelity as judged by someone without a hearing impairment, and this can be achieved. BTE aids with the K-amp (Killion, 1979b), intentionally operated in their worst-case operating range (from the standpoint of measured distortion) but in their flat frequency response mode, received average fidelity ratings across subject groups that were insignificantly different (2.5% higher) than the ratings given the BTE hearing aids themselves (Killion, 1979a), verifying not only that high-fidelity compression amplification circuitry operating on a 1.5 V hearing aid battery was practical, but that the tested compression characteristic was acceptable from the standpoint of fidelity.

Time Response Requirements

In this section, the transient response of a hearing aid is considered.

Transient Wave Form Response

There are two common interpretations of the term "poor transient response." One is the difference between the output and input wave forms viewed on an oscilloscope screen (transient wave form response) when a transient is applied to a sound reproduction system. In general, this difference is an inevitable consequence of any frequency response shaping in the system under test. By the above definition, for example, the ear itself has poor transient response because of the resonances in the external ear.

To a reasonable first approximation, a hearing aid system can be represented as a minimum-phase network. Under those circumstances, the transient response can be predicted directly from the frequency response. The frequency response tailoring of a particular hearing aid may or may not be useful, but its effect on "transient response" is inevitable. Indeed, the inverse procedure—obtaining the frequency response of a hearing aid by analyzing its transient wave form response to short clicks—is now routinely used in one commercial probe microphone system for obtaining the real-ear response of hearing aids.

Two papers should be read by anyone interested in poor transient response. A comprehensive set of frequency response curves and their corresponding transient response wave form resultants was given in the classic paper by Mott (1944). The surprisingly large changes in wave form due to phase shifts that are nonetheless completely inaudible (or audible only under what F. V. Hunt used to call "carefully contrived listening tests") have often been discussed. Bauer (1974) described some of the more rigorous experiments along those lines, which indicated that introducing even 90° per octave phase shifts does not produce audible effects. (Many contaminated experiments exist. Loudspeaker manufacturers selling "time aligned" loudspeakers have been some of the worst offenders, demonstrating readily audible changes that are claimed to be caused by phase changes alone when in fact large, readily audible changes in the amplitude frequency response accompanied the manipulations.)

Transient Amplifier Overload

The other type of "poor transient response" generally involves an amplifier that exhibits a slow recovery from overload. As mentioned above, instantaneous peak sound pressure levels of 110 to 115 dB at the hearing aid input are not uncommon. Such peaks can easily cause sufficient amplifier overload to upset the bias levels on the internal coupling capacitors, causing a condition of high amplifier distortion lasting much longer than the transient itself (Ingelstram, Johanson, Pettersson, and Sjogren, 1971). This "blocking distortion" was more often a problem with older amplifier designs and is much less of a problem now that the majority of hearing aids use some form of fast-acting compression limiting or AGC system.

AGC Time Constants

The attack and release time constants of the AGC system used to obtain the desired input-output characteristics throughout the operating range are an important consideration in any sound processing system. As extensively discussed by Lippman (1978), the proper choice of time constants depends a great deal on the goal set for the AGC system of the hearing aid. When the goal is to maximize speech discrimination, for example, the results of Ahren and colleagues (1977) and Schweitzer and Causey (1977) indicate the attack time should be as short as possible and the release time between 30 and 100 ms, but conclusive findings on this subject have not yet been made. When the goal is to maximize sound quality, on the other hand, the situation is much less clear. Even under ideal conditions, such as those found in professional recording studios, the optimum choice of attack and release time for minimum perceived distortion is highly dependent on the program material. Thus, any choice will be "wrong" at least part of the time. These issues were discussed at some length by Blesser and Ives (1972), who reported that values of 10 ms and 150 ms for attack and release times, respectively, have found common acceptance in equipment designed for the broadcast industry. In the absence of reliable research findings on the optimum values for hearing aids (with sound quality as the goal), these values would presumably represent a reasonable first choice for the AGC system of a high-fidelity hearing aid.

A way out of this dilemma has been recently implemented following an earlier RCA development (Singer, 1950) that has been used for some time in the broadcast industry (Smriga, 1986). This "Adaptive Compression" or "Variable Recovery Time" technique automatically varies the release time dependent on the duration of the high-level signal that engaged the compression action.

In the case of compression-limiting circuits that employ high compression ratios to prevent high-level inputs from producing outputs exceeding the loudness discomfort of the wearer, the use of variable recovery time can increase intelligibility in noise. Fikret-Pasa (1993) compared two 8:1 low-distortion compressors (using basic K-AMP circuitry) with eight subjects having moderate to severe hearing loss. Two of her subjects, Harry Teder and Larry Revit, are well-known engineers in the industry. Listening to a female speak in four-talker babble (the forerunner of the SIN test), each subject obtained the worst SNR with peak clipping and the best with variable recovery time compression. The industry-typical 50 ms recovery time compression was in between. The average SNRs that required for 50% correct in noise were:

Peak clipping	20 dB SNR
50 ms compression	14 dB SNR
Variable recovery time compression	9 dB SNR

The presumed explanation (Teder, 1991) is that a 50 ms recovery time brings the background noise quickly up to the level of the desired speech, making it more difficult for the listener with hearing impairment to use envelope cues to help separate the two.

In the case of wide dynamic range compression circuits using relatively low compression ratios (and increasing gain for quiet sounds rather than limiting gain for loud sounds), the known benefit of variable recovery time (VRT) is better subjective fidelity. VRT increases the steady-state recovery time to 500 ms or so, substantially reducing the "pumping" sound of typical 50 ms recovery, while reducing the recovery time after short transients (hand clap, knife on plate, etc.) to only 20 ms. Intelligibility may or may not be improved (it has not been studied to the author's knowledge), but sound quality certainly is.

IMPLEMENTATION OF THE GUIDELINES IN PRACTICAL HEARING AIDS

Success of Wide Dynamic Range Hearing Aids

In the first article on the new K-AMP amplifier, the final sentence read "The ultimate test of this amplifier design will be the degree of its acceptance by hearing-impaired wearers." The acceptance has been good: There have now been some 3 million of these devices sold, and several times that many Class D receivers. In 1990, wide dynamic range compression (WDRC) processing was found mostly in ReSound (two-channel) and K-AMP (one-channel) circuits. It is now found in nearly all digital hearing aids and in many modern analog circuits, such as the DynamEQ2.

CIC Hearing Aids

Two developments made high-fidelity hearing aids more practical: soft-tip, deeply sealed earmolds and completely-in-the-canal (CIC) fittings.

The practicality of deeply sealed eartips has been demonstrated in the tens of thousands of Musicians Earplugs® sold around the world, which typically use a deeply sealed eartip to reduce the occlusion effect to, in the best cases, less than zero. Zwislocki (1953) first observed the elimination of the occlusion effect with a deep seal; Killion, Wilber and Gudmundsen (1988) demonstrated its effectiveness and practicality. By sealing in or near the bony portion of the ear canal, the canal-wall vibration caused by speaking, chewing, or blowing on a horn can be isolated from the eardrum. The evidence from Musicians Earplugs indicates that deeply sealed BTE earmolds are entirely practical. (They also reduce the likelihood of feedback by improving the seal and reducing the sound-producing vibration of the earmold.) Soft-tip or soft-shell canal aids were first introduced by Voroba and often eliminated the occlusion effect as discussed in the Killion et al. paper above. Since that time, a steady search for practical, durable materials and construction methods has brought us close to the time when soft-shell or soft-tip ITE, canal, and CIC aids may become routine.

The CIC aid is a special case, because many wearers report little occlusion effect. That was the first author's experience with a pair made for him years ago by Randolph Giller. A deeply sealed hard-shell ITE aid has the disadvantage that any bump to the aid or wiggling of the ear can cause intense pain in the bony portion of the ear canal, where the skin is extremely thin and the bone extremely hard. The CIC construction has the advantage that nothing sticks out into the ear canal to be bumped or wiggled so that a snug fit is practical even with hard materials. It may also be that part of the occlusion effect with shallow-tip ITE hearing aids comes from concha vibration transmitted to the shell, causing the shell to pump in the ear canal. Whatever the cause, it is usual to obtain, initially or after a remake, a CIC aid with low occlusion effect and, perhaps for similar reasons, surprisingly low problems with feedback.

Until recently, one problem in smoothing out the real-ear frequency response of hearing aids was the fact that available hearing aid receivers (earphones) had their primary peak at about 3.5 to 4 kHz. Knowles has recently introduced two Class D receivers, the EP-series and the even smaller ES-series, whose primary peaks are near the 2.8 kHz resonance of the external ear.

Musicians as Judges

One of the sternest tests of a hearing aid is whether or not a musician can wear it while performing. For one thing, the circuit of a hearing aid must be capable of handling the peak

SPLs created by the musicians themselves. In the case of virtuoso violinists, this amounts to 115 dB at the left ear (closest to the violin body). As an amateur violinist, it has been gratifying to the first author that several violinists in the Chicago Symphony Orchestra now wear K-AMP hearing aids during rehearsal and performance. (The old stigma is finally gone; it is now well understood that a loss of sensitivity for quiet sounds does not have to interfere with a musician's ability to play; one of the best violinists in the symphony has been wearing a K-AMP hearing aid for years.)

In contrast, one author as choir director has tried a wide variety of popular all-digital hearing aids with disappointing results. Most overload (distort) so badly with the live choir and piano levels that it is impossible to listen for choral balance and intonation: The errors introduced by the hearing aids overwhelm those of the choir!

The problem of handling performance-level SPLs without distortion may explain the comment made by Chasin (personal communication, June 7, 1999): "Out of the last 200 hearing aid fittings on musicians, 180 of them were K-AMPs. Musicians seem to like the low distortion levels of the K-AMP in high-volume environments—perhaps it has to do with the high input limiting level of the K-AMP that distinguishes it from other hearing aids, including digital products."

A Persistent Wax Problem

There is one remaining problem in CIC applications. The damping mesh that must be placed in the receiver outlet to provide a smooth frequency response tends to clog fairly quickly because it is, of necessity, exposed to ear wax. An electronic damping chip is being developed as this chapter is being completed. The use of electronic damping—inverse filtering to remove peaks in the frequency response—should permit wax-free operation of CIC hearing aids with full fidelity.

FIDELITY AS A RETURN TO "HOW WELL I USED TO HEAR IN NOISE"

Performance in Noise

Signal-to-Noise Ratio Loss

As discussed in the introduction of this chapter, "high-fidelity" hearing aids have enabled listeners with hearing impairment to hear speech in quiet at all input levels without adding distortion (Benter & Duve, 1997). The same study, however, showed that today's circuits still do not improve the ability to understand speech in high-level noise. Recently tests that quantify a listener's ability to hear in noise have become an important part of evaluating a patient for amplification (Killion, 1997a, 1997b). These measures (the Speech-in-Noise [SIN] test and the Hearing-in-Noise Test [HINT]) will determine the SNR required for a listener to understand 50% of words-in-sentences. Listeners with normal hearing typically need a 2 dB SNR on the SIN test to understand 50% of words-in-sentences. In other words, the listener with normal hearing requires the signal to be 2 dB louder than the noise to understand 50%. Listeners with hearing impairment usually require a greater SNR to understand 50%. The SNR required is poorly correlated with the audiogram, however, and therefore needs to be measured on all listeners with hearing impairment. Once the SNR required for 50% correct identification of words-in-sentences is determined, the patient's SNR loss is calculated by subtracting 2 dB (the SNR required by a listener with normal hearing). Therefore, a listener with a measured SNR of 8 dB has a 6 dB SNR loss

Figure 5–14 shows a plot of hearing loss (pure-tone average) by the SNR loss. Each dot represents an individual listener with hearing impairment. Note that the regression line does not fit the data well, except showing that in general the more hearing loss, the greater the SNR loss. There is a wide range of SNRs

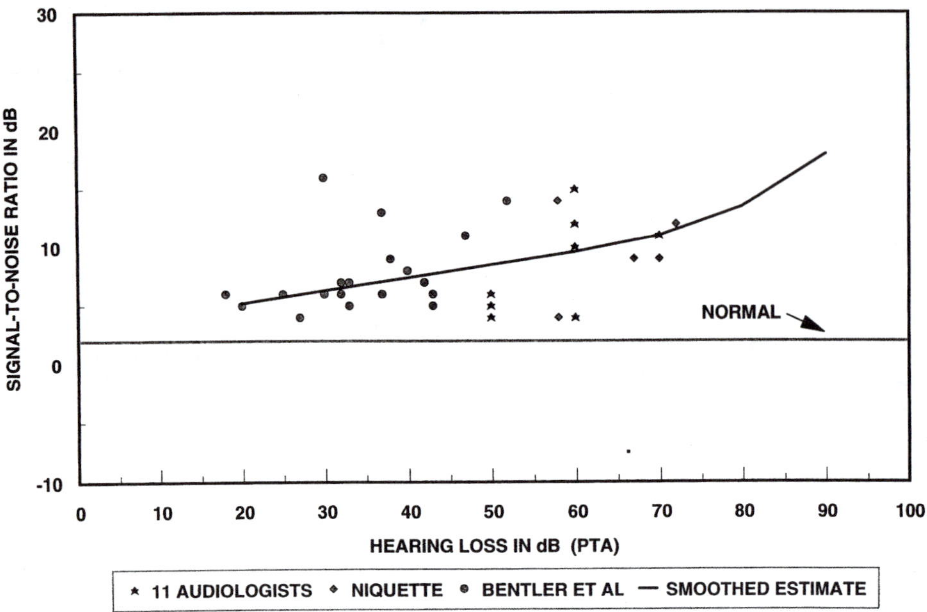

Figure 5–14. SNR required for 50% correct identification of words-in-sentences plotted by average hearing loss (pure-tone average).

for individual listeners with the same average hearing loss, for example, look at the average loss of 60 dB HL. Data from four subjects are plotted on the graph. For these four subjects, the SNR required for 50% correct ranges from 4 dB to 16 dB.

Figure 5–15 shows another way to look at these results. Plotted in this figure is the SNR required for 50% correct for a subject with normal hearing and a subject with a 40 dB average hearing loss. For the listener with normal hearing, the SNR required for 50% correct is approximately 2 dB when listening at a comfortable suprathreshold level. Below 30 dB HL, the SNR required increases because many speech sounds will be missed at this low level. The curve for the individual with a 40 dB average hearing loss is shifted by the amount of the hearing loss, but in addition, this individual will require a greater SNR than normal even at a comfortable supratheshold level. For this hypothetical listener, a 7 dB SNR is required to produce 50% correct. Thus, this patient with a 40 dB average loss has a 5 dB SNR loss. Figure 5–16 illustrates what happens with a 1960's peak clipping hearing aid and a modern hearing aid. The curve for the 1960's hearing aid shows that while the aid does provide somewhat better audibility (represented by the shift in the curve to the left), the SNR requirements substantially increase with this aid. In other words, this individual will have greater trouble understanding in noise with the hearing aid than without it due to distortion in the hearing aid. The high-fidelity aid of the 1990s does not increase the SNR requirement for 50% correct, but it does not improve the SNR requirement either. The patient with the 40 dB average loss still has a 5 dB SNR loss with this modern hearing aid. Figure 5–17 shows Bentler and Duve's (1997) SNR results for each hearing aid used in their study. With those subjects, all of the modern hearing aids required an SNR of approximately 6 dB for 50% correct.

Directional Microphones

Given that hearing aid circuitry has not solved the hearing-in-noise deficit experienced by lis-

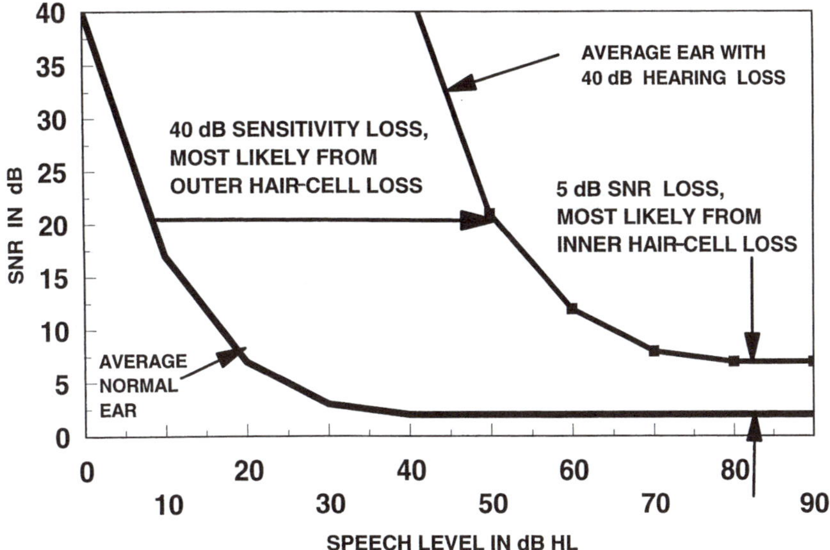

Figure 5–15. SNR required for 50% correct identification of words-in-sentences plotted by presentation level. Results for a normal-hearing listener and a listener with a 40 dB average hearing loss are shown.

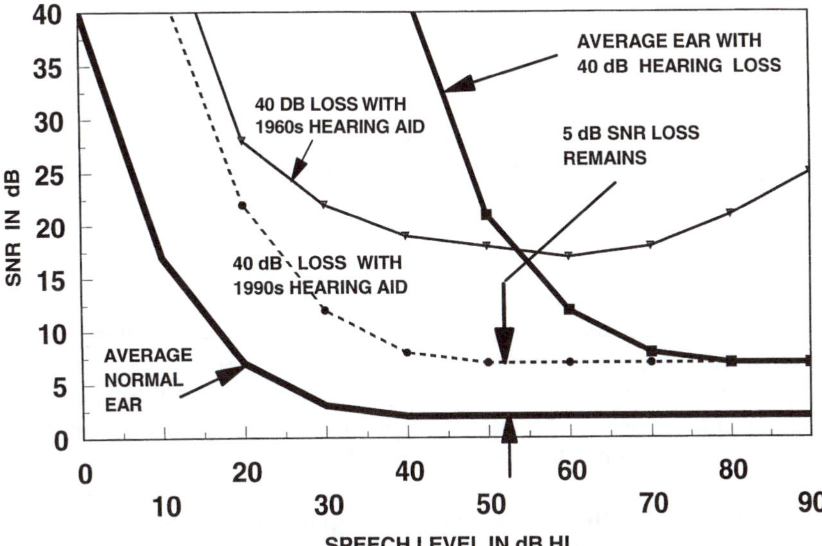

Figure 5–16. SNR required for 50% correct identification of words-in-sentences plotted by presentation level. Results for a normal-hearing listener and a listener with a 40 dB average hearing loss are shown. The performance of two hearing aids (1960s peak clipper and a 1990s modern high-fidelity aid) are given for the listener with the 40 dB average hearing loss.

teners with hearing impairment, engineers have looked for solutions to improve the signal-to-noise ratio for these listeners. The oldest such solution was the speaking tube. Because the talker speaks directly into the mouthpiece and the level at the lips is typically 105 to 115 dB

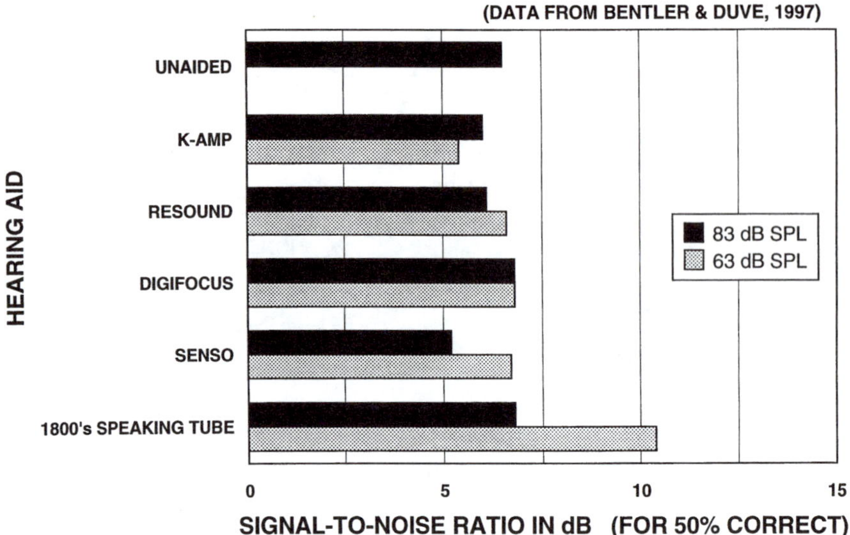

Figure 5–17. SNRs measured using the technologies evaluated in the Benter and Duve (1997) study. (Data are from *Progression of hearing aid benefit over the twentieth century*, by R. A. Bentler and M. R. Duve, 1997, poster presented at the American Academy of Audiology Convention, Ft. Lauderdale, FL. Reprinted with permission.)

SPL, the SNR with a speaking tube can easily reach 20 to 40 dB. (The losses in the tube bring the listening level down to comfortable levels.) FM systems can provide similar SNR improvements with the advantage of wireless operation.

Less dramatic but more convenient SNR improvements can result from using directional microphones in hearing aids. Directional microphones improve the SNR for sounds coming from the front of a listener by attenuating arriving sounds from the sides and the back. Directional microphones in hearing aids are not a new development, although today's microphones provide substantially more benefit than the pre-1990s directional microphones (Killion et al., 1998).

A full chapter in this book is dedicated to directional microphones so this discussion on directional microphones will be limited to the benefits that these microphones can provide listeners.

Today's directional microphones are designed in two ways: (1) electrically subtracting the outputs of two omnidirectional microphones and (2) using a single directional microphone with two ports and acoustically subtracting the signals at these two ports following a delay (called a single cartridge approach). Both methods will provide good directivity if designed correctly.

Killion and colleagues (1998) evaluated the performance of a single-cartridge directional microphone (D-MIC™) in real-world environments. In this study, recordings were made from hearing aids equipped to record from the outputs of both the omnidirectional and the directional microphones simultaneously. Recordings in a variety of environments were accomplished, and results indicated SNR ratio improvements in the directional condition ranging from 4 dB in reverberant environments such as restaurants and cocktail parties to 11 dB in outdoor (nonreverberant) environments. These improvements in SNR ratio translated to significant improvements in speech recognition scores in noise ranging from 30 to 60%.

Appropriately designed directional microphones finally provide listeners help when listening in noisy environments. Thus, coupling a directional microphone with a high-fidelity hearing aid amplifier will provide listeners with mild-to-moderate hearing loss substantial benefit when listening in both quiet and noisy environments.

SUMMARY AND CONCLUSIONS

This chapter has attempted to present the design characteristics required for high-fidelity amplification. An understanding of these characteristics is essential for making decisions about proper amplification for listeners with hearing impairment. Modern hearing aids have eliminated the major problems with older technologies. These problems included distortion, narrow bandwidths, and peaks in the response. High-fidelity hearing aids are available that provide the listener who has hearing impairment with excellent speech understanding in quiet environments for both soft and loud input levels.

Unfortunately, modern high-fidelity hearing aids have not solved the speech understanding problems experienced by listeners with hearing impairment in noisy environments. The problem of hearing in noise has shifted to attention on improving the SNR for the listener. This can be done in a variety of ways but most conveniently by using a directional microphone coupled with a high-fidelity hearing aid.

Future developments in amplification will likely include microphone options that provide greater SNR improvements for listeners with hearing impairments. These improvements will allow hearing aids to provide excellent speech understanding in both quiet and noisy environments. A goal that has taken many decades to achieve.

REVIEW QUESTIONS

Principles of High-Fidelity Hearing Aid Amplification

1. In the Bentler and Duve study (1997), hearing aid technologies over the last 50 years were evaluated. Which of these technologies performed the best?

a. Two channel WDRC (ReSound)
b. WDRC in the high frequencies (K-Amp)
c. Digital signal processing (Digifocus and Senso)
d. Ear trumpet
e. Linear processing with peak clipping
f. a, b, and c above performed equally

2. What are the deficits mentioned in the chapter that were characteristic of older hearing aid technologies that have now been overcome by modern hearing instruments (circle all that apply)?

a. Narrow bandwidth
b. Background noise
c. Distortion
d. Low hearing aid gain
e. Peaks in the frequency response
f. Low SSPL90s

3. A WDRC circuit is one in which:

a. Amplification is only provided in frequency regions where hearing loss is present
b. Compression is applied at high input levels so that the signal does not get clipped
c. Amplification is given for soft- and mid-level inputs but is transparent for high-level inputs
d. Digital signal processing is used to mathematically manipulate the output of the hearing aid to just below the patient's uncomfortable loudness level (ULL)

4. The principal beneficiaries of high-fidelity amplification include:

a. Individuals with profound hearing impairment
b. Individuals with severe-to-profound hearing impairment in the high frequencies
c. Individuals with a loss of sensitivity for low-level sounds and normal hearing for high-level sounds
d. Individuals with poor discrimination abilities

5. One of the most important factors that determines the success of a hearing aid fitting is the:

a. Hearing aid
b. Motivation of the patient
c. Patient's type and degree of hearing loss
d. Counseling given to the patient by the hearing aid dispenser
e. Patient's age

6. What should the minimum bandwidth of a high-fidelity hearing aid be?
a. 250–4000 Hz
b. 125–6000 Hz
c. 60–8000 Hz
d. 500–6000 Hz

7. The input noise level of a modern hearing aid is determined almost entirely by the:
a. Receiver
b. Type of signal processing
c. Size of the hearing aid
d. Style of the hearing aid

8. What should be the maximum total harmonic distortion of CCIF intermodulation distortion for a high-fidelity hearing aid for output levels between 50 and 90 dB eardrum SPL?
a. 1%
b. 2%
c. 5%
d. 7%
e. 10%

9. Normal-hearing listeners typically need a ______ dB SNR to understand 50% of words-in-sentences in noise.
a. +1 dB
b. +2 dB
c. 0 dB
d. +5 dB
e. −2 dB

10. Today's directional micophones can be expected to provide a _____ dB SNR improvement in a typical room:
a. 2
b. 4
c. 5
d. 10
e. 11

REFERENCES

Ahren, T., Arlinger, S., Holmgren, C., Jerlvall, L., Johansson, B., Lindblad, A. C., Persson, L., Pettersson, A., & Sjogrem, G. (1977). *Automatic gain control and hearing aids* (Report TA No. 84). Stockholm: Karolinska Institutet, Technical Audiology.

Barfod, J. (1972). *Investigations on the optimum corrective frequency response for high tone hearing loss* (Report No. 4). Technical University of Denmark, Acoustic Laboratory.

Barfod, J. (1976). *Multichannel compression hearing aids* (Report No. 11). Technical University of Denmark, Acoustics Laboratory.

Barfod, J. (1978). Multichannel compression hearing aids: Experiments and consideration on clinical applicability. Sensorineural hearing impairment and hearing aids. C. Ludvigsen & J. Barfod (Eds.), *Scandinavian Audiology*, Suppl. 6, 315–340.

Bauer, B. B. (1974, March). Audibility of phase distortion. *Wireless World*, pp. 27–28.

Bentler, R. A., & Duve, M. R. (1997, March). Progression of hearing aid benefit over the twentieth century. Poster presented at the American Academy of Audiology Annual Convention, Ft. Lauderdale, FL.

Berland, O., & Nielsen, E. (1969, Summer). Sound pressure generated in the human external ear by a free sound field. *Audecibel*, 103–109.

Berlin, C. I., & Gondra, M. I. (1976). Extratympanic clinical cochleography with clicks. In R. P. Rubin, C. Eberling, & I. Salomon (Eds.), *Electrocochleography*. Baltimore, MD: University Park Press.

Blesser, B. A., & Ives, F. (1972). A reexamination of the S/N question for systems with time-varying gain or frequency response. *Journal of Audiologic Engineering Society, 20*, 638–641.

Bucklein, R. (1962). Horbarkeit von Unregelmakigkeiten in Frequenzgangen bei akustischer Ubertragung. *Frequenz, 16*, 103–108.

Burkhard, M. D., & Sachs, R. M. (1975). Anthropometric manikin for acoustic research. *Journal of the Acoustical Society of America, 58*, 214–222.

Consumer Reports. (1977). How CU's auditory lab tests loudspeaker accuracy. *Consumer Reports TNG-3*. Mount Vernon, NY.

Consumer Reports. (1977). Low-priced loudspeakers. *Consumer Reports, 42*, 406–409.

Dallos, P., Ryan, A., Harris, D., McGee T., & Ozdamar, O. (1977). Cochlear frequency selectivity in the presence of hair cell damage. In E. F. Evans & J. P. Wilson (Eds.), *Phychophysics and physiology of hearing*. London: Academic Press.

Dalsgaard, S. C., & Jensen, O. D. (1974). Measurement of insertion gain of hearing aids. *Eighth International Congress on Acoustics, 1*, 205.

Davis, M. (1978, June). What's really important in loudspeaker performance? *High Fidelity*, 53–58.

Dillon, H., & Macrae, J. (1984). *Derivation of design specifications for hearing aids* (NAL Report No. 102). Australia: National Acoustical Laboratories.

Dunn, H. K., & Farnsworth, D. W. (1939). Exploration of pressure field around the human head during speech. *Journal of the Acoustical Society of America, 10*, 184–199.

Dunn, H. D., & White, S. D. (1940). Statistical measurements on conversational speech. *Journal of the Acoustical Society of America, 11*, 278–288.

Fikret-Pasa, S. (1993). *The effects of compression ratio on speech intelligibility and quality* (Doctoral dissertation, Northwestern University, 1990). University Microfilms, Ann Arbor, MI.

Filler, A. S., Ross, D. A., & Wiener, F. M. (1945). *The pressure distribution in the auditory canal in a progressive sound field* (Report PNR-5, Contract N5ori-76, to Office of Research and Inventions, U.S. Navy). Cambridge, MA: Harvard University.

Flanagan, J. (1957). Difference limen for formant amplitude. *Journal of Speech and Hearing Disorders, 22*, 205–212.

Fletcher, H. (1931). Some physical characteristics of speech and music. *Bell Systems Technology Journal, 10*, 349–373.

Fletcher, H. (1942). Hearing, the determining factor for high-fidelity transmission. *Proceedings of the Institute of Radio Engineering, 30*, 266–277.

Gengel, R. W. (1973). Temporal effects in frequency discrimination by hearing impaired listeners. *Journal of the Acoustical Society of America, 54*, 11–15.

Goldberg, H. (1960). *A new concept in hearing aids.* Flushing, NY: Dynaura, Inc.

Goldberg, H. (1965). Psychological adaptation to hearing correction. *Analog of MPLS dealer bulletin.*

Goldberg, H. (1966). *Hearing aid.* U.S. Patent No. 3229049. Filed Aug. 4, 1960.

Goldberg, H. (1972). The utopian hearing aid: Current state of the art. *Journal of Auditory Research, 12*, 331–335.

Hogan, C. A., & Turner, C. W. (1998). High-frequency audibility: benefits for hearing-impaired listeners. *Journal of the Acoustical Society of America, 104*, 432–441.

Hoth, D. F. (1941). Room noise spectra at subscriber's telephone locations. *Journal of the Acoustical Society of America, 12*, 499–504.

Ingelstram, R., Johansson, B., Pettersson, A., & Sjogren, H. (1971). *The effect of non-linear amplitude distortion, an investigation by variation of the quadratic and the cubic components* (Report TA No. 64). Stockholm: Karolinska Institutet, Tech. Audiology.

Jerger, J. F., Tillman, T. W., & Peterson, J. L. (1960). Masking by octave bands of noise in normal and impaired ears. *Journal of the Acoustical Society of America, 32*, 385–390.

Killion, M. C. (1979a). *Design and evaluation of high-fidelity hearing aids* (Doctoral dissertation, Northwestern University, 1990). University Microfilms, Ann Arbor. MI.

Killion, M. C. (1979b). *AGC circuit particularly for a hearing aid.* U.S. Patent No. 4,170,720.

Killion, M.C. (1993). The K-Amp Hearing Aid. *America Journal of Audiology, 2*, 52–74.

Killion, M. C. (1997a). SNR Loss: "I can hearing what people say, but I can't understand them." *The Hearing Revue, 4*(12), p.8–14.

Killion, M. C. (1997b). The SIN report: Circuits haven't solved the hearing-in-noise problem. *The Hearing Journal, 50*(10), 28–32.

Killion, M. C., & Monser, E. L. (1980). CORFIG: Coupler response for flat insertion gain. In G. A. Studebaker & I. Hockberg (Eds.), *Acoustical factors affecting hearing and performance.* Baltimore, MD: Park Press.

Killion, M. C., Schulein, R., Christensen, L., Fabry, D., Revit, L., Niquette, P., & Chung, K. (1998). Real-world performance of an ITE directional microphone. *The Hearing Journal, 51*, 24–38.

Killion, M. C., & Studebaker, G. A. (1978). A-weighted equivalents of permissible ambient noise during audiometric testing. *Journal of the Acoustical Society of America, 63*, 1633–1635.

Killion, M. C., Wilber, L. A., & Gudmundsen, G. I. (1988). Zwislocki was right. . . . a potential solution to the "hollow voice" problem. *Hearing. Instruments, 39*(1), 14–17.

Kuhn, G. F., & Burnett, E. D. (1977). Acoustic pressure field alongside a manikin's head with a view towards in situ hearing-aid tests. *Journal of the Acoustical Society of America, 62*, 416–423.

Levit, H., & Neuman, A. (1990). A Sentence Test. In: *Proceedings of the 13th annual RESNA Conference.* Washington, DC: RESNA Press.

Licklider, J. C. R. (1949). Basic correlates of the audiotry stimulus. In S. S. Stevens (Ed.), *Handbook of experimental psychology.* New York: Wiley.

Lindblad, A. C. (1982). *Detection of nonlinear distortion on speech signals by hearing impaired listeners* (Report TA105). Stockholm: Karolinska Institutet Technical Audiology.

Lippman, R. P. (1978). *The effect of amplitude compression on the intelligibility of speech for persons with sensorineural hearing loss* (Doctoral dissertation, Massachusetts Institute of Technology 1978). University Microfilms, Ann Arbor, MI.

Lybarger, S. F. (1944). U.S. Patent Applications S.N. 543,278. Filed July 3, 1944.

Macrae, J., & Dillion, H. (1986). *Updated performance requirements for hearing aids* (NAL Report No. 109). Australia: National Acoustical Laboratories.

Madaffari, P. L. (1974). Pressure variation about the ear. *Journal of the Acoustical Society of America 56*, S3(A).

Marsh, R. C. (1975, August). Tweeters in the grass, alas. *Chicago*, pp. 76–78.

Martin, M. C. (1973). Hearing aid gain requirements in sensorineural hearing loss. *British Journal of Audiology, 7*, 21–24.

Mathes, R. C., & Wright, S. B. (1934). The compandor—an aid against static in radio telephony. *Bell Systems Technology Journal, 13,* 315–322.

McGee, T. (1978). *Psychophysical tuning curves from hearing impaired listeners.* (Doctoral dissertation, Northwestern University). University Microfilms, Ann Arbor, MI.

Miller, J. D. (1974). Effects of noise on people. *Journal of the Acoustical Society of America, 56,* 729–764.

Milner, P. (1977, June). How much distortion can you hear? *Stereo Review,* 64–68.

Moir, J. (1958). *High quality sound reproduction* (p. 51). New York: Macmillan.

Mott, E. E. (1944). Idicial response of telephone receivers. *Bell Systems Technology Journal, 23,* 135–150.

Muraoka, T., Iwahara, M., & Yamada, Y. (1981). Examination of audio-bandwidth requirements for optimum sound signal tranmission. *Journal of Audio Engineering Society, 29,* 2–9.

Olson, H. F. (1957). *Acoustic engineering.* New York: Van Nostrand.

Olson, H. F. (1967). *Music, physics, and engineering.* New York: Dover.

Palmer, C. (1991). *The influence of individual ear canal and eardrum characteristics on speech intelligibility and sound quality judgments* (Doctoral dissertation, Northwestern University 1991). University Microfilms, Ann Arbor, MI.

Palva, T., Goodman, A., & Hirsh, I. J. (1953). Critical evaluation of noise audiometry. *Laryngoscope, 63,* 842–860.

Peters, R. W., & Burkhard, M. D. (1968). *On noise distortion and harmonic distortion measurements* (Industrial Res. Prod. Report No. 10350-1). Franklin Park, IL: Knowles Electronics.

Punch, J. D. (1978). Quality judgments of hearing aid-processed speech and music by normal and otopathologic listeners. *Journal of the American Audiology Society, 3,* 179–188.

Rankovic, C. M. (1991). An application of the articulation index to hearing aid fitting. *Journal of Speech and Hearing. Research, 34,* 391–402.

Sachs, R. M., & Burkhard, M. D. (1972). Earphone pressure response in ears and couplers. *Journal of the Acoustical Society of America, 51, 140*(A). (Available as Industrial Research Products Report No. 20021-2 to Knowles Electronics.)

Scharf, B. (1978). Comparison of normal and impaired hearing. I. Loudness, localization: II. Frequency analysis, speech perception. In C. Ludvigsen & J. Barfod (Eds.), Sensorineural hearing impairment and hearing aids. *Scandinavian Audiology,* Suppl. 6, 4–106.

Scharf, B., & Hellman, R. P. (1966). A model of loudness summation applied to impaired ears. *Journal of the Acoustical Society of America, 40,* 71–78.

Schulein, R. B. (1975). In situ measurement and equalization of sound reproduction systems. *Journal of Audio Engineering Society, 23,* 178–186.

Schweitzer, H. D., & Causey, G. D. (1977). The relative importance of recovery time in compression hearing aids. *Audiology, 16,* 61–72.

Seacord, D. F. (1940). Room noise at subscriber's telephone locations. *Journal of the Acoustical Society of America, 12,* 183–187.

Shaw, E. A. G. (1974). The external ear. In W. D. Keidel & W. D. Neff (Eds.), *Handbook of sensory physiology. (Vol. 7).* Berlin: Springer-Verlag.

Shaw, E. A. G. (1976). Diffuse field sensitivity of the external ear based on the reciprocity principle. *Journal of Acoustical Society of America, 60,* S102(A).

Singer, G. A. (1950, November 18-19). New limiting amplifiers. *Audiologic Engineering,* 69–70.

Skinner, M.W. (1976). *Speech intelligibility in noise-induced hearing loss: Effects of high-frequency compensation* (Doctoral dissertation, Washington University). University Microfilms, Ann-Arbor, MI.

Skinner, M. W. (1980). Speech intelligibility in noise-induced hearing loss: Effects of high-frequency compensation. *Journal of the Acoustical Society of America, 67,* 306–317.

Snow, W. B. (1931). Audible frequency ranges of music, speech, and noise, *Bell Systems Technology Journal, 10,* 616–627.

Steinberg, J. C., & Gardner, M. B. (1937). The dependence of hearing impairment on sound intensity. *Journal of the Acoustical Society of America, 9,* 11–23.

Stevens, S. S. (1972). Perceived level of noise by Mark VII and decibels (E). *Journal of the Acoustical Society of America, 51,* 575–601.

Teder, H. (1991). Hearing instruments in noise and the syllabic speech-to-noise ratio. *Hearing Instruments, 42,* 15–18.

Termin, F. E., & Pettit, J. M. (1952). *Electronic measurements* (p. 341). New York: McGraw-Hill

Toole, F. E. (1981). Listening tests—turning opinion into fact. *Journal of the Audio Engineering Society, 30,* 431–445.

Toole, F. E. (1984). Subjective measurements of loudspeaker sound quality and listener performance., *Journal of the Audio Engineering Society, 33,* 2–32.

Toole, F. E. (1986). Loudspeaker measurements and their relationship to listener preferences: Part 2. *Journal of the Audio Engineering Society, 34,* 323–348.

Villchur, E. (1973). Signal processing to improve speech intelligibility in perceptual deafness. *Journal of the Acoustical Society of America, 53,* 1646–1657.

Villchur, E. (1978). A critical survey of research on amplitude compression. In C. Ludvigsen & J. Barfod (Eds.), Sensorineural hearing impairment and hearing aids. *Scandinavian Audiology,* Suppl. 6, 305–314.

Wallach, H. (1940). The role of head movements and vestibular and visual cues in sound localization. *Journal of Experimental Pshychology, 27,* 339–368.

Wang, C. Y., & Dallos, P. (1972). Latency of whole nerve action potentials: Influence of hair cell normalcy. *Journal of the Acoustical Society of America, 52,* 1678–1686.

Wegel, R. L., & Lane, C. E. (1924). The auditory masking of one pure tone by another and its probable relation to the dynamics of the inner ear. *The Hearing Review, 23,* 266–285.

Wiener, F. M., & Ross, D. A. (1946). The pressure distribution in the auditory canal in a progressive sound field. *Journal of the Acoustical Society of America, 18,* 401–408.

Zwislocki, J. J. (1953). Acoustic attenuation betwen the ears. *Journal of the Acoustical Society of America, 25,* 752–759.

Zwislocki, J.J. (1970). *An acoustic coupler for earphone calibration* (Report LSC-S-7). Syracuse, NY: Syracuse University, Laboratory of Sensory Communication.

CHAPTER 6

The Many Faces of Compression

THEODORE H. VENEMA, PH.D.

OUTLINE

INTRODUCTION

Compression often is referred to as automatic gain control (AGC) because it changes the gain of the hearing aid as the input intensity SPL changes. In this chapter, the use of the word "compression" is maintained. Compression is *the* big word today in the realm of hearing aids. At almost every conference that has to do with hearing, there is some presentation that deals specifically with the issues of compression. Hearing aid specifications abound with all types of compression. Many types of compression hearing aids are produced by most hearing aid manufacturers.

Many clinicians readily admit that they do not have a firm understanding of the many types of compression, nor do they know what type is clinically relevant. Indeed, we find ourselves searching the "specs" sheets, trying desperately to find those little, but important, words that will tell us what a specific compression type is for and when to fit it. In colleges and universities, hearing aid science courses do not offer a comprehensive coverage of compression. This is because compression technology has outpaced the clinical experiences of the instructors. There was a time when the clinical requirements and demands for fitting hearing aids drove the technological development of hearing aids. Now, things are the other way around. Clinicians are struggling to keep up with the rapid pace of technological development. The reality of clinical practice is that we must keep current with the constantly changing terminology manufacturers use to promote their products.

Even the most advanced hearing aid technology does not restore "normal hearing." The human cochlea, with the differential roles played by the outer and inner hair cells, is a magnificent nonlinear sensory organ. All of our recent developments in compression technology are but tiny steps toward the goal of imitating the cochlea and its functions. Still, however, they are steps in a positive direction.

This chapter reviews the application of compression in hearing aids. We begin with a preliminary discussion of input/output graphs, reflecting the performance of linear hearing aids. We start here because basic concepts must be understood before discussing nonlinear (compression) hearing aids. Compression has many "faces"; that is, there is no one simple way to describe it. To appreciate compression function, we can liken it to a piece of sculpture. We need to walk around and view it from several different angles to appreciate the entire piece. Accordingly, compression in hearing aids will be reviewed from three separate dimensions: input versus output compression, two very different types of compression controls, the regular versus the "TK" control, and output limiting compression versus wide dynamic range compression (WDRC). The popular concepts of bass and treble increases at low level input (BILL & TILL) will be discussed as two subsets or types of WDRC. In other words, all BILL and TILL are WDRC but not all WDRC is BILL & TILL. Similarly, all WDRC is input compression but not all input compression is WDRC.

Common clinical combinations of the three separate dimensions of compression are discussed mainly to summarize the types of compression that were discussed, and to show that these compression characteristics often are found in clusters, intended for two different degrees of hearing loss: mild-to-moderate and severe-to-profound. Individuals with mild-to-moderate sensorineural hearing loss often are fit with input compression WDRC hearing aids, which utilize a TK control. Those with severe-to-profound hearing loss often are fit with output compression with output limiting, and these hearing aids use a regular compression control. Not to be overlooked are some clinical obstacles that arise when fitting WDRC hearing aids to a hearing-impaired person who is accustomed to wearing linear hearing aids.

Multi-channel and programmable hearing aids recently have achieved a good deal of market share and they are discussed later on in this chapter. Although some hearing aids are both multi-channel and programmable, it is important to understand how these functions exist separately. Only then can we appreciate how they are bound together.

Expansion (as opposed to compression) is reviewed because it is a relative newcomer to the field of compression in hearing aids. Although expansion is not commonly used in analog hearing aids, its popularity is increasing because it presents a unique solution to microphone noise associated with WDRC hearing aids. This is especially true in quiet listening environments.

Lastly, dynamic, as opposed to static, compression characteristics are reviewed. The concepts underlying attack/release times often are poorly understood by clinicians. Some of the more popular applications of attack/release times in hearing aids will be discussed, including adaptive compression, syllabic compression, and automatic volume control. There is also some interaction between attack/release times and actual compression ratios. To that end, some discussion is devoted to this topic.

INPUT/OUTPUT GRAPHS AND LINEAR HEARING AIDS

Input/output graphs are common to all specification sheets from hearing aid manufacturers. One should become familiar with them. Ideally, clinicians should be able to cover up the specs sheet data from any hearing aid manufacturer, look at the graphs, and be able to tell what type of compression is being shown and for whom it is intended.

The graphs in Figures 6–1, 6–2, and 6–4 are input/output graphs. The horizontal axes show input sound pressure level (SPL). The vertical axes show output SPL. The lines on each graph are the "functions" and literally represent the performance of the hearing aid. The functions on each graph indicate the gain of a hearing aid for different SPL input levels.

To understand any hearing aid (linear or compression), it is important to be familiar with the most basic formula for hearing aids: Input + Gain = Output. Input is that sound entering a hearing aid. Gain is the amount of amplification given to the input sound by the hearing aid. Output is the sum total of sound energy that travels from the hearing aid into one's ear.

When fitting a hearing aid, it is important to keep the maximum power output (MPO) below the uncomfortable loudness level (UCL) of the client. For example, an output of 120 dB (SPL) usually is uncomfortably loud for those with normal hearing as well as for those with a sensorineural hearing loss. The level for normal conversational speech is about 70 dB SPL. If a hearing aid yields 50 dB of gain to a 70 dB input signal, its output is 120 dB SPL. For a person with a UCL of 120 dB SPL, maximum acceptable gain has been reached with conversational speech, and any further increases would be contraindicated. As long as input sounds are 70 dB or less, the hearing aid output will remain below the uncomfortable listening level. If input levels rise above 70 dB, the added gain of 50 dB will result in an output exceeding 120 dB SPL, thus inducing discomfort.

A hearing aid circuit that provides the same amount of gain for all input levels is known as "linear" (see Figure 6–1). The straight diagonal function or line represents linear gain, and it shows that the hearing aid

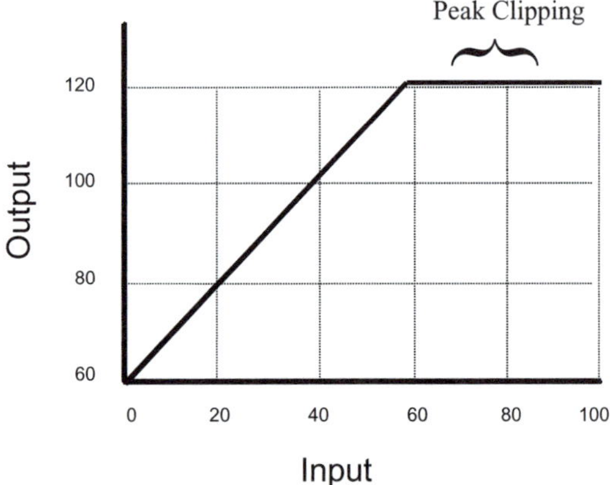

Figure 6–1. With linear hearing aids, the output increases at the same rate as the input increases. In this example, the gain of the linear hearing aid is 60 dB. For 20 dB inputs, the output is 80 dB; for 60 dB inputs, the output is 120 dB; for 100 dB inputs, the output would be 160 dB (if not for output limiting). People with sensorineural hearing loss usually cannot stand much more than about 120 dB SPL, and so linear circuits introduce "peak clipping." This means that any output more than 120 dB SPL gets clipped, or "cut off." Peak clipping means that the diaphragm inside the receiver is actually "slapping" against the sides of the receiver walls, which in turn, produces a very distorted sound quality for the listener.

output increases by 1 dB for each added dB of input (a 1:1 ratio). This continues until a maximum output is achieved. The maximum output of the hearing aid is shown as the horizontal function or line on the figure. Consider the following: If a hearing aid has a gain of 60 dB, then a 20 dB SPL input will result in an 80 dB SPL output, a 40 dB SPL input will result in a 100 dB SPL output, and a 60 dB input will result in an output of 120 dB SPL. The first two output levels would be tolerable for most hearing-impaired individuals, but the third probably would not. When hearing aid output exceeds a wearer's UCL, the remedy of choice for linear circuitry is to "clip the peaks" of the output signal. This usually is accomplished with an MPO, or peak clipping control.

The primary problem with limiting the output by peak clipping is that when the output sound exceeds the established MPO, the hearing aid distorts the signal and the *quality* of listening is degraded. If a hearing aid provides 60 dB of gain and the MPO is set at around 120 dB SPL, then typical speech inputs of 70 dB SPL will constantly drive the hearing aid into saturation. This will result in poor sound quality caused by the distortion. Linear hearing aids were the "state of the art" in technology during the mid 1970s. Even in the 1980s most hearing aid dispensed were those having linear circuitry.

Now, examine the compression input/output graphs in Figure 6–2. For each graph in these figures, gain is represented by the diagonal lines. The point where each gain line

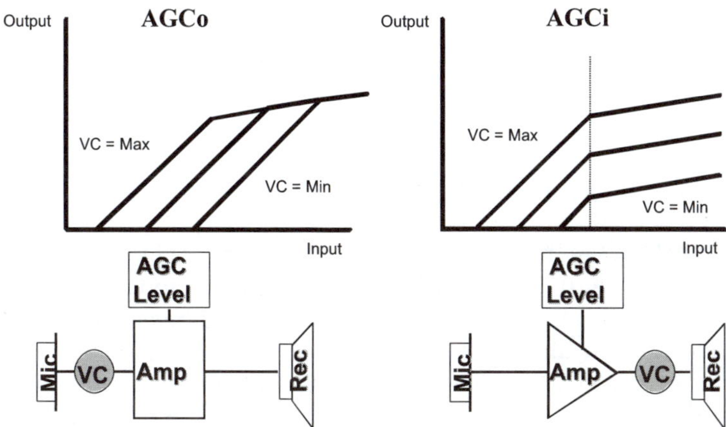

Figure 6–2. Input/output graphs and simple circuit schematics showing relative volume control positions for output compression (left) and input compression (right). For each graph, the parallel diagonal lines rising from the X axis represent linear gain, the corners represent the threshold kneepoint of compression, the line(s) to the right of the kneepoints represent the maximum power output (MPO). The position of the volume control in the circuits determines its effect. For output compression (left), the volume control affects gain and kneepoint, but not MPO. For input compression (right), the volume control affects gain and MPO, but not kneepoint.

suddenly takes a bend is called the compression threshold, or *kneepoint*. It is at this point that compression begins. The kneepoint of compression above the input axis shows the input SPL where compression is initiated. The term *kneepoint* is used to describe the point at which compression begins.

With compression, gain is "nonlinear" because it changes as a function of input SPL. In short, compression hearing aids give different gains for different input levels, whereas linear hearing aids give the same gain for different input levels. Referring to the graph, gain is linear to the left of the kneepoint. This means that for any increase of input SPL there is an equal increase of output SPL. The slope of any line to the right of the kneepoint changes and this shows the effect of compression on the gain of the hearing aid. A compression kneepoint, for example, at an input of 70 dB SPL means that the hearing aid provides linear gain until input levels of 70 dB SPL are reached; above this level, compression is activated. When there is compression, an increase in input SPL does not result in the same increase in output SPL. The gain for input SPL "above" or to the right of the kneepoint is less than the gain for input SPLs "below" the kneepoint.

The maximum power output (MPO) is shown by the "height" of any line that is to the right of the compression kneepoint. For input sound pressure levels to the right of the kneepoint, compression determines the MPO of the hearing aid.

Compression *ratios* are the amount of compression provided by the hearing aid once the compression circuit is activated. Compression ratios can be visualized on an input/output graph by the slant (slope) of the line after the kneepoint. The first number in a compression ratio typically refers to the input, and the second number refers to the output. A 10:1 compression ratio means that, for every 10 dB increase of input SPL, there is only a 1 dB corresponding increase of the output SPL. A 2:1 compression ratio means that, for every 10 dB increase of input SPL, there is a corresponding 5 dB increase to the output SPL of the hearing aid.

Some hearing aids provide "curvilinear compression." This refers to the shape of the input-output line or function. Instead of having a sharp bend, the kneepoint has a more broad curve. Curvilinear compression means that the hearing aid *gradually* goes into its full degree or amount of compression. That is, the amount of compression increases gradually over increasing input levels until it "flattens out" to its maximum.

INPUT COMPRESSION VERSUS OUTPUT COMPRESSION

When the clinician is confronted with compression, the first division that becomes apparent is the issue of input versus output compession. What is the difference and, furthermore, when does one fit which type?

An oft-mentioned concept used to separate input from output compression is that input compression hearing aids have a compressor located between the microphone and the amplifier and output compression hearing aids have a compressor located between the amplifier and the receiver. For the clinician (and the client), however, the major difference between input and output compression is where the *volume control* sits in the circuit (see bottom of Figure 6–2). Manipulation of the volume control has very different effects on the performance of the hearing aid, depending on whether it has input or output compression.

For output compression hearing aids, the VC is situated "early on" in the circuit. It is located between the microphone and the amplifier and the compressor. For input compression hearing aids, the VC is situated just in front of the receiver.

Different VC locations lead to dramatic differences in hearing aid performance. The graphs in Figure 6–2 show the different effects of the VC with output and input compression hearing aids.

Output Compression

For output compression hearing aids (Figure 6–2, left), the VC affects the gain but not the MPO. The three diagonal gain lines in each graph show the effects of three different VC positions. The right-most line shows minimum gain, with the volume control position *lowered* to a minimum position. The left-most line shows maximum gain, with the volume control *raised* to its maximum position.

To clarify, it may help to draw some more lines here. From the right-most kneepoint, draw a vertical line down to the input axis. From the same kneepoint, draw a horizontal line to the output axis. This shows that, at the minimum volume control setting, an X amount of input is needed to give a Y amount of output. If similar vertical and horizontal lines are drawn from the left-most kneepoint, it becomes clear that for the maximum volume control position, less input is needed to give about the same amount of output. Therefore, if a low-volume position, a lot of input is required to result in a specific output, at high-volume positions, less input is needed to give about the same amount of output. This means that the gain is increased as the volume control position is raised. The concept of the left-most gain line, corresponding to the greatest amount of gain, is true for any input/output graph. It will be encountered later in the section on the TK compression control in this chapter.

The left input/output graph also shows that, once beyond, or to the right of the kneepoint in the region of compression, there is only one MPO line that is common to all three diagonal lines. This shows that, for output compression hearing aids, the volume control does not affect the MPO.

Note that the VC also changes the compression kneepoint. This is because the compression kneepoint is adjusted later in the circuit and after the volume control. The compressor is always set to respond to some steady voltage that will tell it to compress. The volume control affects the amount of input signal that will arrive at the compressor of the hearing aid. If the amount of input voltage is not sufficient to tell the compressor to compress, then it will not act at all. Only when the VC rotation sends the required input signal voltage that the compressor is waiting for will the compressor be activated.

Input Compression

For input compression hearing aids, the effects of the VC are completely different (Figure 6–2, right). For input compression, the volume control affects both the gain *and* the MPO.

Again, three diagonal gain lines for three different volume control positions are shown. The right-most diagonal gain line shows the lowest volume control setting, and the left-most gain line shows the highest or maximum volume control setting. It is obvious that the MPO also is affected by the volume control because, once beyond, or to the right of, the kneepoint, the height of three gain lines also changes.

Note also that, for input compression hearing aids, the VC does not affect the kneepoint of compression. As Figure 6–2 (bottom right) shows, the compressor is situated before the VC. This means that the VC does nothing to the kneepoint because the compression kneepoint has already been determined.

Input/output graphs are not the only way to assess differences in the VC effects. The clinician may be familiar with the frequency responses curves (gain as a function of frequency) seen on a hearing aid test box screen or printout, as shown in Figure 6–3. The effects of the VC on gain and MPO are readily apparent for output compression (left graph), as compared to input compression (right graph). For output compression, the VC increases and decreases the gain. For input compression, gain and MPO are affected by the VC.

Clinical Utility of Input and Output Compression

Input and output compression are not superior or inferior to one another. They are just different, and they have different clinical applications.

Output compression may be more appropriate for severe-to-profound hearing losses in which the dynamic range is very restricted. For these patients, the clinician may be concerned that excessive VC settings might cause additional damage to remaining hair cells or residual hearing. Here, an output compression circuit will ensure that the VC affects only the gain and not the MPO of the hearing aid. Output compression also may be good for hearing-impaired children for the same reason; the parent, teacher, or caregiver need not worry about excessive MPO when the little person comes running into the house with the VC in a full-on position.

Input compression may be more appropriate for mild-to-moderate sensorineural hearing loss for which the dynamic range is larger and there is consequently more room to manipulate the MPO. Because mild-to-moderate presbycusis is the most common type of hearing loss, input compression hearing aids have greater potential for clinical fitting.

COMPRESSION CONTROLS: CONVENTIONAL VERSUS "TK"

Here we turn to view another face of compression: the effect of manipulating the compression kneepoint control. There are two types of compression kneepoint controls: 1) the conventional compression control and 2) that referred to as the threshold kneepoint (TK) control. The effect of each of these is presented in Figure 6–4. Both graphs in the figure represent input/output functions similar to those shown in Figure 6–2.

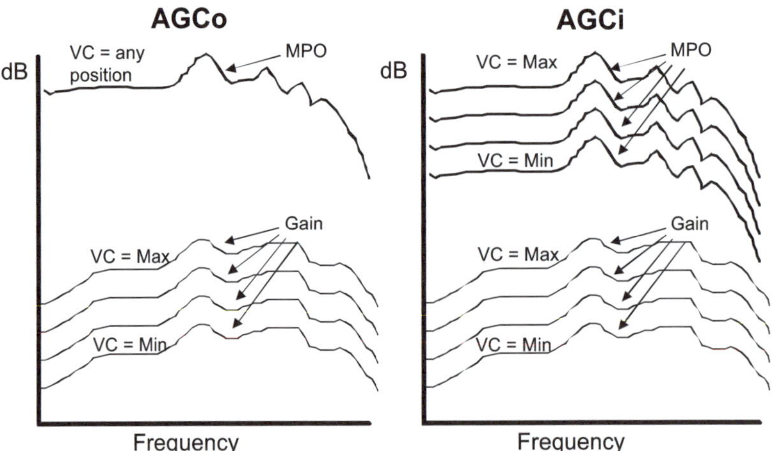

Figure 6–3. Frequency responses showing relative volume control positions for output compression (left) and input compression (right). The volume control for output compression adjusts the gain, but not the MPO; for input compression, the volume control adjusts the gain along with the MPO.

The Conventional Compression Control

The left graph in Figure 6–4 shows the effects of the conventional compression kneepoint control. Typically, it is found on output and on some input compression hearing aids. Most other input compression hearing aids, however, have the TK control.

The conventional compression control affects the compression threshold kneepoint, as well as the MPO. This is accomplished by adjusting the voltage level the compressor circuit needs to begin compressing. As the control is turned to its maximum position, the compressor requires a higher voltage to begin compressing, or the compression kneepoint is raised along with the MPO. At the maximum kneepoint setting, the compression hearing aid is in a "linear gain mode" for a wide-range of input SPL. Compression will not occur until input sounds that are higher than the intensity level specified by the kneepoint are reached. At the maximum kneepoint setting, the MPO also is increased. Referring to Figure 6–4 (left-most graph), note that the conventional compression control does *not* affect the gain; the diagonal, linear gain line does not change with different compression control settings.

The acoustic effects of this control can easily be heard by the clinician, as the cochlea is an excellent acoustic analyzer. Acoustic changes also can be measured in a hearing aid test box. To hear the effect of a typical compression control, one must speak *loudly* into the microphone of the hearing aid. Only then will the input signal (speech) plus the gain reach the established MPO. A low-intensity input, such as a soft voice, plus the gain of the hearing aid may not result in an output that approaches the MPO. As the compres-

Different Ways of Adjusting AGC

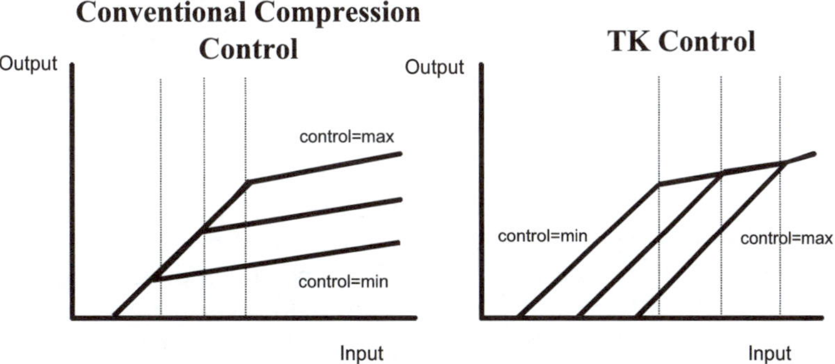

- Compression Control: Affects Kneepoint & Output
- "TK" Control: Affects Kneepoint & Gain

Figure 6–4. Input/output graphs showing effects of two different types of compression controls (volume control is assumed to be held constant at some position). For both graphs, the diagonal line(s) rising from the X axis represent the linear gain; the corners represent the threshold kneepoint of compression; the line(s) to the right of the kneepoints represent the maximum power output (MPO). Both controls adjust the kneepoint of compression, but that is where the similarity ends. The conventional compression control affects MPO, and the TK control affects gain for soft input sound pressure levels only.

sion control is rotated from its maximum to minimum position, the kneepoint of compression, as well as the MPO, is reduced. At this point, one should perceive that the amplified loud voice becomes softer. This is because the compression control affects the MPO, not the gain.

TK Control

The right-most graph in Figure 6–4 shows the effect of the TK control. Technically, any compression control affects the kneepoint of compression, but electrical engineers probably will be quick to note that the term "threshold kneepoint" is an input-related term, and is rarely encountered with output compression hearing aid circuitry. At any rate, the TK control is almost always found on input compression hearing aids. The term TK control is associated most often with K Amp™ hearing aids, and it has become known as a separate entity from regular compression controls.

The TK control affects the threshold kneepoint of compression, as well as the gain for soft input SPLs. This is because the TK control adjusts the kneepoint of compression over a range of relatively low input levels, from about 40 to 55 dB SPL. Like all compression hearing aids, those with the TK control provide linear gain below the threshold kneepoint of compression. However, because this kneepoint is found at relatively soft inputs, the TK control can be seen as a gain booster for soft sounds. Unlike the conventional compression control, the TK control does not affect the MPO.

When listening to a hearing aid with a TK control, it is important to speak softly into the microphone to hear the effect of rotating the control. With loud speech, the effect of the TK will seem minimal or not audible at all. This is very different from the conventional compression control in which the sound becomes louder as the kneepoint is raised and the MPO is increased.

The input/output graph for the TK control (Figure 6–4, right) looks similar to the graph showing the volume control effect for output compression (Figure 6–2, top left). This is because the TK control operates in a similar manner to the volume control for output compression hearing aids. The TK control is located at the input stage of the hearing aid before the compressor and amplifier, just like the VC for output compression (Figure 6–2, bottom left). Therefore it affects the amount of input signal that arrives at the compressor of the circuit, just like the VC does for output compression hearing aids.

Many clinicians have not clearly understood the TK control and how it works. It is important to note that the left-most gain line, where there is greatest gain, shows the TK set to the lowest kneepoint position (Figure 6–4, right graph). The right-most gain line, where there is the least amount of gain, shows the TK set to the highest kneepoint position. As the compression kneepoint with the TK control is lowered, the gain for low-intensity input sounds is increased. Similarly, as the compression kneepoint with the TK control is raised, the gain for low-intensity input sounds is decreased.

Clinical Application of Conventional and TK Compression Controls

Because the conventional compression control affects the MPO and not the gain, it can be used to limit the MPO as a means of protecting the client from further hair cell damage. This type of compression control is useful especially for those clients who have a severe or profound hearing loss and a limited dynamic range. As mentioned earlier, this compression control most often is found on output compression hearing aids, which also are more suited for severe-to-profound hearing loss.

The purpose behind the TK control is an attempt to partially mimic the function of the cochlear outer hair cells (OHCs). The OHCs amplify soft sounds (below 40-50 dB SPL), enabling the inner hair cells to sense these sounds (Killion, 1996b). Damage to OHCs frequently results in the commonly encountered mild-to-moderate sensorineural hearing loss. Use of the TK control therefore is most appropriate for mild-to-moderate SNHL.

The TK control is most often associated with the KAmp™, a type of *input* compression hearing aid (to be discussed further in the following section. Here is some food for thought: It is interesting that two things became clinically popular at around the same time—late 80s and early 90s—and both of these are related specifically to the OHCs: The KAmp™, and the measurement of otoacoustic emissions.

OUTPUT LIMITING COMPRESSION VERSUS WIDE DYNAMIC RANGE COMPRESSION (WDRC)

Two important compression issues have been discussed so far: 1) input versus output compression and 2) the conventional compression control versus the TK control. A third "face" of compression is the issue of "output limiting" compression versus wide dynamic range compression (WDRC). These are actually two different philosophical approaches to compression methods, not specific controls. The effects of output limiting compression and WDRC can be seen in Figure 6–5. Once again, both graphs in the figure are input/output functions, similar to those presented in Figures 6–2 and 6–4.

Output Limiting Compression

Output limiting compression is most often associated with output compression hearing aids that use a conventional compression

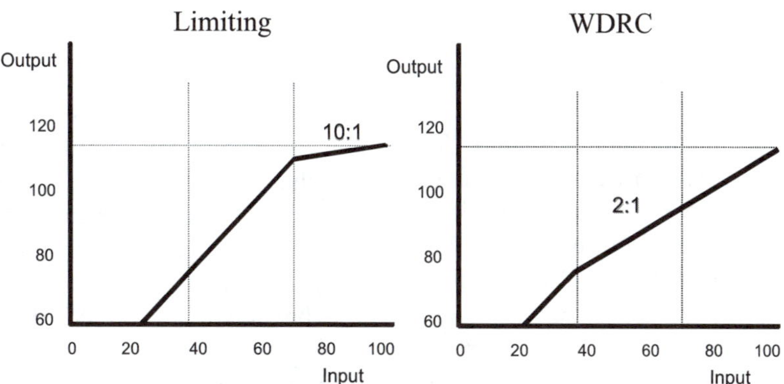

Figure 6–5. Input/output graphs showing effects of output limiting compression (left) and wide dynamic range compression (right). For both graphs, the diagonal lines rising from the X axis represent the gain; the corners represent the threshold kneepoint of compression, the lines to the right of the kneepoint represent the MPO. The hearing aid gain is the same (60 dB) for each type of compression. The gain function, however, is very different for each type of compression. Output limiting compression has a high kneepoint and a high compression ratio, wide dynamic range compression has a low kneepoint and a low compression ratio.

control. Output limiting compression can be found also in some input compression hearing aids, in which compression is used for limiting the output.

The salient features of output limiting compression are shown in the left-most graph of Figure 6–5. Output limiting compression hearing aids have two main features: 1) a "high" compression kneepoint and 2) a high compression ratio. A high kneepoint means that the hearing aid begins to compress at relatively high input SPL (i.e., 55 to 60 dB SPL or more). Below the kneepoint, the hearing aid provides linear gain. A high compression ratio usually is defined as being greater than 5:1 (Dillon, 1988). Higher compression ratios indicate more compression of the input signal.

Output limiting compression hearing aids provide a strong degree of compression over a narrow range of inputs (Figure 6–5, left graph). Below the threshold kneepoint, the output limiting compression hearing aid provides linear gain for a wide range of input SPLs. In other words, it takes a fairly high input SPL signal to activate the compression function; however, once it goes into compression, it *really* goes into compression.

Output limiting compression hearing aids have some similarities to linear hearing aids. Both give a fixed amount of gain over a wide range of different SPL inputs. Also, both provide a sudden limit to the output SPL. The main difference between them is that linear hearing aids use peak clipping to limit the output, whereas output limiting compression hearing aids use a high ratio of compression to limit the output. The advantage of limiting with compression is that it introduces less distortion at the maximum output stage than does peak clipping.

Wide Dynamic Range Compression (WDRC)

WDRC hearing aids have become extremely popular during the past several years. It is important to categorize where WDRC properly fits in the overall spectrum of the many faces of compression. Only then can it be appreciated for what it is and what it is not.

The function of WDRC is shown in Figure 6–5 (right graph). The TK control is used to adjust WDRC and, like the TK control, WDRC almost always is associated with input compression hearing aids. Recall, however, that not all input compression is WDRC. Some input compression uses output limiting compression, which is adjusted by a conventional compression control.

WDRC is associated with low threshold kneepoints (below 55 dB SPL) and low compression ratios (less than 5:1). As the right-most graph of Figure 6–5 shows, the WDRC hearing aid is almost always in compression. It can be seen that many different input levels, from very soft speech to very loud speech, will put the hearing aid into compression. Perhaps it is called "wide dynamic range compression" because of its low kneepoint, which allows compression to take place over a wide range of input levels.

Once the WDRC hearing aid goes into compression, however, it does not provide a greater ratio or degree of compression (Figure 6–5). Basically, a WDRC hearing aid provides a weak degree of compression over a wide range of inputs. The effect of WDRC is very different from output limiting compression or linear hearing aids. Unlike hearing aids that suddenly reduce the gain once the input SPL exceeds a certain amount, WDRC gradually reduces the gain for a wide range of input SPL.

It has been suggested that the use of WDRC along with fast attack/release times can degrade some of the cues necessary for speech recognition (Kuk, 1999). The reasoning is that, although WDRC amplifies soft speech more than loud speech, the use of fast attack/release times can reduce the differences between the "peaks" and "valleys" of the input speech sound wave. More on this topic is discussed in the section on "Syllabic Compression" in this chapter.

Clinical Applications of Output Limiting Compression and WDRC

When comparing output limiting compression to WDRC, it is helpful to look closely at their names. The main clinical difference between the two is that output limiting compression does its work above its kneepoint, where its compression serves to reduce or limit the output for high input sound levels. On the other hand, WDRC does its work below its kneepoint; it is in compression for most input levels, but offers greatest (linear) gain for soft input sounds below the kneepoint (Johnson, 1993; Killion, 1996a). In other words, the focus of output limiting compression is to prevent the "ceiling" of sound output from becoming too loud, whereas the focus of WDRC is to lift or amplify the "floor" or soft input sounds so they become audible.

Why would clinicians want a choice between these types of compression? To answer this question, let us look at the loudness growth phenomenon. The client who has OHC damage usually has a mild-to-moderate SNHL, in which the "floor" of hearing sensitivity is elevated compared to normal, although the "ceiling" of loudness tolerance may be near normal. The appropriate goal of amplification is to restore normal loudness growth. To accomplish this goal, we need to amplify soft sounds by a lot, and loud sounds by little or nothing at all.

Figure 6–6 shows output limiting compression (left) and WDRC (right) superimposed on two identical graphs of loudness growth.

Loudness Growth
&
Types of Compression

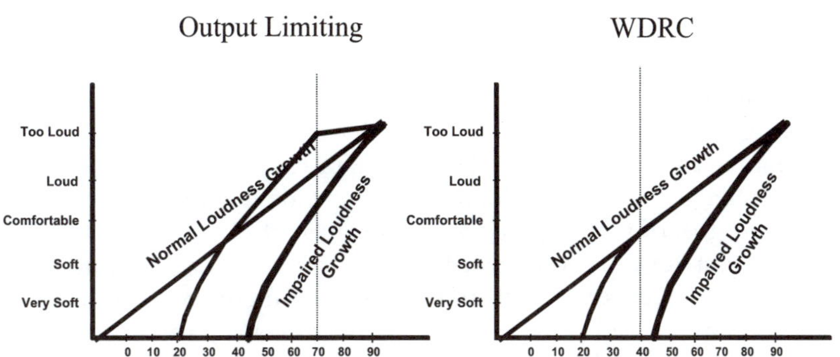

Figure 6–6. Re-establishing normal loudness growth with output limiting compression and wide dynamic range compression (WDRC). The X axis represents the physical dimension of input sound intensity to the hearing aid; the Y axis represents the psychoacoustic dimension of loudness perception. In this example, both output limiting compression and wide dynamic range compression make 90 dB inputs sound "too loud." But the high kneepoint and high compression ratio for output limiting compression make inputs of 70, 80, and 90 dB all sound "too loud," as well. This does not occur for WDRC because it has a low kneepoint and a low compression ratio.

Both graphs show loudness growth functions of a normal hearing person, compared to one with a mild-to-moderate SNHL.

Figure 6–5 showed that both output limiting compression and WDRC may function in the same manner for inputs of 90 dB SPL. They both may reach the point where output sounds are perceived as being "too loud," but the *way* that each arrives at this common point is completely different. At a compression seminar at the American Academy of Audiology conference in 1996, F. Kuk provided a very illustrative analogy. Output limiting compression was compared to a teenager speeding down the road in a car who sees a stop sign at the end of the road, slams on the brakes and screeches to a stop. WDRC was compared to an elderly person who starts out at a normal speed, but on seeing the stop sign far ahead, ever-so-cautiously applies a foot gently to the brakes and slows to a stop over a longer distance. In this analogy, normal loudness growth is the road, linear gain is the gas pedal held down for speed, and compression is the brakes.

Some problems arise when restoring normal loudness growth utilizing output limiting compression (Figure 6–6 left-most graph). First, there is an "overshoot" of normal loudness growth. The greater problem, however, is that 70, 80, and 90 dB inputs, when aided, give the same loudness sensation and are perceived as being "too loud." This is not a restoration of normal loudness growth. The right-most graph of Figure 6–5 shows WDRC applied to the same goal of restoring normal loudness growth. If restoring loudness growth is the goal, then the lower kneepoint and lower compression ratio provided by WDRC are clearly a much better fit. This is because soft input sounds are given most gain, whereas increasingly intense input sounds are given progressively less and less gain. Unlike output limiting compression, the focus of WDRC is to lift the "floor" of hearing sensitivity rather than prevent the "ceiling" of sound from becoming too loud.

Perhaps another reason for the term "WDRC" is that the low kneepoint and low compression ratio reduce a normally large dynamic range into the smaller one associated with mild-to-moderate SNHL. For example, a low compression ratio of 2:1 will compress a dynamic range of 100 dB into one of 50 dB.

Referring to Kuk's (1996) statement, does this mean that we should all drive like the elderly person? Not really. A client with mild-to-moderate hearing loss may be accustomed to wearing linear hearing aids. For this person, a sudden switch to WDRC might be too great a hurdle, and WDRC might be rejected because it is not loud enough. Although WDRC will amplify soft inputs by a considerable amount, it will not amplify average intensity inputs by the same amount, and it is this hearing aid performance that the client accustomed to linear amplification may find frustrating. Output limiting compression may result in the "overshoot" of normal loudness as seen in the left graph of Figure 6–6, but the client may have become accustomed to the sound. In this case, WDRC must be introduced gradually, and with considerable counseling about what to expect from WDRC hearing aids. Many hearing-impaired persons can adjust to WDRC, but others cannot overcome their "perceived" need for more power and may refuse to make the change.

For those with severe-to-profound hearing loss, output limiting compression might be a better choice than WDRC. These individuals may prefer a powerful, linear gain amplifier over a wide range of input sound levels, until the output SPL becomes close to their loudness tolerance or uncomfortable loudness levels. Furthermore, these clients often have worn powerful linear hearing aids in the past. Output limiting compression hearing aids, like their old linear hearing aids, will give lots of gain for soft and average input sounds, and these similar gain characteristics will be appreciated.

Hearing aids with output limiting compression do offer a significant advantage over linear hearing aids. For instance, for high input levels, output limiting compression does not produce the same degree of distortion that is associated with peak clipping, linear hearing aids. As such, they may be more preferable by those clients with severe-to-profound hearing loss.

More is discussed concerning the clinical considerations of fitting linear, output limiting compression, and WDRC hearing aids in a later section of this chapter, "A Clinical Spectrum of Compression."

BASS AND TREBLE INCREASES AT LOW LEVELS (BILL AND TILL)

It has been difficult to miss the recent deluge of advertisements concerning multichannel hearing aids with WDRC. These systems have become *the* high-end hearing aids that promise maximum fitting flexibility, normal loudness growth for different hearing loss configurations, and a natural; high quality of sound. Many manufacturers have their own version of these types of hearing aids. These need not be listed here; readers can review the rather vast amount of literature provided by the manufacturers to see for themselves.

BILL and TILL: Two Types of WDRC

Bass increase at low levels (BILL) and treble increase at low levels (TILL) are two types of WDRC. There are other names that pertain to these categories, such as LDFR (level-dependent frequency response), FDC (frequency-dependent compression), and ASP (automatic signal processing). Basically, these terms can be reduced to one common denominator: Compression in these circuits is more dominant in some frequency ranges than in others. Where compression occurs the most, it will be WDRC, with a low kneepoint and a low compression ratio. The simplest classification of these types of compression is that of BILL and TILL (Killion, Staab, & Preves, 1990).

To understand BILL and TILL, it is important to know that in any compression hearing aid, the compression kneepoint often occurs at a different input SPL for different frequencies. BILL and TILL, however, are hearing aids where the kneepoint of compression occurs at *very* different input SPL for different frequencies.

The fact that compression may occur more at some frequencies than at others, is not evident from the input/output graphs on hearing aid specs sheets. When hearing aid specs sheets in North America show the compression kneepoint, they adhere to the standards established by the American National Standards Institute (ANSI, S3.22). This set of standards shows the compression kneepoint on input/output graphs as we have seen in Figures 6–2, 6–4, and 6-5, and these graphs do not show frequency. The ANSI standard specifies that the kneepoint of compression is to be shown on input/output graphs at one frequency, 2000 Hertz (Hz).

BILL hearing aids have a low kneepoint for the low frequencies and a higher kneepoint for the high frequencies. Low frequency input will not have to be very intense to set the BILL hearing aid into compression, but high-frequency input will have to be greater to cause compression. This means that the BILL circuit will go into compression very often with low-frequency inputs, and not as often with high-frequency inputs.

Figure 6–7 shows a simple set of gain and frequency curves for BILL (left graph) and TILL (right graph) circuits. The BILL hearing aid (left graph) has a very broad, or flat frequency response, with soft inputs (e.g., 40 dB SPL). If input sound is produced so that it is at 40 dB SPL all across the frequency range, then the gain and frequency response of the BILL hearing aid will look something like the top, flat line on the graph. As the input across frequencies is increased in intensity to 60 dB SPL, the gain and frequency response will show a decrease in gain for the low frequencies. As the input intensity is increased to 80 dB SPL, the gain for the low frequencies will drop even more.

The main idea behind the BILL circuit is to provide better listening for speech while in

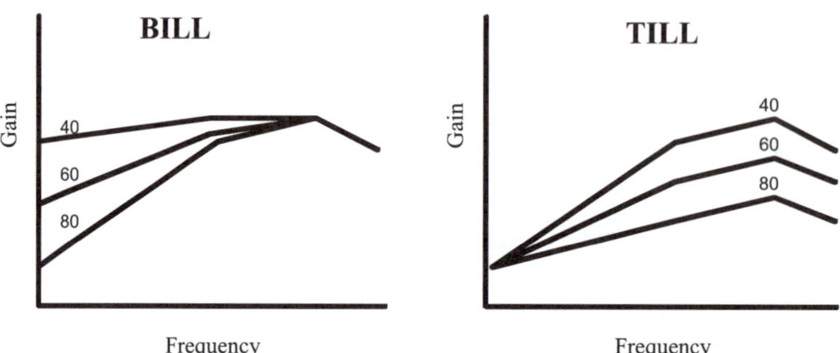

Figure 6–7. For each graph, the gain (Y axis) across a frequency range (X axis) is shown for three different input levels. The left graph shows bass increases at low levels (BILL). As inputs decrease in intensity, low-frequency gain increases. Examples of BILL are the Manhattan circuit™ and the Oticon Multifocus™. The right graph shows treble increase at low levels (TILL). As inputs decrease in intensity, high-frequency gain increases. The KAmp™ is an example of a TILL circuit.

background noise. That is, the "hubbub" of low-frequency background noise will be suppressed by compression, while high-frequency sounds that render clarity for speech still receive a full measure of gain. BILL was originally associated with the Argosy Manhattan™ circuit. The hearing aid most commonly brought to mind when BILL is mentioned today is the Oticon Multifocus™.

The TILL hearing aid (right graph) has an entirely different function. The kneepoint is set at a high input SPL for the low frequencies and at a lower kneepoint for the high frequencies. For the TILL hearing aid, high-frequency input will not need to be very intense to cause compression. Low-frequency input, however, will need to be much more intense to cause compression. This means the TILL circuit will go into compression very often with high-frequency inputs, and not as often with low-frequency inputs.

Figure 6–7 (right graph) shows a TILL response, in which low-intensity inputs of 40dB SPL across the frequency range will result in a gain and frequency response that has more of a high-frequency emphasis. As the input is increased to 60 dB SPL, the high-frequency emphasis will decrease relative to the gain for the low frequencies. With inputs of 80 dB SPL, the gain for the high frequencies will decrease even more. In some TILL in-the-ear hearing aids, the 80+ dB SPL response is intended to resemble the resonance of the open, unaided ear, thus providing an acoustic "transparency" for intense inputs when the hearing aid is not needed, anyway.

The main idea behind TILL is to emphasize the high-frequency sounds of speech for the listener who most typically has sensorineural high-frequency hearing loss. Those with this type of hearing loss will have a reduced dynamic range for the high frequencies. Compared to that for normal hearing, the "floor" of hearing sensitivity will be elevated, although the "ceiling" of loudness tolerance will not be. The hearing aid most commonly thought of when TILL is brought up today is the K Amp™.

MULTICHANNEL HEARING AIDS

Today, BILL and TILL commonly are combined into one hearing aid that has two or more channels (Figure 6–8). A multichannel hearing aid is like having two or more hearing aids in one. A big advantage of multichannel circuits over a single-channel WDRC circuit involves clinical fitting flexibility. Either the BILL or TILL channel can be adjusted to provide an optimal fitting for particular configurations or shapes of mild-to-moderate hearing loss. In essence, only one hearing aid circuit may be required to fit many different hearing losses. Because of the preponderance of presbycusis and other mild-to-moderate SNHL, the flexible multichannel WDRC circuits potentially can be fit on many people.

The term "multichannel" should not be confused with "programmable"; these two terms are mutually exclusive, representing very different systems. Multichannel hearing aids can be programmable, but so can single-channel hearing aids. More will be discussed about programmable hearing aids in the next section. For now, multichannel hearing aids are discussed without relationship to programmability. Because most analog multichannel hearing aids have two channels, the following discussion pertains to two-channel hearing aids, with WDRC in each channel.

Multi-channel circuits often use input compression, which can be determined from the position of the VC in the circuit (see Figure

Multichannel Amplification
with
BILL & TILL

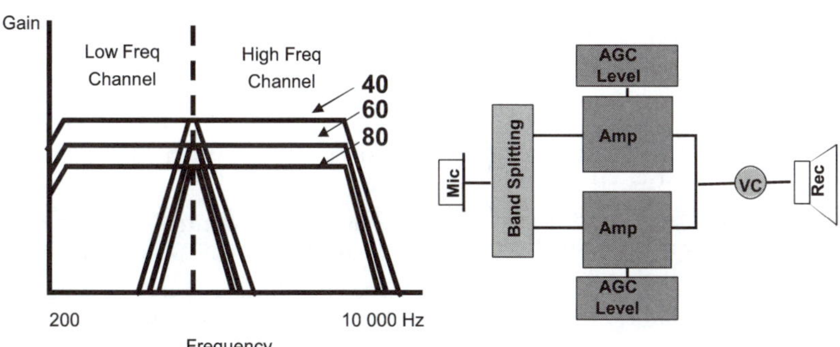

Figure 6–8. A two-channel WDRC hearing aid can be set up to produce a response of BILL, TILL, or both. If both channels have independent WDRC circuits, then the gain for both the low-frequency and high-frequency channels will increase at low-intensity input sound levels. On the right, a schematic for a two-channel compression hearing aid is shown. Following the microphone, a band splitter separates the inputs into a low-frequency band and a high-frequency band. Each frequency band is amplified and compressed separately. The end result is reunited into one receiver. There is also only one volume control. The gain and frequency graph on the left shows a two-channel WDRC hearing aid that is set up for both BILL and TILL. In this example, the client may have a "flat" hearing loss configuration.

6–8, right side). This figure shows that there is one microphone, followed by a band splitter, which separates the incoming input sound into two frequency bands, or channels. Each separate channel has its own amplifier and compressor.

The same circuit is also WDRC, with a TK control to adjust the kneepoint of compression for both channels. Figure 6–8 shows that the circuit combines BILL and TILL into one hearing aid. A BILL response is obtained if the gain of the low-frequency channel is turned up while that of the high-frequency channel is turned down. This could be an appropriate setting for a "reverse" hearing loss configuration. A TILL response is obtained if the gain of the low channel is turned down while that of the high channel is turned up. This could be a good setting for a high-frequency hearing loss. Lastly, if the gain of both channels is turned up equally, then the circuit provides a BILL and a TILL response, which could be a good setting for a flat hearing loss.

Due to the recent popularity of multichannel WDRC hearing aids, it may be helpful to illustrate an example of the BILL and TILL used in the popular DynamEQII™ circuit, built by a Canadian company, the Gennum Corporation of Burlington Ontario. This circuit is used by many manufacturers to create their own two-channel WDRC hearing aids. Some unique features of this circuit and its controls or trimmers are described briefly here. An especially interesting feature of the circuit is that the gain controls for each channel actually adjust the compression ratio within each channel. In most hearing aids that use this circuit, a single threshold kneepoint can be adjusted for both channels together, whereas the compression ratios can be adjusted separately for each channel.

Steep dB/Octave Slope Between the Channels

The DynamEQII™ circuit allows for a 12 dB/octave slope or a more steep 24 dB/octave slope between its two channels (see Figure 6–9). The term "slope" for a multi-channel hearing aid refers to the steepness of the "sides" or "skirts" of the channels. Both channels provide gain over a range of frequencies and, at the crossover frequency region where the two channels "meet," the gain of each channel decreases by a rate of up to 24 dB/octave.

For analog (nondigital) technology, 24 dB/octave is a relatively steep slope that contributes greatly to fitting flexibility. Fitting flexibility is enhanced further when the crossover frequency between the two channels can be adjusted. The circuit has an F control that adjusts the frequency crossover point where the channels come together. Probe microphone, or "real ear," measures of ear canal sound pressure levels reveal that the F control can be used to adjust the frequency crossover from about 500 Hz to about 2000 Hz.

Fitting flexibility is maximized when the gain of the low and high channels can be adjusted independently, along with the crossover frequency. The gain of the low-frequency channel (GL control) can be turned up without much effect on the frequency regions of the high-frequency channel; similarly, the gain of the high-frequency channel (GH control) can be turned up without much effect on the frequency regions of the low-frequency channel. It is thus as if there are two "vertical" gain controls and a "horizontal" crossover control.

These three controls enable one to fit difficult hearing loss configurations. Consider these conditions: 1) the "reverse" hearing loss where the client has hearing loss for the low frequencies and better hearing for the high frequencies or 2) the precipitous hearing loss where the hearing is normal up to 2000 Hz, and then suddenly drops off in the high frequencies. When fitting precipitous high-frequency hearing losses with single-channel hearing aids, high-frequency gain typically is provided, along with a maximum degree of low cut. A common problem, however, is unavoidable, unwanted gain for the mid frequencies at which the person may have no hearing loss. The fitting flexibility of two-channel hearing aids enables the frequency

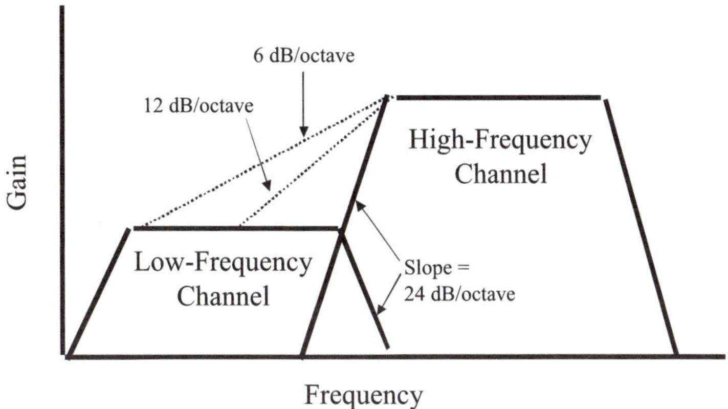

Figure 6–9. "Passive" low-cut or high-cut trimmers usually have a 6 dB/octave slope. "Active" trimmers have a 12 or 18 dB/octave slope, which enables them to have more dramatic effects on the frequency response. A steep 24 dB/octave slope between two channels of a hearing aid enables even more independence between the channels and, consequently, even more flexibility in shaping the frequency response. It also helps to eliminate unwanted mid-frequency gain when this is desired. Two channels divided by a steep slope provide low- and high-frequency "plateaus" that can be raised or lowered with low-frequency and high-channel gain trimmers. In this example, the low-frequency channel gain is turned down whereas the high-frequency channel gain is turned up.

response to be "sculpted" around the "corner" of an audiogram.

Adjustable Compression Ratios

The clinician should know that for these two-channel WDRC hearing aids, an adjustment of the GL (gain for low channel) and GH (gain for high channel) control is really an adjustment of the compression ratios. Input/output graphs show that each channel has two kneepoints, which allows for adjustable compression ratios (see Figure 6–10). This feature is very useful for restoring normal loudness growth. The two-channel DynamEQII™ circuit is by no means the only circuit that has these features. For example, ReSound, Inc. has long been known for restoring normal loudness growth by means of a WDRC circuit with two kneepoints and adjustable compression ratios.

Figure 6–10 illustrates how the concepts of compression kneepoints and ratios are related to the restoration of normal loudness growth. The right side shows the reduced dynamic range and abnormal loudness growth that occurs with sensorineural hearing loss. It also shows the required gain to restore normal loudness growth. The smaller dynamic range will require a greater amount of gain at soft input levels to restore normal loudness growth.

Loudness Growth
&
Compression Ratios

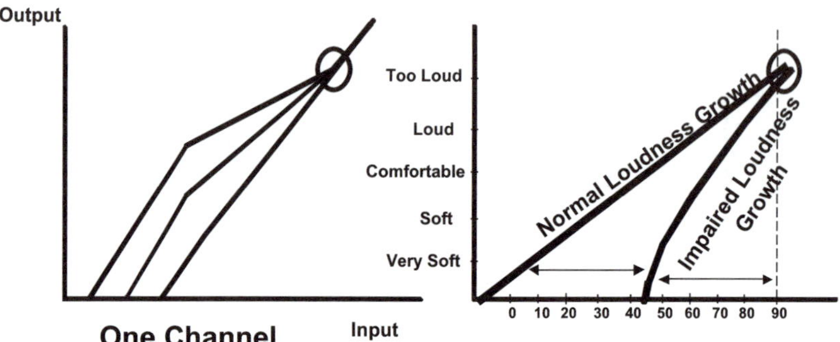

Figure 6–10. The relationship between the concepts of loudness growth and compression ratios are shown. In the right graph, the right arrow shows the dynamic range for an individual's hearing loss at some frequency; the left arrrow shows required gain to restore normal loudness growth. The circle shows the "ceiling" of loudness tolerance for both SNHL and normal hearing. On the left is an input/output graph for one channel of the two-channel DynamEQII™ circuit, the circle shows the output that corresponds to the "ceiling" of loudness tolerance on the right. The diagonal lines rising from the X axis show the linear gain below the kneepoint of compression, which is adjusted by a TK control. The higher kneepoint is fixed at about 95 dB SPL. The compression ratios hinge from this point. The lines sloping to the left of the second kneepoint show the adjustable ratios of compression needed to restore normal loudness growth.

The left side of Figure 6–10 shows an input/output graph that features two kneepoints and adjustable compression ratios. It can represent any one channel of the DynamEQII™ circuit. The lower kneepoint shows the input SPL where compression begins. Below this input level, the gain is linear. A TK control adjusts this lower kneepoint for both channels together because the DynamEQII™ circuit has only one TK control. Between the two kneepoints, the compression ratio can range from 4:1 to 1:1 (recall that these low ratios are typical with WDRC). Note that the compression ratios hinge from the second, higher kneepoint, not from the first, lower kneepoint. With this in mind, it becomes clear that, as the compression ratio increases, so does the gain. This is contrary to most other types of compression, in which an increased compression ratio is associated with decreased gain.

The higher kneepoint shows where compression ends. Beyond this input SPL, the hearing aid has reached a point of *unity gain*. Here, the compression ratio once again becomes linear, but there is no gain whatsoever. For example, a 95 dB input results in a 95 dB output, a 96 dB input results in a 96 dB output, and so on. It is at this point that the hearing aid becomes truly acoustically "transparent."

The feature of adjustable compression ratios separately for both channels is a strong tool for restoring normal loudness growth. The TK control, at one time the only control available to adjust the compression of WDRC hearing aids, now can be relegated to a "rear seat" in the theater. When it comes to restoring normal loudness growth, adjusting compression ratios is a stronger tool than adjusting compression kneepoints (see left graph of Figure 6–10).

Adjustment of the kneepoint and compression ratios, however, should be seen as two parts of a team. The GL and GH controls, which adjust compression ratio, should be adjusted to best restore normal loudness growth for the client. To explain in the broadest terms, this means that, if the client's dynamic range is one-fourth that of normal for some frequency range, then the compression ratio should be adjusted to 4:1 (the maximum gain position for either the GL or the GH control). If the client's dynamic range is half that of normal, then the compression ratio should be adjusted to 2:1. Compression ratios for specific GL or GH control positions are provided by the manufacturer.

The TK control should be adjusted to provide as much gain for soft input sounds as possible, without resulting in feedback or the client's perception of a background "hiss." Recall from the previous discussion on the TK control that a "minus" position lowers the kneepoint of compression and actually increases the gain for soft input sounds. Setting the TK at a "plus" position raises the kneepoint and reduces the effectiveness of the WDRC. For more information on the typical "hiss" sound perceived by some clients when the TK is set to a "minus" position, see the subsequent section in this chapter on "Expansion."

PROGRAMMABLE HEARING AIDS

A discussion of compression and multi-channel hearing aids would be incomplete without some reference to programmable hearing aids, and how compression is utilized in these types of circuits. Almost every hearing aid manufacturer produces at least one programmable hearing aid. The pace of hearing aid technology development has quickened, and there is healthy competition among the manufacturers. In this section, the general aspects of programmable hearing aids are discussed, along with their advantages. Programmable, and also digital, hearing aids have gained considerable popularity. Digital hearing aids are being developed by most manufacturers just about as fast as this chapter is being written. A complete discussion of digital hearing aids is beyond the scope of this chapter; however, the reader should know that many of the types of compression that have been reviewed here are also used in digital hearing aids.

In this section, the term "programmable" is used for analog (nondigital) hearing aids. Digital hearing aids, which actually use digital signal processing (DSP), are a completely separate entity. Thus, the terms "programmable" and "digital" should not be confused. Many hearing aids are "digitally programmable," but this does not necessarily mean that the circuit of the hearing itself provides DSP. Many conventional analog hearing aids are digitally programmable. This simply means that, instead of requiring a screwdriver to adjust the trimmers, the hearing aid trimmer settings (and/or VC) can be programmed by a hand-held programmer or by a computer with appropriate software. (Computers are digital in that they use a complex series of binary mathematical sequences, i.e., a series of 0s and 1s.) In general, programmable hearing aids can provide essentially the same compression characteristics as non-programmable hearing aids; the main difference is in the way that the controls or trimmers are accessed.

Analog, programmable hearing aids appeared in the late 1980s. Many of these were single-channel hearing aids in which the clinician adjusted (i.e., programmed) the hearing aid trimmers with a computer or a hand-held programming unit. Many programmable hearing aids offer two or more memories (i.e., programs). These provide clients access to different frequency responses with the flick of a switch, located on either the actual hearing aids, or on a hand-held remote-control device. By accessing different frequency responses, clients can personally adjust the hearing aids for optimal use in different listening environments.

Programmable Hearing Aids Versus Multichannel Hearing Aids

Just as the terms "digital" and "programmable" represent essentially different concepts, so do the terms programmable and multichannel. When *programmable* and *multi-channel* hearing aids are understood as distinct from each other, it can be appreciated how the properties of multichannel and programmability often intersect or are combined (see Figure 6–11). Programmable hearing aids can be single-channel or multi-channel. Similarly, single-channel and multichannel hearing aids can be programmable or non-programmable. Features like multiple channels and programmability can be combined, however, and investigation of the offerings by manufacturers will quickly verify that combinations of programmable, multi-channel hearing aids abound.

As Figure 6–11 shows, some programmable hearing aids are single-channel and some are multi-channel. Single-channel, programmable hearing aids may have circuitry simi-

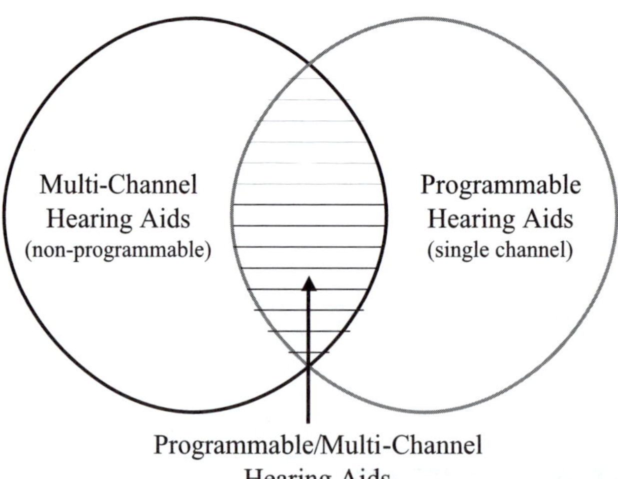

Figure 6–11. The terms "multi-channel" and "programmable" are separate concepts which may or may not be found in combination. Multi-channel hearing aids may or may not be programmable; programmable hearing aids can be single channel or they can have more than one channel. In general, the clinician determines the settings (frequency response/compression characteristics) for each channel in a multi-channel hearing aid. Programmability means that the hearing aid settings are adjusted by a computer. Programmable/multi-channel hearing aids are hearing aids with more than one channel, which can be programmed by a computer.

lar to their non-programmable counterparts; the only difference between them is that the clinician can adjust the trimmers by a computer or hand-held programmer. In the previous section, it was mentioned that, in multi-channel hearing aids, a band splitter divides the input sound into two or more frequency bands, and each band has its own amplifier (and perhaps, compressor). In a single-channel, programmable hearing aid, the incoming sound input is not split into two or more bands.

Single-channel and multi-channel programmable hearing aids may have programmable trimmer settings and, in some of these hearing aids, the VC also may be programmable. Some examples of programmable trimmer settings include MPO, gain, low-cut, high-cut, various compression threshold kneepoints, ratios of compression, and attack/release times. The software provided by various manufacturers might suggest some practical trimmer settings that work well with each other, depending on the degree and slope of the hearing loss. As mentioned earlier, the VC can be programmed at any particular position.

Programmable hearing aids, whether single-channel or multi-channel, also can have more than one memory or program. Figure 6–12 shows a single-channel programmable

Programmable versus Multi-channel

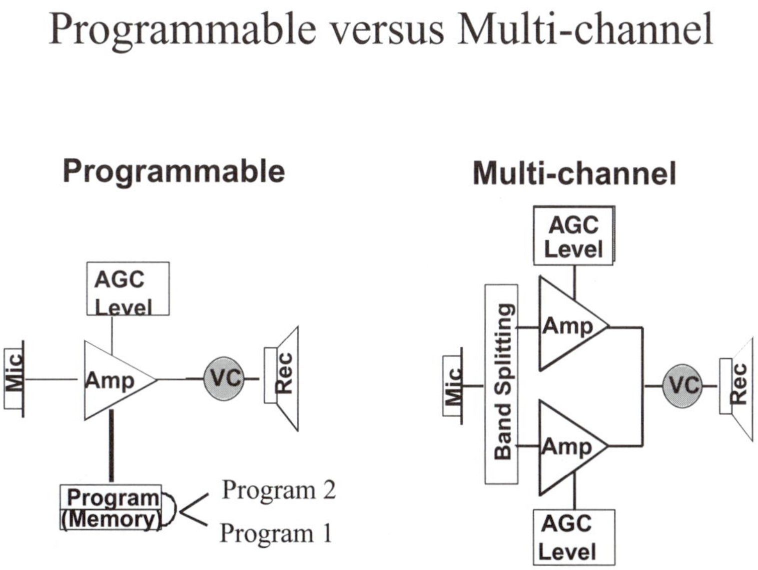

Figure 6–12. Programmable circuits can be single-channel or multi-channel. The programmable circuit (left) is a single-channel circuit with two memories or programs. This means that the trimmer settings can be adjusted by either a hand-held programmer or computer software. The listener can toggle between the two programs. One program might offer a more flat frequency response for listening in quiet, and the second program might offer less low-frequency gain and more high-frequency gain, which may be better for listening in background noise. The multi-channel circuit (right) is available from some manufacturers in either a programmable or a nonprogrammable format. If it is programmable, the trimmer settings can be adjusted by a hand-held programmer or computer software. The multi-channel circuit shown above may also have one or more memories.

circuit with two programs (left), compared to a nonprogrammable multi-channel circuit described earlier (right). The "high-end" analog hearing aids are programmable multi-channel hearing aids that have more than one memory or program.

A programmable hearing aid with two or more programs enables the listener to manually choose (by a switch on the hearing aid or by remote control) among the different programs. Figure 6–13 shows a two-program, single-channel hearing aid set to meet the needs of a client who wants to choose between two different types of sound qualities. One program will provide optimal gain for listening in quiet or listening to music and here, the widest frequency response may be desired. This program might be set to provide the necessary gain to meet target gain dictated by a fitting method. A second program will provide an appropriate frequency response for difficult listening situations, such as discriminating speech in a noisy background. This second program might be set to provide less low-frequency gain to reduce background noise, and more high-frequency gain to increase audibility for the normally less intense, high-frequency consonants of speech.

To provide different frequency responses for the client, programmable hearing aids with more than one memory (multi-memory) typically provide different clusters of trimmer settings for different listening situations. In the example above (the Sigma™ by Unitron), the trimmer settings for Program 1 would

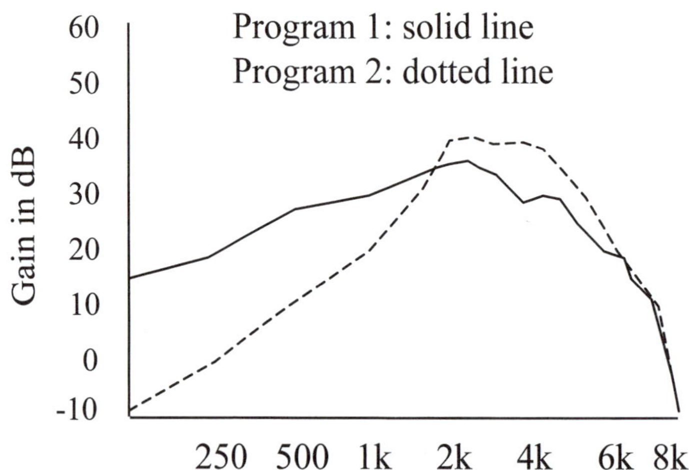

Figure 6–13. A single-channel, two-memory (two-program) hearing aid. The response for Program 1 is set to most closely reach the target gain (for soft speech) for a hearing loss. Program 2 is set to enable "better," perhaps more comfortable, listening to speech in noise. Program 1 has broader, flatter frequency response than Program 2. Program 2 provides more gain for the high frequencies and less gain for the low frequencies than Program 1. Theoretically, this should make the high-frequency consonants more audible to the listener and the low-frequency of background noise less audible. The listener can toggle voluntarily between the two programs, to best meet the need of each listening situation.

be programmed optimally to meet some fitting method target(s). For Program 2, the trimmers could be set to provide more overall gain along with less low-frequency gain (more low-cut). This would create the "teeter-totter" effect in the frequency response: Program 1 would provide more lows and less highs, whereas Program 2 would provide less lows and more highs.

Multi-memory hearing aids are not limited to providing different clusters of trimmer settings for different frequency responses. Different programmed memories can provide also alternate compression characteristics, or permit the client a choice between using directional versus omni-directional microphone characteristics. The Audiozoom™ by Phonak is an example of a single-channel programmable hearing aid in which the programmed memories each provide different microphone characteristics. One program provides omnidirectional sound, while another program provides directional sound. Directional microphones are not a new development in the hearing aid industry, but they are experiencing a revival and are lately receiving a lot of attention. For further reading on directional microphones, the reader is referred to Chapter 7 and encouraged to consult Preves (1997), Killion (1997a, 1997b), and Killion et al. (1998).

Advantages of Programmable Hearing Aids

One advantage of programmable hearing aids is that many parameters (e.g., low-cut, high-cut, gain, MPO, compression kneepoint, etc.) can be accessed through a single port hole or one area on the faceplate of the hearing aid, and these can be programmed by way of the computer or the hand-held programmer. Most non-programmable ITE hearing aids cannot have more than three or four trimmers because the space or "real estate" on the faceplate cannot accommodate more than this number. If changes in some parameters are required that are not accessible through the faceplate, the non-programmable hearing aid may not be able to meet the needs of the client. Programmability permits changes to any possible parameter or trimmer setting in the office, without sending the hearing aids back to the manufacturer for modifications. A hand-held programmer allows easy access and is especially convenient when programming the hearing aids in acoustic environments other than the clinician's office.

Another advantage of programmability is that it enables more interaction between clinician and client. Visual and auditory feedback are available to clients when they watch the programmed changes on the computer screen and, at the same time, they can hear changes take place through the hearing aids. The visual input on the computer screen helps to explain and illustrate the performance and benefits of the hearing aids.

Computer use has gained public acceptance in the public eye. Demonstrating that hearing aid technology has kept in step with computer technology may prompt clients to accept their hearing aids more readily. Clients can be provided with graphic evidence that the hearing aid has been programmed to meet their individual needs.

COMMON CLINICAL COMBINATIONS OF COMPRESSION

Let's pause for a moment and review how the various compression types we have discussed often are combined to provide the best possible hearing aids for the client. After all, it is not as if each type of compression is an island unto itself. On the contrary, when choosing hearing aids for clients, there are some combinations of compression that are encountered commonly by clinicians. Although there are no absolute maxims calling for the endorsement of one type of compression over another, there are some very definite trends. These are described below.

Three dimensions of compression were woven together earlier in this chapter: (1) output versus input compression, (2) conventional compression controls versus the TK control, and (3) output limiting compression versus WDRC. These six aspects of compression often are found in two predictable compression combinations, and each combination can serve a different clinical population (see Figure 6–14).

A Compression Combination for Severe-to-Profound Hearing Loss

Output compression and output limiting compression work well together in the same circuit. This combination has several features for clients with severe-to-profound hearing loss. Severe-to-profound hearing loss usually results in a narrow dynamic range (i.e., about 20 dB) and protection of residual hearing is critical for these clients. With output compression, the client can be assured that although the volume controls of these hearing aids change the kneepoint of compression, they affect only the gain and not the MPO. A conventional compression control in the hearing aid (independent from the VC) also changes the compression kneepoint, and this adjusts the MPO. The output limiting compression in the hearing aid means that the compression kneepoint occurs at a relatively high input level, along with a high ratio of compression. If the hearing aid has a power circuit, the client receives a significant amount of linear gain for soft to at least conversational speech input levels; however, once the output reaches the individual's loudness tolerance level, the hearing aid provides a high degree of compression to limit the output. Although normal loudness growth has not been achieved for these clients, they do get a strong degree of amplification and an output that is limited without peak clipping distortion.

Summary: Applying Compression

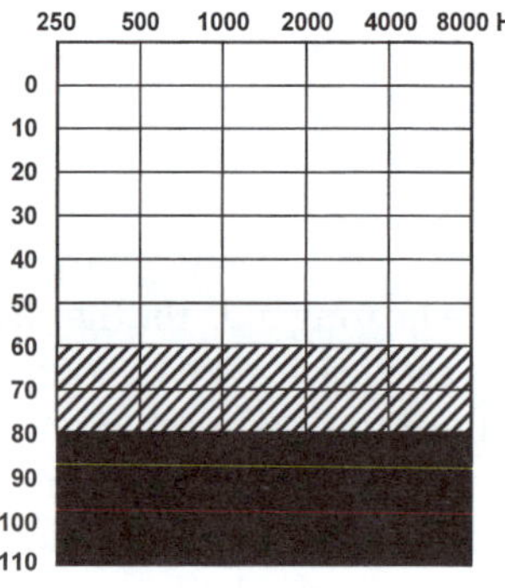

➡Input Compression

➡Wide dynamic range compression

➡ TK control

➡Output Compression

➡Compression Limiting

➡Conventional compression control

Figure 6–14. WDRC, which is a type of input compression, is well suited for fitting mild-to-moderate SNHL. Output limiting, which is almost always used with output compression circuits, is suited for fitting severe-to-profound hearing losses. The diagonal lines in the range from 60 to 80 dB hearing losses represents a "gray" area of intersection for the fitting of either type of hearing aid.

A Compression Combination for Mild-to-Moderate Hearing Loss

Input compression and WDRC work well together in the same hearing aid circuit. This combination has several features useful for those persons with mild-to-moderate SNHL. Compared to that for severe-to-profound hearing loss, mild-to-moderate hearing loss usually presents with a larger dynamic range of 40 to 60 dB. WDRC hearing aids usually have a medium power circuit that is appropriate for these mild-to-moderate hearing losses. With input compression, the VC does not affect the kneepoint of compression, but it does affect the gain and the MPO together. A TK control changes the kneepoint of compression, and it also specifically affects the gain for soft input sounds. Recall from our earlier discussion that, in hearing aids with the TK control, the gain for soft input sounds is increased as the kneepoint is lowered. In hearing aids with WDRC, the kneepoint of compression occurs at a relatively low input level, along with a low compression ratio. The low kneepoint in a WDRC hearing aid means it provides linear gain for only very soft input levels. The hearing aid is otherwise in minimal compression over a wide range of input levels. Given these features, clients get more amplification for soft input sounds and less amplification for sounds that are well within their dynamic range. Recall that for clients with a reduced dynamic range, the "floor" of hearing sensitivity is raised, whereas the ceiling of loudness tolerance is similar to that of normal hearing.

Input compression with WDRC is applicable to a large clinical population (i.e., those persons with mild-to-moderate SNHL). It is important to categorize the increasingly popular types of input compression. Input compression with WDRC can be further divided into two subsets: 1) bass increases at low levels (BILL) and 2) treble increases at low levels (TILL). Recall that BILL hearing aids offer the most compression for the low frequencies and TILL offers most compression for the high frequencies. A straight WDRC hearing aid that is neither BILL nor TILL offers a more similar degree of compression across the amplified frequency range.

A visual categorization of input compression is shown in Figure 6–15. WDRC is a type of input compression, but not all input compression is WDRC. Similarly, BILL and TILL are two types of WDRC, but not all WDRC is specifically BILL or TILL. For example, the K Amp™ hearing aid is TILL, and this is a type of WDRC, which in turn is also a type of input compression. The Oticon Multifocus™ hearing aid is BILL, and this is, also a type of WDRC, which in turn is, again, a type of input compression.

CLINICAL SPECTRUM OF HEARING AIDS

Linear peak clipping, output limiting compression, and WDRC can be placed on a spectrum (see Figure 6–16). Linear peak clipping hearing aids are more similar to output limiting compression hearing aids than they are to WDRC hearing aids. Thus, output limiting is like a bridge between linear peak clipping and WDRC.

Linear Hearing Aids

Linear hearing aids have enjoyed a wide, but diminishing, range of fitting applicability. They can provide a lot of gain for severe-to-profound hearing losses or less gain for mild-to-moderate hearing losses. Their most salient feature is that they give the same gain for all input levels. Note on the left-most graphic of Figure 6–16, that soft, average, and loud inputs are all "elevated" by the same amount. The worst thing about linear hearing aids is that the MPO is limited with peak clipping. Amplified sound that is limited in this manner often is distorted and can result in poor quality for the listener.

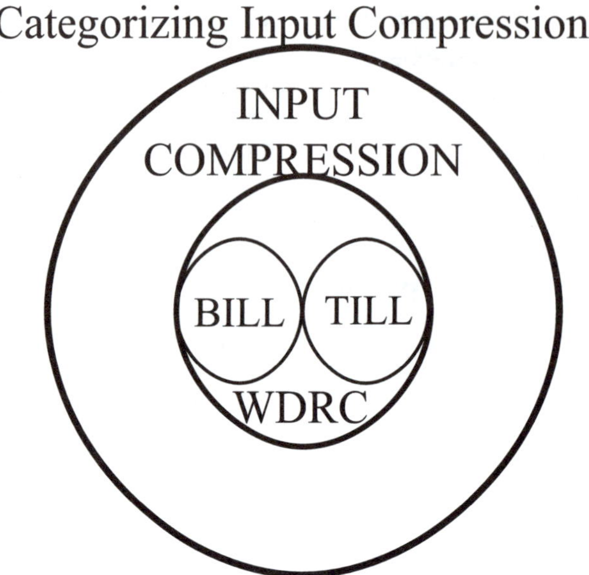

Figure 6–15. Because input compression can be applied to a large segment of the hearing aid fitting population, clinicians may find some categorization helpful. As shown, all WDRC is input compression, but not all input compression is WDRC. Input compression that is not WDRC probably has compression kneepoints and ratios that are more like those of output limiting compression. Bass increases and treble increases at low levels (BILL and TILL) are WDRC, but not all WDRC is BILL or TILL. For WDRC that is neither BILL nor TILL, low inputs result in an equal amount of gain increase at all frequencies.

Output Limiting Hearing Aids

The output limiting compression hearing aid (usually found with output compression) also can be applied to a wide clinical fitting range; however, often is associated with high-power circuitry, which provides a lot of gain for the client with severe-to-profound hearing loss. The middle graphic on Figure 6–16 shows that, with its high kneepoint of compression and high compression ratio, the output limiting compression hearing aid "elevates" soft and average input levels by the same amount; in this way, it is like the linear hearing aid on the left side of the figure. Unlike the linear hearing aid, however, the output limiting compression hearing aid has a conventional compression control that enables compression to limit the output. This is accomplished without the degree of signal distortion often associated with linear peak clipping.

WDRC Hearing Aids

The WDRC hearing aid (found with input compression) can be applied to many different hearing losses, but often it provides less gain than the output limiting hearing aid. The right-most graph on Figure 6–16 shows

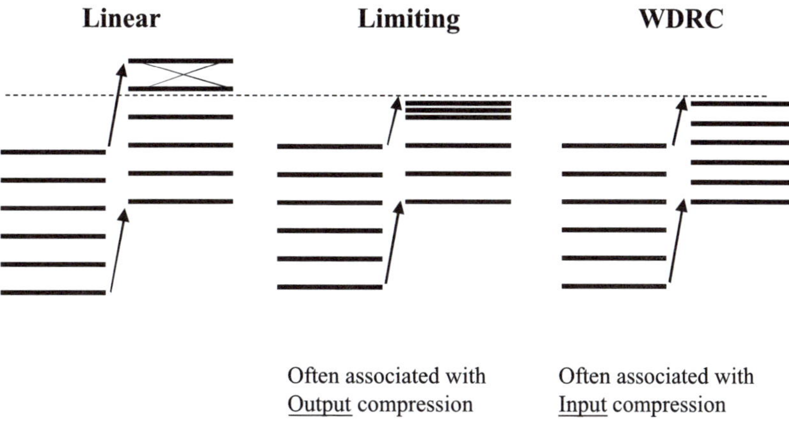

Figure 6–16. For each of three types of hearing aids, two sets of horizontal lines and arrows are shown with the left lines representing the input, the arrows representing the gain, and the right lines representing the output. The dotted line represents the loudness tolerance level for some particular client. For linear hearing aids, the gain is the same for all input levels. When the output reaches the "ceiling" of loudness tolerance, the output is clipped, resulting in distortion of sound quality. For output limiting hearing aids, only the top "output" lines are squeezed together, because the gain is linear for soft and average input sound, and is reduced dramatically for high-intensity input sounds. For WDRC hearing aids, both the input and output lines are spread apart evenly because the gain is reduced gradually as the input intensity increases. A large dynamic range is "evenly" shrunk into a smaller one, which restores normal loudness growth. (Figure courtesy of Huup Van den Heuvel, personal communication).

that, with a low threshold kneepoint and low compression ratio, the WDRC hearing aid gives progressively less and less gain as the inputs increase. Recall from our earlier discussion that the focus of WDRC is to restore normal loudness growth by reducing a large dynamic range to a smaller one. The gain, however, does not decrease to the same degree as the input SPLs increase. If such were true, the output would remain the same for all input levels. The gain must be reduced more slowly than the increase in SPL.

When attempting to fit WDRC hearing aids on clients accustomed to wearing linear hearing aids, they may find initially that WDRC hearing aids are "not loud enough." For soft input sounds, the WDRC hearing aids may be satisfactory to these clients because it is for these sounds that they provide the most gain; however, with their low compression kneepoint and low ratio of compression, the WDRC circuit will not provide as much gain as their older linear hearing aids did for average-to-intense input sounds.

Clients who are accustomed to linear peak clipping may, therefore, initially reject WDRC. For some, it may be a good idea to fit them with output limiting compression, because this type of compression is closer to linear peak clipping. For new clients with mild-to-moderate SNHL who have never worn hearing aids before, WDRC may provide a very good fit.

EXPANSION (AS OPPOSED TO COMPRESSION)

"Expansion," to reduce microphone noise, is a newcomer to compression. Figure 6–17 shows the concept of expansion. Expansion, if seen on an input-output graph, would show a function or line that increases at an angle that is greater than 45° (left panel). Expansion means that the hearing aid is providing *more* than linear gain; and seen in this context, expansion is the opposite of compression. Note how expansion differs from WDRC: Whereas WDRC provides a constant output (linear gain) up until the kneepoint of compression, expansion provides an output that increases dramatically up to the kneepoint. From the kneepoint and on, into compression, WDRC and expansion are similar. The gain functions for expansion and WDRC also are compared in the right panel of Figure 6–17. Expansion has a gain function that is shaped like a diamond. That is, the gain is *not* the same for all input levels below the kneepoint. Unlike WDRC, the greatest amount of gain is found only at the kneepoint of compression, and not for all input levels below

Expansion Versus WDRC

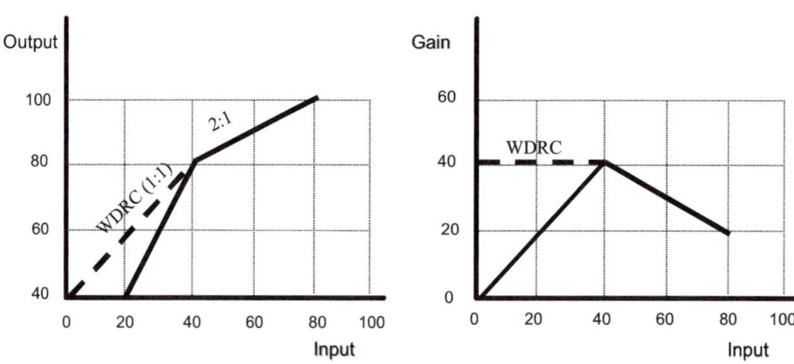

Some DSP hearing aids use expansion

- Reduces microphone noise in quiet
- Addresses typical noise complaint of K Amp & WDRC

Figure 6–17. The concept of expansion is shown and, in both graphs, expansion is compared to WDRC (dotted lines). The graph on the left shows output as a function of input, or a typical input-output type of graph. WDRC typically has a steady, linear gain for all input levels below the kneepoint. In this case, the same linear gain of 40 dB is applied to all inputs below 40 dB. Expansion, in this case, does not apply any gain to input levels below 20 dB, but there is a rapid increase of gain from 20 dB to 40 dB input sounds. After the kneepoint, a typical 2:1 compression ratio applies to both the expansion and the WDRC. The graph on the right shows gain plotted as a function of input. For WDRC, the gain is 40 dB for all inputs below 40 dB. For expansion, however, there is very little gain for 0 to 20 dB input levels. For 40 dB inputs or louder, the gain is the same for expansion and WDRC.

the kneepoint. This implies that very soft sounds (around 10 to 20 dB input levels) are not given as much gain as 40 dB inputs.

The advantage of expansion is that it overcomes the problems noted by many clients who wear WDRC or the KAmp™ hearing aids; namely, that when there are normal environmental sounds present, the hearing aid sounds fine. When things are very quiet in the environment, however, the hearing aid makes a "hissing" sound. This is noted especially by those who have relatively good low-frequency hearing. Some of this "hiss" in quiet environments comes from the amplification of internal microphone and circuit noise of the hearing aid. Because expansion provides very little gain for the very soft inputs, the soft internal circuit and microphone noises are amplified very little. Expansion is well suited for digital hearing aids because it can be implemented with digital algorithms. In conventional analog hearing aids, expansion may require large, more cumbersome, complicated circuitry.

DYNAMIC ASPECTS OF COMPRESSION

Compression has been discussed in terms of threshold kneepoint and compression ratio. These sometimes are known as the "static" aspects of compression, because they involve the input SPL when compression begins and the degree of compression once it occurs. Sound in the environment, however, is changing constantly in intensity over time and a compression hearing aid has to respond to these changes. The "dynamic" aspects of compression hearing aid performance are known as the "attack" and the "release" times.

The attack and release times are the lengths of time it takes for a compression circuit to respond to changes in the intensity of an input SPL (see Figure 6–18). When the input SPL exceeds the kneepoint of compression, the hearing aid "attacks" the sound by reducing the gain. Once the input sound falls below the kneepoint of compression, the hearing aid "releases" from compression and restores the gain. The attack time is the amount of time it takes for a hearing aid to go into compression and reduce the gain; the release time is the length of time it takes for it to come out of compression and restore the gain.

An electrical circuit cannot mirror instantly the changes that take place in the environment, because it requires time to respond to these changes (Dillon, 1988). For example, if a compression circuit is to respond to a sudden increase in input SPL, it has to wait for at least one cycle of the sound wave to "know" if the increased SPL will remain. A change in gain that occurs faster than the longest cycle or period of incoming sound can change the fine details of the sound waves and result in the generation of distortion products.

Hearing aids are not the only electrical devices that use compression and have attack/release times. Audiovisual equipment has used input and output compression for many years. Recall, for example, television broadcasts in which the sports announcer is talking and the background noise is changing in intensity over time. When a score is made and the sport fans suddenly increase the intensity of their cheers, the background noise increases in intensity. It may take a short time for the compression of the audiovisual equipment to attack and reduce the gain of the noise. This also temporarily reduces the gain for the announcer's voice. When the cheering stops, it takes some time for the system to release from compression. The level of the announcer's voice takes some time to return to a normal level.

Most attack and release times are set to achieve a best compromise between two undesirable extremes. Times that are too fast will cause the gain to fluctuate rapidly and this may cause a jarring, "pumping" perception by the listener. Times that are too slow may make the compression act too slowly and cause a lagging perception on the part of the listener. Quick attack times (i.e., 10 ms or less) prevent sudden, transient sounds from becoming too loud for the listener. In general,

Dynamic Characteristics of Compression

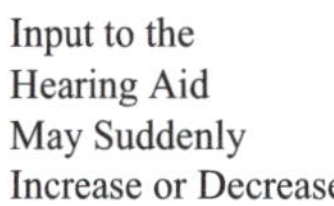

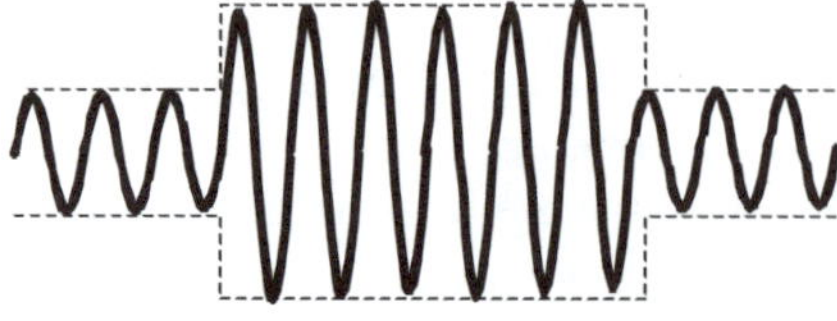

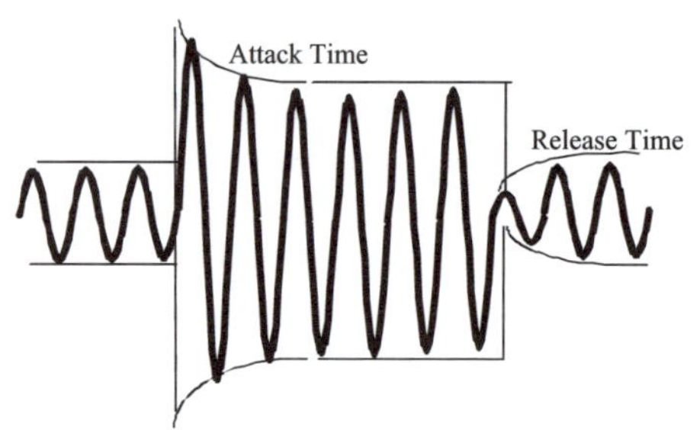

Figure 6–18. The top shows a simple description of *input* sound changing in intensity (vertical dimension) over time (horizontal dimension). The sound has increased suddenly in intensity and, after a while, the sound suddenly decreases in intensity. The bottom shows the *output* response of a compression hearing aid to the changes in sound input intensity over time. The compression circuitry takes some amount of time to respond or compress the incoming signal that has suddenly increased in intensity. This is the "attack" time. Once the input sound has decreased in intensity, the circuit takes some time to stop compressing. This is the "release" time.

release times need to be longer than attack times to prevent a "fluttering" perception on the part of the listener (Staab, 1996). Longer release times (i.e., up to 150 ms) tend to prevent severe distortions that occur with fast release times. Inordinately fast release times can cause the hearing aid to track the amplitude of individual cycles of sound waves (Staab, 1996). Such a rapid modulation of sound can cause a "breathing" or "pumping" perception on the part of the listener (Armstrong, 1996).

Just as we have seen with the static aspects of compression, there are many buzz words used when the dynamic aspects of compression are discussed. Different attack and release times sometimes are used to categorize different types of dynamic compression. Different methods of providing attack/release times also separate one type of dynamic compression from another. These are discussed briefly below.

Automatic Volume Control (AVC)

A type of compression known as "automatic volume control" (AVC) is used in broadcast audiovisual equipment. AVC is known to have relatively long attack and long release times, and it contributes to the time lag or delay in loudness changes in the announcer's voice relative to the sudden-onset cheers of the audience. Its release times are usually more than 150 ms and may be as long as several seconds (Hickson, 1994). Because of long attack/release times, it does not respond to rapid fluctuations of sound input and reduces the need for the listener to adjust the volume control manually, hence, its name.

Syllabic Compression

"Syllabic compression" is identified by relatively short attack and release times. Its release times vary from less than 50 ms to 150 ms. The attack/release times are specifically intended to be shorter than the duration of the typical speech syllable, which is about 200 to 300 ms (Hickson, 1994). Short attack/release times allow the hearing aid to compress or reduce the gain for the peaks of more intense speech (usually the vowel sounds). This provides more uniformity in the intensity of ongoing speech syllables. In other words, syllabic compression reduces the differences between the normally more-intense vowels and the softer unvoiced consonants such as /s/. The premise underlying syllabic compression is to allow the hearing aid to make softer sounds of speech more audible without simultaneously making the normally louder parts of speech from becoming too loud.

Syllabic compression is somewhat controversial and not everyone agrees with its use. Because syllabic compression compresses the peak amplitudes of speech and makes the waveform of ongoing speech more uniform, noise can easily fill in the small gaps that remain (Johnson, 1993). In noisy situations, a hearing aid might amplify the noise that is situated between the peaks of speech. According to Killion (1996a), fast attack/release times of 50 ms can distort the waveform of speech, and, thus, compromise speech intelligibility. As mentioned in the earlier section in this chapter on WDRC, Kuk (1999) suggests that the use of fast attack times (less than 10 ms) and short release times (less than 100 ms) will compromise the intensity differences between the various phonetic elements of speech. Specifically, in the time waveform of speech, the differences between the "peaks" or loud elements and "valleys" or soft elements are compromised or lessened by fast attack/release times. Such a reduction, in turn, can distort the spectral content of speech cues. It is interesting to note that the opposites of AVC and syllabic compression are used presently in current hearing aids, and a firm conclusion has not been reached. Obviously, the jury is still out.

Peak Detection

Most compression hearing aids use a technique called peak detection to "track" the peak amplitude of incoming sound waves. If the peak is greater than the compression threshold kneepoint, the circuit attacks and compresses the signal, which reduces the gain. Once the peak is below the kneepoint, the compression releases and the gain increases once again. Peak detection allows for a wide variety of times that can separately be specified and assigned as attack and release times; however, these times are constant and fixed for any incoming sound intensity patterns (Armstrong, 1993). Most peak detection systems in hearing aids are adjusted to provide quick attack times and longer, slower release times.

An advantage of peak detection is that it reacts very quickly to increases in environmental sound levels. Unfortunately, it can react inappropriately to very short intense sounds, because the longer release times will keep the gain down after the short intense sound has stopped. This may reduce unnecessarily the gain of input sounds the listener might want to hear.

With fixed attack/release times, the hearing aid cannot respond differently to different patterns of sound input intensities when needed. It should be appreciated that speech is a remarkably unique acoustic signal, that changes rapidly over intensity, frequency, and time. The dynamic acoustic sounds of speech within the world of ever-changing (dynamic) background noise, for example, the sudden slamming of a door or the constant roar of traffic, can pose real problems for the peak detection method and the listener.

Adaptive Compression™

This type of compression has fixed, quick attack times, but release times vary with the duration of the intense, incoming sound. For sudden, intense, transient sound inputs, the release time is short. For sound inputs that are longer in duration, the release times are longer. The desired result is a reduction of compression "pumping" heard by the listener. Adaptive compression™ was originally patented by Telex and is now most commonly associated with the K Amp™ circuits.

Average Detection

Average detection is most commonly associated with the DynamEQII™ circuit by Gennum (see the previous section on multichannel hearing aids). Unlike the peak detection method that tracks the peak amplitude of incoming sound waves, the average detection method looks at the average of the incoming signal over a given length of time. When the average exceeds the kneepoint of compression, the gain is reduced.

The DynamEQII™ has "twin" average compression detectors; one is a fast detector and the other is a slow detector (see Figure 6–19). The slow average detector averages sound inputs over a 220 ms time interval (i.e., about 1/5 of a second) and is in control of the com-

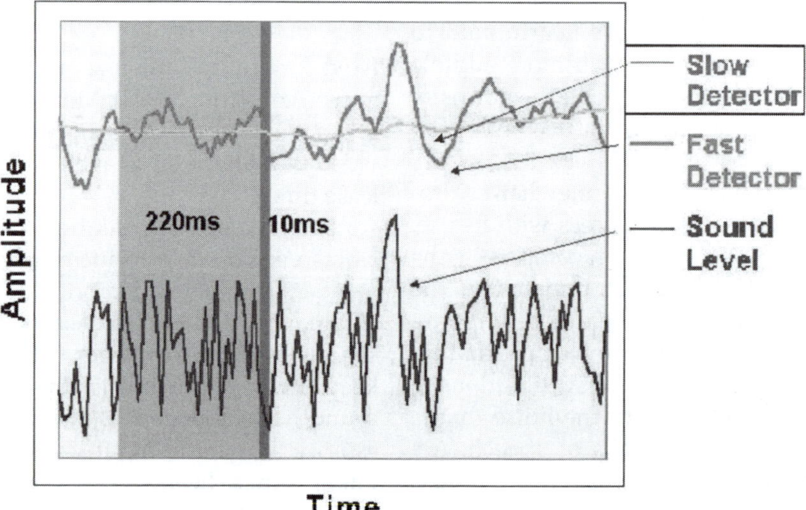

Figure 6–19. The actions of the slow average detector, which averages sound over time intervals of about 220 ms, and the fast average detector, which averages sound over time intervals of about 10 ms. The bottom line represents sound intensity as it occurs over time. The top smooth line represents the input signal when averaged by the slow average detector. Note that the slow average is very flat over time. The top bumpy line represents the input signal when averaged by the fast detector. Note the fast average changes significantly more over time than the slow average.

pression system most of the time. When the slow average of incoming sounds exceeds the threshold kneepoint of compression, the gain is reduced slowly and is hardly noticeable. Very often, however, sudden loud sounds occur in the environment, and the gain should be reduced for these sounds as well. For example, with the slow detector alone, a short spike of intense sound may be averaged into the overall body of sound that takes place over 220 ms. This slow average may not be enough to tell the hearing aid to go into compression and reduce the gain. This is where the fast average detector comes into the picture. The fast average detector averages sound inputs over time intervals of about 10 ms (i.e., 1/100 of a second) and it acts when intense transients are not caught by the slow detector. When the "fast" average is 6dB greater than the "slow" average, the fast average detector takes over and reduces the gain for the spike of intense sound.

The main result of twin average detection is that both the attack and release times vary with the length of the incoming intense sounds. This is in direct contrast to the peak detection systems that give constant, fixed, quick attack and slow release times for all incoming stimuli. As long as the incoming sounds are below the compression threshold, both types of circuits provide uncompressed gain. With sudden, transient, loud sounds, such as a door slam, the twin average detection system will provide quick attack and quick release times. On the other hand, the peak detector will provide its usual quick attack and slow release times. Because of the reduction of gain and the long recovery of the peak detection circuit, soft speech spoken right after the door slam may be temporarily inaudible to the listener. The twin average detection circuit will enable a quick recovery of gain after the door slam, because its release time will be quick for short sounds.

The benefit to the listener is that there is less "pumping" perception. So far, the twin average detection system is the best compromise between compression that reacts to every short intense sound and compression that may react too slowly for some sounds that should be compressed. Clients often are annoyed by audible byproducts of compression, which should not be allowed to become a nuisance. Dynamic aspects should be considered when trying to make hearing aids acoustically "transparent" to listeners.

Interaction Between Static and Dynamic Aspects of Compression

Compression consists of static aspects in one dimension and dynamic aspects in a separate dimension. With incoming sounds, the attack/release times of a hearing aid interact with the ratio of compression (Armstrong, 1996). The input/output graphs on hearing aid specs sheets show compression ratios that are obtained with constant pure tones, not with the stops and starts of sounds like speech. Static compression ratios on specs sheets thus do not accurately represent the actual compression ratios experienced in real life by clients who wear the hearing aids. Fast attack/release times have the effect of temporarily *reducing* the ratio or amount of compression for any given sound stimulus.

Attack and release times interact with compression ratios and these interactions affect the sound quality for the listener. In general, a combination of short attack/release times (e.g., 10 ms) and high compression ratios (e.g., 10:1) cause distortion. If the same short attack/release times are used with low compression ratios (e.g., 2:1), then the sound quality is not quite so compromised (Armstrong, 1996). On the other hand, long attack/release times can be combined with either high or low compression ratios.

Dynamic and static aspects of compression often are found in predictable combinations today. Syllabic compression, with its relatively short attack and release times, is most often associated with WDRC hearing aids that have a low compression kneepoint and a low compression ratio of less than 5:1. It also is sometimes encountered with output limiting compression hearing aids in which the kneepoints and ratios of compression are high. AVC, with its relatively long attack/release times, is most often seen in hearing aids that offer a low threshold kneepoint of compression and high compression ratio (Dillon, 1988; Hickson, 1994).

SUMMARY

In this chapter, we reviewed some of the fundamental concepts that are necessary to comprehend before any discussion of compression: input/output graphs and linear hearing aids. Compression was explored along three dimensions:

1 - Clinically, the main difference between input and output compression is the effect of the volume control. With output compression, the volume control affects the gain but not the MPO. With input compression, the volume control affects both the gain and the MPO.

2 - The conventional compression control affects the threshold kneepoint of compression and also the MPO. The TK control affects the kneepoint and the gain for soft inputs only.

3 - Output limiting compression has a high kneepoint and a high compression ratio. WDRC has a low kneepoint and a low compression ratio. Output limiting acts above its kneepoint to limit the output. WDRC acts below its kneepoint to provide most gain for soft input sounds. Output compression with output limiting, adjusted by a conventional compression control, can be very appropriate for severe-to-profound hearing loss. Input compression, often associated with WDRC, is adjusted with a TK control, and can be appropriate for mild-to-moderate SNHL. Two types of WDRC are BILL and TILL. Multichannel hearing aids that can combine BILL and TILL into one hearing aid are very flexible, and are becoming very popular. The DynamEQII™ is an example of a two-channel WDRC circuit with BILL and TILL.

Programmable hearing aids can be single channel or multi-channel. They also can have one or more memories or programs. It is important not to confuse the term "digitally programmable" with "digital."

Dynamic aspects of compression and different types of attack/release time parameters were discussed. Peak detection (fixed fast attack times and longer release times), adaptive compression (variable release times), and twin average detection (variable attack and release times) were discussed, along with syllabic compression (short attack/release times) and automatic volume control (long attack/release times).

REVIEW QUESTIONS

1. On input/output graphs, input is always on the vertical axis T F

2. On an input/output graph, the left-most diagonal line indicates the most gain T F

3. Treble increases at low levels (TILL) is often associated with the KAmp™ T F

4. The term "programmable" means the hearing aids has two or more channels T F

5. Output minus input equals gain T F

6. Output limiting compression hearing aids came first; WDRC came later T F

7. If 10 dB of increased input results in 2 dB of increased output, this is a compression ratio of:
   a) 5:1
   b) 2:1
   c) 4:1
   d) 1:1

8. For hearing aids with input compression, the volume control affects the:
a) gain, not the MPO
b) MPO, but not the gain
c) both the gain and the MPO
d) input to the hearing aid

9. For hearing aids with output compression, the volume control affects the:
a) gain, not the MPO
b) MPO, but not the gain
c) both the gain and the MPO
d) input to the hearing aid

10. Which of the following is intended basically to imitate the outer hair cells?
a) output limiting
b) WDRC
c) linear gain with peak clipping
d) none of the above

11. For severe hearing losses, ____ with ____ are usually recommended
a) input compression with output limiting
b) output compression with WDRC
c) input compression with WDRC
d) output compression with output limiting

12. For mild to moderate sensorineural hearing losses, ____ with ____ are usually recommended
a) input compression with output limiting
b) output compression with WDRC
c) input compression with WDRC
d) output compression with output limiting

13. WDRC is associated with the following two things:
a) high kneepoint and a high compression ratio
b) low kneepoint and low compression ratio
c) low kneepoint and a high compression ratio
d) high kneepoint and a low compression ratio

14. Output limiting compression is associated with the following two things:
a) high kneepoint and a high compression ratio
b) low kneepoint and low compression ratio
c) low kneepoint and a high compression ratio
d) high kneepoint and a low compression ratio

15. The following statement is true:
a) all input compression is WDRC, but not all WDRC is input compression
b) all WDRC is input compression, but not all input compression is WDRC
c) all output compression is WDRC, but not all WDRC is output compression
d) all WDRC is output compression, but not all output compression is WDRC

16. The TK control affects the:
a) gain for soft input sounds
b) maximum power output
c) gain for loud input sounds
d) none of the above

17. To hear the effect of a regular compression control, you should:
a) talk softly into the hearing aid
b) talk loudly into the hearing aid
c) adjust the volume control to adjust the MPO up and down
d) adjust the volume control to adjust only the gain

18. To hear the effect of a TK control, you should:
a) talk softly into the hearing aid
b) talk loudly into the hearing aid
c) adjust the volume control to adjust the MPO up and down
d) adjust the volume control to adjust only the gain

19. For mild-to-moderate SNHL, the following compression combination is often found:

a) input compression, with output limiting, and a TK control
b) output compression, with WDRC, and a regular compression control
c) input compression, with WDRC, and a TK control
d) output compression, with output limiting, and a regular compression control

20. For severe-to-profound HL, the following compression combination is often found:
a) input compression, with output limiting, and a TK control
b) output compression, with WDRC, and a regular compression control
c) input compression, with WDRC, and a TK control
d) output compression, with output limiting, and a regular compression control

ADDITIONAL READING

Compression handbook: An overview of the characteristics and applications of compression amplification. Eden Prairie, MN: Starkey Marketing Services, Starkey Labs, Inc. 1996.

Dillon, H. (1996). Tutorial. Compression? Yes, but for low or high frequencies, for low or high intensities, and with what response times? *Ear & Hearing, 17*(3); 287–307.

Killion, M.C. (1997). A critique on four popular statements about compression. *The Hearing Review, 4*(2), 36–38.

Mueller, G.H., & Killion, M. C. (1996). *The Hearing Journal, 49*(1), 10–46.

Venema, T.H., (1998). *Compression for clinicians,* San Diego Singular Publishing Group.

REFERENCES

Armstrong, S. (1996, September). *Chips and dips—an engineering perspective of hearing aid circuits, power supplies, and the like.* Paper presented at Jackson Hole Rendezvous, Jackson Hole, WY.

Armstrong, S. (1993). The dynamics of compression: Some key elements explored. *The Hearing Journal, 46*(11), 43-47.

Dillon, H. (1988). Compression in hearing aids. In R. E. Sandlin (Ed.), *Handbook for hearing aid amplification* (Vol. 1). Boston: College Hill.

Hickson, L. M. H. (1994). Compression amplification in hearing aids. *American Journal of Audiology, 3,* 51-65.

Johnson, W. A. (1993). Beyond AGC-O and AGC-I: Thoughts on a new default standard amplifier. *The Hearing Journal, 46*(11), 37-42.

Killion, M. C., Staab, W., & Preves, D. (1990). Classifying automatic signal processors. *Hearing Instruments, 41*(8), 24-26.

Killion, M. C. (1996a). Compression distinctions. *The Hearing Review, 3*(8), 29-32.

Killion, M. C. (1996b). Talking hair cells: What they have to say about hearing aids. In C. I. Berlin (Ed.), *Hair cells and hearing aids* (pp. 125-172). San Diego: Singular Publishing Group, Inc.

Killion, M. C., (1997a). "I can hear what people say, but I can't understand them." *The Hearing Review, 4*(12), 8-14.

Killion, M. C. (1997b). The SIN report: Circuits haven't solved the hearing-in-noise problem. *The Hearing Journal, 50*(10), 28-34.

Killion, M. C., Schulein, R., Christensen, L., Fabry, D., Revit, L., Niquette, P., & Chung, K. (1998). Real-world performance of an ITE directional microphone. *The Hearing Journal, 51*(4), 24–38.

Kuk, F. K. (1996). Compression technology. Paper presented at the meeting of the American Academy of Audiology, Salt Lake City, UT.

Kuk, F. K. (1999) Hearing aid design considerations for optimally fitting the youngest patients. *The Hearing Journal, 52*(4), 48-55.

Preves, D. (1997, July). Directional microphone use in ITE hearing instruments. *The Hearing Review, 4,* 21-27.

Staab, W. J., (December, 1996). Limiting systems in hearing aids. *AAS Bulletin, 21*(3), 23-31.

CHAPTER 7

Use of Microphone Technology to Improve User Performance in Noise

MICHAEL VALENTE, PH.D.

OUTLINE

One of the major complaints of patients with hearing loss is increased difficulty understanding speech in noise (Kochkin, 1993, 1994). The reader might have difficulty recalling any patient reporting hearing well in noise, but who experienced great difficulty in quiet!

Research has shown that listeners with hearing loss require signal-to-noise ratio (SNR) improvements of 4 to 18 dB, depending on the magnitude of hearing loss, to achieve word recognition scores equal to normal listeners when the signal is presented at 70 dB HL (Killion, 1997a, 1997b, 1997c; Roberts & Schulein, 1997). Furthermore, one of the major reasons patients report dissatisfaction with hearing aids is their inability to improve understanding of speech in noise (Kochkin, 1994). Again, can the reader recall any patient returning hearing aids for credit because he or she felt their performance was fine in noisy situations, but unsatisfactory when communicating in quiet environments? If the only goal of hearing aid fittings aids was to improve the understanding of speech in quiet, then the number of dispensed hearing aids would explode. Unfortunately, the relatively poor performance of hearing aids in noisy environments is one of the major reasons consumers do not pursue amplification (Kochkin, 1994). Patients report that hearing aids often make sounds louder, but not clearer, and this problem becomes greater when listening in noise. Thus, a logical conclusion, from the viewpoint of our patients, is that hearing aids are not adequately addressing their needs.

Solving the issue of consumer dissatisfaction with hearing aids can *partially* be resolved by improving our counseling skills. Some patients rationalize that, because "X" dollars were spent for hearing aids, then their performance in a noisy restaurant should be equal to their performance in the quiet of their living room. Patients need to be reminded that even the most technologically advanced hearing aids cannot restore normal hearing and that even normal listeners do not understand speech as well in noise as they do in quiet. Patients need to remind themselves that, if normal listeners have increased difficulty understanding speech in noise, then why should they expect to perform the same as normal listeners under the same conditions?

In the opinion of the author, patients need to be counseled that their well-fitted hearing aids should accomplish *at least* four goals: First, understanding speech in a quiet environment will be significantly better (the patient decides what is significant) with hearing aids than without hearing aids. If this goal cannot be achieved, then little hope remains that any other goals can be achieved. Second, understanding speech in a *noisy* environment will be significantly better with hearing aids than without hearing aids. If the major reason patients seek our services is to improve understanding of speech in noise, then why would they want to keep their hearing aids if the hearing aids do not adequately resolve this problem?

There is ample evidence within your own clinic that patients do, in fact, report better aided performance in noise. For example, as part of my hearing aid fitting protocol, I have the patient complete the Abbreviated Performance of Hearing Aid Benefit (APHAB) (Cox & Alexander, 1995) questionnaire. The author cannot remember any patient whose *aided* BN (aided listening in background noise) or RV (aided listening in a reverberant environment) problem scores were equal to or *poorer* than his *unaided* BN or RV problem scores. That is, the patients are reporting fewer problems with their hearing aids in noise or reverberation than they experience unaided. Whether the difference between the aided and unaided problem score (i.e., benefit score) is significant enough for the patient to keep the hearing aids is another question.

Third, and most important, performance with the hearing aids in noise probably will not be as good as the performance in quiet. As emphasized earlier, patients need to be reminded that listeners with normal hearing do not hear as well in noise as they do in quiet. Therefore, there is no reason for the user to expect to do better than a person with normal hearing in the same listening situation. Having said this, sections of this chapter will illustrate that technology is available, or may soon be available, so that aided performance in the restaurant may in fact, be equal to or better than the performance of normal listeners! Finally, the user should find that input levels of low intensity (less than 50 dB SPL) should be judged as "soft, " input levels of average intensity (60 to 70 dB SPL) should be judged as "comfortable," and input levels of "high" intensity (greater than 80 dB SPL) should be judged as not uncomfortably loud.

Recently, the professional community has been excited about the introduction of digital signal processing (DSP) as a means to improve the understanding of speech in noise. Although DSP has the ability to improve significantly the flexibility of hearing aid fittings and diminish the deleterious effects of feedback, there has been no research demonstrating that DSP, alone, has significantly improved the understanding of speech in noise when compared to analog signal processing (Valente, Fabry, Potts & Sandlin, 1998; Ricketts & Dhar, 1999). However, there has been research to indicate that DSP, in combination with directional microphones, can provide significant improvement in the understanding of speech in noise relative to analog or DSP hearing aids using omnidirectional microphones (Valente, Sweetow, Potts & Bingea, 1999).

One area of hearing aid research that consistently has reported improved understanding of speech in noise is the *directional microphone.* This chapter will provide a comprehensive overview of microphone technology and its impact on improving the understanding of speech in noise for listeners with hearing loss.

MEASURING MICROPHONE PERFORMANCE

It is important for the audiologist to be able to determine if one microphone design may address the needs of a patient better than another microphone design. For example, does one design provide greater attenuation of signals arriving directly from behind? Does the attenuation extend to a higher frequency range than another design? Is the attenuation greatest when signals arrive from the side? Which hearing aid style (i.e., BTE or ITE) provides greater attenuation in noise? Are differences in performance present when directional microphones are used with analog or DSP hearing aids? To help answer these questions, this section will address how microphone performance is measured.

Microphone performance can be measured in a number of ways, but the most common are polar sensitivity plots, front-to-back ratio (FBR), directivity index (DI), and the articulation index-directivity index (AI-DI).

Polar Sensitivity Plots (Directivity Pattern)

A polar sensitivity plot is a graphic "picture" of how the output of the hearing aid changes in response to a single frequency or several discrete frequencies as the signal source arrives from different directions (i.e., azimuth). A polar plot is presented as a circle with concentric reference lines emanating from the center. The outer circle represents 0 dB attenuation and each inner circle typically represents 10 dB of attenuation. Usually, the top of the circle represents 0° azimuth, the right is 90°, the bottom is 180°, and the left is 270°. Often, there are lines in 10° increments. Typically, this measure is performed in an anechoic chamber with the hearing aid suspended in the free field. A polar plot also can be measured with the hearing aid coupled to the Knowles Electronics Manikin for Acoustic Research (KEMAR). The polar plots from these two measures with the same hearing aid will be quite different. When the hearing aid is coupled to KEMAR, the interaction between azimuth and the role played by the torso and head takes place. For example, when a hearing aid with an omnidirectional microphone is suspended in free field, the polar plot will reveal no attenuation as the signal source is rotated from 0° to 360°. When the same hearing aid is placed on the right ear of KEMAR, however, the polar pattern will show greater sensitivity at ~ 30° to 90° (e.g., greater amplification) due to head effects, and less sensitivity (e.g., greater attenuation) at ~ 270° due to the head shadow effect. When a hearing aid with a cardioid directional microphone is suspended in free field, the polar plot will reveal attenuation (i.e., null) at 180°. When the same hearing aid is placed on the right ear of KEMAR, however, the polar pattern will reveal greater sensitivity at ~ 45° to 60° due to the head effects and less sensitivity at ~ 210° due to the head shadow effect. Maximum sensitivity (i.e., less attenuation) will occur when the signal source is in front of the user.

Polar plots typically are reported as being indicative of either *omnidirectional* or *directional* microphone designs. The directional plots are further divided into *cardioid, hypercardioid, supercardioid,* or *bi-directional* designs. (Figures 7-3 and 7-8).

Omnidirectional

As discussed in the previous section, this plot typically shows a solid line hovering around the 0 dB line as the signal source rotates from 0° to 360°. This indicates that no degree of attenuation is provided at any azimuth. This is shown in Figure 7–1.

Cardioid

This plot typically shows a solid line hovering around the 0 dB line as the source is rotated between 0° to 150° and again from approximately 210° to 360°. However, there is significant attenuation (i.e., the polar plot line is moved inward and crosses the –20 dB inner line showing at least 20 dB attenuation) of signals arriving from the rear). This relatively narrow "inversion" from behind is referred to as the "null." The cardioid design attenuates signals maximally when they arrive directly from the rear (i.e., 180°) and appears to resemble a "heart" or "apple." Figure 7–2 illustrates a cardioid polar plot for a dual-microphone DSP BTE.

Hypercardioid

This plot typically shows a solid line hovering around the 0 dB line as the source is rotated between 0° to 100° and again from approximately 260° to 360° (see Figure 7–3). However, there is significant attenuation when the signal arrives from between 130° to 230°. This design has two nulls (110° and 250°) and a "lobe" at 180°. The lobe illustrates that this design provides some amplification when signals arrive from behind when compared to the response provided by a cardioid design. Figures 7–4 and 7–5 illustrate polar

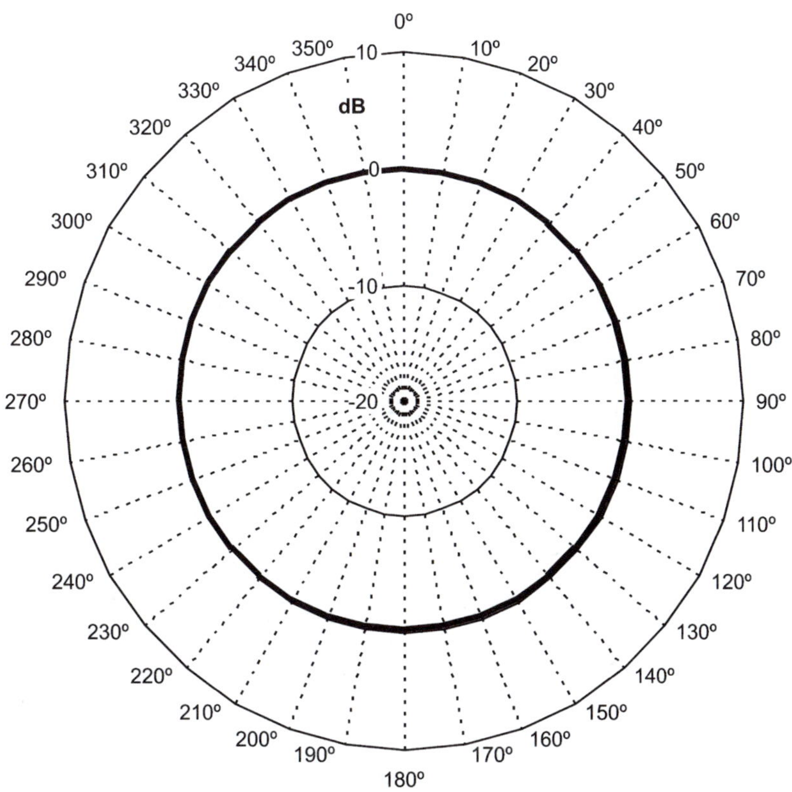

Figure 7–1. Free-field polar sensitivity plot for an omnidirectional microphone. (Reproduced with permission from ReSound Corporation.)

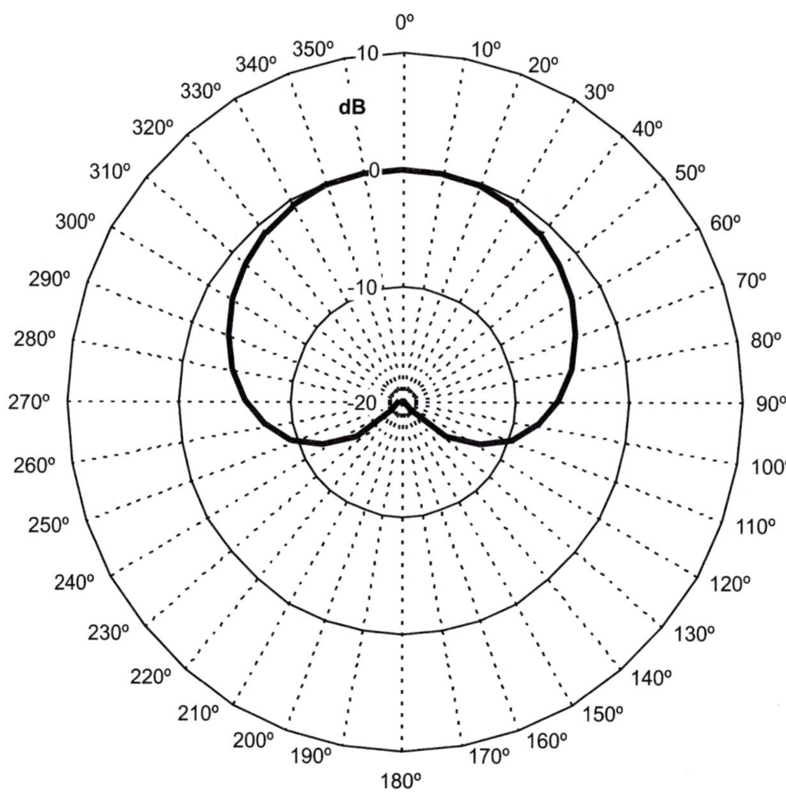

Figure 7–2. Free-field polar sensitivity plot for a cardioid directional microphone. (Reproduced with permission from ReSound Corporation.)

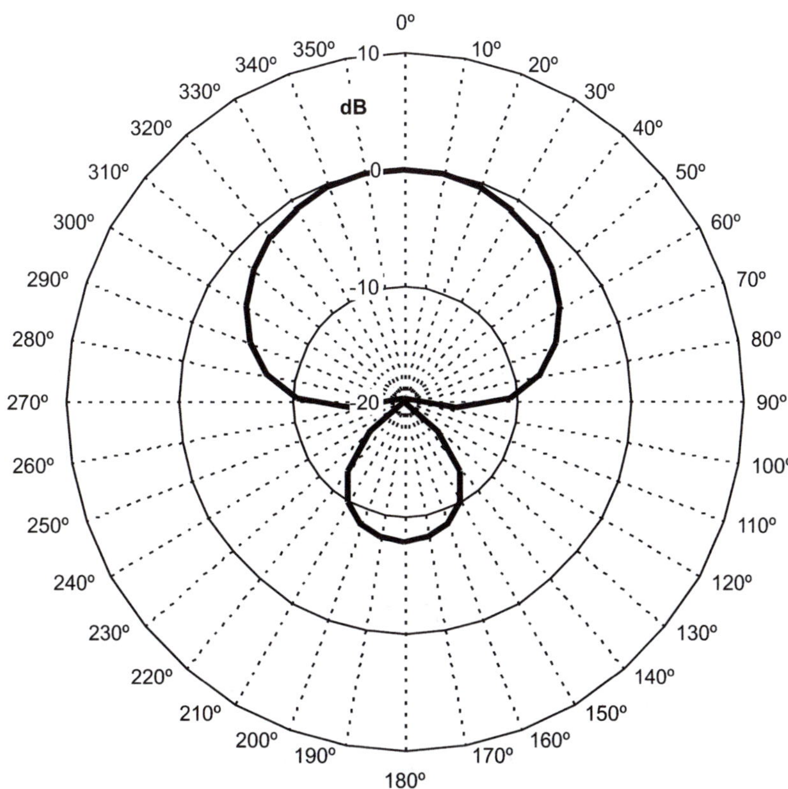

Figure 7–3. Free-field polar sensitivity plot for a hypercardioid directional microphone. (Reproduced with permission from ReSound Corporation.)

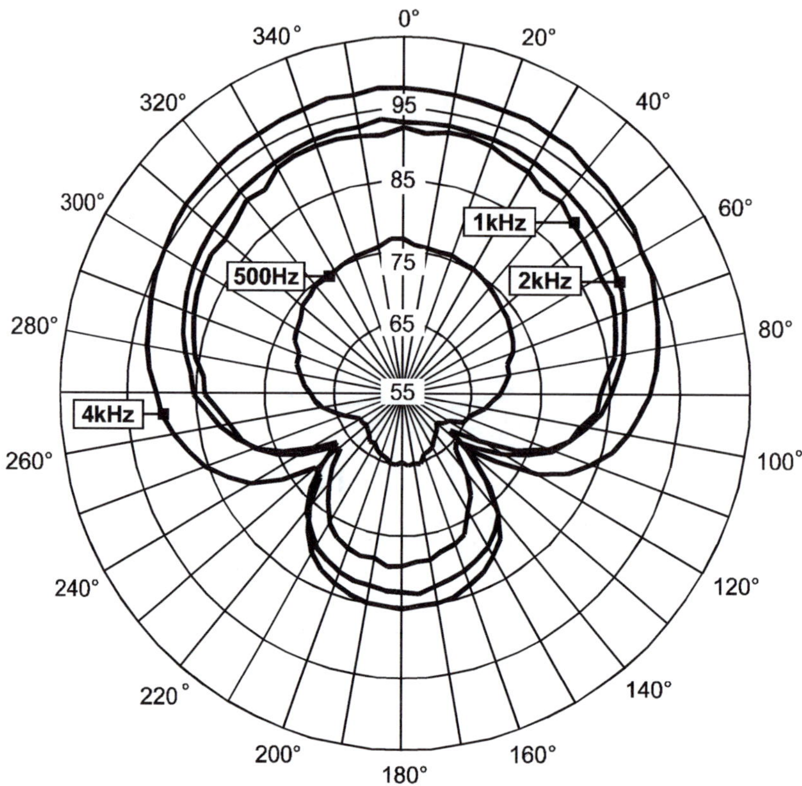

Figure 7–4. Polar sensitivity plot at 500, 1000, 2000, and 4000 Hz of a dual-microphone ITE measured in a free-field. (Reproduced with permission from Siemens Hearing Instruments, Inc.)

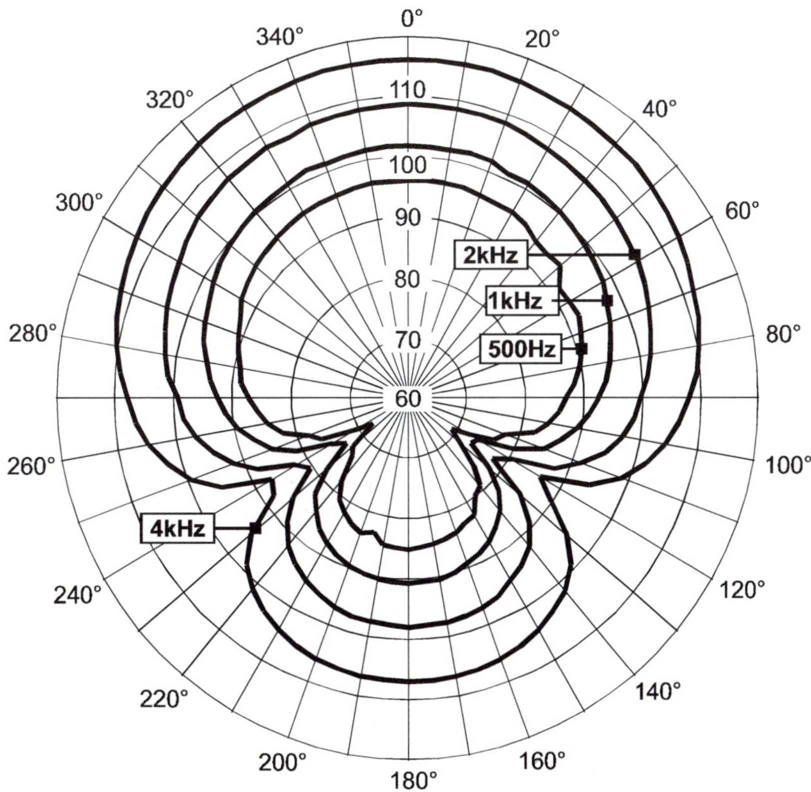

Figure 7–5. Polar sensitivity plot at 500, 1000, 2000, and 4000 Hz of a dual-microphone BTE measured in a free-field. (Reproduced with permission from Siemens Hearing Instruments, Inc.)

plots at 500 to 4000 Hz for a hypercardioid dual-microphone DSP ITE (Figure 7–4) and DSP BTE (Figure 7–5) measured in free field. Notice that, for both styles, attenuation is greatest at 500 Hz and least at 4000 Hz. This is especially true for the ITE. Also, notice that the amount of attenuation for the ITE is very similar at 1000 to 4000 Hz (i.e., the lines are close together), but equally separated for the BTE. Finally, notice that the attenuation at 130° and 230° provided by the ITE is greater than provided by the BTE.

Figures 7–6 (ITE) and 7–7 (BTE) illustrate the polar sensitivity for the same hearing aids, but the measurement performed on KEMAR. Notice how the attenuation seen at 130° and 230° when the aids were measured in free field has virtually disappeared. Also notice that for the BTE, the null appears at ~270° for the lower frequencies and virtually disappears at the higher frequencies. This illustrates why directional polar plots should be reported on KEMAR to provide a more realistic picture of the performance of the hearing aids when worn on a patient.

Supercardioid

This plot typically shows a solid line hovering around the 0 dB line as the source is rotated between 0° to 120° and again from approximately 240° to 360°. However, there is significant attenuation when the signal arrives from between approximately 130° to 230°. This design also has two nulls and a "lobe" at 180°. However, the lobe in this design is considerably shallower and narrower when compared to the lobe of the hypercardioid design. Also, because of the narrow and shallower lobe for signals arriving from directly behind, this design should provide greater improvement in noise than either the cardioid or hypercardioid designs.

Bidirectional

This plot typically shows a solid line hovering around the 0 dB line as the signal source is rotated between 0° to 360°. However, nulls are present when the signal arrives from 90° and 270° (see Figure 7–8). This design is created by *not* incorporating a delay between the front and rear openings. One example in which this design might be helpful would be for a taxi driver who needs to hear conversations from the rear, but requires signals from the sides (windows) to be attenuated. Another potentially useful situation is when a husband and wife are communicating across a kitchen table and their in-laws are to the left and right at the ends of the table.

Front-to-Back Ratio (FBR)

The FBR is reported as the frequency response of the microphone with the signal presented from the front and a second frequency response illustrating performance when the signal is presented from the rear. The difference between these two frequency responses is the FBR. If it is an omnidirectional microphone, the two frequency response curves essentially will superimpose upon each other showing that signals from the rear are amplified in a manner similar to when the signal arrives from the front. In this situation, the FBR is 0 dB. In the case of a directional microphone, the frequency response for signals arriving from the rear will separate from the frequency response of signals presented from the front. The greater the separation, the greater the FBR. Clearly, the FBR would not be an accurate representation of the performance of hypercardioid, supercardioid, and bidirectional microphones because of their reduced attenuation of the signal from behind. In conventional directional microphones (single microphone with a front and rear port), the FBR is greatest in the low-frequency region and the separation decreases as the frequency increases. In dual-microphones, the magnitude of the separation between the front and rear frequency response is greater than a conventional directional microphone and the frequency range for where the separation occurs is wider (i.e., the separation between front and rear frequency response occurs beyond 2000 Hz). Thus, as

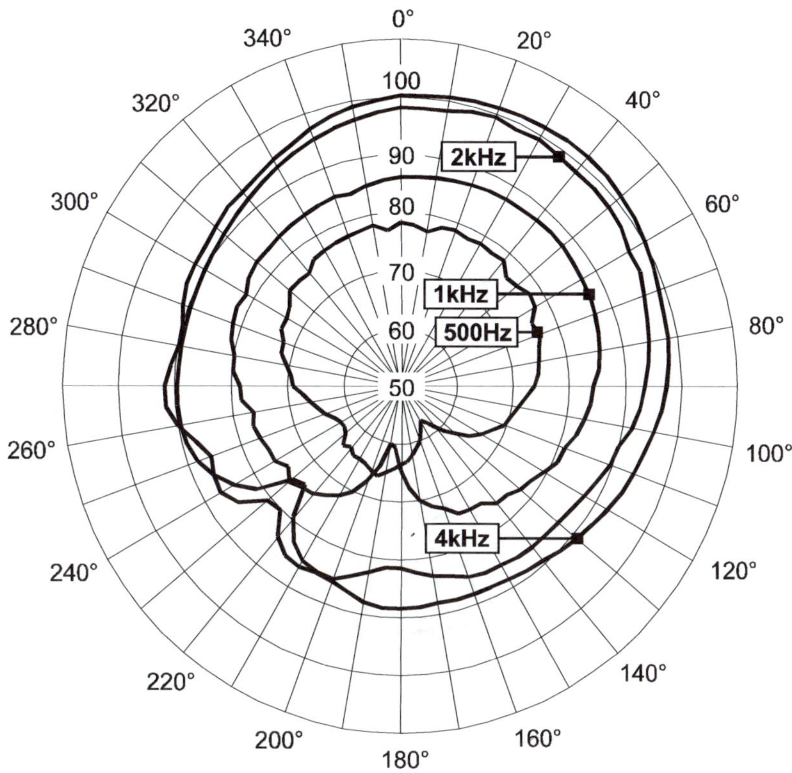

Figure 7–6. Polar sensitivity plot at 500, 1000, 2000, and 4000 Hz of a dual-microphone ITE measured on the right ear of KEMAR. (Reproduced with permission from Siemens Hearing Instruments, Inc.)

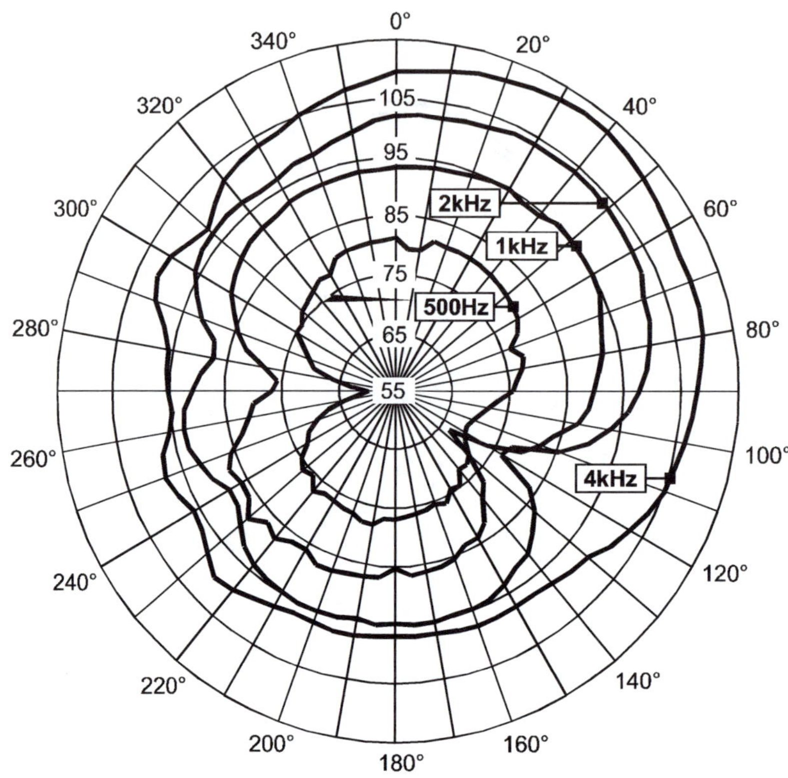

Figure 7–7. Polar sensitivity plot at 500, 1000, 2000, and 4000 Hz of a dual-microphone BTE measured on the right ear of KEMAR. (Reproduced with permission from Siemens Hearing Instruments, Inc.)

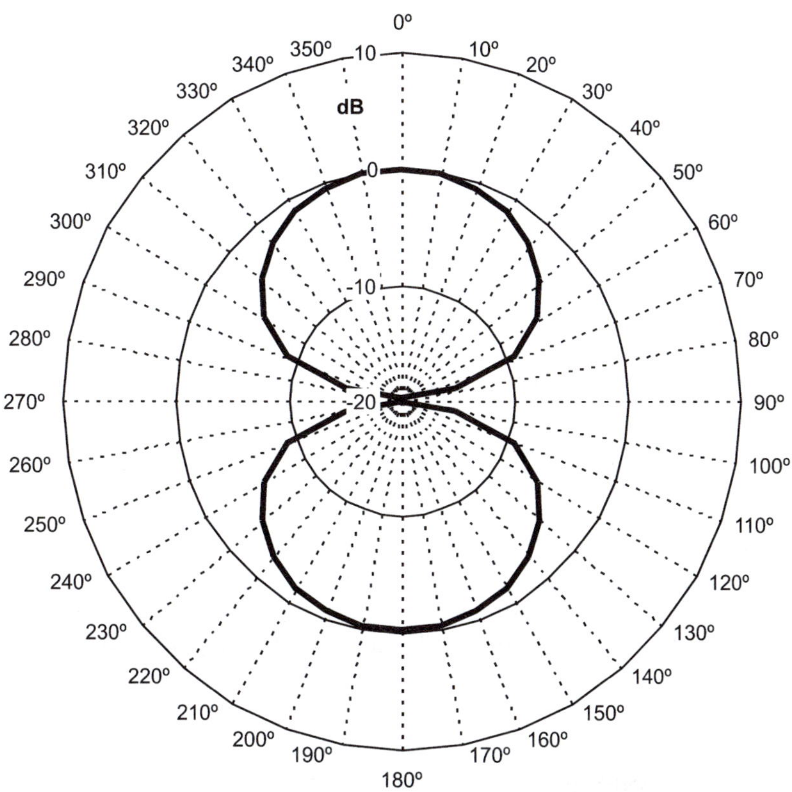

Figure 7–8. Free-field polar sensitivity plot for a bidirectional directional microphone. (Reproduced with permission from ReSound Corporation.)

will be shown later, the dispenser may expect greater directional performance (i.e., greater improved SNR) from hearing aids using dual-microphones than from hearing aids using conventional first-order (i.e., cardioid) directional microphones. Figure 7–9 illustrates the relative frequency-gain response of a dual-microphone hearing aid in its omnidirectional (upper curve) and dual-microphone (lower curve) positions.

Directivity Index (DI)

The DI is a single number (in dB) and represents the ratio of the microphone output for signals from the front (0°) to sounds originating from all directions (diffuse). The DI correlates closely with the predicted improvement in SNR provided by the microphone. For example, the DI of an omnidirectional microphone can be 0 or 1.0 dB (or even less than 0 dB), whereas the DI for a well-designed directional microphone will be between 4 and 6 dB. As will be reported later, the DI for some multiple-array microphone designs can be 12 to 14 dB. The DI provides a good estimate of how helpful the directional microphone will be in difficult listening situations (i.e., with the listener surrounded by sound and trying to understand the talker directly ahead.) The higher the DI, the greater the ease of communication in difficult listening situations. When looking at the DI for a directional microphone, it is important to observe the DI for the open ear and omnidirectional microphone. For example, the open ear DI can be negative in the lower frequencies and positive above 2000 Hz due to pinna effects. It is not uncommon for the DI for the open ear and omnidirectional microphone to be similar (~ −1.5 dB). For example, for an omnidirectional BTE, pinna effects for the high-frequency region do not exist and it is not uncommon to see a negative DI. Figures 7–10 and 7–11 illustrate the DI for a dual-microphone ITE (Figure 7–10) and BTE (Figure 7–11) measured in free field (upper curve in Figures 7–10 and 7–11) and on KEMAR (middle curve). The lower curve in Figures 7–10 and 7–11 represents the unaided response of KEMAR. Notice how the DI is slightly greater for the ITE than the BTE (due to head effect). Also notice, as mentioned earlier, that for each hearing aid design, the DI decreases when the measure is performed on KEMAR due to head and

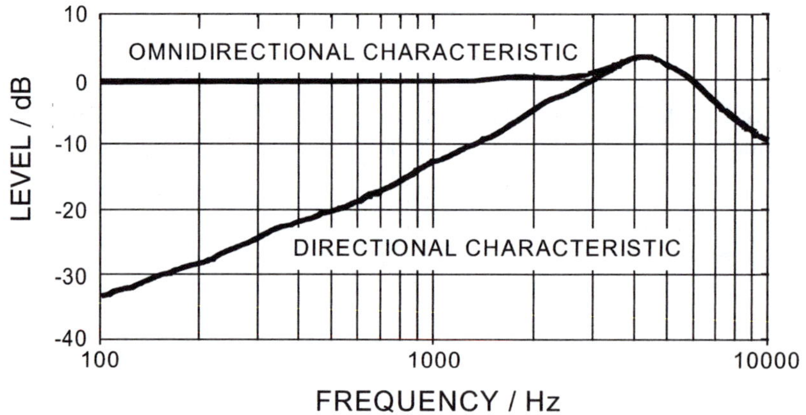

Figure 7–9. Relative frequency-gain response of omnidirectional and dual-microphone positions with a dual-microphone hearing aid. Notice the significant decrease in amplification in the low frequencies when the dual-microphone is activated. (Reproduced with permission from Siemens Hearing Instruments, Inc.)

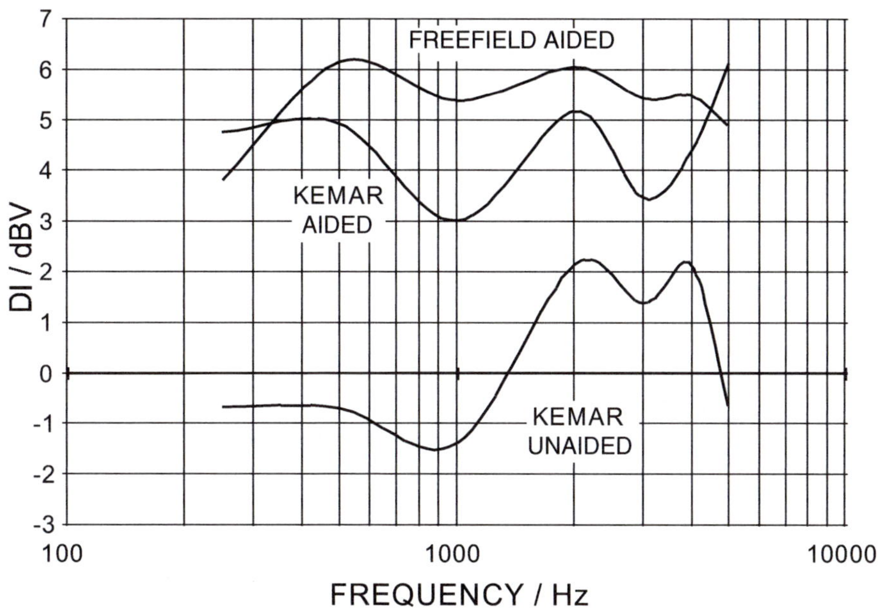

Figure 7–10. Directivity Index (DI) of a dual-microphone ITE measured in free-field (upper curve), on KEMAR (middle curve), and on KEMAR unaided (lower curve). (Reproduced with permission from Siemens Hearing Instruments, Inc.)

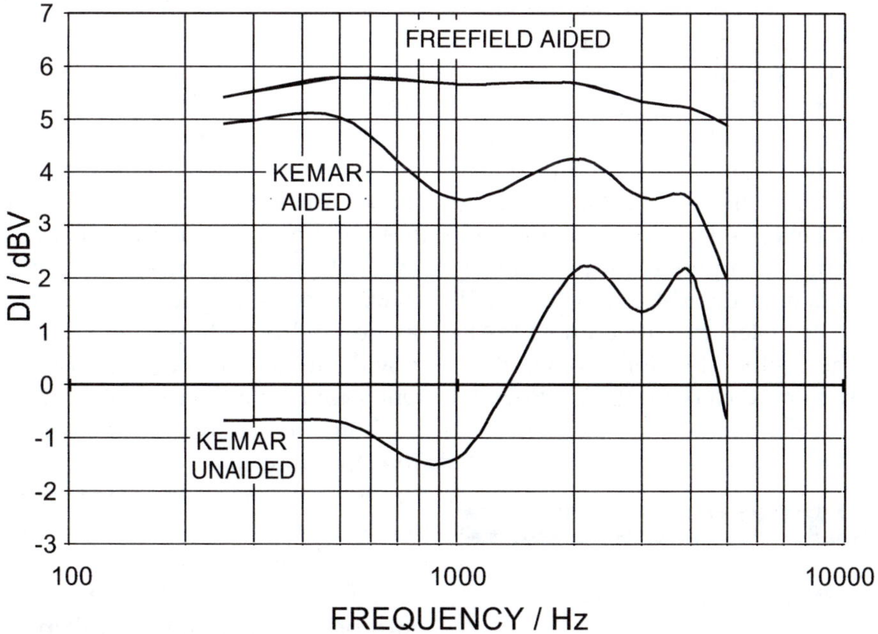

Figure 7–11. Directivity Index (DI) of a dual-microphone BTE measured in free-field (upper curve), on KEMAR (middle curve), and on KEMAR unaided (lower curve). (Reproduced with permission from Siemens Hearing Instruments, Inc.)

torso effects decreasing the low (torso) and high (head) frequency response of the hearing aid.

Articulation Index-Weighted Directivity Index (AI-DI)

The Articulation Index (AI) (ANSI-1969) provides a measure of the percentage of speech energy that is audible (i.e., above threshold or above the level of background noise). The AI provides different weights to the contribution of each individual frequency band to the overall intelligibility of speech. For example, the AI applies a weight of .0010 for 250 Hz and .0024 at 1000 Hz. This increases to .0038 at 2000 Hz and .0034 at 3150 Hz. That is to say that the speech energy at 2000 to 3000 Hz contributes more to overall speech intelligibility than the speech energy at 250 to 1000 Hz. In the AI-DI procedure, the Directivity Index (DI) at each frequency is calculated by multiplying the AI weight and then performing a root mean square (RMS) sum of the resulting products to arrive at one number. Thus, a directional microphone in which the DI extends to the high-frequency region will have a higher AI-DI than a directional microphone in which the DI does not extend beyond 2000 Hz. Theoretically, the directional microphone with a higher AI-DI will provide significantly better performance in noise than the directional microphone with the lower AI-DI. For example, the AI-DI of the D-Mic™ (to be presented later) measured on KEMAR is 4.5 dB whereas the AI-DI for an omnidirectional microphone on a ITE is 0.3 dB (Roberts & Schulein, 1997).

TYPES OF MICROPHONES

Omnidirectional

An omnidirectional microphone has one sound inlet (Figure 7–12) and signals are processed equally regardless of azimuth.

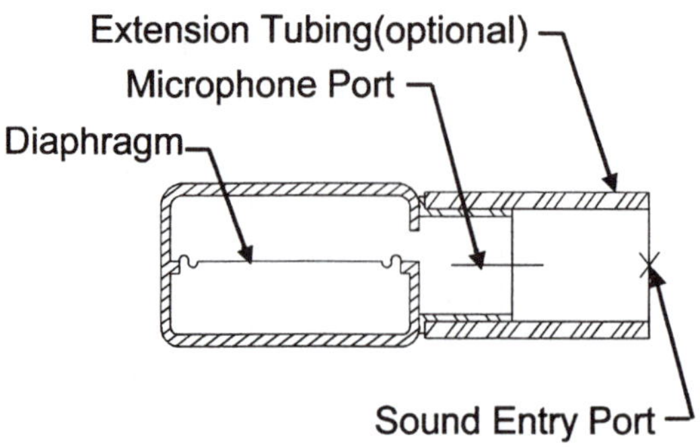

Figure 7–12. Schematic drawing of a omnidirectional microphone. (Reproduced with permission from Knowles Electronics.)

Thus, signals arriving from the 0° azimuth are handled as efficiently as those arising from any other direction. As will become apparent in the remainder of this chapter, this microphone design, although the most widely used, has been shown repeatedly to provide the poorest performance in noise.

Conventional Directional

Directional microphones have been available since 1972 (Arentsschild & Frober, 1972), but Mueller (1981) reported that only 20% of dispensed BTEs contained directional microphones. This microphone has two sound inlets (front and back) leading to separate cavities, divided by a diaphragm. The diaphragm senses differences in air pressure between the two cavities and transduces these differences to provide an electrical output signal. To prevent sound from the rear inlet activating the diaphragm before being activated by signals from the front inlet, an *acoustical time delay network* is placed in the rear inlet to assure that the sound waves from both inlets reach the diaphragm at the same time (Figure 7–13). Equivalent sound pressure on opposite sides of the diaphragm simultaneously results in sound cancellation because the diaphragm cannot move. Therefore, engineers can design different directional microphone

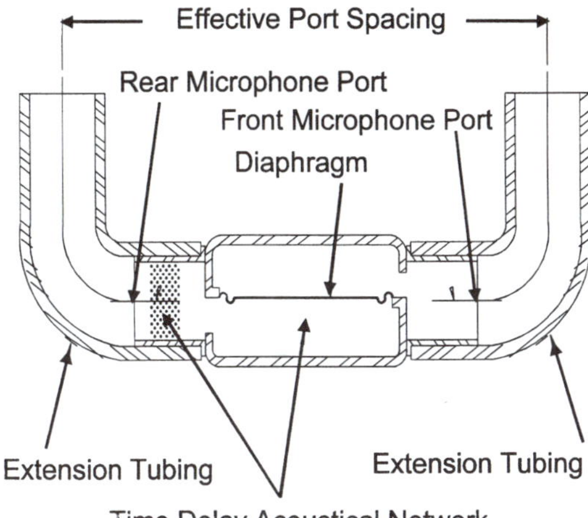

Figure 7–13. Schematic drawing of a directional microphone. (Reproduced with permission from Knowles Electronics.)

patterns by manipulating the magnitude of the delay for the sound arriving from the rear port. In the past, horse or camel hair was used to create the delay. Currently, fine metal mesh acoustical dampers are used to achieve accurate and reliable delays (Preves, 1997). The effectiveness of the time delay network is primarily dependent on the:

1. magnitude of the time delay (in microseconds) in the rear port,
2. distance (in mm) between the front and rear sound inlets (e.g., port spacing),
3. dimensions of the extension tube from each sound inlet, and
4. location of the microphone ports on the hearing aid case.

According to Skinner (1988), the typical time delay incorporated in directional microphones is 58 microseconds. This corresponds to a port spacing of approximately 19.7 mm (i.e., delay × velocity of sound in air, or 58 × 344 mm/s). However, Bachler and Vonlanthen (1995) reported that the time delay can be between 25 to 43 microseconds. According to Nielsen (1973), for the delay network to be most effective, it must be equal to the length of the microphone case. For example, if the length between the front and rear port is 13 mm (1/2 in.) then the delay must be 40 µs because that is the time it will take a sound wave to travel 13 mm. The velocity of sound is 344 m/s (or 1 mm in 3 µs). Thus, it will take sound nearly 40 µs to travel the 13 mm (3 × 13) from the rear to the front inlets and vice versa. If the distance between the front and rear inlets is 15 mm, then the time delay would need to be 45 µs. If this can be accomplished, then the familiar cardioid pattern will appear. If the microphone has a rear port, but no time delay network, the polar pattern is bidirectional. Bachler and Vonlanthen (1995) revealed that it is possible to convert a cardioid design to a hypercardioid design by reducing the time delay from 43.2 µs to 24.9 µs while keeping the port spacing constant at 14 mm. In addition, an engineer may convert a hypercardioid design to a cardioid design by decreasing the port spacing (14.4 mm to 8.3 mm) while keeping the time delay constant (24.9 µs). Due to the continued miniaturization of microphones, hearing aids now can be produced with port spacing as small as 4 mm. One can see that, as inlet spacing is decreased, the acoustic delay in the rear inlet needs to be decreased to maintain the same polar pattern. As inlet spacing is increased, the delay needs to be increased to maintain the same polar pattern.

Another consideration is varying the port spacing via the length of the extension tubing from the inlets to the hearing aid case, but leaving the delay constant. Buerkli-Halevy (1986) illustrated that, by increasing the inlet spacing from 8 mm to 14 mm but leaving the time delay constant at 24.9 microseconds, the directional pattern resulted in greater attenuation from 135° and 225°, but poorer attenuation from 180°.

Finally, directional microphones usually provide less low-frequency gain than omnidirectional microphones due to greater similarity in the amplitude and phase at the two microphone ports for the low-frequency waveform.

Dual-Microphone

In this design, two perfectly matched omnidirectional microphones are placed with the housing of BTE or ITE hearing aids. Figures 7–14, 7–15, and 7–19 illustrate commercially available dual-microphone BTEs, while Figures 7–16, 7–17, 7–18 and 7–19 illustrate commercially available dual-microphone ITEs. In a BTE, size constraints allow the maximum distance between the two microphone ports to be approximately 15 mm, whereas the distance is reduced to 4 mm to 10 mm for an ITE.

In a dual-microphone BTE fitting, it is important that the tubing be short enough so that the two microphone ports are horizontal (Mueller & Wesselkamp, 1999) above the ear. In an ITE, it is important for the dispenser to mark the impression with a horizontal line indicating the proper placement of the two microphone ports for the individual ear. If the horizontal alignment is off by 20° or more, it can reduce the DI by 0.5 dB (Mueller & Wesselkamp, 1999). In either type of fitting, the presence of venting can diminish the performance of dual-microphones. For example, a closed vent fitting provided a DI of 4.2 dB in a dual-microphone ITE. This DI was reduced to 2.9, 1.9, and 1.6 dB for 1, 2, and 3 mm vents, respectively (Mueller & Wesselkamp,

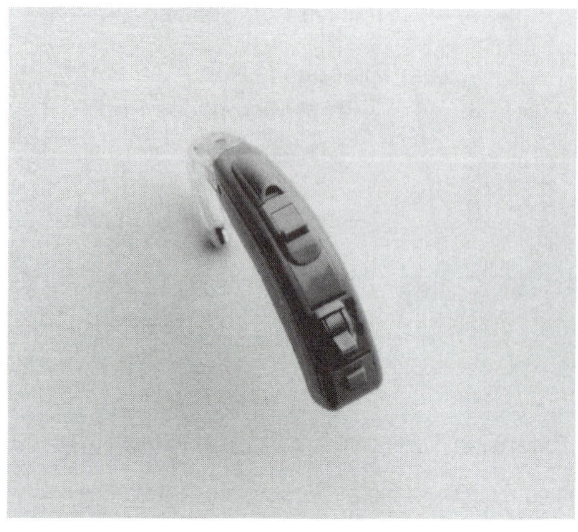

Figure 7–14. Photo of a dual-microphone BTE. (Reproduced with permission from Siemens Hearing Instruments, Inc.)

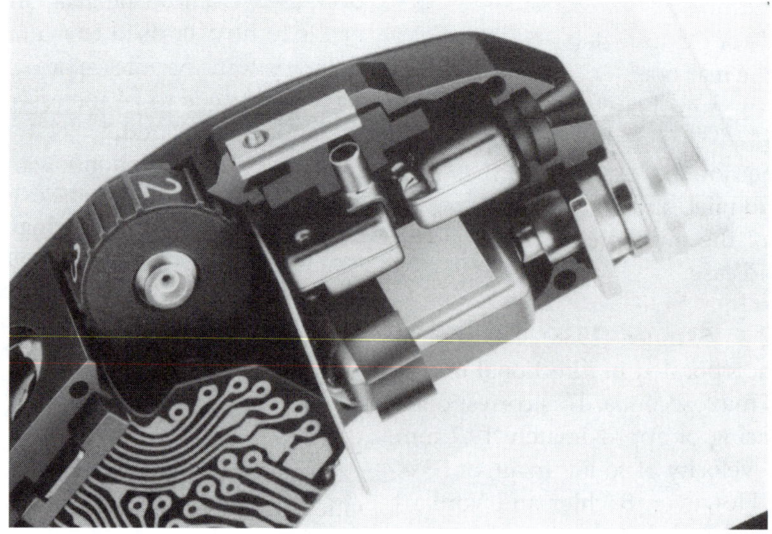

Figure 7–15. Photo illustrating the placement of two omnidirectional microphones in a BTE case. (Reproduced with permission from Phonak, Inc.)

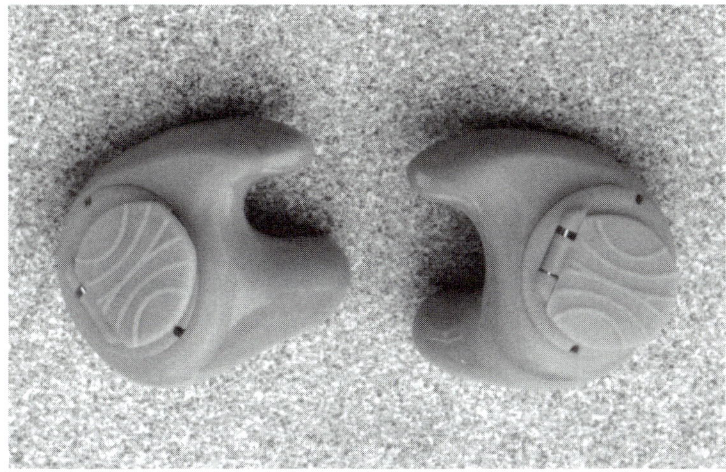

Figure 7–16. Photo of a dual-microphone ITE. (Reproduced with permission from Phonak, Inc.)

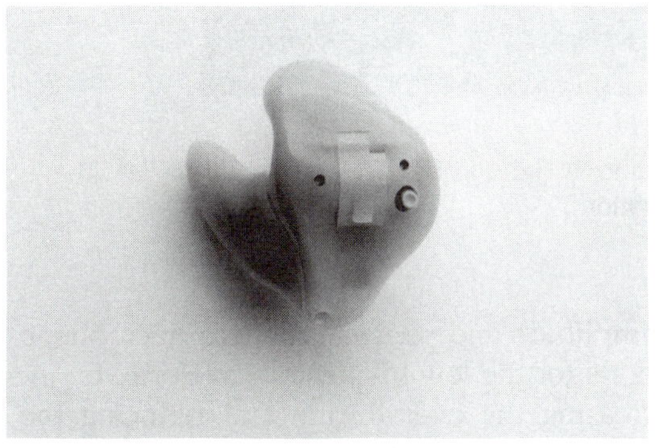

Figure 7–17. Photo of a dual-microphone ITE. (Reproduced with permission from Siemens Hearing Instruments, Inc.)

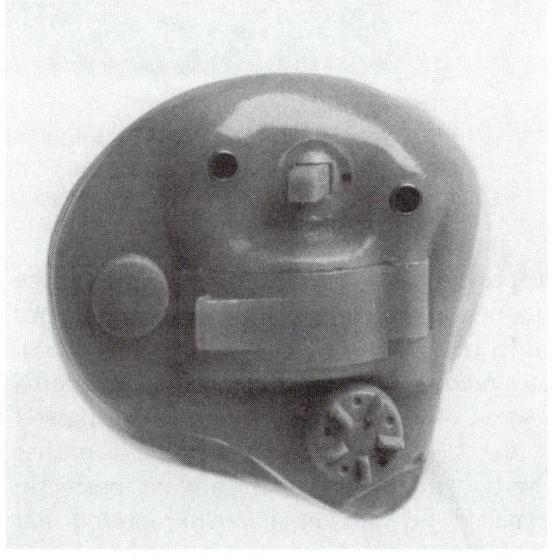

Figure 7–18. Photo of a dual-microphone ITE. (Reproduced with permission from Micro-Tech Hearing Instruments, Inc.)

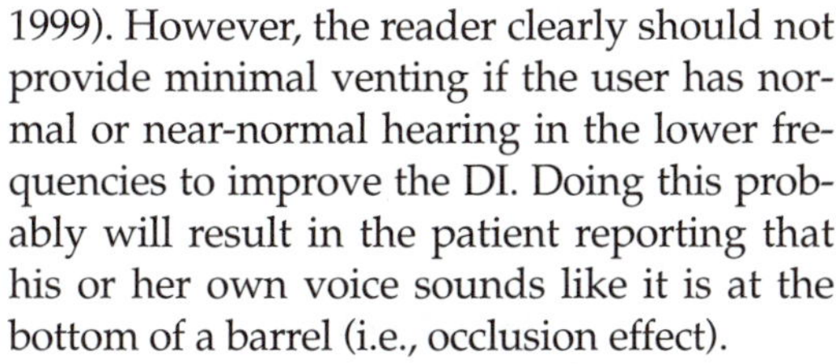

1999). However, the reader clearly should not provide minimal venting if the user has normal or near-normal hearing in the lower frequencies to improve the DI. Doing this probably will result in the patient reporting that his or her own voice sounds like it is at the bottom of a barrel (i.e., occlusion effect).

Improved performance of dual-microphones is provided by subtracting the output of the rear microphone from the output of the front microphone and adding an electronic time delay to the output of the rear microphone. The magnitude of the delay to the signal from the rear microphone is determined by the distance between the two microphones. In some hearing aids, analog to digital (A/D) converters are added so that the output from each microphone is sampled and digitized. Then the rear microphone signal is delayed and subtracted from the front signal digitally

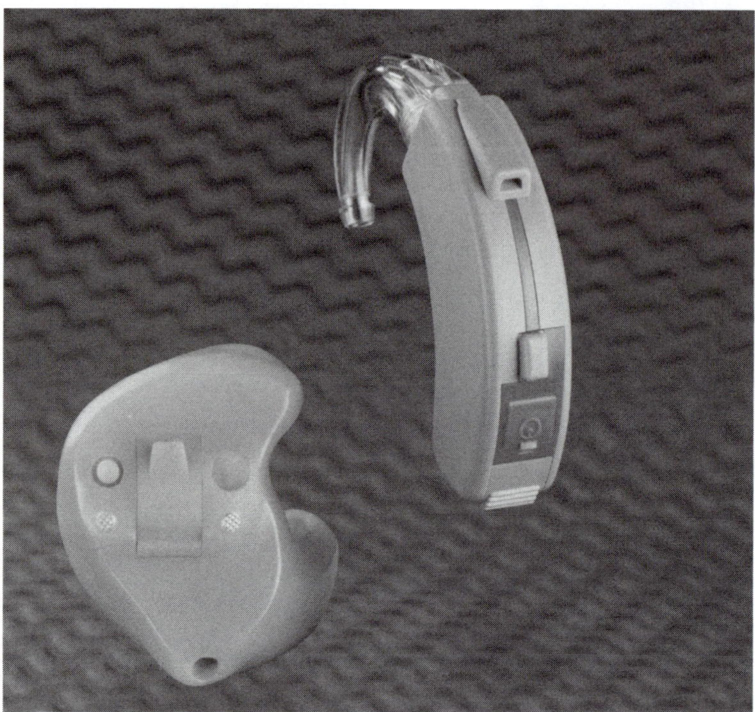

Figure 7–19. Photo of a dual-microphone ITE and BTE. (Reproduced with permission from ReSound Corporation.)

to provide more precision in controlling the frequency response of the two microphones (Edwards, Hou, Struck, & Dharan, 1998). Subtracting the two microphones digitally, instead of electronically, before being passed to the A/D converter is done to assure that the two microphones are always perfectly matched. Edwards et al. (1998) reported that as much as a 1 to 2 dB mismatch in phase and amplitude between the two microphones can convert a hypercardioid response to a near-omnidirectional response. Edwards et al. (1998) went on to report that the effect of mismatched microphones becomes greater as the distance between the two microphones decreases (i.e., greater problem created by mismatched microphones in a ITE).

Finally, as in the conventional directional microphone, in a dual-microphone there is usually less low-frequency gain for signal arriving from behind due to the greater similarity in the amplitude and phase at the two microphone ports for the low-frequency waveform. By increasing the overall gain and reducing the high-frequency gain, it is possible to "equalize" the dual-microphone response so that the response is equal to the response for signals arriving at the front. By equalizing the dual-microphone response, the amplified signal sounds louder (equal loudness between the omnidirectional and dual-microphone positions) and there is less need for the user to increase the overall gain when switching to the dual-microphone position

D-Mic™

One of the more recent advances in microphone technology for ITEs (1/2 or full-shell with a port spacing of 4 mm) is the introduction of the D-Mic™ by Etymotic Research in late 1997. The D-Mic™ is a dual microphone design (one omnidirectional and one hypercardioid directional microphone are within the capsule) with three port openings that are glued into a 6.34 mm opening of an ITE faceplate. Figure 7–20 illustrates two views of the D-Mic™ (left and middle). The right panel of Figure 7–20 illustrates the D-Mic™ capsule with the faceplate removed. Here it is easy to see the single center opening for the omnidirectional microphone and the two openings for the hypercardioid (also called 2nd order) directional microphone. The lower panel shows the various three-opening faceplate colors than can be ordered for this microphone design.

The D-Mic™ can be configured two ways. First, the D-Mic™ can be ordered with a *double-throw switch* allowing the user to switch between omnidirectional (rear position) and either directional *flat* (i.e., equalized) or *low-cut* (i.e., nonequalized) (forward position). When in the omnidirectional mode, the AI-DI is 0.3 dB and only one of the three ports is active. When switched to the directional flat response, the AI-DI varies from 3.3 dB at 1000 Hz to 6.3 dB at 4000 Hz, the two horizontal ports are activated, and the remaining port is deactivated. Second, the hearing aid also can be ordered with a *triple-throw switch* that allows the user access to all three responses. In addition, the dispenser can order a potentiometer to adjust the D-Mic™ low-cut response even further. Reportedly, the directional flat response (equalized) provides a more natural sound quality than the directional low-cut response (nonequalized). However, Preves, Sammeth, and Wynne (1997) reported no significant differences in performance between equalized and nonequalized frequency responses.

Multiple-Microphone Arrays

These experimental hearing aids use two to 17 omnidirectional or directional microphones. As will be reported later, research has shown that additional benefit is not achieved when the number of microphones exceeds five. These devices are sometimes referred to as *"beamformers"* because of their ability to "beam onto" the wanted signal and "beam out" the unwanted signals. Some beamformers have a *fixed* null(s), whereas other beamformers sense the direction of the noise and adaptively move the beam to reduce the effects of the noise by placing a null at the direction of the noise. In a fixed array, the processing is time invariant. Data-dependent weights are applied to the microphone signals to create maximum amplification for signals arriving at the front (target), while reducing amplification for signals arriving off-axis (away from the target). In an adaptive design, the weights are adjusted continually to achieve optimum performance based on some criterion or algorithm (Stadler & Rabinowitz, 1993). This is accomplished by using an adaptive filter to "steer" the array. In general, beamformers can yield up to "N –1" nulls, where N is the number of microphones. Thus, a beamformer with three microphones will have two nulls.

One example of a *fixed* beamformer would be two omnidirectional microphones with an electronic delay built into the hearing aid between the front and rear microphone to obtain a cardioid response. Another example would be using four to five omnidirectional microphones to achieve a response with greater attenuation from the sides and rear (i.e., hyper- or supercardioid response). Still another example would be a hearing aid with two omnidirectional microphones in which the user, by pressing a button on the hearing aid, can obtain cardioid, hypercardioid, or bidirectional responses. In this case, different electronic delays are introduced to the hearing aid via the programming software to achieve the desired directional response. The consistent factor with the scenarios described here is that the microphone design applies amplification for signals arriving from one direction and attenuation for signals arriving from other directions and the design is fixed into what it can achieve.

An example of an adaptive beamformer is provided by a manufacturer who recently in-

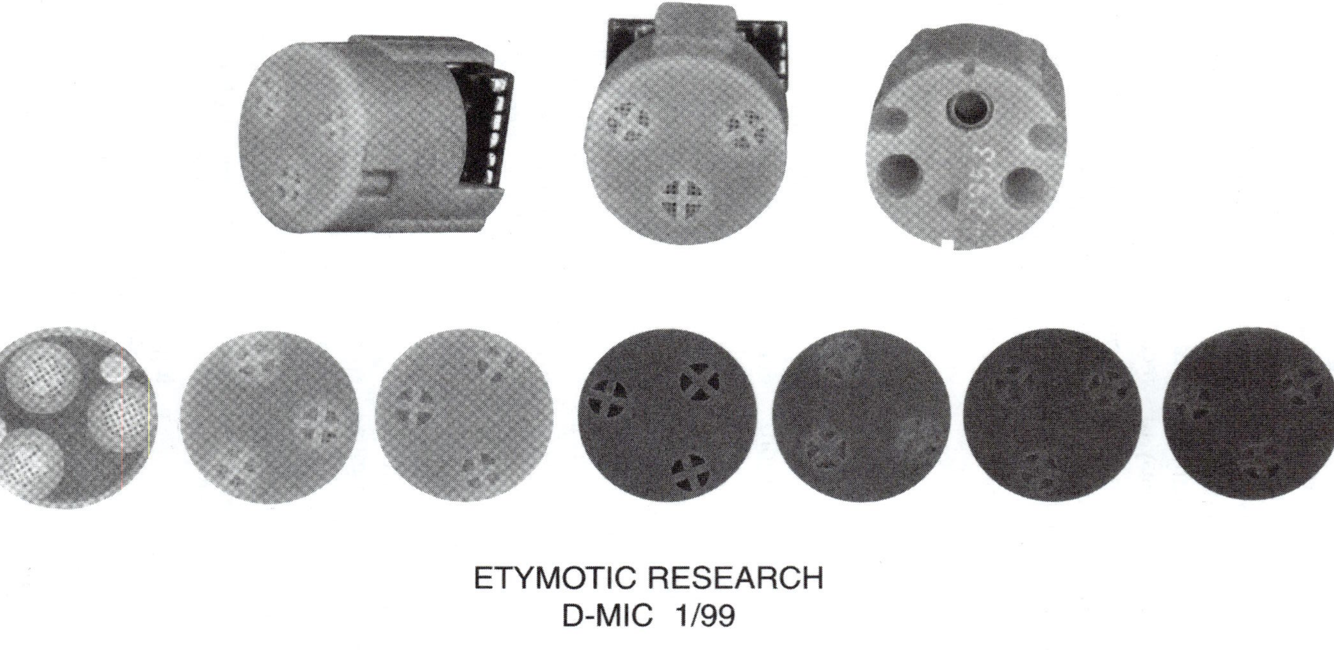

Figure 7–20. Photo illustrating three angles of viewing the D-Mic™ capsule and various faceplate options. The illustration to the right depicts the capsule with the faceplate removed showing the one upper opening for the omnidirectional microphone and the two lower openings for the hypercardioid directional microphone (Reproduced with permission from Etymotic Research.)

troduced a hearing aid that operates in a omnidirectional fashion when the input signal is 50 dB SPL and gradually converts to "full" directionality when the input signal is greater than 75 dB SPL. Figure 7–21 illustrates a polar plot at 2000 Hz for this D-Mic™ hearing aid measured on the right ear of KEMAR for input levels of 50 to 80 dB SPL in 5 dB increments. Notice how the attenuation provided by this hearing aid design at ~ 270° increases as the input signal increases.

Several experimental multiple-microphone arrays have been designed as *broadside* or *end-fire arrays*. In a broadside array, five omnidirectional microphones are spaced equally along the *forehead* using an eyeglass or headband. In some broadside arrays, the output from each microphone is summed and then forwarded to an analog-to-digital (A/D) converter for signal processing. This is why broadside designs sometimes are referred to as "summing" arrays. In an end-fire array, five omnidirectional microphones are spaced equally along the *side* of the head. In the end-fire array, sound from 0° impinges first on the most forward microphone and last on the

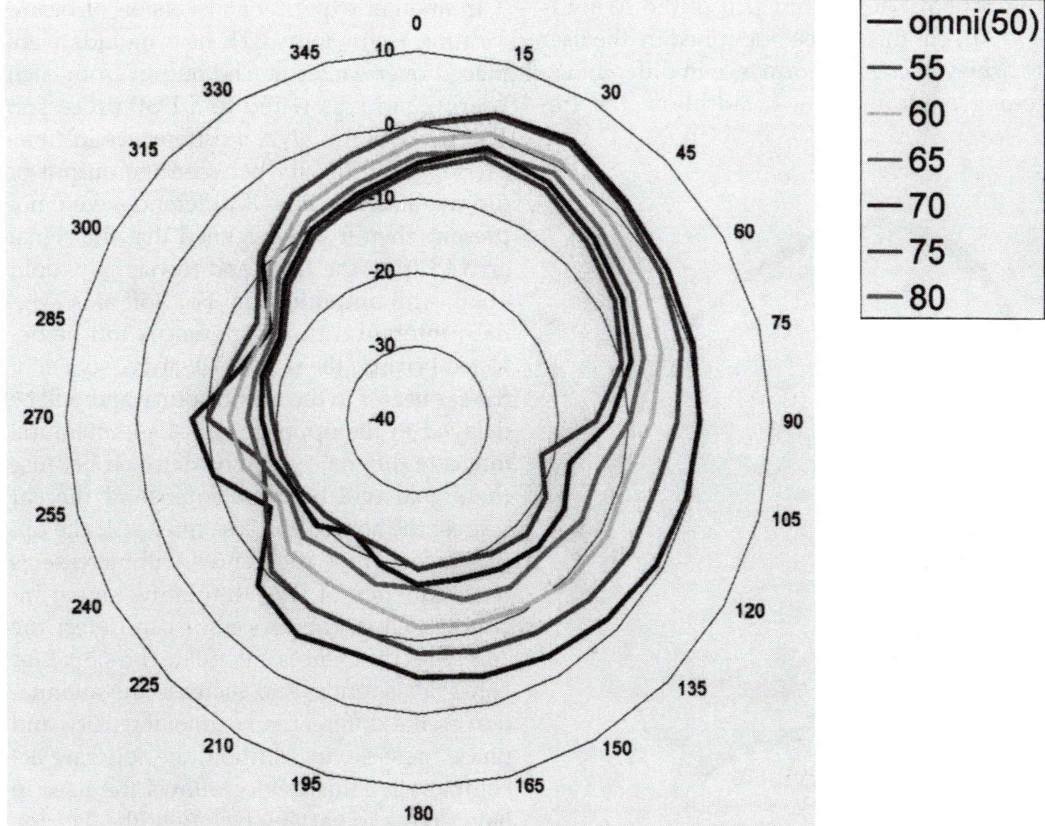

Figure 7–21. Polar sensitivity plot at 2000 Hz of a D-Mic™ ITE measured on the right ear of KEMAR in which the microphone response is omnidirectional at low input levels and becomes more directional as the input level increases. (Reproduced with permission from Audio 'D'.)

most rear microphone. When sound arrives from behind, the process is reversed. Thus, in the end-fire design, increasingly smaller amounts of delay, going from the front to the rear microphone, are incorporated before the output from the five microphones is summed. This is why endfire arrays sometimes are referred to as "delay + sum" arrays.

A commercial product (the "Array") has recently been introduced by one hearing aid manufacturer that contains six omnidirectional microphones (Figure 7–22). This device is worn around the neck and placed under the user's clothing. The output from the Array is transmitted inductively (wireless) to the telecoil of any hearing aid. If the user does not have hearing aids or hearing aids with a telecoil, completely-in-the-canal (CIC) hearing aids with a telecoil can be ordered for the patient. The beamwidth of the Array is +/- 30°, but this can be fine-tuned by the user to achieve better performance in different listening environments. In addition, the frequency response of the Array is divided into twelve independent channels between 200 to 6100 Hz and each channel reportedly can be independently programmed by the dispenser. Results of a pilot study (signal at 0°, noise via eight loudspeakers in the four corners of the ceiling and floor) on nine subjects revealed an average SNR improvement of 10.8 dB when the Array was coupled to the subject's hearing aid relative to the performance with the subject using the hearing aid alone. In addition, the mean word recognition score in noise with the Array was 72.6%, whereas the mean word recognition score was 22.3% for the hearing aid alone condition. Of course, it has yet to be decided if the benefit provided by the Array will be sufficient to overcome the obvious cosmetic disadvantage created by the Array design.

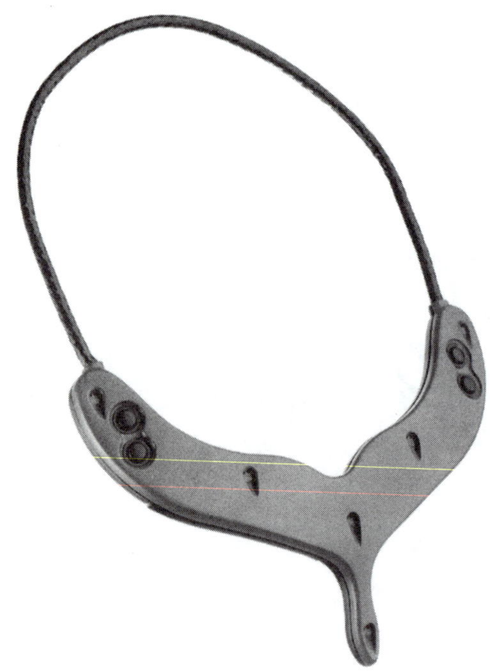

Figure 7–22. Photo of "The Array." (Reproduced with permission from Starkey Laboratories.)

In another experimental version of beamforming technology, BTE hearing aids were placed over each ear. The output from each hearing aid was wired to a DSP processor. The processor analyzed differences in time, phase, and intensity between the output of the two hearing aids. If differences were not present, then it was assumed that the signal arrived from the front and the signal would obtain full amplification. For "off-axis" signals, interaural time differences can be detected because the signal will arrive sooner at the ear nearer to the sound source and will be delayed to the opposite ear. Also, interaural intensity differences can be detected because the signal will be more intense at the ear nearest the source and less intense at the opposite ear. These differences will increase as the frequency of the stimulating signal increases. Thus, the processor can detect the "off-axis" differences, attenuate the signal for "off-axis" sounds, and increase the attenuation as the differences in time, intensity, and phase increase. In addition, the software accompanying this device allows the user to have access to varying beam widths (i.e., the width of accepting signals from the front and attenuating signals off-axis) that can be accessed by the touch of a button on a remote control. For example, the user might need a

10° width for difficult listening situations in which signals arriving +/- 10° from the front will be amplified whereas all other signals would be attenuated. On the other hand, the user might want to implement a wider beam (± 45°) when the signals from a wider section in front of the user are important. In this case, signals arriving ± 45° from the front will be amplified whereas all other signals would be attenuated. Finally, the user might want a "no-beam" response (i.e., omnidirectional) for when signals arriving from any direction are equally important.

OBJECTIVE AND SUBJECTIVE PERFORMANCE OF MICROPHONE DESIGNS

Conventional Directional

Lentz (1972)

This was one of the earliest studies reporting on the improvement provided by directional microphones. In this study, 20 experienced hearing aid users with mild to moderately severe hearing loss were evaluated using omnidirectional and directional hearing aids. Monosyllabic words (CID W-22) were presented at 0° and white noise was presented at 180° and fixed at 62 dB SPL. Word recognition scores were evaluated between the two microphone conditions under conditions of quiet (signal at 62 dB SPL), 0 dB SNR (signal and noise at 62 dB SPL), and –6 dB SNR (signal at 56 dB SPL; noise at 62 dB SPL). The mean directional advantage in was 0.9%. At 0 dB SNR, the mean directional advantage increased to 17.5% and at –6 dB SNR, the advantage increased to 24.9%. This was the first study to illustrate that the directional advantage increased as the listening situation became more difficult.

Frank and Gooden (1973)

This study reported the results of three experiments with 20 normal listeners in each experiment. In each experiment, the signal (Rush Hughes PB-50) was presented at 45° and at 55 dB SPL, while multi-talker babble ("student chatter") was presented at 0° (Experiment 1), 180° (Experiment 2), and 0° and 180° (Experiment 3). The listening conditions were "quiet," and SNRs fixed at +6, 0, –6, –12, and –18 dB. In the first study (noise at 0°) the results revealed no significant difference in mean performance between the omnidirectional and directional hearing aids in quiet or any of the SNRs. In the second study (noise at 180°) results revealed significant difference in mean performance between the omnidirectional and directional hearing aids (~15%) at –18, –12, –6, and 0 dB SNRs. No significant differences were present in "quiet" or at +6 dB SNR. In the third study (noise at 0 and 180°), results revealed a significant difference in mean performance between the omnidirectional and directional hearing aids (~15%) at –12, –6, and 0 dB SNRs. Again, no significant differences were present between the two microphone designs in "quiet," or at –18 or +6 dB SNR. This latter finding points to the fact that directional microphones would not be expected to provide significantly better performance than omnidirectional microphones when the listening situation becomes either too easy (quiet or +6 dB SNR) or too difficult (–18 dB SNR).

Nielsen (1973)

In this study, 22 experienced hearing aid users with mild to moderately severe hearing loss were evaluated using omnidirectional and directional hearing aids. Unspecified monosyllabic words were presented at 0° azimuth at 55 dB SPL, and cafeteria noise was presented at 90°, 180°, and 270° at +5, +10, +15, and +20 dB SNR. At +5 and +10 dB SNR, the average directional advantage was 17.2% and 18.2%, respectively. Significant differences were not present for the +15 and +20 dB SNR conditions. In a second part of the study, the subjects were asked to specify which microphone design they preferred when a male voice was presented at 0° along with three noise sources (young female voice at 90°, cafeteria noise at 180°, and older female voice at 270°). Of the 22 subjects, 15 (68%) stated a preference for the directional design, 5 (23%) preferred the omnidirectional design, and 2 (9%) stated no preference for either design. Finally, the subjects had the opportunity to wear each hearing aid design in their environment for 3 weeks. Based on these experiences, 9 (41%) stated a preference for the directional design, 5 (23%) preferred the omnidirectional design, and 8 (36%) did not prefer either microphone.

Sung, Sung, and Angelelli (1975)

In this study, 32 subjects experienced with monaural amplification and mild to moderate hearing loss were fitted monaurally with three different directional hearing aids and one omnidirectional hearing aid. The signal (CID W-22) was presented at 62 dB SPL at 45°, and the noise (cocktail party) was presented at 62 dB SPL at 225°. Results revealed directional hearing aid #3 provided an average 8.9% better performance than the omnidirectional hearing aid and 6.13% and 14.81% better performance than directional models #2 and #1, respectively. There were no significant differences in performance between directional hearing aid #2 and the omnidirectional hearing aid. Finally, the average performance for directional model #1 was 5.87% poorer than the performance for the omnidirectional hearing aid. The results of this study point out the variability in performance of hearing aids with directional microphones.

Mueller and Johnson (1979)

In this study, 24 experienced adults with mild to moderately severe sensorineural hearing loss were evaluated, with four directional hearing aids that differed between 6 (Aid A) to 20 dB (Aid D) in front-to-back ratio (FBR) measured at 1000 Hz. The signal (Synthetic Sentences) was presented at 55 dB SPL at 0° and the noise (connected discourse) was presented overhead and varied to yield SNRs of 0, –10, and –20 dB. Results revealed directional hearing aid D (FBR of 20 dB) provided significantly better performance (mean of 11.7%) than directional hearing aid A (FBR of 6 dB) at 0 dB SNR. All other comparisons between directional hearing aid B (FBR of 10 dB) or directional hearing aid C (FBR of 16 dB) were not significant. Similar results were reported for the –10 (8.3%) and –20 dB (8.3%) SNR conditions. The results of this study point out that significant improvement provided by a directional microphone is dependent on the degree in which the directional microphone attenuates signals from behind. In this study, a FBR of 16 dB (Aid C) was not sufficient to create significant differences in performance. The FBR needed to be on the order of 20 dB for significant differences to emerge. However, some care must be used in interpreting the results of this study when compared with other studies because the noise source was presented from above as opposed to being presented from behind the listener.

Madison and Hawkins (1983)

In this study, the SNR required to repeat NU-6 words correctly (0° azimuth) embedded in multi-talker babble (180° at 65 dB SPL) was evaluated for 12 normal hearing adults listening, under earphones, to recordings made through omnidirectional and directional hearing aids. Recordings were made in an anechoic chamber (reverberation time = 0.0 second) and a reverberant room (reverberation time = 0.6 second). Results revealed an average advantage for the directional microphone of 10.7 dB in the anechoic room and 3.4 dB in the reverberant room. One might ask what the advantage is of improving the SNR by 3.4 dB. The answer lies in the performance-intensity (PI) functions of the speech signal. For example, for every decibel in improved SNR, the listener, under ideal listening situations, can achieve an average of 8.5% improvement in recognizing sentences correctly. Thus, if the SNR improves by 3.4 dB, one might expect the performance of understanding sentences correctly to improve by 28.9% relative to the same listening situation with an omnidirectional microphone.

Hawkins and Yacullo (1984)

In this study, the SNR required to repeat correctly NU-6 words (0° azimuth) embedded in multi-talker babble (180° at 65 dB SPL) was evaluated on 12 normal hearing and 11 hearing impaired subjects listening, under earphones, to recordings made through monaural and binaural omnidirectional and directional hearing aids. Recordings were made in rooms yielding reverberation times (Rt) of 0.3, 0.6, and 1.2 seconds. For the monaural hearing-impaired condition, results revealed average advantages for the directional microphone of 6.3, 4.7, and –0.6 dB for the Rt of 0.3, 0.6, and 1.2 seconds respectively. For the binaural hearing-impaired condition, results revealed average advantages for the directional microphone of 3.6, 5.5, and 1.5 dB for the Rt of 0.3, 0.6, and 1.2 seconds respectively. For the monaural normal hearing condition, results revealed average advantages for the directional microphone of 3.8, 3.8, and 1.3 dB for the Rt of 0.3, 0.6, and 1.2 seconds. For the binaural normal-hearing condition, results revealed average advantages for the directional microphone of 3.6, 3.6, and 2.6 dB for the Rt of 0.3, 0.6, and 1.2 seconds. These results revealed a directional advantage when Rt was less than 1.2 seconds and the directional advantage was equal at 0.3 and 0.6 second for monaural and binaural listening. Finally, the range of the directional advantage for the hearing-impaired subjects ranged from 1.6 to 7.3 dB.

Table 7–1 was prepared to aid the reader who prefers a brief synopsis of the studies described in this section.

Dual-Microphone: BTE Design

Valente, Fabry, and Potts (1995)

Valente et al. (1995) evaluated the performance of a three-memory programmable dual microphone BTE. Fifty experienced users of binaural hearing aids with mild to moderately severe sensorineural hearing loss were evaluated at two sites under four experimental conditions. First, there was the "basic" program with the omnidirectional microphone and the hearing aids programmed so that the real ear insertion response (REIR) "matched" the NAL-R (Byrne & Dillon, 1986) prescriptive target. Second, there was the "basic" program with the dual-microphones activated. Third, there was the "party" comfort program with only the omnidirectional microphone active. Finally, there was the "party" program with the dual-microphone active. Differences in performance among the four experimental conditions were assessed using the HINT (Soli and Nilsson, 1994) in which the signal was presented at 0° and the noise, set at 65 dBA, was presented at 180°azimuth. Results revealed a mean improvement of 7.4 dB (Site I) to 7.8 dB (Site II) in the "basic" program when the dual-microphone was activated in comparison to omnidirectional performance. In addition, the dual-microphone "party" condition improved the performance by 7.7 dB (Site I) and 8.5 dB (Site II) relative to the basic omnidirectional condition. Finally, there was only a 0.3 dB improvement at Site I and 0.7 dB at Site II for the party dual-microphone condition in comparison to the "basic" dual-microphone condition. This difference was not statistically significant.

Lurquin and Rafhay (1996)

These authors evaluated 20 normal and 20 hearing-impaired subjects to determine differences in signal-to-noise ratio (SNR) necessary to achieve 50% intelligibility. Then they evaluated 15 subjects with a mild to moderately severe sensorineural hearing loss wearing hearing aids with directional microphones to determine differences in performance between normal and unaided performance. Finally, they evaluated 18 subjects with the hearing aids in the omnidirectional and dual-microphone configurations. The speech signal was bisyllabic word lists presented at 0°

Table 7–1. Review of studies using conventional directional microphones (see text for details)

Study	*Subjects*	*Signal/Level/Azimuth*	*Noise/Level/Azimuth*	*Directional Advantage*
Lentz (1972)	20 adults Experienced w/HA Mild to mod-severe	W-22 at 0° azimuth quiet; 0 and –6 dB SNR	White noise at 62 dB SPL 180° azimuth	17.5% at 0 dB 24.9% at −6 dB
Frank/Gooden (1973)	20 normal in three studies (N = 60)	Rush-Hughes at 45° azimuth at 55 dB SPL quiet; +6; 0; –6; -12; –18 dB SNR	MTB at 0° azimuth MTB at 180° azimuth MTB at 0° and 180° azimuth	No directional advantage 15% at 0, −6, −12, −18 dB SNR 15% at 0, −6, and −12 dB SNR
Nielsen (1973)	22 adults Experienced w/HA Mild to mod-severe	PB words at 55 dB SPL at +5,+10,+15, +20 dB SNR	Cafeteria noise at 90°, 180°, and 270° azimuth	17.2% and 18.2% at +5 and +10 dB SNR No advantage at +15 and +20 dB SNR
Sung/Sung/Angelelli (1975)	32 adults Experienced w/HA Mild to mod-severe	W-22 at 45° azimuth at 62 dB SPL	Cocktail noise at 225° azimuth at 62 dB SPL	DHA #3 = 8.9% re: Omni DHA #3 = 14.81% re: DHA #1
Mueller/Johnson (1979)	24 adults Experienced w/HA Mild to mod-severe	SSI at 0° azimuth at 55 dB SPL	Connected discourse presented overhead at 0, –10, and 20 dB SNR	11.6% Aid D > Aid A at 0 dB SNR 8.3% Aid D > Aid A at −10 dB SNR 8.3% Aid D > Aid A at −20 dB SNR
Madison/Hawkins (1983)	12 adults normal hearing	NU-6 at 0° azimuth Adjusted in 2.5 dB steps for 50% performance	MTB at 0° azimuth at 65 dB SPL Rt= 0 and 0.6 second	10.7 dB at 0.0 sec Rt 3.4 dB at 0.6 sec Rt
Hawkins/Yacullo (1984)	12 w/normal hearing 11 w/ HL Experienced w/HA Mild to mod-severe	NU-6 at 0° azimuth Adjusted in 2.5 dB steps for 50% performance	MTB at 0° azimuth at 65 dB SPL Rt = 0.3, 0.6, and 1.2 sec monaural and binaural	MHI= 6.3, 4.7, −0.6 dB at 0.3, 0.6, 1.2 sec Rt BHI= 3.6, 5.5, 1.5 dB at 0.3, 0.6, 1.2 sec Rt MNH= 3.8, 3.8, 1.3 dB at 0.3, 0.6, 1.2 sec Rt BNH= 3.6, 3.6, 2.6 dB at 0.3, 0.6, 1.2 sec Rt

MTB = Multi-talker babble
BHI = binaural hearing impaired
SSI = Synthetic Sentence Identification
MHI = monaural hearing impaired
DHA = Directional hearing aid
BNH = binaural normal hearing
SNR = Signal-to-noise ratio
MNH = monaural normal hearing
Rt = Reverberation time

and the competition was cocktail noise presented at 180° azimuth. The noise level was increased to determine the SNR necessary to achieve 50% intelligibility of the words. Results revealed the mean SNR to be –12.2 dB for the normal group and –4.8 dB for the unaided hearing-impaired group. That is, the hearing-impaired group required, on average, 7.4 dB greater intensity of the signal than the normal hearing subjects to maintain the same level of intelligibility (50%). When the conventional hearing aid with the omnidirectional microphone was placed on the ear, the mean SNR was –4.9 dB. That is, amplification did not improve the recognition of speech in noise (–4.8 unaided versus –4.9 dB aided). When comparing the performance of the dual-microphone, the mean improvement was 6.6 dB relative to the SNR required when only the omnidirectional microphone was active. Also, the average SNR for the dual- microphone was –11.6 dB, which was not significantly different from the –12.2 SNR required for the normal population to correctly recognize the words 50% of the time. That is, the aided performance with the dual-microphone was statistically equivalent to the performance of the normal subjects.

Voss (1997)

Voss (1997) evaluated 13 experienced hearing aids users with mild to moderately severe sensorineural hearing loss. The speech signal was DANTALE (Danish Speech Test) monosyllabic words presented at 0° azimuth and babble noise was presented at 45°, 135°, 225°, and 315° azimuths. The level of the signal and noise was adjusted to create SNRs of 0, –10, and –15 dB. The authors investigated differences in mean performance in word recognition scores at these three SNRs when the dual-microphone hearing aids were programmed to provide the "basic" omnidirectional, "party" omnidirectional, and "party" dual-microphone conditions. Results revealed no significant differences among hearing aid conditions at 0 dB SNR. However, at the –10 dB SNR condition, the activation of the dual-microphone improved the mean score by 16% relative to the "basic" omnidirectional and 11% relative to the "party" omnidirectional. Both of these differences were significant at the <0.05 confidence level. When the listening situation deteriorated further to –15 dB SNR, the activation of the dual-microphone improved the mean word recognition score by 30% relative to the "basic" omnidirectional condition and 22% relative to the "party" omnidirectional condition. Again, these differences were significant at the <0.05 confidence level.

Agnew and Block (1997)

These authors evaluated the performance of a dual-microphone BTE using 20 subjects with bilateral symmetrical sensorineural hearing loss. The subjects were situated equidistant from two loudspeakers. The front loudspeaker presented HINT sentences and the rear loudspeaker presented HINT noise, temporally and spectrally shaped to match the sentences, fixed at 65 dBA. The signal was adjusted in 2 dB steps to find the SNR necessary to obtain 50% performance using hearing aids that allowed switching between omnidirectional and dual-microphone conditions. Results revealed a mean improvement in SNR of 7.53 dB when the hearing aids were placed in the dual-microphone position as compared to the omnidirectional position.

Larsen (1998)

This study reported differences in performance between an analog dual-microphone BTE and an omnidirectional BTE with DSP. Nineteen adult subjects with prior experience with binaural amplification were fitted with a dual-microphone analog BTE and a commercially available omnidirectional BTE with DSP. The subjects wore the aids for two months. The subjects were asked to repeat back DANATALE monosyllabic words presented at 0° azimuth. The intensity level of the signal was adjusted to provide 50% performance when ICRA (International Colloquium of Rehabilitative Audiology) noise was presented at 45°, 135°, 225°, and 315° azimuth. In addition, the subjects were asked to complete the APHAB and a questionnaire requiring answers of "very good, good, or very bad" to twelve questions pertaining to performance of the hearing aids in quiet and noise.

Results revealed an average improvement of 3.6 dB for the dual-microphone BTE when compared to the average performance for the omnidirectional BTE with DSP. Neither of the two questionnaires revealed significant differences between the two hearing aid conditions.

Gravel, Fausel, Liskow, and Chobot (1999)

This study evaluated the advantages provided by a dual-microphone BTE on a group of 20 children (10 younger children between the ages of 4 to 6 years and 10 older children between the ages of 7 to 11 years). For both groups, differences in the SNR necessary to repeat back words and sentences correctly (Pediatric Speech Intelligibility Test; Jerger & Jerger, 1984) 50% of the time was the dependent variable. The signal, presented at 0°, was fixed at 50 dB HL and the noise (multi-talker babble presented at 180°) was varied in 2 dB steps. SNRs were measured for the omnidirectional and dual-microphone positions. Results revealed an overall mean improvement of 4.7 dB for the words and sentences for the dual-microphone position in comparison to the omnidirectional position. For the younger group, the mean advantage provided by the dual-microphone was 4.6 dB for words and 5.1 dB for sentences. For the older group, the improvement was 5.3 dB for words and 4.2 dB for sentences.

Ricketts and Dhar (1999)

This study evaluated differences in performance between three hearing aids. One hearing aid was a dual-microphone BTE with analog signal processing (Phonak Audio-Zoom). The second hearing aid was a dual-microphone BTE with DSP (Siemens Prisma). The third hearing aid was a BTE with DSP and a conventional directional microphone (Senso C9). Twelve subjects with mild to moderately severe sensorineural hearing loss were included in the study. For these subjects, two speech recognition tests (HINT and Nonsense Syllable Tests were administered under anechoic and reverberant (0.6 second) conditions. For each speech test, the signal was presented at 0°, and the competition was presented at 90°, 135°, 180°, 225°, and 270°. Results for the anechoic condition revealed an overall mean improvement of 6.5, 7.5, and 5.0 dB in HINT thresholds for the C9, AZ, and Prisma, respectively. These differences between hearing aids were not statistically significant. Under the reverberant conditions, the mean improvement in HINT thresholds was 4.5, 6.5, and 5.0 dB for the same three hearing aid conditions. Again, differences among hearing aids were not statistically different. For the NST (presented at +8 dB SNR) under reverberant conditions, the mean speech recognition score was 64%, 64%, and 62% for the C9, AZ, and Prisma, respectively. Once again, the differences among hearing aids were not significantly different. The results of this study revealed that the mean performance of a hearing aid with dual-microphone analog signal processing was equal to or better than the mean performance provided by DSP hearing aids with conventional directional or dual-microphones.

Dual-Microphone: ITE Design

Directional microphones have been available in ITEs since the 1970s, but have not been used widely. This probably is due to difficulties in accurately placing the large directional microphone case that was manufactured more than 20 years ago (Preves et al., 1997). However, microphone size has decreased significantly over the past decades and dual-microphones are now available in ITEs. Currently, the user can switch from omnidirectional or dual-microphone performance by either pressing a button on a remote control or changing the position of a user-operated switch on the faceplate. Recently, one manufacturer (Audio-D) introduced a D-Mic™ design in which the hearing aid operates in an omnidirectional mode for input signals below 55 dB SPL and automatically switches to a directional mode when the input signal is 75 dB SPL or greater. For input signals between 55 and 75 dB SPL, the hearing aid operates in a "quasi-directional" mode.

Preves, Sammeth, and Wynne (1997)

In this two-part study, 10 subjects with symmetrical mild to moderately severe bilateral sensorineural hearing loss were evaluated with a dual-microphone ITE (port spacing of 6 mm). In the first study, the low-frequency response in the dual-microphone position provided significantly less low-frequency (125 to 2000 Hz) amplification than with the hearing aid in the omnidirectional position. As noted earlier, this is the typical difference in frequency response between the omni and directional modes reported for directional microphones. This was the "unequalized" condition. In the second study, the low-frequency response in the dual-microphone position was increased to match the low-frequency response in the omnidirectional condition. This was the "equalized" condition. One argument for providing an equalized frequency response is that users might prefer the quieter omnidirectional microphone response in quiet listening situations and have access to the directional response for noisy listening situations in which the noise of the microphone is not likely to be a problem due to the masking effects of the background noise. For both studies, differences in the SNR necessary to repeat correctly HINT sentences 50% of the time was the dependent variable. The sentences were presented at 0° azimuth and HINT uncorrelated noise, fixed at 65 dB SPL, was presented at 115° and 245° azimuth. HINT thresholds were measured for the omnidirectional position and the unequalized and equalized dual-microphone positions. Results revealed a mean improvement of 2.8 dB for the unequalized dual-microphone position and 2.4 dB for the equalized dual-microphone position. This difference was not statistically significant. In addition, 60% to 70% of the subjects stated a preference for the dual-microphone mode. Finally, the majority of subjects preferred to keep the switch so they could toggle between the omnidirectional and dual-microphone positions because, in noisy situations (+8 dB SNR), the majority preferred the dual-microphones, but in quiet situations (65 dB SPL of male connected discourse), they preferred the omnidirectional microphone.

Dual Microphone: BTE Versus ITE

Pumford, Seewald, Scollie, and Jenstad (1999)

This study evaluated differences in performance between a dual-microphone ITE and a dual-microphone BTE hearing aid manufactured by the same company. Twenty-four subjects with mild to moderately severe sensorineural hearing loss were included in the study. For these subjects, HINT thresholds were measured with the signal presented at 0° and the competition presented at 72°, 144°, 216°, and 288°. Results revealed an overall mean improvement of 3.3 dB and 5.8 dB for the ITE and BTE, in the dual-microphone position relative to omnidirectional performance, respectively. In looking at the advantage provided by the ITE microphone location (pinna effect) relative to the BTE microphone location, the study revealed a mean improvement in HINT thresholds of 2.4 dB for the omnidirectional ITE re: omnidirectional BTE. Finally, no significant differences were found in dual-microphone performance between the ITE and BTE (–0.56 dB for the ITE; –0.68 dB for the BTE).

Table 7–2 was prepared to aid the reader who prefers a brief synopsis of the studies described in this section.

Table 7–2. Review of studies using dual-microphones (see text for details).

Study (Type of Aid)	*Subjects*	*Signal/Level/Azimuth*	*Noise/Level/Azimuth*	*Dual-Mic Advantage*
Valente et al. (1995) (BTE)	50 adults Mild to mod-severe	HINT sentences at 0° azimuth	HINT noise at 65 dBA at 180° azimuth	7.4–7.8 dB for "basic" 7.7–8.5 dB for "party"
Lurguin et al. (1996) (BTE)	18 adults Mild to mod-severe	Bisyllabic word list at 0° azimuth	Cocktail noise adjusted to 50% correct at 180° azimuth	6.6 dB
Voss (1997) (BTE)	13 adults Mild to mod-severe	Danatale monosyllabic words at 0° azimuth	Babble noise at 45°, 135°, 225°, 315° azimuth at SNR of 0, –10, and –15 dB	2% at 0 dB SNR 16% at –10 dB SNR 30% at –15 dB SNR
Agnew et al. (1997) (BTE)	20 adults Mild to mod-severe	HINT sentences at 0° azimuth	HINT noise at 65 dBA at 180° azimuth	7.5 dB
Preves et al. (1997) (ITE)	10 adults Mild to mod-severe	HINT sentences at 0° azimuth	HINT noise at 65 dB SPL at 115° and 245° azimuth	~ 3.0 dB for unequalized ~ 2.5 dB for equalized
Gravel et al. (1998) (BTE)	10 young (4–6 yrs) 10 old (7–11 yrs) Mild to mod-severe	Pediatric Speech Intelligibility at 0° azimuth at 50 dB HL	Multi-talker babble at 180° azimuth varied in 2 dB steps	young: 4.6 dB for words 5.1 dB for sentences old: 5.3 dB for words 4.2 dB for sentences
Larsen (in May, 1998) (BTE)	19 adults Mild to mod-severe	Danatale monosyllabic words at 0° azimuth	ICRA noise at 45°, 135°, 225°, and 315° azimuth	3.6 dB re: performance of omnidirectional BTE w/DSP
Ricketts/Dhar (1999) (BTE)	12 adults Mild to mod-severe	HINT sentences at 0° azimuth (.6 ms reverb)	HINT noise at 65 dBA at 90°, 135°, 180°, 225°, and 270°	Senso C9 (directional/digital) = 4.5 dB Phonak AZ (dual/analog) = 6.5 dB Siemens Prisma (dual/digital) = 5.0 dB
		HINT sentences at 0° azimuth (anechoic)	HINT noise at 65 dBA at 90°, 135°, 180°, 225°, and 270°	Senso C9 (directional/digital) = 6.5 dB Phonak AZ (dual/analog) = 7.5 dB Siemens Prisma (dual/digital) = 6.0 dB
Pumford et al. (1998) (ITE and BTE)	24 adults Mild to mod-severe	HINT sentences at 0° azimuth (anechoic)	HINT noise at 65 dBA at 72°, 144°, 216°, and 288° azimuth	ITE = 3.27 dB BTE = 5.77 dB

D-Mic™

Roberts and Schulein (1997)

These authors measured the AI-DI for a D-Mic™ ITE, dual-microphone BTE, omnidirectional ITE, and omnidirectional BTE under anechoic and diffuse-field conditions. Under anechoic conditions, they reported AI-DIs of –0.3 dB for the omnidirectional ITE, –0.7 dB for the omnidirectional BTE, 3.8 dB for the dual-microphone BTE, and 4.8 dB for the D-Mic™ ITE. Under the diffuse test conditions, they reported AI-DIs of 0.8 dB for the omnidirectional ITE, 0.1 dB for the omnidirectional BTE, 2.4 dB for the dual-microphone BTE, and 4.6 dB for the D-Mic™ ITE. Interestingly, the AI-DI in the diffuse-field condition was within 0.3 dB for the two dual-microphones and within 1.1 dB for the two omnidirectional microphones in comparison to the same measures under anechoic conditions. More importantly, the D-Mic™ ITE can provide an AI-DI that is 4.4 dB greater than ITE omnidirectional performance under anechoic measuring conditions and a 3.8 dB advantage under diffuse measuring conditions. The higher AI-DI for the D-Mic™ ITE in both the anechoic and diffuse test conditions was related to the greater DI in the higher frequencies for the D-Mic™ ITE design. According to these authors, directional microphones in ITEs can improve the SNR by 3 to 5 dB indoors and 4 to 8 dB outdoors, where there is less reverberation when compared to ITEs with omnidirectional microphones. In addition, by taking advantage of the pinna effects, ITE directional microphones can provide improvements in the SNR of 3.2 to 8.7 dB for high-frequency sounds when compared to the performance of directional microphones in BTE hearing aids.

Multiple-Microphone Arrays

The major findings from the multitude of research on multiple-microphone array technology are:

- Multiple-microphone arrays can improve SNR by ~ 7–8 dB (re: omnidirectional) for both broadside and endfire designs for normal hearing listeners and listeners with impaired hearing (Schwander & Levitt, 1987; Bilsen, Soede, & Berkhout, 1993; Soede, Bilsen, & Berkout, 1993a, 1993b; Stadler & Rabinowitz, 1993). Kates and Weiss (1996) reported 9 to 11 dB of improvement with a 5 microphone endfire design.
- A five-microphone broadside array will yield a DI of 4.9 dB using omnidirectional microphones (Bilsen et al., 1993; Soede, Bilsen, & Berkout, 1993a, 1993b).
- A five-microphone endfire array will yield a DI of 7.6 dB using omnidirectional microphones (Bilsen et al., 1993; Soede, Bilsen, & Berkout, 1993a, 1993b).
- The "mainbeam" (target @ 0°) is narrower for a broadside design than it is for an endfire design (Bilsen, et al., 1993a, 1993b; Soede, Berkhout, & Bilsen, 1993).
- An endfire design may be more advantageous for diffuse noise suppression (Bilsen, et al., 1993; Soede, Berkhout, & Bilsen, 1993). Also, an endfire design may provide slightly greater DI than broadside (Stadler & Rabinowitz, 1993). On the other hand, Greenberg and Zurek (1992) reported slightly better performance for the broadside design.
- Use of cardioid microphones can increase the DI by 2 to 3 dB relative to omnidirectional microphones. The DI for a cardioid design can be as great as 5 dB in the low frequencies and as great as 10 dB at 4000 Hz (Bilsen et al., 1993a, 1993b; Soede, Berkhout, & Bilsen, 1993). Kates and Weiss (1996) reported that cardioid microphones can improve the DI by 5 dB relative to performance with omnidirectional microphones.
- Adding an endfire + endfire design (10 microphones with 5 on each side) or an endfire + endfire + broadside design (15 microphones with 5 on each side and 5 in the front) can improve the DI by 2 to 3 dB relative to the DI for an endfire design on one side (Bilsen et al.,1993; Soede, Berkhout, & Bilsen, 1993a).

- No further improvement in performance occurs with greater than five microphones (Bilsen et al., 1993; Soede, Berkhout, & Bilsen, 1993a).
- The performance of cardioid and hypercardioid microphones is similar (Stadler & Rabinowitz, 1993).
- Use of multiple microphone arrays can lead to "tunnel hearing" in which the listener's ability to hear "off-axis" signals is greatly diminished (Stadler & Rabinowitz, 1993).
- Use of binaural fit can improve SNR by 2 to 3 dB (Soede, Bilsen, & Berkhout, 1993a).
- Noise reduction capability of multiple microphone array is diminished by 1 dB when the target is off (i.e., "target misalignment") by 10° (Greenberg & Zurek, 1992; Peterson, Wei, Rabinowitz, & Zurek, 1990).
- The addition of a second microphone can improve the SNR by 30, 14, and 0 dB, respectively, in anechoic, living room, and conference room listening situations, relative to performance with a single microphone (Peterson, Durlach, Rabinowitz, & Zurek, 1987).
- For each additional noise source, one additional microphone is required to maintain the performance of the array (Peterson et al. 1987). Thus, if there were four loudspeakers surrounding the listener, a five microphone array would result in the same performance as an array with two microphones with one noise source.
- Moderate head movement (±13° horizontal and ±10° vertical) will diminish performance only slightly (10% decrease in speech recognition relative to when no head movement is allowed) (Schwander & Levitt, 1987).

SUBJECTIVE PREFERENCE BETWEEN MICROPHONE DESIGNS

Typically, most users prefer the response provided by an omnidirectional microphone when listening in quiet environments and a directional microphone when listening in noisy environments (Nielsen, 1973; Sung et al., 1975; Preves et al., 1997). However, there are some environments where using an omnidirectional microphone may provide better performance. For example, an omnidirectional microphone may be more beneficial in a room where several people need to share the same microphone (conference). Another example may be in a lecture or classroom where the listener needs to hear the speaker from the front as well as a speaker from the rear or sides of the room. A third example would be a taxi driver or teacher. Mueller et al. (1983) reported reduced directional advantages if the distance between the listener and talker is between 3 to 6 feet and does not exceed 14 feet.

Mueller, Grimes and Erdman (1983)

These authors reported on two experiments looking at differences in subjective preferences between omnidirectional and directional microphones. In the first experiment, 24 subjects without prior hearing aid experience were fit monaurally with a hearing aid capable of being switched between omnidirectional and directional listening. Using a questionnaire designed to determine if differences were present in microphone designs, no clear preference for either microphone was present when listening in quiet situations. However, when responding to preferences in noisy situations, there was a clear preference for the directional microphone (47% for directional versus 22% for omnidirectional). In the second experiment, 30 subjects with high-frequency hearing loss and without prior experience with amplification were fit with the same hearing aid as was fit in experiment 1. As in the first experiment, as listening situations became more adverse, preference for the directional microphone increased.

Kuk (1996)

Kuk (1996a) surveyed 100 users of a hearing instrument incorporating multiple microphone technology. In 10 quiet environments (e.g., TV, radio, familiar talker, next room, quiet restaurant, small group), 65% preferred the omnidirectional microphone, 25% preferred the dual-microphone, and 10% reported no preference. In noisy environments (e.g., restaurant, large store, large group, car), there was a strong preference for the dual-microphone. Interestingly, more of the subjects preferred the omnidirectional microphone when communicating in a car with the passenger next to or behind them. When listening to nonspeech signals, the listeners stated a preference for the omnidirectional microphone when listening to nature sounds, warning sounds, music, their own voices, and while eating, but preferred the dual-microphones when listening to "annoying sounds." In addition, 67% of the users stated they sometimes or frequently switched between microphone designs. Only 15% of the users stayed in the dual-microphone position all the time.

As stated above, Mueller et al. (1983) reported that most of their listeners used the directional microphone most of the time. In this study, users had to manually switch between omnidirectional and directional responses. However, in the Kuk (1996a) study, users simply pressed a button on a remote control to accomplish the switching. This may account for why 67% of the subjects in the Kuk (1996a) study reported switching between the two microphone designs. To address the concern expressed in the Mueller et al. (1983) study, one hearing aid manufacturer recently introduced a hearing aid that changes directional patterns automatically (adaptive). In this case, the response of the hearing aids is omnidirectional when the input signal is 50 dB SPL or below, quasi-directional when the input signal is 65 dB SPL, and fully directional when the input signal is 75 dB SPL or higher. This concept is based on the assumption that low input levels would represent a quiet environment (i.e., preference for omnidirectional) and the higher input levels would be more typical of a noisy listening situation (i.e., preference for directional).

Kochkin (1996)

Kochkin (1996) performed a consumer survey of 3289 subjects across 13 hearing instruments to determine if the advanced hearing aid features (programmability, multiple memory, multiple bands, dual-microphones, etc.) impacted consumer satisfaction and subjective benefit. In his survey, there were four single-band single-memory hearing aids (Class 1), two single-channel multiple-memory hearing aids (Class 2), three multiple-channel single-memory hearing aids (Class 3), and four multiple-channel multiple-memory hearing aids (Class 4). The hearing aid receiving the highest user satisfaction (90%) was the dual-microphone BTE (Class 2; #5). This is considerably higher than the 64% MarkeTrak norm. The second highest rating was a multiple-channel multiple-memory hearing aid that had an overall satisfaction rating of 83% (Class 4; #10). In addition, the dual-microphone BTE out-performed the other hearing aids and the MarkeTrak norms in almost all the questions related to improved quality of life, hearing, clearness of tone/sound, naturalness of sound, and directionality. Finally, consumers reported that the dual-microphone BTE significantly improved listening in noise, with one-on-one communication, when watching TV, in small groups, when outdoors, in a car, at a concert or movie, in a restaurant, and in a large group. Kuk (1996b) reported similar results for 213 users of a dual-microphone hearing instrument.

RECENT INTRODUCTION OF DUAL-MICROPHONE HEARING AIDS

Because of the improvement in SNR reported for dual-microphones in the studies reviewed in this chapter, it is felt that a greater number of manufacturers will be releasing products containing dual-microphone technology in the near future. For example, at the time this chapter was prepared, Siemens, ReSound, and Danavox introduced dual-microphone

BTE and ITE hearing aids with DSP. Micro-Tech also recently released an ITE with dual-microphones. Oticon recently introduced an ITE with DSP and a D-Mic™. It is clear that more manufacturers will introduce hearing aids with dual-microphones or the D-Mic™ in the years ahead.

CONCLUSION

It is the belief of the author that significant efforts will continue by manufacturers to produce products that will improve the recognition of speech in noise because this is the primary reason patients pursue amplification. Unfortunately, the inability of many current hearing aids (analog or digital) to consistently improve recognition of speech in noise is also the primary reason patients have rejected amplification. Current research has not been able to demonstrate that the current generation of DSP technology, by itself, has improved the recognition of speech in noise significantly.

The one area of hearing aid technology that has consistently demonstrated improved recognition of speech in noise is directional microphones (conventional, dual-microphone, D-Mic™, multiple microphones). It is suspected that hearing aid manufacturers will continue their efforts to improve the performance of directional microphones because this is the area that provides the greatest opportunity for providing improved performance in noise.

Acknowledgments

The author would like to thank Steve Thompson of Knowles Electronics; Robert Wolf of Siemens Hearing Instruments, Inc.; Tim Trine and Diane Van Tassell of Starkey Laboratories; Lynne Murakami, Tina Papke, Chris Struck and Brent Edwards of ReSound Corporation; Ted Gauthier of Audio 'D'; Kurt Trede of Etymotic Research; Dave Preves and Mary MacRae of Micro-Tech Hearing Instruments; and Laura Voll of Phonak, Inc. for going through the trouble of making the figures and photos used in this chapter. In addition, the author would like to thank the hearing aid manufacturers for investing their resources into the development of the technology presented in this chapter. This technology has had a major impact on the listening abilities of our patients with hearing loss.

REVIEW QUESTIONS

1. A patient with hearing loss will require a signal-to-noise ratio of _____ dB in order to hear as well as a person with normal hearing
a. 0 dB
b. 25 dB
c. 3 dB
d. 10 dB

2. The directivity index (DI) measures the performance of a directional microphone relative to when competing signals are originating from
a. the front
b. all around (diffuse)
b. the rear
c. the sides

3. For a taxi driver, who typically needs to hear signals from the rear, but signals from the sides (i.e., windows) can be distracting, a ___________microphone design might be the most appropriate
a. bidirectional
b. cardioid
c. hypercardioid
d. supercardioid

4. The microphone design with the greatest DI is:
a. cardioid
b. hypercardioid
c. supercardioid
d. omnidirecitonal

5. In a conventional directional microphone, the acoustic delay between the front and rear sound inlet is:

a. ~ 4 μsec
b. ~ 50 μsec
c. ~ 125 μsec
d. ~ 500 μsec

6. In D-Mic™ applications, the capsule contains:
a. two omnidirectional microphones
b. one omnidirectional and one hypercardioid microphone
b. two cardioid microphones
c. one omnidirectional and one supercardioid microphone

7. A broadside array consists of multiple microphones along:
a. front of the head
b. side of the head
c. front and side of the head
d. back of the head

8. An endfire array uses ________ to attenuate signals:
a. sum the outputs from the microphones
b. sum the output from only the second through last microphone
c. sum the output from only the last microphone
d. delay and sum the output from the microphones

9. A well-designed dual-microphone BTE can improve the SNR by approximately:
a. 14 dB
b. 10 dB
c. 6 dB
d. 3 dB

10. A well-designed directional BTE can improve the SNR by approximately:
e. 14 dB
f. 10 dB
g. 6 dB
h. 3 dB

REFERENCES

Agnew, J., & Block, M. (1997). HINT thresholds for a dual-microphone BTE. *Hearing Review, 4*(9), 26, 29–30.

American National Standards Institute. (1969). *American National Standard Methods for the Calculation of the Articulation Index* (ANSI S3.5-1969). New York: ANSI.

Arentsschild, O., & Frober, B. (1972). Comparative measurements of the effect of a directional microphone in the hearing aid. *Journal of Audiological Technique, 11*, 204–229.

Bachler, H., & Vonlanthen A. (1995). Audio-zoom processing for improved communication in noise. *Phonak Focus, 18*, 3–18.

Bilsen, F. A., Soede, W., & Berkhout, A. J. (1993). Development and assessment of two fixed array microphones for use in hearing aids. *Journal of Rehabilitation Research and Development, 30*, 73–81.

Buerkli-Halevy, O. (1986). The directional microphone advantage. *Hearing Instruments, 38(8)*, 34, 36–38.

Byrne, D., & Dillon, H. (1986). The National Acoustics Laboratory (NAL) new procedure for selecting gain and frequency response of a hearing aid. *Ear and Hearing, 7*, 257–265

Cox, R. M., & Alexander, G. C. (1995). The abbreviated profile of hearing aid benefit. *Ear and Hearing, 16*,176–186.

Edwards, B., Hou, Z., Struck, C., & Dharan, P. (1998). Signal-processing algorithms for a new software-based, digital hearing device. *Hearing Journal, 51*, 44, 46–47, 50, 52.

Frank, T., & Gooden, R. G. (1973). The effect of hearing aid microphone types on speech discrimination scores in a background of multi-talker noise. *Maico Audiologic Library Series, 11(5)*, 1–4.

Gravel, J. S., Fausel, N., Liskow, C., & Chobot, J. (1999). Children's speech recognition in noise using omnidirectional and dual-microphone hearing aid technology. *Ear and Hearing, 20*, 1–11.

Greenberg, J. E., & Zurek, P. M. (1992). Evaluation of an adaptive beamforming method for hearing aids. *Journal of the Acoustical Society of America, 91*,1662–1676.

Hawkins, D. B., & Yacullo, W. S. (1984). Signal-to-noise ratio advantage of binaural hearing aids and directional microphones under different levels of reverberation. *Journal of Speech and Hearing Disorders, 49*, 278–286.

Kates, J. M., & Weiss, M. R. (1996). A comparison of hearing aid array processing techniques. *Journal of the Acoustical Society of America, 99*, 3138–3148.

Killion, M. C. (1997a). The SIN report: circuits haven't solved the hearing-in-noise problem. *Hearing Journal, 50*(10), 28–30,32.

Killion, M. C. (1997b). SNR loss: I can *hear* what people say, but I can't *understand* them. *Hearing Review, 4*(12), 8, 10, 12, 14.

Killion, M. C. (1997c). Hearing aids: past, present, future: Moving toward normal conversation in noise. *British Journal of Audiology, 31*, 141–148.

Kochkin, S. (1993). MarkeTrak III identifies key factors in determining customer satisfaction. *Hearing Journal, 46*(8), 39–44.

Kochkin, S. (1994). MarkeTrak III: Why 20 million in U.S. don't use hearing aids for their hearing loss. *Hearing Journal, 46*(1), 20–27, 46(2), 26–31, 46(4), 36–37.

Kochkin, S. (1996). Customer satisfaction and subjective benefit with high performance hearing aids. *Hearing Review, 3*(12), 16–26.

Kuk, F. (1996a). Subjective preference for microphone types in daily listening environments. *Hearing Journal, 49*(4), 29–30, 32–35.

Kuk, F. (1996b). Hearing aid survey tests user satisfaction. *Hearing Instruments, 47*(1), 24–26, 29.

Lentz, W. E. (1972). Speech discrimination in the presence of background noise using a hearing aid with a directionally-sensitive microphone. *Maico Audiologic Library Series, 10*(9), 1–4.

Lurquin, P., & Rafhay, S. (1996). Intelligibility in noise using multi-microphone hearing aids. *Acta Oto-laryngology-Rhinology-Laryngology (Belgium), 50,* 103–109.

Madison, T. K., & Hawkins, D. B. (1983). The signal-to-noise ratio advantage of directional microphones. *Hearing Instruments, 34(2),* 18, 49.

May, A. (1998). Multi-microphone instruments, DSP and hearing-in-noise. *Hearing Review, 5*(7), 42–45.

Mueller, H. G. (1981). Directional microphone hearing aids: A 10-year report. *Hearing Instruments, 32*(11), 18–20,66.

Mueller, H. G., Grimes, A. M., & Erdman, S. A. (1983). Subjective ratings of directional amplification. *Hearing Instruments, 34*(2), 14–16, 47–48.

Mueller, H. G., & Johnson, R. M. (1979). The effects of various front-to-back ratios on the performance of directional microphone hearing aids. *Journal of the American Auditory Society, 5,* 30–34.

Mueller, H. G., & Wesselkamp, M. (1999). Ten commonly asked questions about directional microphone fittings. *Hearing Review, 3*(1), 26–30.

Nielsen, H. B. (1973). A comparison between hearing aids with a directional microphone and hearing aids with conventional microphone. *Scandinavian Audiology, 2,* 45–48.

Peterson, P. M., Durlach, N. I., Rabinowitz, W. M., & Zurek, P. M. (1987). Multimicrophone adaptive beamforming for interference reduction in hearing aids. *Journal of Rehabilitation Research and Development, 24*(4), 103–110.

Peterson, P. M., Wei, S. M., Rabinowitz, W. M., & Zurek, P. M. (1990). Robustness of an adaptive beamforming method for hearing aids. *Acta Otolaryngology, 469,* 85–90.

Preves, D. A. (1997). Directional microphone use in ITE hearing instruments. *Hearing Review, 4*(7), 21, 24–27.

Preves, D. A., Sammeth, C. A., & Wynne, M. K. (1997). Field trial evaluations of a switched directional/omnidirectional ITE hearing instrument. Poster presented at NIDCD/VA Hearing Aid Conference, Bethesda, MD.

Pumford, J. M., Seewald, R. C., Scollie, S., & Jenstad, L. M. (1999). Speech recognition in diffuse noise using in-the-ear and behind-the-ear dual-microphone hearing instruments. *Manuscript submitted for publication.*

Ricketts, T., & Dhar, S. (1999). Comparison of performance across three directional hearing aids. *Journal of the American Academy of Audiology, 10,* 180–189.

Roberts, M., & Schulein, R. (1997, October). *Measurement and intelligibility optimization of directional microphones for the use in hearing aid devices.* Paper presented at 103rd Meeting of the Audio Engineering Society, New York.

Schwander, T. M., & Levitt, H. (1987). Effect of two-microphone noise reduction on speech recognition by normal-hearing listeners. *Journal of Rehabilitation Research Development, 24*(4), 87–92.

Skinner, M. W. (1988). *Hearing aid evaluation.* NJ: Prentice-Hall.

Soede, W., Bilsen, F. A., & Berkhout, A. J. (1993a). Assessment of a directional microphone array for hearing-impaired listeners. *Journal of the Acoustical Society of America, 94,* 799–808.

Soede, W., Berkhout, A. J., & Bilsen, F. A. (1993b). Development of a new directional hearing instrument based on array technology. *Journal of the Acoustical Society of America, 94,* 785–798.

Soli, S. D., & Nilsson, M. (1994). Assessment of communication handicap with the HINT. *Hearing Instruments, 45,* 12,15–16.

Stadler, R. W., & Rabinowitz, W. M. (1993). On the potential of fixed arrays for hearing aids. *Journal of the Acoustical Society of America, 94,* 1332–1342.

Sung, G. S., Sung, R. J., & Angelelli, R. M. (1975). Directional microphones in hearing aids. Effects on speech discrimination in noise. *Archive of Otolaryngology, 101,* 316–319.

Valente, M., Fabry, D., & Potts, L. G. (1995). Recognition of speech in noise with hearing aids using dual microphones. *Journal of the American Academy of Audiology, 6, 440–449*

Valente, M., Fabry, D., Potts, L. G., & Sandlin, R. (1998). Comparing the performance of the Widex Senso digital hearing aids with analog heairng aids. *Journal of the American Academy of Audiology, 9,* 342–360.

Valente, M., Sweetow, R., Potts, L., & Bingea, B. (in press). Digital versus analog signal processing: Effect of directional microphone. *Journal of the American Academy of Audiology.*

Voss, T. (1997). Clinical evaluation of multi-microphone hearing instruments. *Hearing Review, 4(9),* 36, 45–46, 74.

CHAPTER 8

DSP Hearing Instruments

INGA HOLUBE, PH.D.
THERESE M. VELDE, PH.D.

OUTLINE

Today three general classes of hearing instruments are available. Until the end of the 1980s, hearing health care professionals dispensed analog hearing instruments that were adjusted according to the degree of hearing loss with screwdriver-controlled potentiometer trimmers. Then the advent of integrated circuit chip technology allowed for the development of analog hearing instruments that could be programmed digitally with dedicated programming devices or with personal computers. In 1996, the third class of hearing instrument was introduced, they were digitally programmable and offered digital signal processing. It is this third category of hearing aids that will be the focus of this chapter. The first part of this chapter will describe the principles of digital technology, and the second part will discuss different digital signal processing algorithms. The user benefit of these algorithms will be addressed in the respective sections.

PRINCIPLES OF DIGITAL TECHNOLOGY

Analog and Digital Hearing Instruments

Digital hearing instruments have several fundamental differences from analog instruments. Figure 8–1 shows a block diagram of an analog hearing aid. Analog devices consist of a microphone, a preamplifier, a means processor (such as a tone control or an AGC), an amplifier, and a receiver. An acoustic input signal (a sine wave in Figure 8–1) is converted by the microphone to an electronic input signal. This electronic input signal is amplified by the preamplifier, and the frequency response is shaped by the tone control. After this shaping, the signal is again amplified and then converted back to an acoustic output signal by the receiver. Both the acoustic and electronic signals in the processing path are analog.

In analog hearing instruments that are digitally programmable, parameters of the means of processing, such as the tone control or the compression ratio of the AGC, are stored in a memory and can be modified for different hearing instrument users.

Figure 8–2 shows a block diagram of a digital hearing instrument. In contrast to an analog instrument, a digital instrument has an analog-to-digital converter, a digital signal processor, and some method of digital-to-analog conversion. The amplified electronic signals are converted into digitized signals that are processed by the digital signal processor before they are converted back to analog electronic signals. The following section will focus on the difference between analog and digital signals and the principles and advantages of digital signal processing.

Analog Signals

All physical signals, such as the sound pressure at the microphone or the voltage of the electronic signal at the receiver of a hearing instrument, are continuous in time and in amplitude. Figure 8–3 shows the time waveform of a sinusoidal electronic signal. Analog signals can have any amplitude value at any particular moment in time, and the level measured at any moment may differ slightly from that immediately preceding or following it. Thus, with this continuously varying signal, there are no "steps" in the signal curve.

Digital Signals

The purpose of the digital signal processor in hearing instruments is to derive, by a series of calculations, an output signal based on the input signal to the instrument. The input signal has to be converted into numbers for the calculations, and these numbers can then be added, subtracted, multiplied, or divided. A program that is composed of a series of calculations is called an algorithm. Several reference sources offer a review of digital signal

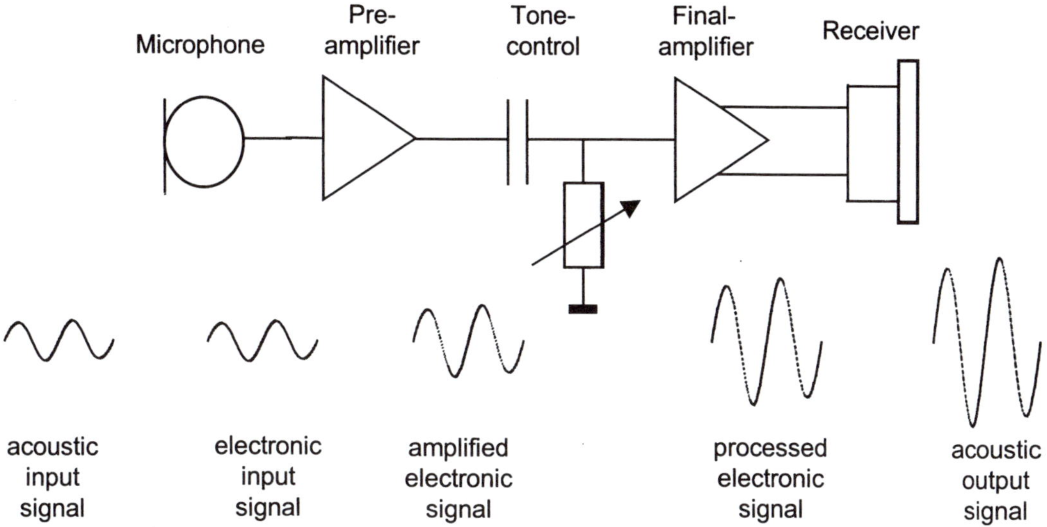

Figure 8–1. Block diagram of an analog hearing instrument.

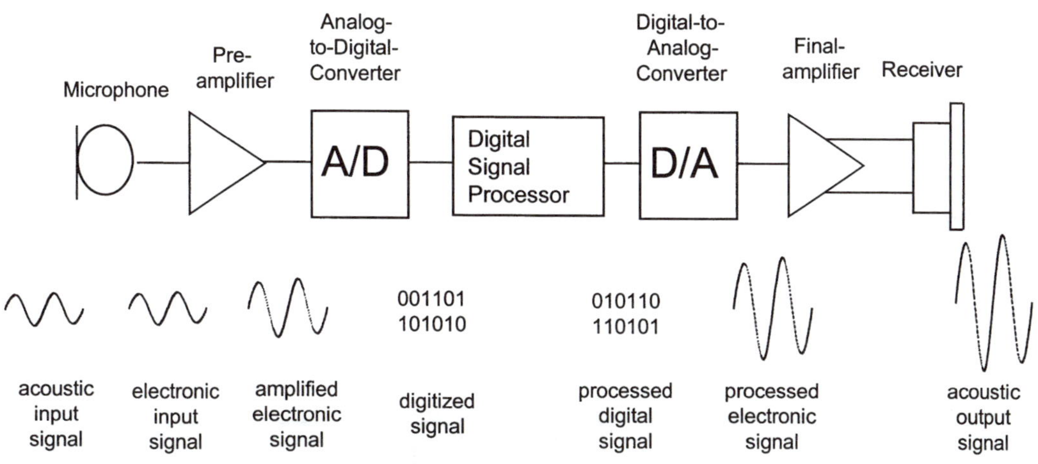

Figure 8–2. Block diagram of a digital hearing instrument.

processing (e.g., Lyons, 1997; Oppenheim & Schafer, 1975).

Sampling

The input signal is sampled at discrete points in time. In Figure 8–4, an analog signal is being sampled every 0.05 second. Only these sampled points or samples are used by the digital signal processor. The rest of the input signal is not considered.

This sampling of the input signal is done in the analog-to-digital (A/D) converter. As is suggested in Figure 8–4, it is important to sample the input signal frequently enough to have a good representation. This requirement will be discussed in greater detail later in this chapter.

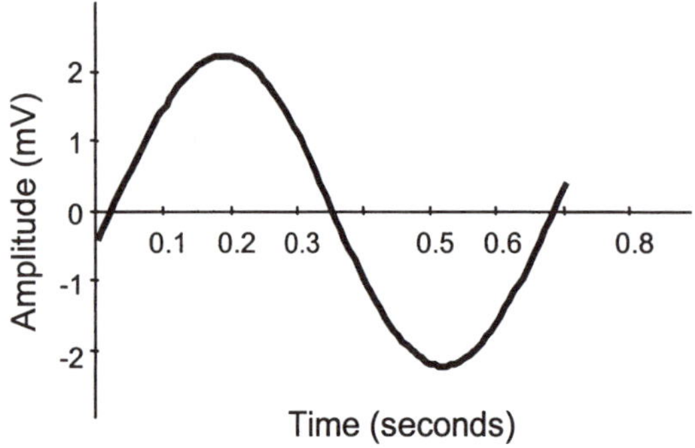

Figure 8–3. An analog signal with different levels at any given point of time.

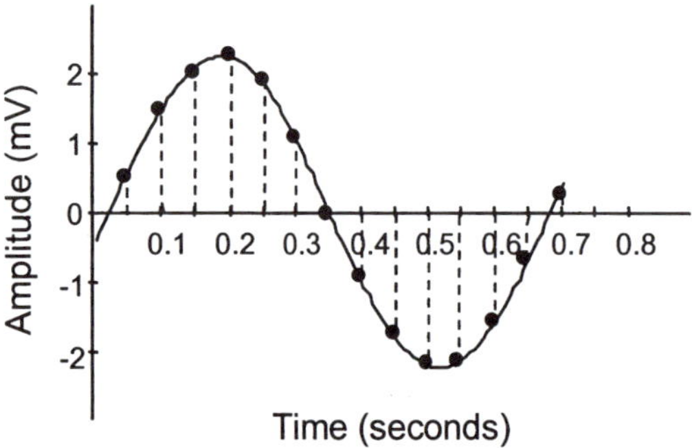

Figure 8–4. An analog signal sampled at discrete points in time.

Quantization

The digital signal processor cannot use numbers with infinite precision for calculation. Therefore, each sample must be either truncated or rounded to a specific precision. This results in a less idealized representation of the analog input signal and is called quantization. The quantized signal is characterized by bit values. A single bit can have two values. These numbers correspond to the two states at its input (i.e., voltage switched on or voltage switched off). In Figure 8–5, we see a digital signal in the upper panel. The signal is either on, with a value of 1, or off, with a value of 0. In the lower panel, the binary code or quantization value corresponding to the signal is given. Numbers that contain only such binary digits (bits) are called binary numbers. The number of bits in a binary number is known as the word length. In this figure, the quantization values are either zero or one. Signals also can be described with greater resolution.

An increase in the word length increases the number of potential values that can be given to a sampled signal. A one-bit A/D converter has 2 (that is, 2^1) values available to assign a sampled point. A two-bit A/D con-

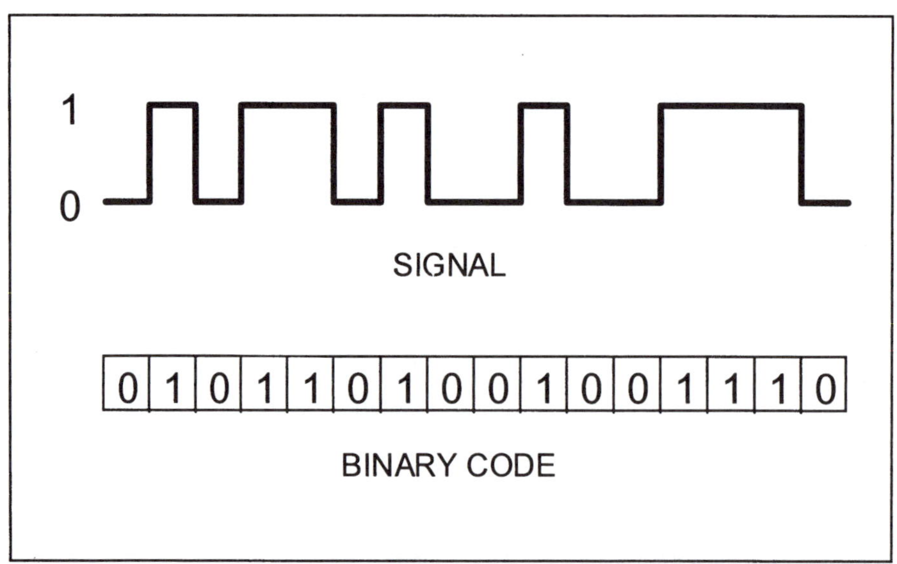

Figure 8–5. A digital signal with only two states, or 1 bit, and its corresponding binary code.

verter has 4 (that is, 2^2) values available to assign to a sampled point. A four-bit A/D converter has 16 (that is, 2^4) values available, and so on.

Figure 8–6 shows the 3-bit digital output (heavy line) for a linear input signal (light line) over time. In this example, the quantization step is 1 mV. When the analog signal is between 0.5 and 1.5 mV, the digital value is 001. Likewise, an analog input signal of 6 mV is converted to the digital value 110. Note that the shape of the digital signal is not linear like the analog signal. Instead, the digital signal remains at one value until it jumps to the next digital value.

The more bits that are available, the better the analog input signal can be represented by the digital numbers. Figure 8–7 shows two examples of analog signals and their digital representation with different numbers of bits. In panel A, two bits are used. In panel B, four bits are used. The sampled value is held constant until the next sample is taken. When a sample is made, the sample is assigned a value. In panel A, only four values are possible to represent the signal because only two bits are used. In panel B, 16 values are possible because four bits are used. The level of the analog signal is rounded to the nearest binary number. The more bits that are used the

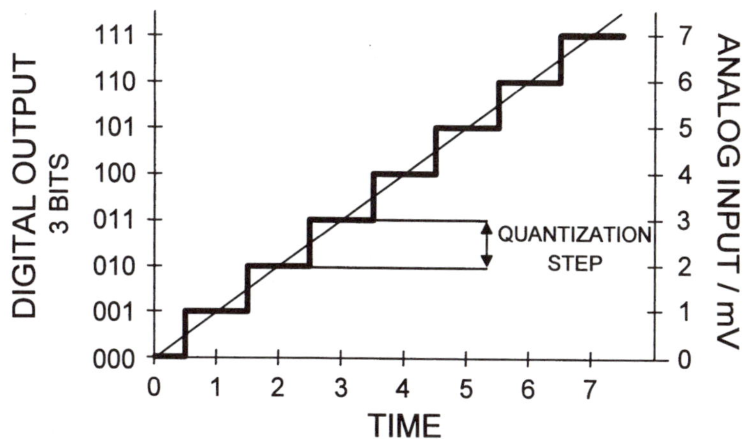

Figure 8–6. Conversion of an analog input signal into a digital signal with 3 bits.

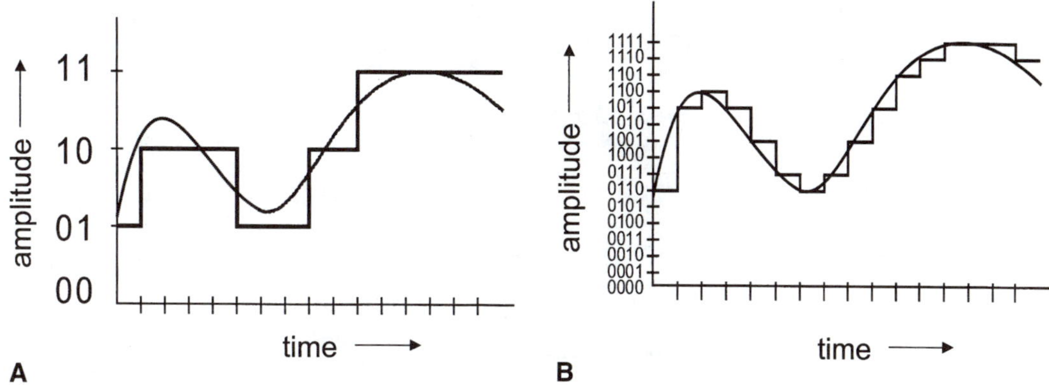

Figure 8–7. A. Analog signal and the corresponding digital signal sampled at 2 bits. **B.** Analog signal and the corresponding digital signal sampled at 4 bits.

smaller the error between the analog and the digital signal.

Quantization Error

An analog signal and its digitized signal are again shown in Figure 8–8. In panel A, the analog signal was sampled with 3 bits as is indicated by the 8 possible values of the digital signal. The difference between the original and the digitized signal is the quantization error. This error signal is shown in the back waveform. Panel B shows the same original signal and the digitized signal that is sam-

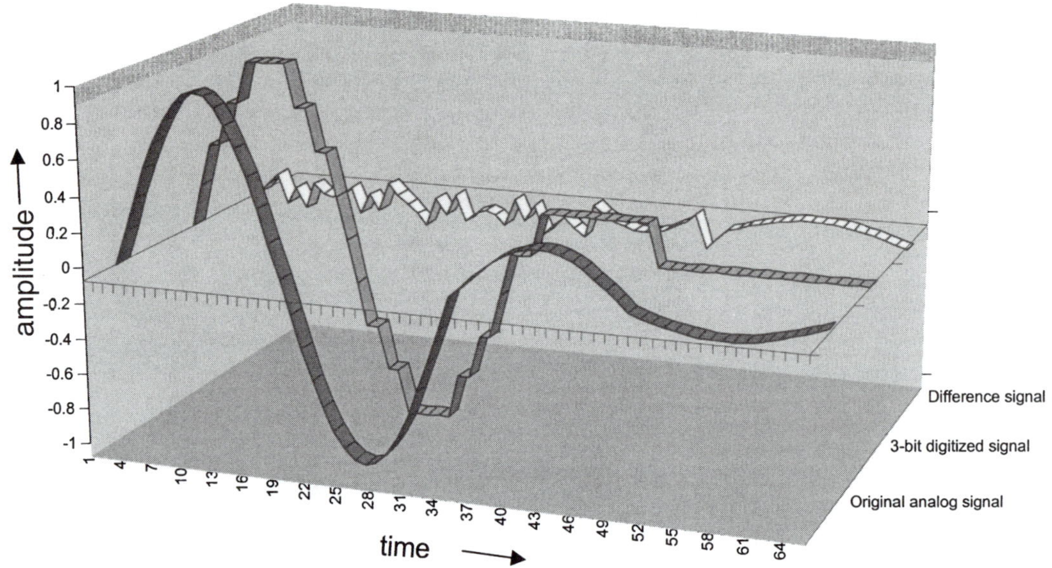

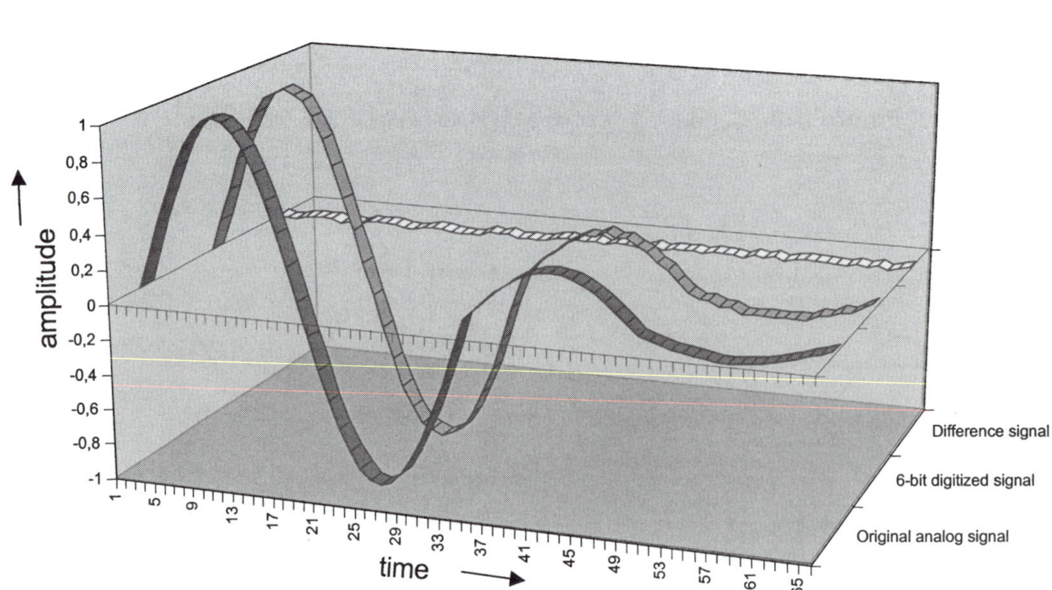

Figure 8–8. **A.** Original signal, digitized signal with 3 bits, and the difference signal. **B.** Original signal, digitized signal with 6 bits, and the difference signal.

pled with a resolution of 6 bits. Note how the digitized signal more closely approximates the original signal, resulting in the quantization error being nearly zero at all points. The error signal shows that the analog signal is better approximated by the digital signal when more bits are used.

Why is quantization error important to hearing instruments? The quantization error is a random noise with its maximum amplitude at one-half the amplitude of the quantization step. Soft input signals to the hearing instrument, which have smaller amplitude than the amplitude of the quantization noise, cannot be distinguished from the noise. Therefore, the quantization noise determines the noise floor for the digital signal processing. Because the maximum output of the hearing instrument is fixed by the selected receiver, the noise floor determines the dynamic range of the digital system. Each bit increases the dynamic range by 6 dB. A digital signal processor with 3 bits has a dynamic range of only 18 dB. When using 6 bits, the dynamic range is increased to 36 dB. Audio compact-disc players normally use 16 bits of resolution and therefore have a dynamic range of 96 dB.

Aliasing

Let's return to the issue of how frequently a signal is sampled. In addition to the quantization error, a digital system can demonstrate an additional error that is not found in analog systems. This error is related to the sampling frequency of the analog signal. Figure 8–9 shows as an example a sine wave, labeled "Input signal" that is sampled at four different discrete points in time. Note that only one or two points are sampled within each cycle. The same four sample points can also represent a different sine wave with a lower frequency, labeled "Aliasing signal." This ambiguity results in the presence of a sine wave, which was not present in the original input, at the output of the digital system. This type of error is called aliasing. In an acoustic system, such as a hearing aid, an aliasing error introduces distortions.

A visual example of aliasing error is when automobile wheels appear to rotate backward in movies. The camera samples the wheel's movement at a specific frequency, but the wheel completes a cycle of movement at a frequency faster than the sampling frequency. Our eyes see a lower frequency of

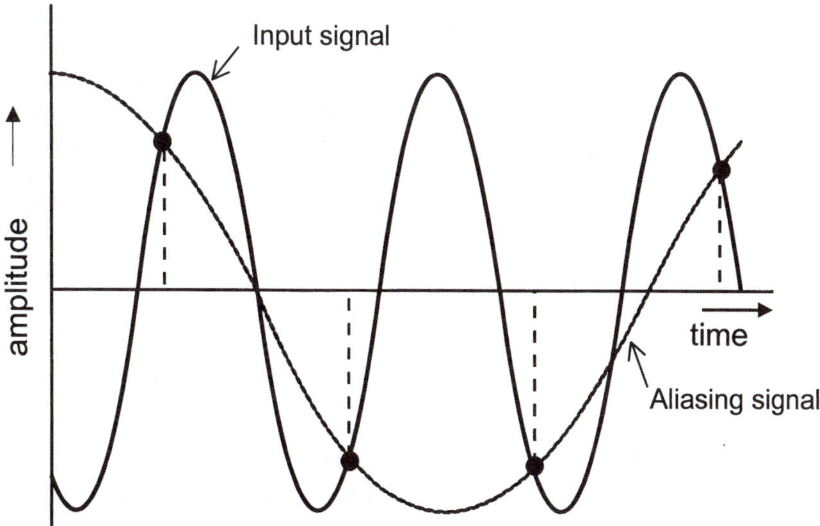

Figure 8–9. Two sine waves of different frequencies that can be represented by the same samples.

movement (as indicated by the wheel turning backward) that fits the camera's samples.

To avoid this aliasing error in a sine wave, it is necessary to sample the input signal with a minimum of two samples per period of the sinusoid. This minimum sample rate is called the Nyquist frequency, named after Nyquist (1928) for his work with telegraph transmission theory. For speech signals, the sampling rate must be at least twice the highest frequency to be processed in a digital system. If an individual wants to hear signals with a frequency content up to 10 kHz, for example, it is necessary to use a sampling rate of 20 kHz. If frequency components above 10 kHz are present in the signal, the person wearing the hearing instrument would hear a false sound. To avoid this aliasing error, the input signal has to be filtered. This low-pass filter, called an anti-aliasing filter, should have an edge frequency of half the sampling frequency or less.

Principles of Digital Signal Processing

Using the principles we have established in the previous sections about digital signals, we can now examine the digital signal processor. We will first describe an analog-to-digital (A/D) converter, then we will discuss some examples of algorithms used in a digital signal processor.

A/D Converter

Figure 8–10 shows the components of an A/D converter. The analog input signal is first low-pass filtered with a cutoff frequency appropriate for a hearing instrument (e.g., 10 kHz). Then, the analog signal is sampled at a rate at least twice the cutoff frequency of the low-pass filter to avoid aliasing. In this last step, quantization of the samples is dependent on the number of bits available in the A/D converter.

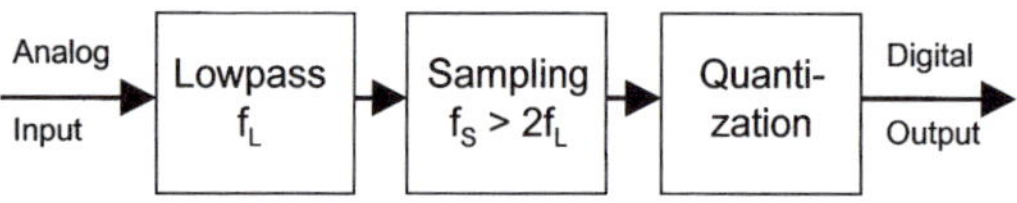

Figure 8–10. Components of an A/D-converter.

Because each additional bit used in an A/D converter increases the space and the power consumption of a hearing instrument, the maximum number of bits is usually restricted to 14. The dynamic range of hearing instruments is 84 dB (14 × 6 dB). The dynamic range in input signals into hearing instruments is greater than 84 dB. Additional precautions to avoid distortion from this difference in dynamic range will be discussed later.

Sigma-Delta Converter

One A/D converter commonly used in hearing instruments is a Sigma-Delta converter. In this converter, the analog input signal is not directly converted to a digital signal with 14 or 16 bits and a sampling rate of 20 kHz. Instead, the difference in voltage from one sampled point to the next is quantized, as opposed to quantizing the absolute value of the sampled point. In addition, the number of bits is reduced to one, and the sampling rate is increased to a frequency many times greater than the Nyquist frequency used in conventional A/D conversion. For example, a frequency of 1000 kHz (1 MHz) is commonly used for audio applications. By increasing the sampling rate and digitizing only the incremental differences between samples, this system can reduce the inherent noise and increase the dynamic range of a system, even when using only 1 bit for conversion. The increase in the sampling rate is also called oversampling.

Processing Algorithms

After A/D conversion of the input signals, the digital signal processor can now use the digitized signals to process the algorithm with a predefined calculation procedure or algorithm (see Figure 8–11).

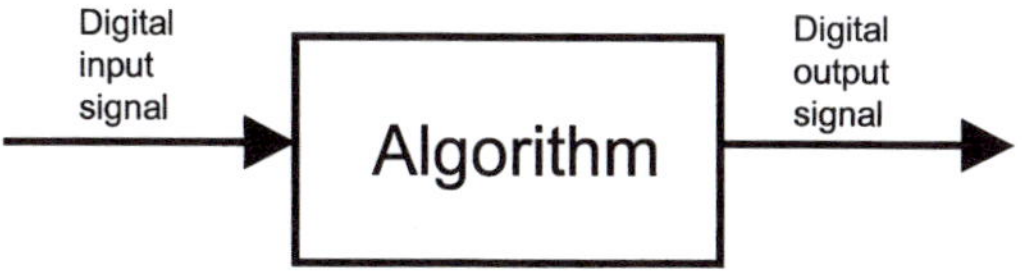

Figure 8–11. Digital signal processor.

A simple example of a signal processing algorithm is multiplication of a digital number, resulting in amplification or attenuation of the input signal. For example, multiplication with a factor of 4 results in a gain of 12 dB.

Another example is a digital filter shown in Figure 8–12. In the digital domain, a filter can be constructed by delaying the input signal by a certain time and adding it back to the original signal. By introducing different time delays and multiplying the input signal and the delayed signals by specific values, filters with a variety of characteristics can be created. A high-pass filter can be constructed by subtracting the delayed signal from the input signal, for example. For steady or slowly changing signals, this results in an output that is zero or very small. For fast-changing signals, the difference between the samples is larger, and therefore the output is also larger. This yields a high-pass characteristic.

When processing digital signals, an adequate number of bits should be used in the calculations. In other words, it is important to perform the signal processing calculations with a high word length. This is particularly true for multiplication or division. Within these algorithms, very small binary numbers can be combined with very large binary numbers. To keep a high precision in these calculations, the number of bits (or the word length) within a digital signal processor is often increased relative to the number of bits used in the A/D converter.

Digital-to-Analog Conversion

After creating the desired output by processing the input signal, the digital signal must be converted back to an analog signal. This procedure is called Digital-to-Analog (D/A) conversion. Let us examine two different methods of D/A conversion.

In the first method, the analog signal is derived by converting the digital value into an analog voltage. This voltage is kept constant until the next digital value is presented, resulting in a stepped signal as seen in Figure 8–7. The stepped function is low-pass filtered with a maximum bandwidth of one half of the sampling frequency. Low-pass filtering results in smoothing the steps of the signal, and the analog signal is reconstructed.

The second type of D/A converter is based on similar principles as the Sigma-Delta A/D converter. This method uses short pulses that are output at a fast rate; the digital number of the signal determines the density of the pulses. This is shown schematically in Figure 8-13. When this pulsed signal is low-pass filtered, an analog signal is output. When this method is used in hearing instruments, the

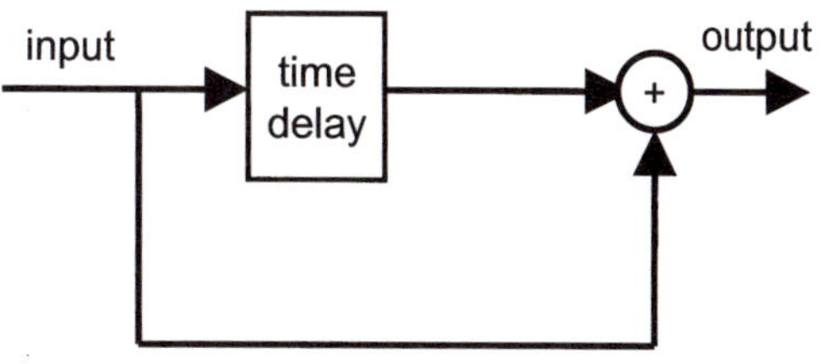

Figure 8–12. Digital filter.

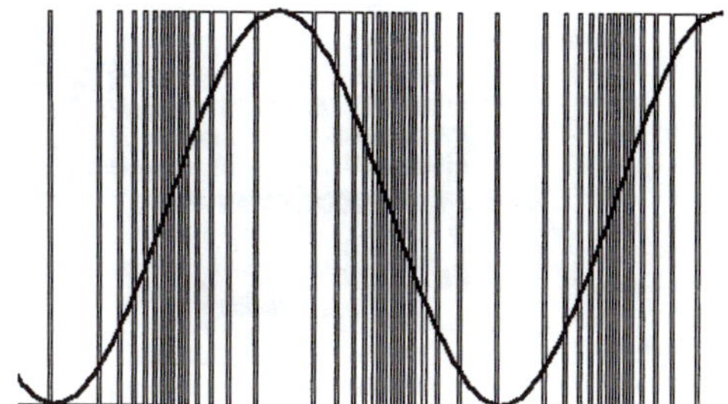

Figure 8–13. Schematic representation of pulse-density modulation. (From "Grundlagen digitaler Signalverarbeitung," by V. Hohnmann, 1998, *Zeitschrift für Audiologie, 37,* p. 124. Copyright 1998 by Median-Verlag Reprinted with permission.)

receiver can act as a low-pass filter. Therefore, an additional low-pass filter may not need to be implemented in the circuit design.

Chip Technology

Today's digitally programmable analog hearing instruments generally contain one integrated circuit chip that contains its electronic parts. These electronic parts are simply small geometric patterns on the chip.

Integrated chips can be characterized by their "structure size," which refers to the spacing between the features. The structure size determines the necessary area on the chip to implement the electronic parts. The smaller the structure size (i.e., the closer the features can be placed), the more electronic parts that can be integrated on the chip; the chip can be smaller but still have the same number of electronic parts. Circuit chips allow digital hearing instruments to be much smaller than analog instruments.

The chips used in hearing instruments must be as small as possible to produce cosmetically desirable instruments. The structure size of the chips has decreased from 3 μm to 0.5 μm within the last 10 years. Figure 8–14 shows progress in miniaturization of the integrated circuit chip technology in hearing instruments.

The difference between analog and digital chip technology can be viewed in terms of the complexity of the signal processing algorithms, and therefore in terms of the possible user benefit. This comparison is shown schematically in Figure 8–15. As depicted by the dashed curve, with analog technology, electronic circuits can be manufactured with little effort and low cost. Unfortunately, these electronic circuits permit only rudimentary

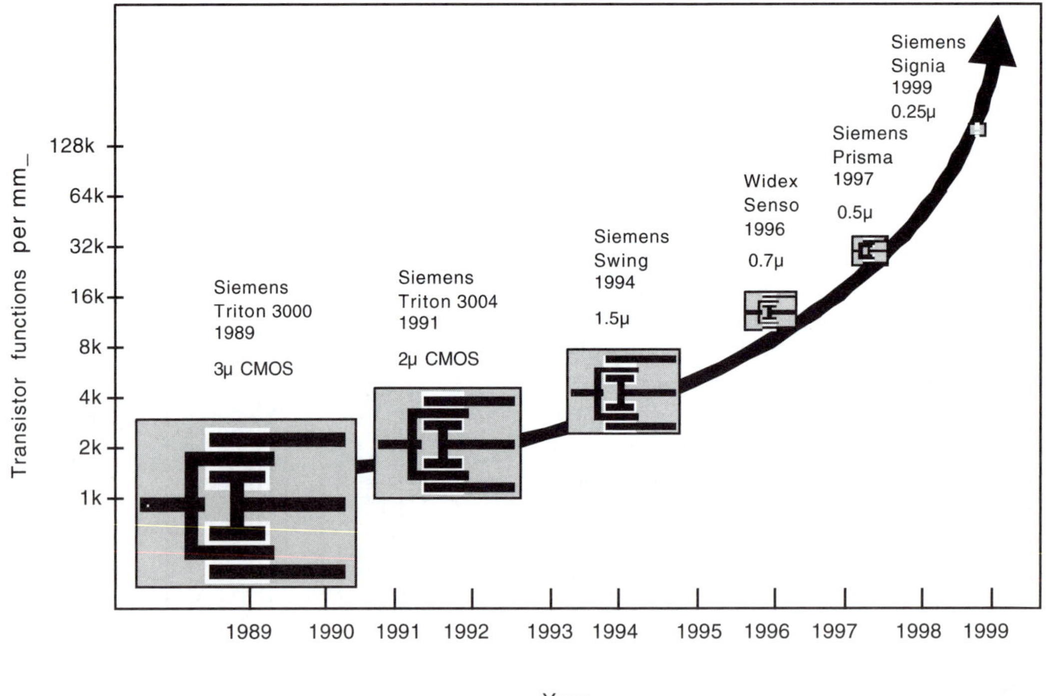

Figure 8–14. Miniaturization progress in the chip technology. (From "Signalverarbeitungs Algorithmen für digitale Hörgeräte," by I. Holube, 1998, *Zeitschrift für Audiologie, 37*, p. 176. Copyright 1998 by Median-Verlag. Adapted with permission.)

signal processing features with limited user benefit. As we strive to increase benefit, the complexity of the electronic circuit and the costs increase. With digitally programmable analog technology, illustrated by the dotted curve, the initial effort required to develop new circuits is higher than with analog technology. With this technology, however, meeting the increasingly complex requirements of the signal processing algorithms occurs before the user benefit plateaus. With digital technology, shown by the solid line, the minimum effort and cost for development of simple signal processing algorithms are the highest. The payoff, however, is demonstrated by the small increases in complexity of the circuits that permit large increases in the quality of the processing and potential user benefit. Therefore, high-value modern hearing instruments can be developed most efficiently with digital technology.

Advantages of Digital Signal Processing

Digital signal processing has several advantages over analog signal processing including miniaturization, low power consumption, low internal noise, reproducibility, stability, programmability, and signal processing complexity.

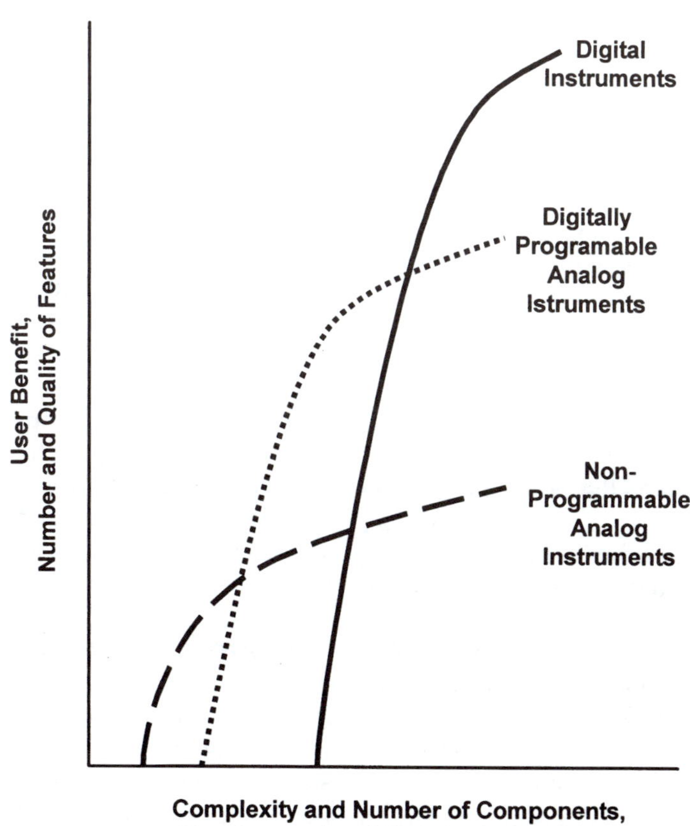

Figure 8–15. Cost vs. user benefit for analog and digital hearing instruments. (From "Signalverarbeitungs Algorithmen für digitale Hörgeräte," by I. Holube, 1998, *Zeitschrift für Audiologie, 37*, p. 177. Copyright 1998 by Median-Verlag. Adapted with permission.)

- Miniaturization: Integrated circuit chip technology allows for small-sized digital signal processors. Complex signal processing algorithms can be implemented on a very small chip. This is especially important for the design of cosmetically appealing hearing instruments. If the current signal processing contained in a digital CIC could be implemented using analog technology, the hearing instrument would be the size of a body-worn instrument.
- Low power consumption: Along with miniaturization comes the advantage of reduced power consumption. For example, a dynamic compression algorithm using digital technology requires only 5 μA, compared to 100 μA for analog instruments. Reduced power consumption permits the use of smaller batteries, which is again advantageous in the design of cosmetically desirable instruments.
- Low internal noise: The number of bits in the system can control the internal noise of digital signal processors. Internal noise is dependent on word length, not on the algorithms, so with analog technology, internal noise increases with increasing complexity of the signal processing.
- Reproducibility: In a digital system, signal manipulation is performed with numbers. Thus, the algorithms always perform the same precise calculations, in contrast to analog technology where the output can vary depending on the exact values of the components in the instrument. Analog components can exhibit differences in performance due to discrepancies in the production process.
- Stability: Digital signal processing is stable because the technology resists external influences. Performance of analog instruments can vary in response to external influences, such as temperature.
- Programmability: With a single chip, the signal processing and its parameters can be widely altered. In analog technology, such flexibility could only be achieved by changing components.
- Complexity: Digital signal processing allows implementation of complex signal processing algorithms. One example is the analysis of the input signal and appropriate signal modification based on the result of this analysis. Other examples of processing algorithms will be discussed later.

SIGNAL PROCESSING ALGORITHMS

Frequency Processing

Hearing instruments must be able to separate incoming signals into different frequency regions to compensate for the variety in the frequency configurations seen in hearing impairment. Thus, the first function performed by the digital signal processor is a frequency analysis of the signal. The wideband input signal is separated into frequency bands, typically done with a bank of filters. The filter bank is characterized by the number of output channels, the crossover frequencies between the channels, and the steepness of the filter slopes. The more frequency channels, and the steeper the filter slopes are, the finer the control of the signal manipulation in later processing can be. The frequency response function is adjusted by the gain in the frequency channels, allowing for better individualized compensation for a hearing loss via variable crossover frequencies of the filters.

Dynamic Range Compression

A characteristic of sensorineural hearing loss is reduced dynamic range, which is the intensity range between threshold sensitivity and the loudness discomfort level (LDL). The general goal of a hearing instrument is to amplify soft sounds until they are audible and to amplify loud sounds to be perceived as loud by the individual listener, but not to exceed the listener's LDL. The target amplification is based on a fitting rationale, which may be adapted from published literature, such as DSL 4.1 or NAL-NL1, or it may be proprietary to an instrument's manufacturer.

To compensate for the reduced dynamic range, compression algorithms that automatically adjust the gain for different input levels are implemented. This adjustment may be based on the amplitude in individual frequency bands or on the broadband signal level. Multichannel compression instruments are advantageous because the reduced dynamic range in most listeners with hearing-impairment varies as a function of frequency. In the analog realm, this compression process would be equivalent to having a SPL meter in each frequency band and turning the gain trimmer according to the reading of the SPL meter in real time. For a summary of the research on multichannel compression systems see Braida, Durlach, De Gennaro, Peterson, & Bustamante (1982), Hickson (1994), and Moore (1995).

Typically, there are three main approaches to compression in hearing aids (Moore, 1990):

1. Compression limiting is implemented with high compression thresholds, high compression ratios, and short time constants. In this way, the amplification at high levels is restricted.
2. As a means to replace the volume control, automatic volume control (AVC) implements a low compression threshold, low-to-medium compression ratios, and long time constants.
3. Syllabic compression utilizes a low compression threshold, low-to-medium compression ratios, and short time constants to adjust the gain for different speech syllables.

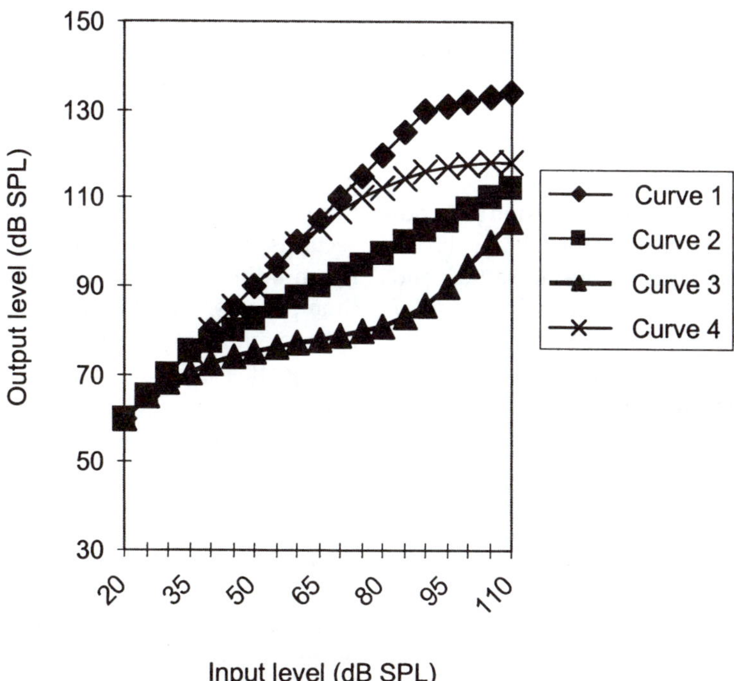

Figure 8–16. Sample input-output functions of different compression schemes.

In addition to selectable compression kneepoints and the compression ratios, the shape of the compressed input-output function can be selected. Figure 8–16 shows a schematic example of different input-output curves. In the function labeled 1, a linear input-output function with a high compression kneepoint is shown. In the function labeled 3, a linear function with a low compression kneepoint is depicted. In functions 2 and 4, we see curvilinear functions with varying kneepoints and varying function shapes. These curves are transforming the levels of the input signals to levels of the output signals dependent on the dynamic range characteristics of the individual listener.

Temporal Behavior

Next, we will examine the temporal characteristics of dynamic compression. The time course of compression is characterized by the attack and release time. In general, there are two implementations of dynamic compression, syllabic compression and automatic volume control, which differ in their temporal behavior. For a complete review, see Dillon, 1996.

Syllabic Compression

The purpose of syllabic compression is to adjust different levels within the syllabic structure of the speech signal. Thus, the attack and release times are very short. Figure 8–17 shows schematically the output signal with syllabic compression engaged. The input signal is rectangular in shape. With the short attack time, the level of the output signal is reduced quickly when a high input signal arrives. Likewise, with the short release time, the output signal quickly returns to the original level. One advantage of syllabic compression is that it can quickly reduce the gain when sudden loud sounds are presented. In addition, syllabic compression responds to level variations within the speech signal that reduce the dynamic range, which may be advantageous for individuals with a narrow dynamic range. A final advantage is quick recovery from gain reduction when a loud signal is no longer present. The disadvantage of syllabic compression is that the variations within speech are reduced, which might result in poorer speech intelligibility (Plomp, 1988).

Automatic Volume Control

Automatic Volume Control (AVC) has relatively long attack and release times compared to syllabic compression, as shown schematically in Figure 8–18. Consequently, fast changes in the amplitude of the input signal are better preserved because adjustments to the output signal occur over a longer time course.

While syllabic compression responds to the level variations within speech signals, the AVC responds only to the average speech level. This preserves the level variations within speech, which is one advantage over syllabic compression. On the other hand, the disadvantage of AVC is that the LDL may be exceeded because the reduction in gain is slower.

Panels A and B in Figure 8–19 show the effect of syllabic compression and AVC on a single sentence. The syllabic compression algorithm adjusts the signal amplitude in short time slices, increasing the gain during the soft sections and pauses in speech. The AVC algorithm adjusts the volume slowly over long time periods, and the fluctuations of the signal remain nearly unchanged from the original signal.

Dual Compression

A compromise combining both compression algorithms is dual compression (Moore, Glasberg, & Stone, 1991). In this algorithm, short and long attack and release times are used depending on the level and time course of the input signal. The dual compression exploits the advantages of both compression procedures. A gain reduction with a short time con-

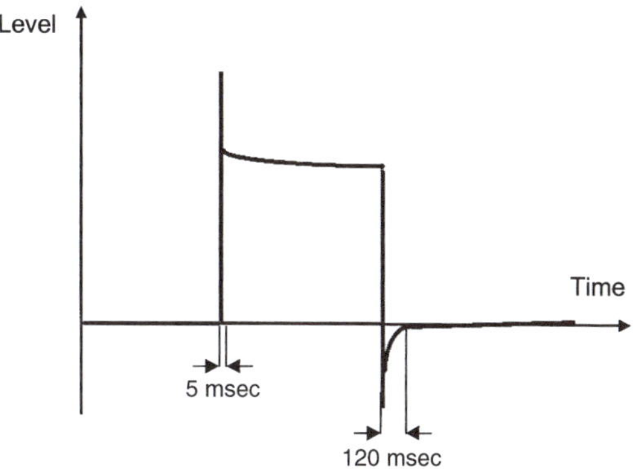

Figure 8–17. Temporal behavior of the syllabic compression algorithm.

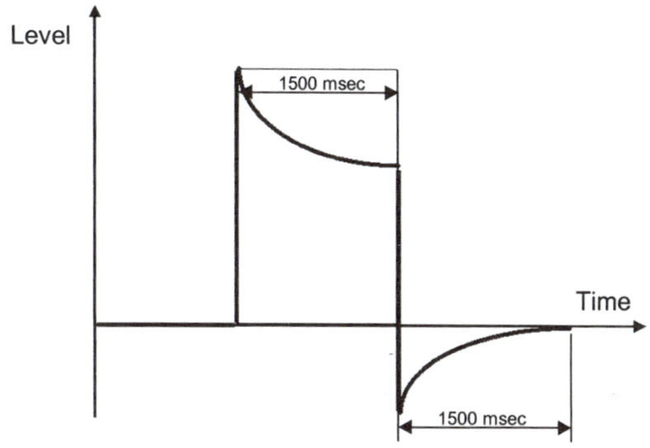

Level
1500 msec
Time
1500 msec

Figure 8–18. Temporal behavior of the AVC algorithm.

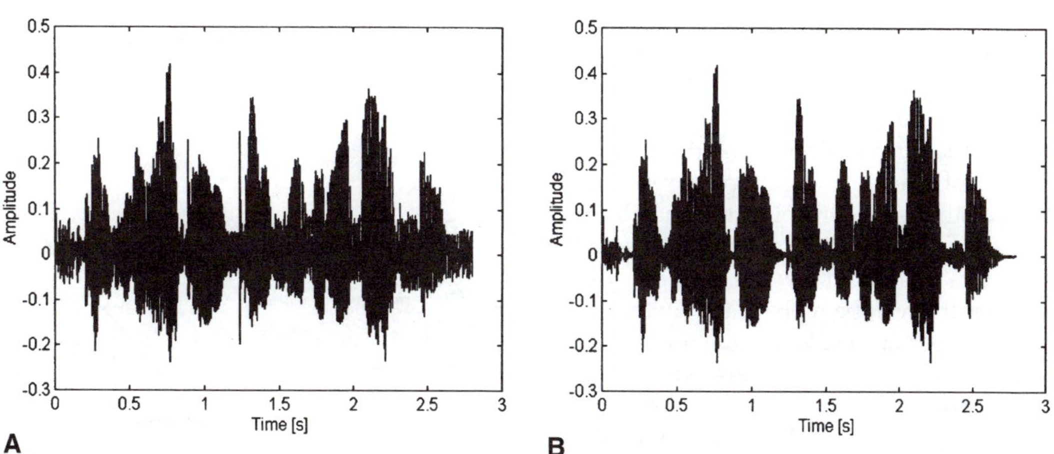

Figure 8–19. A. Effect of syllabic compression on a sentence. **B.** Effect of AVC on a sentence.

stant reacts quickly to sudden, loud sounds. The gain quickly turns to the original level after the loud sound is over. Thus, a desired soft signal occurring after a loud sound is not affected. In contrast, if a criterion sound level is present for a longer time, the long time constants are activated. The gain of the hearing instrument is adjusted only to slow changes of the average input level, and the natural loudness variations in speech levels are preserved.

Reduction of Distortions

As discussed earlier, increasing the number of bits in the A/D converter increases the dynamic range, the size, and the power consumption. Thus, the number of bits is typically reduced to 14. With 14 bits, the dynamic range of the A/D converter is smaller than the dynamic range of the acoustic input signals and the dynamic range of the microphone. To avoid distortions at high input levels, the dynamic range of the input signals is restricted with a high-level compressor. This compressor system has a high compression kneepoint (e.g., 90 dB) and a high compression ratio (e.g., 10:1). With this high-level compression, input signals up to 110 dB SPL can be processed with minimal distortion.

In conventional analog hearing instruments, the output level of the device is normally restricted by peak clipping, resulting in high distortions of the output signal. In digital hearing instruments, the upper level of the device is restricted by the highest digital number that can be represented by the available number of bits. When the amplification of the hearing instruments exceeds this number, distortions will be audible. The sound quality of these digital distortions is worse than the distortions resulting from peak clipping in analog hearing instruments. Therefore, it is important that an output compression algorithm is also incorporated into digital hearing instruments.

The high-level compressor at both the input and the output compressor have short time constants. The gain must be reduced quickly when loud sounds occur, and the gain must be increased quickly after loud sounds diminish to maintain speech intelligibility.

User Benefit

A primary goal of dynamic compression algorithms is normalization of loudness perception, which can be measured with loudness scaling procedures (e.g., Allen & Jeng, 1990; Cox, Alexander, Taylor, & Gray, 1997; Pascoe, 1978). The result of a theoretical loudness scaling procedure is shown in Figure 8–20. For this procedure, listeners are asked to rate the loudness of narrow-band noise on a categorical scale (inaudible, very soft, soft, medium loud, very loud, too loud). This categorical scale was converted into a numerical scale from 0 to 50 categorical units (CU). Zero CU corresponded to inaudible and 50 CU corresponded to too loud. A linear function was fit to the loudness ratings for different input levels and defined by two parameters: the slope and the zero crossing. The zero crossing of this function was an estimation of threshold. The slope and threshold can be used to compare different loudness scaling between listeners with normal hearing and

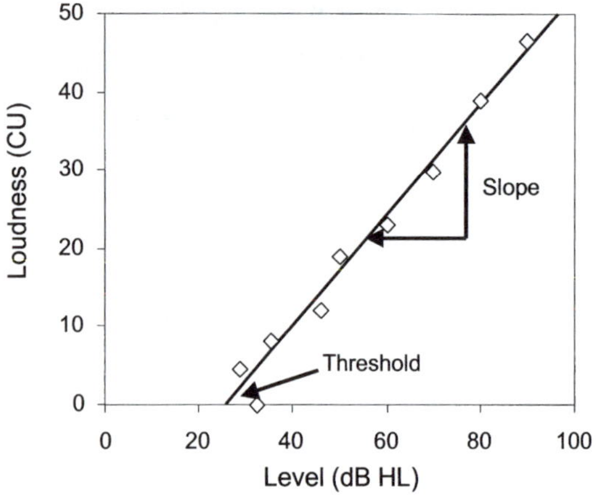

Figure 8–20. Loudness scaling function.

listeners with hearing-impairment and between aided and unaided conditions.

In Figure 8–21, the average slope of the loudness scaling function of 21 listeners with high-frequency hearing loss is shown at 500, 1000, 2000, and 4000 Hz in unaided and aided condition. For the unaided condition, the slope increases with increasing frequency. This result is expected because recruitment in the presence of high-frequency hearing loss increases with frequency. When fit with a digital hearing instrument with dynamic compression (in this example, Siemens PRISMA), the slope differs from the unaided condition dramatically. The aided slope is essentially normalized for all frequencies. The slope of the loudness scaling function of normal-hearing listeners is shown as norm and is independent of the frequency.

In Figure 8–22, the threshold estimate is shown as a function of signal frequency. As expected, the threshold increases as a function of frequency for listeners with high-frequency hearing loss. In the aided condition, the threshold estimate was within the normal range. The threshold for normal hearing listeners is indicated on the graph.

A second goal of dynamic compression is to improve speech understanding, especially when background noise is present. Laboratory experiments have shown that the best temporal characteristics of the dynamic compression algorithm cannot be predicted for all listeners with hearing impairment and all sound environments. Listeners tend to prefer different types of compression, syllabic or dual compression, in different environments. When we studied the different temporal characteristics for the Siemens Prisma for different settings in a paired comparison test, no overall winner emerged for all listeners and all conditions. Although no clear winner was found for understanding speech in different types of noise, an overall loser was determined to be syllabic compression in all four channels. To determine the effects of hearing loss and specific compression conditions, additional studies are needed.

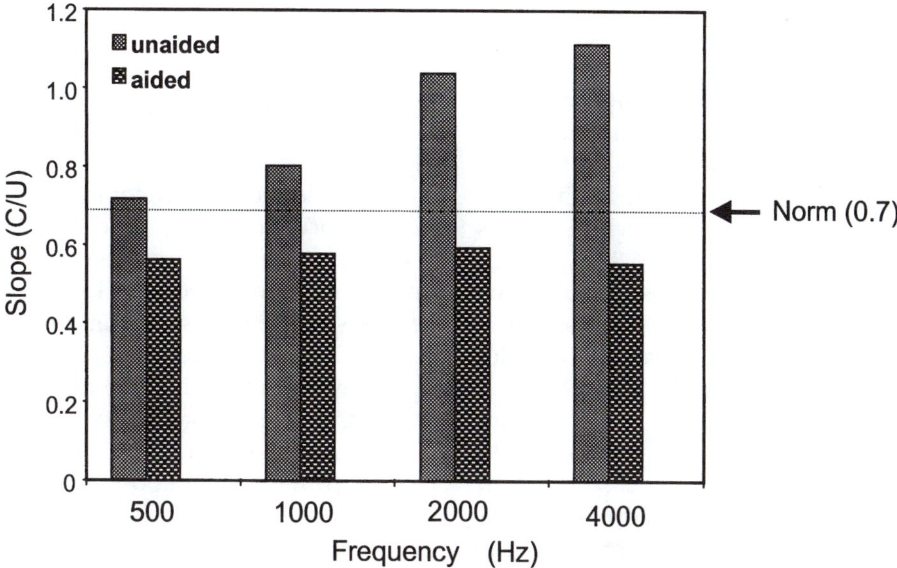

Figure 8–21. Slope of loudness scaling as a function of signal frequency in unaided and aided conditions.

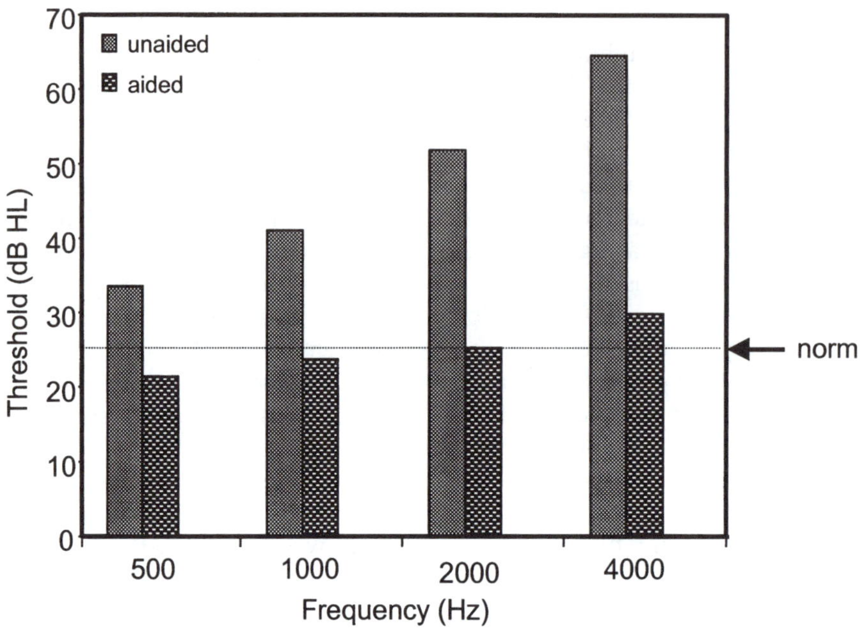

Figure 8–22. Threshold of loudness scaling as a function of signal frequency in unaided and aided conditions.

Noise Reduction

Individuals with hearing impairment often report that speech is difficult to understand in listening situations when background noise is present. In the past several years, a variety of programmable circuits have been developed and evaluated that attempt to improve performance in this difficult listening environment (e.g., Cudahy & Levitt, 1994; Fabry, 1991; Graupe, Grosspietsch, & Basseas, 1987; Stein & Dempesy-Hart, 1984; van Tasell, Larson, & Fabry, 1988). These circuits have met with varying degrees of success, both in reports of patients' benefit and satisfaction and in terms of commercial success.

In the first part of this section, we will limit our discussion to digital processing strategies that can be used to tackle the problem of unwanted background noise with a single microphone. Recently, multimicrophone hearing aids have demonstrated that they are an effective solution for improving the signal-to-noise ratio and thus, improving speech intelligibility in noisy listening environments. A discussion of the design and benefits of multimicrophone directional hearing instruments is reported in the second part of this section.

Single-Microphone Noise Reduction

The introduction of digital hearing instruments has led to the development of unique signal processing that provides advantages over analog instruments. Several manufacturers have introduced signal processing algorithms that detect speech and noise independently and process the two types of signals differently. While the underlying algorithms of these systems may vary, the expected result is the same: improved user listening comfort and possibly improved speech intelligibility in background noise. Additional algorithms identify internal sources of noise, such as microphone noise, and minimize its effects when the user is in a quiet environment. The first algorithm described below is a method of identifying speech and noise based on their modulation spectrum and applying digital control logic to reduce the level of the noise. Secondly, we will discuss an algorithm that has been developed for reducing the potential upward spread of masking effects in multichannel processors. Finally, we will review an algorithm that has been found successful in reducing the effects of internal microphone noise.

Modulation-Based Noise Reduction Algorithms

Two important goals in fitting hearing instruments are improving speech intelligibility in noise for individuals with hearing impairment by improving the signal-to-noise ratio and improving the quality of the overall signal to make listening more comfortable. One processing strategy that attempts to improve the quality of speech employs the modulation spectrum (Powers, Holube, & Wesselkamp, 1999). In this scheme, the speech and noise are identified according to rules based on the fluctuations of their respective amplitude envelopes. Once identified, the negative impact of the noise can be reduced through frequency-specific gain reduction.

The audible frequency range we typically consider is from 20 Hz to 20 kHz. Auditory signals are some composite of frequencies within that range. Figure 8–23 shows a 1 second segment of a sinusoidal signal. For this signal, the maxima are the same amplitude throughout the sinusoid. When the maxima of the signal change over time, the signal is referred to as amplitude modulated, and this is illustrated by the waveform labeled A in Figure 8–24.

The wave form that is defined by the maxima of the sinusoid is called the envelope of the signal, depicted by the wave form labeled B in Figure 8-24. The rate of the change in the signal envelope is the modulation frequency. In this example, the modulation frequency is 5 Hz. Note the modulation frequency is always much lower in value than the original signal frequency.

A sample of speech is shown in Figure 8–25. Typically, the spectrum of speech shows frequency components between 100 Hz and 8 kHz. In addition to the time wave form, this speech signal can be described by its envelope or modulation of the signal amplitude.

The phonemes, syllables, words, sentences, and pauses of speech determine the "envelope" of speech. A human speaker can normally articulate about 12 phonemes, 5 syllables, or 2.5 words per second. A typical sentence is several seconds in duration. The envelope of speech shows a characteristic temporal behavior independent of the speaker or the spoken language. The envelope is an

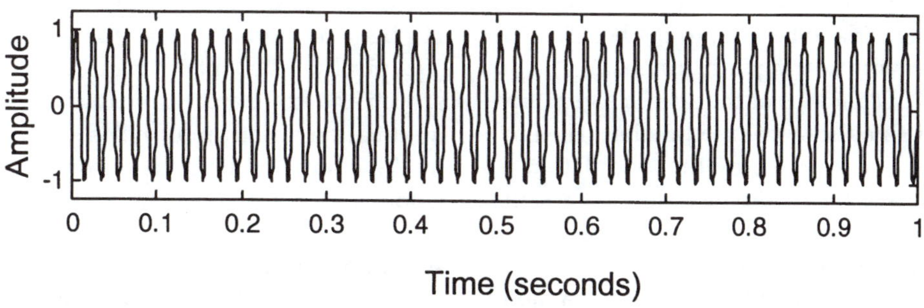

Figure 8–23. Sinusoidal signal.

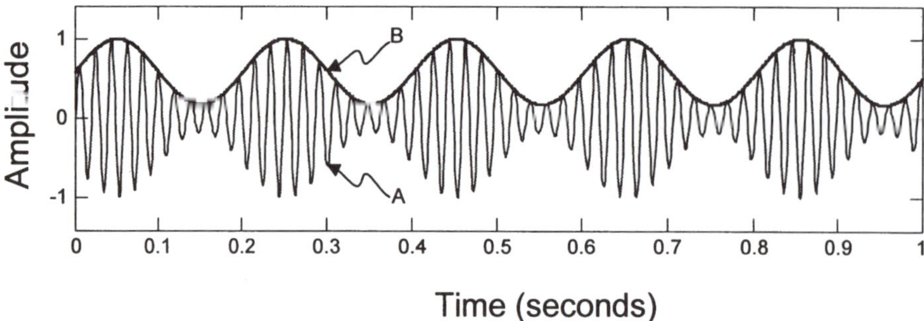

Figure 8–24. Sinusoid modulated at 5 Hz.

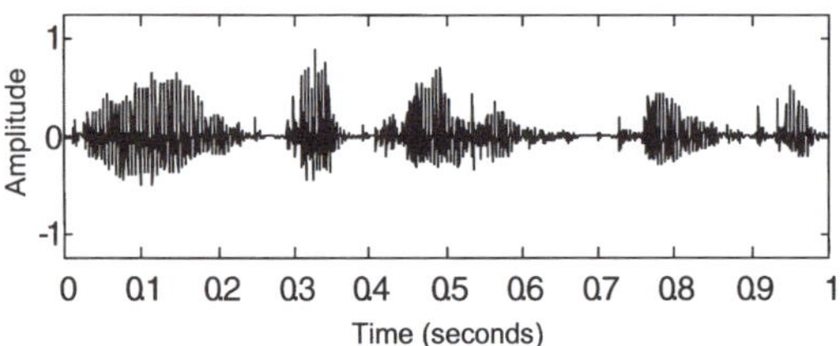

Figure 8–25. Speech signal of a female speaker.

intrinsic and well-defined feature of the speech signal. The importance of the speech envelope has received increasing attention in the speech perception and speech recognition literature (e.g., Drullman, Festen, & Plomp, 1994; Houtgast & Steeneken, 1985). It is only with the advent of the digital signal processing in hearing instruments that this feature has been able to be used to the benefit of the listener with hearing impairment.

The fluctuations of the speech signal envelope define the signal modulation. The envelope is characterized by the modulation frequency and the modulation depth of a signal. The modulation frequency is defined by the rate of change of the fluctuations. Twelve phonemes per second correspond to a modulation frequency of 12 Hz. Syllables yield a modulation frequency of 5 Hz, words yield a modulation frequency of 2.5 Hz, and sentences a modulation frequency of 0.3 Hz. The modulation depth is the difference between the maxima and the minima of the envelope. The modulation depth of speech is maximum during speech pauses when the signal value is zero.

The modulation spectrum is a plot, which graphically illustrates the relative modulation as a function of the modulation frequency of a signal. Figure 8–26 shows the modulation spectrum calculated from speech of a female speaker (see Ostendorf, Hohnmann, & Kollmeier, 1997). In this example, we see the greatest modulation occurring between 3 and 4 Hz.

Plomp (1983) calculated the average modulation spectrum over different listeners. The result was a smoothed curve with a maximum around 3 to 4 Hz. Modulation frequencies of speech are present up to about 15 Hz. His figure is reproduced here as Figure 8–27.

Typically, the modulation spectra for speech and noise are distinctly different. The modulation spectrum of noise shows faster modulations, and thus the maximum modulation is seen at higher modulation frequencies. Figure 8–28 and 8-29 show the time structure of a jet engine noise and its modulation spectrum (Ostendorf et al., 1997). The envelope of the signal in Figure 8-28 does not show the slow fluctuations of the envelope of

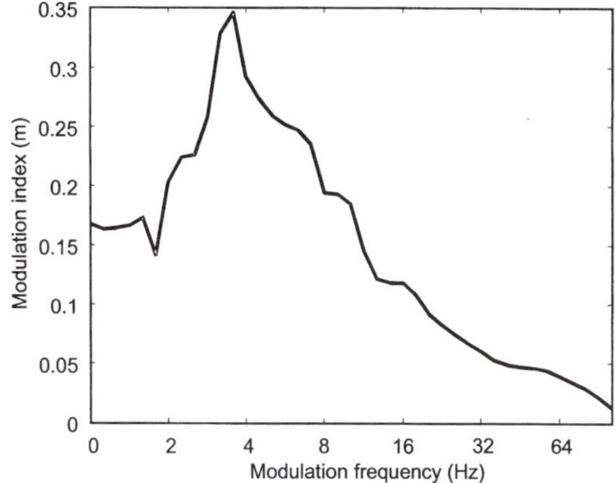

Figure 8–26. Modulation spectrum of a single sentence. (From "Signalverarbeitungsalgorithmen für digitale Hörgeräte" by I. Holube, 1998, *Zeitschrift für Audiologie,37*, p. 177. Copyright 1998 by Median-Verlag. Adapted with permission.)

the speech-time wave form in Figure 8–25. Therefore, little energy is present at low modulation frequencies in the modulation spectrum in Figure 8–29. In this example, the maximum at modulation frequencies of around 30 to 60 Hz is the result of the faster fluctuations in the envelope.

Hearing Aid Applications. This difference in the modulation spectrum between speech and noise can be used to detect speech and to reduce the noise in the signals. A reduction in noise can result in a more comfortable sound, a reduced listening effort, and increased speech intelligibility. In the application to hearing instruments, the envelope of the signals is analyzed in different frequency channels. If modulation frequencies characteristic of speech are detected (i.e., modulation frequencies of 1 to 12 Hz), the gain in the channel is kept constant. If modulation frequencies characteristic of speech

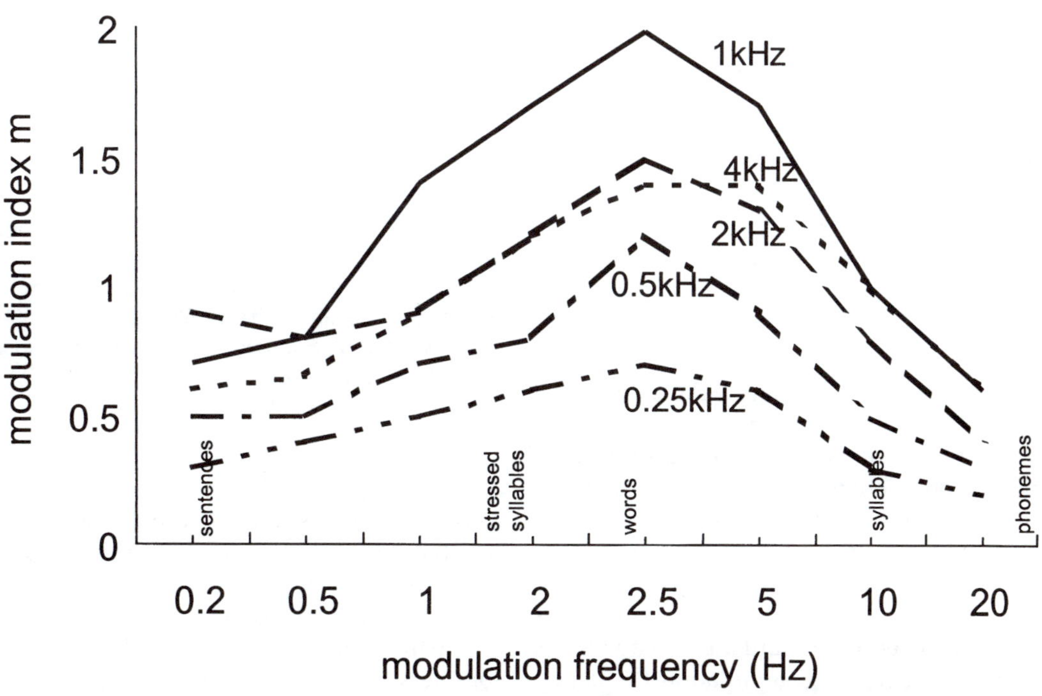

Figure 8–27. Modulation spectrum of running speech (From "Perception of Speech as a Modulated Signal" by R. Plomp, 1983: Proceedings of the 10th International Congress of Phonetic Sciences. Copyright© by R. Plomp. Adapted with permission.)

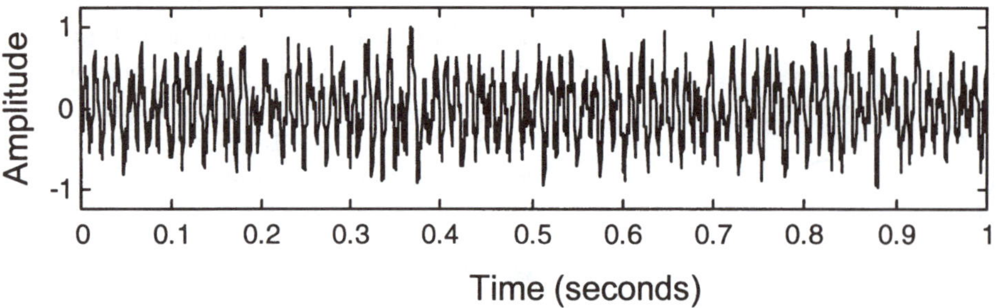

Figure 8–28. Time waveform of jet engine noise.

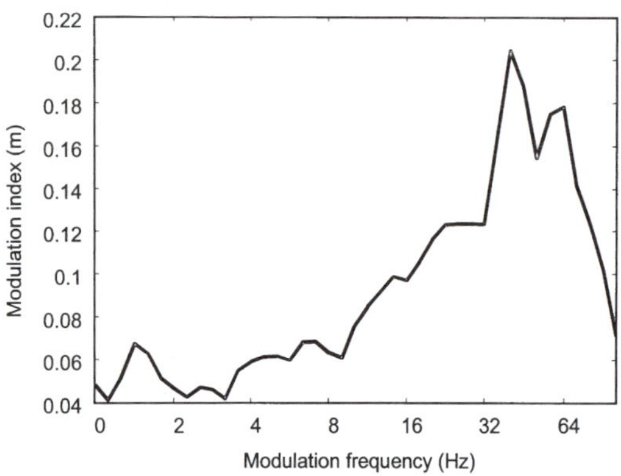

Figure 8–29. Modulation spectrum of jet engine noise. (From "Signalverarbeitungs Algorithmen für digitale Hörgeräte," by I. Holube, 1998, *Zeitschrift für Audiologie, 37*, p. 177. Copyright 1998 by Median-Verlag. Adapted with permission.)

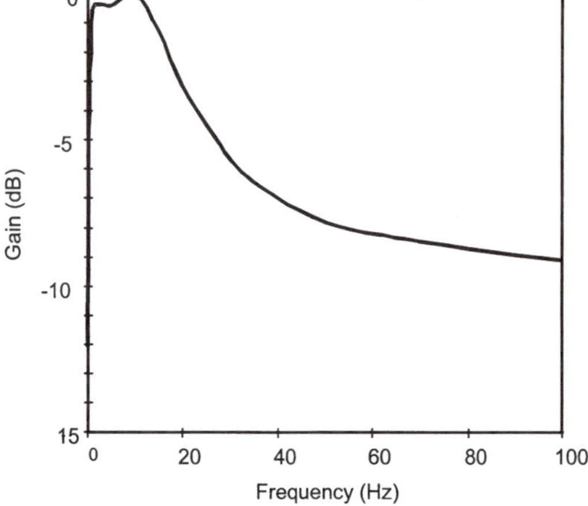

Figure 8–30. Gain reduction as a function of the modulation frequency in modulation-based noise reduction algorithm. (From "The Use of Digital Features to Combat Background Noise," by T. Powers, I. Holuta, and W. Wesselkamp, 1999. *Hearing Review Supplement, High Performance Hearing Solutions, 3. Hearing in Noise*, 36–39.)

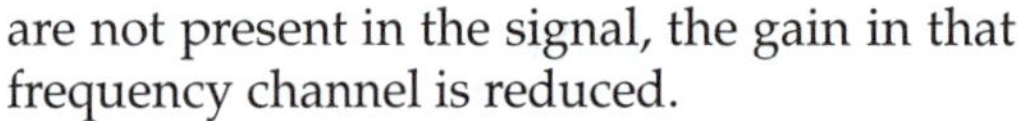

are not present in the signal, the gain in that frequency channel is reduced.

The amount of gain reduction is dependent on the modulation frequencies and the modulation depths. Figure 8–30 depicts the change in gain in a given channel as a function of the detected modulation frequency. Figure 8–30 shows that the change in gain is minimal when the modulation frequency is low; with increasing modulation frequency, however, gain is increasingly reduced.

Figure 8–31 depicts the degree of gain reduction as a function of modulation depth. This figure shows that when the modulation depth is low, the reduction in gain is greatest. As the modulation depth increases, the reduction in gain decreases.

The time constant of the modulation detector refers to the duration required to examine the signal for modulation and return the answer to the processor. Recall that the modulation frequencies we are looking for can be as

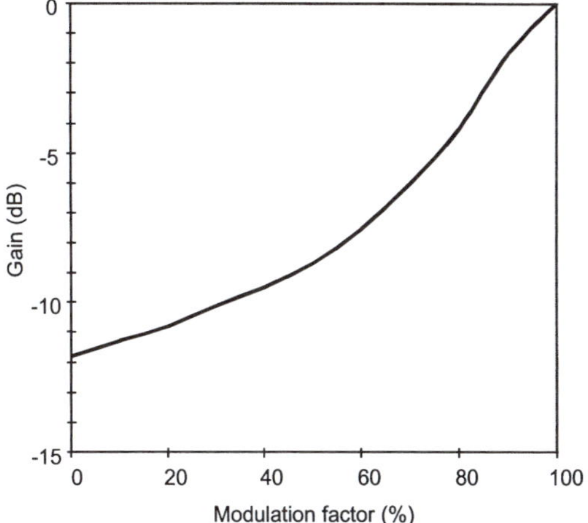

Figure 8–31. Gain reduction as a function of the modulation depth in modulation-based noise reduction algorithm. (From "The Use of Digital Features to Combat Background Noise," by T. Powers, I. Holuta, and W. Wesselkamp, 1999. *Hearing Review Supplement, High Performance Hearing Solutions, 3. Hearing in Noise*, 36–39.)

low as 2 Hz. The period of 2 Hz is 0.5 second. Thus, detection of 2 Hz requires a minimum of 0.5 second of sampling. To reliably examine the incoming signal for modulation, the signal processor requires several seconds. To avoid an audible "pumping" effect, the gain reduction should occur within approximately 2 to 3 seconds of the onset of the noise signal. If speech is detected as the primary signal, as defined by the modulation spectrum within a given channel, gain should be quickly restored (e.g., within 500 ms) to the original gain values.

There may be some listening situations when a gain reduction is not desired. Some signals processed as "noise" by the hearing aid may indeed be viewed as a "desired signal" by the hearing aid user. One example is music. The modulation spectrum of music is different than the modulation spectrum of speech, therefore the gain in the channels where the music is present will be reduced. For this type of situation, it is possible to deactivate the processing algorithm in each frequency channel. Also, noise-reduction algorithms should be turned off when electroacoustic or probe-microphone measurements are conducted unless the purpose of the testing is to assess the effects of the noise-reduction system.

The modulation spectrum provides an effective processing tool for distinguishing between speech and noise signals. In a multichannel system, incoming signals can be broken up into different frequency channels, allowing speech to be distinguished from disturbing noise in specific channels. The gain in the channels with high modulation is reduced, reducing the overall noise contained within the complex signal.

User Benefit. This modulation-based algorithm is implemented in some form in commercially available hearing instruments. In the Siemens PRISMA hearing instrument, it is known as Voice Activity Detection (VAD). This feature can be assessed in the clinic using either 2-cc coupler measurements or probe-microphone measurements at the time of the hearing instrument fitting. Not only does this provide verification that the digital signal analysis system is working properly, but it also provides an opportunity to demonstrate this capability to the instrument user. The user can see the real-time effects of the noise reduction, including the compression attack and release time, on the monitor of the probe-microphone system.

These algorithms can be demonstrated to the user by turning off all noise reduction, and then implementing the signal processing strategy one channel at a time. An example of this is shown in Figure 8–32. Panel A shows the insertion gain and target gain for an instrument using speech-shaped input and without the signal processing activated. In the subsequent panels (B-E), the effects of the noise reduction can be seen as the algorithm activated for channels 1 through 4 respectively.

How does this processing affect speech understanding? It has been established that reduction of noise, especially low-frequency noise, provides more "relaxed listening" for

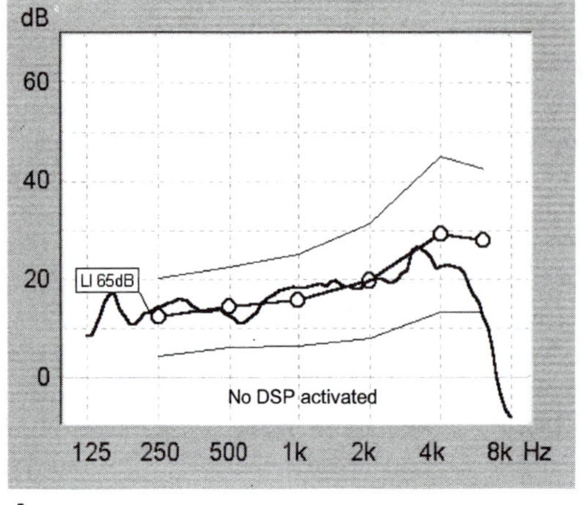

A

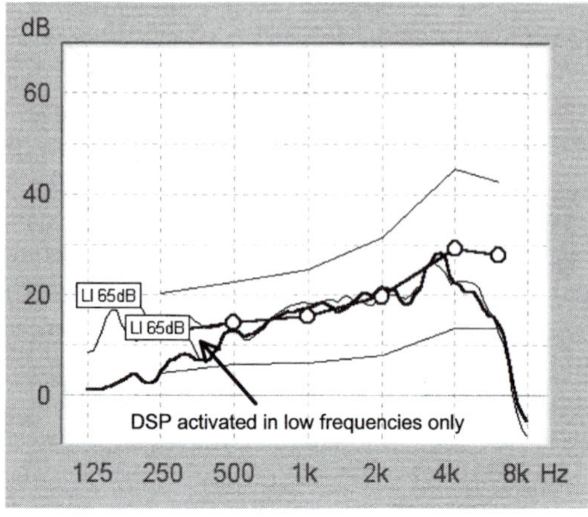

B

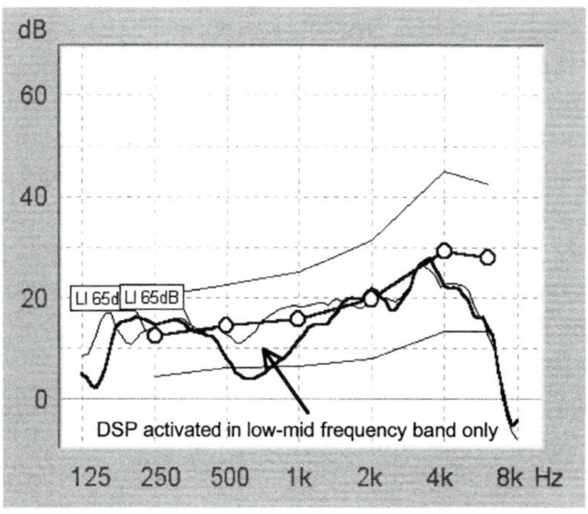

C

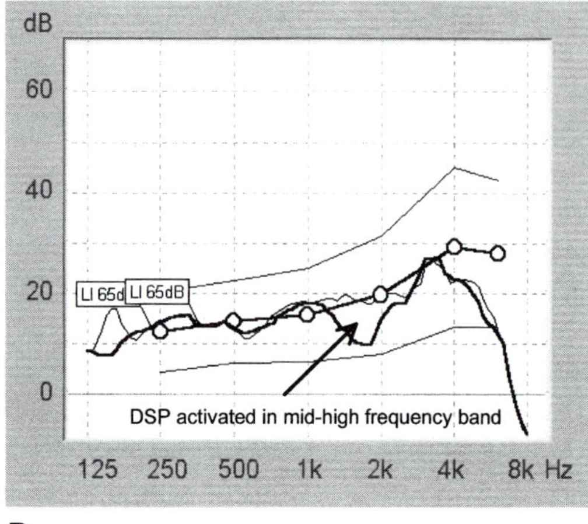

D

E

Figure 8–32. A-E. Target and insertion gain without signal processing activated (A) and with signal processing activated in channels 1–4 (B-E).

the hearing aid user. Because modulation-based processing has only recently become available in hearing instruments, little study has been conducted on the effects on speech intelligibility. Ricketts and Dhar (1999), however, have addressed this issue in a recent publication. These authors evaluated the Siemens PRISMA (with directional microphone capability), fitted binaurally on 12 subjects. Two different speech-in-noise measures, the Hearing in Noise Test (HINT; Nilsson, Soli, & Sullivan, 1994) and the Nonsense Syllable Test (NST; Resnick, Dubno, Hoffnung, & Levitt, 1975), were used. The results of the HINT are shown in Figure 8–33.

Aided performance was evaluated for three different conditions: omnidirectional microphone with VAD off, omnidirectional microphone with VAD on, and directional microphone with VAD off. The best performance, as expected, was for the directional microphone setting. (Directional microphones are discussed later in this chapter.) Observe from Figure 8–33, however, that for the omnidirectional conditions, the average HINT was improved by 2 dB when the VAD was activated. A 2 dB improvement can result in a substantial improvement in speech understanding in many listening situations. A similar finding also was observed for the average NST scores.

Reduction of Low-Frequency Masking Effects

Masking occurs when the detection of one signal is affected by the presence of a second signal. In speech, masking often occurs when other sounds that have a dominant low-frequency content are present. This masking effect can significantly influence speech recognition because the listener will not perceive the speech components below the masked threshold. The process of low-frequency sounds affecting the detection of higher frequency sounds is referred to as the "upward spread of masking."

The detection of higher frequency speech components can be improved by reducing the level of the low-frequency masking signals (Dreschler & Verschuure, 1996). Consider that in a multichannel instrument, compression acts independently for different frequency regions. Independent channel processing has

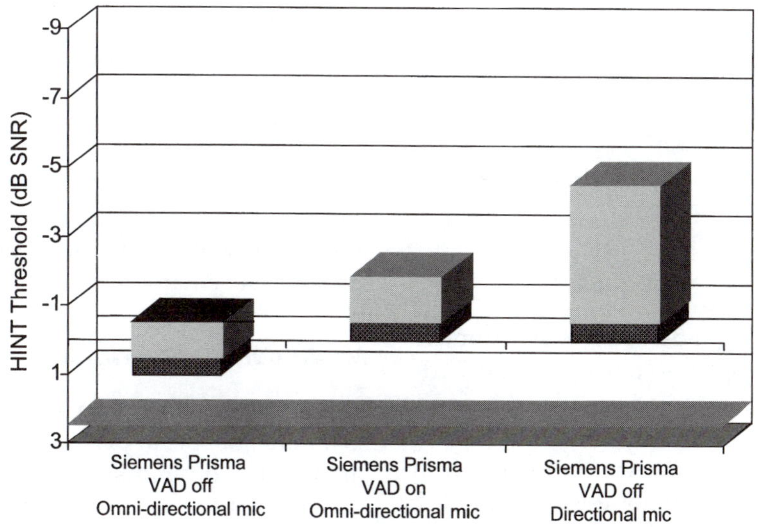

Figure 8–33. HINT results for three conditions of DSP and microphone directionality mode. (From "Comparison of Performance Across THree Directional Hearing Aids," by T. Ricketts and S. Dhar, 1999, *Journal of the American Academy of Audiology, 10*, 184. Copyright by B.C. Decker, Inc. Adapted by permission.)

the advantage that a low frequency noise will not activate compression in the higher channels. Audibility of high-frequency speech sounds is maintained more effectively because the potential low-frequency maskers are reduced.

Totally independent processing could work against speech intelligibility in some situations. When a loud signal is present in a high-frequency channel, the high-frequency channel compression circuit is activated, and the gain in that channel is reduced. If the gain in the lower frequency channels is not affected, the higher gain in the lower channel can potentially mask the speech signal in the high-frequency channel.

The potential detrimental effect of upward spread of masking can be reduced with an algorithm called channel coupling. This process involves the coupling or interaction of a high-frequency channel and its adjacent lower frequency channel. Interchannel communication influences the gain in the lower channels when compression is active in a higher frequency channel. If channel coupling is activated, the gain reduction caused by the compression circuit in a higher channel prompts a gain reduction in the lower frequency channel. Interchannel communication provides the user with better overall shaping of the frequency response. Controlling the gain in the lower frequency channels minimizes the negative effects of upward spread of masking, making channel coupling a desired feature of digital hearing instruments.

Microphone Noise Reduction

Modern hearing aids use low-noise microphones. Microphone noise, typically described as an unwanted constant hissing in the hearing aid, still troubles many hearing-instrument users, however. In today's hearing aids, microphone noise is only about 20 dB, but in quiet environments, this can be noticable for people with hearing thresholds at or near normal for some frequency regions. This complaint is observed most frequently when minimal venting is used, as this low-level noise cannot escape from the ear canal.

If we consider the input signals to the hearing aid amplifier, we note that both the input signal to the microphone and microphone noise are present. In most listening environments, the microphone noise will not be audible to the hearing aid user. Microphone noise is masked when an input signal is present because gain is applied to that signal. Unfortunately, the noise may be audible in some situations.

Microphone noise reduction is achieved using a squelch function, or a reduction of gain, using nonlinear processing of signals that have intensities below a certain level. If the intensity of the input signal to the microphone is below a set value, the microphone noise reduction, or squelch, is engaged. We have found that the best level to use for this digital noise reduction is about 30 dB.

The signal processor continuously monitors intensity of the input signal in each channel of the hearing aid. If the intensity of a signal is below the squelch threshold, the gain of that channel is reduced. The signal processing reduces the remaining low-level microphone noise below the patient's threshold. If the hearing instrument user moves from the quiet environment to one with higher intensity background noise or useful signals, the microphone noise reduction function releases within a short time constant, and the original gain in the channel is returned. Because of the short release time, the user does not miss any components of the useful signal, yet can enjoy a quiet environment.

Multimicrophone Noise Reduction

The algorithms for noise reduction described so far are not able to distinguish between desired and undesired speech signals because most often, the speech one wants to hear and the speech one does not want to hear have the same spectrum and the same time structure. Therefore, these algorithms have no benefit in so called cocktail party situations.

To provide benefit in these difficult situations, other options are necessary.

Multimicrophone noise reduction systems are an effective method for improving the intelligibility of speech in noisy situations. They act essentially as spatial noise reduction systems by enhancing the hearing instrument's sensitivity to sound from desired directions over sound from other directions. The sound from "other directions" is normally considered noise and is deemed as not desirable. The general goal of the multimicrophone systems is to improve the signal-to-noise ratio (SNR).

While audibility of the primary signal is essential, SNR (expressed in dB), determines overall intelligibility. Directional microphones, with a primary design aimed at enhancing the SNR, will nearly always yield improvements in intelligibility (Mueller & Wesselkamp, 1999; Wolf, Hohn, Martin, & Powers, 1999).

Commercially Available Products

Omnidirectional microphones utilize a single microphone and single sound inlet and are equally sensitive to sound from all directions. Directional microphones also utilize a single microphone with two sound inlets and an acoustic damper to shift the phase or to introduce an internal time delay respectively. In commercially available products with two omnidirectional microphones, the outputs of the two separate microphones are coupled with electronic time delay and subtraction components.

Specific directional patterns are determined by the exact values of the time delay corresponding to the microphone distance and the internal time delay. The directionality of a microphone, as shown on a polar plot, can be modified by changing the time delays externally and internally between the two microphones. Figure 8–34 shows the polar plots of different ratios between external and internal time delays, Ti/Te, of the two microphones. In addition, the Directivity Index (DI) is shown. The DI characterizes the strength of the microphone directivity, relating the amplification for the frontal direction and the amplification to all other directions. It suggests the improvement in signal-to-noise ratio that can be expected from a microphone system in a diffuse sound field. As can be seen in Figure 8–34, the hyper-cardioid gives the best directionality with a DI of 6 dB.

To achieve the 6 dB advantage in directivity with a two-microphone system, precise matching of the microphones in amplitude and phase is imperative. When a stronger directivity than 6 dB is desired, more than two microphones are necessary.

While it is not clear if the recent commercially available two-microphone systems are better than the conventional directional microphones, there is one important advantage of the two-microphone systems. Because it is controlled electronically, the directional effect can be a programmable parameter that can be selected or deleted, depending on the user's needs, for different listening situations.

Figure 8–35 shows an example of a directionality pattern for a two-microphone system mounted to the right ear of the KEMAR. Compared to Figure 8–34, which shows the behavior in the free field, the KEMAR exhibits a considerable influence on the polar plots. With the omnidirectional microphone, the signals from all directions are amplified by the same value. Only the head shadow effect of the mannekin has an influence on the directionality pattern. When the two omnidirectional microphones are combined, the largest amplification is achieved for signals from the front, whereas signals from the other directions are attenuated relative to the frontal direction.

A primary advantage of digital signal processing using the two-microphone systems is that the matching of the two microphones can be accomplished in the digital domain. In addition, with digital signal processing, the directivity pattern can be adjusted to the wishes of the hearing instrument user by changing the phase between the two microphones (e.g., if it is important for the user to listen in a variety of specific listening situations).

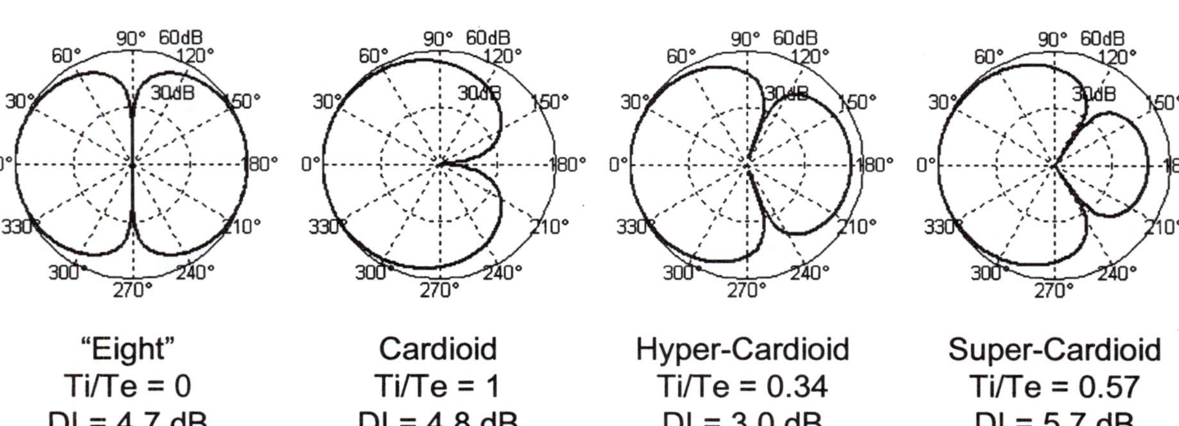

Figure 8–34. Polar plots and DIs for different ratios between internal and external delays in a two-microphone system.

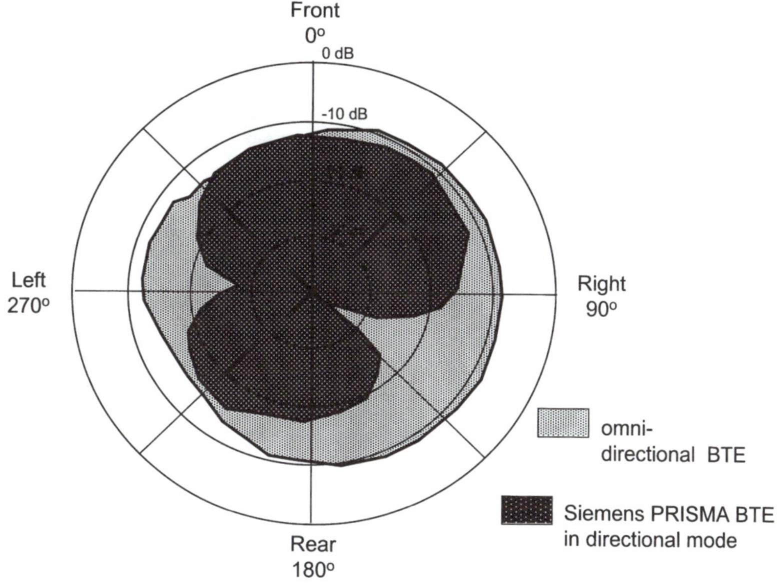

Figure 8–35. Directionality patterns of an omnidirectional microphone and a two-microphone system mounted on KEMAR. (From "Signalverarbeitungs algorithmen für digitale Hörgeräte," by I. Holube, 1998, *Zeitschrift für Audiologie, 37*, 181. Copyright by Median-Verlag. Adapted with permission.)

The benefit of hearing instruments with a directional microphone characteristic has been shown in several studies. To briefly illustrate the benefits of directional microphone technology, we will review one study of unaided and aided speech intelligibility for a hearing instrument with a two microphone directional system (Siemens PRISMA) conducted by Arlinger, Billermark, and Slattengren (1999). Speech intelligibility in noise was measured by determining the speech recognition threshold for speech in noise in a sound field. The speech test material was the low-redundancy, five-word sentences test from Hagerman (1982), recorded on CD. The speech-to-noise ratio corresponding to 40% of correctly recognized test words was determined by means of an adaptive method (Hagerman & Kinnerfors, 1995). The speech was presented with a level of 70 dB SPL. The noise was speech-weighted random noise. In Figure 8–36, speech intelligibility is shown for unaided condition and for aided conditions with a hearing instrument in omnidirectional or in directional mode. In the left panel, speech and noise were presented from the front, 0° azimuth. In the right panel, the speech signal was presented at 0°, and noise was presented at 90° and 270°. This spatial configuration is comparable to everyday listening conditions with diffuse noise.

In the left panel, we see aided performance superior to unaided performance. When both the signal and noise are from the same direction, however, little difference is observed between omnidirectional and directional microphone conditions. In the right panel, a small difference is seen between unaided and aided with an omnidirectional microphone instrument. Performance with a directional microphone shows marked improvement over the other conditions in diffuse noise. Research by Ricketts and Darr (1999) has shown that this directional benefit also is present for the Siemens Prisma in everyday listening environments, such as a living room and classroom settings.

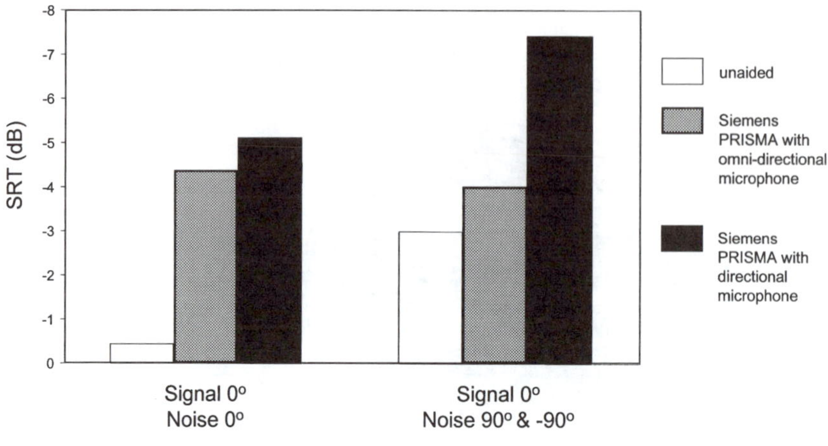

Figure 8–36. Speech intelligibility for the unaided condition and for aided conditions with omnidirectional and directional modes for two spatial listening conditions.

Future Developments

Several improvements in digital technology can be expected in the coming years. One intriguing example is the possibility of a wireless communication link between a listener's right and left hearing instruments. If both hearing instruments can communicate and share received signals, a beam-forming algorithm could be implemented. The assumption upon which beam-forming is based is the same as directional microphone systems. Desired signals originate from the frontal direction, whereas the sounds from all other directions should be attenuated. There are in general two different approaches for beam-forming.

The first approach is based on the capabilities of the human auditory system (Bodden, 1992; Kollmeier, Peissig, & Hohnmann, 1993). Figure 8–37 shows a simplified block diagram of the algorithm. The input signals of the left and right hearing instrument are transformed from the time domain into the frequency domain. Then the interaural phase and level differences are compared by calculating the differences between the two signals in different frequency bands. If the differences are zero or very small, then the signal is assumed to come from the frontal direction or from within the beam angle. A difference greater than a specified criterion would indicate that the signals are originating from outside the beam angle. In this case, the corresponding frequency channels are attenuated by a weighting function. Because this system strives to improve speech intelligibility by attenuating unwanted signals from surrounding directions, it is known as a "Cocktail-Party-Processor."

The adaptive beam former reaches the same goal by a more technical approach, as seen in Figure 8–38 (Griffiths & Jim, 1982). With this approach, the signals from the left and right microphone are subtracted and added to each other. The reference channel is the result of the subtraction of the two inputs. On the preconditions that the target source is in the frontal direction, no reverberation is present, and microphone sensitivities are matched, the reference channel contains only noise because the signal coming from the frontal direction is the same in the left and right microphone. The primary channel is the result of the addition of the two sides. The primary channel contains a doubling of the target signal. The remaining noise components in the reference channel are transformed by

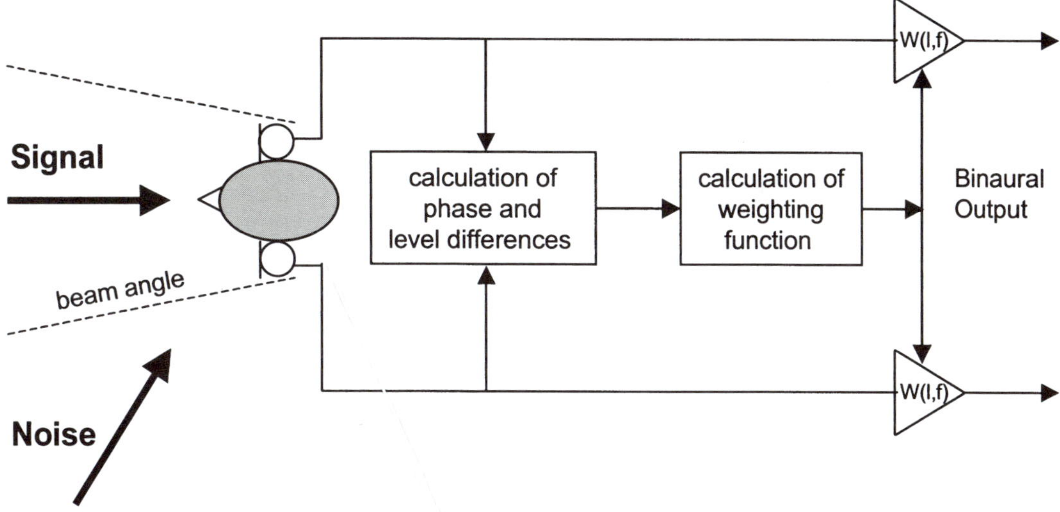

Figure 8–37. Block diagram of binaural "Cocktail-Party-Processor."

an adaptive filter such that they estimate the remaining noise in the primary channel. The output of the adaptive filter is subtracted from the primary channel, canceling out the noise.

Both algorithms offer good user benefit under ideal conditions, e.g., no reverberation. Their benefit in everyday life still must be investigated.

Feedback Reduction

An important quality issue for hearing instruments is acoustic feedback. The ringing sound that signifies acoustic feedback often bothers hearing instrument users or their conversation partners. In the feedback condition, the output signals from the receiver are fed back into the microphone and amplified again in the signal processor which causes acoustic feedback or ringing. In some instances, feedback can be avoided by reducing the amplification of a certain frequency region while fitting the hearing instrument. This approach can sometime have a deleterious effect of reducing speech intelligibility, however. Another possible feedback reduction technique is narrow band-reject filters, also called notch filters. These notch filters are positioned at the critical feedback frequencies to selectively reduce the amplification at those frequencies.

The static adjustments are useless if the feedback occurs suddenly at a different frequency due to changes in the acoustical conditions. The acoustical conditions can be changed in a variety of ways, for example, by wearing a hat, putting the hand to the ear, or sitting in a moving car next to the window. It can be resolved using adaptive algorithms. A feedback-reduction algorithm constantly analyzes the input signal, searching for feedback. A notch filter or a compensation filter changes the frequency response, but this filter constantly must be adjusted to the actual condition. A block diagram of a feedback-reduction algorithm is depicted in Figure 8–39. Shown is a digital hearing instrument with microphone, preamplifier, A/D converter, digital signal processor, D/A converter, end amplifier, and receiver. In the digital signal processor, the input signals are amplified and adjusted to the individual hearing loss. To avoid feedback, the feedback path is estimated, and an adaptive filter is adjusted within the signal processor to compensate for this feedback path.

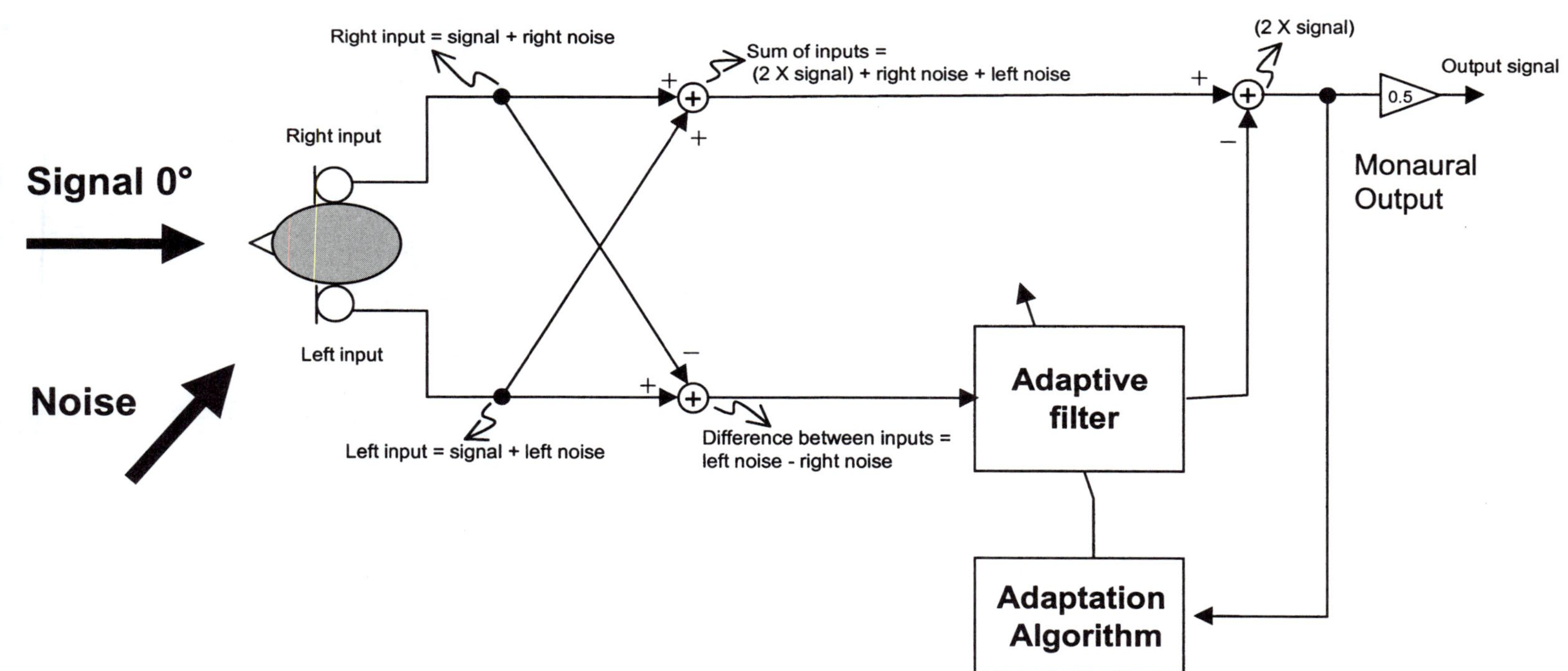

Figure 8–38. Block diagram of the adaptive beamformer.

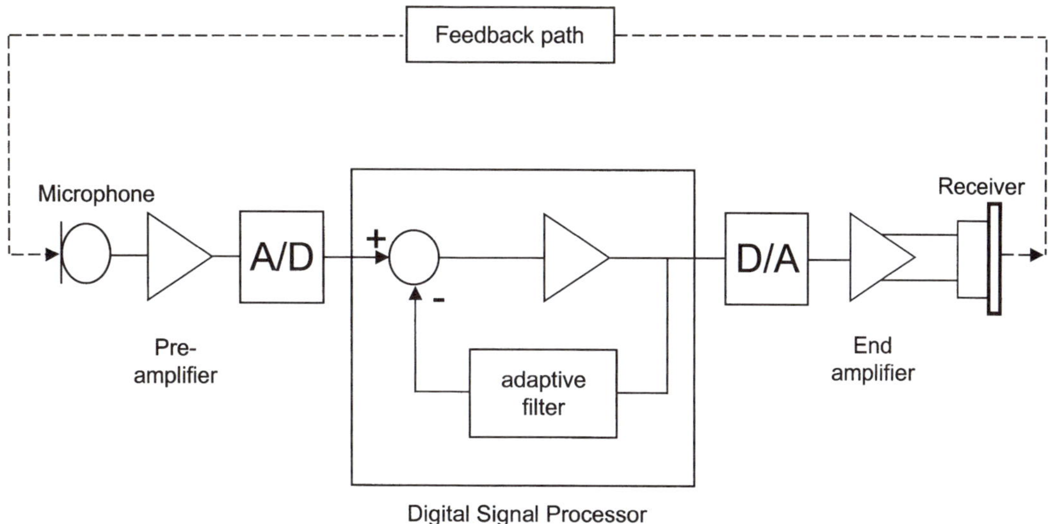

Figure 8–39. Block diagram of a feedback reduction algorithm. (From "Signalverarbeitungs algorithmen für digitale Hörgeräte," by I. Holube, 1998, *Zeitschrift für Audiologie, 37*, 182. Copyright 1998 by Median-Verlag. Adapted with permission.)

Overall Benefit of Digital Hearing Instruments

Digital hearing instruments are not necessarily better than analog hearing instruments. The limitations of digital signal processing have to be considered when developing a digital instrument. Many DSP algorithms could be conceived for hearing instruments, but only those that are beneficial should be included in the hearing instrument. At times, a benefit can be shown in subjective measurements, such as questionnaires, but speech intelligibility test scores show only minimal improvement. While it is beyond the scope of this chapter to give a detailed overview of all published research with digital hearing instruments, one qualitative measurement of hearing instrument benefit will be highlighted.

Arlinger (1999) rated hearing instrument benefit with different instruments after a 4-week period of use. A 10-point scale from "worthless" to "like normal hearing" rated perception of benefit by the hearing instrument user. The users completed a questionnaire for each hearing instrument examining perceived benefit in different situations. Table 8–1 lists the situations in which subjects rated the benefit of the respective instrument on a 10-point scale.

Results of benefit ratings are shown in Figures 8-40. Benefit was estimated by the difference in ratings between a digital hearing instrument with directional microphone (Siemens PRISMA) and two reference hearing instruments. In Figure 8–40A, the reference was an analog hearing instrument with directional microphone, and in Figure 8–40B, the reference was a digital hearing instrument without directional microphone, but using an active noise reduction algorithm.

The differences between the benefit scaling for the hearing instruments show results favoring the directional DSP instrument. They indicate a tendency toward higher subjective benefit for a digital hearing instrument with a directional microphone compared to both an analog hearing instrument with directional microphone and a digital hearing instrument alone.

Table 1. Hearing Instrument Benefit after Four Weeks of Use (Arlinger, 1999).

Listening conditions for which hearing instrument benefit was rated	
a	Speech in a quiet environment
b	Speech at a distance
c	Speech on the street or in traffic noise
d	When listening to someone talking among many others, e.g., at a party
e	General sound quality
f	Loud sounds in background noise
g	Own voice
h	Changing sound environment

Scale used for the rating of hearing instrument benefit	
0–1	worthless
3	acceptable sometimes
5	acceptable
7	good most of the time
9–10	like normal hearing

SUMMARY

This presentation outlines the principles of digital signal processing and processing algorithms for digital hearing instruments and their benefit for the users of those instruments. Whereas analog signals are continuous in time and in level, digital signals are sampled at discrete points in time and are quantized and represented by binary numbers. Both the sampling and the quantization can result in artifacts, which have to be avoided. In general, digital hearing instruments have several advantages over analog hearing instruments. These are miniaturization, low power consumption, low internal noise, reproducibility, stability, programmability, and signal processing complexity. Several signal processing algorithms can be implemented in digital hearing instruments. They normally include the possibility of frequency specific processing, several possibilities of dynamic range compression, noise reduction, and feedback reduction algorithms. The noise reduction algorithms can be divided into single-microphone systems, which separate speech and noise by their different temporal structure, and multi-microphone systems that separate speech and noise by assumptions about their spatial location. All algorithms are beneficial for the user of hearing instruments.

REVIEW QUESTIONS

1. An analog sine wave:
   a. Is sampled at 25,000 Hz.
   b. Is continuously varying in amplitude.
   c. Looks like stair steps.
   d. All of the above.

2. A digital sine wave:
   a. May be sampled at 25,000 Hz.
   b. Is not continuous.

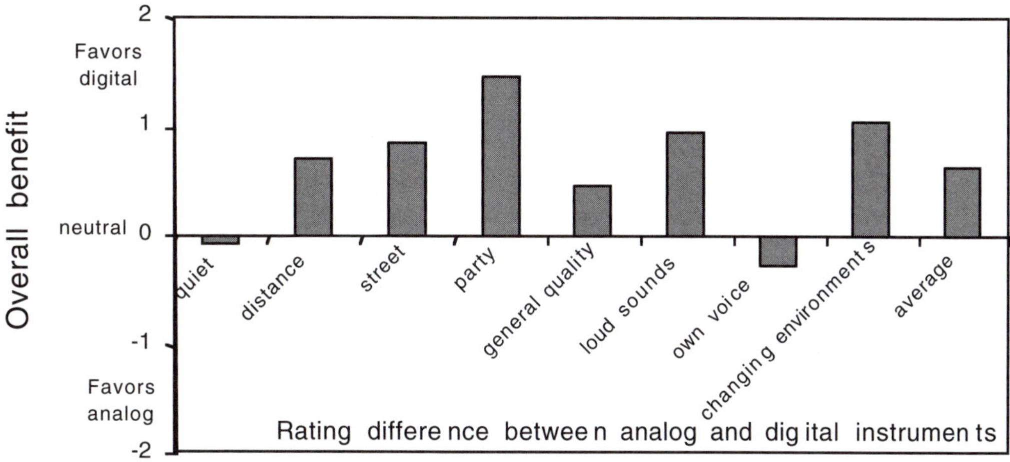

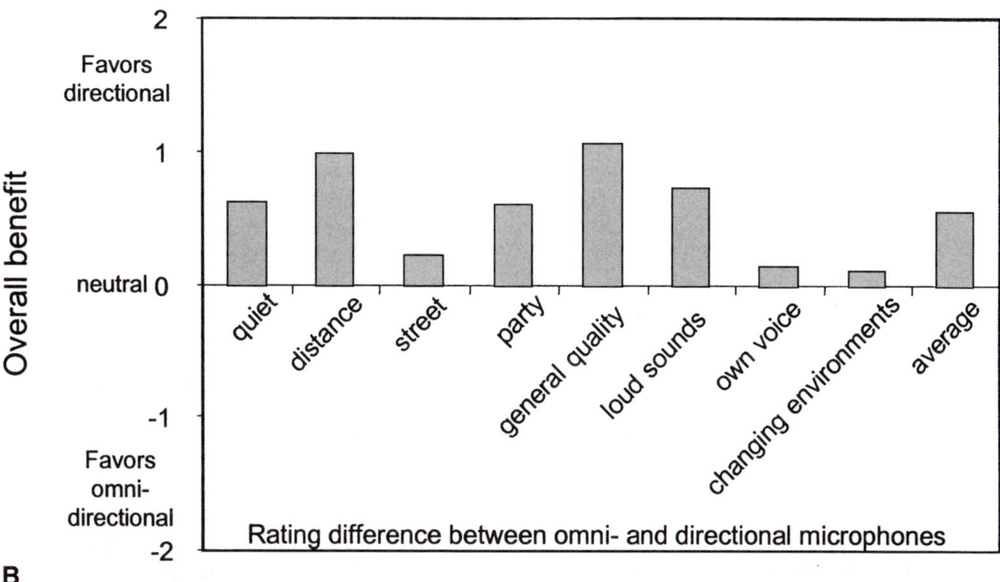

Figure 8–40. A. Benefit of digital hearing instrument over an analog hearing instrument, both with directional microphone. **B.** Benefit of a digital hearing instrument with directional microphone over a digital hearing instrument with omnidirectional microphone.

c. Looks like stair steps.
d. All of the above.

3. Aliasing occurs when:
a. A 5000 Hz sine wave is sampled at 8000 Hz.
b. The sampling frequency is less than the Nyquist frequency.
c. The input signal is sampled at an insufficient number of points.
d. All of the above.

4. Which was not discussed as a source of error in a digital hearing instrument?
   a. Aliasing.
   b. Quantization.
   c. Integrated chip structure size.
   d. None of these contribute to error.

5. Which statement is true?
   a. In syllabic compression, the attack and release times are short.
   b. Syllabic compression does not affect the dynamic range of speech.
   c. Compared to syllabic compression, automatic volume control has a short attack time and a long release time.
   d. Automatic volume control has a greater effect on the envelope of speech than does syllabic compression.

6. The modulation spectrum of speech:
   a. Has a broad peak at 3 kHz.
   b. Has a sharp peak at 30 Hz.
   c. Reflects the frequencies of sentences, words, and speech sounds.
   d. Is an essential measure for the calculation of the directivity index.

7. What is the goal of the following algorithms: microphone noise reduction, directional microphones, and channel coupling?
   a. Feedback reduction.
   b. Noise reduction.
   c. Reduction of the occlusion effect.
   d. Instrument size reduction.

8. The relation between the amplification for frontal sounds and the amplification for sounds from all other directions is called:
   a. The squelch effect.
   b. The Nyquist frequency.
   c. The upward spread of masking.
   d. The directivity index.

9. Feedback reduction can be:
   a. Achieved using adaptive filters.
   b. Achieved by modulating the Nyquist frequency.
   c. Achieved with dual compression.
   d. Alas, feedback cannot be affected by digital technology.

10. Name five advantages of hearing instruments with digital technology over hearing instruments with analog technology.

a. ______________________

b. ______________________

c. ______________________

d. ______________________

e. ______________________

REFERENCES

Allen, J. B., & Jeng, P. S. (1990). Loudness growth in ½ octave bands (LGOB); a procedure for the assessment of loudness. *Journal of the Acoustical Society of America, 88,* 745–753.

Arlinger, S., Billermark, E., & Slättengren, I. (1999). Internal report. [Unpublished]

Braida, L. D., Durlach, N. I., De Gennaro, S. V., Peterson, P. M., & Bustamante, D. K. (1982). Review of recent research on multiband amplitude compression for the hearing impaired. In G. A. Studebaker & F. H. Bess (Eds.), *The Vanderbilt Hearing-Aid Report* (pp. 122–140). Upper Darby, PA: Monographs in Contemporary Audiology.

Bodden, M. (1992). Beurteilung der Störgeräuschunterdrückung mit einem Cocktail-Party-Prozessor. *Fortschritte der Akustik—DAGA 1992* (pp. 649–652). Bad Honnef: DPG-Kongreß-GmbH.

Cox, R. M., Alexander, G. C., Taylor, I. M., & Gray, G. A. (1997). The Contour Test of Loudness Perception. *Ear & Hearing, 18,* 388–400.

Cudahy, E., & Levitt, H. (1994). Digital hearing instruments: A historical perspective. In R. Sandlin (Ed.), *Understanding digitally programmable hearing aids.* Needham Heights, NY: Allyn and Bacon.

Dillon, H. (1996). Tutorial: Compression? Yes, but for low or high frequencies, and with what response times? *Ear & Hearing, 17,* 287–307.

Dreschler, W. A., & Verschuure, H. (1996). Psychophysical evaluation of fast compression systems. In B. Kollmeier (Ed.), *Psychoacoustics, speech and hearing aids* (pp. 183–191). Singapore: World Scientific.

Drullman, R., Festen, J. M., & Plomp, R. (1994). Effect of temporal envelope smearing on speech reception. *Journal of the Acoustical Society of America, 95,* 1053–1064.

Fabry, D. A. (1991). Programmable and automatic noise reduction in existing hearing instruments. In G. A. Studebaker & F. H. Bess (Eds.), *The Vanderbilt Hearing Aid Report II* (pp. 65–78). Parkton, MD: York Press.

Graupe, D., Grosspietsch, J. K., & Basseas, S. P. (1987). A single-microphone-based self-adaptive filter of noise from speech and its performance evaluation. *Journal of Rehabilitation Research and Development, 24*(4), 119–126.

Griffiths, L. J., & Jim, C. W. (1982). An alternative approach to linearly constrained adaptive beamforming. *IEEE Transactions: Antennas Propag, AP-30,* 1662–1672.

Hagerman, B. (1982). Sentences for testing speech intelligibility in noise. *Scandinavian Audiology, 11,* 79–87.

Hagerman, B., & Kinnerfors, C. (1995). Efficient adaptive methods for measurements of speech reception thresholds in quiet and in noise. *Scandinavian Audiology, 24,* 71–77.

Hickson, L. M. H. (1994). Compression amplification in hearing aids. *American Journal of Audiology, 3,* 51–65.

Hohmann, V. (1998). Grundlagen digitaler Signalverarbeitung. *Zeitschrift für Audiologie, 37,* 121–130.

Holube, I. (1998). Signalverarbeitungsalgorithmen für digitale Hörgeräte. *Zeitschrift für Audiologie, 37,* 176–182.

Houtgast, T., & Steeneken, H. J. M. (1985). A review of the MTF concept in room acoustics and its use for estimating speech intelligibility in auditoria. *Journal of the Acoustical Society of America, 77,* 1069–1077.

Kollmeier, B., Peissig, J., & Hohmann, V. (1993). Binaural noise-reduction hearing aid scheme with real-time processing in the frequency domain. *Scandinavian Audiolology, Suppl. 38,* 28–38.

Lyons, R. G. (1997). *Understanding digital signal processing.* Reading, MA: Addison-Wesley Publishing Company.

Moore, B. C. J. (1990). How much do we gain by gain control in hearing aids? *Acta Otolaryngologica, Suppl. 469,* 250–256.

Moore, B. C. J. (1995). *Perceptual consequences of cochlear damage.* Oxford; England: Oxford University Press.

Moore, B. C. J., Glasberg, B. R., & Stone, M. A. (1991). Optimization of a slow-acting automatic gain control system for use in hearing aids. *British Journal of Audiology, 25,* 171–182.

Mueller, H. G., & Wesselkamp, M. (1999). Ten commonly asked questions about directional microphone fittings. *Hearing Review Supplement, High Performance Hearing Solutions, Hearing in Noise, Vol. 3.* 25–30.

Nilsson, M. J., Soli, S. D., & Sullivan, J. (1994). Development of a hearing in noise test for the measurement of speech reception threshold. *Journal of the Acoustical Society of. America, 95,* 1085–1099.

Oppenheim, A. V., & Schafer, R. W. (1975). *Digital signal processing.* Englewood Cliffs, NJ: Prentice-Hall.

Ostendorf, M., Hohmann, V., & Kollmeier, B. (1997). Empirische Klassifizierung verschiedener akustischer Signale und Sprache mittels einer Modulationsfrequenzanalyse. *Fortschritte der Akustik, DAGA-97.*

Pascoe, D. P. (1978). An approach to hearing aid selection. *Hearing Instruments, 29,* 12–16.

Plomp, R. (1983). Perception of speech as a modulated signal. *Proceedings of the 10th International Congress of Phonetic Sciences,* Utrecht, The Netherlands.

Plomp, R. (1988). The negative effect of amplitude compression in multichannel hearing aids in the light of the modulation-transfer function. *Journal of the Acoustical Society of America, 83,* 2322–2327.

Powers, T., Holube, I., & Wesselkamp, M. (1999). The use of digital features to combat background noise. *Hearing Review Supplement, High Performance Hearing Solutions, 3. Hearing in Noise,* 36–39.

Resnick, S. B., Dubno, J. R., Hoffnung, S., & Levitt, H. (1975). Phoneme errors on a nonsense syllable test. *Journal of the Acoustical Society of America, 58,* 114.

Ricketts, T., & Dhar, S. (1999). Comparison of performance across three directional hearing aids. *Journal of the American Academy of Audiology, 10,* 180–189.

Stein, L., & Dempesy-Hart, D. (1984). Listener-assessed intelligiblity of a hearing instrument self-adaptive noise filter. *Ear & Hearing, 5,* 199–204.

Van Tassel, D. J., Larsen, S. Y., & Fabry, D. A. (1988). Effects of an adaptive filter hearing instrument on speech recognition in noise by hearing-impaired subjects. *Ear & Hearing, 9,* 15–21.

Wolf, R. P., Hohn, W., Martin, R., & Powers, T. A. (1999). Directional microphone hearing instruments: How and why they work. *Hearing Review Supplement, High Performance Hearing Solutions, Vol. 3. Hearing in Noise,* 14–25.

CHAPTER 9

Technical Considerations for Sound Field Audiometry

GARY WALKER, PH.D.

OUTLINE

Audiologists use the term *sound field audiometry* to refer to procedures in which the test signal is presented through a loudspeaker rather than through headphones. Sound field audiometry has long been used to estimate the auditory thresholds of young children and other clients who will not tolerate earphones. In the last decade or so, sound field aided and unaided threshold testing has been used increasingly as part of the hearing aid selection and fitting process. This has followed from the realization that the gain provided by the hearing aid, while being worn by the particular client, is essential information that cannot be accurately estimated from coupler-based measurements. This chapter examines the scientific basis of sound field audiometry as it relates specifically to hearing aid selection, fitting, and evaluation.

ROOM ACOUSTICS

A sound field is any area in which sound waves are present. Sound field audiometry is carried out in a variety of acoustic environments ranging from anechoic chambers, audiometric test booths, and specifically modified rooms to rooms that have little or no special treatment. The sound field is bounded by the walls, floor, and ceiling of the room. The sound field within a room is not uniform, but exhibits different characteristics at different locations. The sound field can be divided into the near and far fields, and the far field can, in turn, be divided into direct and reverberant fields.

If a small sound source is placed in a room and activated, sound waves will move away from it in all directions, with the wave fronts forming a spherical pattern. If sound intensity is measured at 0.5 m and at 1 m from the source, so that the distance of the second measuring point from the source is double that of the first, it will be found that the sound intensity has decreased fourfold. That is, the intensity of the sound is inversely proportional to the square of the distance from its source. The sound is then said to be obeying the inverse square law. A simple rule to remember is that the intensity of such sounds will decrease by 6 dB for each doubling of the distance between the source and the measuring point.

If this rule were to be applied back to the source, the calculations would indicate that an infinite sound pressure level must exist at the source. This is absurd: In fact, the operation of the inverse square law relies on the assumption that the sound's wavefront is spherical. This does not apply in close proximity to the source, and the sound pressure level in this region is almost constant. The term *near field* refers to that area that is so close to the source that the inverse square law does not apply, and the term *far field* refers to all other points in the sound field. At some distance from the source, the spherical wave front becomes so large that, for all practical purposes, it can be considered to be flat. The wave is then described as a *plane wave*.

Up to now, it has been assumed that the sound has traveled directly from its source to the measuring point. In reality, direct sound is by no means the only contributor to the field. When a sound wave strikes an object in a sound field, it may be refracted, reflected, absorbed, or transmitted.

If a large object (e.g., 1 m × 1 m × 2 cm thick) is placed facing a plane sound wave at a frequency of 3 kHz, the successive wave fronts passing the object will be deformed in the manner shown in Figure 9-1. For simplicity, it is assumed that no sound is absorbed or

Editor's note: The chapter submitted by Gary Walker for the first edition of the *Handbook of Hearing Aid Amplification* needs little, if any, modification. Unfortunately, he was unable to revise his excellent chapter. A number of diagnostic procedures conducted in sound field have been greatly expanded over the past decade to assess hearing aid performance. Reverberant sound fields have been utilized to assess the affect on speech recognition as a function of reverberating time. The technical considerations have not changed sufficiently to lessen the contribution of his chapter, however. It is included therefore in the revised edition as it originally appeared in the first edition.

transmitted by the object. The wavelength of a 3 kHz tone is 0.115 m, so the long dimensions of the object are much larger than 1 wavelength.

Waves that pass to the side of the obstacle are diffracted around it. That is, their direction of motion is changed so that some sound actually reaches all points on the back of the obstacle. Because the sound that covers the back comes from wave fronts near the edges, however, the pressure fluctuation reaching most of the back is greatly diminished relative to that at the front, and a "sound shadow" is created.

By contrast, the pressure in front of the obstacle will actually be greater than at its surface. This occurs because waves hitting a solid heavy object reflect off the object and travel back toward the source. Immediately adjacent to the surface of the object, the incoming and reflected waves are still in phase with each other, so their contributions to the total pressure add consecutively (see Figure 9–1). As a result, the pressure is double what it would be if the obstacle was not there, and the sound pressure level (SPL) is thus increased by 6 dB over that in the surrounding field. After the reflected wave has traveled back one quarter of a wavelength toward the source, it has then traveled a half wavelength farther than the incoming wave it is currently meeting head-on. Consequently, they are 180° out of phase and add destructively, creating a pressure minimum one quarter of a wavelength in front of the obstacle. Thus, the pressure increase observable on the surface exists for only a small fraction of a wavelength in front of the obstacle.

For the opposite situation, when a low-frequency, long-wavelength sound wave hits a very small obstacle, any buildup of pressure on the front surface is prevented because the entire surface of the obstacle is immersed in a relatively large region of uniform pressure. There can be no significant departure from the "natural" pressure of the wave at that point of its travel because there is a sufficient time before the next part of the wave arrives for the molecules to redistribute themselves uniformly around the obstacle. Thus, the pressure on the front, back, and sides of the obstacle is the same as that which would be present in the incoming wave in the absence of the obstacle.

When an incoming sound wave meets a solid obstacle, such as a wall, some sound en-

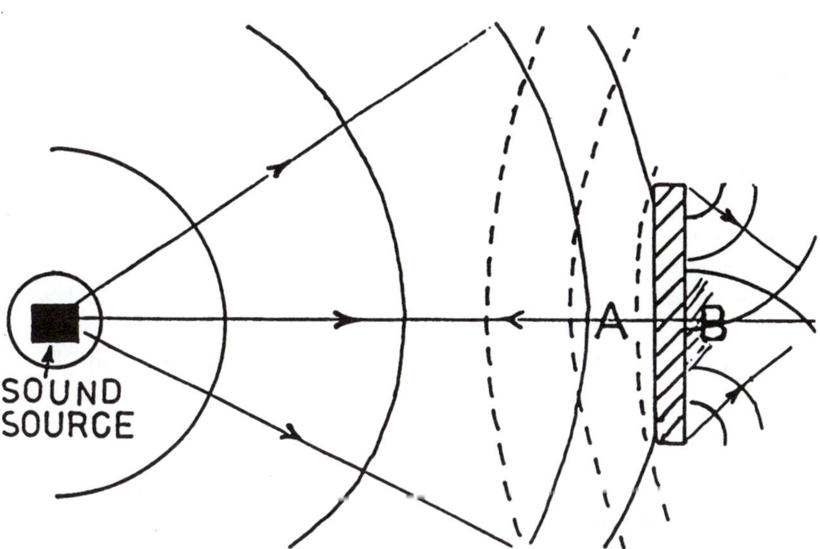

Figure 9–1. Sound propagation.

ergy may be transmitted through the obstacle to the far side. This transmission can occur in two ways. First, a genuine acoustic wave (i.e., a progression of compressions and rarefactions) can be set up in the obstacle. The magnitude of the sound radiated into the air on the other side of the obstacle by this transmission mechanism is usually insignificant for walls of typical construction. The amount transmitted decreases as the density and thickness of the wall increases and also as the frequency of the incoming wave increases. The second way in which transmission occurs is when the wall as a whole vibrates, much like the diaphragm of a loudspeaker. Just as with acoustic wave transmission, the amount transmitted decreases as the mass of the wall increases and as frequency increases. Thus, irrespective of the type of transmission, the attenuation provided by a wall can be increased by making the wall thicker or by using a denser material. Unfortunately, doubling the mass-per-unit area of a wall (e.g., by doubling the thickness) only results in a 5 or 6 dB decrease in the sound intensity transmitted. It thus quickly becomes uneconomical to continue to increase wall attenuation in this way. An alternative that is usually used when high wall attenuation is required is to use a double wall construction. Provided there is no coupling between the two walls (such as by having them rest on a common, nonabsorbing support or by using too small an air space between them), the total attenuation in dB is twice that of either wall alone. It should be remembered that the attenuation provided by an entire room (such as an audiometric test booth) is often limited by leakage around joints between panels or around windows or doors. That is, air conduction paths provide much better transmission than paths that truly transmit sound through solid obstacles. This occurs because the density of solid objects is many times greater than that of air so that transmission from air to a solid is inefficient. This density change is sometimes described as an impedance mismatch.

Sound, in addition to being reflected from, transmitted through, or diffracted around the obstacle, can also be absorbed at the surface of the obstacle. Soft or porous substances absorb sound more than hard or dense substances. The amount of absorption is characterized by the substance's *absorption coefficient*, which is defined as the proportion of sound intensity that is absorbed when the wave hits a surface. Absorbed sound energy is neither transmitted nor reflected but rather is converted into a small amount of heat energy at the surface of the obstacle. Often the absorption is greater for high frequencies than for low frequencies. When the surface of an obstacle has a high absorption coefficient, the pressure buildup on the front face, which was described earlier, will not occur to the same degree. Recall that the pressure increase occurs when the obstacle is large enough compared to the sound's wavelength to cause a reflected wave to travel back toward the source. It is the in-phase addition of the incident and reflected waves that produces the pressure increase.

If the sound wave is completely absorbed (absorption coefficient = 1.0) by the obstacle, there can be no reflected wave and consequently no pressure increase. The pressure at the surface of the obstacle would then be exactly the same as if the obstacle was not there at all. Intuitively, this seems reasonable because the sound wave travels on past the surface of the obstacle into the absorbent material in just the same way as it would if the absorbent obstacle was absent. For objects with more realistic absorption coefficients (i.e., neither completely absorbing nor completely reflecting), the SPL increase at the surface still occurs, but is of diminished size. It is worth remembering that the SPL increase for a wave hitting a large object wall always be between 0 dB (for complete absorption) and 6 dB (for complete reflection). From an audiological point of view, the major reason for interest in the pressure increase at the surface of obstacles is that it affects the pressure detected by microphones mounted on the body, such as hearing aid microphones or noise dosimeters.

If a sound source produces a single brief impulse (e.g., a click), an observer will first hear the direct wave, followed shortly by a series of echoes as the sound waves hit the walls of the room and are reflected back into the room, some of them eventually to reach the observer. Because of absorption, each echo will individually be weaker than the direct wave but the total intensity of all of the reflected sound waves may well be greater than that of the original wave. It is now possible to define the terms *direct* and *reverberant* sound fields. A *direct field* is dominated by directly radiated sound, whereas a reverberant field is dominated by reflected sound. Figure 9–2A, which shows the sound pressure level

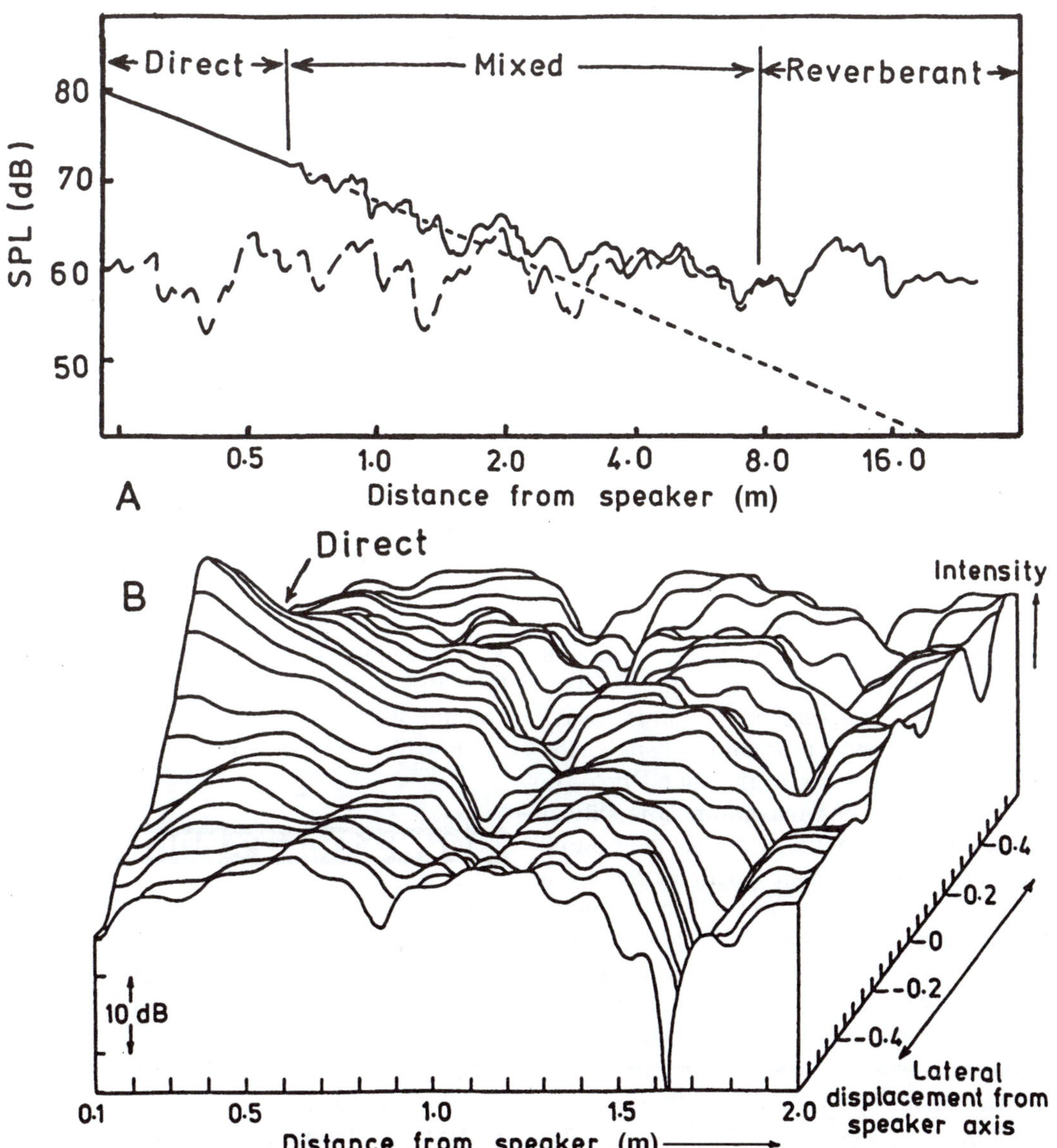

Figure 9–2. Sound fields generated in a room. Panel **A** shows the sound pressure level of a pure tone in a room as a function of distance from the sound source. Panel **B** is a three-dimensional (length x width x intensity) representation of a pure tone sound field generated in a room.

in a room versus the distance from the sound source, illustrates how the fields combine in a room. The dotted line shows the direct field component, the dashed line the reverberant component, and the solid line the combined field. Note that the logarithmic distance axis used results in a straight-line relationship in the direct field region.

At any particular point in the room, the various reflected waves arriving at that point may tend to add together constructively (i.e., in phase) or may partially or even completely cancel one another out. The combined field is simply the sum of the two individual components (i.e., direct and reverberant). Close to the source, the total field is dominated by the direct component, which varies smoothly by 6 dB for every doubling of distance. Far away from the source, the reverberant field dominates, so small movements by the observer can result in large changes in sound pressure. At intermediate distances both fields contribute. The distance at which the level of the direct field equals the average level of the reverberant field is called the *critical distance*. In a typical living room with carpets and drapes plus hard and soft furnishings, the critical distance is likely to be less than 1 m. Other rooms, such as kitchens and bathrooms, would typically have more hard surfaces, so their critical distances would be even less. It is concluded, therefore, that in indoor listening situations, the reverberant field is always a significant contributor, and is usually the dominant contributor, to the sound field. In panel A of Figure 9–2 maximum variability of the reverberant field is of the order of 6 to 8 dB. For the three-dimensional plot shown in panel B, however, one "trough" in the reverberant field is more than 20 dB "deep." Both parts of Figure 9–2 are based on measurements made in real rooms. The ultimate reverberant field is one in which there is an equal likelihood of the sound arriving at the measurement point from any direction, including above and below. This is called a *diffuse field*.

Two measurements that are basic to architectural acoustics are a room's reverberation time and its absorption coefficient. The *reverberation time* is defined as the time taken for any sound to decay in level by 60 dB. Reverberant sound can have both beneficial and detrimental effects. Although reflected sound can decrease the intelligibility of the original signal by merging one part of the sound into the next, it can add "warmth" to the tonal quality of speech, and, especially, music. Reverberation is often simulated by recording studios for just this purpose. Also, the reverberant sound helps to even out the range of intensities to which people are subjected. Consider what would happen in a lecture theater if only the direct field were present. Although the audience at the front may only be 2 m from the speaker, those at the back may be 20 m away. This 10:1 distance ratio would mean that those at the front received a signal 20 dB more intense than those at the back. By contrast, the reverberant component of the sound field fills the entire theater uniformly. Thus the people at the back of the theater have the relatively weak direct field considerably augmented by the reverberant sound. Arriving at the correct ratio of direct sound (often described as crisp, clear, or dry) to reverberant sound (often described as smooth, warm, or full) is always a compromise between the conflicting demands of high intelligibility and pleasant tonal quality. It should not be surprising that the optimum amount of reverberant sound depends on the use to which the room or theater is to be put.

SOUND FIELD AUDIOMETRY

When contemplating the practice of sound field audiometry, a number of important questions must be addressed. Walker, Dillon, and Byrne (1984) listed seven such questions:

1. What type of stimulus is most suitable for sound field audiometry?
2. What are the optimal characteristics (e.g., bandwidth) of such a stimulus?
3. What are the relative merits of testing in the direct versus the reverberant field?

4. What test room characteristics are important?
5. How should calibration be performed?
6. What other aspects of testing technique or test room arrangements are important?
7. What limitations apply, and how can they be minimized, if testing has to be performed with a less than optimal stimulus or technique?

Of these questions, the first four will be dealt with at length in this chapter, while the others, which are essentially practical, will be touched on only briefly.

The Stimulus

Problems arise for sound field audiometry as a result of the variation in the sound pressure level of the signal at different places within the room, and because it is impractical to keep the client's ears in exactly the same position for the duration of the test and in exactly the same position assumed during calibration. The problem exists even when the clients are alert and cooperative adults but is much greater when the client is an infant. It is difficult if not impossible to restrain the child's movement without jeopardizing cooperation or inhibiting natural response to the stimulus.

Figure 9–2 should make it clear why pure tones are not considered to be appropriate stimuli for sound field testing in a reverberant field. Small movements of the client's head or drifts in the signal's frequency can result in large variations in the sound pressure level at the test ear. This problem has been noted by many authors (e.g., Morgan, Dirks, & Bower, 1979) and was confirmed by this author and a colleague in an extensive series of measurements (Dillon & Walker, 1982a).

Figure 9–3 shows the sound pressure levels of three tones, 5 Hz apart in frequency, as a function of distance from the sound source. It illustrates how large errors can be introduced by small shifts in the frequency of the tone. It also illustrates how one could be misled regarding the variability of a sound field if judgments are made on the basis of measurements taken at too few frequencies, too few positions in the field, or both.

Dillon and Walker (1982a) listed four attributes that a suitable sound field stimulus should possess:

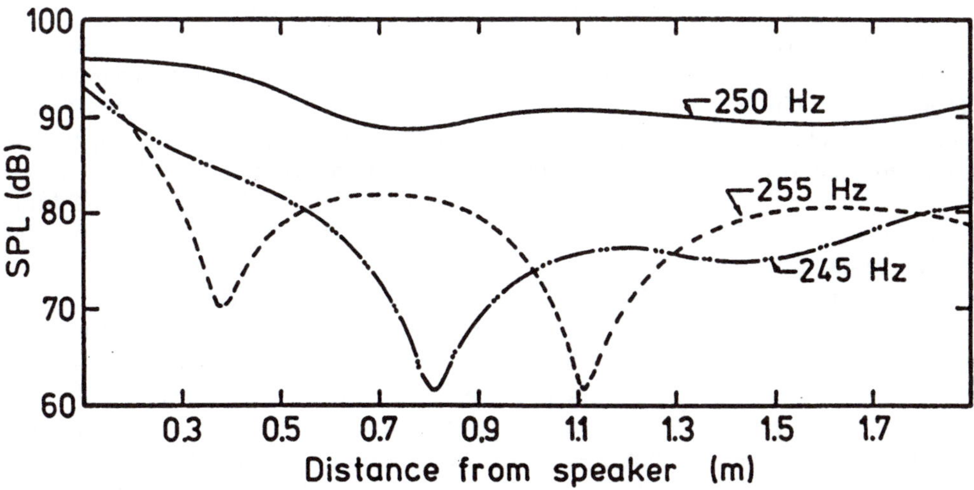

Figure 9–3. The sound pressure levels of three pure tones, 5 Hz apart, as a function of distance from the loudspeaker.

1. It must be reasonably frequency specific because frequency-specific information is needed for a satisfactory definition of the client's hearing status and amplification needs.
2. The sound pressure level generated in the field must be stable over the whole region that the client's head could occupy during testing.
3. The sound pressure level generated at the client's ear must be stable for small shifts in frequency, such as may occur in an oscillator's output between calibrations.
4. The results obtained in the sound field must be relatable to similar measurements made with pure tones under earphones.

Various complex signals have been promoted as suitable for sound field testing. Frequency modulated (warble) tones and narrow bands of noise are in common clinical use, although their specific parameters vary widely among audiometers. Other stimuli that have been proposed include amplitude modulated tones (Goldberg, 1979) and damped wavetrains (Victoreen, 1974). The common feature of these stimuli is that they contain energy in a band of frequencies around the nominal frequency. The rationale for their use is that the auditory system averages the sound energy within the pass band, thereby reducing the effects of the energy at any one frequency. The perception of a complex stimulus should therefore be relatively unaffected by a null in the room's response if the stimulus contains significant energy within a frequency band that is wider than the null.

Dillon and Walker (1982c) examined the uniformity of sound fields generated by various complex stimuli in a typical audiometric test room. They concluded that, given a relatively uniform distribution of sound energy within its frequency pass band, the factor determining the variability of the sound field generated by a complex stimulus is its bandwidth.

Figure 9–4 shows how the variability of a pure-tone sound field can be reduced by the introduction of frequency modulation. It is clear that the variability of the sound field is inversely related to the bandwidth of the FM tone.

It follows that any comparison of the effectiveness of different types of stimulus must be done with stimuli of equal bandwidths. A number of studies have compared warble tones with bands of noise that were not equal in this respect (e.g., Morgan et al., 1979; Orchik & Rintlemann, 1978; Stephens & Rintlemann, 1978). Their findings and comments may be valid for the particular stimuli investigated but should not be generalized to include all stimuli of the same type. The noted limitations of the various types of stimuli may not apply when they have optimal characteristics.

As all of the types of complex stimulus discussed so far can be produced with a range of bandwidths, this characteristic alone cannot be used to choose between them.

Dillon and Walker (1982a) used a variety of grounds to argue against the use of amplitude modulated tones, damped wave trains, and very narrow bands of noise.

Amplitude-modulated tones do not have as uniform a distribution of energy within the pass band as the other candidates and, in the absence of any unique virtue to balance this shortcoming, they were eliminated from further consideration.

Dillon and Walker (1982b) also argued against the use of damped wave trains on the grounds that the results obtained with this type of stimulus cannot be compared with other audiometric data. Audiometry is normally carried out with stimuli whose duration is sufficiently long that it does not affect the results (i.e., >200 ms). Damped wave trains on the other hand are exponentially decaying sinusoidal tone bursts in which the number of cycles in each burst remains constant. For practical bandwidths, the stimulus duration is shorter than the integration time of the normal human ear, and the thresholds obtained with them will thus be a function of stimulus duration. The problem is made worse by the fact that the temporal integration function may be

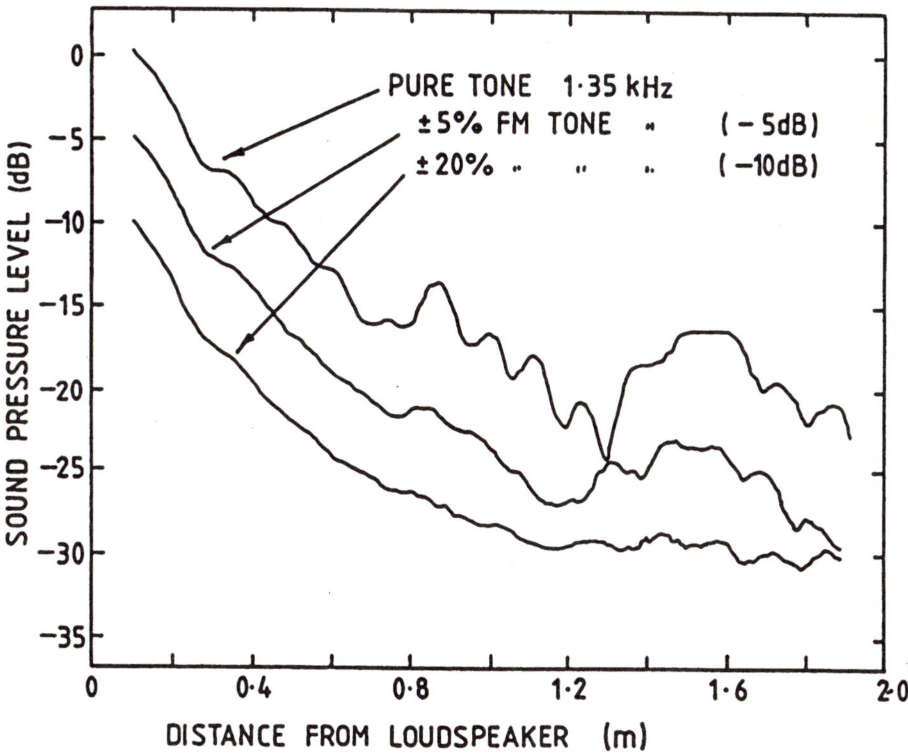

Figure 9–4. The sound pressure levels generated by an unmodulated tone and two modulated tones with the same center frequency but different bandwidths, as a function of distance from the loudspeaker. To facilitate comparison the overall levels of the tones have been arbitrarily separated by 5 dB.

grossly disturbed in cases of sensorineural hearing loss (Wright, 1968).

Dillon and Walker's (1982c) results show that band-pass-filtered random noise is inferior to all other stimuli for bandwidths up to and including 5% of the center frequency. They explained this in terms of the random amplitude fluctuations, which are a characteristic of noise. These fluctuations are relatively slow at the smallest bandwidths and consequently are not smoothed out by the lowpass filter to the same extent that more rapid fluctuations are. For higher center frequencies, the absolute bandwidth of a 5% noise band will be larger. The temporal fluctuations in intensity will therefore be faster and so will increasingly be smoothed by both the ear and the calibrating device.

Audiometric stimuli that contain significant sound energy over a range of frequencies will always underestimate the size of a hearing loss unless that loss is constant across frequencies. The reason is that some of the energy of the stimulus will be at frequencies where the client has better hearing than at the nominal center frequency. This is illustrated in Figure 9–5. Dillon and Walker (1982c) measured the differences between pure tone and warble tone thresholds as a function of the differences between the pure tone thresholds for frequencies at the band center and band edge of the warble tone. This revealed that the threshold differences between the pure and warble tones were about 0.75 times the band center to band edge threshold difference. In other words, a broadband stimu-

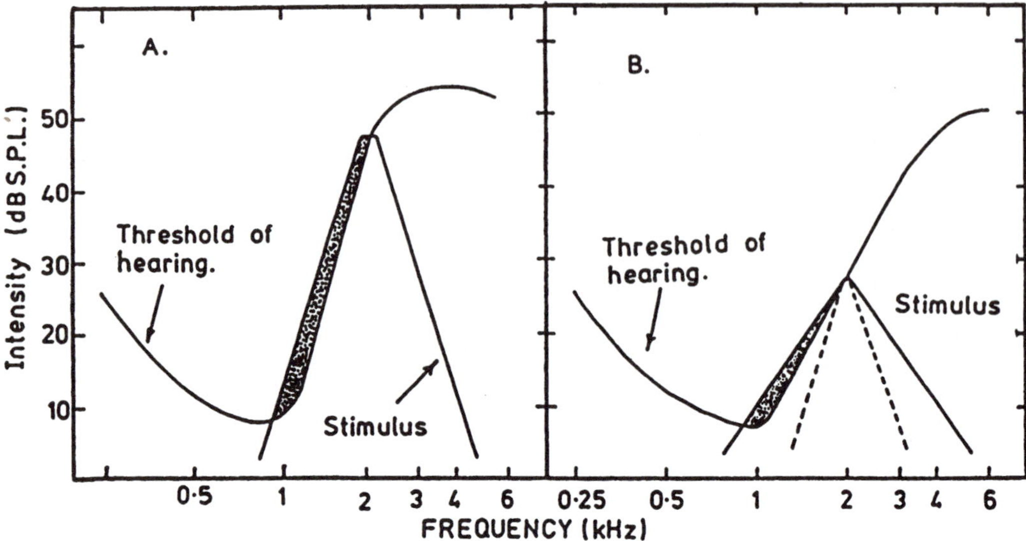

Figure 9–5. Panel **A** shows why the use of complex signals results in underestimation of the threshold. Some of the stimulus energy (shaded area) falls at frequencies where the client has better thresholds. Panel **B** shows that maximum error will result when the "skirts" of the stimulus are less steep than the threshold (solid lines) and minimized when they are steeper than the threshold function (broken lines).

lus will underestimate a hearing loss in the presence of a sloping threshold curve by an amount equal to three-quarters of the difference between the pure tone thresholds at frequencies corresponding to the center and band edge of the stimulus. The problem is worse at high frequencies where the thresholds of many people with sensorineural hearing loss change rapidly across frequencies. It is desirable that the stimulus not only have as narrow a bandwidth as practicable but that energy outside the band limits falls off as rapidly as possible. Orchik and Mosher (1975) demonstrated that filter slopes can have a marked effect on the thresholds obtained with narrow bands of noise. Figure 9–5B shows how the error is increased when the out-of-band slope of the stimulus is less than the slope of the threshold function but not when it is greater. Threshold functions can be steep. Rosler and Anderson (1978) found slopes as great as 250 dB/octave in the frequency range 2000 to 4000 Hz whereas Dillon and Walker reported that slopes of 120 dB/octave or more could be expected in this frequency range in 1% of persons with sensorineural hearing loss.

Warble tones do not require filtering for their generation, their spectral slope depending on the modulate rate, waveform, and frequency deviation. Very steep slopes can be obtained, especially at the higher frequencies where they are most required. On the other hand, narrow bands of noise with steep filter slopes are not readily available as simple low-order filters will not provide sufficiently steep filter slopes. Furthermore, the use of complex higher order filters is not desirable in a clinical instrument because they require careful alignment. Lippman and Adams (1982), however, have described an inexpensive method of generating suitable noise bands, although the one-third octave bandwidth that they suggest would not be optimal for all frequencies. There are also ways of producing bands of noise with the desired characteristics that do not involve bandpass-filtering broadband noise. The noise can be synthesized by adding together a number of discrete components, or it can be produced by means of the modulation technique proposed by Zwislocki (1951). With the advent of microprocessors in audiometers, it is now also possible to generate a noise waveform with any desired spectral properties by cyclically accessing a waveform stored in computer memory.

It is concluded that frequency modulated (warble) tones and suitably generated narrow bands of noise are the stimuli of choice for reverberant sound field audiometry.

The Required Bandwidths of Sound Field Stimuli

The selection of the bandwidths of stimuli for sound field audiometry necessarily involves a compromise. On the one hand, large bandwidths are required to obtain uniform sound fields; on the other hand, small bandwidths are needed to measure a frequency dependent hearing loss. These clearly are conflicting requirements. The size of errors arising from both sources must be quantified before a reasoned decision can be made about the appropriate stimulus for a particular client. If there is reason to believe that the client has a very steep threshold slope, a narrow bandwidth may be chosen for high frequencies, even though this results in a more variable sound field. If the testing is being carried out in an area with poor acoustic characteristics, however, a broader band stimulus may be needed. In this case, the clinician should be aware of the likely size of the introduced error. The author and his colleagues (Dillon & Walker, 1982c; Walker et al., 1984) have considered this issue in detail and have made specific recommendations about the stimuli that should be made available to clinicians.

The Required Modulation Waveform and Modulation Rate of FM Tones

For FM tones, the modulation waveform and rate must also be specified. The modulation waveform describes the manner in which the instantaneous frequency of the signal moves back and forth about the center frequency. Dillon and Walker (1982b) addressed the question of the most desirable waveform. In electronics, sinusoidal, triangular, ramp, and rectangular (square) waveforms are commonly used. These are shown in Figure 9–6.

Ramp and square wave modulation both involve very rapid frequency changes during their cycles and this results in a "splattering" of energy to out-of-band frequencies. As can clearly be seen in Figure 9–6, the result is a less-steep, out-of-band characteristic. It is concluded that they are not suitable for use in sound field audiometry. There is little to choose between sinusoidal and triangular modulation. As can be seen in Figure 9–7, sinusoidal modulation produces a steeper "edge" than triangular modulation; however, triangular modulation produces a more uniform in-band spectral density (because in sinusoidal modulation, the signal "dwells" longer at the frequency extremes). Both are acceptable, but because triangular modulation has an acceptable out-of-band characteristic and superior in-band characteristic, it is the waveform of choice.

Modulation rate or *modulation frequency* refers to the rate (in Hz) at which the instantaneous frequency is swept across the frequency band. Walker and Dillon (1983) examined the question of which modulation rate or rates are suitable for use in sound field FM tones. Two factors must be considered. First, if the modulation rate is too low, the ear will respond to individual fluctuations as the signal sweeps over the various peaks and troughs in the rooms' response. Consequently, the obtained threshold will depend on the highest peak occurring within the modulation cycle. Second, if the modulation rate is too high, field uniformity will decrease because there will be insufficient spectral components to ensure reasonable averaging within the band. The reason for this is that in the spectrum of an FM tone the energy of the signal is confined to discrete frequencies, and the spacing between these spectral components is a function of the modulation rate. Hence, for a fixed bandwidth signal, as the modulation rate increases, fewer and fewer spectral components will fall within the pass-

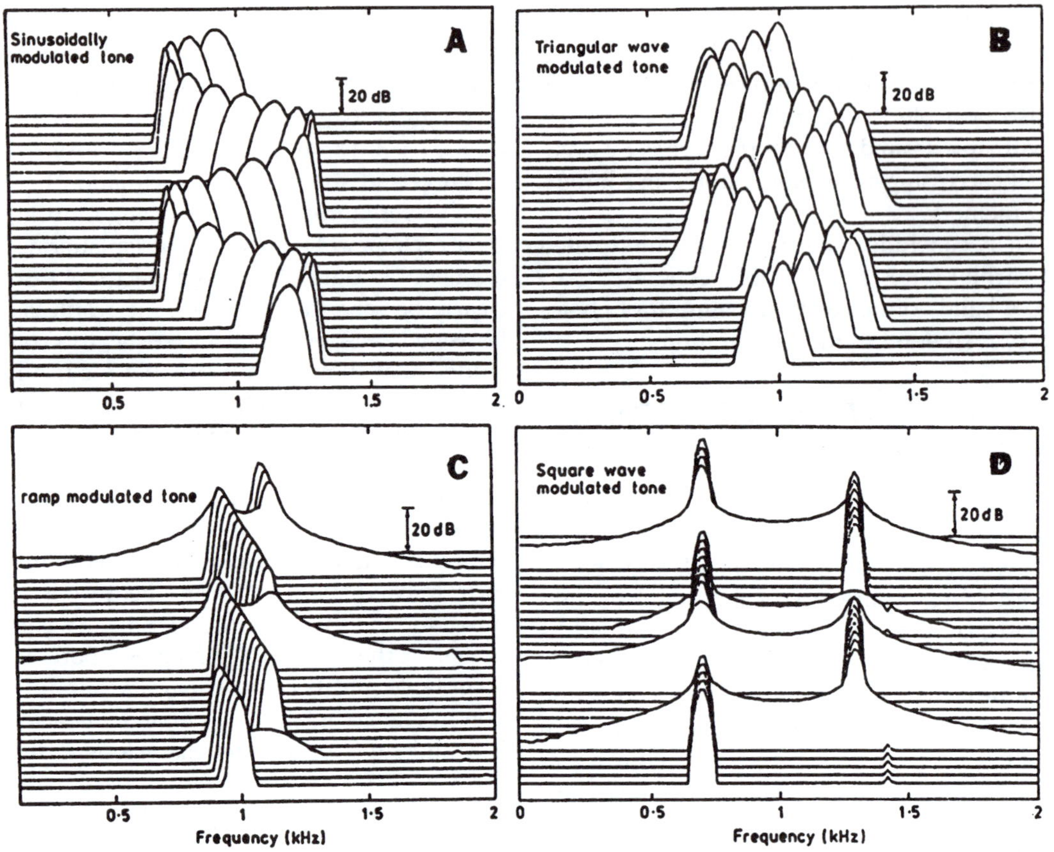

Figure 9–6. The spectra of a 1 kHz frequency modulated tone, as a function of time for **(A)** sinusoidal, **(B)** triangular, **(C)** ramp, and **(D)** square wave modulation.

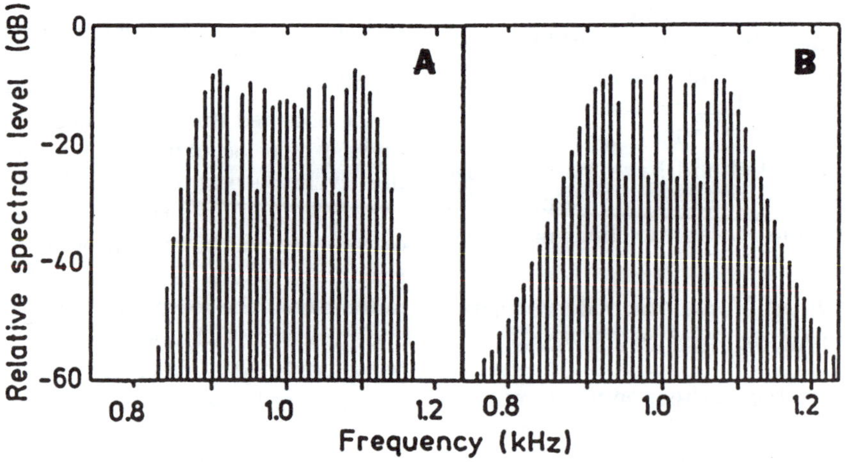

Figure 9–7. Spectra of **(A)** a sinusoidal modulated tone and **(B)** a triangularly modulated tone. Note the broader "skirts" but more uniform distribution of energy in **(B)**.

band. The physical basis of this phenomenon will not be discussed here. The important point is that Walker and Dillon's measurements indicate that if, as is usual, the signal bandwidth is a fixed percentage of the center frequency, the upper limit of the range of modulation rates will vary from frequency to frequency. More importantly, the fall off in energy beyond the band edges of FM tones is partly determined by the modulation rate, being steeper for lower modulation rates. Therefore, the maximum permissible modulation rate is not particularly important because, as steep out-of-band slopes are very desirable, the modulation rate should be kept as low as possible.

The modulation rate at which individual peaks in the response begin to be perceived will depend on the temporal integration properties of the listening ear. For persons with normal hearing, the threshold and loudness of a pure tone are independent of the duration of the tone as long as that duration is greater than 200 ms. For briefer tones, the threshold of hearing increases with decreasing duration at a rate of about 10 dB per decade of duration. The threshold for a tone of 10 ms duration, for example, will be 10 dB higher than that for the same tone of 100 ms duration. In other words, the normal ear integrates sound energy over a period of about 200 ms (see Figure 9–8).

It has been shown by investigators that persons with hearing losses of cochlear origin have abnormal auditory temporal integration with the integration time greatly reduced (e.g., Wright, 1968). The breakpoint in some cases may be as low as 10 ms.

From Walker and Dillon's (1983) measurements, it is clear that although the 5 Hz modulation rate commonly encountered in audiometers may be adequate for persons with normal hearing, it is not adequate for those with sensorineural hearing losses. It is concluded that the preferred modulation rate depends on the center frequency and band-

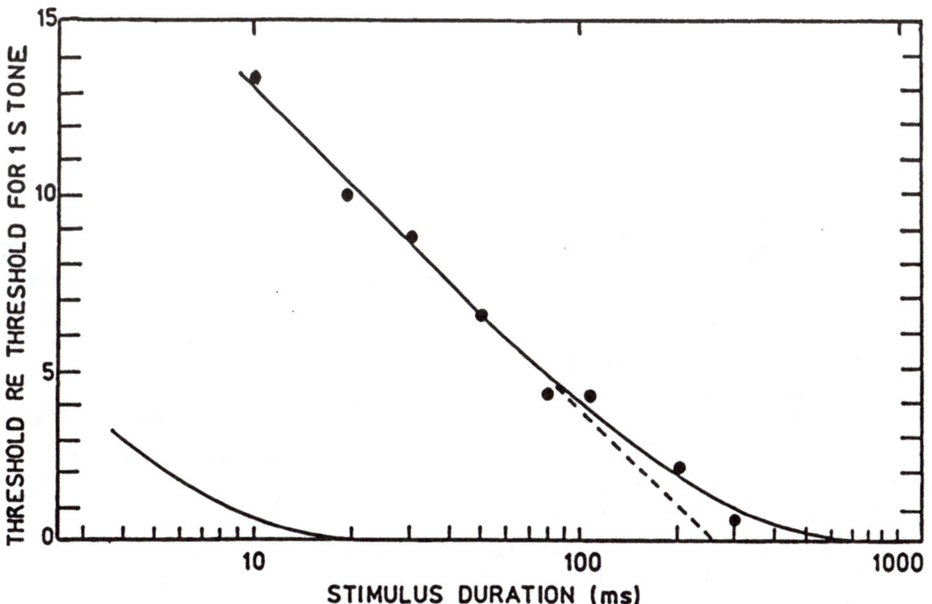

Figure 9–8. The threshold-duration function of a person with normal hearing. The threshold increases at about 10 dB per decade of time for stimulus durations less than about 200 ms. This indicates that a normal ear integrates sound energy over a 200 ms period. The curve on the left is for a subject with severe sensorineural hearing loss.

width of the tone. For the amplitude fluctuations to be fully integrated by ears with abnormal temporal integration functions, the modulation rate should be at least 20 Hz. As other considerations indicate that the modulation rate be kept as low as possible within the permissible range, if a single modulation rate is chosen to cover all frequencies, 20 Hz appears to be the best choice.

In summary, the preferred stimuli for reverberant sound field audiometry are triangularly or sinusoidally modulated FM (warble) tones or suitably generated narrow bands of noise. The optimal bandwidth of the stimulus, expressed as a percentage of the center frequency, will vary with frequency, ranging from about 30% at 0.25 kHz to 10% at 4 kHz. Stimuli with longer and smaller bandwidths than this may be needed in some circumstances, however. For FM (warble) tones the optimum modulation rate will also vary with frequency but, if a single modulation rate is required, 20 Hz is acceptable at all frequencies.

These recommendations have been adopted for use in National Acoustic Laboratory Hearing Centres throughout Australia. Evidence suggests that their use has improved the reliability of sound field audiometry (Byrne & Dillon, 1981; Cichello, 1987).

Reverberant Versus Direct Sound Field Audiometry

Discussion up to this point has been focused on reverberant field testing. It is also possible, of course, to carry out testing in the direct field; that is, in that part of the field where the inverse square law is operating. It has been demonstrated that acceptably reliable results can be obtained from direct field testing so long as certain precautions are taken (Walker, 1979; Woodford & Tecca, 1985). The crucial question is that of validity. As discussed earlier in this chapter, in most rooms, the direct field would only extend for about 0.5 to 1 m around the sound source. It is argued, therefore, that most listening is carried out under reverberant or mixed field conditions. "Face validity" would seem to favor the reverberant field. It remains an open question as to whether or not direct field testing provides useful information about aided hearing.

In direct field testing, complex stimuli have no advantages over pure tones as stimuli. Because the use of pure tones is convenient and avoids the errors associated with multifrequency stimuli, they are the stimuli of choice. It must be recognized, however, that as soon as the client's head is introduced into the field, it ceases to be a direct field. Thus, for direct field testing, the functional gain and frequency response will be influenced by the azimuth of the incident sound because of head baffle and shadow effects. The choice of testing arrangement (orientation of subject to the loudspeaker) thus becomes a significant issue. Indeed, testing with more than one arrangement may be needed to obtain an adequate description of the performance of hearing aids, especially those with directional microphones or CROS (contralateral routing of signals) fittings.

To minimize errors resulting from small movements of the subject's head toward or away from the sound source, the client should be positioned as far away from the sound source as possible (while staying in the direct field). Even so, a headrest or other restraining device should be used to restrict head movement. Even changes in the positioning of the client's shoulders can result in small changes in the signal reaching the ear (Walker, 1979).

Desirable Characteristics of the Test Room

In this section, the desirable characteristics of the room in which sound field audiometry is to be conducted will be discussed.

Absorption Characteristics

In truly anechoic conditions, the direct field extends throughout the room. Anechoic chambers, therefore, provide the ideal conditions for direct field testing as the test position can be a long way from the sound source, thus minimizing the effects of head movement. Few, if any, clinicians have access to such facilities, however.

If testing is to be carried out in a reverberant field, the question is: Should the room's surfaces be designed to maximize or minimize the amount of reflected energy? Recall the earlier comment that a highly reverberant room reinforces the sound field at the back of the room. Because the answer to the previous question was not clear on theoretical grounds, Dillon and Walker (1981) examined it experimentally. The sound field variability of pure-tone and warble-tone sound fields was measured at a large number of positions within a special room which reverberation time and absorbivity could be systematically varied. As expected for pure tones measured in the reverberant field, the peaks and troughs that occurred at any one frequency sweep became greater in number and amplitude but lesser in bandwidth as the room was made more reflective. This is illustrated in Figure 9–9, which shows the frequency-response curves for frequencies between 1 and 2 kHz as a function of distance from the loudspeaker in rooms having short, moderate, and long reverberation times. This finding supports the theoretical prediction of Schroeder and Kuttruff (1962) that the average frequency spacing between adjacent maxima is equal to 3.9 divided by the reverberation time. Remember that warble tones and bands of noise result in more uniform fields because they average the intensity over the frequencies within their passbands. This averaging is most effective when the troughs are not too deep and when they are narrower in bandwidth than the stimulus. Thus, highly reflecting rooms have the advantage of narrower troughs but the disadvantage is that these are deep and many. The measurements made with warble tones made two things clear. First, irrespective of the room's reflectivity, the stimuli with the larger bandwidths provided the more uniform fields. Second, the more reflective rooms produced fields that were inferior at all stimulus bandwidths but particularly for the narrower band stim-

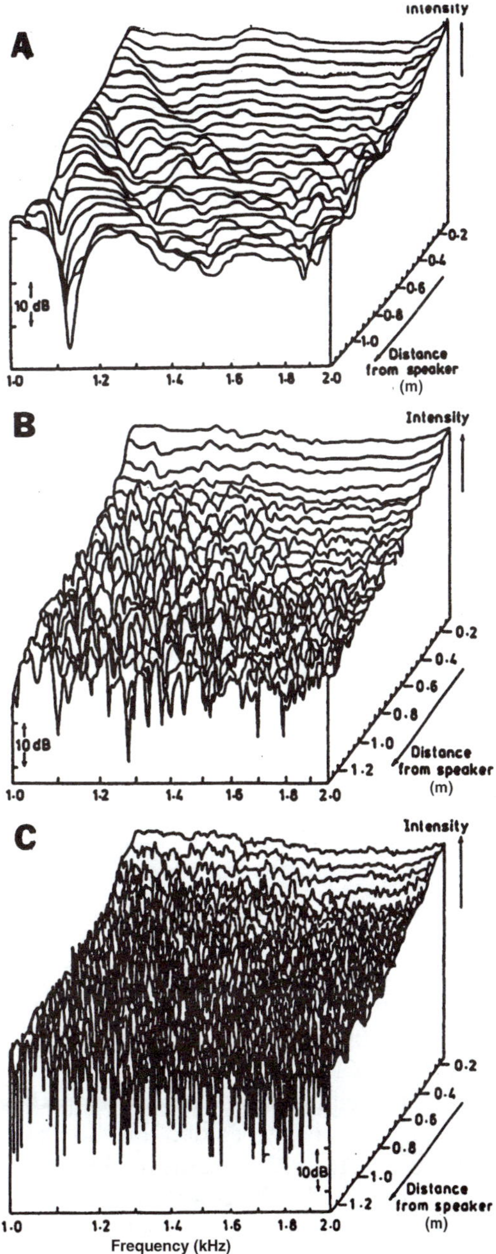

Figure 9–9. Pure tone frequency response curves for frequencies between 1 and 2 kHz as a function of distance from the sound source for **(A)** a highly absorbent audiometric test booth, **(B)** a moderately reverberant room, and **(C)** a highly reverberant room.

uli. The obvious practical implication is that the reverberation times of test rooms should be made as short as possible by making all surfaces within them as absorbing as possible.

Background Noise

Various standards specify the maximum background noise that is permissible in audiometric test rooms (e.g., ANSI S3.11977). The aim is to ensure that the background noise does not mask the stimulus and result in spuriously high thresholds. Background noise levels need to be lower for sound field testing than for testing under earphones because the earphones themselves to some extent act as attenuators. As mentioned earlier, complex construction techniques are used by booth manufacturers in order to meet standard specifications, particularly if the test room must be located in a noisy part of the building.

Macrae and Frazer (1980) have pointed out that invalid aided thresholds often result, not because of masking by background noise but because of masking by the internal noise of the hearing aid itself. Valid aided thresholds cannot be obtained if the actual threshold is lower than the equivalent input noise level (EINL) of the aid. Beck (1980) measured the EINLs of 251 different models of hearing aids and reported that the mean EINL averaged over three frequencies (1, 1.6, and 2.5 kHz), was 21.1 dB SPL with a standard deviation of 3.3 dB. Procedures have been developed for checking the validity of aided thresholds (see Macrae, 1981, 1982; Macrae & Frazer). It should be readily obvious that background noise in the test environment of the EINLs of specific hearing aid models can yield unacceptable threshold measurements.

Size and Shape of the Room

Sound wave patterns are influenced by the shape of the room. Anderson (1979) applied basic acoustic theory to devise two practical sizes for audiometric booths. Walker and colleagues (1984) cautioned, however, that test rooms having optimized dimensions may reduce, but will not eliminate, intensity irregularities in the sound field. They also stated that, to the best of their knowledge, the hypothetical advantages of rooms with such dimensions have never been quantified. They further cautioned that rooms having nonrectangular shapes will not eliminate standing wave effects. So, the only requirement regarding room size and shape is that it must be large enough to permit the subject to be seated at a sufficient distance from the loudspeaker and walls.

Test Arrangements

There are theoretical advantages to placing the loudspeaker in a three-way corner of the room, that is, the conjunction of two walls and floor or ceiling, and this is an arrangement favored by many. It must be cautioned that the advantages would be expected to be small, and several investigations have been unable to demonstrate any advantages at all (Davy, 1981; Walker & Dillon, 1984). It is concluded that the position of the loudspeaker in the room is not critical.

Calibration

A discussion of the practical issues involved in calibration of a sound field does not fall within the scope of this chapter; however, several issues need to be discussed.

Calibration serves two purposes. First, it establishes the relationship between sound pressure level, measured at some point in the field, and the corresponding attenuator setting on the signal generator. Second, it establishes the sound pressure levels corresponding to normal thresholds so that an individual's hearing level may be compared to this standard. This second type of calibration is important for diagnostic audiology but less so for hearing aid evaluation, where interest focuses on the change in threshold that results from the use of a hearing aid and upon the absolute level of sound that can be heard through the aid.

Sound field stimuli have normally been calibrated by measuring the sound pressure levels at the point in the sound field that is later to be occupied by the client's head. With this technique, the acoustic effects resulting from the introduction of the client's head into the field are automatically taken into account when thresholds are measured.

These effects are, to some extent, dependent on the particular test position, however. It can be argued that only those components of head diffraction that are constant across diverse acoustic environments should be included in the measurements. Also, any movement by the client away from the calibration point will result in an error. Use of the complex stimuli discussed in this chapter will minimize such errors, but it will not totally eliminate them. The alternative technique is to place a control microphone on or near the client's head. The output of this microphone is used to automatically control the attenuator of the signal generator in order to maintain an invariant sound pressure level at that point occupied by the microphone. Unfortunately, some error will remain because the control microphone cannot be exactly at the position of interest, that is, the hearing aid microphone post for aided testing or the client's eardrum for unaided testing. Also, head diffraction effects are not included at all in the measurements so that if one wishes to refer the measurements to the sound pressure level in the undisturbed field, average head diffraction effects must be assumed. Again, errors will be minimized by the use of complex stimuli. Dillon (1982) quantified the errors associated with both calibration procedures and concluded that, on average, the errors were less when the control microphone technique was used.

One other issue remains to be discussed. For all complex stimuli used in sound field testing, intensity at the client's ear will vary with time. Even those stimuli such as warble tones that do not contain temporal intensity fluctuations when generated will do so at the client's ear as a result of peaks and troughs in the room's frequency response being sequentially excited as the tone sweeps across its frequency band. Earlier it was suggested that it is desirable that sound field thresholds be relatable to pure tone thresholds obtained with audiometric earphones. For this to be achieved, the sound field stimulus must be measured in a way that mimics the temporal integration function of the human ear. From an experiment in which Plomp and Bauman's (1959) "leaky integrator" model of threshold detection was applied, Dillon and Walker (1980) devised just such a method. Unfortunately, this method is not clinically feasible, as it involves the derivation of individual calibration figures for each client. Fortunately, an acceptably accurate approximation can be obtained by reading the peak deflections of a sound level meter in the "RMS fast" mode.

SUMMARY

This chapter has examined the acoustic properties of rooms, with specific reference to the practice of sound field audiometry. A major impediment to accurate audiometric testing in a reverberant or diffuse sound field is the variability of the sound pressure level of the field as a function of both the frequency of the sound and the measurement position in the field. Methods for minimizing these errors have been discussed. Frequency-modulated tones with optimized parameters or suitably generated narrow bands of noise, again with optimized parameters, are proposed as stimuli for reverberant field testing. Direct field sound field audiometry has also been discussed, and it is concluded that in this case, complex stimuli offer no advantages over pure tone. Accurate testing in the direct field is only possible if the client's head can be sufficiently immobilized or if the testing is performed under anechoic conditions, however. Desirable room characteristics and suitable calibration procedures have been considered. If the materials and techniques described in this chapter are employed, it is possible to achieve the same degree of reliability in sound field audiometry as is achieved in traditional audiometry under earphones.

REVIEW QUESTIONS

1. What is sound field audiometry and why has it come to be more widely used as part of the hearing aid selection and fitting process?
2. What is a reverberant sound field?
3. Describe what happens to a sound wave that is absorbed by an object.
4. Describe the four qualities of a suitable sound field stimulus.
5. What are some of the arguments against the use of damped wave trains as stimuli?
6. Why are ramp and square wave modulation not suitable for use in sound field audiometry?
7. What is the preferred stimuli for reverberant sound field audiometry?
8. Why might the validity of direct sound field audiometry be questioned?
9. Describe the ideal characteristics of the test room in which sound field audiometry is to be conducted.

REFERENCES

Anderson, C. D. (1979). New ideas in sound field systems. *Hearing Instruments, 30,* 12–13, 43.

ANSI. (S3.11977). *American standard criteria for background noise in audiometer rooms.* New York: American Standards Association, Inc.

Beck, L.. (Ed.). (1980). *Handbook of hearing aid measurement.* Washington, DC: Veterans Administration.

Byrne, D. J., & Dillon, H. (1981). Comparative reliability of warble tone thresholds under earphones and in sound field. *Australian Journal of. Audioliology, 3,* 12–14.

Cichello, P. (1987). Sound field visual reinforcement orientation audiometry revisited. *Australian Journal of Audiology, 8,* 12–17.

Davy, J. L. (1981). The relative variance of the transmission function of a reverberation room. *Journal of Sound and Vibration, 77,* 455–479.

Dillon, H. (1982). The use of a control microphone in reverberant sound field audiometric testing. *Journal of the Acoustical Society of America, 72*(Suppl. 1), S108.

Dillon, H., & Walker, G. (1980). The perception of normal hearing persons of intensity fluctuations in narrow band stimuli and its implications for sound field calibration procedures. *Australian Journal of Audiology, 2,* 72–82.

Dillon, H., & Walker, G. (1981). The effect of acoustic environment on the reliability of sound field audiometry. *Australian Journal of Audiology, 3,* 67–72.

Dillon, H., & Walker, G. (1982a). Comparison of stimuli used in sound field audiometric testing. *Journal of the Acoustical Society of America, 71,* 161–172.

Dillon, H., & Walker, G. (1982b). The selection of modulation waveform for frequency modulated sound field stimuli. *Australian Journal of Audiology, 4,* 56–61.

Dillon, H., & Walker, G. (1982c, November). *An optimum bandwidth for audiometric sound field stimuli.* Paper presented at the annual American Speech and Hearing Association convention, Toronto, Canada.

Goldberg, H. (1979, March). Discrete sound field audiometry. *Hearing Journal,* pp. 42–43.

Lippman, R., & Adams, D. (1982). A 1/3 octave band noise generator for soundfield audiometric measurements. *Journal of Speech and Hearing Disorders, 47,* 84–88.

Macrae, H. J. (1981). *Invalid aided thresholds and equivalent input noise levels* (NAL Informal Report No. 81). Sydney, Australia: National Acoustics Laboratories.

Macrae, H. J. (1982). The validity of aided thresholds. *Australian Journal of Audiology, 4,* 48–54.

Macrae, H. J., & Frazer, G. (1980). An investigation of variables affecting aided thresholds. *Australian Journal of Audiology, 2,* 56–62.

Morgan, D. E., Dirks, D. D., & Bower, D. R. (1979). Suggested threshold sound pressure levels for frequency modulated (warble) tones in the sound field. *Journal of Speech and Hearing Disorders, 44,* 37–54.

Orchik, D., & Mosher, N. (1975). Narrow band noise audiometry: The effect of filter slope. *Journal of the American Audiology Society, 1,* 50–53.

Orchik, D., & Rintelmann, W. (1978). Comparison of pure-tone, warble-tone and narrow band noise thresholds of young normal hearing children. *Journal of the American Audiology Society, 3,* 214–220.

Plomp, R., & Bouman, M. (1959). Relation between hearing threshold and duration for tone pulses. *Journal of the Acoustical Society of America, 31,* 749–758.

Rosler, G., & Anderson, H. (1978). Maximum steepness of slopes in hearing threshold curves. *Audiology, 17,* 299–316.

Schroeder, M. R., & Kuttruff, K H. (1962). On frequency response curves in rooms. Comparison of experimental, theoretical and Monte Carlo results for the average spacing between maxima. *Journal of the Acoustical Society of America, 34,* 76–80.

Stephens, M., & Rintelmann, W. (1978). The influence of audiometric configuration on pure tone, warble-tones, and narrow band noise thresholds of adults with sensorineural hearing losses. *Journal of the American Audiology Society, 3,* 221–226.

Victoreen, J. (1974). Equal loudness pressure determined with a decaying oscillatory waveform. *Journal of the Acoustical Society of America, 55,* 309–312.

Walker, G. (1979). The pure tone in sound field testing. Experimental results and suggested procedures. *Australian Journal of Audiology, 1,* 49–60.

Walker, G., & Dillon, H. (1983). The selection of modulation rates for frequency modulated sound field stimuli. *Scandinavian Audiology, 12,* 151–156.

Walker, G., Dillon, H., & Byrne, D. (1984). Sound field audiometry: Recommended stimuli and procedures. *Ear and Hearing, 5,* 13–21.

Woodford, C. M., & Tecca, J. (1985, June). The use of pure-tone stimuli in a sound field. *Hearing Journal,* 21–27.

Wright, H. H. (1968). The effect of sensorineural hearing loss on threshold-duration functions. *Journal of Speech and Hearing Research, 11,* 842–852.

Zwislocki, J. (1951). Eine verbesserte Vertaubungsmethode für die Audiometric. *Acta Oto-Laryngologica, 39,* 338–356.

CHAPTER 10

Sound Field Assessment: Hearing Aids and Related Issues

ROBERT E. SANDLIN, PH.D.

OUTLINE

HISTORICAL PERSPECTIVE

SUBJECTIVE ASSESSMENT IN HEARING AID FITTING

OBJECTIVE MEASURES IN HEARING AID FITTING

APPLICATION OF FITTING FORMULAE

SOUND FIELD ACOUSTIC CONDITIONS

PATIENT PLACEMENT IN A SOUND FIELD

SPEECH OR SPEECHLIKE STIMULI IN A SOUND FIELD

- Magnitude Estimation
- Phoneme Recognition
- Paired Comparison

DETERMINING MOST COMFORTABLE LISTENING LEVEL

More than 10 years have passed since the introduction of the first edition of the *Handbook of Hearing Aid Amplification*. In addition to the more conventional procedures involved in sound field assessment, a number of subjective scales for determining satisfaction, acceptance, and benefit have been developed. Some of these are administered in a sound field to assist in the proper selection of hearing aid devices and the subsequent determination of benefit. For example, the Speech Intelligibility Rating (SIR) test developed by Cox and McDaniels (1984) has been useful in assessing differences among hearing aids when speech stimuli are presented in a noise background. The use of various scales to assess satisfaction, benefit, and acceptance represents a positive step involving the person with hearing impairment in the decision-making process.

For any professional discipline, change is inevitable. The absence of change results in intellectual stagnation and a downward spiraling of the effectiveness of a discipline or a professional organization. Depending on the underlying motivation for change, it may be orderly or random. Orderly change suggests that one builds on the level of knowledge available to enhance the performance and benefit of hearing aid amplification. Random change suggests that new technologies are introduced, or new and innovative clinical procedures are developed, that contribute to the skills of the hearing health care professional. There have been significant changes over the past 10 years or so in how audiologists and clinicians assess the benefits of amplification. Many of these changes have been related to objective clinical methods, suggested either by various fitting formulae or in instrumental measurement exemplified by real-ear (probe microphone) assessment.

In this revision, the major task is to review the value of sound field assessment in the hearing aid selection and fitting process. In the truest sense, sound field assessment includes procedures that use acoustic stimuli presented through a calibrated loudspeaker system in a sound-level-controlled environment rather than through calibrated headphones. In a much larger sense, however, this chapter stresses subjective assessment in hearing aid selection and fitting. It may appear very basic to suggest that only through subjective measurement can one obtain hard data on the processing capabilities of the auditory system. To fit hearing aid devices without some assessment of the patient's ability to utilize hearing aid amplification in communicative situations is untenable. The contributions of sound field measurements are not a panacea, nor do they replace or render obsolete the contributions of more objective measures. The sound field does not have to be anechoic to be of significant clinical value. As a matter of fact, anechoic conditions may be contraindicated when evaluating a patient's performance with hearing instruments because they eliminate acoustic conditions encountered in the real world of communicative function.

HISTORICAL PERSPECTIVE

In the late 1930s, the Speech and Hearing Center at the University of Wisconsin was among the first to introduce the clinical value of sound field evaluation. The Speech and Hearing Center was under the direction of Dr. Robert West, a prominent figure of the time and a frequent contributor to the scientific literature. During and after World War II, it was not uncommon for university- and hospital-based speech and hearing centers to use sound field testing in rehabilitation programs for veterans with hearing loss. Many World War II veterans incurred hearing impairment due to their war experiences. The underlying principle dictating the use of sound field assessment was that of providing information about the patient's response to acoustic stimuli with and without a hearing aid. Although the validity of some sound field measurement was questioned by some, information gained contributed to the value of the hearing aid selection process.

A number of investigators reported on the applications, contributions, and value of some form of sound field assessment (Carhart, 1946; Cox & McDaniel, 1992; Duffy, 1967, 1978; Farby & Schum, 1994; Gabrielson et al., 1988; Goldberg, 1981; Preves, 1984; Punch & Parker, 1978; Ross & Duffy, 1961; Sandlin, 1990; Studebaker & Sherbecoe, 1988; Sweetow, 1994; Valente et al., 1994, 1994, 1996; Victoreen, 1973; Walker, 1981; Walker et al., 1984; Zelnick, 1982).

In hearing instrument dispensing, early attempts to reasonably conclude that a given hearing aid was appropriately fitted utilized some form of sound field assessment. Patients were placed in a sound-controlled environment and instructed to respond to one or more acoustic stimuli. By carefully selecting the stimuli, the clinician could be certain that differences between the patient's aided and unaided responses were strong indicators of probable success with the hearing aid. An acoustic stimulus might have been a phonetically balanced word, connected discourse, pure tone, warble tone, narrow bands of noise, amplitude modulated signal, damped wave train, or a variety of other signals. The patient's response to the stimulus was the final arbiter in deciding the value of the amplification system under test. Even though hearing aid selection procedures differed from one facility to another, clinicians generally assumed the instrument that performed best, by whichever criteria, was the instrument of choice.

Many investigators have reported the utility of sound field assessment, but the introduction and utilization of probe tube microphone measurements provided a means for a stable, objective, and repeatable assessment of hearing aid performance. More definitive control over the electroacoustic response parameters of the hearing aid is possible through use of a probe microphone system (see Chapter 3).

Over the past several years, there has been a movement among many hearing health care professionals to embrace new, challenging, and exciting procedures, which provide useful clinical information not available prior to the introduction of the technology. Unfortunately, there is also a tendency for some to discard older procedures that have provided useful information. One would hope that objective measures of hearing aid performance do not entirely replace subjective measures of performance and patient acceptance. The exclusive use of objective measures, to the exclusion of a more subjectively based assessment protocol, may deny the clinician a wealth of information that contributes significantly to the successful use of hearing aid amplification.

A number of years ago, the author asked Dr. James Jerger (1987) what he thought about the clinical utility of sound field assessment. The following is his reply to that question:

> Although systems for the measurement of real ear gain of hearing aids represent a significant technologic advance over analogous closed coupler measurements in quantifying the frequency response of a hearing aid system, it is important to remember that successful fitting of a hearing aid involves much more than the determination of the optimal frequency response. The audiologist must answer the following questions:
>
> 1. Is the use of any hearing aid appropriate?
> 2. What is the best arrangement and configuration of the hearing aid system (e.g., BTE, ITE, canal aid; monaural vs. binaural; CROS, BICROS, etc.)?
> 3. Does the patient perform adequately with the recommended aid in the sense of understanding speech in realistic environments?
> 4. Is there a better solution than a hearing aid (i.e., assistive listening device)?
>
> To answer these questions, a thoughtful and responsible audiologist must necessarily incorporate into the evaluative system measures that go far beyond the real ear frequency response. They will typically involve some measure of the patient's ability to understand real speech in a realistic environment. They may involve quality judgements, paired comparison, adaptive measures of signal-to-noise ratio, or more traditional speech audiometric measures. Whatever their nature, however, they will broaden the evaluative spectrum beyond the narrow confines of frequency responses.

Dr. Jerger's remarks are just as appropriate now as they were in 1987. In essence, his message is that one must not abandon clinical procedures that assist the hearing health care professional in making decisions about the appropriateness of selected hearing aid systems. This is not to suggest that audiologists and others have completely abandoned sound field assessment to determine performance and benefit, but rather that absolute reliance on real-ear assessment may not be the complete answer to the hearing instrument selection process.

One can safely argue that sound field and probe tube measurements provide distinctly different kinds of performance information. Sound field measures provide information about the patient's response to acoustic signal(s) processed by the auditory system. The patient judges whether the signal is present or absent, loud or soft, distorted or undistorted, intelligible or unintelligible. Sound field measures determine, in part, the degree to which patient satisfaction, acceptance, and benefit have been achieved. Sound field assessment involves the patient in the decision-making process and also provides critical information to the dispenser relative to changes that need to be made to achieve maximum benefit, acceptance, and satisfaction.

Probe microphone measurements provide objective electroacoustic information about the performance characteristics of an acoustic signal impinging on the eardrum. This chapter does not attempt to pit one assessment protocol against the other, which contributes little to understanding the needs of persons with hearing impairment. It has not conclusively been demonstrated that one assessment method is more valid than another in determining the hearing aid of choice. There is sufficient evidence to suggest that both methods provide specific information about the performance of the hearing aid under test.

The reader may question why a portion of this chapter devoted to sound field assessment deals with objective measurement of hearing aid performance. The purpose is to demonstrate that both objective and subjective measurements contribute to the determination of "optimal" amplification needs for the individual with hearing impairment. This chapter, in part, reviews the advantages and limitations of sound field testing in determining hearing aid performance and its appropriateness for the patient with hearing impairment. More importantly, it emphasizes subjective assessment and its contribution to the decision-making process, suggesting that when used intelligently the principles underlying sound field assessment can be of clinical value. It is not intended to provide "how-to" information, but rather to stress the utility of sound field assessment as an integral part of the fitting of hearing aid devices.

SUBJECTIVE ASSESSMENT IN HEARING AID FITTING

Subjective assessment is defined as the testing of the manner in which individuals perceive and process acoustic information. It involves the physical event (the sound) and the psychological events (perception and processing). It includes psychoacoustics, which has been defined as the branch of psychophysics which *deals with the quantification of sensation and the measurement of the psychological correlates of the physical stimulus. Psychoacoustics thus embraces the study of the psychological response to acoustical stimulation* (Durrant & Lovrinic, 1984, p. 214).

Subjective assessment implies more than just the perception of acoustic stimuli. It involves

- Judging the contribution of perceived sounds to the intelligibility of the intended message.
- Measuring sound quality by the introduction of rating scales, which reflect patients' perception of sound quality. It involves a process through which the patient determines whether a complex, amplified acoustic signal enhanceS speech intelligibility.
- Evaluation and determination of whether or not two or more acoustic signals can be discriminated when delivered to the ear at the same time.

(Obviously, some of these measurements can be made through calibrated earphones.) The point to be emphasized, however, is that the measurements referred to here are made with the hearing aid in place. It signifies appraising whether or not the auditory system perceives loudness changes in a normal or abnormal manner. Some type of subjective sound field assessment has been used for a number of years by engineering laboratories to make some differentiation among sound transmission circuitry (McDermott, 1968; Munson et al., 1962).

Sound field assessment refers to responses to acoustic signals produced in a sound field. Audiologists and hearing instrument dispensers of a decade ago used sound field assessment in some form to make the final determination of successful hearing aid use more frequently than do audiologists and dispensers today. The introduction and clinical application of probe tube measurements and the subsequent emphasis placed on its "objective significance" lessened reliance on sound field assessment. Sound field measures fall into the behavioral category of subjective measurement known as psychoacoustics—the study of human perception and response to acoustic events.

The following are some psychoacoustic measures that have been used in evaluating the response of the human auditory system to acoustic stimuli. Normally, these procedures are presented in the aided and unaided condition in a sound field:

- *Preferred listening level:* the level at which the patient judges speech to be at its optimal level for attending to sustained discourse. It is a form of the most comfortable listening level (MCL).
- *Uncomfortable listening level (UCL):* the level at which the patient judges speech or other acoustic signals to be uncomfortably loud. That is, any further increase in the acoustic energy might result in the rejection of amplification. UCLs predicted by a fitting formula need to reassessed to meet patient acceptance.
- *Word recognition score:* the percentage of selected words correctly identified when presented at an optimal listening level in a variety of listening environments. Although word recognition scores do not guarantee hearing aid acceptance, they do represent a beneficial assessment tool.

- *Binaural performance:* the contribution to the perception and discrimination of acoustic signals presented to both ears, as opposed to one ear only. Normally, binaural amplification offers additional benefit to the hearing instrument user. Such benefits include, but are not limited to, location of sound in space, the squelch affect, circumferential hearing, improvement in threshold sensitivity, and spatial separation of signal and noise.
- *Word recognition in noise:* the discrimination of words in the presence of background noise at some specified signal-to-noise ratio (SNR).
- *Dynamic range:* the subjective assessment of the level at which a given acoustic signal violates the uncomfortable listening level subtracted from the level at which the patient is barely able to detect the presence of that signal.
- *Rollover phenomenon:* the phenomenon occurring when, above a certain input intensity level, word identification is degraded. Obviously, this can be assessed through earphones; however, this chapter is concerned with the assessment of acoustic stimuli processed through a hearing aid device when fitted to the ear of the patient.
- *Central processing disorder:* a disorder in which the peripheral auditory system is functioning adequately, but other, more central, structures such as the brainstem, midbrain, and the auditory cortex are incapable of normal processing of speech and other acoustic signals.
- *Speech reception threshold:* the presentation level at which the patient is able to correctly identify 50% of the bisyllabic words presented.
- *Difference limen for frequency (pitch):* the point at which the patient can just detect differences between two signals of different frequencies when presented at the same level.
- *Difference limen for intensity (loudness):* the point at which the patient can just detect differences between signals of different intensities.
- *Loudness growth:* the rate of perceived loudness growth as the intensity of the input signal increases.
- *Magnitude estimation:* the subjective intelligibility rating (usually expressed as a percentage) of speech or speechlike material presented at specified output levels.
- *Pure tone threshold sensitivity:* the point at which the individual perceives the presence of a pure tone signal (sinusoid).

Obviously, not all of these tests are performed in a sound field all of the time on all patients fitted with hearing instruments, but the length of the list reflects the value of psychoacoustic measures conducted in a sound field to evaluate auditory processing function. Most who select and fit hearing aids conclude that the patient is the final arbiter of perceived benefit. This is true regardless of the method(s) employed to determine the electroacoustic properties of the hearing aid. The reasoning is quite obvious. Regardless of the objective means by which hearing instruments are evaluated, the patient determines whether an instrument is acceptable. Although the clinician may have selected an instrument that met all of the objective, electroacoustic criteria (audibility, comfort, ease of listening, loudness growth, frequency range, etc.), there is that unknown "X" factor of human behavior that, for some patients, dictates against the use of amplification.

OBJECTIVE MEASURES IN HEARING AID FITTING

Objective measures do not require an overt response from the patient during the hearing aid assessment process or, more accurately, they do not require some intentional or cognitive processing of the acoustic signal(s) to which the patient is asked to attend. A patient's threshold response to a pure-tone signal submitted in a sound field is considered by some to be objective. The person either hears it or does not. In another sense, it is subjective. The patient decides whether the signal was heard. The same is true when a patient is asked whether a signal is too loud or too soft. It is an either-or response. Additionally, because the patient either does or does not correctly identify the word, some argument can be made that a word recognition score is also an objective assessment. One may argue that the essential difference is that subjectivity implies some central processing of any acoustic event preceding a voluntary response.

Among the methods used in objective assessment is real-ear probe tube measurement. In real-ear measurement, the examiner places a probe tube close to the tympanic membrane, presents a sound, and measures its acoustic characteristics. The examiner judges if the acoustic signal at the eardrum meets predetermined criteria. Mueller, Hawkins, and Northern (1992) have written an excellent textbook to which the reader is referred to gain a better understanding of probe tube measurement and its contribution. A number of acronyms have been proposed to reflect the utility of real-ear probe tube measurements. Among them are the following:

- **REIG** (real ear insertion gain): the real ear response in which gain is a value expressed in dB at a specific frequency
- **REAR** (real ear aided response): the real ear response in an occluded ear canal with the aid turned on
- **REUR** (real ear unaided response): the real ear response without a hearing aid or earmold inserted into the ear canal
- **REIR** (real ear insertion response): the real ear difference between the REUR and the REAR to the same stimulus under the same sound field condition
- **REOR** (real ear occluded response): the real ear response in an occluded ear canal with the instrument turned off
- **RESR** (real ear saturation response): the real ear response to a stimulus intensity to cause the hearing aid to function at its maximum output
- **RECD** (real ear coupler difference): the real ear response expresses the difference in gain function between real ear and 2-c coupler.

Each measurement provides information about the acoustic signal(s) at the eardrum and whether predetermined criteria are met. Furthermore, probe tube measurements are conducted in a sound field, in which the ambient conditions of that field are held constant. Nonreverberant and reverberant sound field conditions affecting measurement reliability have been reported by Hawkins and Mueller (1986) and Tecca (1990). Mueller and Hawkins reported significant differences between reverberant and nonreverberant conditions affecting test-retest reliability. Tecca reported no significant differences between the two conditions. It is highly probable that test conditions were not the same for each study, thus the differences in the results reported. Reverberation is best explained as the persistence of sound waves generated in a sound field to reflect off hard surfaces and the walls of the sound chamber. The time it takes for a sound to decrease by 60 dB in level is referred to as the *reverberation time.*

APPLICATION OF FITTING FORMULAE

There have been a number of individual efforts over the past several decades to develop an effective and objective fitting method to determine the hearing aid performance requirements to meet patients' acoustic needs. These efforts have resulted in a number of fitting formulae. Most methods suggest that recommended target gains for selected frequencies, based on pure tone thresholds, are those best suited to meet the amplification demands of the patient (see Chapter 11). The following list of fitting methods is not exhaustive. It may serve, however, to underscore the continuing search for quasi-objective methods to be employed in the successful selection and fitting of hearing aid devices:

- Balbi (1930)
- Watson and Knudsen (1940)
- Lybarger (1944)
- Carhart (1946)

- Davis (1954)
- Redell and Calvert (1966)
- Key (1972)
- Victoreen (1973)
- Pascoe (1975)
- Byrne and Tonnison (1976)
- Skinner (1976)
- Berger (1977)
- McCandless and Lyregaard (1983)
- Cox (1985)
- Byrne and Dillon (1986), National Acoustics Laboratory of Australia (NAL) *Note:* There have been revisions to the NAL procedure that have contributed to its effective use.
- Libby (1986).

For the most part, the intent of each fitting method was to make the speech spectrum audible to the person with hearing impairment. Most approaches suggested the degree to which specific frequencies should be amplified (insertion gain) to achieve audibility of the speech spectrum. For example, in Figure 10–1, recommended insertion gains for three divergent fitting methods for a moderately sloping high frequency hearing loss are shown. The gain response for each method has been normalized at 1000 Hz. The fitting methods shown here are those of Berger, Libby, and Lybarger. They do not predict the same recommended insertion gain values for the same target frequencies. Although these differences exist, it does not mean that such methods cannot be useful. It suggests, rather, that the clinician should select the method best representing the acoustic needs of the patient, and therein lies the problem. Because each fitting method recommends different insertion gain values, how does one determine the fitting strategy best corresponding to an individual patient's acoustic needs? Furthermore, does the clinician want to normalize the acoustic response or equalize the response to achieve the desired goal? Normalization can be defined as the restoration of normal loudness for an impaired auditory system by assigning the same gain for the same degree of hearing loss. In this case, one assumes that the goal of amplification is the restoration of normal loudness. On the other hand, the goal of most prescriptive formulae is that of equalization. Equalization can be defined as an attempt to make each frequency region equally loud by providing different gain functions for the same degree of hearing loss. Equalization is the end goal of most fitting methods using linear amplifiers.

Normally, some clinical experimentation is needed to determine if one fitting method is superior to another. To some extent, all of the fitting methods listed here compromise the ideal amplification needs for different listening environments. That is, most fitting formulae specify the best output response for quiet listening environments. None recommends the appropriate responses for listening in various types of environmental backgrounds such as crowd noise, traffic noise, industrial noise, speech babble, and so forth.

Most of the currently accepted fitting protocols to determine insertion gain requirements are based on sensorineural losses, occluding earmolds, and linear amplifiers. Linear amplifiers do not change their acoustic gain response as the listening environment changes. A digital signal processing instrument or a nonlinear analog, multimemory hearing aid are probably instruments of choice to meet amplification needs as a function of listening environment. With the myriad of digitally programmable and digital signal processing hearing aids available, the clinician is faced with the task of deciding the electroacoustic response best suited for a given listening condition. The reader is referred to Valente, Valente, and Potts' definitive work (1996) for an overview of analog programmable hearing aid instrumentation and their utility.

Regardless of the fitting method employed, real-ear probe tube measurement is an effective tool in measuring and validating response parameters, such as insertion gain. It is a reasonably rapid and accurate measurement of insertion gain at selected target frequencies. It offers positive confirmation of whether target gains have been achieved. The closer the actual gain of the hearing aid is to

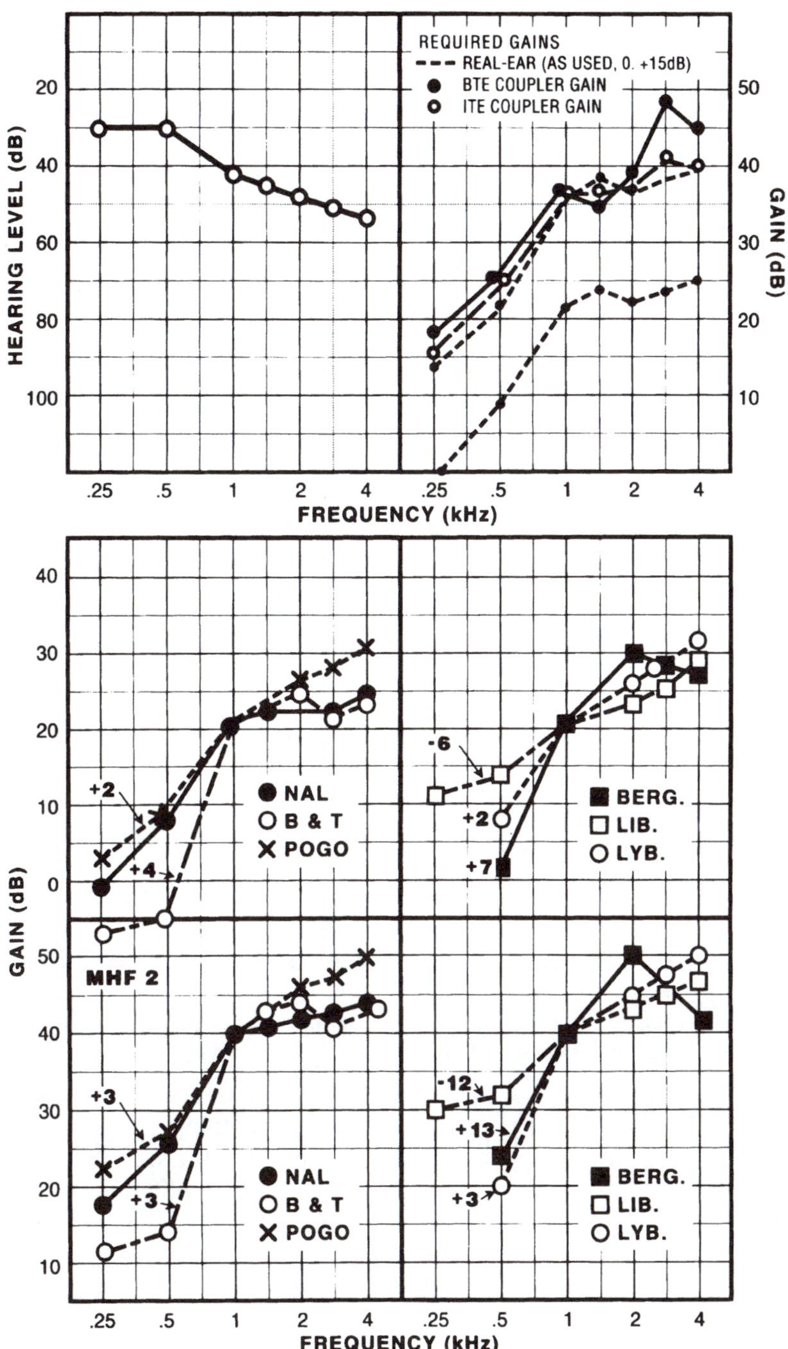

Figure 10–1. Recommended insertion gain for a moderately sloping high frequency hearing impairment using three different fitting methods. Note that required target gain differs from one method to another.

the target gain, the more appropriate the hearing aid.

Current prescriptive methods define what the insertion gain should be for a linear hearing device. They fail to accurately define hearing aid response when the input is increased or when nonlinear hearing aids are used. There is no broadbased acceptance of selection and fitting guidelines for setting the electroacoustic parameters for instruments with compression or other automatic signal processing functions. Fabry and Schum (1994, p. 136) made the following comments regarding the utility of probe microphone assessment and the application of fitting formulae:

> . . . other problems hamper this approach, including (1) there are nearly a dozen published prescriptive threshold formulae, and none has been demonstrated to be clearly superior to all others; (2) it is difficult to quantify what is meant by an "adequate " match to target gain; (3) many prescriptive formulae do not include prescription of maximum hearing aid output levels; and (4) these methods do not suffice for many of the advanced circuits such as automatic signal processing (ASP) or programmable hearing aids that have low compression thresholds (i.e., 45–55 dB SPL) and variable compression ratios.
>
> A primary issue becomes the accuracy of a hearing aid fitting model that uses only puretone thresholds and probe tube measurements for prescription and assessment of hearing aid performance, respectively. This strategy disregards the preferences of the person who ultimately provides the final determinant of hearing aid effectiveness.

The issue is not whether objective or subjective procedures can be clinically defended. The issue is whether the acoustic needs of the patients are met by the clinical method employed. One would like to think that when insertion gain requirements are met at target frequencies, acceptance is guaranteed. Unfortunately, there is no consensus as to how closely the target gain must be met for a patient to accept the hearing aid. Interestingly, when the clinician is unsure of the appropriateness of the instrument based on the obtained insertion gain function, some type of sound field assessment is employed in making the final determination. Let us assume, for example, that the patient is unsure of the benefit received based solely on meeting target gain requirements. In some instances, a simple paired-comparison procedure may be employed. That is, the clinician will modify the insertion gain at selected target frequencies and then ask the patient to make some determination of perceived benefit based on some predetermined criteria. Even though assessment of instrument function in the aided mode is an objective procedure, subjective measures often are used to gain patient acceptance.

SOUND FIELD ACOUSTIC CONDITIONS

To achieve reliable and repeatable psychoacoustic measurements in a sound field, it is necessary to place the patient in an area where ambient noise levels are controlled. A sound-treated test chamber is bounded by the walls, floor, and ceiling. The construction of such a test environment should not permit ambient sounds to interfere with the patient's ability to respond to acoustic stimuli presented by the examiner or to interfere with the assessment of benefit. To create an optimal test environment, the sound field should be acoustically treated to reduce sound reverberation (standing waves) to a minimum. If the acoustic stimulus from a sound field speaker becomes highly reverberant, it may interfere with the patient's recognition or with accurate assessment of the test signal(s). To create permissible test conditions, the use of sound-absorbing materials that dampen sounds in the test chamber and reduce standing waves to a negligible amount is necessary. In the "real world," some sound reverberation is present in the listening environment and constitutes part of a normal listening condition. Nonetheless, the task is one of constructing a test chamber in which standing waves or reverberation do not create acoustic conditions that degrade the patient's ability to respond appropriately to the test stimuli. (This statement does not imply that some investigative approaches may not measure reverberation times and their effect on word or speech recognition.)

Sound field acoustics have been defined as being reverberating or direct. A direct sound field is dominated by directly radiated sound. Sound generated at the source (the sound field speaker) radiates directly to the listener, or the individual under test. A reverberant sound field is dominated by the reflected sound from surfaces within the test chamber. The degree to which a reverberating sound field can be controlled will determine the accuracy of acoustic measurements conducted in that field. One doesn't need to create an anechoic chamber to conduct sound field tests to select and fit hearing aids. A direct field is present throughout an anechoic test chamber. There is no reflected sound that alters the sound pressure at the eardrum of the test subject. To create an anechoic environment would be expensive and of questionable clinical value for the evaluation of hearing aids when worn by the patient. Few professionals have access to, need, or can afford such a test facility.

The dispenser should be aware of the need to control sound levels within the test chamber. External ambient sounds must not interfere with the patient's ability to properly assess test signals generated within the chamber. To attenuate outside sounds, the test chamber is constructed of materials that provide stiffness and mass. The degree to which external sounds are attenuated depends on the types and amount of material used in the construction of the sound room. The level of sound attenuation is frequency specific. Low frequencies, having longer wavelengths, are more difficult to attenuate than higher frequencies having shorter wavelengths.

Ambient noise levels in the test chamber might interfere with measuring organic thresholds (Macrae & Frazer 1980; Zemplenyi, Dirks, & Gilman, 1985). As mentioned previously, unless one can afford the expense of constructing something that approaches the characteristics of an anechoic chamber, the hearing health care professional must accept some minimal error in threshold assessment, regardless of its magnitude. It is generally accepted that, as long as the ambient noise in the sound chamber is at or below 45 dB(A), the effect on reliable measures of hearing aid performance is minimal.

Figure 10–2 shows the average hearing threshold sensitivity to selected pure tones in a sound room. The ambient noise level is at or below 45 dB(A). All threshold measures are expressed in sound pressure level (SPL). Measurements were made with the sound source at 90° azimuth. The sound field speakers were placed approximately 9 in. from a Type 2 sound level meter, positioned where the person's head would be during the various tests.

A 45 dB(A) ambient level may interfere with audibility as the azimuth or distance from the speaker-to-ear is altered. Most patients tested in a sound field have a bilateral hearing impairment. For these patients, a 45 dB(A) ambient noise level would seldom create a problem in obtaining reliable threshold measurements over a broad frequency range.

PATIENT PLACEMENT IN A SOUND FIELD

Accurate sound field measurement of an individual's response to acoustic stimuli is not without problems. Patients must be positioned so that the desired signal level at the ear is not greatly influenced by sound room characteristics. Placement of the patient in a sound field, in part, is determined by the test to be performed. (Harford 1969; Hodgson 1986: Pollack 1988; Skinner 1988; Valente et al., 1994). The sound pressure level of a given signal at the patient's ear should be constant and not influenced by standing waves. If a stable sound field cannot be accomplished, signal intensity at the eardrum can vary

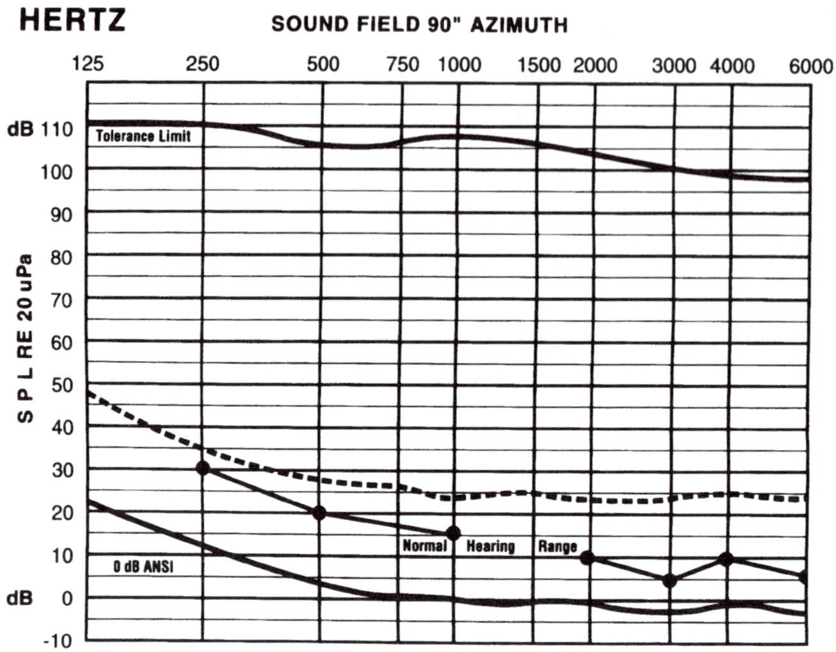

Figure 10–2. Shown here is the average hearing threshold sensitivity to selected pure-tone stimuli for six normal hearing individuals. The averaged ambient noise level is 45 dBA and the signal source is 90°. The solid and dashed lines indicate the range of thresholds for monaural presentation.

greatly and lead to erroneous measurements. To achieve stability, the patient must be placed far enough from reflecting surfaces so that there is no disturbance from changes in sound pressure (D'Antonio, 1986; Preves & Sullivan, 1987). The distance of the patient from the sound field speaker is influenced by the signal level variability at the eardrum. Figure 10–3 shows signal intensity variability as a function of distance from the sound source. As the distance from the sound source increases, the more pronounced is the variability of test signal level. Most investigators recommend that the patient be placed approximately 1 m from the sound field speaker to reduce the influence of standing waves. The patient's head must be held as steady as possible. The patient's orientation to the sound field speakers is shown in Figure 10–4. Note that the sound field speaker, in this instance, is about 9 in. from the person's ear. The type of signal generated in the sound field will determine the degree of variation in sound pressure when the head is moved only slightly. In general, pure tones are not the most appropriate stimuli to use in a sound field assessment. Depending on the frequency of the pure tone, slight movements of the head may create rather marked changes in signal intensity. Goldberg (1979), however, reported that pure tones can be employed successfully if the sound source (signal) is only 9 to 12 in. from the ear. Also, restricting the source-to-listener distance greatly reduces the deleterious effects of standing waves within the field.

Woodward and Tecca (1985, p. 22) reported: "If use of pure tones in a sound field yield reliable measures of auditory sensitivity, the application of these stimuli in assessment of functional gain for various modes of amplification may prove more accurate than alternative stimuli. When a hearing aid is introduced, the potential for client response to

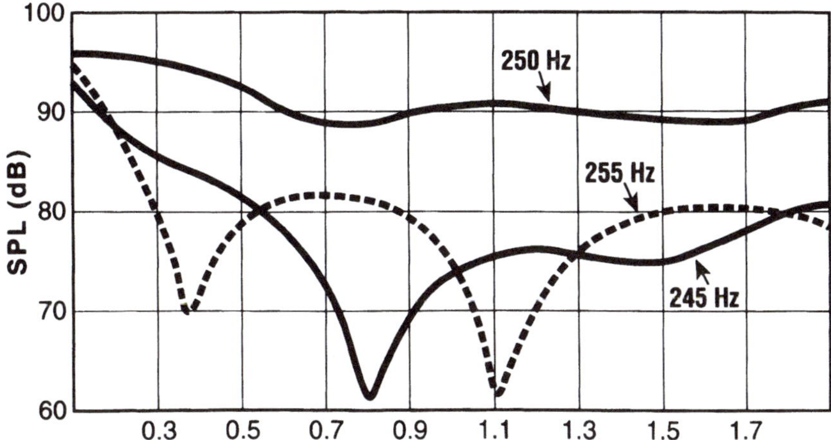

Figure 10–3. Signal intensity variability in level for three pure tones, 5 Hz apart, as the distance increases from the sound source.

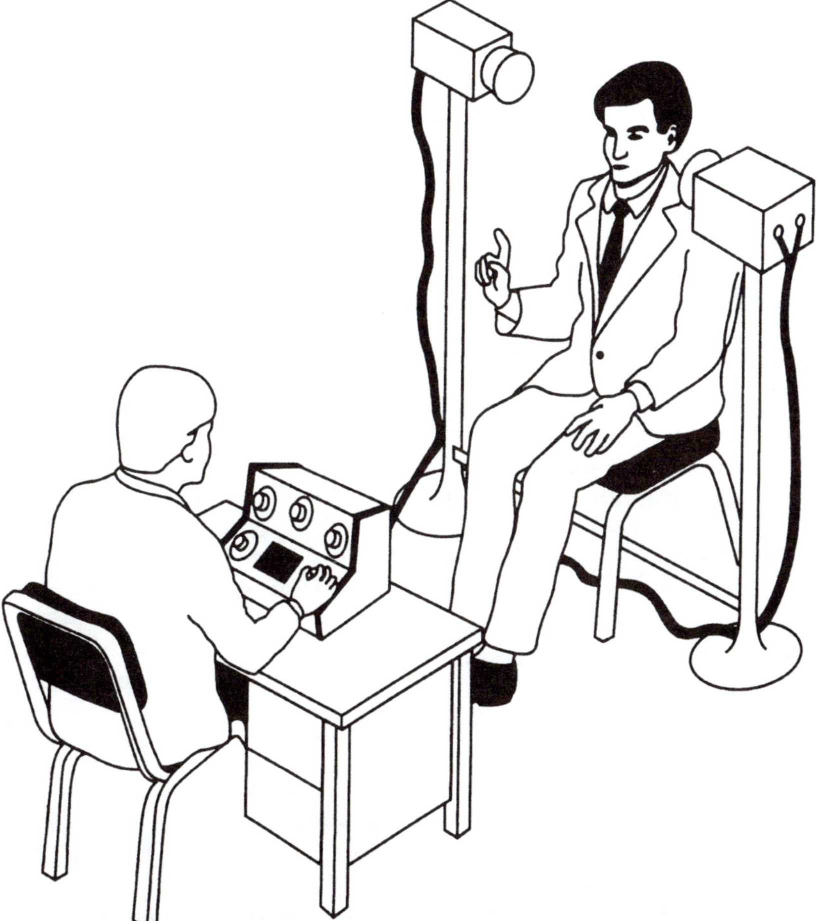

Figure 10–4. Subject position in a sound chamber for obtaining pure-tone threshold measurements. Note that the sound source is at a 90° azimuth, and the speaker is about 9 in. from the ear under test.

components of frequencies other than the normal test frequency or any alternative stimuli may be affected not only by the slope of an individual audiogram. It may be affected, also by the frequency response of the hearing aid and the interaction of these two variables. For example, if one uses a "warble tone" signal in assessing organic thresholds in a sound field, the frequency deviation and modulation rate constitute two parameters that must be controlled, or at least recorded. As mentioned by Lundeen (1988, p. 32), frequency deviation refers "to that difference between an unmodulated carrier frequency and the lowest or the highest instantaneous frequency attained by the waveform during modulation." Modulation rate simply refers to the rate at which frequency/intensity change occurs.

Depending on the acoustic stimuli presented and what is intended to be measured, more than one sound field speaker may be necessary to acquire the desired information. In assessing the patient's binaural response to acoustic signals, for example, more than one sound field speaker is needed. When different signals are presented simultaneously, for example, one signal may come from one speaker and another from a different sound field speaker. In general, if only one sound field speaker is used, it is placed at 0° azimuth when assessing aided and unaided monaural response. When assessing binaural response, two speakers are used and should be placed at about 45° azimuth, relative to the patient's head position in the sound field.

A number of complex signals other than speech have been suggested as suitable for sound field measurement. Commonly used, complex signals include frequency modulated (warble tone) signals, and narrow bands of noise. Their spectral characteristics may vary depending on the signal generator used, however. Other types of complex signals include amplitude modulated tones (Goldberg, 1979) and damped wavetrains (Victoreen, 1974). The rationale for the use of these test signals is that they have acoustic energy centered around a nominal frequency. Figure 10–5 shows the response of a pure tone and two modulated tones (5% and 20%, respectively) as a function of distance from the sound source. Note the significant differences among the various sounds. The 20% modulated tone had the least variability of the three stimuli measured.

Care must be exercised in selecting the slope of the filter skirts. If the filter skirts are not "steep" enough, a distinct possibility exists that frequency specificity may be sacrificed. This is especially true for patients who have rapidly falling hearing loss. That is, the filter skirts should be steep enough to prevent loss of frequency specificity.

In selecting the appropriate test stimulus, the hearing health care professional should consider the suggestions of Dillon and Walker (1982, p. 153):

- It must be reasonably frequency specific because frequency specific information is needed for a satisfactory definition of the client's hearing status and amplification needs.
- The sound pressure level generated in the field must be stable over the whole region that the client's head could occupy during testing.
- The sound pressure level generated at the client's ear must be stable for small shifts in frequency, such as may occur in an oscillator's output between calibrations.
- The results obtained in the sound field must be relatable to similar measurements made with pure tones under earphones.

The acoustic stimuli employed by the clinician must contribute to making a decision about the amplification needs of the patient and permit determination of whether desired psychoacoustic performance has been achieved.

SPEECH OR SPEECHLIKE STIMULI IN A SOUND FIELD

There is common agreement that the single most compelling reason for hearing aid amplification use is to improve the individual's

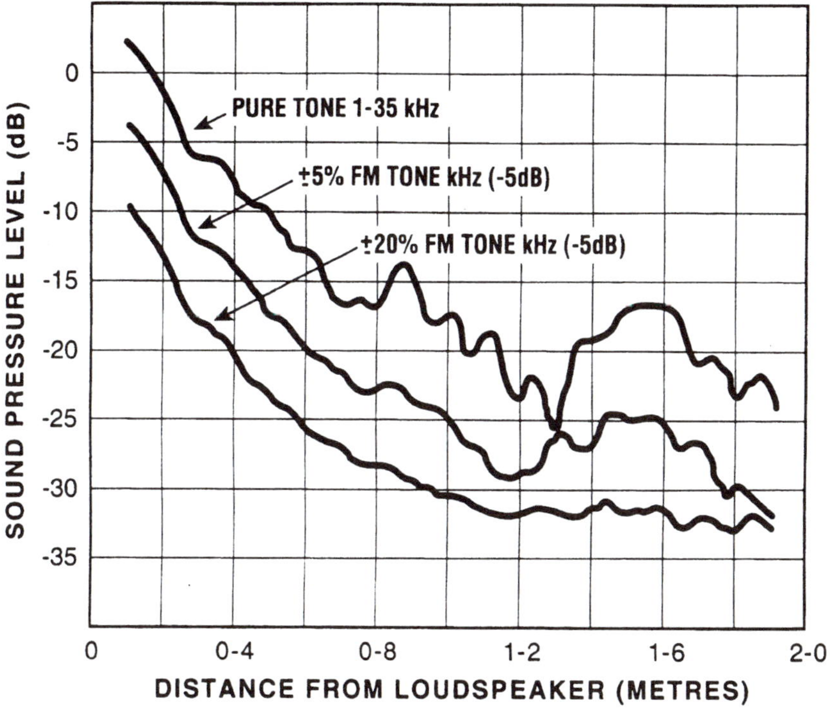

Figure 10–5. The sound pressure levels generated by an unmodulated and two modulated tones with the same center frequency but different bandwidths, as a function of distance from the speaker. The overall levels have been arbitrarily separated by 5 dB.

ability to understand conversational speech under a variety of listening conditions. There is considerable disagreement, however, regarding the speech stimulus of choice in the evaluation process. Regardless of the stimulus employed, improved speech discrimination is one of the desired goals. An important evaluative task is determining the most appropriate speech stimulus to use when assessing the clinical contributions of a hearing aid. In 1946, Carhart recommended that when word recognition scores differed by only 8%, the hearing aid yielding the better score was the instrument of choice. Unfortunately, the use of monosyllabic, phonetically balanced words to define real differences among two or more hearing aids is fraught with error (Thornton & Rafin, 1978). The total number of monosyllabic words needed to consistently and reliably differentiate among hearing aids, depending on the level of confidence desired, far exceeds the amount of time one can devote to the evaluation and selection process. Shore, Bilger, and Hirsch (1960) reported that word recognition scores do not consistently differentiate among the contributing electroacoustic features of two or more hearing aids. Schwartz and Walden (1983) demonstrated that word recognition scores for eight patients, extending over a 5-day period, varied as much as 30%.

Other than using monosyllabic words to assess word recognition scores between or among hearing aids, a number of other speech-based or speechlike procedures have been recommended to determine hearing aid performance. Such tests as the Nonsense Syllable Test (NST) developed by Levitt and Resnick (1978), the Synthetic Sentence Identification (SSI) reported by Speaks and Jerger (1965), and the Speech Perception in Noise (SPIN) created by Kalikow, Stevens, and Elliot (1977) have contributed to the clinician's ability to determine the best hearing aid from a number of instruments evaluated.

There are other speech-based procedures that can be used in sound field assessment to quantify the performance value of hearing aids. Nonetheless, determining speech performance is only one of a host of clinical procedures to select and fit hearing instruments.

Magnitude Estimation

It is possible for individuals to judge the intelligibility of a paragraph or selected sentences by the process of magnitude estimation (Lawson & Chial,1982; Purdy & Watson, 1990). *Magnitude estimation* is defined as the task of subjectively rating the intelligibility of selected discourse, or other speech samples, presented at a specified level to the ear(s) under test. The patient simply estimates what he or she determines to be the percentage of intelligibility of a spoken passage. There is a close approximation between magnitude estimation and actual measures of intelligibility expressed in percentage.

Magnitude estimation is useful in assessing the intelligibility of speech material in the presence of background noise or competing messages at specified signal-to-noise ratios. In a sound field, the hearing health care professional can determine differences between aided and unaided performance for one or more hearing aids when the same acoustic stimuli are presented. In this manner, the only variable affecting magnitude estimation is the electroacoustic response of the hearing aid(s). The reader is referred to the pioneering work of Cox and McDaniels (1989, 1992, 1994) in their germinal studies of intelligibility rating of connected discourse and its application to hearing aid selection. Also, the study by Studebaker and Sherbecoe (1988) should be appreciated for its contribution to the application of magnitude estimation measures.

Not only is magnitude estimation useful in assessing the intelligibility of connected discourse, it is also valuable in determining quality judgments, signal sharpness and clarity, and the comfort (ease of listening) of connected speech. Each of these measures can be instrumental in helping the hearing health care professional judge overall hearing aid performance.

Phoneme Recognition

Duffy (1987) presented a cogent argument for phoneme recognition testing. A phoneme is defined as any speech sound associated with a family of sounds having identifying acoustic characteristics that distinguish it from all other phonemes. There are 44 different phonemes in the English phonological system. To delineate the acoustic characteristics of a phoneme, it must be audible and identifiable by the listener if it is to be correctly perceived. Tests of phoneme recognition in aided and unaided conditions require some type of sound field assessment. Sound field testing to determine phoneme recognition contributes to the decision-making process in hearing instrument selection. Obviously, the extent to which a hearing aid device can reinstate essential acoustic information contained in any phoneme, and the extent to which the auditory system is capable of processing this information, contributes to validity of the selection process. Such an assessment is valuable for both monaural instrument function and binaural function.

Paired Comparison

Since the introduction of the first edition of the *Handbook of Hearing Aid Amplification*, development in computer hardware and software has begun to permit paired comparison of two or more hearing instruments simply by manipulating various commands or selecting appropriate controls (Kuk, 1994). Computer commands can change the acoustic response of the hearing aid(s) from one program to another so the patient may select which of the two acoustic responses best meets some specific, predetermined criteria. The response criterion is one of limited choice in that the patient must make a decision base on paired comparisons, such as "Which sound is clearer? This one or this one?" The advantage of conducting comparison tests in a sound field is that acoustic environments can be controlled. Such control eliminates sound conditions that would interfere with the reliability of the paired-comparison tests administered. As such, the variable to which the patient responds is the change in instrument response, not unwanted acoustic changes in the field. Aided paired-comparisons conducted in a sound field have been used for many years to determine the hearing aid of choice. The advantage of using computer-assisted paired comparison is that the time between comparisons is much shorter and, the patient's auditory memory of the response characteristics of hearing aid A and B is not overly challenged.

Kuk (1994) described a number of other paired-comparison procedures used in hearing aid fittings. The common thread that binds these procedures is that the patient must choose which of the instruments best meets the performance criteria. Normally, performance criteria are predetermined by the investigator.

Round-Robin Tournament Format

The round-robin tournament is an extension of the paired comparison procedure. The purpose of the round-robin tournament is to have the patient judge which instruments, or which settings of a given instrument, conform best to established criteria. The investigator determines the number of instruments to be employed in the tournament or the number of different settings of an individual hearing aid. A number of instruments or settings may be evaluated to determine which most closely corresponds to the desired criteria established by the investigator. In the round-robin format, the evaluation process is continued until one instrument or a given setting(s) of a single instrument is determined to be the "winner." Regarding the clinical utility of the round-robin tournament, Kuk (1994, p. 115) made the following statement: "the round-robin tournament may be practical only if (1) specific ranking information is needed among the comparison hearing aids and (2) the number of comparison hearing aids (or settings) is small (e.g., under four). Other methods may be more efficient to verify the appropriateness of a selected frequency-gain response."

One of the major drawbacks to the utility of a round-robin tournament is that it is time consuming. It is not unusual to take 80 to 85 minutes to complete the process.

Single-Elimination Tournament Format

In the single-elimination tournament, the goal is to evaluate two or more hearing aid devices. To determine the "winner" every hearing aid is compared with one other instrument. If several hearing aids are evaluated, a number of comparison rounds may be needed to determine the ultimate winner. As with most tournaments, the clinical time needed to complete the tournament may be more than most hearing instrument dispensers are willing to give, thus rendering the single-elimination procedure impractical.

Other Techniques

In the simple up-down procedure, the clinician estimates the settings of a hearing aid device to yield the best response. Having done this, the subject makes subjective judgments about the performance of the hearing aid as electroacoustic changes are made, which deviate from initial estimates.

Another technique—the Modified Simplex Procedure (Box, 1957)—is based on an assumption that only one set of conditions or combination of instrument settings will create optimal listening for a specific condition. At the outset, the patient's hearing aid is adjusted to achieve some preferred setting, for example, the initial setting may be based on some prescriptive formula. The initial setting is compared to modified settings until the patient reports that a single combination of setting reflects the patient's preference for a given listening condition.

DETERMINING MOST COMFORTABLE LISTENING LEVEL

Whenever possible, persons with hearing impairment will adjust hearing aid gain to maintain the most comfortable listening level (the level at which a person listens to connected discourse for extended periods of time without adjusting the hearing aid volume or sensing the need for volume change to maintain sound comfort). The hearing loss type, hearing loss magnitude, the signal processing capabilities of the hearing, aid and the environment in which listening takes place help to determine the preferred listening, or most comfortable, listening level.

To determine the most comfortable listening level, the patient must make some judgment based on the electroacoustic performance of the hearing aid under test. Fitting formulae assume that, if the hearing aid achieves recommended target gain, a most comfortable listening level results (Leijon, Eriksson-Mangold, & Berch-Karlsen, 1984). Current fitting methods utilizing a half-gain rule, for example, may not be valid in setting hearing aid gain for mild hearing impairments. Other fitting protocols, such as that proposed by Libby (1986), recommend that the one-third gain is more appropriate for mild to moderate hearing losses and two-thirds gain is recommended for more severe losses. Furthermore, various fitting methods do not always accurately predict insertion gain requirements to achieve most comfortable listening for patients with severe to profound hearing impairment. Attention has been given to fitting criteria for individuals with severe to profound hearing loss, based on the patient's psychological assessment of the gain required, to achieve a comfortable level of listening. Subsequently, some fitting methods have been revised to more closely reflect the insertion gains needed to achieve acceptable levels (Byrne, Parkinson, & Newall 1991; Libby, 1986; Schwartz, Lyregaard, & Lundh, 1988).

The patient determines the acceptability of the hearing aid relative to listening comfort. The hearing health care professional can best confirm the listening comfort level in the sound field. Assuming that current fitting methods provide a first approximation of the most comfortable listening, the task is *to fine tune* the hearing aid response to achieve patient acceptance and use. Fine tuning requires a subjective response from the person being evaluated.

The clinician should be aware that there is a difference between the amplification needed to achieve the most comfortable listening level and what is required to best understand the intended message. In an early study, Posner and Ventry (1977) found that "subjects with sensorineural loss did not achieve PB max (maximum intelligibility of monosyllabic, phonetically balanced words) . . . when listening at the most comfortable loudness (MCL). While the mean MCL for their subjects was 14.6 dB SL, PB, max did not occur until a mean SL of 37.2 dB" (p. 117).

Whether the issue is one of a most comfortable listening level or a level to achieve maximum word or speech recognition, such determining measures are properly administered through some type of sound field assessment. The dilemma is whether to set the response of the hearing aid to provide an acceptable comfort level or set the response of the hearing aid to gain the best discrimination function for a given listening environment. A reasonable compromise may be to counsel the patient regarding the limitations and advantages of adjusting the volume level to meet comfort or intelligibility needs. For some patients, appropriate counseling can result in acceptance of the hearing aid response offering maximum understanding without violating the comfort listening level.

An unrelenting challenge for the hearing health care professional is to determine how to maintain a comfortable listening level when there is noise or a competing message in the background. Current fitting formulae do not provide for the best electroacoustic response when the patient is exposed to environmental conditions other than quiet. The reason for this is straightforward. Most fitting formulae are based on the use of a linear hearing aid. Because linear systems do not change acoustic behavior as a function of ambient noise levels, it is of little consequence. As a result, the recommended hearing aid response is a deliberate compromise. The acoustic parameters of the hearing aid are set to yield a response that is "as adequate as possible" for listening conditions to which the person may be exposed on a frequent basis.

With the number of nonlinear hearing aids available today, however, comfortable listening levels may be more closely approximated for a number of listening environments. This is especially true for multimemory, digitally controlled, analog-programmable hearing aid systems. Such hearing instruments permit the manipulation of the electroacoustic response of two or more programs to provide an appropriate interface with specific background conditions. Even with analog multimemory hearing aids, the clinician must determine what the response of the instrument should be for each of the available memories. Some hearing aid manufacturers have attempted to assist the dispenser by providing fitting guidelines for multiprogrammable systems. The Widex Hearing Aid Company, for example, developed a fitting guide for their analog multimemory hearing aids that recommended the necessary changes in the output response to maintain comfortable listening level for a number of listening environments.

Regardless of the linear or nonlinear characteristics of today's hearing aids, realistically clinical assessment of a most comfortable level as a function of the listening environment can only be confirmed in a sound field. Sound field assessment provides clinically useful information relative to the patient's determination of his or her comfort level as the listening environment changes. Sound field measurement provides equally useful information of the effects of nonlinear hearing aids on the determination of a most comfortable listening level.

Since the introduction of the first edition of this textbook in 1988, digital signal processing (DSP) hearing aids have been introduced into the marketplace. The sophistication of DSP systems permits a much greater control of amplification factors contributing to a most comfortable listening level. The ability of DSP systems to reduce the negative effects of environmental noise, through the application of an appropriate algorithm, has contributed greatly to maintaining a comfortable listening level in a host of environmental backgrounds.

DETERMINING LOUDNESS DISCOMFORT LEVELS

Should the author ever be limited to a single criterion for gaining hearing aid acceptance, it would be the direct measurement of loudness discomfort. Those involved in the selection, fitting, and follow-up care of patients with hearing impairment will attest to the advantage of correctly determining loudness discomfort levels. The error many practitioners commit is providing an SSPL90 function that unrealistically represents the maximum sound pressure the user is willing to accept. In the author's opinion, it has been incorrectly assumed by many hearing aid dispensers that changes in sensorineural hearing impairment required higher SSPL90 values. Subsequent studies have indicated that this may not be the case, that is, the SSPL90 values do not differ greatly from those of normal hearing persons.

Some fitting formulae assume that loudness discomfort can be predicted from target frequency thresholds. McCandless (1994, p. 4) reported: "Although the use of prescriptive procedures has become popular, no general agreement has been reached as to what measurements should be used to calculate the prescribed gain (e.g., hearing thresholds, MCL or UCL). However, most dispensers and manufacturers currently use threshold-based procedures for calculation of the prescribed frequency-gain response since the pure-tone audiogram is easily obtained and always available.

McCandless suggested that there may be other ways to obtain a more accurate assessment of functions such as loudness discomfort. Moreover, Mueller (1992, p. 60) stated: "One of the primary goals of the hearing aid fitting procedure is to assure that maximum output of the hearing aid is both comfortable and safe. While this can be accomplished with some degree of accuracy with adult patients without using probe-microphone measurements, by combining the RESR [Real Ear Saturation Response] with aided LDLs [Loudness Discomfort Levels], more precise fitting of the hearing aid's output can be obtained" (p. 60). This statement suggests that combining objective measurement with subjective responses from the patient may contribute more useful information than any one single measurement.

Obtaining reliable and subjective estimations of loudness discomfort in a sound field is not without some difficulty. Most clinicians concede that the subjective assessment of loudness discomfort is, in part, a function of the instruction given to the patient. If the instruction asks the patient to determine when the sound level creates a sensation of tickle, pain, or dizziness, for example, it is unlikely that the attending result approximates a realistic SSPL90. Conversely, if the instruction is asking the patient to determine when the sound is "just" becoming annoying, it may underestimate the SSPL90 required for optimal listening performance. The most appropriate instruction, therefore, may be determining at what point the sound level is acceptable for specified periods of time without violating the discomfort level of the patient.

Problems encountered by patients fitted with hearing aids providing excessive SPL90 are twofold, relative to predictable behaviors. In the first instance, the patient will adjust the volume control downward to guard against sudden exposure to overly loud sounds. When this happens, certain speech sounds (primarily the consonants) may become inaudible, thus creating a loss of speech cues needed to understand the intended message. When the patient turns the volume up to clearly understand the message, sudden loud sounds violate comfort levels. In this case, the patient may turn the hearing aid off during those moments of discomfort. Such activity may ultimately lead to limited use or rejection of amplification.

THE ARTICULATION INDEX

The popularity of a simplified articulation index (AI) (Humes, 1991; Mueller & Killion, 1990; Pavlovic, 1991) is based on the ease with which a threshold audiogram can be obtained. Having measured organic thresholds for selected frequencies, one can "count the dots" (Mueller & Killion, 1990) that fall below the unaided thresholds and predict articulation function. The dots have weighted values depending on their location within a given frequency range. Additional impetus was given to the use of some form of AI by the clinical report of Humes who found that there was a positive correlation between the articulation function predicted by an AI procedure and sound recognition scores obtained by a nonsense syllable test. That is, if one can determine the extent to which the speech spectrum is made audible by hearing aid devices, a reasonable estimation of actual intelligibility performance can be predicted from the AI.

When one reports word recognition scores for a group of individuals, the assumption is that an individual within that group will produce a score consistent with the average of the group. Although the use of some AI may yield a reliable predictor of function, and thus reflect accurately the articulation skills of the patient with hearing impairment, this is not always the case. Again, such statements are not intended to indict the use of some AI function, but rather to caution against the tendency to assume that the obtained AI accurately represents the patient's ability to perform speech discrimination tasks in all cases.

A number of factors may influence the patient's ability to understand the intended word message. For example, the ability of the auditory system to process information, even though the speech spectrum may be audible, may be highly compromised. Regardless of the amplification device provided, the auditory system cannot correctly process enough incoming acoustic information to correspond to the predicted function of an AI procedure. Central auditory processing disorders (see Chapter 14), which often accompany the aging process, influence the ability to discriminate acoustic events. Various cochlear distortions degrade the kinds of neural input to the processing system needed to correctly identify the intended message. Furthermore, distortion products produced by the hearing aid (e.g., intermodulation distortion, harmonic distortion, internal noise, symmetrical and asymmetrical peak clipping) may provided barriers to understanding the intended signal or message.

The value of "first approximation" of need provided by current hearing aid fitting formulae was mentioned earlier in this chapter. The first approximation concept may come into play when discussing the application of an Articulation Index based on the probability of speech discrimination performance. It gives the hearing health care professional some indication of probable word recognition function. No audiologist or hearing instrument dispenser is unaware of this possibility. One is cautioned, however, not to accept as an absolute the predicted function of speech intelligibility based on an Articulation Index.

This extended overview of the value of an Articulation Index suggests that sound field assessment of word recognition skills is still a viable clinical procedure. There is considerable concern about what kind of speech material should be used when testing the individual's ability. Such tests as the CID W22 word lists, NU 6, or perhaps other recognized word lists and measures of speech recognition performance may fall short of yielding totally reliable scores. In some cases, the value of such measures may be more clinically useful than predicted measures, however. Studebaker (1991) presented a provocative overview of the limitations of measures of intelligibility using monosyllabic words.

FOLLOW-UP SOUND FIELD ASSESSMENT

Almost any fitting procedure or protocol, subjective or objective, is to be considered a "first approximation" of the appropriateness of the electroacoustic response of the recommended hearing aid(s). There is often a need to modify the acoustic response parameters of the hearing aid to achieve optimal performance in a number of listening environments. Justification of change is based on the individual's experiences with hearing aid amplification under daily listening conditions. Modification of hearing aid response dictated by patient reports such as excessive SPL90, minimal improvement in word recognition function, significantly reduced discrimination in the presence of noise, or signal distortions produced by the hearing aid, are best determined under sound field conditions.

If the patient complains of poor speech intelligibility, sound field testing will reflect changes in intelligibility performance as specific instrument settings are modified. It is possible, for example, to determine which phonemes are unintelligible and which are correctly identified as the instrument response is modified. If the patient complains of poor speech recognition performance in the presence of specific noise environments, sound field assessment indicates whether a positive change is demonstrable following changes in frequency/gain response. If the patient feels that monaural performance is more acceptable than binaural performance, sound field assessment identifies the magnitude of difference in performance. If the patient complains that the hearing aid is too loud or too soft to be acceptable, subsequent sound field testing confirms whether electroacoustic changes in hearing aid performance have satisfied the complaint. It should be self-evident that successful fitting of hearing aids must involve the patient's assessment of perceived benefit.

One of the problems encountered by the hearing health care professional is meeting the patient's acoustic needs without violating the patient's acceptance of amplification. Unfortunately, determining appropriate acoustic performances to meet the needs of individuals with hearing impairment is not the same as the individual's acceptance of the recommended hearing aid. Experienced hearing instrument dispensers know that patients reject the hearing aid(s), even though the electroacoustic response meets all reasonable criteria.

Among the advantages of sound field testing is using test results to counsel patients regarding what is needed and what is acceptable. If the patient is aware that improved performance is possible with the recommended hearing aid, management strategies can be developed that permit acceptance of the recommended response change. That is, the clinician can compare optimal acoustic performance with that which the patient is willing to accept and suggest that he or she is best served by adapting to the recommended changes.

PROGRAMMABLE AND DIGITAL SIGNAL PROCESSING HEARING AIDS AND SOUND FIELD ASSESSMENT

No textbook dealing with hearing aid amplification selection and use-value would be complete without some comment on the utility of analog, digitally programmable, and digital signal processing hearing aid systems. This chapter will review only the need for subjective, sound field assessment relating to how one decides on the most appropriate hearing aid response for different listening environments. The clinical concern is not only what the output response is of the hearing aid, but whether some form of signal processing is indicated, compared to conventional, linear hearing aid systems

It is difficult to arrive at some absolute standard by which one sets the various acoustic parameters for specific listening conditions. This is so because one cannot replicate all of the acoustic environments to which an individual with hearing impairment may be exposed. It would seem appropriate to get information from the patient about the listening environments to which he or she is frequently exposed. Having done so, one may then attempt to replicate in a sound field the acoustic conditions of those environments as nearly as possible. The extent to which a number of environments can be managed successfully may depend, in part, on whether the instrument is a single or multimemory unit or whether it is analog or digital. If an analog, multiple-memory system is the instrument of choice, the task is gathering appropriate patient information to set the various acoustic responses for two or more listening conditions to best meet individual needs. If a DSP instrument is selected, the task is determining if appropriate algorithms are present to offer the best solution to the processing of information in a number of listening environments.

Based on the degree of hearing impairment and the auditory processing capabilities, it may not be possible to meet all of the patient's acoustic needs for all possible listening conditions. Sound field assessment offers the best method at this time to approximate optimal amplification needs in a specific background environment. This statement is not intended to indict efforts to provide a "cookbook" or "recipe" for presetting the hearing aid performance parameters to provide predicted response, but rather to state that such methods offer only a first approximation of need. The "fine tuning" of the hearing aid response demands some patient input, preferably obtained in a sound field. This is true regardless of the hearing aid device selected.

CONCLUSION

Even though reliance on sound field assessment has lost some of its luster because of the introduction and use of objective tests (such as probe tube measurements), it continues to be a useful tool in the selection, fitting, evaluation, and verification of hearing aid performance. Sound field assessment provides a clinically viable tool for assessing unaided and aided responses to acoustic stimuli in a sound-treated chamber or appropriate enclosure. By comparing patient performance in the aided and unaided conditions, the hearing health care professional is able to determine some of the advantages and limitations of the hearing aid(s) under test.

Sound field assessment does not imply that other measurement protocols are not appropriate in the selection and fitting of hearing aids. Rather, it suggests that one should use the clinical contributions of each to assess hearing instrument(s) benefit in a number of listening environments. It would be a mistake to deny the contributions made by objective measurements of hearing aid performance. Measurements using probe microphone systems have been and continue to be beneficial in determining amplification benefit. To minimize the objectivity of current fitting methods would be an error in clinical judgment. Even though there is no consensus regarding the desired insertion gain to achieve optimal performance, such objective fitting methods do provide a valuable first approximation of need. Nonetheless, it would be less than astute for one to reject the contributions of sound field assessment.

Based on advances to date, the audiologist and dispenser are advised to utilize objective and subjective measurement protocols, which assist in determining the selection of hearing aids. By doing this, the patient's ability to respond more appropriately in his or her acoustic environment is elevated significantly. It is the author's opinion that the patient must be an active player in the decision-making process regarding hearing aid amplification and its perceived benefit.

Clinicians who hesitate to adopt more advanced methods to fit hearing aid devices place themselves in a kind of professional limbo. In all probability, there remains a small group of hearing health care professionals who continue to select and fit amplification system without relying on any organized assessment method. For some, the approach to validation and verification of hearing instrument success is to ask the patient, "How do you like it?" or "Does this sound better to you?" If the patient responds in the affirmative, the hearing aid fitting is a success. If the patient responds in the negative, the hearing aid is modified until an affirmative answer is received. Using this approach, the dispenser does not know what electroacoustic response changes were responsible for the acceptance or rejection. This type of evaluation should be abandoned.

Hearing health care professionals cannot predict the future development of optimal measurement criteria that will be used to determine the best hearing aid. Future requirements must measure, in part, the patient's utilization and acceptance of hearing aid amplification and the extent to which speech recognition and the use-value of other acoustic stimuli are enhanced. Today, the value of sound field assessment cannot be overlooked. Although new and useful assessment tools may be developed to measure subjectivity, some form of an acoustically controlled environment in which to conduct such tests will always be needed.

REVIEW QUESTIONS

1. What is the primary difference between subjective and objective assessment of hearing aid benefit?

2. What is the relationship between psychoacoustics and subjective measurements conducted in a sound field?

3. What are (at least) four psychoacoustic measures commonly used in a sound

field assessment when evaluating hearing aid amplification benefit?

4. What is the role of the real-ear measurement in the selection and validation of hearing aid devices?

5. What are some of the advantages of utilizing hearing aid fitting formulae?

6. What are some of the disadvantages of utilizing hearing aid fitting formulae?

7. What type of measure error may be introduced by unwanted standing waves generated in a sound field?

8. What is the primary rationale for using magnitude estimation when assessing intelligibility of speech or speechlike stimuli in a sound field?

9. What is the clinical value of paired-comparison tests in the determination of the "best" hearing aid?

10. What is the probable behavior of patients with hearing impairment if the UCL violates their sense of comfort?

REFERENCES

Box, G. (1957). Evolutionary operation: A method for increasing industrial productivity. *Applied Statistics, 26*, 679–685.

Byrne, D., Parkinson, A., & Newall, R. (1991). Modified hearing aid selection procedures for severe/profound hearing losses. In G. Studebaker, F. Bess, & L. Beck (Eds.), *The Vanderbilt Report HearingAid Report II* (pp. 295–300). Parkton, MD: York Press.

Carhart, R. (1946). The selection of hearing aids. *Archives of Otolaryngology, 44*, 1–18.

Cox, R. M., & Alexander, G. C. (1992). Maturation of hearing aid benefit: Objective and subjective measurements. *Ear and Hearing, 143*, 131–141.

Cox, R. M., & McDaniel, D. M. (1984). Intelligibility ratings of continuous discourse: Application to hearing aid selection. *Journal of the Acoustical Society of America, 76*, 758–766.

Cox, R. M., & McDaniel, D. M. (1992a). Intelligibility rating of continuous discourse: Application to hearing aid selection. *Journal of the Acoustical Society of America, 92*, 758–766.

Cox, R. M., & McDaniel D. M. (1992b). Evaluation of the speech intelligibility rating (SIR) test for hearing aid comparisons. *Journal of Speech and Hearing Research, 35*; 686–693.

Dillon, H., & Walker, J. (1992). Comparison of stimuli used in sound field audiometric testing. *Journal of the Acoustical Society of America, 91*, 161–172.

Duffy, J. K. (1967). Audio-visuals speech audiometry and a new audio-visual speech perception index. *Maico Audiological Library Services, 5*(9), 1–3.

Duffy, J. (1978). Sound field audiometry and hearing aid advisement. *Hearing Instruments, 29*(2), 6–12.

Duffy, J. K. (1987). Sound field audiometry and hearing aid selection. In E. Zelnick (Ed.), *Hearing instrument: Selection and evaluation* (pp. 179–215) Livonia, MI: NIHIS.

Durrant, J. D., Lovrinic, J. H. (1981). *Bases of hearing science* (2nd ed.). Baltimore, MD: Williams & Wilkins.

Fabry, D. A., & Schum, D. J. (1994): The role of subjective measurement techniques in hearing aid fittings. In M. Valente (Ed.), *Strategies for selecting and verifying hearing aid fittings* (pp 136–155). New York: Thieme Medical Publishers, Inc..

Hawkins, D., & Mueller, G. (1992). Test protocols for probe-microphone measurements. In D. Hawkins, G. Mueller, & J. Northern (Eds.), *Probe microphone measurements* (pp. 269–278). San Diego, CA: College-Hill Press.

Harford, E. (1969). Is a hearing aid ever justified in unilateral hearing loss? In L. Boles (Ed.), *Hearing loss — Problems in diagnosis and treatment* (pp. 153–173). Otolaryngology Clinics of North America.

Hodgson, W. R. (1986). Special cases of hearing aid assessment. In W. R. Hodgson (Ed.), *Hearing aid assessment and use in audiologic habilitation* (3rd ed., pp. 191–216). Baltimore: Williams and Wilkins.

Kuk, F. K. (1994). Use of paired comparisons in hearing aid fittings. In M. Valente (Ed.), *Strategies for selecting and verifying hearing aid fittings* (pp. 108–135). New York: Thieme Medical Publishers, Inc.

Lawson, G. D., & Chial, M. R. (1982). Magnitude estimation of degraded speech quality by normal- and impaired-hearing listeners. *Journal of the Acoustical Society of America, 72*, 1781–1787.

Mueller, H. G. (1992). Terminology and procedures. In G. Mueller, D. Hawkins, & J. Northern (Eds.), *Probe microphone measurements: Hearing aid selection and assessment* (pp. 41–66). San Diego, CA: Singular Publishing Group.

Mueller, H. G., Hawkins, D., & Northern, J. (1992). *Probe microphone measurements: Hearing aid selection and assessment*. San Diego, CA: Singular Publishing Group.

Munson, W. A., & Karlin, J. E. (1962). Isoreference method of evaluating speech transmission circuits. *Journal of the Acoustical Society of America, 34,* 762–774.

Pavlovic, C. (1991). Speech recognition and five articulation indexes. *Hearing Instruments, 42,* 20–24.

Pollack, M. C. (1998), Special applications of amplification. In M. C. Pollack (Ed.), *Amplification for the hearing impaired* (3rd ed., pp. 295–328). New York: Grune & Stratton.

Posner, J., & Ventry, I. (1977). Relationships between comfortable loudness levels for speech and speech discrimination in sensorineural loss. *Journal of Speech and Hearing Disorders, 42,* 370–375.

Preves, D. (1990). Principles of signal processing. In R. E. Sandlin (Ed.), *Handbook of hearing aid amplification* (Vol. 1, pp. 81–120). San Diego, CA: College-Hill Press.

Punch, J. L., & Parker, C. A. (1981). Pairwise listener preferences in hearing aid evaluation. *Journal of Speech and Hearing Research, 24,* 366–374.

Purdy, S. C. (1990). *Reliability, sensitivity, and validity of magnitude estimation, paired comparisons, and category scaling.* Unpublished doctoral dissertation, University of Iowa, Iowa City.

Ross, M., & Duffy, J. (1961, November). *Report on sound field audiometry.* Paper presented at the American Speech and Hearing Convention, Chicago, IL.

Sandlin, R. E. (1995). Clinical application of sound-field audiometry. In R. E. Sandlin (Ed.), *Handbook of hearing aid amplification* (Vol. 2, pp. 257–278). San Diego, CA: College-Hill Press.

Sandlin, R. E. (1996): Principles of sound field audiometry. In R. E. Sandlin (Ed.), *Hearing instrument science and fitting practices* (pp. 597–626). Livonia, MI: National Institute of Hearing Instrument Studies.

Schwartz, D., Lyregaard, R., & Lundh, R. (1988). Hearing aid selection for severe-to-profound hearing loss. *Hearing Journal, 41,* 13–17.

Shore, I., Bilger, R., & Hirsh, I. (1960). Hearing aid evaluation: Reliability of repeated measurements. *Journal of Speech and Hearing Disorders, 25,* 142–170.

Skinner, M. W. (1988). *Hearing aid evaluation* (pp. 212–219). Englewood Cliffs, NJ: Prentice-Hall.

Speaks, C., & Jerger, J. (1965). Method for measurement of speech identification. *Journal of Speech and Hearing Research, 8,* 185–194.

Studebaker, G. A. (1991). Measures of intelligibility and quality. In G. Studebaker, E. Bess, & L. Beck (Eds.), *The Vanderbilt hearing-aid report 11* (pp. 185–195). Parkton, MD: York Press.

Studebaker, G. A., & Sherbecole, R. L. (1988). Magnitude estimations of the intelligibility and quality of speech in noise. *Ear and Hearing, 9,* 259–267.

Sweetow, R. (1994): Fitting strategies for noise induced hearing loss. In M. Valente (Ed.), *Strategies for selecting and verifying hearing aid fittings* (pp. 156–179). New York. Thieme Medical Publishers, Inc.

Tecca, J. (1990) Clinical applications of real-ear probe tube measurement. In R. Sandlin (Ed.), *Handbook of hearing aid amplification.* Vol. II: Clinical considerations and fitting practices (pp. 225–255). San Diego, CA: College-Hill Press.

Thorton, A., & Rafin, M. (1978). Speech discrimination scores modeled as a binomial variable. *Journal of Speech and Hearing Research, 21,* 507–518.

Valente, M., Valente, M., Meister, M., Macauley, K., & Vass, W. (1994). Selecting and verifying hearing aid fittings for unilateral hearing loss. In M. Valente (Ed.), *Strategies for selecting and verifying hearing aid fittings* (pp. 228–248) New York: Thieme Medical Publishers.

Valente, M., Valente, M., & Potts, L. G. (1996). Programmable hearing systems. In R. E. Sandlin (Ed.), *Hearing instrument science and fitting practices* (pp. 647–693). Livonia MI: National Institute for Hearing Instrument Studies.

Victoreen, J. (1973). *Hearing enhancement.* Springfield, IL: Charles C. Thomas.

Walden, B. E., Schwartz, D. M., & Williams, D. L. (1983). Test of the assumptions underlying comparative hearing aid evaluations. *Journal of Speech and Hearing Disorders, 48,* 264–273.

Walker, G., Dillon, H., & Byrne, D. (1984). The use of loudness discomfort levels for selecting the maximum output of hearing aids. *Australian Journal of Audiology, 6,* 23–32.

Walker, G. (1981). Technical considerations for sound field audiometry. In R. Sandlin (Ed.), *Handbook of hearing aid amplification* (Vol. 1, pp. 146–164). San Diego, CA: College-Hill Press.

Woodward, C. M., & Tecca, J. E. (1985). The use of pure tone stimuli in a soundfield. *Hearing Journal, 38,* 21–27.

Zelnick, E. (1982). Selecting frequency response. *Hearing Journal, 35*(3), 31.

CHAPTER 11

Principles and Clinical Utility of Hearing Aid Fitting Formulas

PHILLIP T. MCCANDLESS, PH.D.

OUTLINE

Questions often asked regarding hearing aid evaluation procedures are related to what are fitting formulas and what do they do? At a minimum, hearing aid formulas estimate electroacoustic amplification requirements for individuals with hearing loss. To that end, all modern fitting methodologies are considered to be successful to some degree as all specify at least *some* corrective gain to the ear. While it is true that simply providing amplification will lessen hearing impairment, an arbitrary amount may not always prove to be satisfactory. To provide a satisfactory fitting, a hearing aid must amplify sufficiently to maximize speech recognition at a wide range of inputs within the loudness constraints of normal listeners, provide good overall sound quality, and do this in an instrument that is both physically and acoustically comfortable. The trivial application of important electroacoustic features may result in less than optimum speech understanding, poor accommodation of loudness, and increased returns of hearing aids due to patient dissatisfaction. It is interesting to note that this practice is common despite the abundance of advanced fitting software available from various manufacturers and hearing aid research laboratories. Without the benefit of rational and valid scientific methods applied to the fitting process, each patient functions as a unique experiment with variable and unpredictable outcomes. Although some patient dissatisfaction will persist no matter what fitting method is used, there is wisdom in implementing at least one of the many proven procedures to better estimate the final fitting requirements of the individual.

Nearly all rationales used in the various modern fitting procedures seek to satisfy many amplification goals to meet the needs of the individual. Although not yet developed, the optimum fitting method would seek to specify all salient electroacoustic parameters required to restore all dynamic acoustic properties lost through cochlear and conductive causes. Such an optimum formula assumes a hearing aid capable of compensating for all the necessary amplification properties such as one that would compensate reduced frequency and temporal discrimination of the impaired ear. It is evident from recent user satisfaction studies and modest industry-side return rates that the technology has not yet achieved that goal. Wide dynamic range compression (WDRC), available in nearly all programmable and digital instruments, improves our ability to deliver proper loudness compensation to the pathologic cochlea, and future improvements in technology will certainly continue to improve patient satisfaction. With these improved instruments, there has been a certain impetus for developing a formula that will sufficiently address all the variables contained in the new technologies. It will be seen in this chapter that the thrust of fitting formulas has been to satisfy loudness needs of the impaired ear by restoring pure tones, bands of noise, or speech frequencies to their proper loudness relationships enjoyed by normal listeners. Each of these rationales enjoys a unique path to satisfy those loudness requirements and are discussed below.

FOUNDATIONS OF MODERN HEARING AID FITTING

Fitting methods can be classified into three general categories: comparative approaches, prescriptive approaches, and combination prescriptive-comparative approaches (McCandless, 1985). Comparative approaches recommend that the optimum hearing instrument is ultimately chosen from a number of "appropriate" models, each judged by measures of speech intelligibility and subjective quality estimates made by the patient. The comparative approach generally does not implement psychoacoustic data (such as threshold or suprathreshold loudness scaling data) to formulate an optimum fitting recommendation.

Conversely, the prescriptive approaches derive optimum fitting recommendations based on individual threshold and/or loudness scaling procedures with little regard to formal speech intelligibility tests or subjective ratings. Some prescriptive approaches *predict* optimum electroacoustic parameters from the audiometric threshold data alone; other approaches claim that between-subject differences are significant enough to warrant *direct* loudness scaling measurements be obtained from each individual. The advocates of the predictive approaches make the assumption that calculations for nonlinear gain can be based on average data of individual hearing loss and any deviations can be corrected for in the clinic by "tweaking" response, gain, or other parameters, or simply by adjusting the volume control. Most manufacturers continue to use threshold-based algorithms largely because of the difficulties associated with incorporating individual loudness data for each instrument. That is not to say that manufacturers use thresholds exclusively, as some may incorporate measures of MCL or UCL or they may estimate the anticipated speech spectrum through various proprietary speech optimization protocols. The comparative-prescriptive methods use some features common to both comparative and prescriptive categories but will not be discussed in this chapter.

Early Comparative Approaches

Formal fitting recommendations emerged as early as the late 1920s and 1930s, as can be seen in the works of West (1937) as well as various other U.S. Patents in the 1930s. In 1946, Carhart developed the popular "comparative fitting approach" that ranks or prioritizes hearing aids from a limited number of models without regard to response gain, maximum output, or other electroacoustic parameters. Still in widespread clinical use, the comparative approach selects the "best" hearing aid from a number of appropriate "candidate" hearing aids that would produce best aided speech reception thresholds, most comfortable levels, and discrimination scores measured in quiet and in noise. Some comparative approaches allowed little more than the subjective impression from the user to be applied toward the final selection.

Several problems have been identified with this approach. First, it was considered by some to be too time consuming for practical use, and the final acoustic parameters are not identified with any particular set of electroacoustic parameters that have been demonstrated to contribute to improved performance (McCandless, 1995). Second, poor reliability and to some extent poor validity of word recognition used in the comparative method were identified (Shore, Bilger, & Hirsch 1960; Resnick & Becker, 1963). Another drawback is that the final response characteristics may or may not resemble the optimum prescription for the ear and the comparative method is used with little regard to scientific rationale. Harris (1976) also pointed out that the hearing aids used in comparisons provided no significant measurable differences among various hearing aids. As a result, hearing aids were often chosen by very small differences in actual performance without regard to electroacoustic characteristics. It is interesting to note that the utility of the comparative method was limited, in part by the need to stop the test to change instruments. This tested the auditory memory of the individual between relatively long breaks in the evaluation process.

Despite these limitations, the comparative approach continues as a favorite fitting method made more convenient by today's modern programmable instruments. Instantaneous adjustments with memory storage capabilities allow immediate subjective A/B comparisons within the same instrument. Through this expedient, fitting comparisons are made easier and reduce the demands and difficulties associated with long-term auditory recall during the evaluation process.

Prescriptive Approaches

West (1937) was the first to describe a prescriptive formula, shortly followed by Watson and Knudsen (1940), that popularized the "audiogram mirror-fitting" technique. This technique essentially provided gain to the ear that "mirrored" the magnitude of loss seen in the audiogram. The rationale simply states that the greatest amount of gain should be delivered to the regions of greatest loss. While at first glance the mirrored-audiogram approach seems logical, the approach has been criticized, as it tended to overamplify at higher sound inputs. This reason for overamplification has been related to the nature of loudness perception contours that tend to normalize at suprathreshold levels (Ross, 1978).

The evolution of the early prescriptive fitting strategies was advanced in 1942 by Lybarger to include a mathematical scaling factor of 0.5 that was applied against the magnitude of threshold loss at each frequency. For example, a hearing loss of 60 dB at 2000 Hz would receive 30 dB of gain in the hearing aid. Whether it was intentional or not, this ½ gain approach had the positive effect of limiting the overamplification seen in the "mirror-fitting" approach, while having a negative effect of providing too little amplification at low levels or with distant conversation. This was not entirely the fault of the procedure, rather it is an unfortunate characteristic of all linear amplifiers available at the time. This ½ gain rule applied to linear hearing aids struck what turned out to be an effective compromise between the undesirable effects relating to overamplification and the desirable benefits of acoustic gain. Interestingly, all subsequent traditional linear approaches utilize some mathematical variation of the ½ gain rule, ranging between ⅓ to ⅔ gain according to the specific fitting rationale and frequency of interest.

About the same time that Lybarger introduced the ½ gain rule, Davis, Hudgins, and Marquis (1946) suggested that optimum frequency responses did not seem to be related to patterns that could be seen in the individual's audiometric threshold. The "Harvard Report" emerged from these data suggesting that the frequency response of a hearing aid cannot be prescribed for any individual. The Harvard Report recommended that a flat or gradually rising "6 dB per octave" high pass response characteristic would be sufficient and would satisfy the amplification requirements for most subjects. Some modifications of that 6 dB rule recommendation were implemented at later dates to accommodate the calibration differences between real-ear and hearing aid coupler data. The Harvard Report suggested that the "one-size-fits all" approach would satisfy most hearing aid candidates without the need for formal calculations.

It was not until the late 1970s and 1980s that prescriptive fitting formulas regained widespread acceptance. Among the most popular formulas are the Prescription of Gain and Output, or POGO (McCandless & Lyregaard, 1983), the National Acoustic Laboratories' NAL and the revised version known as NAL-R (Byrne & Dillon 1986); Berger's method (Berger, Hagberg, & Rane, 1977), and Byrne and Tonisson (1976). As stated earlier, these formulas were best suited to the currently available state-of-the-art linear instruments utilizing abrupt peak clipping or compression limiting. These traditional prescriptive formulas (POGO, NAL, Berger, etc.) were relatively simple, utilizing easily calculable response characteristics. All traditional linear approaches provided a single gain recommendation at various frequencies and maximum output sound pressure level estimated from easily obtainable audiometric threshold or MCL and UCL measures.

Prescription of Gain and Output (POGO)

McCandless and Lyregaard (1983) developed a prescriptive fitting strategy that provides gain and maximum power output (MPO) recommendations for mild to severe sensorineural hearing losses. The predictive gain recommendations used in POGO are derived from the audiometric threshold, similar to Lybarger's approach (Lybarger, 1946). POGO also applied a mathematical scaling factor of 0.5 to the magnitude of threshold loss to derive recommended gain. McCandless and Lyregaard proposed a slight reduction in low frequency gain values to optimize speech intelligibility in noise due to the undesirable effects of the upward spread of masking. The POGO prescriptive formula was developed from a series of studies designed to carefully define the optimum listening levels for various degrees and types of hearing impairment (McCandless, 1987). Other factors such as speech intelligibility and overall pleasantness were incorporated into the design.

POGO is one of the simplest linear formulas to implement clinically. In addition, POGO was designed to (1) avoid the relative complexity and time demands of the comparative approaches, (2) be easily implemented, and (3) be accurate for a large number of users based on routine audiometric threshold data. It was designed to provide a complete, comprehensive method of selection, implementation, and verification for losses of cochlear and conductive origin with proper computational corrections. POGO provides recommendations for hearing aid selection using 2 cc coupler data provided by the manufacturer.

POGO claims that, although ideal gain may be calculated from threshold values, the resultant gain does shift speech and other sounds correctly into the patients' MCL range. Small corrections to the volume control alter the intensity of these sounds to meet the patients' MCL requirements. Insertion gain and ease of implementation is evident by the formulas shown in Table 11–1. Suggested verification of the POGO is through the use of insertion gain measurements obtained at the eardrum using *in situ* probe tube measurements. It is interesting to note that POGO also includes general, but not specific, recommendations, for reserve gain when the formula is used to choose an appropriate fitting circuit from published manufacturer data. POGO accommodates binaural fittings by allowing the user to adjust gain through use of the volume control, rather than specifying *a priori* compensation values. This is because of the potentially wide variations in loudness discomfort reported among patients.

Revised NAL (NAL-R)

Among the most popular linear amplification formulas still in use today are the National Acoustic Laboratories (NAL) and the revised (NAL-R) procedures (Byrne & Dillon, 1986). Similar to POGO, the NAL-R is calculated from the audiometric thresholds and verified preferably through real-ear procedures. NAL-R employs relatively simple formulas (shown in Table 11–2) that attempt to make all bands of speech equally loud. In doing so,

Table 11–1. POGO procedures for insertion gain.

Frequency (Hz)	*Formula*
250	(½ * HL) – 10 dB
500	(½ * HL) – 5 dB
1000	½ * HL
2000	½ * HL
3000	½ * HL
4000	½ * HL

POGO Procedures for determining MPO

$$\text{MPO} = \frac{(\text{UCL 500 Hz}) + (\text{UCL 1000 Hz}) + (\text{UCL 2000 Hz})}{3}$$

Table 11–2. Revised NAL procedure.

Step 1. Calculate X where:

$X = 0.05\ (H500 + H1000 + H2000)$

Step 2. Calculate gain at each frequency:

$G\ 250 = X + 0.31\ H\ 250 - 17$

$G\ 500 = X + 0.31\ H\ 500 - 8$

$G\ 750 = X + 0.31\ H\ 750 - 3$

$G\ 1000 = X + 0.31\ H\ 1000 + 1$

$G\ 1500 = X + 0.31\ H\ 1500 + 1$

$G\ 2000 = X + 0.31\ H\ 2000 - 1$

$G\ 3000 = X + 0.31\ H\ 3000 - 2$

$G\ 4000 = X + 0.31\ H\ 4000 - 2$

$G\ 6000 = X + 0.31\ H\ 6000 - 2$

Where:

G is the required gain at the specified frequency

H is the hearing threshold level obtained from the audiogram

this approach hopes to maximize audibility and speech intelligibility. The NAL-R applies frequency-specific calculations based on the long-term average speech spectrum, whereas POGO and other linear prescriptive formulations assume a flat response characteristic. The NAL-R utilizes mathematic scaling corrections slightly different than the straightforward ½ gain rule used in the Lybarger and POGO approaches, but they are simple enough to incorporate manually without the need for computer software. The NAL-R shares a similar low frequency attenuation rationale with POGO and many other linear formulas to optimize speech information delivered to the ear. The NAL procedure also supplies a formula for correction to a 2 cc coupler so that an appropriate hearing aid may be chosen from published data.

Berger Method

Another popular, linear approach is the Berger prescriptive method initially described in 1976 and again in 1979 by Berger, Hagberg, and Rane. It was updated in 1988. The formula shown in Table 11–3 is relatively simple to

Table 11–3. Berger procedure for calculating full-on 2cc gain.

	Formula	
Frequency (Hz)	***BTE***	***ITE***
500	$\frac{HL\ 500}{2.0} + 10$	$\frac{HL\ 500}{2.0} + 10$
1000	$\frac{HL\ 1000}{6} + 10$	$\frac{HL\ 1000}{1.6} + 10$
2000	$\frac{HL\ 2000}{5} + 12$	$\frac{HL\ 2000}{1.5} + 10$
3000	$\frac{HL\ 3000}{6} + 13$	$\frac{HL\ 3000}{1.7} + 10$
4000	$\frac{HL\ 4000}{9} + 10$	$\frac{HL\ 4000}{1.9} + 10$
6000	$\frac{HL\ 6000}{2.0} + 10$	$\frac{HL\ 6000}{2.0} + 10$

implement, yet like the NAL-R, it is derived from a series of comparatively sophisticated rationales based on several key acoustic conditions and observations of normal speech intensities. A key assumption in the Berger approach is that speech is presented at an average sound pressure level of 55 to 70 dB. The desired gain to amplify these levels of speech, therefore, would require amplification of slightly more than ½ the magnitude of the audiometric threshold loss. The Berger approach contends that the most important frequency spectrum relating to speech intelligibility is contained from 2 to 4 KHz. The speech spectrum reveals these high frequencies also have the lowest energy, making amplification in these regions most critical. The contribution of speech discrimination declines after approximately 4 KHz; therefore, these frequencies are not emphasized. Below 500 Hz, voiced vowels and voiced consonants produce a significant amount of low-frequency energy, yet contribute relatively little to overall speech intelligibility. Therefore, frequencies below 500 are also de-emphasized in the Berger approach.

Gain is applied according to measures obtained from the audiometric thresholds and thus is considered to be a predictive prescriptive method. Maximum gain is specified in the final recommendations rather than the typical operating or use gain. This is because the operating gain is usually variable according to individual preference and particular listening situation. As such, the maximum gain is set according to the formula: maximum gain = operating gain + reserve gain ± correction factors for BTE vs. ITE microphone settings.

For conductive losses, an additional ⅕ gain factor is added to the operating and maximum gain values. Saturation sound pressure levels (SSPL) and binaural correction are also suggested.

Byrne and Tonisson

The Byrne and Tonisson (1976) rationale is based on maximizing speech intelligibility by presenting all of the frequency components of speech presented to the impaired ear at equal loudness levels. To implement this prescriptive method, tables were used to indicate the relationship between the audiometric threshold levels and the user's recommended gain at various critical frequencies. Other modifications of this procedure used MCLs and LDLs of speech to specify the recommended gain at various frequency regions (Byrne & Murray, 1985).

THEORETICAL LIMITATIONS OF LINEAR AMPLIFICATION APPROACHES

The traditional formulas described in this chapter are characterized by the single-gain specifications that most often predict insertion or coupler gain values from the audiometric threshold data or from direct measurement of the MCLs or UCLs. Gain recommendations are based on rationales derived from unique perspectives, each having distinct outcomes and characteristic response patterns. The variability can be seen from the examples shown in Figure 11–1. However, similarities do exist. Regardless of the hearing loss, the prescribed gain provided by linear formulas is generally sufficient to optimize speech presented at or near an "ideal" 60 dB sound pressure level. 60 dB correlates to conversational speech levels measured at speaker-listener distances of approximately 3 to 6 feet, and rarely any farther. Linear hearing aids fit with conventional methods continue to overamplify louder environmental and speech inputs, while underamplifying softer speech signals. The result of restoring hearing with single gain recommendations is that the loudness is accommodated at only one moderate intensity input level. Because these formulas are limited in their ability to provide satisfactory amplification for soft speech and too much loudness for loud sounds, this limited the usefulness of the early linear formulas to face-to-face conversations in quiet.

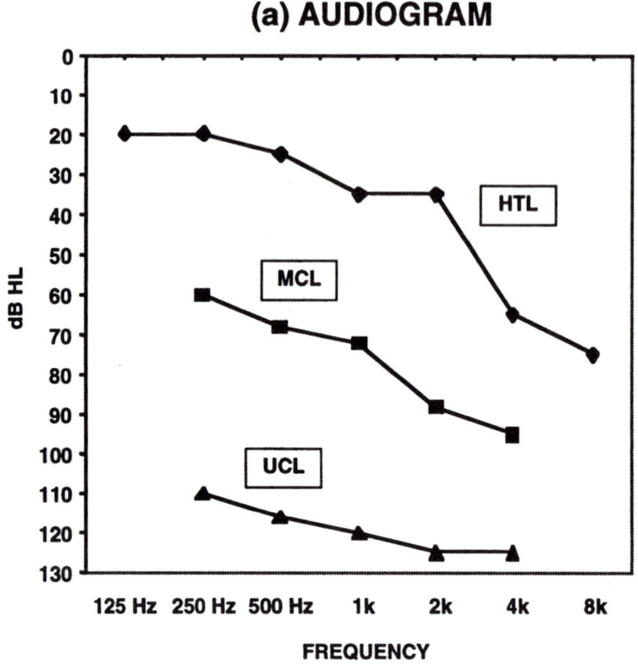

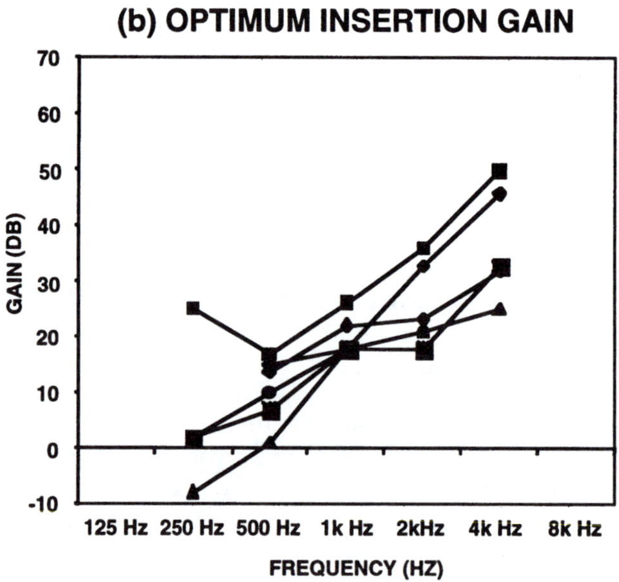

Figure 11–1. Prescribed ideal gain/frequency characteristics **(b)** calculated from seven different procedures for a typical high frequency hearing loss shown in **(a)**. Graph is adapted from McCandless (1987) with permission.

Figures 11–2, 11–3, and 11–4 illustrate this paradoxical overamplification and underamplification problem associated with linear amplifiers and single-gain formulas. Figure 11–2 shows two empirically derived mean loudness-growth functions using a 2 KHz pure tone from 10 normal and 5 subjects with 60 dB unilateral sensory hearing losses. These curves are binaural loudness-balance experiments wherein the loudness estimations of the impaired or "poorer" are ear plotted against a reference level of the unimpaired or "normal" ear. The "better" ear acts as a reference or control ear for the subjects with unilateral losses. An arbitrary ear was chosen to serve as the "better" ear for the normal hearing subjects. The diagonal line extending from 0 to 115 dB represents the loudness-growth function from the subjects with normal hearing. The curvilinear line of Figure 11–2 is the mean loudness curve obtained from the five unilateral, hearing impaired subjects with 60 dB hearing loss. These curves are similar to loudness-growth curves reported by Hell-

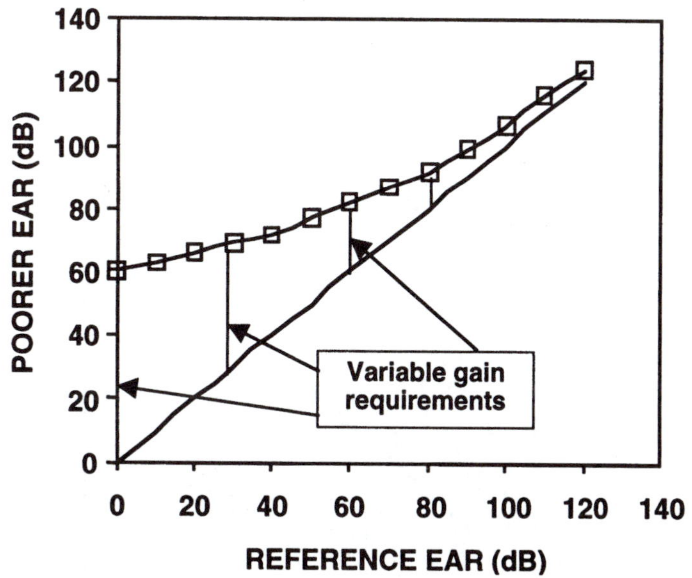

Figure 11–2. Typical I/O plot showing the auditory dynamic range and loudness growth curves for a 2 KHz pure tone measured in 5 individuals with unilateral sensory hearing loss and 10 individuals with normal hearing bilaterally (see text). The diagonal line extending from 0,0 to 120,120 is the binaural loudness balancing function of 10 normal-hearing individuals. The curvilinear line is the mean loudness-growth curves for 5 individuals with a 60 dB hearing loss at 2 KHz. This means that the amount of gain necessary to restore loudness of a 0 dB signal to be judged equally loud by an individual with 60 dB hearing loss, would require 60 dB of gain; 30 dB gain at 60 dB inputs ; and 8 dB gain at 80 dB inputs (see text).

man and Meiselman (1990) and Lyregaard (1988). An interesting side note that bears mentioning is that several recent studies on loudness growth have reported steeper loudness functions than are reported in this chapter. This may be explained from the observation that the newer loudness studies may be using comparatively broad band noise and speech stimuli, which may affect the ear's response to loudness estimates. The steep curves may also be explained simply by differences in the psychoacoustic method used to obtain loudness growth functions (Ricketts, 1997; Elberling 1999).

The gain required to restore the loudness functions to "normal" at each input level for the impaired group is determined by measuring the vertical distance (measured in dB) between the curvilinear loudness-growth function of the impaired ear and the diagonal line of the normal-hearing subjects. In this case, the ideal theoretical hearing aid will require 60 dB of gain to the impaired ear with sinusoidal inputs of 0 dB presented to the better ear, 30 dB gain with a 40 dB input to the better ear, and only 6 dB gain is required at 80 dB.

The line in Figure 11–3 beginning at 30 dB on the ordinate, continuing at a 45° diagonal to asymptote at 115 dB, is a typical I/O curve of a linear hearing aid with a typical ½ gain rule applied. In this case, the I/O curve of the linear hearing aid shows that there is an approximate gain of 30 dB to correct for a 60 dB hearing loss. As stated above, if the ear is to return to normal loudness growth, the amount of gain that should be delivered to the ear is not a constant; rather the amplification requirements are variable as a function of input level. Linear hearing aids provide fixed gain regardless of the input level, therefore the I/O curve of Figure 11–3 can only satisfy loudness requirements of the ear where the I/O curve and loudness growth curves intersect. For inputs below the inter-

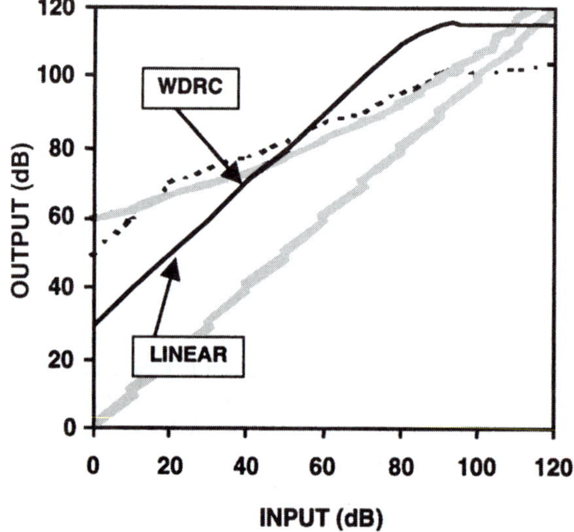

Figure 11–3. I/O performance characteristics of a theoretical linear and WDRC hearing aid superimposed on the loudness-growth curves of Figure 11–2 (*gray lines*). Notice how the WDRC (*dashed line*) best approximates the loudness requirements of the impaired ear.

section (below 60 dB), the linear hearing aid does not provide enough amplification for soft sounds to become audible. For inputs above the intersection (above 60 dB), sound at the output of the hearing aid exceeds the ears' requirements for loudness compensation and is said, therefore, to overamplify.

The mean loudness-growth curve of Figure 11–2 is normalized in Figure 11–4 and is used as a 0 dB reference from which linear and WDRC instruments can be compared. Figure 11–4 is an illustration of amplification error, or the relative overamplification at higher inputs, and underamplification at lower inputs provided by these two types of amplification. The "ideal" hearing aid would provide a response characteristic that would not deviate from this 0 dB reference. It can be seen that the greatest deviation from the normalized recruitment curve in Figure 11–4 occurs in the linear instrument. The WDRC instrument better approximates the normalized loudness growth pattern, and thus better satisfies the requirements of the impaired ear. However, this assumes that the WDRC instrument is set by the clinician to provide correct compensation for the magnitude of the hearing loss. That accuracy is determined by factors used in the fitting procedure and the flexibility of the instrument itself.

FORMULAS AND MODERN FITTING STRATEGIES

The presumption of current noncomparative fitting rationales is that if you can provide certain loudness compensation characteristics you can achieve better audibility. More recent analog and digital signal processing

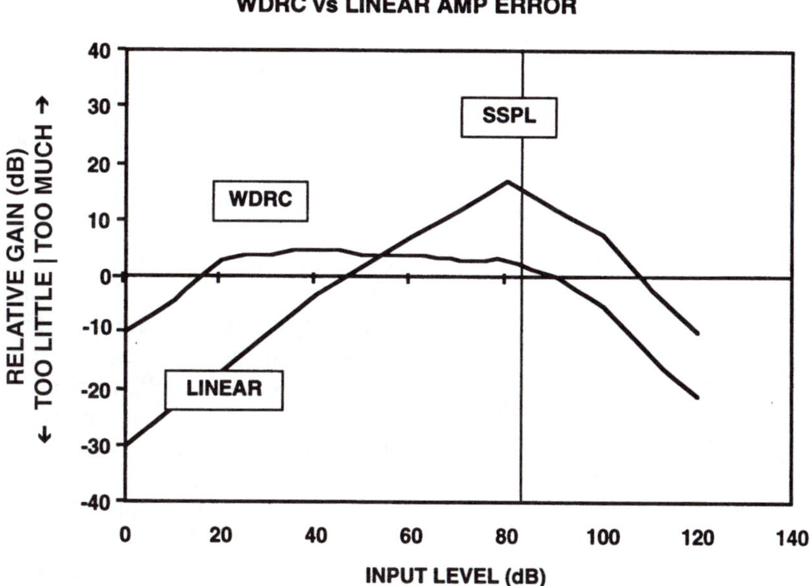

Figure 11–4. Graph illustrating the amount of amplification error (overamplification and underamplification) referenced to a normalized loudness-growth curve for the 5 impaired ears shown in Figure 11–3. An optimum hearing instrument that would correctly accommodate the loudness growth patterns of the impaired ear would demonstrate no deviation from the normalized recruitment (0 dB reference) in the above figure.

technology allows better accommodation for abnormal loudness reconstruction. Currently, compression-class circuitry in modern hearing aids is capable of providing nonlinear amplification characteristics to the ear. Therefore, different gains need to be specified to restore the loudness functions to those more closely approximating normal loudness scaling characteristics.

Further complicating the fitting issue is that hearing loss is not uniform across frequencies. In view of this, the calculation of electroacoustic parameters such as gain and output is not equal at all frequencies. Not only does loudness have to be compensated as a function of input, but calculations of loudness compensation must be duplicated at a wide range of frequencies. Hearing aid manufacturers have responded by providing independent compression function within multiple channels so the hearing loss can be accommodated independently at a relatively large number of frequencies. The following summaries are illustrative of formulas used in modern WDRC instruments. Like their linear counterparts, the nonlinear prescriptions are based on unique rationales and procedures that result in differences in the ultimate fitting.

NAL Non-linear Version 1 (NAL-NL1)

NAL-NL1 refers to the National Acoustic Laboratories Non-linear Version 1. The fitting formula is among the most recent versions available and is designed to provide the gain-frequency response that will maximize speech intelligibility while controlling the overall loudness at a level that is perceived by a normal listener as acceptable (Dillon, 1999). The audiometric data contained on the audiogram were fed to the computer for analysis along with the parameters of modified AI and loudness algorithms to derive the "rules" of selection and recommendation for a wide range of hearing losses. (Dillon, 1999). The computer derived optimum gain characteristics for each of the 51 audiograms. The goal was to provide maximum speech intelligibility without simultaneously exceeding normal loudness for soft speech. The process was repeated for the same audiogram at moderate and high level speech until an optimum fitting was obtained at various input levels.

According to Dillon, the gain-frequency response requirements are variable according to the input level and therefore are suited to nonlinear instruments. Generally speaking, the NAL-NL1 is reported to give more low frequency attenuation than other nonlinear prescriptive formulas so that it can optimize speech cues available to the impaired listener. It is said that it de-emphasizes the low frequencies because it is difficult for most people to extract speech cues in regions of the greatest loss. The NAL-NL1 emphasizes the higher frequencies more than most other fitting formulas. In the case of steep audiometric contours, Dillon claims that the NAL-NL1 prescribes a more flat gain-response pattern than do other formulas. The NL1 also advocates the use of lower compression ratios.

The mathematical formulas derived from these 51 "optimized" audiograms are not utilized directly, as they are reported to be far too complicated for practical use. Therefore, the NAL-NL1 requires the use of proprietary software to arrive at clinically meaningful instructions. The NAL-NL1 allows the user to input the audiometric data, aid type, vent size, tubing type, number of channels, and signal type used in the analysis. Further, it will output the recommended I/O curve, insertion gain curves, REAR curves, coupler responses, crossover frequencies, compression thresholds, compression ratios, and gain for 50 and 80 dB inputs. Finally, the suggested MPO or SSPL 90 levels are recommended (Dillon, 1999). Because this procedure is among the newest of the nonlinear formulas, Dillon suggests that the NAL-NL1 is subject to validation, but the typical recommendations from average input levels of the NAL-NL1 yield similar values recommended by the NAL-RP (an updated revision of the NAL-R) at the same input levels.

FIG6 (1994)

Killion and Fikret-Pasa (1993) described three categories of hearing loss and calculated the amount of gain that would satisfy the loudness requirements for those losses. Figure 6 of that article was an illustration of the gain required to achieve those goals, thus, the name FIG6. The gain recommendations are calculated from audiometric threshold data derived from loudness-growth data published by several research sources (Lipmann, Braida, & Durlach, 1981; Lyregaard, 1988; Hellman & Meiselman, 1993). Like the NAL-NL1, and other modern nonlinear formulas, FIG 6 calculates the gain on a frequency-by-frequency basis for each of the three different input levels (40, 65, and 90 dB). This formula is generally useful for hearing losses up to 60 dB and losses with very little need for amplification at higher inputs. Generally, FIG6 is not recommended for losses over 70 dB HL.

FIG6—Gain for <40 dB Inputs

The FIG6 formula originates gain recommendations for soft speech inputs from the observation that portions of quiet conversational speech are as low as 20 dB HL (Mueller & Killion, 1992). Mueller and Killion's count-the-dot audiogram for calculating the articulation index suggests that, if the aided threshold does not provide enough amplification to include speech frequencies at 20 dB, then some of the speech cues will be missed. Gain that restores hearing below 20 dB HL is considered to be excessive because the room noise, as well as hearing aid noise, may mask out lower speech cues. Therefore, the formula is designed to correct hearing to 20 dB, no more and no less. Thus, the formula for 40 dB inputs and lower becomes: G40 = HL − 20.

FIG6—Gain for 65 dB SPL (Conversational Speech)

Pascoe (1988) studied the mean MCLs found in subjects with normal, mild, moderate, and severe hearing losses. He found that the mean MCL for normal listeners was 65 dB HL, 77 dB for mild loss, 90 dB for moderate losses, and so forth. Using the mean MCL data for each level of hearing loss, one may target the amount of gain necessary to transfer conversational speech into Pascoe's predicted MCL levels. The gain formula appropriate for conversational speech inputs is: G65 = (mean MCL [re HL]) − 65

For example, gain at 65 dB for a hearing impaired listener with a 40 dB HL loss would require, 77 dB − 65 dB or 12 dB of gain for a mild 40 dB hearing loss.

FIG6—Gain for 95 dB Inputs

FIG6 prescribes gain based on loudness-growth work reported by Lyregaard (1988) and Lippman et al. (1977). FIG 6 assumes that mild losses typically demonstrate complete loudness recruitment at high sound levels and thus do not need amplification with high inputs. However, as the amount of hearing loss increases into the moderate ranges and above, the amount of required amplification increases only slightly.

Data for two frequency bands are generated in the software package showing the target insertion gain for low, medium, and high input levels. While the Fig 6 procedure specifies REIG targets, it also provides 2 cc coupler recommendations in tabular and graph form for ITE, BTE, ITC, and deep CIC instruments. In doing this, an appropriate hearing aid may be easily selected from the manufacturers published data specifications. One feature of the software is that it specifies compression ratios for the independent low and high frequency channels found on many of the current two-channel instruments.

Independent Hearing Aid Fitting Forum (IHAFF)

The IHAFF was created by a select forum of researchers, manufacturers, and engineers. The purpose of the forum was to reach a consensus for a standardized and comprehensive hearing aid fitting protocol to be applied to linear and modern nonlinear hearing aids. The rationale for the IHAFF is based on the restoration of loudness perception across a wide frequency range. Cox (1995) states that the goal underlying the IHAFF procedure is that "amplification should normalize the relationship between the environmental sounds and loudness perception. This means that a sound that appears to be soft to a normal-hearing listener should be audible but soft, after amplification, to the hearing aid wearer." The same loudness scaling criteria are applied to medium and loud environmental sounds as well. The IHAFF procedure differs from the NAL-NL1 and FIG6 in that gain recommendations are made according to direct loudness scaling measurements obtained from each listener, instead of predicted gain recommendations predicted from the audiometric thresholds.

The implementation of the IHAFF includes direct measures of loudness scaling estimations using 500 and 3000 Hz warble tones stimuli. A computer program, having the acronym *V*isualization of *I*nput/*O*utput *L*ocator *A*lgorithm (VIOLA) assists in categorization of the loudness estimations at 500 and 3000 Hz. These loudness categories are shown in Table 11–4 (Cox, 1995; Cox, Alexander, Taylor, & Gray, 1997).The responsibility of the VIOLA software is to translate the loudness scaled, warble tone data into categories of loudness estimations ranging from soft to uncomfortably loud. Using these data of loudness scaling, the VIOLA program aligns the categories into a meaningful loudness prescription for the hearing aid so that soft sounds are perceived as soft, and loud sounds are perceived as loud, approaching but not exceeding the user's LDLs. The procedure uses audiometric pure tone threshold data, combined with the loudness scaling data, to derive three input level recommended targets for entry into the nonlinear hearing aid. The software program also assists in setting gain, compression thresholds, and output characteristics. Verification procedures are also available on the software. Provisions are also included to predict gain characteristics for those unable to participate in loudness-scaling tasks.

The IHAFF approach is one of the few procedures that relies strongly on direct loudness measures from the patient. The time-factor has been a major point of criticism, as some suggest that it takes a considerably longer time to implement than other procedures. Although this method may prove to be more accurate for any given patient, the time needed to implement may discourage clinical use.

Table 11–4. Categories of loudness used in the contour test.

7. Uncomfortably loud
6. Loud, but okay
5. Comfortable, but slightly loud
4. Comfortable
3. Comfortable, but slightly soft
2. Soft
1. Very soft

Source: Reprinted with permission from "Using Loudness Data for Hearing Aid Selection," by R. M. Cox, 1995. *Hearing Journal, 47*(2), 39–42.

Desired Sensation Level (DSL) [I/O]

The desired sensation level (DSL) was originally the first comprehensive software-driven hearing aid fitting protocols optimized for the fitting of children and others who cannot participate in advanced psychoacoustic measurements (Seewald, Ross, & Spiro, 1985; Seewald, 1994). It started as a formula of amplified speech targets developed for linear instruments, but evolved into a multi-input specific formula for more modern compression-class instruments. Cornelisse (1995) stated that it was the goal of the DSL to develop a formula that would specify ideal electroacoustic parameters for a wide range of inputs, regardless of the unique hearing device characteristics. The procedure seeks to place amplified speech in the listener's residual auditory dynamic range by using estimated suprathreshold data including estimated UCLs. Essentially, the DSL I/O is designed to maximize the speech information without exceeding the sound pressure levels that would make speech uncomfortable (Cornelisse, 1994).

The approach is a threshold-based design that uses a series of mathematical equations that specify output sound pressure level gains according to a range of input levels. Three electroacoustic amplification "reference points" characteristic of most WDRC instruments are identified as three separate amplification regions: (1) input levels below compression threshold, (2) input levels that will exceed the compression threshold when amplified, and (3) the region between these two limits. Linear gain is assumed for the levels below the compression threshold and aggressive limiting is assumed in the regions near UCL. The mathematical equations are used to construct the distinct low, mid, and high amplification "regions" seen in typical input/output (I/O) curves of WDRC amplifiers at a number of frequencies (see Figure 11–5). The DSL attempts to relate these electroacoustic regions of WDRC instruments to measures of residual hearing capacity from the audiometric threshold to levels of discomfort.

The fitting is made primarily from input of the audiometric thresholds alone. Other data such as the UCL are used, but not required to estimate the maximum output. An "exponent" input is allowed in the current software

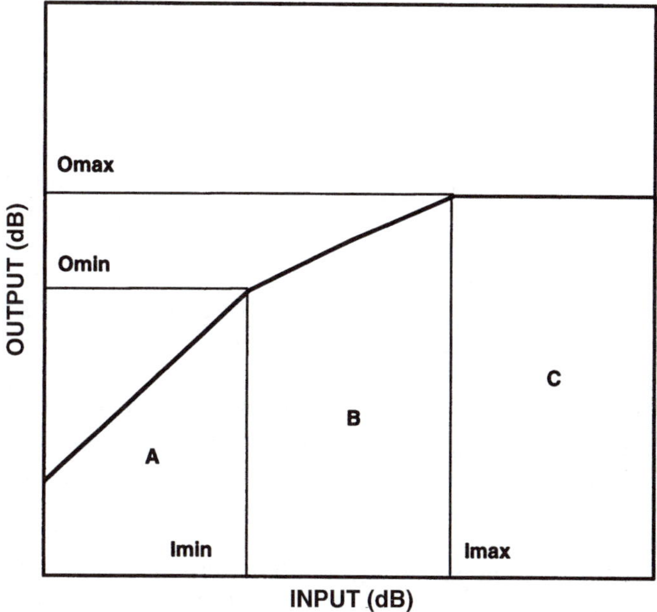

Figure 11–5. I/O function showing regions of (A) linear gain, (B) compression, and C) output limiting of a typical WDRC hearing aid. The DSL I/O approach essentially establishes the lower threshold of compression (intersection of O min and I min) to correspond with threshold levels so that soft sounds become audible, and the upper threshold of compression (intersection of I max and O max) are set to correspond with the patient's UCLs. (Adapted from Cornelisse et al., 1994.)

package, although not required in the calculations, so that a compression ratio of the compression, or mid-amplification region can be more appropriately recommended. Advanced data inputs are allowed for the calculation of real-ear-to-coupler-difference (RECD), real-ear-unaided-gain (REUG), and real-ear-to-dial-differences (REDD). The reader is encouraged to refer to the software package for detailed information relating to features and procedural specifics.

CLINICAL UTILITY OF FITTING FORMULAS

It is necessary to have a fitting protocol that approximates as closely as possible the true fitting requirement that the hearing impaired ear needs and one that the subject finds satisfactory. The objectives are the same as with the linear devices. That is, it is important to get as close a possible to the desired electroacoustic performance before final adjustments are made. Figure 11–6 illustrates the relative difference between the various fitting procedures. Note that some variability is seen with softer (40 dB) and louder (60 dB) inputs. The greatest similarity among the various procedures is found with average (65 dB) inputs with the DSL procedure recommending the most real ear gain at all input levels. This commonality among the three procedures at mid-input levels is probably a good thing, as it would not matter what procedure is used in average listening situations. There may be variability, but all fitting procedures provide benefit to the user. The variability seen with extreme input levels suggests that there may be preferable formulas for certain patients in unique listening environments.

Regardless of the fitting procedure, it is safe to say that all fitting procedures provide at least some, if not a great deal, of benefit to the user. It is not the intent of this chapter to differentiate—or to imply the best formula—but only to educate the reader on the background, rationale, and differences among the most popular fitting strategies. The question of what is the appropriate fitting procedure has been raised many times in the past, and is no less a valid question for modern formulas. Purdy (1999) reported the work of Sullivan, Levitt, Hwang, and Hennessey (1988) who suggested that a significant interaction occurs between the prescriptive method and the subject. It is their contention that, because of this interaction, different methods should be applied to different subjects. But what is the variability seen between the various fitting procedures and subjects that would warrant a change in selecting the fitting procedure? Of course, there is significant variability depending on the type of hearing loss (i.e., conductive, mixed, or sensorineural). Also critical is the presenting pathology contributing to the loss, the survivability and distribution of the hair cell population of the cochlea, and central neural pathways contributing to the conduction and ultimate central processing of environmental sounds. These factors cannot be controlled for in any single fitting formula.

In summary, the latest nonlinear formulas specify gains for a variety of input levels, whereas the linear counterparts are capable of only single-gain level specifications. Not only do the newer formulas consider the need for multiple gain specifications, each calculation must be duplicated across a number of frequencies so that a family of frequency response curves may be generated or assumed in the final fitting. Although it seems astonishing that one may accurately predict a wide range of gains for various inputs from the audiogram alone, this is exactly what most modern prescriptive formulas seek to accomplish. Direct scaling procedures, such as those used in the IHAFF and by a number of select manufacturers such as Resound, arguably provide some assurance that individual variability is not overlooked in loudness compensation. However, threshold-based formulas are seeing a great deal of clinical use, probably due to their relatively time-efficient characteristics and their ease of implementation in everyday clinical use.

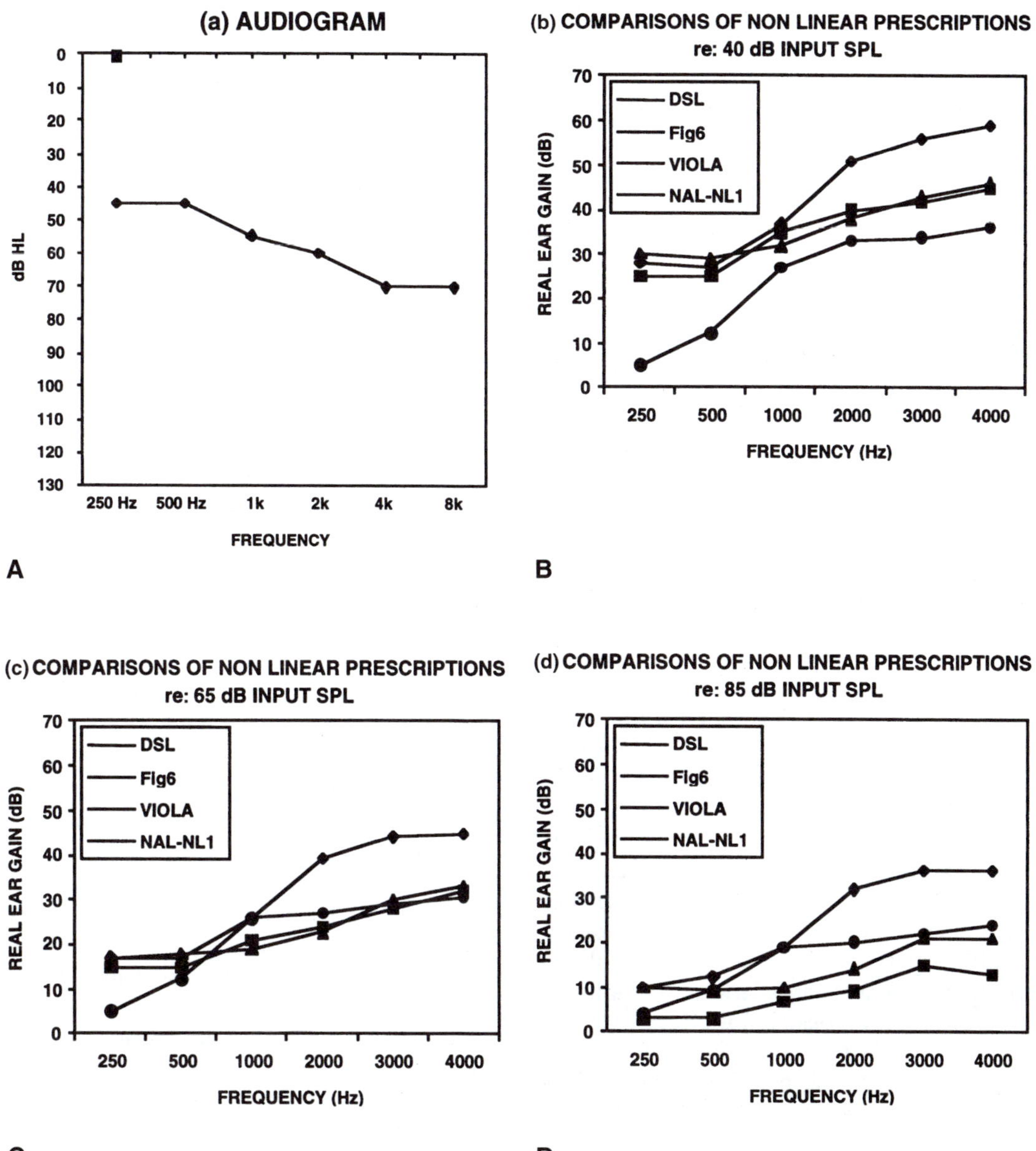

Figure 11–6. Prescribed gain/frequency curves for four nonlinear formulas discussed in chapter. All calculations are based on the audiogram shown in **A.** Gain/response curves of **B**, **C**, and **D** assume inputs of 40, 65, and 85 dB, respectively. All gains are specified as real-ear values, converted in some instances from HA-1 coupler data. Data from 95 dB input specifications were estimated accordingly for procedures where 80 dB input was not specified in the manufacturer's software.

SUMMARY AND CONCLUSION

Ever since the introduction of a commercially available carbon hearing aid developed in 1902 by Hutchinson, there have been valiant efforts to derive a fitting formula that best compensates for the type and magnitude of a given hearing impairment. There have been a number of attempts to develop appropriate fitting formulas, most of which were based on predicting specific gain functions based on threshold data for discrete frequencies. Most, if not all, of the early fitting rationales attempted to compensate for hearing loss using linear amplifiers. It was not until the introduction of nonlinear hearing aid systems that new or modified formulas were introduced to include the advantages offered by these nonlinear instruments.

The rationale underlying any fitting formula is to improve signal audibility and word recognition and to avoid discomfort. With regard to the prescription of gain and output, no two formulas recommended the same values. Bascially, two goals guided the efforts of those who developed a fitting rationale. The first rationale was loudness equalization, the purpose of which was to ensure that each frequency or frequency band had the same loudness perception. The second rationale was to equalize loudness perception for a given range of frequencies or frequency bands. It is evident that normal loudness perception could best be realized through nonlinear ampifiers, whereas linear amplifiers were best suited for loudness equalization. With the introduction of computer-assisted fitting paradigms, innovative methods for determining the "optimal" hearing aid response were introduced and have accelerated the use of fitting formulas.

The purpose of this chapter was to review some of the more popular fitting rationales employed to meet the electroacoustic needs of persons with hearing impairment. Although no one fitting rationale has proved sufficiently compelling to be embraced by all clinicians who select and fit hearing aid devices, a common consensus exists that they are beneficial. That is, a structured approach in arriving at gain and output requirements is far more efficient and utilitarian than some *a priori* approach based on guess, trial, and error.

In the final analysis, as new and more complex signal processing hearing aids are developed, and as we understand more of the behavior of impaired auditory systems, fitting methods will be developed to embrace these new and challenging contributions.

REVIEW QUESTIONS

1. What arguments have some made against the use of the "comparative method" of hearing aid fitting?
   a. It is too time consuming.
   b. It has poor reliability.
   c. It uses too many audiometric frequencies in the calculation of functional gain and output maximums.
   d. b and c
   e. a and b

2. The problem with the "mirrored-audiogram" approach is that it:
   a. Undercompensates hearing by providing too little gain.
   b. Overcompensates hearing by providing too much gain.
   c. Reflects too many sounds from the ear.
   d. None of the above

3. Which linear approaches reported in the article rely solely on audiometric threshold data to arrive at appropriate gain recommendations?
   a. POGO and NAL-R
   b. Berger and NAL-R
   c. POGO, NAL-R, and Berger
   d. None of the above

4. The limitations of linear formulas are seen as:
   a. They specify gain recommendations at only one input level.
   b. They specify gain recommendations at only three (soft, medium, and loud) input levels.

c. a and b
d. None of the above

5. An appropriately fit linear hearing aid better satisfies the loudness requirements of the impaired ear at all input intensities.
a. True
b. False

6. The NAL-NL1 is a complex predictive formula that optimizes speech intelligibility within the constraints of loudness perception for soft, medium, and loud inputs.
a. True
b. False

7. The FIG6 procedure routinely amplifies speech so that sound is audible below 20 dB HL.
a. True
b. False

8. The early version of the DSL was optimized for prescribing electroacoustic hearing aid parameters to children.
a. True
b. False

9. Most nonlinear fitting recommendations appropriate for the use in modern WDRC instruments specify gain for inputs of approximately:
a. 20, 40, and 60 dB
b. 20, 40, and 90 dB
c. 40, 65, and 90 dB
d. 20, 75, and 85 dB

10. Linear formulas assume that loudness accommodation is made with inputs of approximately 60 dB SPL. This sound pressure translates into a typical speaker-listener limitations ranging from _____ feet.
a. 1 to 3
b. 3 to 6
c. 5 to 12
d. 8 to 32

REFERENCES

Berger K., Hagberg, E., & Rane, R. (1977). *Prescription of hearing aids: Rationale, procedures and results.* Kent, OH: Harald Publishing.

Berger, K. W., Hagberg E. N., & Rane, R. L. (1979). *Prescription of hearing aids: Rationale, procedure, and results* (rev. ed.). Kent, OH: Herald Publishing House.

Byrne D., & Dillon, H. (1986). The National Acoustic Laboratories' (NAL) new procedure for selecting the gain and frequency response of a hearing aid. *Ear and Hearing, 7,* 257–265.

Byrne, D., & Murray, N. (1985). Relationships of HTL's, MCL's, LDL's and psychoacoustic tuning curves to the optimal frequency response characteristics of hearing aids. *The Australian Journal of Audiology, 7*(1), 7–16.

Byrne, D., & Tonisson, W. (1976). Selecting the gain of hearing aids for persons with sensorineural hearing impairments. *Scandinavian Audiology, 5,* 51–59.

Carhart, R. (1946). Tests for the selection of hearing aids. *Laryngoscope, 56,* 780–794.

Cornelisse, L. E., Seewald, R. C., & Jamieson, D. G. (1995). The input output formula: A theoretical approach to the fitting of personal amplification devices. *Journal of the Acoustical Society of America, 97,* 1854–1864.

Cox, R. M. Using loudness data for hearing aid selection: The IHAFF approach. *The Hearing Journal, 47*(2), 10, 39–42.

Cox, R. M., Alexander, G. C., Taylor, I. M., & Gray, G. A. (1997). The contour test of loudness perception. *Ear and Hearing, 18,* 388–400.

Davis, H., Hudgins, V., Marquis, R., et al. (1946). The selection of hearing aids. *Laryngoscope, 56,* 85–115, 135–163.

Dillon, H. (1998, June). *Compression sorts of things.* Jackson Hole Rendezvous, Jackson Hole, WY.

Dillon, H. (1999). NAL-NL1: A new procedure for fitting non-linear hearing aids. *Hearing Journal, 52*(4), 10–16.

Elberling, C., & Naylor, G. (1996, May). *Evaluation of nonlinear processing using speech signals.* Lake Arrowhead Conference.

Elberling, C. (1999). Loudness scaling revisited. *Journal of the American Academy of Audiology, 10,* 248–260.

Harris, J. D. (1976). Introduction to hearing aids: Current developments and concepts. In M. Rubin (Ed.), *Hearing aids* (pp. 3–6). Baltimore, MD: University Park Press.

Hellman, R. P., & Meiselman, C. H. (1993). Rate of loudness growth of pure tones in normal and impaired hearing. *Journal of the Acoustical Society of America, 2,* 966–975.

Hellman, R. P., & Meiselman, C. H. (1990). Loudness relations for individuals and groups in normal and impaired hearing. *Journal of the Acoustical Society of America, 88,* 2596–2606.

Killion, M. C., & Fikret-Pasa, S. (1993). The three types of sensorineural hearing loss: Loudness and intelligibility considerations. *Hearing Journal, 46*(11), 31–34.

Lipmann, P., Braida, L., & Durlach, N. (1981). Study of multichannel amplitude compression and linear amplification for persons with sensorineural hearing loss. *Journal of the Acoustical Society of America, 69*(2), 524–534.

Lyregaard, P. (1988). POGO and the theory behind. In J. Jensen (Ed.), *Hearing aid fitting: Proceedings of the 13th Danavox Symposium* (pp. 92–94). Copenhagen, Denmark: GN Danavox.

Lybarger, S. F. (1944). Method of fitting hearing aids. United States Patent Application No. 543,278. Filed July 3, 1944.

McCandless, G. A. (1987). POGO method of hearing aid selection. In E. Zelnick (Ed.), *Hearing instruments: Selection and evaluation* (pp. 95–115). New York: National Institute for Hearing Instrument Studies.

McCandless, G. (1995). Hearing aid formulae and their application. In R. E. Sandlin (Ed.), *Handbook of hearing aid amplification. Volume 1: Theoretical and technical considerations* (pp. 221–238). San Diego, CA: Singular Publishing Group.

McCandless G., & Lyregaard, P. (1983). Prescription of gain and output (POGO) for hearing aids. *Hearing Instruments, 34,* 16–21.

Mueller, H. G., & Killion, M. C. (1992). An easy method for calculating the Articulation Index. *Hearing Journal, 46*(9), 14–17.

Pascoe, D. (1988). Clinical measurements of the auditory dynamic range and their relation to formulas for hearing aid gain. In J. Jensen (Ed.), *Hearing aid fitting: Proceedings of the 13th Danavox symposium* (pp. 81–94). Copenhagen, Denmark: GN Danavox.

Purdy, J. K. (1999). Validation of hearing instruments. Part 3: Non-linear fitting prescriptions. *The Hearing Review, 69*(3), 22–30.

Resnick, D., & Becker, M. (1963). Hearing aid evaluation: A new approach. *Asha, 5,* 596–699.

Ricketts, T. (1997). Clinical use of loudness growth procedures. *Hearing Journal, 50*(3), 10–15.

Ross, M. (1978). Hearing aid evaluation. In J. Katz (Ed.), *Handbook of clinical audiology* (2nd ed., pp. 524–549). Baltimore, MD: Williams and Wilkins.

Seewald, R. C., Ross, M., & Spiro, M. (1985). Selecting amplification characteristics for young hearing impaired children. *Ear and Hearing, 6,* 48–53.

Seewald, R. C. (1994). Fitting children with the DSL method. *Hearing Journal, 47*(9), 10, 48–51.

Shore, I., Bilger, R.D., & Hirsch, I. J. (1960). Hearing aid evaluation: Reliability of repeated measurements. *Journal of Speech and Hearing Disorders,* 25, 152–170.

Sullivan, J., Leavitt, H., Hwang, J., & Hennessey, A. (1988). An experimental comparison of four hearing aid prescription methods. *Ear and Hearing,* 9, 22–32.

Watson, N., & Knudsen, V. (1940). Selective amplification in hearing aids. *Journal of the Acoustical Society of America, 11,* 406–419.

West, R., Kennedy, L. & Carr, A. (1937): *The rehabilitation of speech* (p. 9). New York: Harper Brothers.

Van Vliet, D. (1995). A comprehensive fitting protocol. *Audiology Today, 7,* 11–13.

CHAPTER 12

Ear Canal Resonances

SÖREN WESTERMANN, M.Sc.

OUTLINE

Editor's note: In the first edition of this book, the section on ear canal resonances was part of the Libby and Westermann chapter. In the revised edition, the Westermann chapter on ear canal resonances stands alone. The principles and clinical utility of real ear measurement are discussed in the next chapter by Robert Martin.

Performing real ear measurements may appear to be a straightforward procedure. The measurements, however, are performed in a highly complex and sophisticated acoustic environment that contains many pitfalls. Understanding these acoustic parameters can help considerably in improving the reliability of real ear measurements.

Directional acoustics, external ear acoustics, and earmold acoustics (earmold plumbing) are complex phenomena that one tends to underestimate. What influence on the response does a change from a 2 mm to a 3 mm earmold bore cause? Questions like this seem difficult to answer, and the trend has been to almost ignore them because so few hearing health care professionals possess a thorough understanding of the nature of real ear measurements.

Real ear measurements make possible the verification of an actual acoustic system and also make available the tools to investigate response changes in the acoustic system. This section describes the various acoustic components, their characteristics, and their influence on the final acoustic response. The electroacoustic measurements in this section were performed by the author.

DIRECTIONAL ACOUSTICS

The directional variations of the sound field, caused by the torso, head, and pinna, are factors in real ear measurements. It is important to be aware of these effects to obtain reliable test results. Figure 12–1 shows the sound level variation as measured at the "eardrum" of KEMAR for five different frequencies as a function of the horizontal angle of incidence. Differences on the order of 30 to 40 dB can be

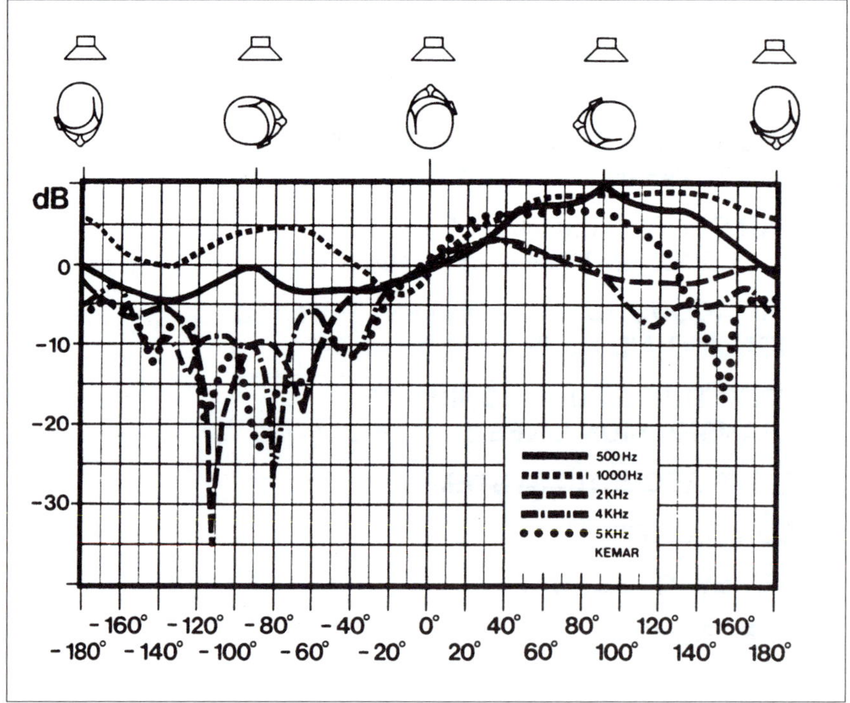

Figure 12–1. The SPL as a function of the horizontal angle of incidence measured on KEMAR (right ear). The five responses at different frequencies are normalized for frontal (0°) incidence.

seen and are most pronounced at the higher frequencies.

Figure 12–2 shows the same measurements taken in the median plane. Each direction in space has its own unique frequency pattern that is exploited in an ingenious way by the brain. The VIIIth nerve nuclei are capable of separating this frequency pattern from the original sound signal, converging it into the corresponding directional information, and presenting it as a conscious directional feeling as suggested by Figure 12–3. Thus individuals do not *hear* the change in frequency pattern, they only *experience* a change in sound direction.

Nevertheless, this frequency coloring does exist at the eardrum and will, therefore, distort real ear measurements if the head is moved during the measuring procedure. Figure 12–4 shows how the insertion gain may vary if the head is turned between measuring the open ear sound pressure level (SPL) and the aided ear SPL.

Ideally, an ITE hearing aid has an insertion gain that is independent of the direction to the sound source due to the fact that an ITE picks up approximately the same directional variations as does the real ear (Westermann & Toepholm, 1985).

In particular, behind-the-ear aids (BTEs), hearing glasses, and body aids pick up the sound at positions where the directional variation is markedly different from the variation at the entrance to the ear canal. Figure 12–5 shows insertion gains of a BTE aid, measured correctly but with the loudspeaker in five different positions. Considerable variations on the order of 30 dB are found and most distinctly at high frequencies.

Figure 12–6 shows similar results for a canal instrument. Clearly, the canal aid picks up exactly the same directional information

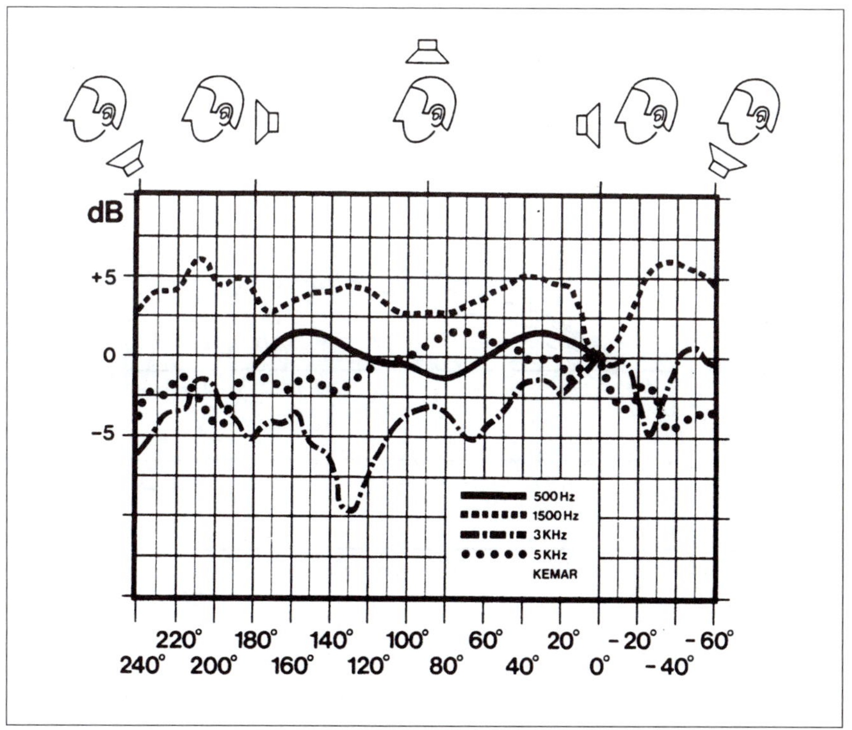

Figure 12–2. The SPL as a function of the vertical angle of incidence (the median plane) measured on KEMAR. The four responses at different frequencies are normalized for frontal (0°) incidence.

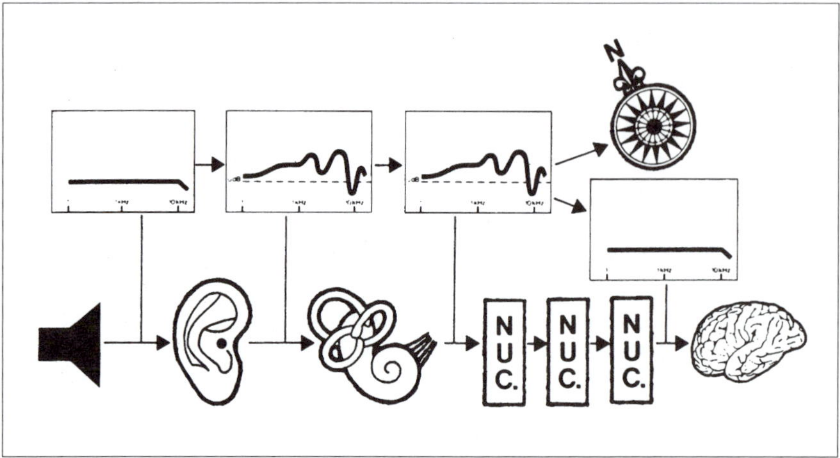

Figure 12–3. The nuclei in the VIIIth nerve separate the frequency coloring pattern caused by the head, pinna, concha, and ear canal from the original signal and convert it into directional information that is experienced as a directional feeling.

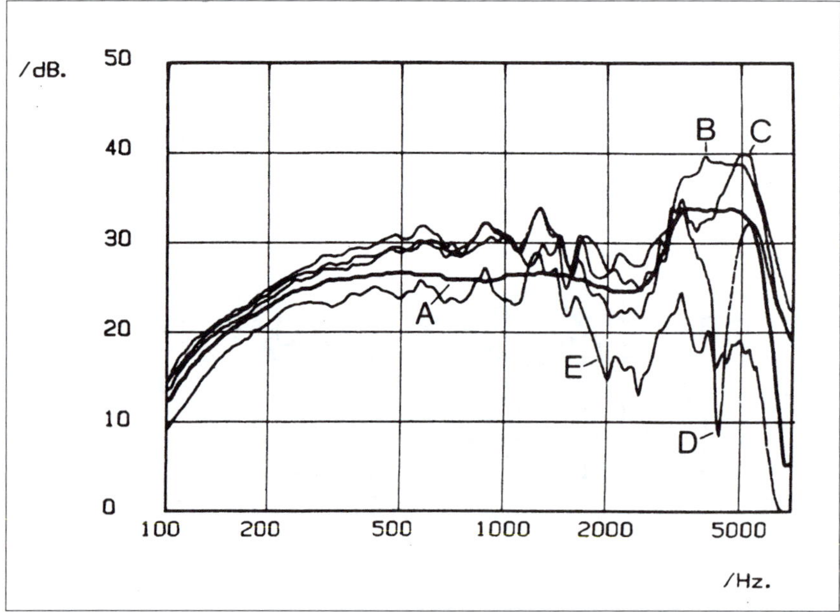

Figure 12–4. The curves show how much the measured insertion gain may vary if the head is turned between the open ear measurement and the aided ear measurement using a canal instrument (KEMAR). The baseline (0 dB) is the open ear calibration curve measured at frontal (0°) incidence, the insertion gains are measured at A: 0°, B: 45°, C: 90°, D: 135°, E: −90°.

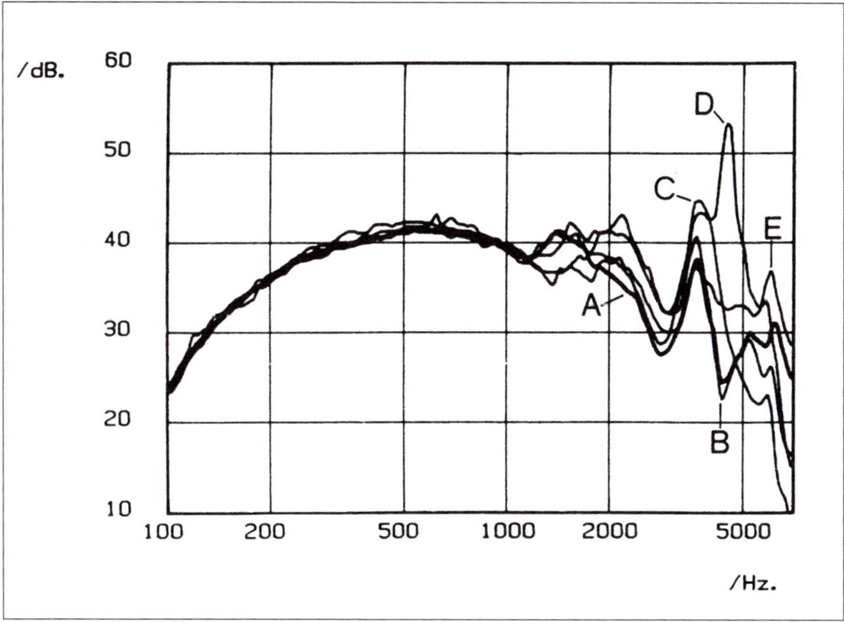

Figure 12–5. True insertion gains of a wide range BTE instrument measured on KEMAR with different horizontal angles of incidence. A: 0°, B: 45°, C: 90°, D: 145°, E: 180°.

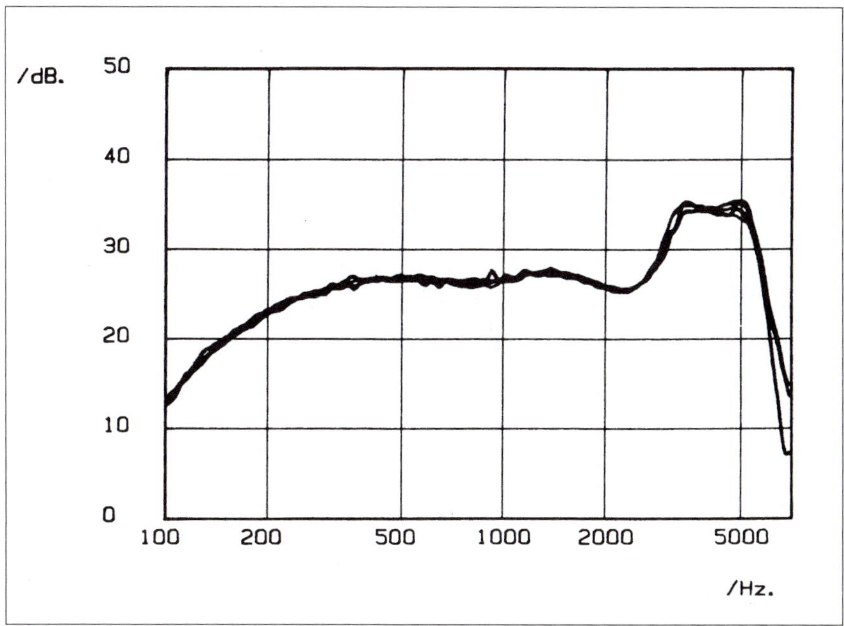

Figure 12–6. True insertion gain of a canal aid measured on KEMAR with horizontal angles of incidence of 0°, 45°, 90°, 135°, 180°.

as the open ear up to at least 6 kHz. A canal aid, and to a certain extent other ITE instruments, can be regarded as having one unique insertion gain. BTEs and other aids have different insertion gains from each angle of incidence. Consequently, as one normally faces the sound source, it is generally suggested that the dispenser always use frontal incidence of the sound when carrying out real ear measurements, particularly with noncanal instruments.

EXTERNAL EAR ACOUSTICS

The external ear consists of the pinna, concha, ear canal, and the eardrum. Although the external ear is individually shaped (normally, symmetry does not even exist between the same individual's two ears) certain common features can be observed (Figure 12–7).

The main function of the pinna is to disturb the sound field around the ear canal opening in a complex manner, enabling the brain to extract directional information from the received sound and thereby make directional hearing possible.

The effect of the concha is also influenced by the direction of the sound source, whereas the ear canal effect is essentially independent of the sound direction. Both the concha and the ear canal produce resonance effects that strongly relate to their physical dimensions. The ear canal is an individually shaped tube starting at the concha cavum, ending at the eardrum, and normally bending twice in between, resulting in a zigzag shape (Figure 12–8). It tilts slightly upward toward the eardrum and has an average length of 25 mm. As the eardrum is tilted approximately 40 to 50 degrees, the walls of the ear canal vary in length between 20 and 30 mm. The ear canal is normally somewhat oval, being higher than it is wide, and its average diameter is 7.5 mm. The residual volume of the ear canal varies between 1–2 cc (children, small canals) and 3 cc (adults, very wide canals), with the average adult having a volume slightly over 1 cc.

Like the ear canal, a terminated tube has the characteristics of a standing wave resonator. There are several standing wave frequencies possible for a specific tube, but the most important one is that of lowest frequency, called the *quarterwave frequency*. This is

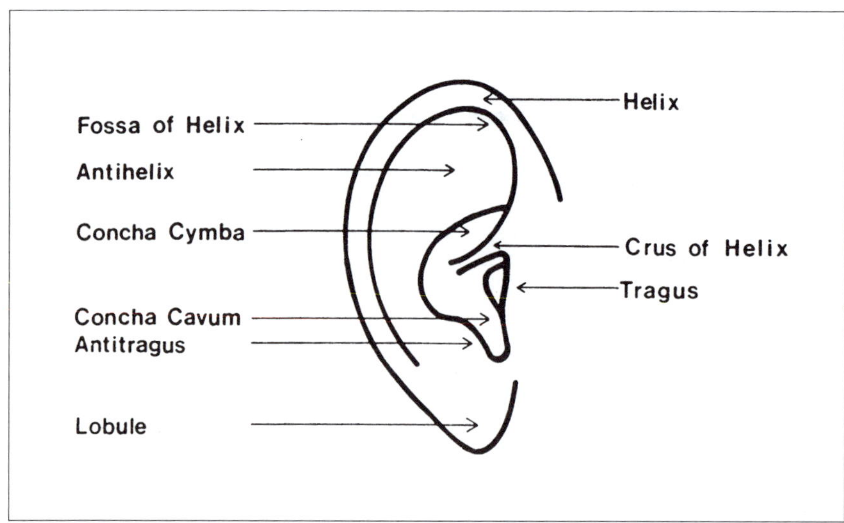

Figure 12–7. Details of the pinna and the concha.

because the length of the canal equals one quarter the wave length of the resonance frequency (Figure 12–9).

In that it is 25 mm in length, the ear canal has a quarterwave frequency (Fc), at approximately 3400 Hz. Combined with the concha (Ic+c), the canal forms a longer resonator (Figure 12–10) having an average length of 34 mm, thus resulting in a quarter wave frequency (Fc+c) of 2500 Hz. The latter resonance (Fc+c) is normally more pronounced than the ear canal resonance (Fc), but often the two resonances merge into broad resonance extending from 2 to 4 kHz. The emphasis of the sound pressure at the eardrum caused by these resonances is normally in the range of 10 to 20 dB.

Two more resonances caused by the ear canal and the ear canal combined with the concha—the three-quarter wave resonances (Figure 12–9)—can be expected at approximately 7.5 kHz and 10 kHz. These peaks often

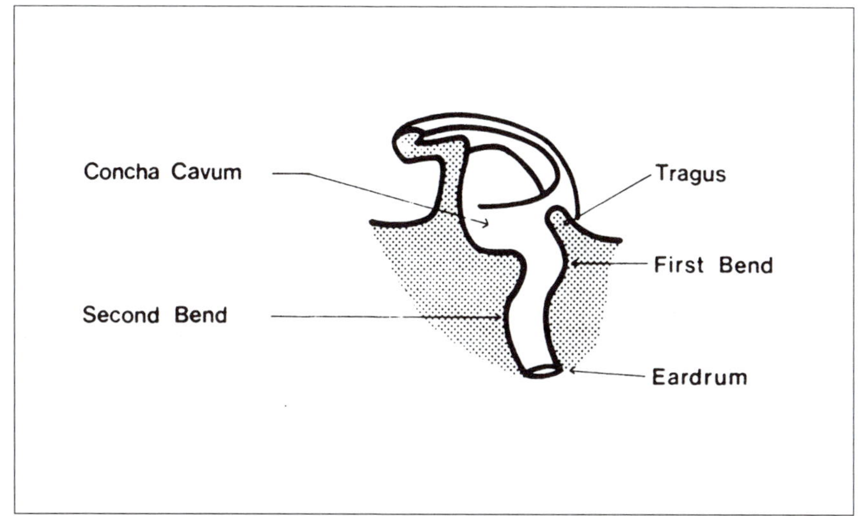

Figure 12–8. Cross-sectional view of the ear canal and the concha.

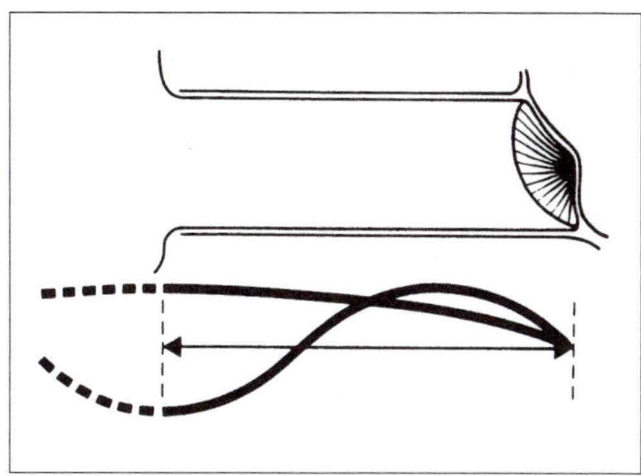

Figure 12–9. The quarter wave and the three-quarter wave resonances' relation to the length of the ear canal.

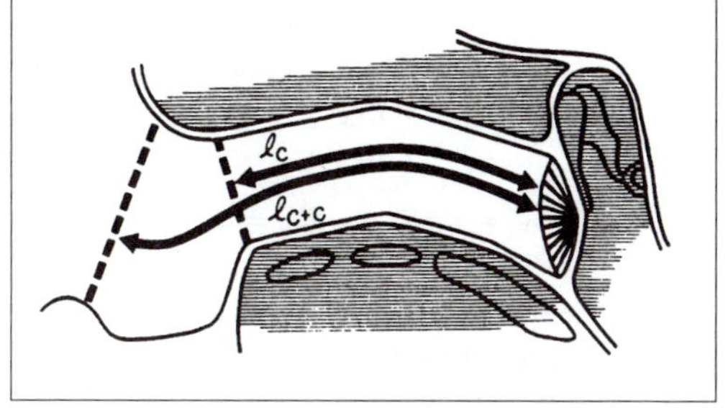

Figure 12–10. Two sets of standing wave resonances involve the ear canal. One set involves the ear canal length (lc) only. The other involves the ear canal combined with the concha (lc+c).

collide with the pronounced directional effects at these high frequencies and with concha resonances that often cannot be recognized or may even vanish in an open ear response. Figure 12–11, taken from Shaw and Teranishi (1968), shows the pressure distribution for (Fc+c), (Fc), and the three-quarter wave resonance relating to the combined canal and cocha length, lc+c.

The concha consists of two open cavities closely connected to each other (see Figure 12–7). The concha cavum is the lower and larger cavity of the two, and at its foremost and deepest part (the tragus), the concha cavum becomes the ear canal. The concha cymba appears just above and is only separated from the concha cavum by the crus of helix.

The concha is individually shaped, but if the crus of helix is left out, the shape approaches that of an ellipse. Burkhard and Sachs (1975) measured 12 male and 12 female ears and found an average concha height of 2.63 cm, concha breadth of 1.30 cm, concha depth of 1.29 cm, and an average volume of 4.30 cc.

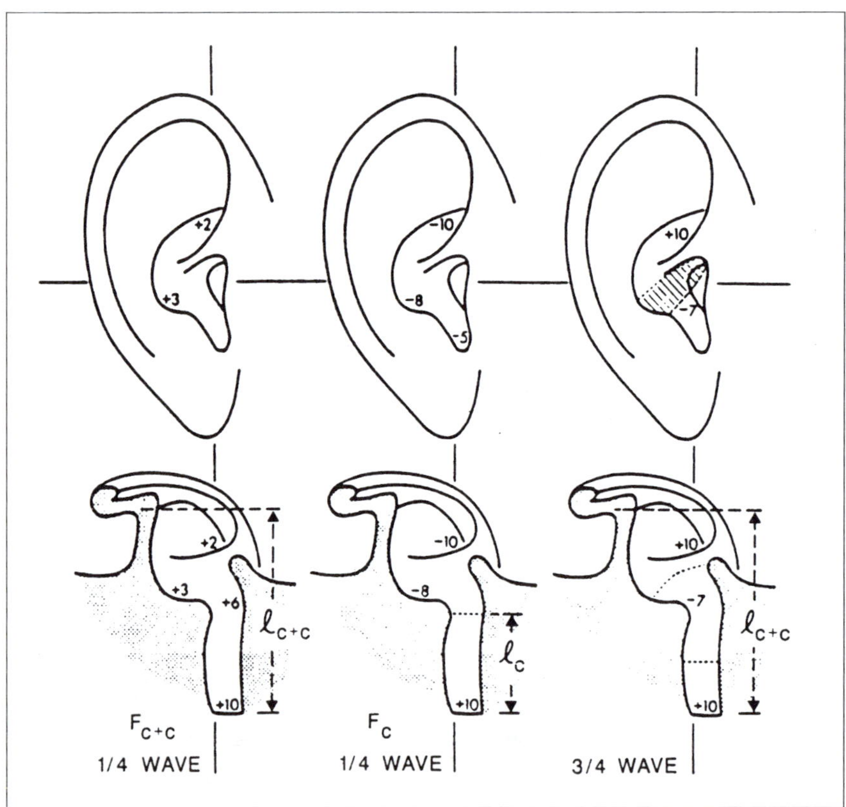

Figure 12–11. Pressure distributions in the concha and the ear canal of an ear replica with hard-wall eardrum at the two quarter-wave ear canal resonances and the three-quarter wave resonance relating to the combined concha and ear canal (lc+c). Dotted lines show standing wave minima, the numerals give relative pressure on a linear scale, and the signs (+, −) indicate phase. Reprinted with permission from "Sound Pressure Generated in an External Ear Replica and Real Human Ears by a Nearby Point Source," by E. A. G. Shaw and R. Teranishi, 1968, *Journal of the Acoustical Society of America, 34.*

Shaw (1975) found that the concha exhibits complex resonance modes, the excitation of which are strongly dependent on the lateral direction to the sound. Six of these modes based on 10 subjects are shown in Figure 12–12 for the "blocked ear canal." These resonances will not necessarily be the same (or present at all) in the open ear canal, but they must closely resemble the resonances present in the concha when a small canal instrument is placed deep in the ear canal.

It appears that at least three different types of resonance modes can be found in the concha (Figure 12–13). Mode 1 at 4.3 kHz is a simple quarter-wave mode related to the depth of the concha, implying an effective concha depth of approximately 1.9 cm for Shaw's subjects. This is shown in Figure 12–12. Modes 2 and 5 appear to be what could be called "bent channel longitudinal resonances," wherein the channel starts at the (blocked) ear canal entrance, goes back and upward in the

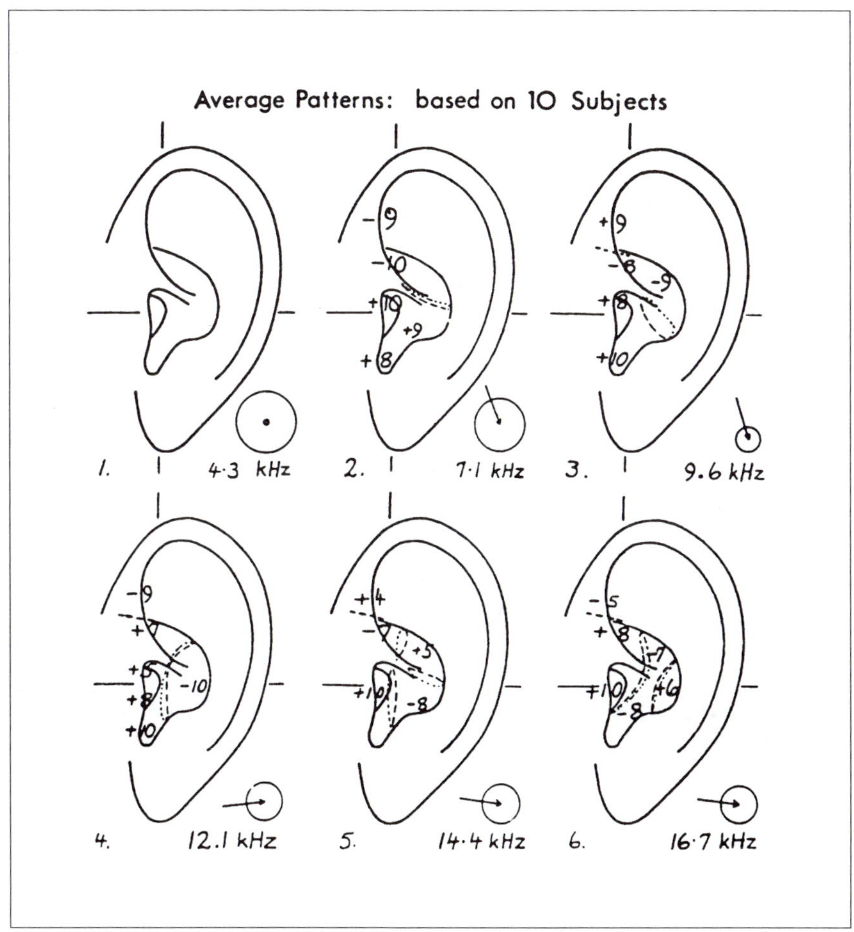

Figure 12–12. Six concha resonance modes measured on 10 individuals with blocked ear canals. The circle to the right of each outline indicates the relative response of that mode at its most favorable angle of incidence as indicated by the arrow. Reprinted with permission from "The external ear: New knowledge," by E. A. G. Shaw, 1975, *Scandinavian Audiology* (Suppl. 5).

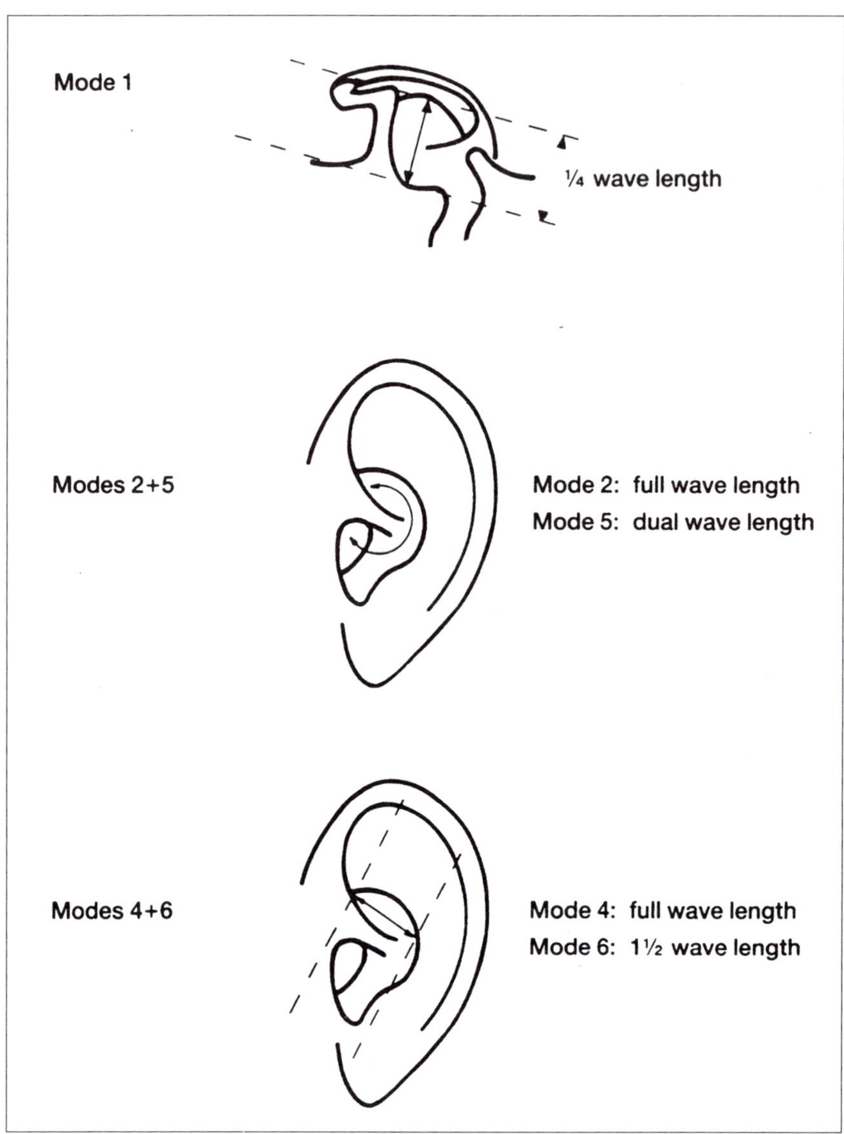

Figure 12–13. Resonance types in the concha, Mode 1: quarter-wave depth resonance. Modes 2 and 5: bent channel longitudinal resonance. Modes 4 and 6: transversal standing waves between two walls of the concha.

concha cavum, and ends in the foremost part of concha cymba. Mode 2 would be a full wave resonance, and Mode 5 (approximately double frequency) would be a dual wave resonance. Modes 4 and 6 are standing waves between two opposite walls in the entire concha. Mode 4 is a full wave standing resonance, and Mode 6 is a 1½ wave standing resonance. Mode 3 is a rather modest resonance, and it is not immediately apparent whether it is a standing wave resonance between two other walls of the concha or another bent channel resonance where the channel may include the fossa or helix.

All six modes produce increased sound levels at the ear canal entrance on the range of 5 to 12 dB. As Figure 12–14 illustrates, this does not imply peaks at the frequencies in the open ear response.

Curve A is a response obtained with a probe tube microphone placed deep in the concha (close to the ear canal entrance) on a real ear with blocked ear canal and frontal sound incidence. Two soft resonances at 3.5 kHz and 6 kHz can be recognized and could be Mode 1 and Mode 2 resonances. Curve B shows the same measurement but with open ear canal and indicates clearly that the ear canal influences the sound pattern in the concha. Curve C is the open ear response as measured close to the eardrum. These curves are quite typical in that the ear canal entrance (curve B) and eardrum (curve C) responses show a certain resemblance up to 5 kHz but with higher levels at the eardrum. When the ear canal is blocked (curve A), the ear canal entrance response changes to a different pattern, which is worth noting in the case of a canal aid that would accept this response as frontal incidence.

The eardrum and the middle ear to which it is coupled show a rather complex behavior and influence on the sound pressure in the ear canal (see Shaw, 1975, for a list of measurements on eardrum impedance).

As the eardrum is somewhat compliant, it adds slightly to the effective length and volume of the ear canal, resulting in lower ear canal resonances than would be found with a hard walled ear canal termination. The eardrum has almost no influence below 1 to 2 kHz.

The residual volume, which is the remaining ear canal volume between an earmold and the eardrum, has a certain impact on the

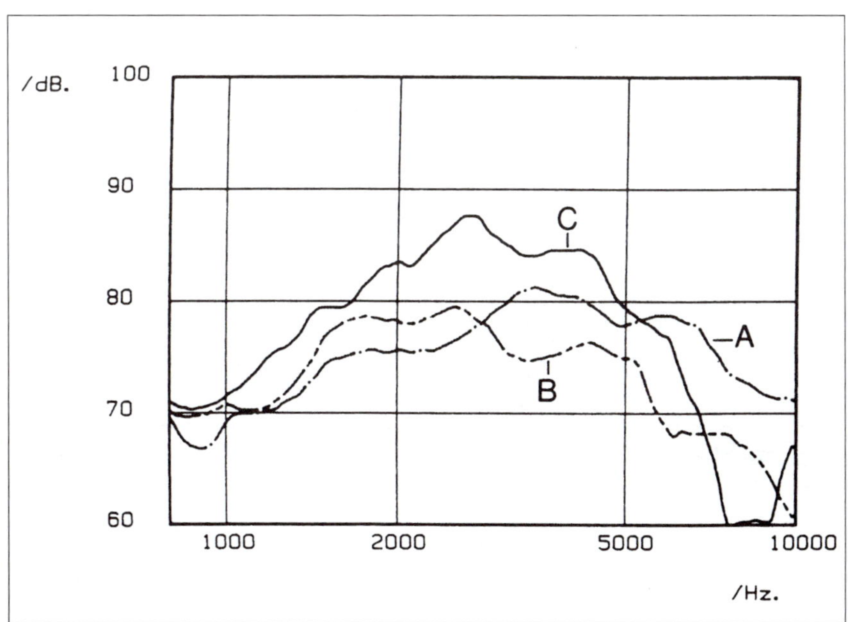

Figure 12–14. SPL measured with probe on one ear by frontal sound incidence (70 dB SPL in free field) at (A) a position deep in concha with ear canal blocked; (B) same position as A but with open ear canal; and (C) a position close to the tympanic membrane with open ear canal (open ear response).

insertion gain. Figure 12–15A and 12–15B show simulated responses for a BTE and an ITE instrument with various residual volumes. As can be seen, a small volume (curve A) results in a high SPL at the eardrum, and a large volume (larger ear canal, curve D) causes the SPL to drop considerably, particularly at high frequencies.

SOUND PRESSURE AT DIFFERENT POSITIONS IN THE EAR CANAL

When using probe measurements on real ears, the position of the probe tube is important to the accuracy and usefulness of measured responses. The situation is quite different for the open ear measurement and the blocked (with an earmold) or aided ear response. The open ear canal acts as a standing wave resonator coupled to the free field, whereas the blocked ear canal is a pressure cavity with essentially uniform sound pressure distribution throughout the residual volume up to 10 kHz. This is true except from the zone close to the sound outlet of the earmold (Sachs & Burkhard, 1972). At frequencies below the combined ear canal and concha resonance (approximately 2500 Hz), the sound pressure distribution throughout the ear canal is quite uniform, resulting in measurements that are essentially independent of probe position.

For the open ear response at higher frequencies, the probe position becomes more critical, and a distance of just a few millimeters from the tympanic membrane may result in errors of several dB.

In the blocked canal case, the major consideration is to position the probe tube outside the near field of the sound outlet from the earmold. Normally a position 5 mm past the earmold tip will guarantee a reliable aided ear response.

For the position of the probe tube, it can be concluded that when taking open ear canal responses, the probe should be positioned as close as possible to the tympanic membrane. For the aided responses, it suffices to ensure a probe-tube position at least 5 mm past the earmold tip. It should be emphasized, however, that the probe must be in the same position if insertion gain is to be accurate.

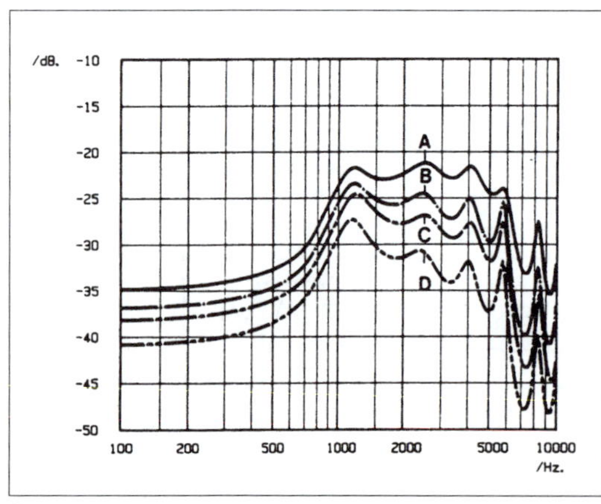

A

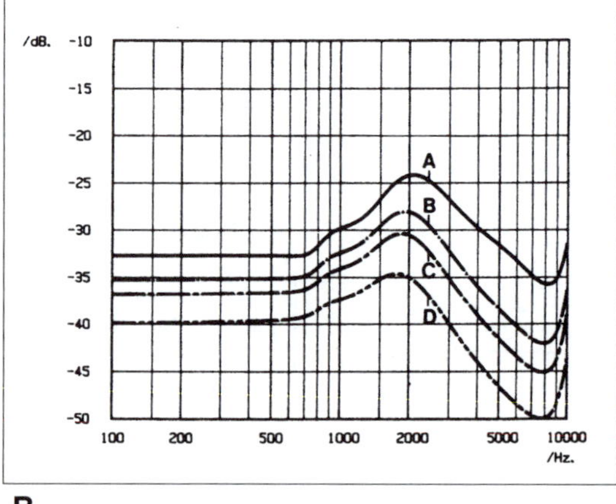

B

Figure 12–15. Simulated responses showing the influence of residual volume on ear simulator response for **(A)** a BTE instrument and **(B)** an ITE instrument: A: residual volume = 1.3 cm × 0.5 cm = 0.26 cc. B: residual volume = 1.3 cm × 0.75 cm = 0.57 cc. C: residual volume = 1.3 cm × 0.9 cm = 0.83 cc. D: residual volume = 1.3 cm × 1.2 cm = 1.47 cc.

EAR CANAL RESONANCES VERSUS RECEIVER AND TUBE RESONANCES

When the open ear canal resonances do not match the receiver resonance and/or the tube resonances for the BTE instrument, undesirable insertion gains may occur. Figures 12–16, 12–17, and 12–18 illustrate this problem. The normal open ear results in an SPL response at the eardrum that exhibits one or more peaks due to various ear canal resonances. Despite the fact that this peaky response is present at the eardrum, one experiences the sound as having a flat or natural response (Figure 12–16). This means that individuals are "used to" the peaky response. When the ear canal is

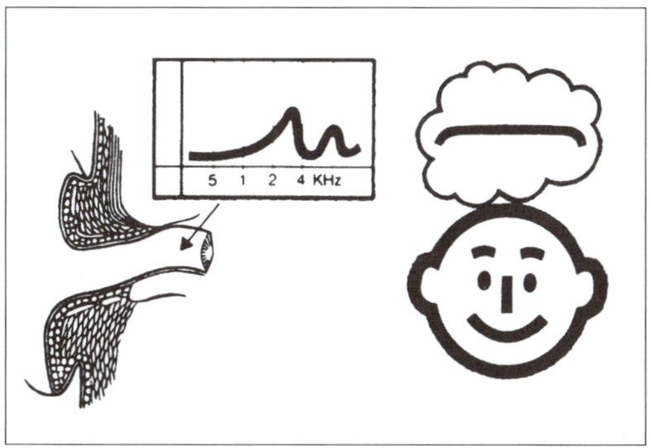

Figure 12–16. The peaks caused by ear canal resonances are not "heard."

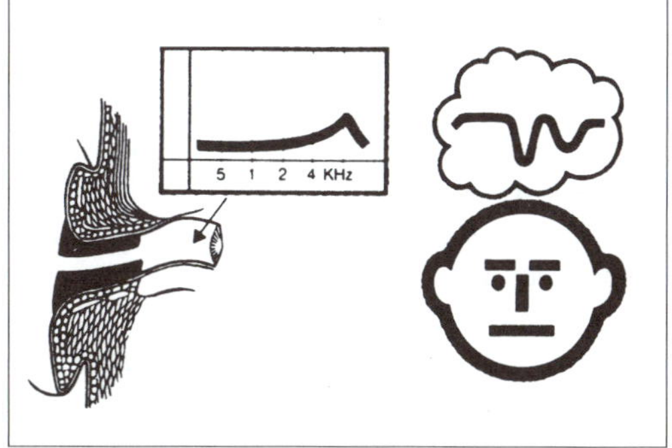

Figure 12–17. Removing the ear canal resonances by inserting an earmold in the canal is experienced as dips in the frequency response.

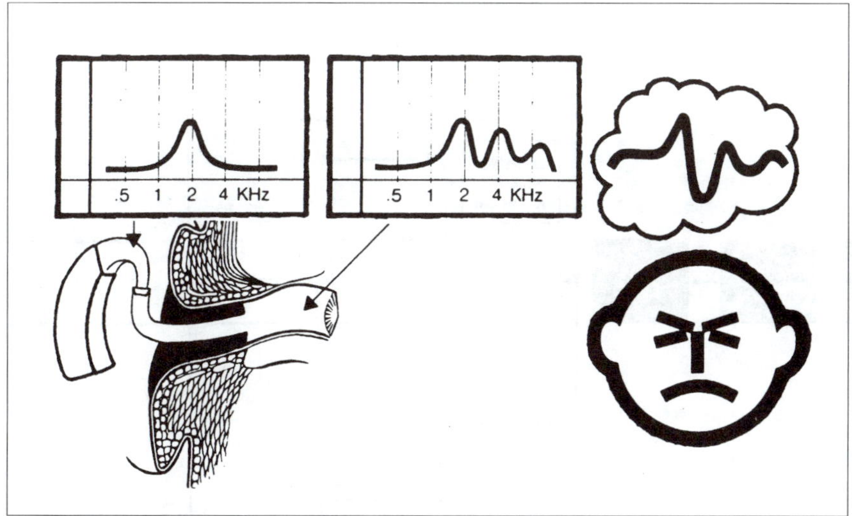

Figure 12–18. Adding a hearing aid system with peaks at frequencies other than the natural ear canal resonances can result in insertion gains with pronounced peaks and valleys.

blocked with an earmold, all these resonances disappear (Figue 12-18). Because individuals are used to the peaky response, they now miss the peaks and instead experience dips or valleys at the frequencies that used to have peaks. If a BTE hearing aid system is added, which has receiver resonances and tube resonance at frequencies that differ significantly from the ear canal resonance frequencies (Figure 12–18), the result is some missing peaks (the ear canal resonances) and some unwanted extra peaks (the receiver and tubing resonances). This situation is quite common and can result in an extremely undesirable insertion gain with pronounced peaks and valleys up to 15 dB in the 1 to 6 kHz range. Apart from obvious drawbacks, such as masking and reduced speech discrimination, it seems that the well-known problems associated with certain annoying types of sounds (e.g., paper rustling and coffee cups clattering) in connection with hearing aids may be traced to this type of insertion gain response. Furthermore, it can be expected that a person with hearing impairment will adjust the instrument volume so that the sound level at those peaks will not feel uncomfortable instead of adjusting the aid to an optimum overall gain. Unfortunately, this is a difficult problem to correct, as it implies the removal of receiver resonance combined with the recreating of individual ear canal resonances.

THE ACOUSTIC ENVIRONMENT FOR A HEARING AID USER

Figure 12-19 is a diagram of all possible sound paths from the sound source to the eardrum of a hearing aid user. The three black boxes to the left and the two boxes to the right constitute the acoustic system of a person with normal hearing. The entire middle section is the hearing aid, the tubing, the earmold, and the possible feedback pathways such as vents, leaks, acoustic couplings, and so forth.

All the elements of the diagram represent acoustic phenomena, except for the hearing instrument. Even though this instrument is mainly electronic, it still contains two com-

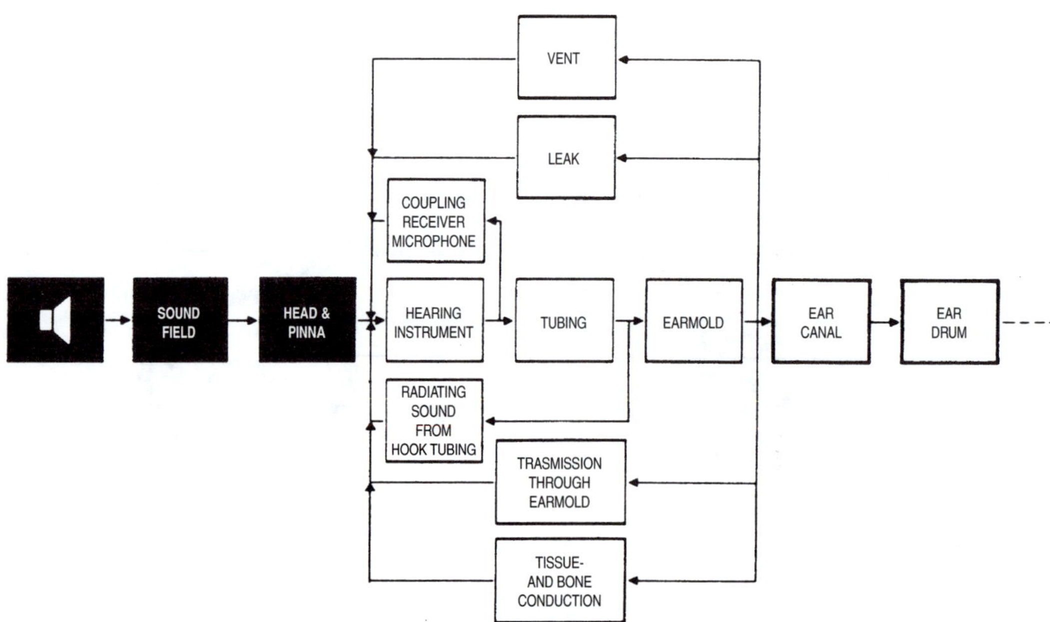

Figure 12–19. All possible sound paths between sound source and eardrum for a hearing aid user.

plex and important electroacoustic elements: the microphone and the receiver.

The two lower boxes (transmission through the earmold proper and tissue and bone conduction) have no influence, at least up to hearing aid gains of 60 to 70 dB. This seems to apply to the sound radiating from earhook and tubing as well. The coupling from the receiver to the microphone is also a "high gain" problem and can only be controlled by the hearing aid manufacturer. The influence of the remaining "boxes" will be discussed in detail below.

Figure 12–20 points out necessary details of a BTE acoustic system and a canal or ITE acoustic system. For the BTE system, a receiver, some tubing, and an earmold, possibly with a vent, can be recognized. For the ITE instrument, the sound path is short. An acoustic leak can occur for both types of systems. Finally, a residual volume and the eardrum can be recognized.

In the acoustic world relevant to hearing aid fitting, acoustic systems are composed of only four basic acoustic building blocks: the cavity, the short tube, the transmission line, and the horn.

A cavity is found, for instance, in the occluded ear as the residual volume (Figure 12–21). The main acoustic characteristic of a cavity originates from the fact that a cavity is filled with air and that air is compressible, causing an increasing short-circuiting of the sound pressure in the cavity toward higher frequencies. Introducing a cavity in the sound path will create a "bend" in the system's response (lower right part of Figure 12–21) with a cutoff frequency that is dependent on the size of the cavity and the acoustic compo-

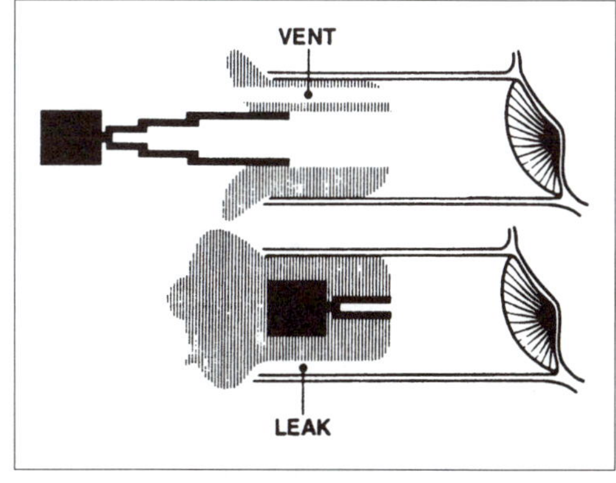

Figure 12–20. Schematic principle of a BTE acoustic system (*top*) and an ITE or canal aid acoustic system (*bottom*).

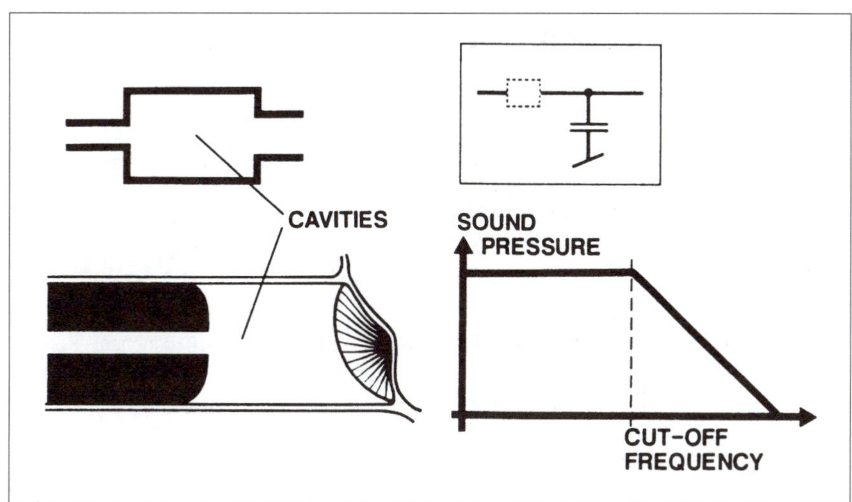

Figure 12–21. Top left: simple cavity. Bottom left: the residual volume is a cavity. Top right: the electronic analogue to a cavity is a capacitor. Bottom right: introducing a cavity in the sound path will cause a drop in the high frequencies starting a cutoff frequency that depends on the size of the cavity.

nents before and after the cavity. This behavior is analogous to the introduction of a capacitor in an electronic circuit as shown in the upper right of Figure 12–21.

Introducing a short tube in the sound path will also result in a cutoff in the high frequencies (Figure 12–22). This is due to the fact that, inside the tube, a column of air has to be accelerated forward and backward at the frequency of the sound. A high-frequency response will thus need more energy than a low-frequency response to overcome the many more accelerations necessary to force the sound through the tube. This behavior is analogous to the introduction of an inductor, or coil, in an electronic circuit (Figure 12–22). Increasing the length or decreasing the diameter of the tube will result in a low cutoff frequency and a consequent further dampening of the high frequencies.

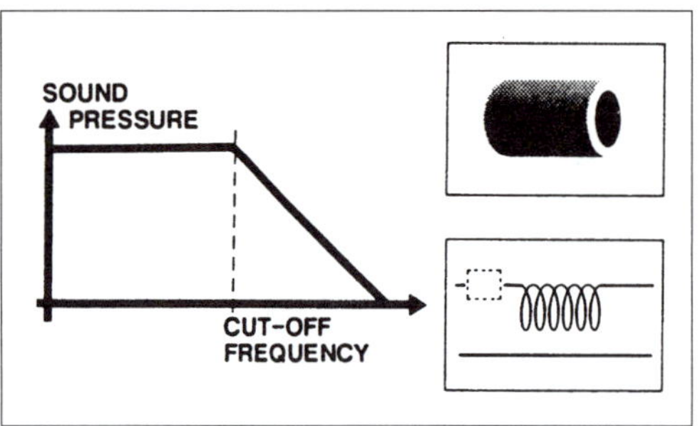

Figure 12–22. Left: a short tube in the sound path cuts off in the high frequencies. Top right: a simple short tube. Bottom right: the electronic analogue to a tube is a series inductor.

LONG TUBES FUNCTIONING AS TRANSMISSION LINES

If a tube exceeds a certain length, depending on how high frequencies are transmitted through the tube, its behavior changes from simple inductor-like behavior to that of a transmission line. A transmission line is a complicated component, the length (tube length) of which has an important impact on the transmitted signal.

Figure 12–23 indicates how long a tube may be when transmitting sounds up to a certain frequency before it is necessary to regard it as a transmission line and not as a simple

Tubes as transmission lines

Frequency	Wave length of frequency	Transmission line when longer than:
100 Hz	340 cm (134 inches)	34 cm (13 inches)
1000 Hz	34 cm (13 inches)	3.4 cm (1.3 inches)
5000 Hz	6.8 cm (2.7 inches)	0.7 cm (0.3 inches)
10000 Hz	3.4 cm (1.3 inches)	0.3 cm (0.1 inches)

Figure 12–23. First and second columns list various frequencies and their corresponding wavelengths. The third column indicates how long a tube may be before it becomes necessary to treat it as a transmission line at each frequency.

short tube. For instance, if frequencies up to 5000 Hz are to be transmitted, any tube longer than 0.7 cm should be treated as a transmission line. Tubes shorter than 0.7 cm can be treated as simple short tubes.

Briefly stated, the complications in connection with a transmission line arise when the wave length of the signal becomes comparable to the length of the tube (Figure 12–24). In these cases, standing wave resonances appear together with time delays. For each standing wave resonance, a peak can be found in the measured hearing aid response (Figure 12–25).

Introducing a transmission line in the sound path will cause low frequencies to just pass through, although they will be somewhat attenuated because of simple losses that occur through the tube and the high frequencies being strongly influenced by the standing wave peaks.

The *horn is* a relatively new component in use with hearing aids (Killion, 1976; Libby, 1981). It is, nevertheless, the ideal means of connecting the small (less than 1 mm in bore size) hearing aid receiver outlet to the eardrum (average diameter 7.5 mm, approximately 60 times the area of the receiver outlet), as it creates a gradual transition between the two (Figure 12–26). The horn thereby acts as an *acoustic impedance transformer,* and it can

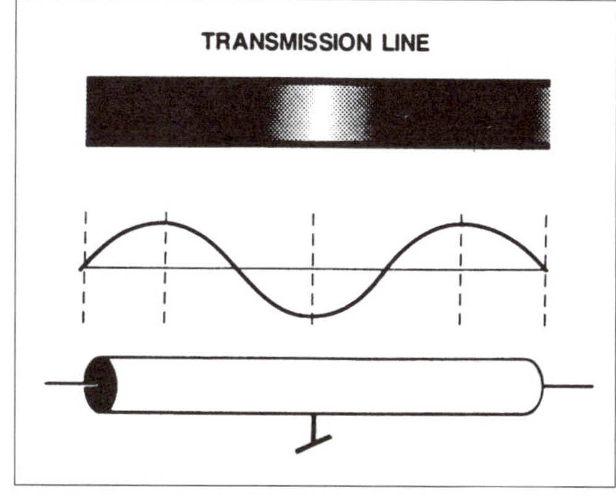

Figure 12–24. Top and middle: standing waves in a long tube. Bottom: the (electric) symbol of a transmission line.

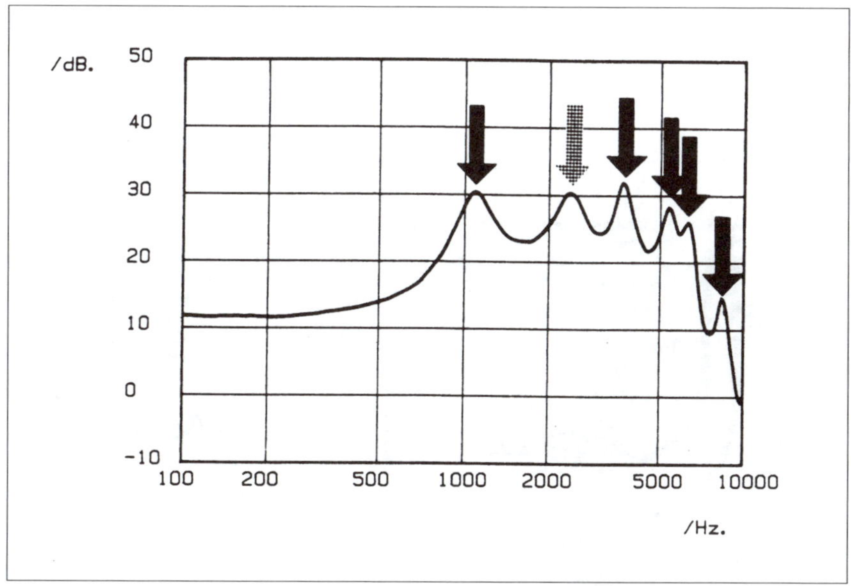

Figure 12–25. Gain response of a BTE aid as measured on an ear simulator. The tubing system consists of a receiver tube (8 mm × 1 mm), a hook (27 mm × 1.5 mm), a tube (25 mm × 2 mm), and an earmold bore (18 mm × 3 mm). All the peaks under the black arrows are standing wave resonances in the various transmission lines. The shaded arrow indicates the receiver resonance.

yield smooth frequency responses with optimal high-frequency performance. Figure 12–27 shows response improvement from 2 mm standard tubing (1) to a damped Libby horn (2).

A BTE ACOUSTIC SYSTEM

The acoustic components of the BTE system shown in the upper part of Figure 12–20 are a receiver, a series of tubes, and the residual volume with the eardrum (the vent is omitted). These four sections are best described as four separate transmission lines in a series, as shown in the lower part of Figure 12–28.

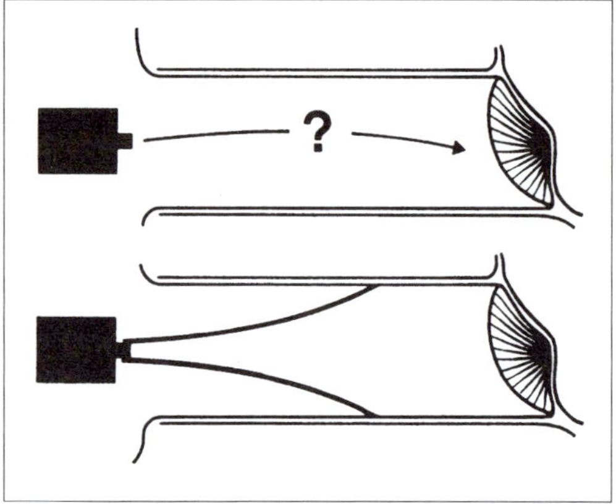

Figure 12–26. The mismatch between the area of the receiver outlet and the area of the eardrum is best remedied by a horn.

The eardrum's residual volume is the most complicated part of the system because of the delicate coupling of the eardrum to the middle ear. The behavior of the eardrum has not been sufficiently investigated and modeled to make possible a meaningful model such as that of the receiver in Figure 12–29. Zwislocki (1970, 1971), however, designed an ear simulator (Figure 12–30) that behaves much like an average human ear. Its residual volume is the same as that of an average human ear (approximately 0.57 cc), but the behavior of the eardrum is simulated by four side branch acoustic resonators (R1-R4) that have no actual parallel in the real ear, but only behave like the eardrum.

As eardrum behavior normally cannot be altered and the coupler closely simulates this behavior, the Zwislocki coupler is often used as a model of the residual volume and eardrum. The left part of Figure 12–30 shows the electronic analogy to the Zwislocki coupler with its four resonators. Figure 12–31 shows a detailed drawing of the system from

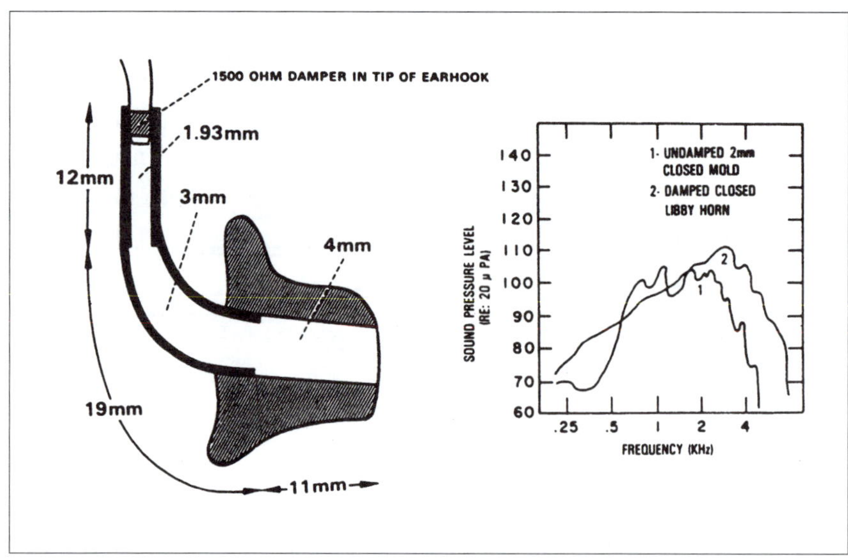

Figure 12–27. Damped Libby horn.

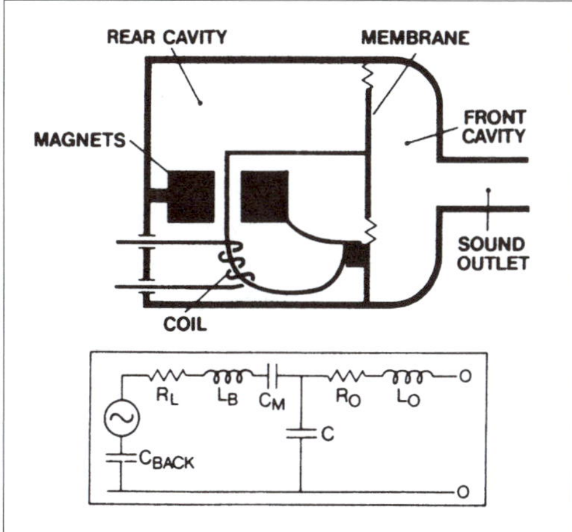

Figure 12–28. Top: the principle of a hearing aid receiver. Bottom: electric analogue to the acoustic system of the receiver.

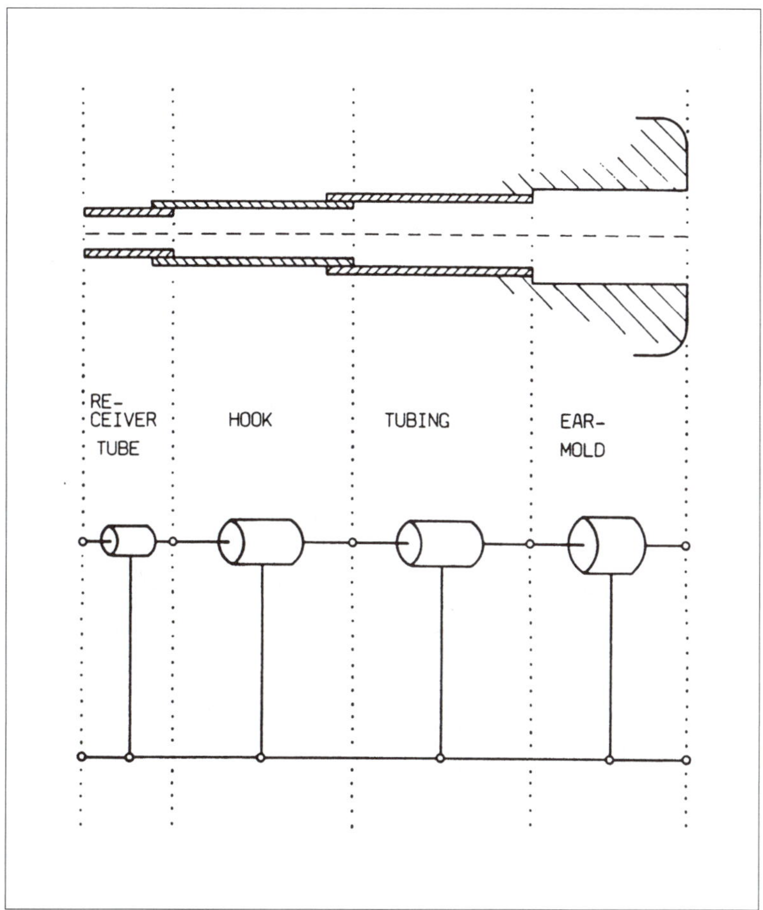

Figure 12–29. The tube system from a BTE to the tip of the earmold typically consists of four transmission lines.

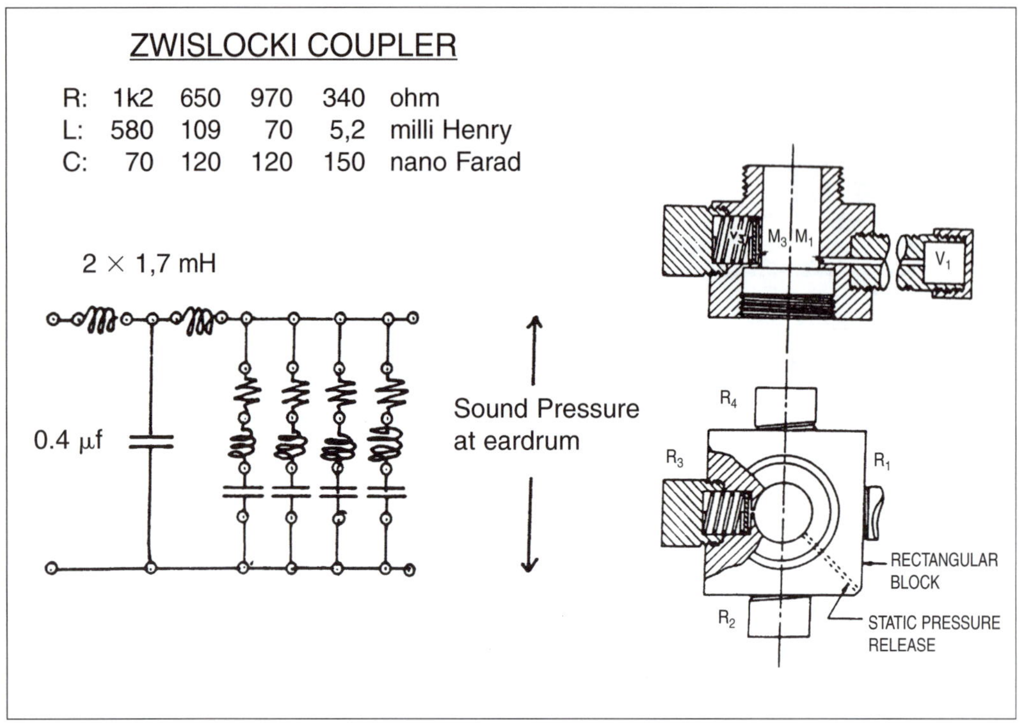

Figure 12–30. Right: the Zwislocki coupler. Left: electric analogue to the Zwislocki coupler.

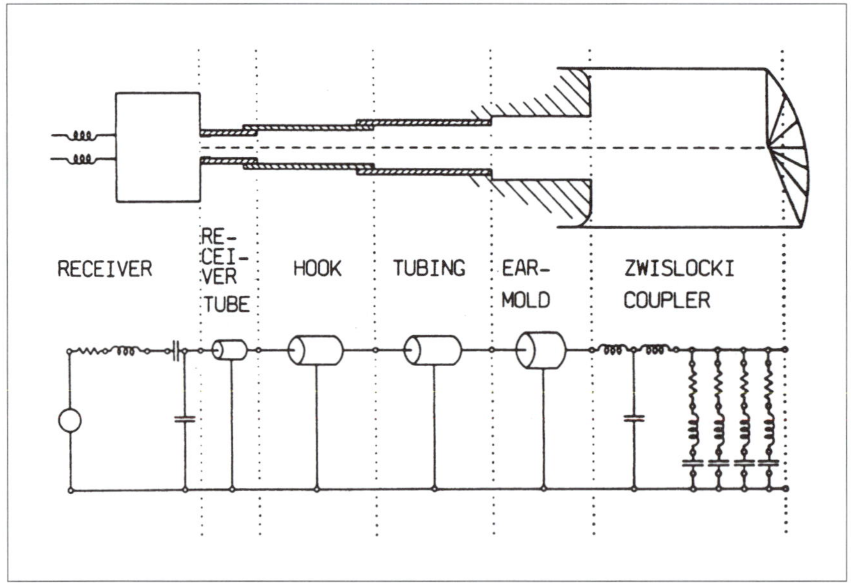

Figure 12–31. Complete BTE acoustic system and electric analogue.

receiver to the eardrum, together with the electronic analogous circuit.

Figure 12–32 (curve A) is a simulated phase and amplitude response of the above described BTE system. Also shown are two examples of what happens if the system is changed. Curve B shows what happens if the entire tubing system is replaced by an ideal horn starting with a diameter of 1 mm and ending with the diameter of the ear canal (7.5 mm). Curve C shows what happens if the tubing in Figure 12–31 is changed to a length of 40 mm and the

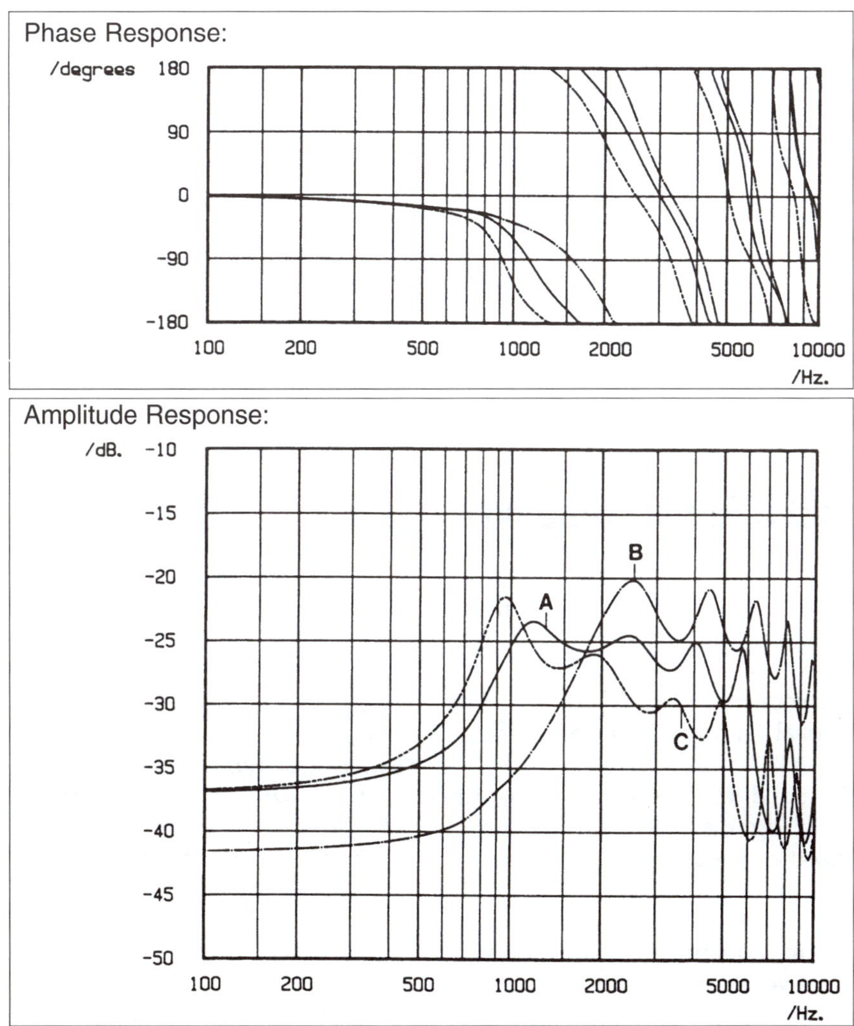

Figure 12–32. Simulated responses of BTE systems. **A.** response of the system shown in Figure 12–31. **B.** response of the system in Figure 12–31 but with a horn (entrance diameter 1 mm, exit diameter 7.5 mm) replacing the entire tube system. **C.** same system as Figure 12–31, but with the tube length changed from 25 to 40 mm and the earmold bore reduced from 3 to 2 mm.

bore of the earmold is reduced to 2 mm, resulting in a 58 mm tube, 2 mm in bore, from the hook to the residual volume.

Vents (and leaks) are acoustic "modifications" of the earmold with significant influence on the low frequency response of the hearing aid system. A vent, as a tube that connects the residual volume with the free field, will short-circuit the low frequencies and leave the high frequencies unchanged at the eardrum.

CONCLUSION

The need for accurate information concerning all the acoustic factors that affect the signal delivered to the cochlea is obvious. This chapter has described the various acoustic elements, their characteristics, and their influence on the final acoustic measurement response. Understanding these complex acoustic characteristics should improve the reliability and clinical expertise of real ear measurements.

REVIEW QUESTIONS

1. What is the clinical utility of real ear measurements?
2. What are some of the factors contributing to directional variations in the sound field?
3. Why do sound level variations at the eardrum vary significantly as a function of the horizontal angle of incidence or in the median plane?
4. What are the advantages of a CIC instrument relative to picking up directional information?
5. Explain ear canal resonances.
6. Why is the positioning of the probe tube so critical in obtaining accurate and reliable measures of sound pressure?
7. Although the SPL response at the eardrum on a normal open ear is "peaky," why is it perceived as a flat or natural response?
8. In a BTE instrument, the sound path is longer than it is in a CIC device. What resonance differences may one expect to find because of this?
9. What is the clinical value of the Libby horn?
10. What was the primary purpose of the Zwislocki coupler?
11. What is the rationale underlying the use of "vents" in modifying the acoustic signal?

REFERENCES

Burkhard, M. D., & Sachs, R. M. (1975). Anthropometric manikin for acoustic research. *Journal of the Acoustical Society of America, 58*.

Killion, M. C. (1976). Experimental wideband hearing aid. *Journal of the Acoustical Society of America, 55*.

Libby, E. R. (1981). In search of transparent insertion gain hearing aid responses. In G. Studebaker & F.H. Bess (Eds.), *The Vanderbilt Hearing Aid Report*. Upper Darby, PA: Monographs in Comtemporary Audiology.

Sachs, R. M., & Burkhard, M. D. (1972). Making pressure measurements in insert earphone couplers and real ears. *Journal of the Acoustical Society of America, 51*, 140(A).

Shaw, E. A. G. (1975). The external ear. New knowledge. *Scandinavian Audiology* (Suppl. 5).

Shaw, E. A. G., & Teranishi, R. (1968). Sound pressure generated in an external ear replica and real human ears by a nearby point source. *Journal of the Acoustical Society of America, 34*, 240–249.

Westermann, S., & Toepholm, J. (1985). Comparing BTEs and ITEs for localizing speech. *Hearing Instrument Technology, 36*.

Zwislocki, J. J. (1970). An acoustic coupler for earphone calibration (Rep. No. LSC-S-7). Syracuse, NY: Syracuse University, Laboratory of Sensory Communication.

Zwislocki, J. J. (1971). An ear-like coupler for earphone calibration (Rep. No. LSC-S-9). Syracuse, NY: Syracuse University, Laboratory of Sensory Communication.

CHAPTER 13

Hearing Aid Measurements and Clinical Applications

ROBERT MARTIN, PH.D.

OUTLINE

Over the past decade or so, there have been many advances in amplifier design. Computer-based fitting algorithms are now routinely used to set the performance parameters of hearing aids. One might question, therefore, whether it is still necessary to place a hearing aid into a test box, or into the patient's ear, and measure the sound produced by the aid.

In this author's opinion, hearing aids cannot be properly fitted without precise, in-office instrumental tests. Electroacoustic measurements—hereafter simply called tests— should be a mandatory part of any hearing aid delivery system. Clinical skill and judgment improve each time objective testing confirms or rejects a fitting. Also, some patients return to the office with complaints, and the clinician must be able to resolve these problems quickly and successfully. Failing to do this, the patient losses confidence in both the clinician and the product.

A professional hearing aid fitting includes measurement of the quantity and quality of the amplified sound. Quantity tests include gain, bandwidth, and input-output measures. Quality tests consider distortion products produced by the hearing aid. Some electroacoustic measurements, such as real ear target studies, check both.

REFERENCE POINTS

After the hearing aids are received from the manufacturer and before the hearing aids are fit on the patient, the initial in-office tests should be done. Common sense suggests that it is better to detect a nonfunctioning or defective instrument before the patient comes to the office.

These preliminary hearing aid tests are invaluable for several reasons. First, the instruments must be adjusted so that the patient hears well initially. Second, these tests serve as reference points because sooner or later the patient will return to the office complaining of increased difficulty in hearing. The clinician needs to be able to quickly ascertain whether the patient's hearing has changed, the hearing aids have changed their electroacoustic response, or both.

Measurements are also important from the patient's point of view. A visit to the eye doctor or heart specialist usually includes a variety of tests to determine appropriate management. Appropriate testing helps to ensure accuracy and inspire patient confidence. In many cases, it adds objectivity to a subjective process. Some patients may place greater faith in the measurements made than in the clinician's professional opinion.

PREDICTING HEARING AID PERFORMANCE

Each new hearing aid comes with a strip chart showing the ANSI (American National Standards Institute) tests. ANSI revises these tests periodically (ANSI 60, 76, 82, 85, 92, 96). These tests are informative, but they do not tell you how the instrument will perform when placed in the patient's ear. According to D. Preves (personal communications, 1995), these tests were developed by the ANSI working group to give manufacturers a quality-control tool. For example, if a hearing aid was wired incorrectly or if a microphone or speaker was nonfunctional, then the ANSI tests would alert the manufacturer to the problem. The persons who wrote the ANSI standard recognize that these tests do not describe how the instrument will function when used by a patient.

Rather than relying on the ANSI data supplied with each new aid, it is recommended that clinicians perform their own hearing aid tests. In-office testing is needed to adjust the amplified sound to the specific level needed by the patient (Berland, 1978). The level of sound required by the patient is called the "use gain" setting, as suggested in the following designation, "the instrument was set to 27 dB use gain."

Tests performed *in situ* are called real ear measurements (Preves, 1987). A small probe tube inserted into the ear canal measures the sound produced at or near the eardrum by the hearing aid.

Real ear testing has advanced the hearing aid science profession by revealing the glaring inadequacies of hearing aid fittings. The need for real ear tests is well documented (McCandless, 1996). It is quite possible that many patients wear hearing aids with unsatisfactory real ear frequency responses in spite of the use of sound field testing and other classic measurements to ensure appropriate fittings.

The development of real ear systems and their associated terminology have been reviewed by Libby and Westermann (1995). The results of real ear tests are described using acronyms beginning with the letters "RE" for real ear and ending with the letters "R" or "G" for response or gain. For example, the Real Ear Unaided Response is referred to as the REUR. The Real Ear Insertion Gain is REIG.

Real ear tests and sound box measurements are essential tools that allow quick documentation of whether or not a hearing aid is performing up to some predetermined goal. These tests are objective and can often be completed in a few minutes.

Finally, patients may be skeptical about the need to replace their current hearing aid(s). If clinical judgement of benefit can be documented with objective hearing aid tests, patients may have more confidence in the recommendation for utilization of technologically advanced instruments.

THE TESTING SEQUENCE

The purpose of hearing aid tests is to gather information that assists in improving the selection and fitting process, as well as the patient's hearing ability. Before testing the hearing aid, an otoscopic examination of the patient's external ear canals is recommended. Also, the magnification and light of the otoscope permits an examination of the microphone opening and the receiver port of the hearing aid to determine whether these openings are completely or partially occluded with debris.

Some patients have great difficulty correctly inserting the aid. When dealing with a feedback problem, it is important to differentiate between an incorrectly inserted hearing aid and one that does not fit correctly or that has internal feedback.

There are a number of different tests done in the sound box and many real ear tests. Some real ear measurements have more practical clinical value than others. The Real Ear Insertion Response (REIR), also called the Real Ear Insertion Gain (REIG), is useful. Other tests, such as attack and release time measurements, are seldom used to evaluate or resolve day-to-day fitting problems. The tests discussed below are those used most often to diagnose or solve problems. Before considering specific tests, we will review the equipment utilized.

Input Signals and Couplers

For years, all objective hearing aid measurements were done in a sound-treated test box. These traditional tests were done by attaching a hearing aid to a measurement microphone with a device called a 2 cc coupler. For an extensive review of couplers, see Stabb (1985). The coupler contains 2 cubic centimeters of air and simulates the human external ear canal volume. A speaker in the test box presents a sound (the input signal) to the hearing aid, and the output (the amplified sound) is routed to the measurement microphone through the 2 cc coupler. The output of the hearing aid is presented on a video monitor. If desired, the output response can be printed.

Traditionally, the basic input signal used to test hearing aids has been the pure tone. Pure-tone input signals create artifacts reflected in the test results (Millin, 1978; Studebaker, 1977). Composite noise or speech-shaped broad-band noise is preferred to pure tone for many tests. There are three main advantages to using a composite noise signal rather than a pure-tone signal. First, the measurements can be obtained in real time. If a pure tone is used, it takes time for the tone to sweep through the frequency range. Use of composite or broad-band noise eliminates this delay. It is possible to adjust the hearing aid and observe as the response instantly changes on the video monitor. Second, the noise signal can be filtered to create a speech-shaped input. Hearing aids are generally used to hear conversation, therefore it is desirable to have the input signal shaped with a balance of frequencies that simulate human speech. Third, broad-band noise signals are needed to obtain valid test results for AGC (automatic gain control) circuits (Purdy, 1999). As the name implies, AGC circuits control the gain function of the hearing aid. Figure 13–1 illustrates the difference between the results obtained using a composite noise and a pure-tone input. Note the 12 dB difference in the lower frequencies. A pure-tone sweep presented to an AGC aid can produce "blooming," an artificial elevation of low frequencies, and possible attenuation of the high frequencies. The lower curve (B) on Figure 13–1 more accurately reflects the amount of amplification produced by this aid when real-world noises are amplified.

The easiest and most accurate way to adjust a hearing aid in the test box is to use the multicurve feature. One response curve is saved in memory and displayed on the video monitor. A second response curve is superimposed on the first curve, usually in a different color. This second curve is called the "real-time" curve, meaning the test unit is constantly measuring and displaying the result in real time. When any adjustment is made to the instrument, the change in response is immediately seen by comparing the real-time curve to the "saved" curve.

Types of Tests

Hearing aid tests fall into four categories: frequency response, distortion, output, and audibility-tolerance measurements.

Frequency response curves can be generat-

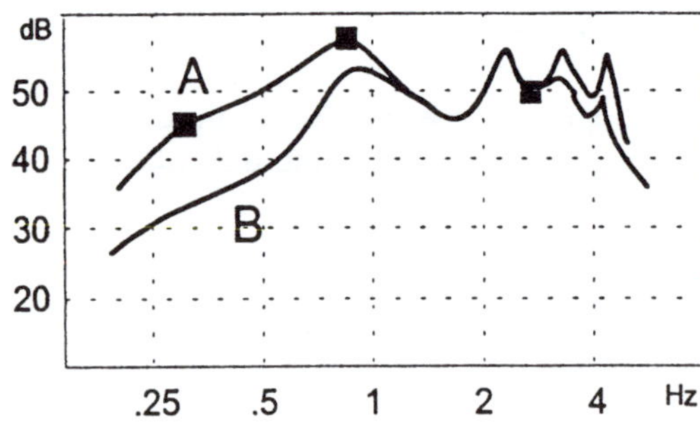

Figure 13–1. Two response curves from the same hearing aid. A 75 dB SPL composite noise input was used for **B**. A 75 dB SPL pure-tone input was used for **A**.

ed in a test box or in the patient's ear. A response curve is executed to see whether the hearing instrument is providing amplification in all frequency zones: (250, 500, 1000, 2000, 4000, and 6000 Hz.) The real ear insertion response (REIR) discussed below, is often compared to a real ear target, which makes it easy to determine whether the aid is providing adequate amplification in each of the frequency zones.

Distortion measurements are made in the sound box and are used to document the amount of harmonic or intermodulation distortion present at a preset input level.

Output measurements show the amount of gain, output, or both gain and output that are produced by the aid at various input levels. These tests are needed to see how well the hearing aid is controlling (reducing) the output. No hearing aid response should expose the patient to sound levels that are intolerably loud.

Audibility and tolerance studies overlie real ear data on the patient's pure-tone thresholds and uncomfortable listening levels (UCL) values. These studies assist in determining whether soft sounds are audible to the patient and whether the amplified sound exceeds the patient's comfortable listening level.

Frequency Response

The most commonly used test is the simple frequency response curve made in a test box using a 2 cc coupler. This is an efficient measurement that shows what the hearing aid is doing and whether it appears to be appropriate for the patient's hearing loss (Kasten, 1967). As an example, suppose a patient with a high-frequency hearing loss is wearing a Class A linear hearing aid and complains that he does not hear clearly. When the aid is tested in the sound box, the response curve shown in Figure 13–2 is generated. The amplification peaks at 1000 Hz and decreases markedly in the higher frequencies. Because clarity is usually improved by amplifying the high-frequency consonants, and this hearing aid does not accomplish that, the sound box test has identified the problem.

Figure 13–3 shows the test box response of a more recent Class D amplifier. Patients with high-frequency hearing loss generally need the additional gain in the 2000–4000 Hz region provided by this type of amplifier. This acoustic gain is needed to compensate for the insertion loss (discussed below) and for the hearing loss. Many older-style aids have inadequate gain in the higher frequencies, and this deficiency is quickly observed in the test box.

Families of Curves

Figures 13–4, 13–5, and 13–6 show examples of a family of curves. A family of curves is created by putting the hearing aid in the test box

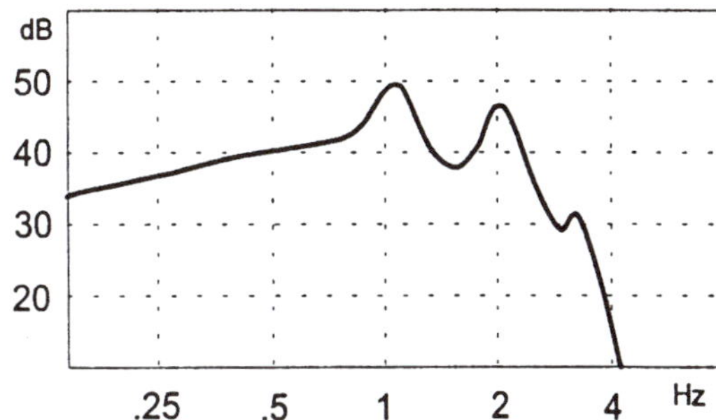

Figure 13–2. Frequency response curve for class A hearing aid.

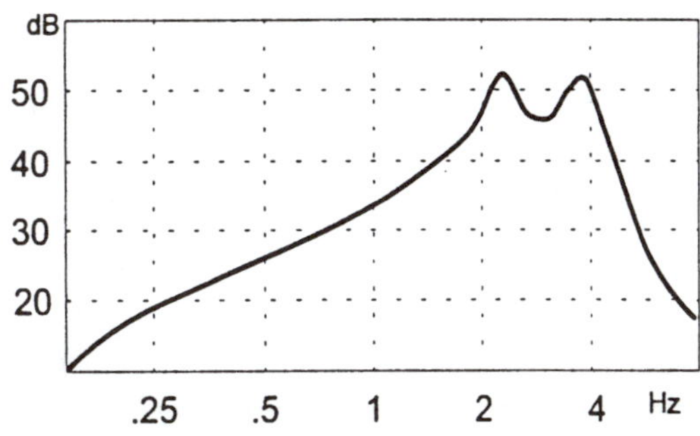

Figure 13–3. Frequency response for class D hearing aid.

and measuring the response at four different input levels, ranging from soft to loud, without changing the volume setting or other instrumental settings. The four response curves are recorded on the same graph, as in Figures 13–4, 13–5, and 13–6, to show the "family." In most cases, the type of amplifier in the hearing aid can be identified by looking at the family of curves.

Figure 13–4 shows four curves evenly spaced approximately 5 dB apart in the higher frequencies. This indicates that the aid is a compression circuit, a wide dynamic range compression (WDRC) amplifier with a 2:1 compression ratio (Killion, 1997). The four input levels of 50, 60, 70, and 80 dB are spaced 10 dB apart. The four curves are 5 dB apart because the compression circuit automatically adjusts the output. It is also possible to identify this as a treble increase at low level (TILL) circuit by noting that most of the change occurs in the high frequencies.

Figure 13–5 shows a family of curves for a hearing aid having a linear amplifier. Notice how the response curves fall on top of each other at input levels of 50, 60, and 70 dB SPL. Only the 80 dB SPL input level creates a different response curve characteristic. With a typical linear amplifier, the gain does not change with changes in the input level until the instrument saturates. When this happens, the amplifier has reached its point of maximum amplification, and increases in input create ragged response curves similar to the lower curve in Figure 13–5. The hearing aid peak clips the input signal and additional increases in input intensity create unwanted distortion products.

Figure 13–6 is an example of a "BILL" circuit. BILL is an acronym for base increase at low level. Study carefully Figures 13–4, 13–5, and 13–6 to observe the differences in their morphology. Look at the low frequency zone

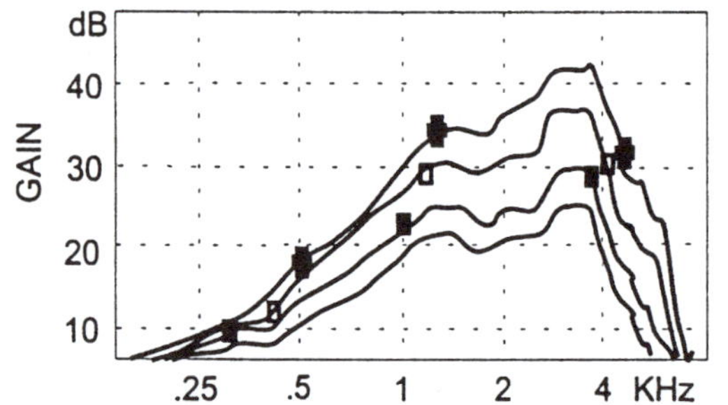

TITLE	INPUT	OUTPUT
CRV 1	80dB	97.4dB
■ CRV 2	70dB	92.3dB
□ CRV 3	60dB	87.9dB
✚ CRV 4	50dB	82.0dB

Figure 13–4. TILL circuit with wide dynamic range compression.

TITLE	INPUT	OUTPUT
CRV 1	80dB	105.7dB
■ CRV 2	70dB	99.4dB
□ CRV 3	60dB	90.5dB
✚ CRV 4	50dB	80.3dB

Figure 13–5. Linear amplifier with peak clipping.

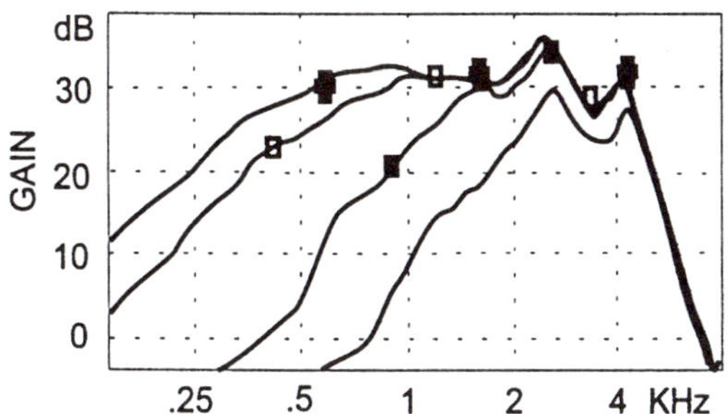

	TITLE	INPUT	OUTPUT
	CRV 1	80dB	100.4dB
▮	CRV 2	70dB	96.5dB
▯	CRV 3	60dB	89.8dB
✚	CRV 4	50dB	80.8dB

Figure 13–6. BILL circuit with compression.

near 250 Hz and compare the spacing of the response curves in the three graphs. In Figure 13–6, the curves are distributed across a wide range of acoustic gain. Notice, as well, that they are close together at 250 Hz in Figure 13–4 and on top of each other in Figure 13–5. Note that the "BILL" circuit in Figure 13–6 essentially mirrors the TILL response in Figure 13–4. The changes are more apparent in the opposite part of the frequency spectrum.

Families of frequency response curves are useful tools to evaluate amplification systems. Studying the curves in a family clearly indicates how the frequency response changes with a change in the input level.

ANSI Testing

Many hearing aid test systems have a button labeled "ANSI". When the button is pressed, the unit automatically performs a specified series of tests (ANSI 92). As discussed earlier, manufacturers use this option to evaluate their hearing aids.

ANSI recommendations are updated periodically. The ANSI 92 option (ANSI S3.42-1992) is useful because it automatically generates a family of response curves, and significant amounts of information are readily available. The new composite noise test signal is used as the input for these tests.

The ANSI 92 option can be used to quickly evaluate any hearing aid before it is fitted to the individual. When fitting digital hearing aids, for example, it is important to check the gain and frequency responses after the aids have been programmed to meet some target gain criteria. Place the aid in the test box, push the ANSI button, then inspect the family of curves to see whether the hearing aid circuits are functioning as intended. Sometimes the computer algorithm programs the aid in an unexpected fashion. The digital circuit may be programmed for linear amplification rather than compression, or, for example, a mechanical filter in the aid may be partially blocked, resulting in weak amplification. The ANSI 92 feature provides a quick, efficient sequence of tests that can be used to identify problems before the hearing aid is placed in the patient's ear.

Real Ear Testing

There is considerable literature on the topic of real ear testing (Preves, 1987; Purdy, 1999), as well as the language and conversions used for these tests (Revit, 1997). Real ear testing involves a simple procedure. A small-diameter probe tube is placed into the ear canal just beyond the earmold tip (at least 5 mm) and a short distance from the eardrum (at least 5–7 mm). The identical placement of the probe should be maintained throughout the entire assessment procedure. A 70 dB SPL composite noise test signal is emitted from a speaker placed 12 in. (30 cm) away from the patient's ear. The hearing instrument's response is viewed on the monitor.

The first real ear test, obtained without the hearing aid in place, measures the contribution of the pinna and the outer ear canal to natural hearing ability. This contribution is called the real ear unaided response (REUR). The terms REUR and REUG (real ear unaided gain) are often used interchangeably. In the earlier literature, REUR was called the ear canal resonance.

Figure 13–7 is a graph that shows REUR as a shaded area. It is helpful to think of the REUR as an area rather than as a line (Martin, 1994). Figure 13–7 inverts the REUR area and superimposes it on the pure-tone audiogram to stress an important concept. Amplification is used to compensate for the hearing loss, and additional amplification is needed to compensate for the loss of the REUR. The loss of the natural advantage (resonance) of the outer ear that occurs when a hearing aid is inserted in it is called the insertion loss.

Real ear aided response (REAR) is the actual sound level expressed in decibels of sound pressure level (dB SPL) produced by the hearing aid in the ear. Real ear insertion response (REIR) is a mathematically generated curve that shows the benefit (improvement in gain) that a hearing aid wearer receives. This definition assumes that the patient has been receiving some natural benefit from his or her outer ear resonance (the REUR values) and that this is eliminated when the aid is placed in the ear (REIR = REAR – REUR).

Real ear measurements should follow soundbox tests. They are critical in showing how the hearing aid functions in the patient's ear (McCandless, 1996). Real ear data often vary markedly from sound box measurements because each ear is unique, and hearing aid configurations vary considerably as a result of differences in canal length, venting, and so forth. It is not possible to look at the ANSI test data and accurately predict the gain for the real ear fitting.

There are many variables that alter real ear performance. The three most important vari-

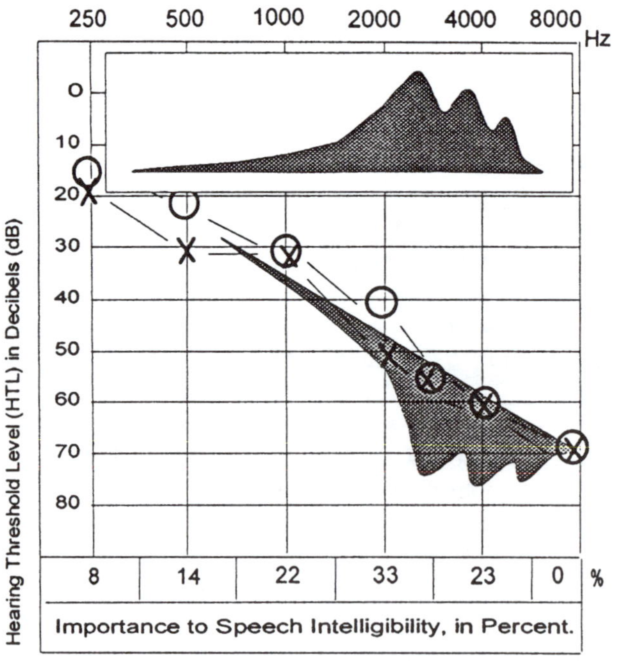

Figure 13–7. The REUR is eliminated (creating a loss) when a hearing aid is inserted so more 2 cc gain is needed.

ables include (a) venting effects, (b) loss of ear-canal resonance, and (c) the influence of the residual volume of air in the ear.

Large diameter vents can allow huge amounts (20 dB or more) of low-frequency gain to escape from an ear. In fact, large vents produce such unpredictable variations in hearing aid performance that they should be used with caution. Real ear tests are needed to determine the actual amount of amplification delivered to the ear.

Loss of the natural ear-canal resonance can reduce or eliminate all of the usable amplification in the higher frequencies. Ears differ in shape and size so the REUR values vary from person to person. The resulting insertion losses vary accordingly. It is relatively simple to study a frequency curve obtained in the test box and mistakenly believe that there is adequate gain in the higher frequencies.

Hearing aids, such as completely-in-the-canal (CIC) aids that extend deep into the ear canal, may have 10 dB more gain than observed in a standard 2 cc test coupler because they operate in a much smaller volume of residual air. These volume effects are discussed below.

Table 13–1 summarizes the differences between test box and real ear measurements. Figures 13–8, 13–9, and 13–10 show the test box and real ear curves for the same hearing aid. The differences shown clearly illustrate the need for real ear tests.

Figure 13–8 is the factory-generated (ANSI) frequency response curve for an ITE hearing aid with a short canal and a large vent. Note the smoothness of the curve and the 30 dB of gain in the higher frequencies. This sound box test was done with vent closed.

Figure 13–9 shows two curves. The lower curve is the real ear unaided response (REUR).

Table 13–1. Real ear versus sound box measurements.

Real Ear Amplification Measurements	*Coupler or "Box" Amplification Measurements*
Gain set at "Use" level	Gain set at Max or ANSI
Exact ear volume included	Volume fixed at 2 ccs
Vent effects included	Vent effects excluded
Ear canal resonance included	Ear canal resonance excluded

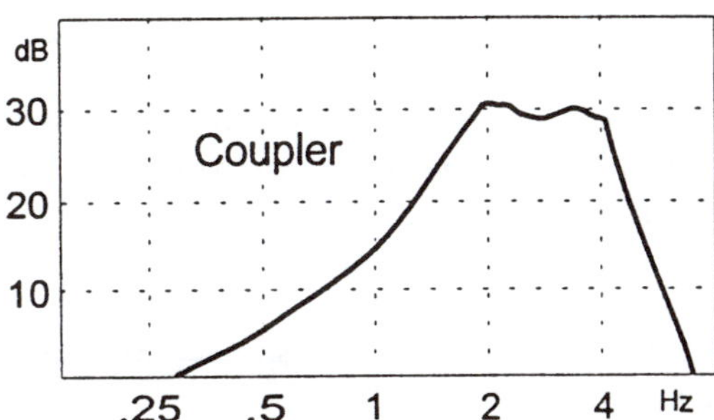

Figure 13–8. Factory-generated frequency response curve made in sound box.

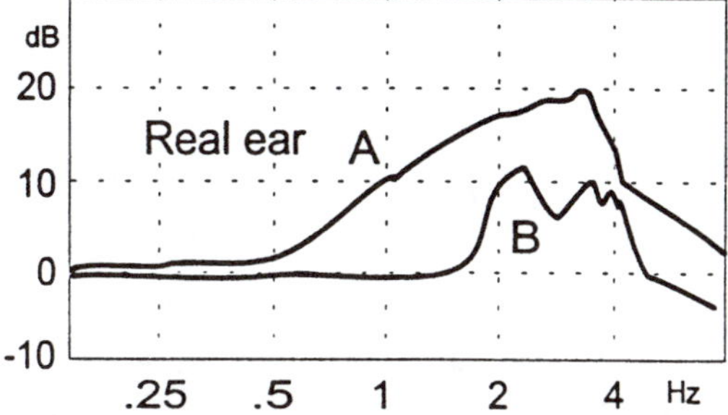

Figure 13–9. Real ear curves for aid shown in Figure 13–8. Upper curve (A) is aided response, REAR. Lower curve (B) is unaided response, REUR.

The upper curve is the real ear aided response (REAR). The volume control was set the same for Figures 13–8 and 13–9. The real ear aided response shows much less gain in all frequencies than the ANSI curve. Most of the sound has been lost through the large vent.

Figure 13–10 is the real ear insertion response (REIR). In this case the aid is only supplying about 12 dB of gain in the zone between 1000 and 2000 Hz and little real ear gain in the higher frequencies. Years ago, hearing aids were fit without real ear tests, and in many cases the results were not unlike these. Data generated in a test box can be misleading if venting, insertion, and volume effects are not considered and accounted for.

ADVANTAGES AND LIMITATIONS OF REAL EAR TESTS

The advantages of real ear tests are numerous. The measurements are made without verbal input from the patient. As such, patient prejudice (pro or con) is not a determining factor. The tests can be done on children of any age. Unlike hearing threshold measurements that must be done in a sound-treated room, these tests can be made in rooms with typical ambient noise. The measurements are efficient and can be made quickly (e.g., a few seconds).

There are several limitations of real ear tests. The ear canal must be clean and free of cerumen and debris, otherwise the probe tube becomes plugged, and severe measurement artifact is observed. The diameter of the probe tube sometimes interferes with the test by breaking the acoustical seal around the hearing aid. UCL testing is difficult because typical input signals exceed the patient's comfort level to the point of causing pain. It is difficult, if not impossible, to test at low input levels, such as 40 dB SPL. It is necessary to stay below the compression kneepoint of the new digital hearing aids.

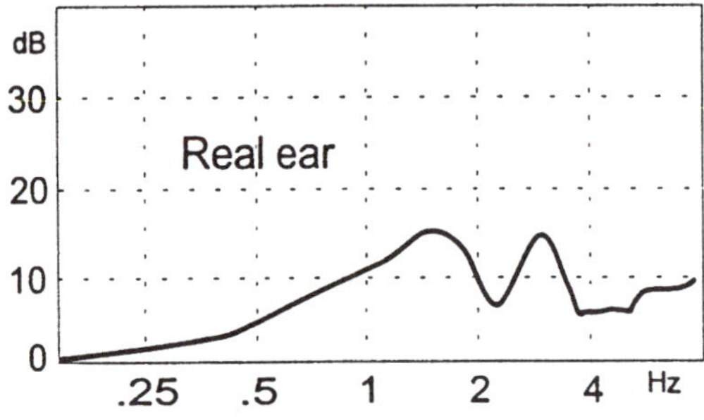

Figure 13–10. The real ear insertion response, REIR, for aid shown in Figure 13–8.

Volume Effects

Figure 13–11 illustrates the effect of the residual volume of the ear canal on hearing aid performance. The diaphragm of a hearing aid receiver (speaker) is tiny compared to that of a stereo speaker. When a hearing aid, such as the CIC in Figure 13–11, operates in a small volume of air, the gain and output are increased (Chasin, 1994). When the same receiver is placed in a BTE aid and operated in a larger volume of air, the gain and output are greatly reduced. This large volume includes the air in the canal plus the air outside the canal that is in contact with the receiver through the vent. This concept is better understood if one considers the high-fidelity headphones of a Walkman-type radio. The sound is bright, clear, and loud when the phones are inserted snuggly into the ear canal. If one pulls the earphones away from the ear only slightly, the sound decreases dramatically in volume and clarity. When a receiver is "loaded" by large volumes of air (as through large vents) its ability to generate sound is markedly reduced.

When hearing aids are placed on children with small residual ear canal volumes, the gain and output are much higher than the 2 cc coupler data indicate (Weber & Northern, 1980). Excessive output may damage the residual hearing. Amplified levels should be measured, not estimated. Because the point of reference for real ear measurements is deep in the ear canal, the effect of the residual air volume is included in the real ear test results.

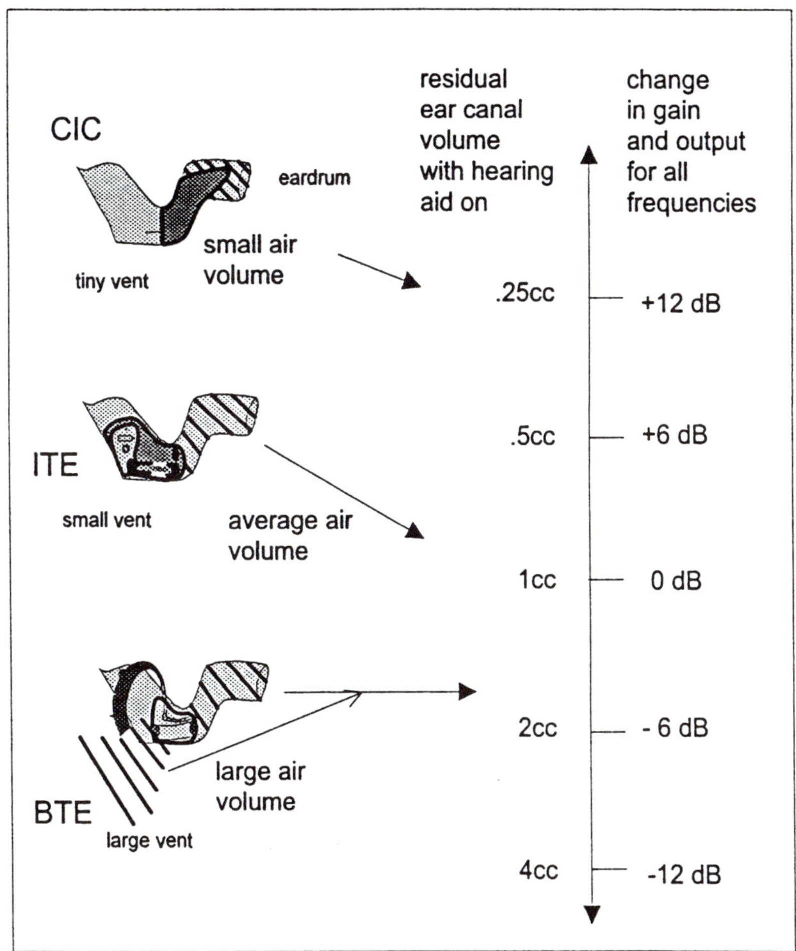

Figure 13–11. The relative effect of residual air volume on the gain and output. CIC instruments operate in small volumes and have increased gain and output relative to 2 cc data.

Target Gain

Target gains are used to evaluate the adequacy of amplification. That is, to check the real ear gain in the low, mid, and higher frequencies. While no single measurement can ensure that the patient has adequate amplification, the match between the REIR and the real ear target gives a reliable estimate of whether there is enough or too much sound available throughout the amplified frequency range. According to Libby (1995), the goal is to achieve good word recognition, as well as acceptable listening comfort. The speech signal should be audible, and the optimal placement of speech energy within the patient's auditory area between 250–6000 Hz should be determined.

Real ear measurements are especially useful in dealing with current hearing aid users who report poor word recognition. In these cases, the REIR-Target match usually shows zones where the amplification needs to be adjusted.

A real ear target is generated by entering the patient's hearing thresholds into the hearing aid test system. The software applies the selected fitting formula to the data and creates a goal or target gain (National Acoustic Labs, 1999). The target appears as a heavy line on the monitor. With the aid inserted into the patient's ear, the volume control is adjusted until the level of the REIR curve approximates the level of the target curve. Inspect the amount of amplification at each point across the frequency spectrum. If the gain is not appropriate, make adjustments. Remember that the octave bands vary in their contribution to word understanding (ANSI 1969). These values are shown on the bottom of Figure 13–7. Because the higher frequencies are most important to word recognition, be sure the REIR is close to the target gain in that area.

Figures 13–12 and 13–13 are two examples of REIR-Target comparisons. Figure 13–13 is clearly a better fit than Figure 13–12. The fitting shown in Figure 13–12 has too much amplification in the low-frequency zone and too little in the higher range.

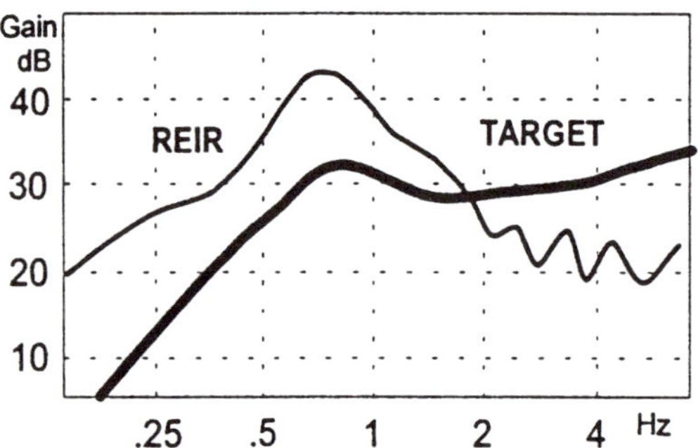

Figure 13–12. REIR-Target comparison. Poor match.

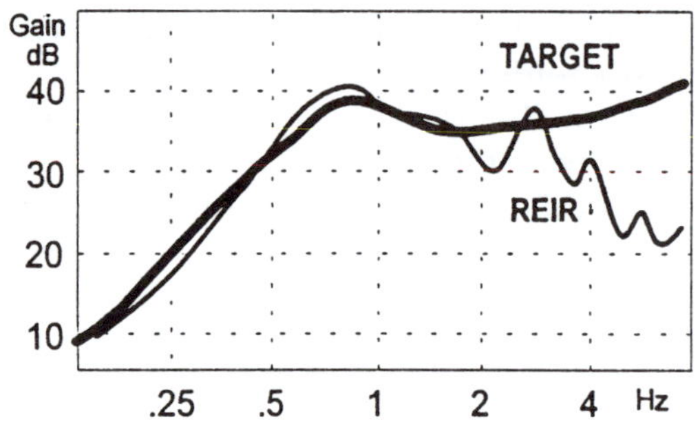

Figure 13–13. REIR-Target comparison. Good match.

The REIR-Target comparison is a powerful tool for both novices and experienced clinicians. A novice can use the target as a fitting guide and make adjustments similar to those illustrated in Figures 13–12 and 13–13. An experienced clinician knows the limitations inherent in target matching and can make subtle changes to improve word recognition over that obtained with a simple target match. In this case, an experienced clinician might increase the gain in the 2000 Hz zone, the 250 Hz zone, or both.

Targets are invaluable because they give a specific real ear reference from which the amplification characteristics can be modified. Trial-and-error adjustments often provide significant improvement in aided performance.

Over the years, there have been many debates about which fitting formula is best (Byrne 1996; Fortune, 1998; Stabb, 1989). Most hearing test systems are equipped with 10 or more fitting formulas. Through trial and observation of results, most fitting formulas were rejected, and only a few, such as NAL-RM, are currently popular choices. Also, the professional clinician is now interested in studying whether the amplification exceeds the patient-comfortable listening zone. Thus, both tolerance (UCL) studies and REIR-Target match studies are needed. The latest NAL formula and the DSL-I/O formula provide "targets" in the three critical zones within the patient's dynamic range. They represent hearing of soft, medium, and loud sounds.

Uncomfortable listening levels may be measured or predicted (Pascoe, 1988). The term "measured" means that the patient was asked to respond to a variety of sounds, and the responses were recorded. The term "predicted" indicates that the patient's hearing thresholds were entered into a computer, and the software "predicted" the UCL values, based on normative data. Measured values are more accurate than predicted values, although predicted levels are often used.

Output Tests

Hearing aid test systems can produce different types of output test data and information. The most simple are the frequency response curve and the RMS-output number (a number shown in the data box). Response curves provide information at specific points across the frequency spectrum, whereas the RMS value is a single number that shows the averaged or "total" energy in the signal. If the patient has a reduced dynamic range in a specific frequency zone, the information provided by a response curve is more helpful than the RMS value. If the overall signal is too loud, the RMS value is useful and easier to modify (Martin , 1995).

Figure 13–14 shows the data summary boxes for two output measurements. The type of signal used (composite noise), the RMS level of the input source (80 dB SPL), and the RMS levels of the outputs (110.5 dB SPL and 94.5 dB SPL) are listed. The upper box shows the output with the AGC circuit set to a high kneepoint (least output reduction), the second with the AGC set to a low kneepoint (greatest output reduction). The change in output made by the change in AGC setting can be easily observed.

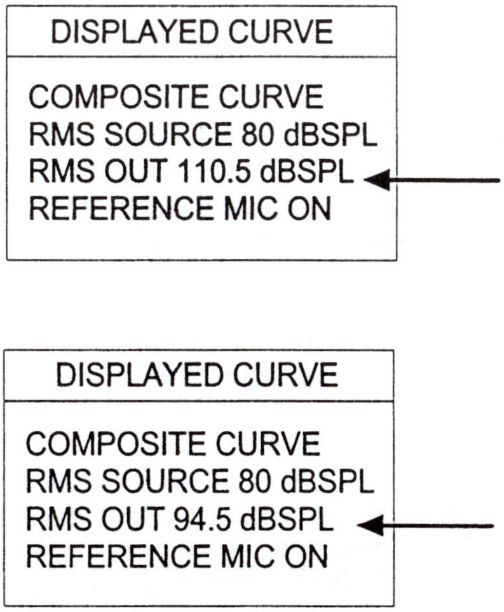

DISPLAYED CURVE
COMPOSITE CURVE RMS SOURCE 80 dBSPL RMS OUT 110.5 dBSPL ← REFERENCE MIC ON

DISPLAYED CURVE
COMPOSITE CURVE RMS SOURCE 80 dBSPL RMS OUT 94.5 dBSPL ← REFERENCE MIC ON

Figure 13–14. Examples of two RMS data boxes.

Select the type of input signal for an output test carefully. Most often, the input signal should have a spectral shape that simulates speech. This activates the compression circuits of the aid in a manner similar to normal conversation. Also, be careful in selecting the input level. Techniques used to evaluate the hearing aid output vary (Purdy, 1999). The author uses an 80 dB composite noise input during the initial adjustment phase of the fitting because this intensity approximates loud speech.

Output tests done by the manufacturer and output tests done in the clinic may provide totally different measurements. When a hearing aid is constructed, the manufacturer does a series of tests to document its performance. The procedure used to find the maximum output is specified by ANSI (S3.22 1987). This value is called the SSPL-90, which stands for Saturation Sound Pressure Level—90 dB input. When an AGC circuit is evaluated using this ANSI protocol, the volume control is adjusted to the full "on" position, and a 90 dB SPL pure-tone sweep is used as the input.

The SSPL-90 number can be used by the manufacturer to separate amplifiers into the various power levels. Most clinicians, however, are more interested in the intensity of output in the patient's ear and how the patient reacts to this sound than in the theoretical "maximum output" levels generated in a test box.

The important question is whether the output-limiting circuit reduces the output response enough to keep amplified sounds within the patient's comfortable listening range. To answer this question, several output measurements are made with the volume control at the "use-gain" position, not at the maximum volume-control setting. One will recall that the volume and tone controls were set in the REIR-Target match, discussed above.

It is helpful to have a "target" use-output RMS value in mind and to make an initial AGC adjustment before placing the aid in the patient's ear. This helps to avoid exposing the patient to sounds that are too loud. Table 13–2 shows four hearing losses and the author's suggested use-output values. These data are presented as guides that the clinician can use when

Table 13–2.

Hearing Level			
500	***1000***	***2000Hz***	***Use Output in dB***
30	40	50 dB HTL	80–90
50	60	70 dB HTL	93–102
70	80	90 dB HTL	103–112
90	100	110 dB HTL	117–127

Note: The left-hand column shows four levels of hearing loss. The values in the right-hand column are suggested initial use-output values in dB. An 80 dB SPL composite noise input is used.

initially setting the hearing aids. Comfortable listening levels vary greatly among individuals, therefore these values should not be taken as absolutes.

When preliminary adjustments are completed, insert the instrument in the patient's ear and proceed with real-ear measurements. Inform the patient that a loud sound will be presented. The instructions given to the patient are important and should be consistent. Hawkins (1987) outlined this procedure. The author presents an 80 dB composite noise for 2 to 3 seconds, records the real ear response, then asks the patient to rate the loudness of the sound according to a Hawkins' loudness rating chart: too loud, very loud, loud, OK, soft, very soft, cannot hear.

Inspect the response curve and the RMS level to see whether the intensity of amplification is within the desired range. Adjust AGC settings according to the patient's response and the observed output level. Be very careful if the observed RMS value is significantly higher than anticipated.

If it is necessary to reduce the output substantially, place the aid in the test box, use an 80 dB composite noise input, watch the "real time" RMS-output values shown in the data box (see Figure 13–14), and change the limiter circuit (AGC). Adjustments at this point will be to AGC, gain, or bandwidth. The effect of the adjustment is seen instantly. Once the values are in the desired range, reinsert the aid in the patient's ear and repeat the test.

Recall that "aided" real ear data show the actual sound levels produced by the hearing aid in the ear canal. When analyzing the patient's hearing-aided response to loud sounds, compare UCL data with real ear "aided" data (Preves, 1987). It is important to use "aided" values, which show the "total" intensity of the sound, not "insertion" values, which show the amount of improvement with the aid. Hearing level (HL) to sound pressure level (SPL) conversions are needed when switching from traditional test data to measurements made in SPL.

REAR data are compared to UCL measurements to see whether the intensity of the sound produced by the aid exceeds the patient's tolerance levels. This comparison and SPL testing is discussed in more detail in the next section.

After these adjustments have been completed, the input is changed to a 90 dB SPL pure tone. This test represents a "worst-case-scenario" measurement and is needed because hearing aid wearers are sometimes exposed to pure-tone-like signals, such as warning bells, intense musical notes, and so forth. Do a pure-tone sweep, record the data, and be sure not to exceed the UCL at any frequency.

There are two references used for real ear tests: gain and SPL. Both measure sound in decibels. Traditional real ear tests, such as the REIG-Target discussed previously, quantify the amount of sound the hearing aid adds to the ear, so the gain reference is used. The other reference for real ear tests is called the "SPL mode." These tests measure and display the actual SPL in the patient's ear.

The SPL Mode for Real Ear Tests

The SPL mode is a new way to do real ear tests (Martin, 1997; Purdy, 1999). Large amounts of information are gathered in just a few seconds. The SPL mode has three parts: (1) an audibility study, (2) a classic target match, and (3) a UCL evaluation. The audibility study indicates whether soft sounds are audible to the patient. The target match shows how well a moderately loud input signal matches the real ear target. The UCL evaluation compares the patient's pure-tone UCL scores to the sound created by a 90 dB pure-tone signal. There is a new patient-friendly input signal called "burst" that can be used for the UCL test.

In SPL mode, the patient's hearing thresholds and UCL values are entered into the analyzer, and the software converts them to SPL and displays them. If no UCL values are available, the software allows the prediction of these levels.

The target seen in the traditional gain mode is adjusted for the SPL mode. Traditional real ear tests use the insertion response (aided minus unaided) as the working response, so REIR (REIG) is compared to the target. In the SPL mode the working responses are REAR curves, not REIR curves.

The target is modified by the software so that the distance between the working curve and the target is the same for gain or SPL measurements. Traditional gain real ear tests use the composite input noise signal, which has a spectrum similar to that of human speech; there is a 6 dB/octave roll-off in the higher frequencies. In the SPL mode, the real ear target is modified (corrected) so that the test results are reported in actual SPL.

Figure 13–15 is an example of real ear tests done in the SPL mode. Three real ear curves (REAR) are displayed. Curve 1 is part of an audibility study. Curve 2 is the classic target match. Curve 3 is the tolerance study. A continuous, composite-noise input was used to make curves 1 and 2. The "Burst" input was used to generate curve 3.

A soft input signal, 50 dB SPL composite noise was used to generate curve 1', a REAR,

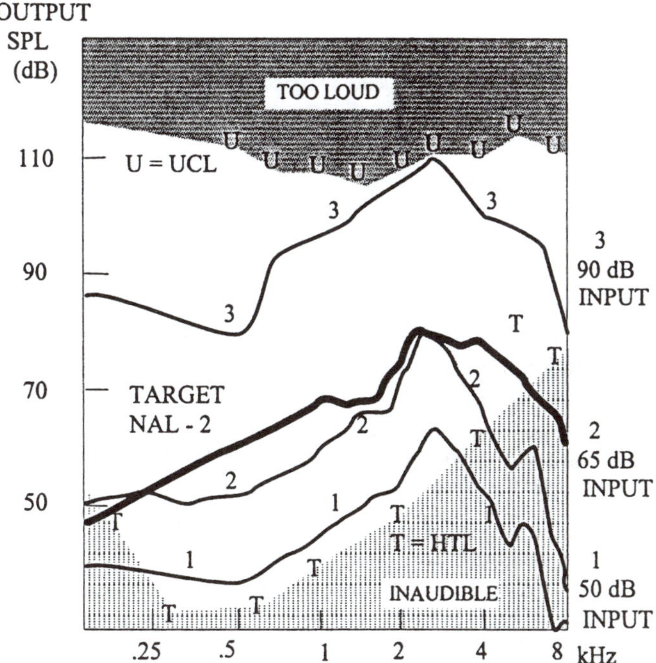

Figure 13–15. The SPL mode for real ear tests using three REAR curves. REAR-1 is compared to hearing threshold levels; REAR-2 is compared to the real ear target; REAR-3 is compared to the patient's UCLs.

which is compared to the patient's hearing thresholds, marked "T." Soft sounds are audible to the patient if curve 1 is higher than "T." This is the audibility study. A 70 dB SPL composite noise input was used to generate curve 2, the traditional REAR, which is compared to the real ear Target (dark line).

Frye Electronics recently created a new input signal called the "Burst" (Frye, 1998). The "Burst" is a brief (0.03–0.05 second) pure tone with a high intensity level (90 dB SPL) used as part of a real ear evaluation. The duration (shortness) of the signal is such that people do not perceive the sound as loud, yet the analyzer can accurately measure and record the real ear output resulting from this intense sound.

The "Burst" was used to generate curve 3, a REAR. Curve 3 values should not exceed the patient's UCL values, marked "U." This comparison is part of the tolerance evaluation.

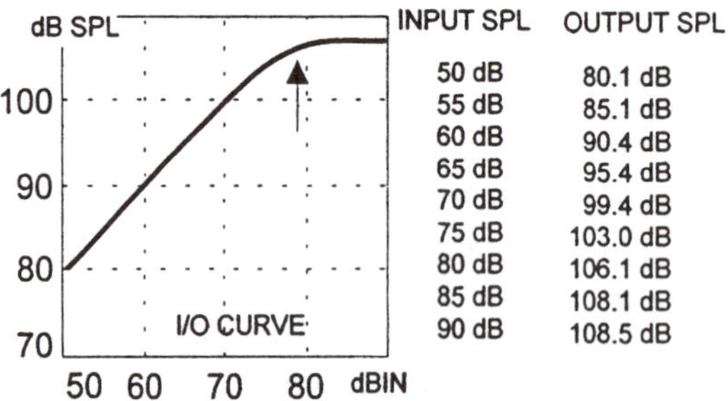

Figure 13–16. Linear amplifier. Peak clipping begins at arrow.

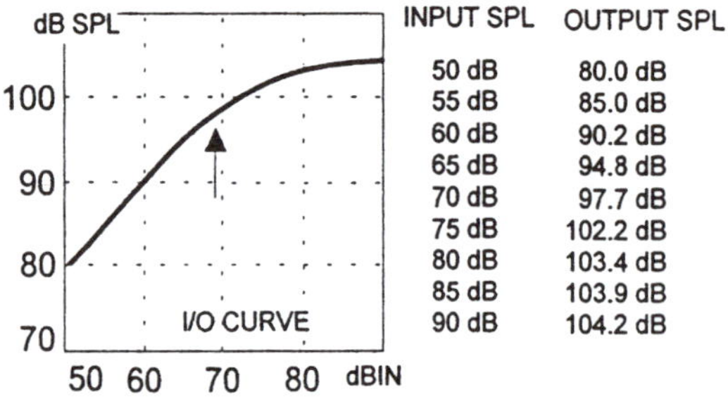

Figure 13–17. Compression circuit. Arrow indicates kneepoint.

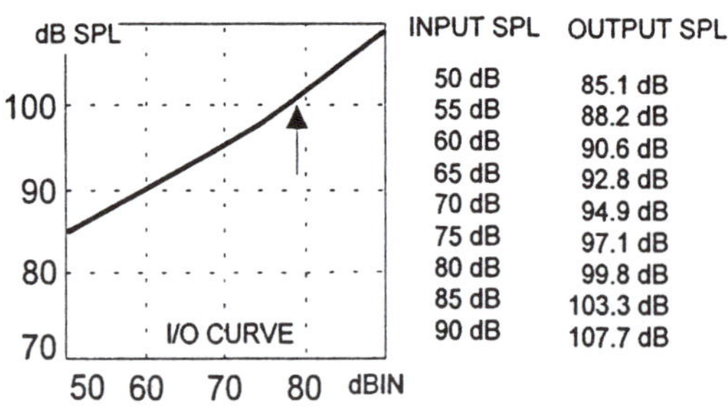

Figure 13–18. WDRC circuit. Compression begins at low levels, ends at arrow.

INPUT/OUTPUT TESTS

Another type of output test routinely done in the clinic is the input/output curve, called the "I/O curve." Input/output studies are used to see the specific compression or peak clipping characteristics of the circuit. The default input signal for these tests is composite noise. Pure tones are sometimes used to study the circuit's compression characteristics in a specific frequency zone, however. Examples of three different hearing aid circuits are shown in Figures 13–16, 13–17, and 13–18.

Figure 13–16 is an example of linear amplification. The output increases 10 dB for each 10 dB increase in the input signal up to the point at which the aid goes into peak clipping, in this case an 80 dB input. The zone of linear amplification is the straight line that crosses the graph at a 45° angle. The curved portion of the graph, to the right of the arrow, is the zone of peak clipping, in which the amplifier is saturated.

Figure 13–17 is a compression circuit with the input kneepoint set at 70 dB. Below the kneepoint, indicated by the arrow, the gain is linear, increasing 10 dB for each 10 dB increase in input. Above the kneepoint, a 5:1 (five to one) compressor is active, so the output only increases 2 dB for each 10 dB increase in the input.

Figure 13–18 is a WDRC circuit (Killion, 1992). The loudness limiting activates at a low level, 40–50 dB. This is useful for patients with recruitment. A 2:1 compression ratio is seen across most of the graph. A linear amplified zone is observed to the right of the arrow, above the 80 dB input level.

EVALUATING DISTORTION

When a hearing aid is utilized in a noisy environment, the circuit must operate cleanly. If not, the patient stands little chance of understanding an ongoing conversation (Killion, 1992). The word "clean" means that the amplified sound is relatively pure, in that the amount of distortion is low or inaudible.

Most hearing aid circuits cleanly amplify soft sounds. The question is whether these hearing aids also cleanly amplify speech in the various environments in which the patient wants to hear, such as in a restaurant. People usually speak loudly in a noisy environment. Also, if a person wears hearing aids, friends and family members may tend to speak more loudly to him or her. One needs to measure the distortion produced by the circuit at levels similar to those typically encountered by the patient in noise-filled environments.

Distortion measurements are done in the sound box rather than in the real ear to obtain a cleaner response. Measurements made in the real ear include the peaks created by the ear, which are not related to distortion in the circuit. Environmental noise also causes high distortion in real ear tests.

Earlier in this chapter, the ANSI tests strips were discussed. These tests include measures of distortion. These measurements have little, if any, clinical value, however, due to the low level at which they are made.

Two distortion tests, harmonic and intermodulation, are easily done in the clinic. The composite noise signal can be used for the intermodulation distortion test. Pure tones are used for the harmonic distortion test. Figure 13–19 is a simple graphic that shows the correct pure-tone input level for the harmonic distortion test. For example, if the clinician wants to know how cleanly a hearing aid will amplify medium-loud speech at 80 dB SPL, pure-tone input should be used for the harmonic distortion test.

Speech can be divided into soft, medium, and loud levels. Soft speech averages about 60 dB SPL, medium speech averages about 70 dB SPL, and loud speech averages about 80 dB SPL. Figure 13–20 shows the relationship between the level of speech and the level of pure-tone input used for the harmonic distortion test (Martin, 1994c).

When the signal is amplified cleanly, the peaks are preserved. This preservation of signal is shown in Figure 13–21A. When a linear amplifier saturates, it flattens the peaks of the amplified sound, as shown in Figure 13–21B. When an amplifier is pushed into saturation by ever-increasing sound levels, the degree of peak clipping rapidly increases and the harmonic distortion values may soon exceed 30–60%. The point of amplifier saturation (the point at which peak clipping increases rapidly) can be found using the harmonic distortion test.

	RMS values		Pure tone input levels used to evaluate harmonic distortion
Select	70 dB SPL	to evaluate	soft speech
Select	80 dB SPL	to evaluate	average speech
Select	90 dB SPL	to evaluate	loud speech

Figure 13–19. Evaluating harmonic distortion.

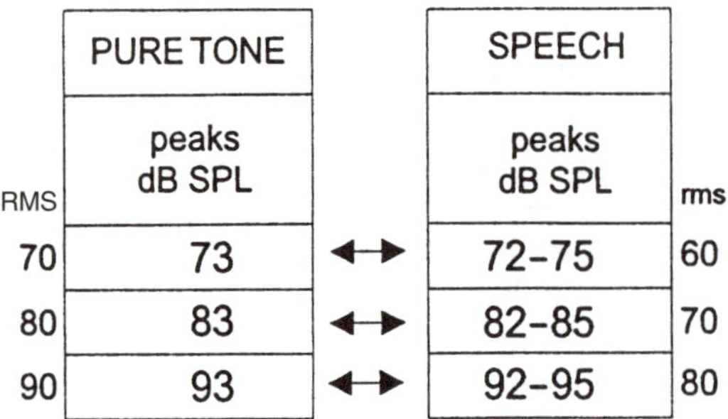

RMS	PURE TONE peaks dB SPL		SPEECH peaks dB SPL	rms
70	73	↔	72-75	60
80	83	↔	82-85	70
90	93	↔	92-95	80

Figure 13–20. When pure-tone peaks are set equal to speech peaks, their RMS values differ by about 10 dB.

Peak energy, not the RMS energy, is considered when studying peak clipping. The hearing aid test unit, however, is set in RMS values. For the harmonic distortion test, one needs to know the peak values of the sounds because one is evaluating the hearing aid's tendency to peak clip. The peak value of the pure tone used as an input must match the peak level of the speech (soft, medium, or loud) the clinician is interested in considering.

The relationship between the peak value and the RMS value is called the crest factor. Pure tones have a fixed 3 dB crest factor. That is, the peak value is always 3 dB higher than the RMS value. When speech is viewed on an oscilloscope, the peaks vary across time. Typically, the peaks of speech are about 12–14 dB higher than the RMS values. Occasionally some peaks may be much higher.

Whenever a patient complains of not being able to understand speech in a noisy listening situation, the harmonic distortion test will show how much sound the hearing aid is able to handle (amplify) before it distorts the input signal.

The harmonic distortion test is done by adjusting the aid to the use-gain setting and placing the aid in a test box. This shows how "cleanly" the aid will amplify soft speech. The input level is increased to 80 dB, then 85 dB, and 90 dB SPL, and the sweep is sequentially repeated. The results are printed for the level one wants to study (see Figure 13–20).

The data are inspected to determine whether the circuit saturates (has high levels of distortion) or is close to saturation. When a circuit saturates, the harmonic distortion values are huge, in the 30–60% range. It is fairly easy to separate hearing aids into two categories, those that distort at moderate to high levels and those that do not.

Figures 13–22, 13–23, and 13–24 show harmonic distortion measurements for a behind-the-ear (BTE) hearing aid. These tests were done with the volume level set at three-fourth capacity, not full on. The output levels are displayed as a curve, with the references for these

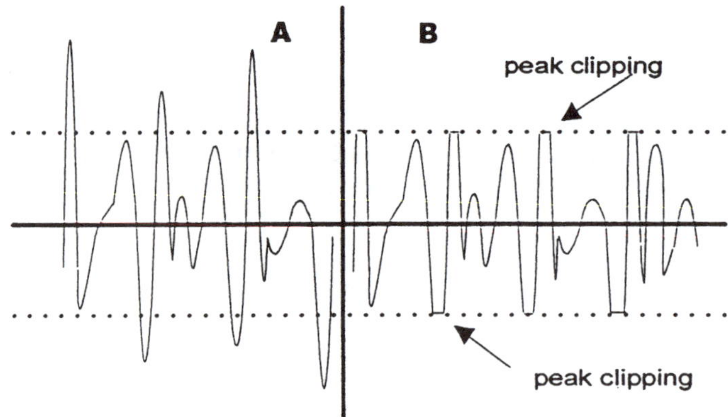

Figure 13–21. **A.** Normal. **B.** A saturated amplifier results in severe peak clipping.

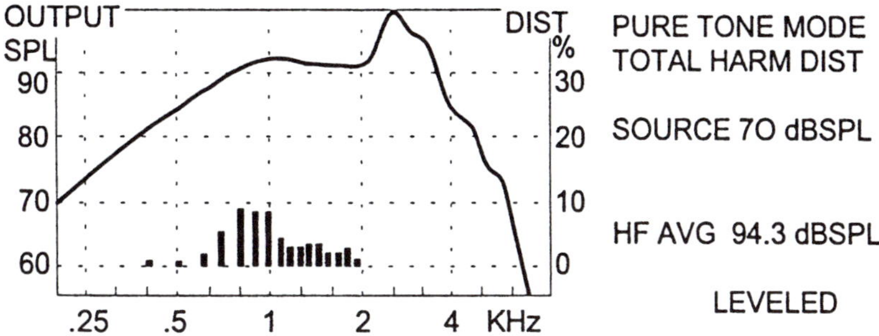

Figure 13–22. Harmonic distortion study, 70 dB input.

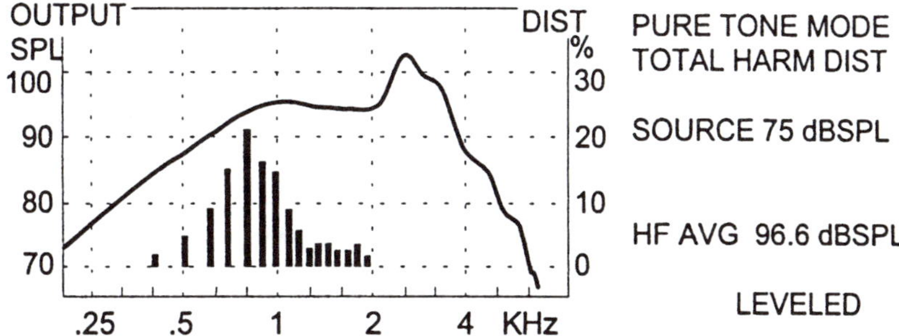

Figure 13–23. Harmonic distortion study, 75 dB input.

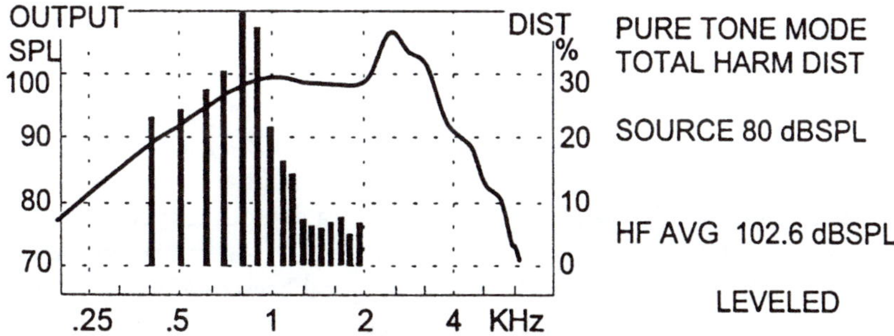

Figure 13–24. Harmonic distortion study, 80 dB input.

levels on the left. The harmonic distortion values are shown as bars, with the references shown on the right. This circuit is a peak clipper and the amplifier saturates at a fairly low level. Any input to this aid over 75 dB, the patient's voice, for example, will cause the output to contain large amounts of distortion.

The "use-gain" harmonic distortion test is a powerful tool. The results show the clinician the point (amplitude) at which the circuit becomes highly distorted. One would not expect the patient to be able to understand much of the speech signal when the aid is worn in a competing noise environment.

A second type of distortion often seen in hearing aids is intermodulation distortion. Bernstein (1966) reported that this distortion is even more destructive to word recognition than harmonic distortion.

According to Frye (personal communication, 1999), when a poorly designed hearing aid amplifies a complex sound, such as a chorus of voices, the input is clipped, and a significant number of inharmonious products are generated. Intermodulation distortion is a condition that occurs when a nonlinear product is introduced into a complex signal. The wave form is distorted, and this resulting distortion can be devastating to word recognition. When one uses poorly designed hearing aids in a noisy dining room, for example, the amplifier attempts to react to all the different voices coming into the input stage of the hearing aid circuit. If this complex input is clipped to avoid overdriving the amplifier, however, a nonlinear product (peak clipping) is introduced into a complex signal (the voice of someone to whom the hearing aid adviser is talking), and the wave form of the desired signal is deformed.

While small amounts of harmonic distortion might be acceptable, this is not the case with intermodulation distortion. According to Bernstein (1966), "as little as 1 percent is noticeable, and 2 percent is definitely objectionable."

Intermodulation distortion can be studied using a composite noise signal. The aid is set to use gain and a soft (50 dB SPL) input level is presented. The output curve should be smooth when a soft input level is used, noise reduction is often employed to make the test results more visible, and the response curve is smoother. If noise reduction is employed and the curve remains rough, suspect intermodulation distortion. The input level is increased in successive steps until the curve appears ragged regardless of noise reduction. Figure 13–25 is an instructional graphic from Martin (1994) created by increasing the input level in 5 dB steps from 70 to 90 dB and recording all responses. The five curves were placed above each other on this graphic to help the reader understand the concept of "smoothness." The response curve for the 70 dB input is smooth. As the input levels increase, there is a noticeable deterioration of smoothness.

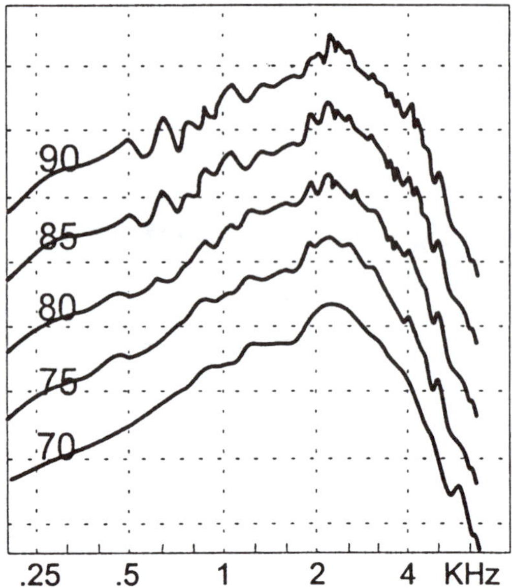

Figure 13–25. Intermodulation distortion study. Input levels increased from 70 to 90 dB.

The author asked George Frye (personal communication, 1999) how to interpret the "smoothness" of a curve to know when the aid exceeded 2% intermodulation distortion. He responded that "whenever any significant change in smoothness is noticed (as the level is increased), the intermodulation distortion level probably exceeds 5 to 10%." In this instance, notice the change in smoothness in Figure 13–25 between the 70 dB and 75 dB curves.

Frye also stated one can quickly screen hearing aids for excessive intermodulation distortion by putting the hearing aid, set to the use gain volume, into the test chamber. Using an 85 dB SPL composite noise input, look at the response curve. If the curve is smooth, the aid is clean. If the curve is ragged, the instrument has distortion that may be caused by microphone signal clipping, output overload, or both.

FLOOR NOISE (EQUIVALENT INPUT NOISE)

Hearing aids have an inherent noise that is created by the circuit transistors, diodes, and other component parts. This noise is sometimes audible when the aid is worn in a quiet environment. It is not unlike the noise a stereo speaker makes when the stereo is on, but nothing is playing. When a noise-producing component is used to build the aid or when a component part goes bad, the floor noise is sometimes elevated and becomes irritating to the patient. In most instances, hearing-aid-produced noise is only bothersome for those whose hearing loss in the lower frequencies is minimal.

The floor noise should be inaudible, or at least not irritating to the patient. Some hearing aid test units can measure this noise. Simply place the aid in the box at the use gain setting, turn the sound off, and record the output (floor noise).

If your unit is equipped with an ANSI test sequence, run the ANSI tests and record the "equivalent input noise" level. Note that either of these measurements can be used to communicate a potential problem to the factory.

TELECOIL MEASUREMENT

Many hearing aid users depend on the telecoil, or T-coil, of the hearing aid for telephone communication. When a patient complains of not being able to hear clearly when using the T-coil, be sure the telephone is held next to the hearing aid, not at the ear. Then use a listening scope to check the T-coil. Set the aid on the "T" position, and listen to a recorded message, such as the weather report, over the telephone. If the T-coil is working and the patient is using it properly but needs more gain, the aid can be returned to the factory and a larger coil added. In some of the more recent DSP hearing aids, however, the telecoil strength can be increased or decreased by an in-office adjustment.

A hearing aid test unit can measure T-coil amplification using a T-coil test unit (ANSI 1996). Some units have the coil built into the test chamber, others use auxiliary units. A T-coil test unit, such as a sound box, is used to generate an input signal for the hearing aid. The hearing aid is attached to the 2 cc coupler and the measurement microphone and placed not in the sound box, but on the test platform. The MTO switch is set in the "T" position. The test unit routes the input signal to the T-coil test platform. The T-coil in the hearing aid receives this input, the hearing aid amplifies the signal, and the output is seen on the video monitor.

New multimemory, programmable hearing aids have made the fitting of T-coils more flexible. Adjustments can be made to all aspects of the sound amplified via the T-coil, including gain, bandwidth, AGC ratios, AGC kneepoints, and any other adjustable parameters built into the hearing aid.

Some patients with severe hearing losses hear better on the phone if the gain in the T-coil response is increased in the lower frequencies, between 250 and 500 Hz. Also, these individuals tend to hear better if the AGC kneepoint in the T-coil circuit is set high (between 75 and 80), rather than low (between 50 and 55).

INCIPIENT FEEDBACK MEASUREMENTS

One persistent problem experienced by hearing aid users is feedback, a condition that occurs when the amplified sound returns to the input of the aid and is reamplified. Hearing aid tests are useful in managing feedback problems. The first task is to differentiate internal from external feedback. With internal feedback, the feedback loop happens inside the case of the hearing aid.

When a patient has a problem with feedback, the hearing aid can be placed on the 2 cc coupler in the test box. Make sure the aid has a good acoustic seal to the coupler and that the vent is closed. The aid should be set to the use-gain level and the analyzer set to spectrum mode. Listen for feedback. An input signal (noise) may be needed to initiate the feedback. If oscillation occurs, it is internal feedback, assuming the clinician has created an adequate acoustic seal with the molding clay. If no feedback is heard, place the aid in the patient's ear, set the volume control to use gain, and listen. If feedback is heard, it is external feedback.

It is difficult to test high gain (70–80 dB) BTE instruments. The gain in these units is high enough to create a feedback path through the tube that connects the earhook to the coupler. This problem can be avoided by using heavy wall #13 tubing.

Each generation of new amplifiers widens the upper frequency bandwidth of sound amplified by the hearing aid. It is not uncommon to see useful gain above 6000 Hz. When an aid amplifies the high frequency range, it may create feedback that the patient cannot hear. In the case of TILL circuits, the feedback may only happen when the room is quiet. Room noise de-activates the TILL circuit, and the feedback disappears.

If initial attempts to eliminate feedback are not successful, real ear tests can be helpful in locating the frequency zone and degree of feedback. Some analyzers have a "smoothing" feature that makes it easy to read the curve. When looking for feedback, it is necessary to reduce or eliminate this "smoothing" function. Figures 13–26, 13–27, and 13–28 show three sets of REIR curves for the same aid. Figure 13–28 is an obvious case of feedback. The aid is producing an audible feedback whistle and a large feedback peak is observed in the real ear data.

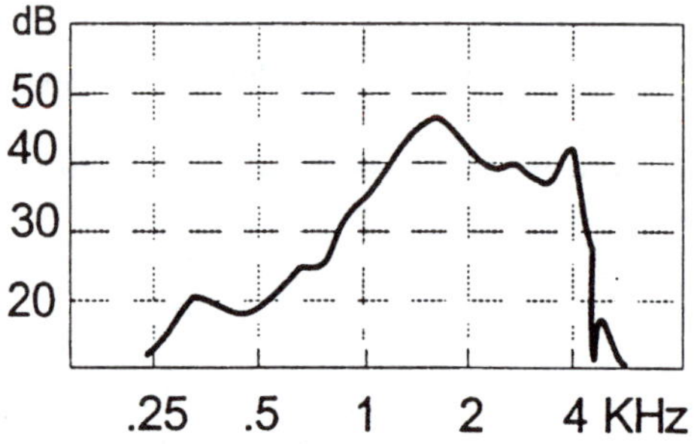

Figure 13–26. Normal real ear curve.

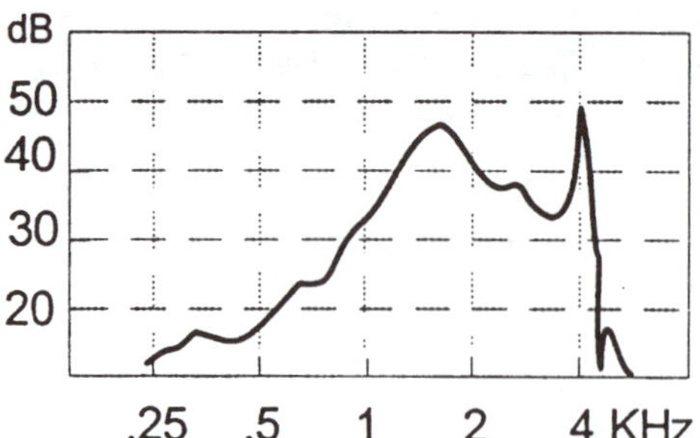

Figure 13–27. Same real ear curve as Figure 13–26, but small feedback peak observed.

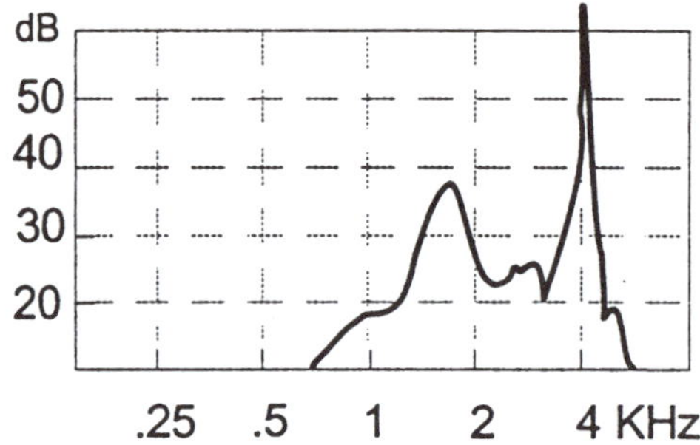

Figure 13–28. Same real ear curve as Figures 13–26 and 13–27, but large feedback peak observed.

Figure 13–27 shows an example of incipient feedback. Incipient feedback is a condition in which the feedback cycle has started, but the intensity of the feedback is low because the amount of sound "leaking back" to the input is small and controlled. Incipient feedback peaks can be seen and studied on the video monitor by putting one's hand near the patient's ear while the test unit is generating a REIR curve. No feedback whistle is heard when the incipient feedback peak is small, but this peak increases in size, and feedback becomes audible, when the aid is forced into oscillation by placing the hand closer to the patient's ear.

Incipient feedback peaks can be used to see whether the amplifier is about to go into feedback. When these peaks are observed, use the conventional tricks, such as changing the earmold, using dampers, or adjusting the response of the amplifier, to eliminate the problem. If the feedback persists, note the location (frequency) and size of the peak to help the factory design the best strategy to eliminate it.

TESTING DIGITAL AND MULTICHANNEL AMPLIFIERS

The advantages of multichannel amplifiers have been known for some time (Villchur, 1978). Some hearing aid test systems have been updated to accurately evaluate the new multichannel digital amplifiers.

New digital signal processing amplifiers attempt to differentiate between "noise" and "speech." When the circuit identifies the input sound as being "noise dominant," the gain in that specific band is decreased. When "speech dominance" is detected, the gain is maintained. The terms "speech" and "noise" are enclosed in quotation marks because these circuits are actually differentiating modulation rates. The modulation rate of noise and speech is markedly different and can be easily detected by the appropriate algorithm. Frye Electronics' DSIN (Digital Speech in Noise) test was developed to test the newest digital amplifiers. The software provides an interrupted test signal that the digital amplifier believes is speech. The frequency response curve is accurately seen. Measurements can be made in the test box or on the real ear.

The new software also provides a bias signal that can be presented simultaneously with the interrupted input signal. The bias signal is used to see how the circuit reduces the level of perceived noise. It should reduce gain only in the specific frequency band associated with the noise.

Figures 13–29, 13–30, 13–31, and 13–32 illustrate the use of this new software. A 60 dB composite noise input was used for all four graphs. This low-level interrupted signal generates the frequency response. Figures 13–29 and 13–30 are measurements of a one-channel AGC amplifier. Figure 13–29 shows a good REIR-Target match. Figure 13–30 shows the change in REIR values when an 80 dB bias pure tone is introduced. This high-level bias signal simulates environmental noise and activates the AGC circuits. The REIR values decrease markedly in all areas. Much of the

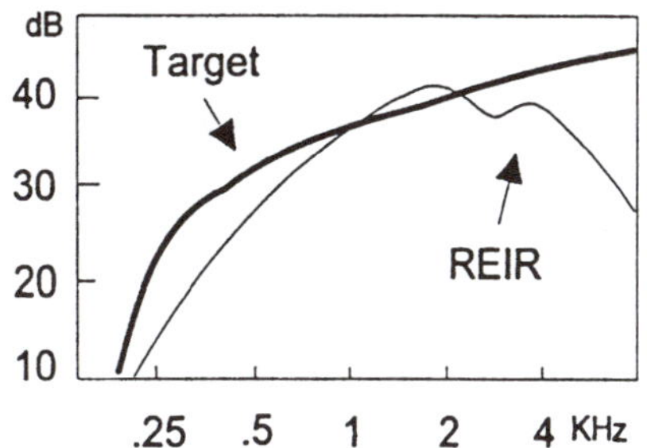

Figure 13–29. One-channel amplifier. A 60 dB composite noise input.

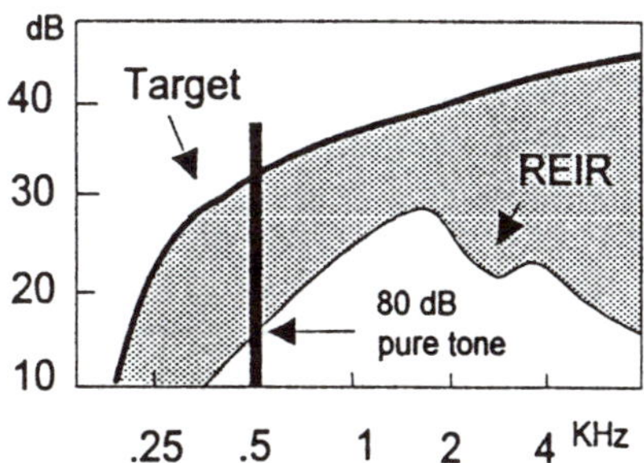

Figure 13–30. One-channel amplifier. A 60 dB composite noise input.

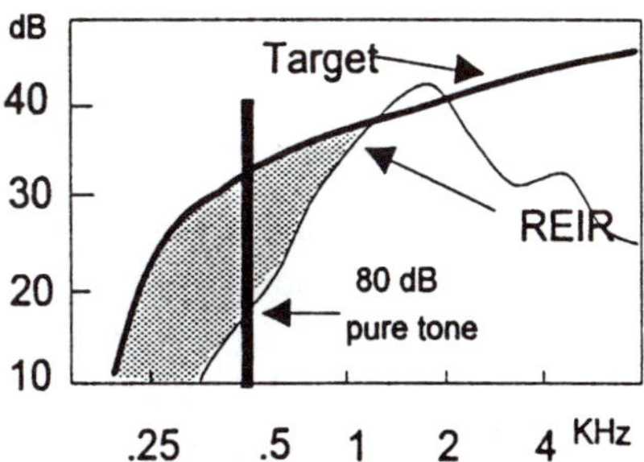

Figure 13–31. Multichannel amplifier. A 60 dB composite noise input.

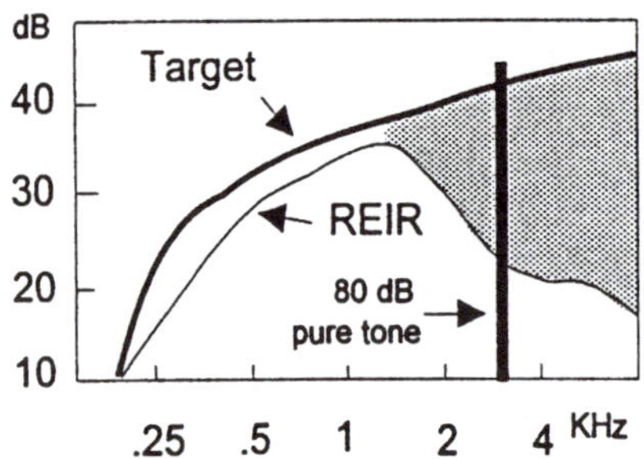

Figure 13–32. Multichannel amplifier. A 60 dB composite noise input.

usable amplification of this aid is lost in a noisy environment because the AGC circuits are easily activated, and amplification is reduced in all zones.

Figures 13–31 and 13–32 illustrate measurements of a four-channel digital amplifier. Figure 13–31 shows the effect of a 500 Hz biasing pure tone. Only the gain in the low-frequency band is reduced. Figure 13–32 shows the effect of a 3000 Hz bias pure tone. Only the gain the high-frequency band is reduced. This aid produces more usable amplification in noisy environments than the aid shown in Figure 13–30.

SOUND CARD MEASUREMENTS

Temporal distortion is the destruction of the natural time patterns of sound. If the AGC circuits of hearing aids are not set appropriately, they can reduce word-understanding cues inherent in speech (Teder 1991, 1992, 1993). This type of distortion cannot be measured with today's hearing aid testing equipment. However, measuring systems are advancing rapidly in their sophistication. As such, measuring such distortions may soon become a reality.

Human speech is a mixture of hundreds of different sounds that are presented in an ongoing stream (Stevens & House, 1972). Some sounds, such as vowels, are relatively long in duration, between 200 and 400 milliseconds. Other sounds, like the plosive consonants, are very short in duration, about 10–20 ms. Figure 13–33 is an illustration that shows the temporal (time) pattern of speech. Intensity (amplitude) is shown on the vertical axis; time is shown on the horizontal axis. The peaks represent high-intensity sounds, the valleys are zones of no sound (absence of sound).

Years ago, if one wanted to study the temporal aspects of human speech, he or she recorded a sample and analyzed it on a storage oscilloscope. An attached camera recorded the exact temporal patterns. This type of analysis was tedious and time-consuming. If one needed to study the spectral and temporal variations simultaneously, a Kay Spectrogram analyzer was used. These high-tech systems cost thousands of dollars, but they did show whether or not the temporal patterns of speech became distorted when amplified by a hearing aid.

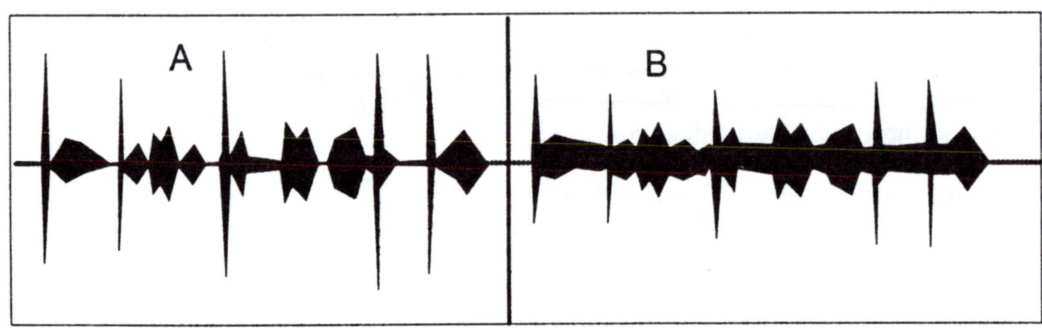

Figure 13–33. Two temporal patterns of the same sample of speech. **A.** Normal. **B.** Peaks reduced and valleys filled in.

The speech sample illustrated in Figure 13–33A is undistorted in its temporal domain. The peaks and valleys are clearly evident. Figure 13–33B shows the same sample of speech, but significant temporal distortion is observed. The valleys have been lost and the peaks reduced because the attack and release times in the hearing aid's AGC circuits were not appropriate.

Teder (1991, 1992, 1993), a hearing aid engineer now retired from Telex, has strongly recommended that one include temporal measurements as part of all hearing aid tests. He believes that the attack and release times of the AGC circuits are critically important variables and should be measured and analyzed when a hearing aid is fit.

Teder suggested that we should look at speech samples before and after they are amplified to determine whether the hearing aid circuit destroys the natural temporal pattern of speech, especially the valleys. His research indicated that the hearing impaired will have much greater difficulty hearing clearly if the circuit modifies the natural time pattern of speech.

Computer add-on boards called "sound cards" are becoming available. These units can measure temporal and spectral aspects of sound. They have not yet made their way into hearing aid test units, but considering the amount of technology built into these boards, it would not be surprising to see them incorporated into testing units in the future.

SUMMARY AND CONCLUSION

Hearing aid measurements are an indispensable part of solving hearing aid problems. Many patients come to the hearing aid clinic with a number of specific complaints. The wise and skilled practitioner listens to the patient, makes appropriate measurements, and adjusts amplification parameters to achieve patient satisfaction and improve performance. This is not to suggest that real ear measurements solve all problems related to hearing aid use but rather that they assist in eliminating some problems before they occur and solving other problems when they do occur.

Without question, one can predict that technological advances in design and performance of real ear measuring systems will add greatly to the clinician's ability to provide a more usable, amplified signal to enhance speech understanding.

REVIEW QUESTIONS

1. A test artifact called "the blooming effect" happens when a pure-tone input signal is used to test:
a. Class A linear circuits
b. Class D linear circuits
c. AGC circuits
d. All of the above

2. If a family of curves is generated for a hearing aid and all the responses have the same level (the curves are on top of each other), the circuit is probably:
a. BILL
b. TILL
c. Linear
d. None of the above

3. The real ear insertion response (REIR) is:
a. REA – REUR
b. Same as REAR
c. REUR – REAR
d. REUR + REAR

4. A variable that alters real ear performance is:
a. Loss of REUR
b. Venting
c. Residual volume of air in the ear
d. All of the above

5. Relative to the 2 cc data, hearing aids placed on children tend to have:
a. More gain, same output
b. Less gain, less output
c. More gain, more output
d. Same gain, more output

6. If the patient says the overall signal is too loud, the author recommends initially working with:
   a. The RMS value using an 80 dB input
   b. The frequency response curve using a 70 dB input
   c. The frequency response using a 90 dB input
   d. The RMS value using a 100 dB input

7. Which of the following sentences is true?
   a. Traditional real ear tests use a "gain" reference
   b. In the SPL mode, the "gain" reference is used
   c. "Gain" refers to the true level of sound in the ear
   d. All of the above are true

8. The advantage of working with the new "burst" signal is:
   a. A 100 dB input level is needed to test UCL
   b. The burst is low intensity
   c. The burst sound does not irritate the patient
   d. All of the above

9. When an input/output test is done, and the line crosses the graph at a 45° angle, the circuit is responding like:
   a. A BILL circuit
   b. A TILL circuit
   c. A linear amplifier
   d. None of the above

10. If a clinician wants to evaluate a hearing aid's ability to amplify medium volume speech, he or she should use a pure-tone input level of:
   a. 60 dB
   b. 70 dB
   c. 80 dB
   d. 90 dB

REFERENCES

ANSI (1960, revised 1976, and 1992). S3.3. *Methods for measurements of electroacoustical characteristics of hearing aids*. New York: American National Standards Institute.

ANSI (1969). S3.5. *Methods for the Articulation Index*. New York: American National Standards Institute.

ANSI (1982). S3.22. *Specifications of hearing aid characteristics*. New York: American National Standards Institute.

ANSI (1985). S3.35. *Performance characteristics of hearing aids under simulated in situ working conditions*. New York: American National Standards Institute.

Berland, O. (1978). The industrial aspect in describing performance characteristics in complex hearing aids. Sensorineural Hearing Impairment and Hearing Aids. *Scandinavian Audiology*, (Suppl. 6), 423–432.

Bernstein, J. (1966). *Audio systems*. New York: John Wiley & Sons.

Byrne, D. (1996). Hearing aid selection for the 1990s: Where to? *Journal of the American Academy of the Audiology, 7*, 377–395.

Carhart, R. (1950). Hearing aid selection by university clinics. *Journal of Speech and Hearing Disorders, 15*, 106–113.

Chasin, M. (1994). The acoustic advantages of CIC hearing aids. *The Hearing Journal, 47*(11), 14.

Fortune, T. (1998, September). Using DSL, FIG6 and NAL for sloping and precipitous losses. *Hearing Review*, 40–43.

Frye, G. (1998). *Manual for the Fonix FP40 portable hearing aid analyzer*. Tigard, OR: Frye Electronics.

Harford, E. R., & Markle, D. M. (1955). The atypical effect of a hearing aid on one patient with congenital deafness. *Laryngoscope, X*, 970–972.

Hawkins, D. B., (1987). Procedure designed to select SSPL-90. *Ear and Hearing, 8*, 162–169.

Kasten, R. N., Lotterman, S. H., & Revoile, S. G. (1967). Variability of gain versus frequency characteristics in hearing aids. *Journal of Speech and Hearing Research, 10*, 377–383.

Killion, M. C. (1992). The K-Amp hearing aid: An attempt to present high fidelity for the hearing impaired. *American Journal of Audiology, 2*, 52–74.

Libby, E. R. (1996). Hearing instrument systems technology and performance standards. In R. Sandlin (Ed.), *Hearing instrument science and fitting practices* (pp. 237–247). Livonia, MI: NIHIS.

Libby, E. R., & Westerman, S. Principles of acoustic measurement and ear canal resonances. In R. E. Sandlin (Ed.), *Hearing aid amplification* (Vol. 1, pp. 188–190). San Diego, CA: Singular Publishing Group.

Lotterman, S. H., Kastenk, R. N., & Majerus, D. M. (1968). Battery life and nonlinear distortion in hearing aids. *Journal of Speech and Hearing Disorders, 32*, 274–283.

Martin, R .L. (1994a, August). Measure distortion for real-world situations. *The Hearing Journal*.

Martin, R. L. (1994c, September). A fitting strategy for understanding speech in noise. *The Hearing Journal*.

Martin, R. L. (1994b, November). Intermodulation distortion: bane of hearing aid wearers. *The Hearing Journal,*

Martin, R. L. (1995, January). Use the rms value to manage output. *The Hearing Journal, 80*

Martin, R. L. (1997, September). New probe-mic systems offer major help in improving fittings. *The Hearing Journal, 82.*

McCandless, G. A. (1979). Real ear measures of hearing aid performance. *Rehabilitation strategies for sensorineural hearing loss.* New York: Grune & Stratton.

McCandless, G. A. (1996). Probe microphone measurements. In R. Sandlin (Ed.), *Hearing instrument science and fitting practices* (pp. 627–643). Livonia, MI: NIHIS.

McConnell, F., Silber, E. F., & McDonald, D. (1960). Test re-test consistency of clinical hearing aid tests, *Journal of Speech and Hearing Disorders, 25,* 273–280.

Millin, J. P. (1978). The electroacoustic dimensions of hearing aids. In P. Yanick & S. Freifeld (Eds.). *The application of signal processing concepts to hearing aids* (pp. 126–131). New York: Grune and Stratton.

NAL. (1999). *NAL Non-linear LAL NAL LN1.* Chatswood, Australia: Author.

Pascoe, D. (1988). Clinical measurements of the auditory dynamic range and their relation to formulas for hearing aid gain. In J. H. Jensen (Ed.). *Hearing aid fitting, theoretical and practical views.* The 13th Danavox Symposium. Copenhagen, Denmark.

Preves, D. (1987). Application of probe microphones for validating hearing aid fittings. In S. Zelnick (Ed.), *Hearing instrument selection and evaluation* (pp. 149–178). Livonia, MI: National Institute for Hearing Instrument Studies.

Purdy, J. K. (1999a). Linear fitting prescriptions. *Hearing Review, 6*(2), 42–45.

Purdy, J. K. (1999b). Nonlinear fitting prescriptions. *Hearing Review, 6*(3), 22–30.

Purdy, J. K. (1999c). Output measurements. *Hearing Review, 6*(4), 24–26.

Revit, L. (1997). The circle of decibels: Relating the hearing test, to the hearing instrument, to real ear response. *Hearing Review, 4,* 35–38.

Shore, I., Bilger, R. C., & Hirsh., I. J. (1960). Hearing aid evaluation: Reliability of repeated measurements. *Journal of Speech and Hearing Disorders, 25,* 152–170.

Staab, W. J. (1985). *Hearing aid handbook.* Phoenix, AZ: Wayne Staab Publisher.

Staab, W. J. (1996). Selecting amplification systems. In R. Sandlin (Ed.), *Hearing instrument science and fitting practices* (pp 431–593). Livonia, MI: National Insitute for Hearing Instrument Studies.

Stevens, K. N., & House, A. S. (1972). Speech perception. In J. V. Tobias (Ed.), *Foundations of modern auditory theory* (Vol. 2). New York: Academic Press.

Studebaker, G. A. (1977). Utilization of real-time spectral analyzers for the electroacoustic evaluation of hearing aids. In V. Larson, D. P. Egof, R. Kirlin, & S. Stile, (Eds). *Auditory and hearing prosthetics research* (pp. 347–376). New York: Grune & Stratton.

Teder, H. (1990). Noise and speech levels in noisy environments. *Hearing Instruments, 41*(4), 32–33.

Teder, H. (1991). Hearing instrument in noise and the syllabic speech-to-noise ratio. *Hearing Instruments, 42*(2), 15–18.

Teder, H. (1993). Compression in the time domain. *American Journal of Audiology, 2,* 41–46.

Weber, J. W, & Northern, J. L. (1980). Selection of children's hearing aids: Colorado Department of Health program. In Libby (Ed.), *Binaural hearing aid amplification.* Chicago, IL: Zenetron, Inc.

Villchur, E. (1978). The rationale for multi-channel amplitude compression combined with host-compression equalization. Sensorineural hearing impairment and hearing aids. *Scandinavian Audiology,* (Suppl. 6), 163–179.

CHAPTER 14

Principles of Postfitting Rehabilitation

ROSE BONGIOVANNI, M.A.

OUTLINE

Before one can successfully manage the hearing aid patient, it is necessary to know something about the patient's hearing handicap (Schow & Nerbonne, 1989). Audiometric findings, a thorough case history, and self-assessment questionnaires will help determine the degree of handicap and the proper course of action. The hearing health care professional, the patient, and the patient's family can then work together to craft the optimal hearing plan.

Postfitting encompasses many things. It is not simply a 6-month follow-up appointment. So much of what we do after we fit the hearing aids is tied into what we do before we fit the hearing aids. We must look at and understand many factors. Individuals with hearing impairment come to us for a variety of reasons. The most straightforward is that they are aware they have a hearing loss and want to hear better. Other people may also motivate the individual to seek assistance, such as a spouse, an employer, or loved ones who insist they "need hearing aids." An effective starting point with each patient is to determine his or her personal motivation for coming to your office. Simple questions such as "Why are you here today?" and "What would you like to accomplish from the visit?" can effectively open this discussion.

The first part of this chapter will discuss how to insert the aid, turn it on, adjust its volume, take it off, change the battery, and take care of it. Although these activities are fundamentally important to hearing aid use, they are only a small part of the postfitting process. The second part of this chapter will address the key skills and concepts necessary to assist the hearing aid wearer develop positive emotional attitudes, communication skills, and other strategies to maximize their communication ability.

It is not the intent of this chapter to offer an exhaustive analysis of follow-up care, but to provide a reasonable and intelligent set of guidelines that have proven beneficial, both to the clinician and to the patient, in achieving maximum benefit from hearing aid amplification. As with most guidelines, they serve as a basis from which additional management strategies can be developed.

THE INITIAL FITTING

Practical tip: To save yourself needless trouble and the patient inconvenience, check the hearing aids before scheduling the fitting appointment. Be sure the aids are functioning properly and that they are the correct hearing aids.

Providing pertinent, usable, understandable information, verbally and in writing, is an essential first step toward successful hearing aid use. Keep your explanations clear and brief. Avoid using highly technical terms with patients. They want to know what hearing aid use means to them and their improved hearing, without inconveniencing their daily living. Written materials to facilitate understanding and acceptance should be used whenever possible.

Delivery tools needed: Operations manual, delivery packet containing the necessary brochures, cleaning tools, working hearing aids, and batteries.

After ensuring a good physical and acoustically appropriate fit of the instruments and before the patient leaves your office, the following procedures should be clearly understood, practiced, and learned.

Hearing Aid Insertion and Removal

This activity is best learned through directed practice. Clinicians should avoid teaching only a single procedure, as patients differ in their physical dexterity and ear anatomy. Each person must find and learn an efficient way to hold and to insert the earmold or the hearing aid. Clinicians may give their patient suggestions and demonstrations and guide their fingers, but hearing aid recipients' best learn by "doing. " Use of a double mirror can be helpful if it gives a clear impression of how the hearing aid or earmold should fit within the concha or sit behind the ear, but further practice should focus on "feeling" the positions and the physical actions required.

Remind the patient to insert the battery and close the battery door prior to placing the instrument in the ear. The hearing aid may whistle (acoustic feedback) if the volume is on. The whistle will continue until the aid is placed correctly in the ear canal.

One common error of insertion is to fit the ITE hearing aid or the earmold shaft into the canal and leave the top "hook" or helix outside of the pinna's front folds, just above the tragus. This position can be uncomfortable and may be the cause of feedback. In this case, the user needs to be taught how to rotate the aid or the earmold back so that it will slide correctly into place.

Removing the aid from the ear can also be a problem if the thumb is inserted behind the rear edge of the aid's faceplate, forcing the hand to turn forward and pull the rear edge out first. This motion makes the aid's canal shaft hook against the ear-canal wall and impedes removal of the hearing aid or earmold. Because most ear canals turn toward the rear of the head, hearing aids and earmolds should be extracted by rotating them toward the rear of the head. In other words, the front edge of the hearing aid or earmold should be removed first.

To avoid feedback, hearing aids should be turned off, if possible, when they are being inserted or removed. Additionally, the battery doors of ITE hearing aids and the tubing of BTE hearing aids should not be used as handles for insertion or removal. To help those individuals with poor manual dexterity, fingernail grooves or removal handles should be specified when ordering these instruments.

The following instructions may be of benefit for inserting or removing the earmold or hearing aid:

- When inserting a CIC instrument, hold the hearing aid by the removal line with your thumb and forefinger. The red hearing aid fits in your right ear, and the blue one fits in your left ear.
- Slowly guide the instrument into your ear canal until you feel resistance. Release the removal line and use your forefinger to gently push the instrument into your ear until it rests comfortably in the canal.
- To ensure that the hearing aid is properly seated, it may be helpful to gently pull the outer ear upward and backward with the opposite hand as you insert the hearing aid.
- If the hearing aid still whistles after insertion, it is probably not placed correctly in the canal. Remove the hearing aid and try again.
- To remove a CIC, gently pull the small removal line with your thumb and forefin-

ger. Sometimes it helps to move the aid from side to side while pulling on the removal line. It may also help to pull the pinna upward and backward with the opposite hand or to apply a little pressure around the ear opening with the opposite forefinger (Widex Hearing Aid Company, 1998).

When necessary, relatives or caretakers should be shown how the hearing aid appears when it is properly inserted so that they can give appropriate help at home. In most cases, the proof of an efficient insertion is the absence of feedback when the volume of the hearing aid is adjusted to achieve a desired loudness level.

Adjusting the Hearing Aid

Practical tip: Before initiating the fitting process, know the type of hearing aid processor you are fitting and which user controls apply for this particular patient. Explain and demonstrate their proper use. Verify that the patient is comfortable with the proper operation.

If There is a Volume Control

Show the patient how to adjust the volume control with the aid(s) in the ear. Arriving at the "best" volume level may not be as simple as one would like. Here are some suggestions regarding an appropriate volume setting:

1. A simple approach is to ask the listener to increase the volume as the clinician speaks to reach a level that sounds louder than desired. Next, reduce the volume slowly until the level is acceptable. Individuals with hearing impairment speak louder than necessary because they can not properly monitor their own voice because of the loss of hearing. It is not uncommon for the client to complain that his or her own voice is too loud. For this reason, suggest that the wearer lower his or her voice and not the volume of the hearing aids.
2. The audiologist or the dispenser can also preadjust an aid's volume in a test box or via real ear measurement by following one of several well-known assumptions, such as the one-half or one-third rules that predict "use" gain from the listener's average hearing levels.
3. The preadjusted levels should not be used to show the listeners where the hearing aid's volume must be set but simply to give them an idea of the levels that can be used after amplified sound becomes more acceptable. Often, users like to know the "number, " or the relative position of the volume control, so that they can set it at the desired level before insertion. Sometimes marking the correct setting with a colored dot can be helpful. Check to be sure that the user can increase the volume without experiencing feedback. The user should have enough volume range to reduce the volume if sounds are too loud and to increase the volume if sounds are too soft.

Adjusting Volume on a Binaural Hearing Aid Fitting

When two hearing aids are adjusted, one approach is to set each aid at the desired target obtained during real ear measurement. For new users, it is not unusual to set the volume on each ear below the prescribed target (approximately 3–4 dB), at least during the initial wearing period. This will help the new wearer to gradually adjust to hearing things they may not have heard for some time while introducing him or her to amplified sound. The volume can be raised by the patient or by the clinician as the patient adjusts to amplified sound.

Another method, when adjusting two hearing aids, is to set the first aid to a lower level than would be chosen if it was worn as a single aid. If the loss is asymmetrical, adjust the better ear first to avoid a combined setting that is too loud. Then the volume of the other hearing aid should be increased until sound is perceived in that ear and then decreased so that sound is perceived in the center of the head. In either event, to verify that a binaural balance has been achieved, do the following:

1. With eyes closed, ask the patient to locate sounds presented around their head. If he or she is unable to correctly locate the sound source, adjust the volume accordingly. This will verify that both aids are working together to improve sound localization, which is one of the primary advantages of binaural amplification.
2. Introduce a noise source (radio, television, compact disc, etc.) and speak to the patient. Verify that he or she is able to separate speech from the noise at a realistic noise level. This will indicate another key binaural advantage—a greater ability to discriminate speech in the presence of noise.

Automatic Volume Control

If the aid does not have a user-adjusted volume control, the clinician must appropriately counsel the patient. Understanding how the hearing aid processor works is essential. Does the aid actually have an automatic gain adjustment, or is it simply a "screw set" volume control? If the aid has an automatic gain adjustment, is it based on frequency of the signal, intensity of the signal, or speech versus noise input? Once these factors are known, the clinician can properly explain to the wearer how the hearing aid functions in a given listening environment. A simple explanation, using a common listening situation that the user reports, should be adequate. For example, the patient is a waiter in a busy restaurant. He or she can expect the hearing aids to reduce gain as the restaurant gets noisier. "The hearing aid is making the adjustment so you do not have to reach up to adjust the volume control or find your remote control to push the appropriate button." This is assuming, of course, that the instrument is capable of changing its response as the environmental condition changes.

If the Hearing Aid Includes Other Controls

If the instrument has an on-off switch or a "phone" or a "tone" position, whether on the aid or on a remote control, these controls should be pointed out. Some hearing aids include an on-off position in the volume control that must be demonstrated by feel or by sound. When hearing aids do not turn off, the user must be shown how the battery door should be opened to interrupt function and thus increase battery life. Some BTE instruments use the battery door as a switch, and the direction of their on-off action (in contrast to the normal opening motion) should be shown to new users. Patients should also practice this operation, while referring to the operation manual.

If the Hearing Aid Includes a Directional Microphone

It is necessary to provide an explanation and demonstration of the directional microphone's operation. If a switch on the hearing aid or a button on the remote control activates the directional mode, this must be demonstrated while referring to the operation manual. A discussion on how to use this feature is critical. Be sure to explain how an automatic directional hearing aid works. As a clinician, knowing the polar plot of the microphone on the hearing aid will assist in explaining to the patient where the aid is more and less sensitive. Emphasize that directional microphones will work best when the desired speech signal can be spatially separated from the background noise.

If the Hearing Aid Includes a Telecoil Switch

An actual demonstration of telephone use should be given. If there is more than one telephone line in the clinician's office, telephone conversations should be carried out for practice. The placement of the telephone handset over the hearing aid must be demonstrated so that the patient can learn the most effective handset placement. In some cases, after the hearing aid has been set to the "T" position, the volume can be increased to improve reception, because feedback will not occur. Some hearing aids allow the clinician to program the sensitivity of the telecoil. In such cases, the telecoil may be set for optimum gain without the presence of an unacceptable "hum" that can occur if the telecoil sensitivity is set too high. Furthermore, when the telephone conversation is over, the user must remember to reset the switch to "M" for normal function. These details may sound overly simple, but their omission, or insufficient emphasis on them in training new hearing aid users, often causes unnecessary problems.

Because many newer telephones and cellular telephones are not compatible with hearing aid telecoil function, other alternatives must be discussed, and the availability of acoustic and electromagnetic couplers should be reviewed (Burwood and Crichton, 1999; Kuk, 1997).

In some cases, telephone reception can be achieved through the hearing aid's microphone (acoustic coupling). This is particularly true for the completely-in-the-canal (CIC) instrument because the microphone is further recessed into the ear canal. For this option, it is important to show the listener how the telephone should be kept close to the ear but not touching the hearing aid and also how the fingers can be used to maintain the handset at a specific distance from the head. The vent, in fact, can be used as a direct path for telephone reception when an individual has sufficient low-frequency hearing.

Sometimes patients spend time and effort to see the audiologist or the dispenser because they think that their hearing aids are not working. They discover, however, that the problem is as simple as a switch in the wrong position. Proper instruction can help patients avoid these undesirable events. When they do occur, they can often be solved over the telephone by asking the caller to move the appropriate switch back and forth, or to take the battery out and put it back in, while the audiologist or the dispenser listens for the onset of feedback.

Understanding Feedback

Even experienced hearing aid users may not understand what feedback is or what causes it. In many cases, that annoying squeal is the guideline people use to set hearing aid volume. People often say, "I raise the volume up until I hear the whistle, and then I set it back a little." Without any doubt, feedback is a major problem in achieving optimal amplification. It must be avoided, not by turning the aid's volume below a desired level, but by solving the acoustic factors that cause it.

A hearing aid that functions well, that fits into the ear canal and concha and makes an efficient closure or seal, does not cause feedback when it is properly inserted. A hearing aid that fits well, by this definition, is one that can be set to a desired loudness level without causing feedback. Nevertheless, even with a hearing aid that fits properly, the user should understand that feedback could still occur in the following situations: if the hearing aid is not inserted properly, if a hand is cupped over the microphone, if the ear canal is partially blocked with earwax, or if the instrument has developed an internal malfunction. BTE hearing aids can generate feedback when the earmold's tubing or the hearing aid's earhook are cracked or allow leakage of sound around their joints. Sometimes a hearing aid feeds back when the ear canal changes shape during the act of chewing or when the mold slips out because of jaw movements.

Never allow the patient to leave your office if feedback is a potential concern. Listeners with hearing impairment should be able to set the volume of the hearing aid as high as required to make voices comfortably loud. If a desired setting cannot be reached because of feedback, the aid does not fit properly. Do not overlook relatively easy fixes, such as reducing the vent size, using thick wall tubing on a BTE, and shortening or tapering the hearing aid tip to direct the sound away from the ear-canal bend. Also one can add mass by applying a coat of hypoallergenic, clear nail polish to the canal portion of the hearing aid. If all else fails, a new earmold or hearing aid cast must be obtained.

New users should realize that feedback is related to the amount of power (gain) needed, so the greater the power used, the tighter the fit of the earmold must be. Furthermore, users should understand that the closer the microphone is to the sound outlet, or the more open the fitting is, the greater the chances of creating feedback. Of course, this means that while a vented or wide-open earmold is more comfortable than a full and closed one, a mold or its vent cannot be more open than is necessary to avoid feedback at the desired use levels.

In cases of profound high-frequency hearing loss, feedback squeal is often inaudible to the user of the device, but it is highly annoying to those persons nearby. Even if no one is bothered by this high-pitched sound, it must be avoided simply because it introduces distortion and consumes power without any positive purpose.

It is important to remember that brief, simple, and clearly written materials, such as the example shown in Figure 14–1, facilitate a clearer understanding of the problem of feedback, its causes, and the solutions available.

The Battery

Another important function that the patient must be able to perform is correctly changing the batteries in the hearing instruments (see Figure 14–2). Use the hearing aid operation manual as a guide to illustrate proper battery removal and insertion. Practice with the patient to be certain that he or she is comfortable performing this task.

> Hearing aids often produce a loud, high-pitched whistle that can be extremely annoying to you and to others around you. This loud noise is produced by amplified sound that escapes from your ear canal and "feeds back" into the aid's mike, becoming amplified again and again.
>
> You may hear that whistle when you touch the aid or place your hand close to it, or when you forget to turn off the aid before taking it out or putting it in your ear. Also, your aid may whistle if it is not correctly inserted in your ear.
>
> If you cannot set your aid's volume to make it sound as loud as you want because it starts to whistle, first check whether you have pushed the aid or the earmold in as far as it should be. If you cannot make the aid stop whistling, let us know as soon as you can.
>
> We may have to remake your earmold or your aid so that a better fit can be achieved, or perhaps a reduction in the vent's diameter will solve the problem. In one way or another, we will have to solve your problem.
>
> You cannot go on using an aid that is constantly whistling!

Figure 14–1. If your aid whistles. Sample of instructional material on hearing aid feedback. (From "Post-Fitting and Rehabilitative Management of Adult Hearing Aid Users," by D. P. Pascoe in R. E. Sandlin (Ed.), *Handbook of Hearing Aid Amplification*, Vol. 2, 1988, p. 65. Copyright 1995 by Singular Publishing Group. Reprinted with permission.)

As you probably know, all batteries have a negative (-) and a positive (+) side. The battery drawer door in your hearing aid shows the (+) side with a small red cross. Be sure to place your battery so that the two (+) signs match. If the battery is placed in the wrong direction, the aid will not work.

The positive side in hearing aid batteries is usually flat and shows the (+), while the negative side has rounded edges.

The bottom or negative side of the battery drawer is also rounded so that the battery fits snugly only when it is inserted in the correct direction. In many aids, if the battery is placed incorrectly, the battery door cannot be closed.

To insert the battery, you can grasp it between your thumb and index finger, with the positive side touching the thumb. Push the battery through the front or through the larger opening. If the battery door does not close easily, do not force it shut! The battery must be in the wrong direction. When the battery is in the correct position, the door should close easily.

In some cases, the battery door may stop just short of being fully closed and you need to give it one more firm push until it clicks in. Otherwise the aid will not work.

Figure 14–2. Changing the batteries. Sample of instructional material on how to change hearing aid batteries. (From "Post-Fitting and Rehabilitative Management of Adult Hearing Aid Users," by D. P. Pascoe in R. E. Sandlin (Ed.),*Handbook of Hearing Aid Amplification, Vol.* 2, 1988, p. 66. Copyright 1995 by Singular Publishing Group. Reprinted with permission.)

Additional information to share with the patient about the hearing aid batteries, as suggested in Figure 14–3, should include the size and type of battery, where to purchase it, how to store it, when to change it, how to discard it and what to do in an emergency (Meier, 1998).

The most commonly used hearing aid battery is the Zinc-Air type. Zinc-Air batteries last longer than mercury batteries and are also much better for the environment. They come with a paper tab glued to the battery. Remove the tab prior to inserting the battery into the hearing aid. Clean the new battery with a dry cloth to remove any remaining adhesive. Once the tab has been removed from the battery, replacing it will not prevent the battery drain.

Store hearing aid batteries in a cool, dry location. Unlike other batteries, hearing aid batteries operate at full power and then go "dead" rather abruptly. Recommend that your patients carry extra batteries and a battery tester. Remove batteries from the aids if they will not be used for an extended period of time. If the battery is exposed to excessive moisture, remove it from the hearing aid and wipe it dry to prevent corrosion.

Practical tip: Use the tab on the back of the battery to mark the date on the calendar that the battery was replaced. Mark the calendar with the tab every time the battery is replaced. This is a handy way to determine how long a battery lasts.

Once the batteries are spent, the hearing aid will not make any sound. Patients should never leave an exhausted battery in the hearing aid, as it may leak. Once they remove the spent battery from the aid, hearing aid users discard it immediately to avoid mixing it in with the good batteries. Used batteries sometimes work after they sit for a while, but it is not a good idea to reuse them

You know that a battery is dead when you turn up the aid's volume and you cannot hear any amplified sound. If your aid is on your hand, the battery is dead if the aid does not "whistle."

You have to be sure, however, that the battery is inserted in the correct position, that the battery door is fully closed, and that the aid is turned full-on. If your aid has an "on-off" switch, it must be set to "M" (for microphone).

If you insert a new battery and the aid still does not work, then the problem is different. Either you have the on-off switch in the wrong position (it may be set to "T" for telephone, or on "O" for off), you placed the battery upside down, or you did not close the battery door completely.

Another possibility is that the sound outlet is plugged with earwax. Look closely at the tip-end of your aid or your earmold and see if it needs cleaning.

Of course, if none of the above conditions exists, the aid may not be working, and you need to call us as soon as possible. Before you give up, try again! Check all of the above-mentioned problems.

Figure 14–3. When to change your batteries. Sample of instructional material on when to change hearing aid batteries. (From "Post-Fitting and Rehabilitative Management of Adult Hearing Aid Users," by D. P. Pascoe in R. E. Sandlin (Ed.), *Handbook of Hearing Aid Amplification, Vol.* 2, 1988, p. 67. Copyright 1995 by Singular Publishing Group. Reprinted with permission.)

because the charge will not last long and the hearing aid will not operate optimally (Earaces, 1999).

Of course, batteries should not be ingested. If someone accidentally swallows a battery, he or she must see a doctor immediately and call National Button Battery Hotline: (202) 625-3333. This warning usually applies to children and pets that are unaware of battery hazards.

Care and Maintenance of Hearing Aids

The following are important points to cover with your patients to ensure optimal performance of their hearing aids.

Cleaning

Wipe the outside of the hearing aid daily with a soft, dry cloth or tissue to remove earwax and body oils. A wax brush, usually provided with the hearing aid, may be used to remove stubborn wax. For a custom-made instrument, clean the receiver opening with great care. Allow the hearing aid to dry out overnight. Gently remove any debris from the opening with a wax loop or brush. Also, clean the vent opening if applicable. The hearing heath care professional should clean hearing aids every 3 to 6 months. Some people tend to develop more earwax than others do, and they should have their ears checked and cleaned regularly to prevent the wax from damaging the hearing aid. They should also have their hearing aids cleaned more frequently. If the patient is wearing BTE hearing aids, instruction on the proper cleaning of the earmold is necessary. Written instructions should also be provided for patient reference (Healthtouch, 1999).

General Tips

Here are some general tips to include in the oral and written instruction regarding cleaning the hearing aids:

- Keep the hearing aids dry. If you accidentally get the hearing aid wet, remove it from your ear, remove the battery, and wipe the aid with a cloth. Never use heat to dry the instrument.
- Do not expose the hearing aids to extreme heat.
- Keep the hearing aid clean. Avoid dusty and dirty environments; do not wear while applying hairspray or perfume.
- Handle with care. Do not drop the aid. Do not leave it where pets or children can reach it. They are attracted to the "whistle" if the instrument is not turned off.
- Avoid losing your hearing aids by keeping them in their case when not in your ears.
- Do not attempt repairs on your own. Do not force parts if they appear to be jammed. If basic troubleshooting does not work, contact your hearing health care professional.
- Visit your audiologist or dispenser regularly, especially before the end of the warranty period (Buchanan, 1996).

Most hearing aid manufacturers include excellent descriptions of the hearing aid, instructions for its use, use of the controls, precautions, and trial strategies. It is important to be aware of their recommendations and to review them with the patient. Patients should be encouraged to read these pamphlets with care within the first few days of wearing their new hearing instruments.

A delivery checklist may be helpful to check off completed items as you go through the orientation process with your patient. Have the patient sign the checklist when you complete it.

Hearing aids are well-built instruments, but they can be damaged if you drop them on hard surfaces. Always handle them when you are sitting down or standing over a rug, never when you are over a tile floor.

Be sure that your hands are dry and clean when you handle your aids. Water can ruin them, and oily creams or Vaseline can plug up their sound inlet or outlet ports. Never spray your hair or powder your face when you have an aid in your ear. Always take off your aids when you take a bath, shave, or wash your face.

Never loan your aid to anyone. It will not fit anybody else's ear correctly. Because of this, it can make a loud squeal or whistle that is not only bothersome, but also dangerous. If your aid is very powerful, it could even damage somebody's hearing.

Do not leave your aid where a child or a pet can grab it. Put it away every night in the same place, preferably, its original box, and leave the battery door open. If it is a very humid time of the year, use a dehumidifier pack. Never leave your aid inside the glove compartment of your car.

Never stick anything into the aid's sound outlet port or into the mike's opening. If you have trouble with earwax, use the brush you were given with a soft tissue.

Keep your ears free of earwax as much as you can. If needed, see your physician regularly and have your ears cleaned.

Figure 14–4. Taking care of your hearing aids. Sample of instructional material on proper care of hearing aids. (From "Post-Fitting and Rehabilitative Management of Adult Hearing Aid Users," by D. P. Pascoe in R. E. Sandlin (Ed.), *Handbook of Hearing Aid Amplification, Vol.* 2, 1988, p. 69. Copyright 1995 by Singular Publishing Group. Reprinted with permission.)

THE TRIAL PERIOD

Most hearing health care professionals offer a hearing aid trial period during (or following) which time the consumer has the opportunity to return the instruments for a refund. The trial period provides an opportunity for the hearing health care professional and the patient to work together to optimally adjust the amplification to meet the individual's listening needs. It is important to counsel patients that their active participation in the trial period is essential for obtaining maximum hearing aid benefit.

Adjusting to Amplification

Opinions vary as to the best method for counseling patients on how to adapt to amplification. Some say wear the hearing aids all the time and only remove them if you think you need to. Others put all their patients on a wearing schedule that "eases" them into amplification. Probably somewhere between the two extremes lies the best approach. Certainly, your approach will vary based on the needs and desires of the individual patient. Therefore, you must develop a trusting, respectful, and honest relationship with your patients. The process starts at the first meeting with the patient and hopefully continues for a lifetime. Use all the tools you can: communication and needs assessments, self-assessment questionnaires (COSI, APHAB, etc.—see Chapter 15), handouts, videos, and aural rehabilitation programs. There is so much information available today to assist clinicians in properly educating our patients. At the end of this chapter, I have included a resource guide to help you get started building your "tools library."

Based on my clinical experience and research, I have found the following tools helpful in facilitating patients' adjustment to hearing aid use:

- If you like the idea of a wearing schedule, Portland State University Audiology Clinic created the "21 Day Hearing Aid Adjustment Program" (1999). It is a comprehensive guide through the first three weeks of hearing aid use, outlining hours of use, listening environments, goals, listening assignments, and a journal in an easy-to-follow-day-by-day format. Some of the goals include identifying familiar sounds, becoming accustomed to one's own voice, becoming positively assertive, and improving communication abilities in noise. Activities include participation of a "hearing partner," a friend or loved one who can participate in the process of gaining maximum benefit from hearing aid use.
- The Veterans Administration Aural Rehabilitation Program lists strategies for improved communication (1997). Their suggestions include:
  1. Be a full-time hearing aid user. It takes 4 to 8 weeks of consistent full-time use for your brain to adapt to the changed way your world sounds and accept that as the "normal state."
  2. Your ability to "focus" on sounds of interest is affected by your capacity to ignore the normal background sounds of life. The ability to hear ordinary sounds in your environment may require a learning period.
  3. You are constantly monitoring your acoustic environment. As you become more proficient at doing this, you will be able to understand what people are saying, as well as attending to other important sounds that provide useful information.
  4. Don't withdraw from society because of your hearing difficulty. It is normal to "tune out" when in deep thought, daydreaming, or just to rest. Do not confuse these times with your hearing difficulty.
  5. Avoid monopolizing conversations as a method of relieving yourself of the need to hear what others say. Realize that there are factors such as loud background noise or a speaker with a heavy

accent that make speech more difficult for anyone to understand.

6. Strategies for managing background noise, hearing distance sounds, and problems associated with riding in a car should be addressed. Importance should be placed on using visual clues or speech-reading skills. Also, being assertive in your communication needs should be encouraged. The assertive person makes requests in ways that show respect to others, as well as to one's self.

Realistic Expectations

Hearing instruments, regardless of the brand or type of technology, can never replace patients' normal hearing in all listening situations. The patient, his or her family, and the dispenser must agree upon realistic expectations. Mark Ross (1999a) suggested ways to guide the consumer from the first visit to the conclusion of the hearing aid selection process with a series of pertinent questions.

When discussing realistic expectations it is important to integrate all the individual factors of the hearing loss to answer the patient's questions, "What will these hearing aids do for me?" and "What can I expect from these hearing aids?" Mormer and Palmer (1999, p. 172) suggested using a patient expectation worksheet to outline how the client functions pretreatment, the patient's goals in order of priority, and how often they expect to accomplish those goals. Then the clinician adds what he/she realistically targets. This method can facilitate an interactive treatment plan where participation of the client and the clinician are equally important.

Sweetow and Valente (1998) summarized realistic expectations from hearing aids:

- Aided performance in quiet should be better than unaided performance in quiet.
- Aided performance in noise should be better than unaided performance in the same listening situation.
- Aided performance in noise will NOT be as good as aided performance in quiet.
- Soft speech should be audible, conversational speech should be comfortable, loud speech should not uncomfortable.
- Earmold should be comfortable; there should be no feedback.
- One's own voice should be "acceptable."

Combine the patient's needs with what they can expect. Hearing aid fitting is a process that requires fine-tuning adjustment and time for the auditory system to adapt to a different world of sound. Be patient with the process. Stress to your patients that they are part of the process. Train them to be good listeners (Sweetow, 1999) and good reporters of their listening experiences. One way to do this is to break down their listening experiences into categories. For example, soft, moderate, and loud environments in which verbal communication takes place are representative of those categories. Is the background noise "too loud," or is the speech they are listening to "too soft"? Are ambient noises too loud? Is speech too soft under quiet listening conditions? Is general conversation too soft? Is speech not clear in the presence of background noise? Is the background noise so loud that even persons with normal hearing have difficulty understanding the spoken word?

If you instruct your patients to report in this fashion, it will make your job infinitely easier when it comes to making programming adjustments and understanding the real problems your patients may be experiencing.

Obtaining Support from Relatives and Friends

Some individuals do not need help from others and may not even want anyone to notice that they are using hearing aids. Others, however, may have trouble inserting the hearing aid correctly or be unable to see well enough to change the batteries. These people need help every day, at least until those tasks are learned. In these cases, someone else should be instructed in the proper procedures so that the hearing aids are used appropriately. Some hearing aid users also need someone there to encourage them, to confirm their impressions, and to provide a friendly voice. Everyone feels awkward when handling a hearing aid for the first time. These difficulties are normal, and it helps to have a friend or relative available for your patients.

Unfortunately, all too often people who are close to a person with hearing impairment not only do not understand the depth of the problem, but also may contribute to the anxiety and the frustration experienced by the patient. These people are important and indispensable factors in successful hearing aid use. They should be included in developing counseling strategies. Tips for people communicating with individuals with hearing loss should be addressed with written reinforcement. They should include the admonition to speak clearly, to use different words if misunderstood, to face the listener when speaking, to attract their attention before beginning and, when possible, to turn off or attenuate room noises.

Acceptance or Rejection of Amplification

Our goal as hearing healthcare professionals is to provide the best possible hearing for each patient we treat. Having said that, it may be a long road to reach this goal. Amplification is the prime strategy used to realize this goal. There are so many factors that contribute to the successful use of amplification. Age, degree and type of the loss, physical factors (such as ear size and manual dexterity), auditory processing ability, previous hearing aid use, and length of the hearing impairment all play a key role in the ultimate acceptance of amplification. Additionally, perceived hearing handicap, cost, patient expectations, satisfaction, performance, and benefit must be addressed successfully if we are to have a happy and satisfied hearing aid user.

AURAL REHABILITATION: IS IT WORTH THE EFFORT?

Although technology is moving along at an incredible pace, market penetration, based on the number of individuals with hearing impairment who could benefit from amplification, is not improving at the same rate. Hearing aid return rates have not decreased: They remain at about 18%. In fact, although hearing instruments with advanced technologies receive higher satisfaction ratings, their return rate is higher than the more conventional technologies. Hearing aids have never performed better in more listening situations in the history of the industry than they do today. Why haven't the numbers followed? Why don't more persons with hearing impairment purchase hearing aids?

Even with all the advancements in circuitry and a marked reduction in the physical size of the instrument, we are still fitting hearing aids on an impaired auditory system and because of the impairment hearing aids alone may not solve all the wearer's hearing needs. We are still fitting them on persons with a set of expectations that are not realistically based on the limitations of the apparatus. So we are left with the compelling need to counsel and educate on the intelligent use of amplification.

Mark Ross (1999b) cited some interesting studies. Abrams and his colleagues (1992) found that the hearing handicap can be reduced more if the selection process includes a short-term aural rehabilitation program than with hearing aids alone. Primeau (1997) reported on persons with hearing impairment who showed significant reductions in handicap after 6 weeks of hearing aid use and those who did not. When he provided additional aural rehabilitation to those who did not, he was able to increase the number who demonstrated a significant reduction in handicap from 78% to 89%. Almost half the people responding to the 1997 AAA marketing study (1997) reported that they would like more information on how to select, wear, and care for hearing aids. Forty percent wanted to learn more about the causes and treatment options for hearing impairments. Northern (1998) found, in reviewing more than 9,000 hearing aid patient records from HearX, that the incidence of returns for those patients completing their 3 hour hearing education and learning program was 3.5%, compared to a 12% return rate for those patients who did not take this program. In another study, DiSarno (1997) found a return rate of only 2% for those patients who completed an 8-hour hearing education program.

Group Sessions

Conducting in-office group sessions, or referring to a local hearing help group is a valuable way to assist your patients in adapting to and maximizing the use of amplification. Postfitting counseling is usually thought of as requiring one-on-one contact. Whenever possible, however, counseling should include family members or other relatives or friends. Counseling should be continued over weeks or even months. Preferably, every individual or couple, whenever possible, should be exposed to some self-help group. New wearers or potential new wearers may benefit from these sessions to have their questions answered and to see the positive effects of amplification. Simply meeting individuals who have similar problems and learning how they cope is often beneficial. To execute a successful group aural rehabilitation program, the clinician must consider many factors. Some basic questions to consider are:

- Who should be included?
- How many attendees are optimal?
- When should the sessions be held and how often?
- How should the sessions be handled?
- What topics should be included?
- What are the objectives in holding such sessions?

Knowing the objectives or "why are we doing this?" is probably the most important factor in conducting such an effort. David Pascoe (1999, personal correspondence) talks about three principal objectives:

1. Acquisition or understanding of concepts or information
2. Development of positive emotional attitudes
3. Development of habits or skills

These objectives include three different areas of concern. The first has to do with learning facts related to sound, hearing, hearing loss, hearing tests, hearing aids, the sounds of speech, assistive listening devices, and whatever other information you find to be of possible help to attendees (wearers, family, friends, potential wearers).

The second objective has to do with knowing how patients feel about themselves, or at least how they appear to feel based on what you see in their behaviors. It has to do with feelings, with self-assurance, with the development of confidence. This is something that cannot be "taught" or "learned" but can be developed or strengthened. It is really something that should flow from a nurturing environment that the AR session must create. It has more to do with each of the participants than with the "teacher."

The third objective is related to doing things, not just talking about them. It is developing habits of good speech, enhancing visual and auditory attention, learning deductive strategies that reflect efficient ways of asking for information.

Suggested Topics for Discussion

Any topic can be of value if it helps the participants to better understand their communication problems. How we hear, fundamentals of sound, hearing loss, hearing aids, language, and speech are all broad topics that can be addressed in many ways. A series of sessions on hearing aids could include care and maintenance, technologies, monaural or binaural, optimal style of the aid, and so forth. An informative presentation on one of these topics could be part of a single session.

Another session could address effective communication strategies. Teach your patients the art of listening, looking, talking, asking questions, choosing their position, and maximizing amplification:

- LISTENING requires knowing the general topic.
- LOOKING requires moving one's body and head to see with comfort, avoiding obstacles, and shifting direction when the talker changes.
- TALKING requires looking up and toward the listener, not covering one's mouth or chewing when speaking, and speaking at a normal rate.
- ASKING QUESTIONS is important. Encourage your patients to say what they have heard even if they are sure that it is not what was said. The talker then knows that the listener was paying attention and knows what the listener missed.
- Remind your patients to CHOOSE their POSITION appropriately in terms of distance, lighting, noise, and environmental backgrounds. They should arrive early to meetings and other events and get a good seat in the front.
- AMPLIFICATION should be checked to be sure that it is functioning appropriately, and spare batteries should always be on hand.

Group sessions provide a unique environment to address important communication issues that may be overlooked or ignored in other counseling settings. The sessions also provide the opportunity for individuals with hearing impairment to be with people in the same situation and to share frustrations and triumphs.

Peer Group Interaction

Patients should be encouraged to participate in groups such as SHHH (Self Help for Hard of Hearing People, Inc.), which was organized by individuals with hearing impairment to achieve the goal stated in the group's name. This national organization promotes the creation of local autonomous groups. These groups meet periodically to discuss and share experiences related to their hearing problems. The primary purpose is to educate themselves, their relatives, and their friends about the causes, characteristics, problems, and possible remedies for hearing loss.

The National Association of the Deaf is another peer group organization. It is directed toward profoundly deaf individuals whose hearing losses are of congenital or prelingual origin. This organization publishes a journal, *Deaf American*.

Contact information for these organizations, as well as for additional resources, are listed in Appendix B.

Supportive Literature

Many pamphlets and books have been written specifically to convey the information discussed here. In addition to manufacturer's pamphlets, there are others materials that can be used. Suggested reading materials and where they may be obtained are presented in Appendix 14B. Use materials to form a "listening packet, " to mail to patients intermittently, to insert portions in a newsletter.

POSTDELIVERY AND FOLLOW-UP CARE

It is suggested that clinicians schedule a recheck with the patient 1 week after the initial fitting. Call the patient, especially for CIC fittings, within the first 48-hour period to identify any existing or potential problems. Check the ear, the hearing aid, and earmold at all office visits. Schedule the next appointment when the patient is in your office. The first hearing aid maintenance visit should be scheduled at 6 months post fitting. Scheduling a visit prior to warranty expiration is advisable. This is an important session in that any uncertainties about hearing aid use can be resolved, and the patient has the opportunity to purchase extended warranties and services if interested.

Troubleshooting, Repairs, and Loaner Hearing Aids

When a hearing aid needs to be returned to the manufacturer for repair, the patient's old hearing aid comes in handy as a "spare" to wear while the new instrument is being repaired. If the patient does not have a "spare," the dispensing office should be able to provide a loaner hearing aid for the patient to wear in the interim period. BTE loaner hearing aids with an "instant" earmold or a foam tip can be provided to clients who are willing to use them.

Awareness of basic troubleshooting strategies should be encouraged. This objective can be pursued through troubleshooting charts, such as those shown in Appendix 16A. These charts are to be used as references by hearing aid wearers to assist them in determining possible causes and solutions to common problems they may encounter. They should be included in the written material you provide to all new hearing aid patients.

Assistive Listening Devices

Assistive listening devices (ALDs) are often underutilized in busy practices, yet they should be an integral part of the overall better hearing picture. Many theaters, auditoriums, and churches have group listening systems that listeners with hearing losses may use. Personal listening systems are also available that are useful for television listening, business meetings, and a variety of difficult listening environments. Depending on the severity of hearing loss and the patient's performance with hearing aids, ALD's are a viable component to better hearing with or without personal hearing aids. Consider creating an ALD display in your reception area where patients may evaluate various devices. For more information, the reader is referred to Chapter 20, which reviews the utility and contributions of assistive listening devices.

SUMMARY AND CONCLUSION

To a large extent, your patient's hearing aid success rests in your hands, and, your success rests on the utilization of an effective "postfitting" program. This chapter was developed to provide a platform for the development of comprehensive postfitting rehabilitation programs.

By no means is this all the information or the only way to approach this broad and important subject. Not only is this a process for patients with hearing impairment, it is also a process for all of us to fine-tune our skills as counselor and educator. A balanced approach of skill, continuous learning, compassion, good listening, and humor will go far in helping more consumers with hearing loss become successful hearing aid wearers.

Our patients are more than just individuals with a degree of acoustic deficit. Often, we look only at the severity of the hearing loss and what the hearing aid must do to meet the individual's needs. We become so intent on fitting the best hearing aid that we forget there is an individual who needs our guidance and compassion. Our fitting programs must treat the whole person. We must take into account both the severity of the hearing loss and the psychological and emotional factors that accompany hearing impairment.

I hope that the message contained in this chapter is one of concern for the total needs of the patient. Those engaged in the selection, fitting, and follow-up care of individuals with hearing impairment face a number of unique challenges. One of the most rewarding professional experiences is to meet those challenges and to know that one has contributed to improving the quality of life of another human being.

REVIEW QUESTIONS

1. What do we need to find out from each of our patients before determining candidacy for amplification?

2. List three things you can do to help your patients learn to insert their earmolds/hearing aids.
a.
b.
c.

3. Describe how caregivers can aid in ensuring that amplification is properly inserted.

4. Describe how you would adjust the volume on a binaural hearing aid fitting.

5. Never allow a patient to leave your office if __________ is a potential concern. The most commonly used battery is the _______ - _______ type because:
a.
b.

6. When discussing realistic expectations, it is important to integrate all the individual factors of the hearing loss to answer the following patient questions:
a.
b.

7. Aural rehabilitation—is it worth the effort? Cite three studies that answer this question.
a.
b.
c.

8. List Pascoe's three principal objectives for an aural rehabilitation program.
a.
b.
c.

9. List three resources you may use to create your aural rehabilitation packet.
a.
b.
c.

10. List two peer groups for individuals with hearing loss (a and b) and then describe their primary purpose (c).
a.
b.
c.

REFERENCES

Abrahmson, J. (1991). Teaching coping strategies: A client education approach. Academy of Rehabilitative *Audiology, 14*, 43–54.

Abrahamson, J. (1997). Patient education and peer interaction facilitate hearing adjustment. High performance hearing solutions. *Hearing Review*, (Suppl.), 19–22.

Abrams, H. B., Hnath-Chisolm, T., Guerreiro S. M., & Ritterman, S. I. (1992). The effects of intervention strategy on self-perception of hearing handicap. *Ear and Hearing, 13*(5), 371–377.

American Speech-Language-Hearing Association. (1999). Hearing aids: Common problems & solutions. Available on the Internet (Healthtouch Online Website): *http://www.healthtouch.com/lvel1/leaflets/ASLHA057.htm*

Atlantic Coast Ear Specialists. (1999). Tell me about hearing aid batteries. Available on the Internet: *http://www.earaces.com*, habaHeries.htm

Buchanan Initial (1996). Hearing aid orientation booklet. Available on the Internet: *http://www.cmh.on.ca*

Burwood, E., & Crichton, W. (1999). Digital telephones and hearing aids. Available on the Internet: *http://www.hearing.com.*

DiSarno, N. (1997). Informing the older consumer—A model. *The Hearing Journal, 50*(10), 49–52.

Kuk, F. K. (1997). Factors affecting interference from digital cellular telephones. *The Hearing Journal, 8*, 1–3.

Meier, G. (1998). "Hearing Help Library. " Available on the Internet (Audiology Awareness Campaign Website): *http://www.audiologyawareness.com/hhelp/lib/htm*

Mormer, E., & Palmer, C. (1999). A systematic program for hearing aid orientation and adjustment.

In R. Sweetow (Ed.), *Counseling for hearing aid fittings* (pp. 165–201). San Diego; CA: Singular Publishing Group.

Northern, J. (1998, April). *Reducing hearing aid returns through patient education*. Paper presented at the American Academy of Audiology Convention, Los Angeles, CA.

Pascoe, D. P. (1991). *Hearing aids, who needs them?*, St. Louis; MO: Mosby.

Portland State University Audiology Clinic. (1999). Revised 21 day hearing aid adjustment program. *http://www.minfox.com*, 1–25.

Primeau, R. (1993, April). *Hearing aid benefit in adults and older adults*. Paper presented at the annual meeting of the American Academy of Audiology, Phoenix, AZ.

Ross, M. (1999). A retrospective look at the future of aural rehabilitation. *http://207.32.121.222/ross/ross-retro.htm*, 1–19.

Ross, M. (1999b). Redefining the hearing aid selection process. Available on the Internet: *http://207.32.121.222/ross/aahaorie.htm*, 1–10.

Ross, M. (1999). Getting through: talking to a person who is hard of hearing. Avaliable on the Internet: *http://audiology.org/ross/getthru.htm*. 1–5.

Ross, M. (1999). Expectations: A consumer checklist. Available on the Internet: *http://audiology.org/ross/expect.htm*

Schow, R., & Nerbonne, M. (1989). *Introduction to aural rehabilitation* (2nd ed.). Austin, TX: Pro-Ed.

Sweetow, R. W. (1999). Counseling: It's the key to successful hearing aid fittings. *Hearing Journal, 52*(3), 10–17.

Sweetow, R., Valente, M. (1998, April). *"I bought some digital hearing aids so I don't have to listen anymore."* Paper presented at the Annual Convention of the American Academy of Audiology, Los Angeles, CA.

Veterans Administration Health Care Services. (1997). Aural Rehabilitation Program. San Diego, CA.

Widex Hearing Aid Company. (1998). User's Instructions the Senso system. Vaerloese, Denmark: Author.

APPENDIX 16A:

Troubleshooting Guide

Symptom	*Possible Causes*	*Solutions*
1. No sound, hearing aid does not seem to work. WARNING! Never ask others to listen to your hearing aid by placing it directly in their ear. Because your hearing aid will not fit anyone else correctly, it will probably "whistle," and this sound may be dangerous to their hearing. It is all right to listen for the whistle when the hearing aid is not in the ear.	A. On-off switch in wrong position. Your hearing aid may or may not have an on-off switch. It may be part of the volume control or be separate. Your hearing aid may use the battery door to turn the hearing aid on and off. To do this, you may have to open the door in a different direction, opposite from when you change the battery.	With the hearing aid in your hand, turn the volume control full-on and flip the on-off switch to "M." Listen for the feedback whistle; or with the hearing aid in your ear, flip the switch back and forth, listen for the sound to appear.
	B. The battery door may not be firmly closed or the battery is in the wrong position.	Be sure you know how your hearing aid's switches work. If you are not sure, ask your hearing-aid counselor.First make sure that the battery is inserted in the correct direction. The battery's "+" side should match correctly with the "+" sign in the battery drawer. Then push the hearing aid's battery door in firmly, until you feel a click. If you cannot see the "+" symbols, either use a mirror or ask someone else to look for them. WARNING! If you force the door shut when the battery is in the wrong position, you can damage the hearing aid!
C. Battery is dead or too weak.	If you have a battery meter, check the battery and see if it still reaches the "green" or acceptable level. Otherwise, simply try a new battery. If the hearing aid works, retire the old battery in the correct manner. (See the special warning about correct ways to dispose of batteries.)	

continued

Symptom	Possible Causes	Solutions
	D. Battery contacts may be dirty, or the battery surfaces may be greasy.	Remove the battery and clean surfaces with a clean cloth. Cleaning the battery contacts is best left for the professional.
	E. The sound outlet hole of your hearing aid or of your earmold may be plugged up with earwax.	Examine the outlet carefully under a good light. Use the tool that came with your hearing aid (a small brush or a wire loop) to remove the wax. Do not insert pins or wires more than one-eighth of an inch into the hole. You may damage the receiver or earphone. If you cannot clean the hearing aid, take it to your hearing aid counselor.
	F. With behind-the-ear or eyeglass hearing aids, the tubing that connects the hearing aid to the earmold may be plugged with humidity, or it may be twisted.	If your hearing aid does not "whistle" when it is in your hand and you turn it on, disconnect the earmold and see if the whistle starts. This means that the problem is either in the earmold or the tubing. Check for dirt, and after washing in warm, soapy water, blow air through the tubing to make sure that it is completely dry. When you replace the earmold, be sure to connect the tubing to the hearing aid correctly so that the earmold faces in the right direction and does not have to be twisted to enter your ear canal.
	G. For pocket or body hearing aids, the cord or wire that connects the hearing aid to the receiver may be broken or defective. It may also be poorly connected at either end.	After making sure that both plugs are well-connected, move the cord up and down to see if the hearing aid whistles. This means that the cord is defective and needs replacement. If you have a spare cord (which you should), try changing it to see what happens.
	H. You ear canal may be totally plugged with earwax.	If you do not hear any sound from your hearing aid, but other people can hear it whistle when

Symptom	*Possible Causes*	*Solutions*
		it is out of your ear, you should see your physisian and ask him or her to check your ears. Do not attempt to clean deep into your ears. If there is enough wax to close the ear canals, they should be cleaned under the supervision of a physician.
	I. Your hearing may have gotten worse.	See your physician or ask your audiologist to retest your hearing. He or she should then make the proper recommendations.
	J. In the case of body hearing aids, the contact between the earmold and the receiver may not be sufficiently tight.	A thin plastic washer can be placed in this joint to improve the seal. If this is not sufficient, either the receiver or the earmold will have to be changed.
2. Hearing aid whistles, squeals, or howls.	A. Hearing aid is turned on and is not in the ear.	This is perfectly normal and shows that the hearing aid is working.
The hearing aid's amplified sound feeds back into the microphone.	B. The hearing aid or the earmold is not fully or properly inserted into the ear.	First, turn the volume down to stop the whistling. Then with your fingers, feel around the rim of the hearing aid or the earmold to see if any parts are sticking out of place. You may have to twist the earmold or pull your ear back while you push the earmold farther in. When you have it reset, turn the volume up again to the level you normally use.
	C. There is too much earwax in your ear canal.	Earwax may force you to set your hearing aid to a stronger level. This may be sufficient to cause "feedback." You should follow the recommendations made in 1H.
	D. The squeal may occur only when you have your hand near the hearing aid or when you lean your head against a pillow. A hat close to the hearing aid can also cause this problem.	If your earmold or hearing aid is correctly inserted and you are bothered by this occasional squeal, consult your hearing aid counselor to see what can be done.

continued

Symptom	*Possible Causes*	*Solutions*
	E. If your hearing aid or earmold has a "vent" (this is a simple hole or tube that goes through the earmold into the ear canal), and the vent had a plug to either close or reduce its size, the vent plug may have fallen out.	You have to take your hearing aid back to the seller, so that the vent plug can be reinserted.
	F. Your ear may have stretched or the earmold may have shrunk so that the hearing aid or earmold do not fit tightly anymore.	You probably need a new earmold impression, unless your hearing aid counselor can improve the fit by increasing the size with a plastic additive.
	G. In the case of "behind-the-ear" hearing aids (also eyeglass aids), the earmold tubing may have sprung a leak. The tubing may have become too stiff and may have cracked.	Your hearing aid counselor will have to replace the tubing. This is a simple procedure and should not take much time. Tubing should be changed periodically.
	H. If none of the above conditions applies, it is possible that the hearing aid is damaged and has an internal problem.	If your hearing aid squeals even when you plug the sound outlet, the feedback is internal and it should be sent for repair.
3. Sound is not strong enough	A. Often the hearing aid has sufficient power, but you cannot raise it to the level you want because it begins to whistle.	Check section 2.
		Consult your hearing aid counselor. If nothing can be done to improve the hearing aid or earmold fit, a new impression may have to be made.
	B. The battery may be getting low.	Try a new battery and see if the problem disappears.
	C. Your ear canal may be plugged with earwax.	See your physician.
	D. Your hearing may have changed.	Have your hearing retested. See your audiologist or your physician.

Symptom	*Possible Causes*	*Solutions*
	E. The entry port to your hearing aid's microphone may be dirty.	Unless you can clearly see some dirt or fuzz over the microphone's entrance that can be cleaned with your small brush, take your hearing aid to your hearing aid counselor.
	F. The weather has been very cold or extremely humid.	Batteries, especially the "air" type, can react both to extreme cold and to excessive humidity. Take the battery out and either wipe it with a clean cloth or let it warm up.
	G. In the case of "behind-the-ear: and "eyeglass" hearing aids, the earmold's tubing may be bent or twisted.	Check this condition and reinsert earmold carefully.
	H. The earmold or the tubing may be plugged, either by earwax or by drops of humidity.	Disconnect earmold from hearing aid and blow through tubing, preferably with the "forced-air bulb" to avoid breath humidity. If needed, wash the earmold with warm soapy water and dry carefully. If you prefer not to deal with this, take the hearing aid to your hearing aid counselor.
	I. The acoustic "damper" inserted into the tubing may be plugged.	This element cannot be washed, so if air alone does not do the job, you must take the hearing aid to your hearing aid counselor.
4. Sound stops and starts intermittently.	A. There may be dirt in the volume control or in the battery contacts.	There are special sprays for electronic circuits. Your hearing aid counselor will be able to take care of this problem.
	B. In the case of "body" or "pocket" type hearing aids, the cord may be defective, or its contacts may be loose.	If you have a spare cord, try to see if the problem disappears. Otherwise, you will have to take your hearing aid to the counselor.
	C. The problem may be a loose internal component.	This will require professional repair.
5. Hearing aid sounds "funny."	A. The battery may be running low.	Change battery and see if problem disappears.

continued

Symptom	*Possible Causes*	*Solutions*
The sound is distorted or scratchy.	B. The switch may be set to "T" and the microphone is thus disconnected.	Check switch position and see if problem disappears.
There is a constant buzz or a hum.	C. Your hearing aid may be working at a level that is too close to its maximum power output.	Your hearing aid counselor will have to deal with this. It may be possible to adjust the hearing aid's power, or the hearing aid will have to be changed.
	D. Dirt in the volume control may produce a scratchy sound when you adjust it.	See 4A above.
	E. Your hearing aid may have too much power in the higher pitch sound region. If your hearing for these sounds is very poor, what you hear may sound distorted.	Your hearing aid's "frequency response," which is the way in which your hearing aid responds to various "tones," may have to be changed. See your hearing aid counselor.
	F. Your hearing aid may be damaged internally.	Take your hearing aid to your counselor, who will check it to decide about needed repair.
Your voice sounds "hollow," or you hear an echo when you speak.	G. Your earmold is probably too tight and does not allow any sound pressure to escape.	This problem may be solved by "venting" your earmold or your hearing aid, but, your hearing aid counselor will have to decide whether this is possible.
6. Your hearing aid or your earmold hurts.	A. The pain or discomfort may be "physical." In other words, your ear canal or your outer ear hurts because your hearing aid or your earmold is too tight or has an edge that pushes against your skin.	If the pain does not seem to decrease with time but gets worse, take the hearing aid off and call your hearing aid counselor. Try to pinpoint the place where it hurts so that your counselor can decide whether it can be fixed by buffing or whether a new hearing aid or earmold must be made.
	B. Your discomfort may be "acoustic," in other words, due to the impact of sound on your hearing.	Your hearing aid counselor will have to test you and measure the sound produced by your hearing aid, preferably in your ear. Your hearing aid or your earmold and tubing may have

Symptom	*Possible Causes*	*Solutions*
		to be adjusted to reduce the source of discomfort. If this cannot be done, you may need to try a new hearing aid.
7. Your batteries are not lasting very long.	A. You may be forgetting to turn off your hearing aid at night or when you are not using it (or them).	In some cases, it is difficult to know if the hearing aid is "off." It is best to open the battery drawer at night and whenever you put your hearing aid away. This disconnects the battery and prolongs its life.
	B. You may have bought a defective batch of batteries.	Batteries that have been kept too long on the shelf may have lost some of their life. If kept in their plastic cases and not opened, "air" batteries will last much longer. Try a battery from a different batch and keep track of the starting date.
8. You cannot use your hearing aid on the telephone.	A. If your hearing aid has a "T" switch, your telephone may not be compatible.	Some telephones do not have enough magnetic field leakage to drive your hearing aid's "T" coil. Ask your counselor about special telephone couplers.
	B. You may not be placing the telephone in the best position over your hearing aid.	Try moving the telephone around your ear and see if the sound increases. Also, once you set your hearing aid on "T," you can increase the hearing aid's volume.
	C. If you do not use or do not have a "T" switch, you may be placing the telephone too close to your ear. This causes feedback.	When you use the telephone through the hearing aid's microphone, you must keep the receiver slightly away from the hearing aid. Use one finger to keep the telephone just away from your ear.

Source: From "Post-Fitting and Rehabilitative Management of Adult Hearing Aid Users," by D. P. Pascoe: In R. E. Sandlin, (Ed.), *Handbook of Hearing Aid Amplification, Vol. 2.* 1988, (pp. 79–85). Copyright 1995 by Singular Publishing Group. Reprinted with permission.

APPENDIX 16B:

Resources

Associations

American Speech-Language-Hearing Association
10801 Rockville Pike
Rockville, MD 20852
301-897-5700
www.asha.org

American Academy of Audiology
1735 N. Lynn Street, Suite 950
Arlington, VA 22209-2022
800-AAA-2336
www.audiology.org

Alexander Graham Bell Association for the Deaf
3417 Volta Place NW
Washington, DC 20007
202-337-5220
www.agbell.org

Better Hearing Institute
1430 K Street NW, Suite 600
Washington, DC 20005
800-424-8576
www.betterhearing.org

International Hearing Society
16880 Middlebelt Road, Suite 4
Livonia, MI 48154
734-522-7200
www.Hearingihs.org

Self Help for Hard of Hearing People, Inc.
7910 Woodmont Avenue, Suite 1200
Bethesda, MD 20814
301-657-2248 (V) 301-657-2249 (TTY)
www.shhh.org

National Association of the Deaf
814 Thayer Avenue
Silver Spring, MD 29010
301-587-1788 (V) 301-587-1789 (TTY)

Telecommunications for the Deaf, Inc.
8719 Colesville Road, Suite 300
Silver Spring, MD 20910-3919
301-589-3786 (V) 301-589-3006 (TTY)

Texts

Richard Carmen (Ed.). *A consumer handbook on hearing loss and hearing aids. A Bridge to healing.* Sedona, AZ: Auricle Ink Publishers, 1998.

Harold Orlans (Ed.). *Adjustment to adult hearing loss.* Boston, MA: College-Hill Press, 1985.

Susan V. Rezen and Carl Hausman. *Coping with hearing loss, A guide for adults and their families.* New York: Dembner Books, 1985.

David P. Pascoe. *Hearing aids, Who needs them?* St. Louis, MO: C.V. Mosby, 1991.

Joan M. Sayre. *Helping the older adult with an acquired hearing loss.* Danville, IL: The Interstate Printers and Publishers, Inc., 1980.

Web Sites

The internet is an invaluable source of information, including handouts that you can use to educate your patients. Following are a few recommended resources.

www.searchwave.com
Search engine for audiology, hearing loss, hearing aids and the ear.

www.audiologyawareness.com
Provides help for persons with hearing loss. Includes a complete list of brochures that provide information in an easy-to-understand manner on hearing, hearing aids, and other audiology-related information.

www.audiology.org
The American Academy of Audiology has a consumer area that offers Dr. Ross articles, frequently asked questions regarding hearing aids, and other consumer related information.

www.betterhearing.org
Better Hearing Institute "Hearing Help-On-Line" provides comprehensive information on hearing loss, tinnitus, and hearing aids.

www.entnet.org
American Academy of Otolaryngology – Head and Neck Surgery.

www.deafchildren.org
American Society for Deaf Children.

www.theearfound.org
The Ear Foundation.

Tap.gallaudet.edu
Gallaudet University Technical Assessment Program (TAP).

www.sertoma.org
Sertoma International.

www.deja.com
Sound Advice.

www.realworldsuccess.com
Provider of custom training programs and success motivation services for deaf and hard of hearing individuals.

www.healthtouch.com
ASHA provides information on hearing through this online resource that brings together valuable information.

www.lawpublish.com/ftchear.htm
Federal Trade commission hearing aid fast facts for consumers

CHAPTER 15

Acceptance, Benefit, and Satisfaction Measures of Hearing Aid User Attitudes

HOLLY HOSFORD-DUNN, Ph.D.
JUDY L. HUCH, M.S.

OUTLINE

"You can't always get what you want.
But if you try sometimes
You just might find
You get what you need."
(Rolling Stones)

Success is getting what you want.
Happiness is liking what you get.
(AAdam, comic strip)

The quest to fit the right hearing aid on the right patient at the right time all of the time is the "Holy Grail" of dispensing audiology. Industry statistics, hearing aid users surveys, and our own experiences confirm the elusive nature of the quest but also give us hope. We know that some patients are more likely to adopt amplification than others, that some clinicians enjoy more successful fitting rates than others, that some hearing aid technologies satisfy more than others, and so forth. In the present milieu, our quest focuses on identifying and quantifying the characteristics of patients, clinicians, hearing aid technologies, and other factors that predict or confirm successful hearing aid fittings. The assumption is that such data will advance our quest for the hearing aid Holy Grail by enabling us to fit the right aid to the right patient at the right time *most* of the time. It will also allow us to learn what steps are needed to perfect the fittings the rest of the time.

This chapter considers a variety of candidate variables that may be associated with successful hearing aid outcomes. The factors of interest are users' perceptions of hearing aid *acceptance, benefit,* and *satisfaction*. Although these terms are not synonymous, there is some confusion with their use in hearing aid outcome measures. In particular, satisfaction is a nebulous term in many applications. It is sometimes used synonymously with benefit (cf. Gerber & Fisher, 1979), but more often it is defined, somewhat tangentially, by attempts to relate a global measure of satisfaction to factors that are thought to underlie user satisfaction (Hosford-Dunn & Baxter, 1985; Humes, 1999; Oja & Schow, 1984). It is not unusual to encounter discussions in which measures of benefit are suggested as predictors of satisfaction (Purdy, 1999). An undifferentiated measure of acceptance, such as return for credit, is sometimes used to reflect a satisfactory or unsatisfactory outcome. There is nothing inherently wrong with assuming that these factors are related; in fact, the multidimensional characteristic of hearing aid outcome makes it almost certain that they *are* related, at least for some aspects of outcome (Dillon, James, & Ginis, 1997). This assumption does nothing to clarify these terms, however. It only makes it more difficult to develop separate discussions of acceptance, benefit, and satisfaction.

In the present situation of imperfect knowledge, clinicians need practical ways to separate these factors to understand and document how patients respond to hearing aids and the hearing aid fitting process. Electroacoustic adjustments that optimize aided benefit do not predict how well a patient will react to amplification in daily life. Acceptance depends on other factors besides hearing aid fitting parameters and should be measured according to more than just whether the aid was returned for credit or sold. Long-term satisfaction is not guaranteed by acceptance. Measuring these outcomes separately and in constellations has value for many reasons. It may help to reduce service and time costs, and reduce manufacturers' returns for credit. It may also improve measures of quality for managed care organizations, increase patient benefit and satisfaction, and demonstrate value to third party payers.

This chapter defines acceptance, benefit, and satisfaction and discusses variables that may underlie these factors. It describes methods of measurement and uses the World Health Organization (WHO) classification scheme to lend structure to clinical implementation of specific measurement tools, which are described in detail in Chapter 16 (Inventory of Self-Assessment Measures of Hearing Aid Outcome).

DEFINITIONS AND EXPLANATIONS OF TERMS

Acceptance

Definition of Acceptance

Accept: *To receive as adequate or satisfactory.*

Acceptance: *The act of accepting (Morris 1973).*

Reduced to its final outcome, acceptance is binary: Patients either keep their hearing aids or reject them. In industry, hearing aid acceptance is measured as the inverse of hearing aid returns for credit, regardless of whether patients use or appreciate aids that they keep. In this sense, acceptance is a passive act and only rejection requires real action on the part of the patient. There are two ways of categorizing returns for credits: either the instrument(s) is returned to the manufacturer and replaced with another type, or the patient rejects amplification entirely. In either case, some combination of factors or events have made some hearing aids unacceptable to some people, even when prescriptive targets are met. Physical discomfort, for example, is a common reason for rejection of otherwise acceptable CIC instruments (Hall & Norton, 1997).

Aside from its use as an accounting tool for tracking aid sales, acceptance is interesting because of the underlying variables that predict success or failure, independent of aided performance. If we could identify and measure some of the variables that underlie acceptance at the time of the hearing aid consultation and in advance of fitting or selling, we might be able to predict which patients would accept (keep) their instruments and which ones would return them. *Not* fitting the wrong patient with an inappropriate aid is just as important as fitting the right patient with the right aid: Successful gamblers always know and play the odds. Resnick (1998, p. 133) commented that "One may, indeed, adopt the position that identification of the variables contributing to an unsuccessful fitting is as useful as identification of those giving rise to a successful one."

Even better, we might use those measures to improve the odds by counseling patients regarding their fears and expectations, the nature of their hearing loss, appropriate and inappropriate coping strategies, and listening tactics for different situations. Such measures may also allow us to tailor available technologies to individual patient's needs and expectations. Audiologists go through sub rosa versions of these processes whenever they evaluate, recommend, and dispense amplification (Dillon, Birtles, & Lovegrove, 1999). Their return-for-credit rates undoubtedly reflect how accomplished and thorough they are at calculating and manipulating the odds to obtain a favorable outcome for their patients and themselves.

Other variables underlying acceptance come into play when the order is received, at the time of fitting, and at follow-up. Successful dispensers check these variables and take action when indicated to reduce the probability of patient rejection. Thus, it is important to objectify and codify the processes that produce high acceptance rates.

Adoption

The preceding discussion of acceptance is couched in terms of audiologist's perceptions and actions that reduce the likelihood of hearing aid rejection. In this view, the patients' role is essentially passive—they will accept the hearing aids as long as there is nothing wrong. But what if there is nothing wrong in the audiologist's estimation, but nothing particularly right in the patient's estimation? Then the instruments are accepted but not satisfactory, and they end up in the proverbial drawer. This is the distinction between acceptance and satisfaction, posing the question, *"What processes or variables predict that instruments that are accepted by patients will subsequently be judged satisfactory by those patients?"*

Acceptance has another meaning in our profession. Beyond keeping or returning a device, acceptance can also mean the psychological process of "getting used to" the idea and sensation of amplification and incorporating hearing aids into one's lifestyle. This meaning shifts the focus away from the audiologist's perceptions and actions and considers the patient's needs, attitudes, and concerns over time. Regardless of how perfectly the audiologist assesses the patient's situation and matches it with the "right" hearing aid(s) and strategic recommendations, the appropriate adoption of the instruments into everyday life is an ongoing accommodation process that remains strictly in the patient's domain. For purposes of clarification, we refer to this construct as *adoption*. Adoption is a synonym for acceptance, but it also implies ownership and assignment of responsibility to the adopter, in this case, the hearing aid acceptor.

The definition of acceptance as nonrejection is a static term that may or may not imply satisfaction. The definition of acceptance as a dynamic process of adoption is similar to the construct of satisfaction because it depends solely on a patient's subjective impressions. Adoption differs from satisfaction because it is an ongoing process that leads to patient satisfaction or dissatisfaction with amplification, whereas satisfaction is a static measurement of how successful the process is at any given time.[1]

There are underlying variables common to both static and dynamic definitions of acceptance. Examples of these variables that may affect hearing aid acceptance and adoption are:

- **Psychological readiness.** Motivation to wear amplification is an important aspect of acceptance and adoption. Patients who do not perceive a hearing problem or who associate hearing aids with aging or with social stigma (Johnson & Danhauer, 1997; Hansen, 1998) are more likely to reject amplification or relegate the instrument(s) to the dresser drawer (Franks & Beckmann, 1985; Hosford-Dunn & Baxter, 1985; Kochkin, 1996).
- **Psychological profile.** Hearing aid acceptance and adoption require adaptation on the part of the user and a willingness to cope with something new in the environment (Cox, 1999). Individuals who demonstrate traits of "learned helplessness" on psychological profiles may be more likely to fail at hearing aid use (Singer, Healey, & Preece, 1997).
- **Expectations.** Unrealistic expectations lead to unreasonable disappointment with or complete rejection of hearing aids. This topic is addressed in the next section.
- **Physical fit.** Acceptance requires aids that do not fall off or out of the ear; custom aids or molds that fit snugly enough to prevent feedback, but do not irritate the surrounding cartilage; receiver channels that are not occluded by the canal wall with jaw motion; volume controls and switches that do not scratch the helix or antihelix; BTEs that do not compete with eyeglasses or oxygen tubes behind the pinna.
- **Cosmetics.** Acceptance requires that custom aids and molds should not extrude beyond the concha; BTEs should not fall off the pinna or push the pinna out from the head. Beyond that, however, most patients have images of what constitutes acceptable cosmetics for hearing aids and remote controls before fitting. Violating that image often results in rejection of the instrument, or failure to adapt it to everyday life.
- **Manipulation.** Patients may not accept or adopt their instruments if they have diffi-

[1]Business-oriented readers may relate the three terms to an accounting analogy in which Acceptance is analogous to setting up or winding down the business, Adoption is analogous to the continuous actions of the business that are reflected on an Income statement, and Satisfaction is analogous to the overall fiscal health of the business at any given moment, as reflected on the business' balance sheet.

culty manipulating manual volume controls or if they find the remote controls confusing. Other patients reject or become disenchanted with automatic instruments because they cannot control them manually.

- **Sound.** Acceptance and adoption are more likely when the patient's own voice is tolerable and overall sound quality is pleasant.
- **Assimilation and Acclimatization.** As they wear their instruments, some new hearing aid users become more accustomed to the aids' physical presence, occlusion effects, or amplification of environmental sounds. They may even demonstrate improvements in aided speech recognition and discrimination over time (Gatehouse, 1992; Horwitz & Turner, 1997; Yung & Buckles, 1995), although perhaps not all patients and perhaps not always at the same time intervals (Saunders & Cienkowski, 1997). It seems plausible that acceptance and adoption are more likely when the instruments are easy to assimilate (Hosford-Dunn & Baxter, 1985), produce acclimatization effects, or both.
- **Credibility and Trust.** It seems likely that patients will accept instruments more willingly if they feel the instruments are high quality, backed by a comprehensive warranty, and provided by a trustworthy hearing health professional (Franks & Beckmann, 1985).
- **Performance.** A hearing aid that repeatedly fails from its inception will usually be returned for credit. An aid that requires frequent repairs at any time in its life may be "unadopted" by its wearer and discarded. (If the aid was satisfactory prior to onset of problems, it will probably be replaced and a new round of acceptance and adoption will commence.)
- **Visual Capability.** Depending on the patient's motivation, age and impaired vision can reduce acceptance and subsequent adoption.
- **Comorbid Conditions.** A patient struggling with cancer, severe heart or kidney disease, or other health problems, may not view hearing aids as a critically important intervention and may not accept or continue to adopt the hearing aids because of his or her preoccupation with the other illnesses.
- **Domestic/Social Background.** Acceptance and adoption are less likely for patients who live alone than for those with spouses or children who live with them or visit often (Noble, 1999). For working patients, peer pressure from other workers may increase acceptance and hasten adoption in much the same way that family pressure affects the hearing aid outcome in the home.
- **Cost.** Patients are likely to reject hearing aids if they cannot afford them or if their perceived value does not equal perceived cost (Franks & Beckmann, 1985). Although cost refers to a financial outlay in this variable, it is worth noting that each of the preceding variables represents a cost to the consumer (e.g., time, frustration, cosmetics, comfort) that tallies with financial cost and must be offset by perceived value to ensure acceptance.

Measures for Predicting Acceptance

Acceptance as purchase is a de facto outcome measure: patients either keep the instruments, or they return them. Beyond the binary outcome measure, and *before* rejection occurs, there are no industry standards and few clinical tools that query underlying variables for purposes of estimating the likelihood of hearing aid acceptance. Most of the following comments are based on clinical intuition and personal opinion rather than hard data or consensus. Scattered reports exist (Franks & Beckman, 1985), but there is no corpus of research that directly measures relationships among the variables described above and the acceptance outcome. Perhaps this is because some of the questions seem mundane or unscientific, while other questions involve constructs such as personality and motivation (Traynor & Buckles, 1997), which are also multidimensional, that are difficult to measure or may seem synonymous with satisfaction.

In clinical settings, appraisals of the important variables underlying acceptance should occur in successive counseling stages, beginning with an in-depth needs assessment performed during hearing aid counseling and selection. Audiologists usually assume that they know why patients have come in and what they need. The audiologists probably do, but they should always be curious and caring enough to confirm their assumptions by asking their patients what they expect to gain from their appointments. Hansen (1998, p. 10) suggested an unintimidating question such as, *"So, Mr. Jones, it is my experience after years of doing this work that people do not come here just to get a day off from work or meet a hearing care professional. What was it that caused you to come to my office today?"* Besides giving the audiologist information, such a question helps patients clarify their needs, expectations, and objections.

At this point, the assessment should survey practical wants as well as communication needs. Instead, the patient encounter often skips the above query and begins with a question-and-answer exchange along the following lines:

> Audiologist (or Questionnaire): *You are scheduled for a hearing test today. If we find through our testing that your hearing could be helped, are you ready to accept that help?*
>
> Patient: *It depends.*

Such exchanges do little to predict acceptance, except to clearly indicate that there are important but unknown variables that will influence the patient's decision regarding acceptance or rejection of amplification. A better assessment approach, if amplification is desired or indicated, is simply to ask, *"Tell me what you don't want or won't accept."* This interview-style question, couched in the negative, almost always elicits several responses that address Acceptance variables explicitly:

- *"I don't want anything hanging over my ear"*
- *"My ear canals are very sensitive, so I don't want anything deep inside my ear"*
- *"My eyes are bad, so I don't want something small"*
- *"I can't feel well with my fingers, so I don't want to have to make adjustments"*
- *"I don't want something that is difficult to maintain or breaks frequently"*
- *"I don't want anything that costs more than $_______"*
- *"I don't want whistling on the telephone"*
- *"I don't want anything that shows"*
- *"I don't want a hearing aid, and I won't wear one"*
- *"I don't care what it looks like or how much it costs, so long as I hear better"*

All of the responses above can be scored using scales for different acceptance variables. This approach is not new. Many years ago, Rupp and colleagues advocated his Feasibility Scale for Predicting Hearing Aid Use in which audiologists rated patients on a number of acceptance variables, based on observation and interview before and at the hearing aid fittings (Maurer & Rupp, 1979; Rupp, 1982; Rupp, Maurer, & Higgins, 1977). This scale is discussed and reproduced in Chapter 16 (Inventory of Self-Assessment Measures of Hearing Aid Outcome).

Precounseling is an important part of securing acceptance and adoption. In addition to identifying what a patient does *not* want, it is also important to get the patient to formulate what he or she *does* expect from amplification. This is important for two reasons. First, unreasonable expectations need to be recalibrated in advance to avoid subsequent disappointment with amplification. Patients' expectations need to be aligned with their hearing capabilities and with appropriate technologies. Second, recording specific expectations at the time of the hearing aid consultation allows subsequent determination of how well amplification is measuring up to expectations. The Client Oriented Scale of Improvement (COSI) (Dillon, James, & Ginis, 1997), is a handy tool that allows patients and clinicians to identify expectations and measure acceptance and adoption (see Chapter 16). As Schumm (Iskowitz, 1998, p. 15) described it, "Everyone has a belief set about what a hearing aid can do. . . . If you just ask a standard set of questions about situations, it's very hard to predict success; but when you tailor the process specifically to what the patient wants out of a hearing aid, you have a very reliable estimate of eventual performance. The COSI helps to customize the hearing aid fitting process to a client's own expectations." The COSI also allows the clinician to identify unrealistic expectations, negotiate reasonable outcomes, and develop a "contract" that, if met, should maximize acceptance.

It is important to use all avenues to stress the adoption process to patients when aids are recommended and again when they are fitted. For instance, Robert Sweetow (Strom, 1998) suggested substituting "Introductory/Adjustment Period" for "30-day trial period." This simple change in language shifts patients' and providers' thinking away from a negative idea (e.g., one can "try" but not succeed; something that is not acceptable can be "trying") to the positive and exciting connotations associated with getting introduced and adjusting to a new experience.

Acceptance measurements should be continued at the hearing aid fitting and at follow-up visits using check lists, rating scales, or both. As an example, two of the authors' homemade checklists are shown in Figure 15–1A and 15–1B, filled out for a hypothetical patient. Checklist A and B are completed in stages: (1) when medical clearance is received or waived; (2) when the aids are received and checked (against the order form, acoustically, electroacoustically) and preset or preprogrammed; (3) when the aids are packaged for delivery with cleaning tools, product information, battery warning, carrying/storage case(s), and accessories; and (4) with the patient during the fitting/orientation appointment. The first three stages are quality control measures aimed at reducing service time and maximizing our credibility with patients. The goals of these steps are to eliminate errors of omission, enhance communications, and reduce technological and professional errors. Checklist A is completed with the patient at the time of fitting. It provides immediate feedback to the patient and the provider regarding acceptance variables such as physical fit, manipulation, and hearing aid maintenance. It also serves as a road map for follow-up appointments, highlighting areas that may inhibit acceptance or adoption (e.g., "feedback may be a problem with jaw motion," "will need to work on left ear insertion," "occlusion may be a problem"). It is worth noting that fitting items on the check list can be rated, even as simply as 1 = OK, 0 = Not OK, for future analysis of variables that contribute to acceptance and adoption.

Singer, Healey, and Preece (1997) used a checklist as a postfitting management strategy. Their Hearing Functioning Profile (HFP) surveys listening categories and potential problem areas that hearing aid wearers may report at follow-up (e.g., listening to TV). Problems are noted according to whether they occur with or without amplification and according to factor(s) that may explain the problems (e.g., visibility, background noise, etc.). Patients are also queried on contextual issues (e.g., living quarters, occupational concerns). Recommendations are made according to a "S.E.T." approach of Strategies, Environmental Manipulations, and Technology. The HFP is reproduced and discussed in more detail in Chapter 16.

A final step in documenting acceptance and adoption is to measure satisfaction. Postfitting measures of satisfaction include some or all of the variables that underlie acceptance and adoption, whether they are made explicit or not.

Benefit

Definition of Benefit

Benefit: *Anything that promotes or enhances well being; advantage (Morris, 1973).*

CHECK IN LIST FOR NEW INSTRUMENTS FOR___________________
patient last name

Initials of person checking in ________ Date checked in ___________

Paperwork:
- ➢ _____ Aid(s) is what was ordered
- ➢ _____ Mold(s) are here and what was ordered
- ➢ _____ Original invoices put in office manager's box
- ➢ _____ Copy of invoices (without pricing) in patient's chart
- ➢ _____ Copy of specifications/settings/matrix put in patient's chart
- ➢ _____ Serial numbers written on Dispensing Transaction Form
- ➢ _____ Hearing Aid Conformity form printout
- ➢ _____ Is signed waiver or Medical clearance in chart?
  If not, fax second request or create waiver; if yes, fill in physician's name on Dispensing Transaction Form
- ➢ _____ Is a Binaural Waiver needed in packet?

Computer:
- ➢ _____ Serial numbers in database?
- ➢ _____ Warranty expiration dates in database?
- ➢ _____ Program aid in NOAH hearing aid module
- ➢ _____ Print out programmed settings and put in patient chart

Aid Check:
- ➢ _____ Do listening check
- ➢ _____ 2 cc coupler and put printout in patient's chart

Presentation Packaging:
- ➢ _____ Aid and case(s)
- ➢ _____ Disinfectant spray
- ➢ _____ Lubricant (if needed)
- ➢ _____ Cleaning tools
- ➢ _____ 1 pack of batteries
- ➢ _____ Patient's name on package

Scheduling:
- ➢ _____ Make sure patient has appointment set at earliest convenient time

A

Hearing Aid Checklist for Acceptance
Audiology Center, 1 Main St., Centerville, USA

ORDER DATE: 2/1/2000
PATIENT: Jack Jones DISPENSING DATE: 2/15/2000, 2:30pm

HEARING AID FITTING: Binaural Quality Sound BTEs
Right Serial Number: R123456789
Left Serial Number: L123456789

ACCESSORIES

*Battery Size: A13 Amount provided: 1 pkg of 6
*Cleaning Tools: 1 Brush 1 Wire Loop 1 Vent Cleaner
1 Spray Cleaner Other: case

DISPENSING CHECK LIST

[√] Medical Clearance (attached)/~~waived/pending~~ (Dr. White, 2/1/2000)

[√] Aid Nomenclature & Maintenance: √ left/right identification
√ microphone √ receiver √ vent √ battery door

[√] Battery Insertion/Removal no manipulation difficulty

[√] Battery Warning (in writing) [√] Manufacturer's Pamphlets

[√] Hearing Aid Insertion/Removal will need practice on left aid insertion

[√] Telecoil/Telephone Use no feedback in mic position

[√] When, where and how to use aid: WEARING SCHEDULE

Comments

may need to buff Right mold in helix area

Day		Environment
1	1	Hr Quiet
2	2	Hrs Quiet
3	4	Hrs Your choice
4	6	Hrs Your choice
5	8	Hrs Your choice

[√] Warranty Expiration: 2/15/2001 Warranty Period: 12 months
*Coverage: Repair, Damage, 1-time Loss

[√] Special Instructions for ~~Patient~~/(Family)/~~Companions~~:

Went over instructions with Mrs Jones – her voice sounds natural to him with aids on.

Total Cost: $2000.00

Balance Due: $1000.00

Date/Method Payment: 2/15/2000, #1111 Amount Paid: $1000.00

Balance Due: $ 0.00

Jack Jones
Patient Signature/Date

Julie Jackson
Audiologist Signature/Date
License #1234

B

Figure 15–1. Example of acceptance checklists that are filled out when hearing aids are received **(A)** and when they are fitted on the patient **(B)**.

The dictionary definition of acceptance implies that acceptance encompasses satisfaction, as only that which is adequate *or* adequate *and* satisfactory will be accepted. Likewise, the dictionary definition of benefit implies that benefit is part of acceptance and satisfaction, because that which does not promote or enhance well-being will not be adequate or satisfactory and will therefore be rejected or not adopted. The problem with this interpretation is that it does not work with real-life instances of hearing aid fittings. This is because our operational definition of benefit is a measurable difference in performance, handicap, or disability (Cox & Alexander, in press). All experienced clinicians can readily call to mind patients who derived substantial benefit from their hearing aids, but rejected them in spite of, or even because of benefit (i.e., "I hear too much. It doesn't sound normal.") (Case 1). Clinicians can also recall the occasional case in which patients derived no measurable benefit but expressed satisfaction with amplification or hearing aid services (Case 2) or accepted the hearing aid(s) even though they did not plan to use them and therefore did not qualify as satisfied by standard measures (Case 3).

The relationship among benefit, acceptance, and satisfaction is one of overlap as shown in the Ven diagram of Figure 15–2. Applying the dictionary definitions respectively to the three cases of mismatch above, benefit can be present in the form of "advantage" but other acceptance factors are not adequate or satisfactory (Case 1), so the hearing aid is either rejected or accepted and put aside. Areas 1 and 2 show these outcomes in Figure 15–2, respectively. The possibilities that explain Case 2 fall into area 4 of Figure 15–2 as follows: A patient may experience a "feeling of well-being" from receiving or wearing a hearing aid even though aided-versus-unaided measures show little benefit; or a satisfied patient may note subjective benefit, but only in a specific situation that is not covered in a questionnaire of benefit (e.g., birdsong). Case 3 can occur with passive acceptance (the patient never got around to returning the instruments) or can be due to a variety of idiosyncratic reasons (e.g., to increase the patient's income tax medical deduction, or to quiet a nagging spouse) (area 3 of Figure 15–2).

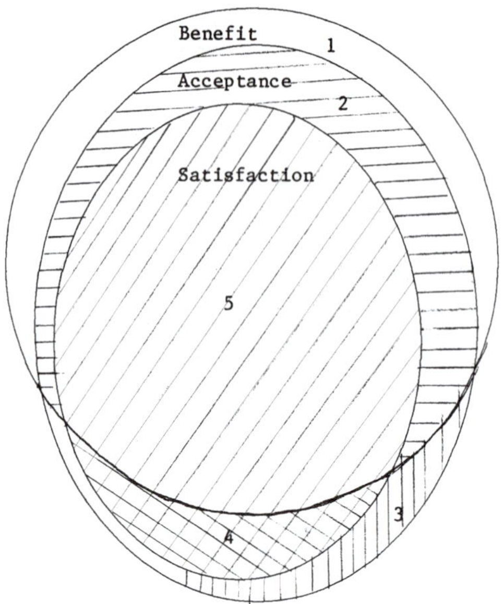

Figure 15–2. Ven diagram of overlapping relationships between Benefit (B), Acceptance (A), and Satisfaction (S) with areas denoted numerically:

- Area 1 = Aid provides measurable benefit, but it is rejected (and therefore not acceptable or satisfactory).
- Area 2 = Aid provides measurable benefit, is accepted, but subsequently does not satisfy.
- Area 3 = Aid is accepted but provides no measurable benefit and does not satisfy.
- Area 4 = Aid is accepted and satisfies, but provides no measurable benefit.
- Area 5 = Aid is accepted, provides measurable benefit, and satisfies.

Clearly, the relationship of benefit to acceptance and satisfaction depends on how benefit is defined. Investigations of the relationship among various measures of benefit and satisfaction suggest that the two are closely linked (Cox & Alexander, in press; Dillon, James, & Ginis, 1997) but not the same. As Dillon et al. (p. 42) commented, "The separation of Satisfaction (with the hearing aid or with the service) from Benefit (measured as a reduction in disability or in handicap) in the minds of clients, and the relative value of each of these concepts to them, must await further study." We would add "in the minds of audiologists" to that statement.

Outcome Measures of Benefit

Unlike acceptance, standardized hearing aid outcome measures of benefit are plentiful. Benefit can refer to an objective measure in which two or more treatments (e.g., aid #1 versus aid #2, aided versus unaided; monaural versus binaural) are compared in a controlled environment with a real ear system or in a calibrated sound field. The amount of benefit that accrues from objective measures is often couched in terms of "efficacy" of the hearing aid's circuitry/algorithm, "performance" on speech-recognition tests, or "improvement" in scores, audibility, or insertion gain. Benefit also refers to subjective ratings of qualitative dimensions (e.g., clarity, sound quality, loudness, overall impression) of different hearing aids in a controlled environment (e.g., Naidoo & Hawkins, 1997). In all cases, benefit is a straightforward, quantifiable concept. It refers to the magnitude of difference between conditions: The larger the difference, the greater the benefit.

These methods of quantifying a hearing aid outcome are appealing because they are performed in the clinic with other variables controlled. The objective methods are especially ideal, because they eliminate "human" factors that can contaminate the measures. An association of "digital" with "high technology" or "expensive," for example, could bias patients to rate the clarity of digital instruments higher than analog instruments because the former is considered "better." Blinding subjects to the study design and hearing aid can control this problem (Bentler & Dittberner, 1998).

Unfortunately, neither objective nor controlled subjective measurements yield device-specific outcomes that are good predictors of how people perform with their hearing aids in daily life. As Cox (1999, p. 1) commented, "Despite our sophistication in computing important hearing aid fitting parameters such as audibility improvement, dynamic range compression, and appropriate maximum output, we still cannot predict with confidence how well anyone will react to amplification until he or she has had the opportunity to try it in daily life."

For this reason, self-report questionnaires have been developed to measure performance and perceived changes over time (e.g., hearing disability or handicap before and after hearing aid fitting) in activities associated with speech understanding in the real world. Examples of such outcome measures are the HHIE, APHAB, COSI, and the PAL (Palmer, Mueller, & Moriarty, 1999) which are described in detail in Chapter 16. In most applications of these measures, the larger the magnitude of pre- and post-treatment difference in scores, the greater the advantage. These questionnaires are widely accepted as preferred measures of hearing aid outcome because they provide reliable and valid measures of users' perceptions of hearing aid treatment (Schum, 1999). They are not without drawbacks, however. Measuring hearing aid benefit may not reflect relevant listening situations in patients' daily lives (Dillon, Birtles, & Lovegrove, 1999; Horwitz & Turner, 1997). Walden, Demorest, & Hepler (1984) have reported an "acquiescence response set" in which the patient's desire to please the clinician results in exaggerated reports of aided improvement. As already noted in Case 2 above, self-reports of benefit may also be influenced by the patient's feelings of satisfaction toward the hearing aids or toward the hearing aid providers (Dillon, James, & Ginis, 1997).

The problem for self-report questionnaires is that it is not clear what variables are contributing to the outcome measurements. Self-report ratings of hearing disability are only weakly correlated with clinical measures of hearing impairment (e.g., speech intelligibility) and objective measures of benefit (Horwitz & Turner, 1997). Perceived benefit from amplification varies a good deal among patients, despite matching for hearing impairment and objective aided benefit. What variables besides hearing aid performance influence a patient's perception of hearing aid benefit in daily life? A number of familiar candidates have been suggested, including:

- **Age.** Older patients report less disability and less hearing handicap than younger patients with matched audiograms (Gatehouse, 1990; Gordon-Salant, Lantz, & Fitzgibbons, 1994), leading to speculation that older patients will also report less aided benefit (Cox, 1993).
- **Personality.** Extroverts report more hearing aid benefit. People who believe that others control events also reacted more negatively to loud environmental sounds. Personality accounted for about 10% of variability in APHAB results (Cox, 1999).
- **Expectation.** In general, patients expect more benefit from hearing aids than they will actually achieve, especially in noisy environments (Schum, 1999).
- **Experience.** Self-reported benefit "matures" in the postfitting period, similar to objective measures of acclimatization. Previous hearing aid users report more hearing aid benefit at follow-up than new users (Cox & Alexander, 1992).

In summary, objective measures of benefit are important for hearing aid fit verification. Self-report measures of benefit are important to validate fittings by gaining an understanding of how useful patients feel their hearing aids are for the speech activities of daily life. User attitudes vary greatly among patients, however, suggesting that there are other factors affecting these judgments that are independent of the excellence of the hearing aid and fitting strategy. These factors include variables that also affect acceptance and satisfaction.

Satisfaction

Definition of Satisfaction

Satisfaction: *The fulfillment or gratification of a desire, need, or appetite (Morris, 1973).*

All measures of satisfaction are subjective, reflect only the patient's point of view, and all are performed postfitting, no earlier than at the time of acceptance.[2] Unlike benefit, which can be referenced to a specific treatment, satisfaction hinges on a host of factors, many of which are marginal to the treatment. Returning to the dictionary definitions, the most obvious difference among acceptance, benefit, and satisfaction is that only satisfaction has to do with active desire on the part of the patient.

The Relationship of Satisfaction to Acceptance and Benefit

From the previous definitions and explanations, we are persuaded that acceptance is a measurable facet of satisfaction that can be stated as follows: Hearing aids that are not acceptable are never satisfactory, and hearing aids that are acceptable may not satisfy completely.[3] In other words, acceptance is necessary but not sufficient to guarantee satisfac-

[2]In almost all cases, satisfaction measures at the time of acceptance should be relatively high. At this time, and only at this time, satisfaction and acceptance are essentially the same construct. The adoption process (or lack of adoption) dictates that satisfaction must be measured postfitting to be clinically useful.

[3]If the aid(s) satisfies in some dimension (e.g., happiness with provider) but is rejected, does this imply satisfaction? No. Acceptance is not exclusive: any single acceptance variable can trigger rejection. But the construct of satisfaction is inclusive: It is measured by the sum of its parts, which is why most investigators refer to a "global" measure of satisfaction in addition to component measures of satisfaction along different dimensions.

tion (see Figure 15–2, area 5). Acceptance is a passive act that occurs when a hearing aid is acceptable (e.g., the instrument that was ordered, an instrument that is functional, an instrument that fits) and sometimes even satisfactory. It bears repeating that the legendary "large number of hearing aids in dresser drawers" demonstrates that acceptance does not always imply subsequent satisfaction (see Figure 15–2, areas 2 and 3).

The situation is more complex with regard to benefit and satisfaction. A common assumption is that satisfaction will more or less covary with benefit. That is, hearing aid wearers are likely to express satisfaction with the instruments that yield the largest improvement, the best performance, the most efficacy, the highest ratings, the largest pre- and post-treatment change, and so forth. This assumption has a good deal of face validity and is probably valid most of the time (cf., Dillon, James, & Ginis, 1997; Hosford-Dunn & Baxter, 1985), but not always (Oja & Schow, 1984). In any case, the earlier discussion shows that the definition of measures of benefit is too narrow to encompass all aspects of satisfaction (Cox & Alexander, in press); see Figure 15–2, areas 2, 3 and 4). Abrams & Hnath-Chisolm (in press) pointed out that benefit is neither necessary nor sufficient to guarantee satisfaction:

> Satisfaction does not always correspond to significant or quantifiable changes in impairment, activity limitations, participation, or health-related quality of life. In addition to improvements in communication and real-world functioning, the domain of satisfaction involves the patient's relationship with service providers, the ease of access to services, as well as the influence of factors such as cosmetics, comfort, expectations and perceived value. *It is a construct that needs independent assessment.* [Italics added.]

Benefit is a measurable enhancement or advancement that occurs independent of whether the thing is desired or wanted (see Figure 15–2, areas 1 and 2) and is therefore a different construct than satisfaction. As Cox and Alexander (in press, p. 3) commented, "Satisfaction is the outcome variable that appears to encompass the full constellation of factors needed for a positive fitting results. . . . We propose that when the overall outcome of amplification provision *from the patient's point of view* is the variable of interest, Satisfaction is perhaps more important than Benefit alone." [Italics added.]

Variables Associated with Satisfaction

A number of studies have looked at many candidate variables that may be related to measures of satisfaction. The results do not always agree, and they are not always comparable because of demographic and procedural differences among studies. Some of the areas of difference are detailed in the following list and discussion:

- sample population demographics (e.g., age range, hearing aid type, fitting environment, hearing aid use, total hearing aid experience, etc.)
- settings and providers (e.g., number of different settings in sample, VA versus private practice, audiologists and/or hearing aid dispensers)
- measurement variables (or definitions of variables)
- statistics (e.g., principle components analysis, factor analysis, logistic regression)
- number of items that measured satisfaction (e.g., single "global" item, multiple items, categorical groups of items)
- methods of measurement (e.g., 5-point Likert scales, 5-point or 7-point equal-appearing linguistic scales)

Kochkin (1993) found four factors that accounted for 96% of the variance in overall satisfaction ratings of hearing aid wearers fitted in many different locations in the United States. Those four factors were value and perceived benefit, sound quality of the aid, reliability of the aid, and satisfaction in multiple listening situations. Humes (1999) looked at some of the same variables and found that items grouped statistically into two independent measures of satisfaction: hearing aid instruments factors (e.g., comfort/fit, cost, performance) and provider-related factors (dispenser knowledge, quality of services). Humes concluded that the hearing aid satisfaction dimension depends on a complex interaction of many factors, including "severity of hearing loss, perceived handicap or need for assistance, aided sound quality, reliability or dependability of the instruments, and the personality of the wearer" (p. 38). Hosford-Dunn and Baxter (1985) found no relationship among severity of hearing loss and satisfaction in a younger sample population but found that user satisfaction was significantly related to aided speech performance in quiet, self-assessed, aided-versus-unaided speech understanding benefit and to two variables that may be associated with the patient's personality (motivation and initial response to amplification at fitting). Patient age was not related to satisfaction in one study (Oja & Schow, 1984) while Smedley (1990) found an inverse relationship between age and satisfaction.

In other studies of hearing aid users, the variables linked to satisfaction include daily use, improved speech understanding in quiet, use in other environments, fit and comfort, sound quality, ease of manipulation, reliability, services and counseling (encompassing what Dillon, Birtles, and Lovegrove, 1999, called "the basics of hearing aid fitting"), and social stigma (Brooks, 1981; Hawes, Durand, & Clark, 1985; Kochkin, 1993; Stock, Fichtl, & Heller, 1997).

Several studies have asked hearing aid owners, nonowners, or both to rate the importance of lists of variables that could contribute to wearer satisfaction (Cox & Alexander, in press; Franks & Beckmann, 1985; Surr, Schuchman, & Montgomery, 1978). Cox and Alexander surveyed the literature and concluded that the relevant variables comprise six satisfaction domains, which they labeled Cosmetics and self-image, Sound quality/acoustics, Benefit, Comfort and ease of use, Cost, and Service.

When to measure satisfaction, or at what intervals, is an important, but largely unknown factor. Many of the variables supporting a satisfactory outcome are contextual in nature, such as overall health and presence of significant other in the household, and therefore subject to change over time (Noble, 1999). Studies report changes in satisfaction-related measures several months post-fitting that may be related to hearing aid adoption (Brooks, 1979, 1996; Dillon, Birtles, & Lovegrove, 1999; Hosford-Dunn & Baxter, 1985). Several of those studies suggested intervention in the form of counseling and satisfaction measures at a minimum of three months postfitting.

Outcome Measures of Satisfaction

Satisfaction is an active demand that is best anticipated by asking patients the flip side of the acceptance question. Rather than "Tell me what you don't want and won't accept," the correct question during hearing aid selection and follow-up is: "Tell me what you want and how I can best satisfy you." Again, this question is likely to result in several answers from the patient. Not all of the answers can be met with satisfaction, but the answers help reveal patient expectations and contextual information, as shown in the following sample answers from prospective and experienced users:

- "I want a tiny hearing aid like the ones advertised on television."
- "I want the best hearing aid there is, regardless of cost."
- "I want the least expensive hearing aid you have."
- "The hearing aid is fine except that I cannot hear the person across the table in our dining room at the retirement center."
- "I want a hearing aid without a battery."
- "I want a hearing aid that I don't have to adjust."

- "I want a hearing aid that I can adjust."
- "I want you to change this hearing aid so I can (or don't have to) adjust it myself."
- "I want the whistling in my hearing aid to stop."
- "I want to go over how to clean my hearing aid again."
- "I just got out of the hospital and lost a lot of weight. My hearing aid is whistling and is loose in my ear. I want it to be like it used to be."
- "I want a guarantee that the hearing aid will work."
- "I want to know why my hearing aid stopped working."

As in the previous discussion of acceptance, all of these responses lend themselves to scoring. For instance, one could construct an in-house assessment tool in which the audiologist rates the importance of different acceptance and adoptions variables to the patient on a Likert scale (e.g., Importance of Cost, Importance of Cosmetics, Importance of Volume Control) as part of the hearing aid consultation. Other variables could be scored at the fitting and again at follow-up appointments (e.g., Manipulation Ability, Occurrence of Feedback, Occlusion Effect). For example, Dillon, Birtles, and Lovegrove (1999) recently reported a rehabilitation program in which a Hearing Aid User's Questionnaire (HAUQ) was used in conjunction with the COSI. The program spanned appointments from assessment to postfitting follow-up, comprising a three-to-four month period. Items in the HAUQ included acceptance, benefit, and satisfaction questions.

Kochkin (1993, 1995, 1996, 1997, 1999) has done some of the most extensive survey work on satisfaction. He used the Knowles Hearing Aid Satisfaction Survey to measure consumer satisfaction with hearing aids on one global item and in others items that survey more than 60 variables that may be related to satisfaction, such as:

- ease of use
- costs and expenses
- dispenser knowledge
- quality of services
- comfort/fit
- battery life
- value
- visibility
- performance in specific listening situations

In Kochkin's MarkeTrak satisfaction surveys, global satisfaction with hearing aids was 16% higher for programmable than for nonprogrammable hearing aids (Kochkin, 1999). Among newer instruments (less than 2 years old), overall satisfaction was greater for higher technology instruments, but not necessarily for difficult listening situations (Kochkin, 1997). Fit type was also associated with differences in satisfaction. Respondents who wore completely-in-the-canal instruments reported higher than average satisfaction ratings for several variables (telephone use, outdoor use, directionality, feedback, visibility) (Kochkin, 1995). Wearing time was associated with satisfaction (most "very satisfied" users wore more than 5 hours per day; only a third of "very dissatisfied" users did so). However, self-reported benefit was not greater for those who wore their hearing aids more hours per day compared to those who wore their instruments 4 hours or less per day (Kochkin, 1995).

Sandridge and Newman (1998) used the Knowles Hearing Aid Satisfaction Survey to compare consumer satisfaction ratings of digital hearing aids with MarkeTrak research norms of consumer satisfaction with high-performance and conventional instruments. Among the 70 subjects, satisfaction was higher for digital than for nondigital instruments, except for difficult listening situations in which digital instruments did not prove more satisfactory.

Cox and Alexander (in press) approached satisfaction in a different manner. Instead of measuring satisfaction to deduce what variables and groups of variables contributed to the measure(s), they defined satisfaction through a series of inductive steps in which hearing aid wearers were interviewed and then completed questionnaires about the relative importance of different variables to their satisfaction with hearing aids. This method is appealing because it represents a formalized, structured version of the *"Tell me what you want and how I can best satisfy you"* strategy advocated earlier in this section. Indeed, Cox and Alexander commented that "relatively few studies have been reported in which subjects experienced with hearing aids have been asked directly 'what things are important to your satisfaction with a hearing aid?'" (in press). The result of their approach is a questionnaire entitled Satisfaction with Amplification in Daily Life (SADL). It measures satisfaction with 15 items that correspond to four dimensions of satisfaction that were ranked high in importance by hearing aid users. The SADL includes several potential cross-validation measures (hearing aid experience, daily use, perceived degree of hearing impairment).

ASHA's Consumer Satisfaction Measure queries patients on aspects of office appearance, provider competence, and service delivery. Martin (1997) published a 20-item checklist to measure the quality of service delivery. Besides these tools, many offices develop their own measures of patient satisfaction, which are either handed to patients at the time of service or mailed at strategic intervals as part of follow-up. Samples of the latter, Martin's Quality Checklist, and the authors' adapted version of the ASHA survey are reproduced in Chapter 16.

USING ACCEPTANCE, BENEFIT, AND SATISFACTION MEASURES IN CONSTELLATION: THE WHO MODEL

The clinician's goals are three-fold with potential and current hearing aid users: (1) assess and appropriately treat hearing impairment with amplification, (2) validate fittings by measuring benefit, (3) validate treatment by postfitting measure(s) of satisfaction. How do measures of acceptance, benefit, and satisfaction fit into this three-step intervention model? How does a clinician decide which measure(s) best appraises each goal of intervention?

One way to conceptualize the process is by applying the World Health Organization (WHO, 1980, 1997) classification scheme for describing the consequences of health conditions to audiology assessment and treatment goals, as shown in Table 15–1. In the WHO nomenclature, the *Impairment* dimension refers to body-level structure and function, as in decreased auditory sensitivity or middle-ear disease. Appropriate selection of amplification aims to correct the loss of auditory sensitivity, which can be verified by objective measures of benefit. The *Disability/Activity* dimension refers to person-level function, manifested by limitations in a patient's daily activities (e.g., cannot hear television unless volume is high). Hearing aid treatment goals for this dimension are to reduce or eliminate limitations, which can be validated by objective and subjective measures of Benefit and performance. The third dimension of the WHO model is Handicap/Participation, which refers to societal-level function (e.g., no longer watches television because it is so loud that the neighbors complain). Here, the goal of amplification is to restore or expand the patient's social involvement, which can be validated by some subjective measures of benefit and other measures of handicap. The fourth dimension was introduced to the WHO model as the result of revisions published in 1997. That dimension, *Contextual Factors*, refers to "features of the physical, social, and attitudinal world" (Abrams & Hnath-Chisolm, in press). This dimension seems most related to measures of acceptance and satisfaction as discussed in this chapter. The amplification goals in this dimension are to increase acceptance by eliminating wearer objections, optimize benefit for user-specific situations, use postfitting counseling to facilitate adoption and optimize wearer satisfac-

Table 15–1. WHO Classification System applied to audiology assessment and treatment by amplification. Examples of subjective measurement tools are show by their acronyms. Refer to Chapter 16 for explanation of acronyms and discussion of these and other measurement devices of the same types.

WHO Dimensions (1980/1997)	*Hearing Aid Goals*	*Hearing Aid Intervention Steps*
Impairment Changes in auditory anatomy or function	I. Audibility of soft sounds II. Normal speech comfortably loud III. Loud sounds tolerable IV. Minimize occlusion effect	Hearing Aid Selection/Verification I. Selection A. electroacoustic characteristics B. fit type (BTE, CIC, etc.) C. monaural/binaural/CROS D. circuit options (linear, compression, etc.) E. user options (t-coil, multimic, etc.) F. patient psychoacoustic profiles ■ PAL II. Verification A. 2cc/REM B. functional gain C. Portions of Acceptance checklists
Disability/Activity Limitations in daily activities	I. Improve patient's ability to understand speech II. Improve communication functioning	I. Fitting and Follow-up A. Orientation B. Acclimatization C. Modifications, adjustment, reprogramming II. Validation A. Objective measures of Benefit B. Subjective measures of Benefit ■ APHAB ■ COSI ■ GPHABP ■ HAPI ■ HHIE
Handicap/Participation Stop participating in social activities Cease some or all job functions	I. Expand patient's participation in social situations II. Maintain or enhance ability to perform job functions	I. Quality of Life Measures A. Measures of handicap ■ HHIE ■ CPHI ■ CSOA ■ SAC ■ SOAC II. Needs Contracts ■ COSI
Contextual Factors I. Environmental A. family structure B. work structure C. social attitudes and habits D. architectural characteristics II. Personal A. gender B. age C. visual ability D. dexterity	I. Increase Acceptance rate II. Maximize Benefit for important listening situations III. Facilitate Adoption IV. Optimize wearer Satisfaction	I. Measure predictors of Acceptance to identify and correct reasons for hearing aid rejection *Prediction Questionnaires ■ FSPHAU ■ HANA A. In-office hearing aid quality control measures B. Match hearing aid recommendations with patient's C. home/work/lifestyle ■ HHIA ■ HPI-R D. needs/desires ■ COSI E. functionality (dexterity, vision, etc.)

(continued)

Table 15–1. *(continued)*

WHO Dimensions (1980/1997)	*Hearing Aid Goals*	*Hearing Aid Intervention Steps*
Contextual Factors ***(continued)***		
E. fingertip sensitivity		F. health status
F. coping style		G. stated financial objectives
G. background		II. Use Benefit measures that reflect patient's needs and expectations
H. education		■ APHAB
		■ HAPI
		■ HHIE
		■ GHABP
		III. Provide follow-up services to adjust programming, ensure comfortable fit, continue training, etc.
		III. Measure Satisfaction at specific intervals
		■ HAUQ
		■ SADL
		■ ASHA Service Satisfaction Questionnaire
		■ In-office Satisfaction surveys

tion over time. These goals are validated by measuring predictors of acceptance, using valid measures of benefit (i.e., those that measure things which happen in the patient's daily life), and measuring satisfaction at appropriate intervals according to that patient's progress with amplification.

Self-report measures of benefit and satisfaction are underused by audiologists (Abrams & Hnath-Chisolm, in press; Mueller, 1997; Schow et al, 1993; Schow & Nerbonne, 1982). Table 15–1 is designed to help clinicians conceptualize how different measurement tools correspond to our clinical goals and "fit" into our intervention strategies. It is also helpful to know what is available and convenient. Toward that end, Chapter 16 describes a number of measurement tools that are available and that are applicable to different stages of intervention in the WHO model of Table 15–1.

CONCLUSION

The chapter began by describing a "Holy Grail" of hearing aid intervention, in which the right patient is fitted with the right hearing aid, at the right time, all of the time. Clinical experience and clinical research suggest that we are more likely to fit the right hearing aid to the right patient at the right time if we develop and use:

- Predictive measures of acceptance to anticipate objections and shape expectations
- Patient-specific measures of benefit to facilitate the adoption process and direct postfitting counseling
- Periodic measures of satisfaction identifying ways that the fitting can be improved or that adoption of the fitting can be enhanced.

In-office procedures can be codified to contribute to measures of acceptance and adoption. A number of clinical researchers have developed good tools for measuring benefit and satisfaction. At present, these measures are underused, perhaps because they are not well understood in terms of how and when they are administered and for what purpose(s). This chapter explains how acceptance, benefit, and satisfaction dimensions are different and how they are related. It describes how measurements are conducted in each dimension and provides a model for how and when to use different measurement tools in the hearing aid intervention process. Even if we do not succeed in every fitting, audiologists can come closer to the Holy Grail of hearing aid fitting if we *learn to apply the right measurement tools to the right patients at the right time and understand the reasons for failure at different steps of intervention the rest of the time.*

REVIEW QUESTIONS

1. Two common measures that are used frequently to estimate hearing aid user satisfaction are:
  a. PTA and SRT
  b. Age and Gender
  c. Daily Use and Return Rate
  d. Daily Use and PTA

2. According to definitions in this chapter, Acceptance is:
  a. Opposite of rejection
  b. Process of getting used to amplification
  c. a and b
  d. None of the above

3. Acclimatization is a phenomenon described by Gatehouse that
  a. Describes improvements in aided speech recognition and discrimination over time
  b. Is a consistent measure because it affects all hearing aid users in the same way
  c. Occurs at the sixth week of hearing aid use
  d. Is universally accepted

4. The COSI
  a. Was developed by researchers in Minnesota
  b. Stands for Customer Options and Satisfaction Inventory
  c. Was developed by researchers in Australia
  d. Allows patients and clinicians to identify expectations and measure Acceptance and Adoption
  e. a and b
  f. c and d

5. Benefit is specified in terms of:
  a. Aided thresholds in sound field
  b. Multiples of hearing sensitivity
  c. Difference scores comparing two conditions
  d. Hearing Handicap

6. Objective measures of benefit are based on measures of:
  a. Circuit or algorithm efficacy
  b. Performance on speech recognition tests
  c. Audibility, or insertion gain
  d. All of the above

7. In looking at satisfaction issues with different measurement tools, Kochkin and also Cox and colleagues found that most of the variance was accounted for by how many factors?
  a. 1
  b. 2
  c. 3
  d. 4
  e. none of the above

8. A preliminary study by Sandridge and Newman comparing satisfaction for digital versus nondigital instruments found that:
  a. Satisfaction was higher for digital than nondigital instruments in most conditions
  b. Satisfaction was poor for all instruments with volume controls
  c. Satisfaction was greatest for digital instruments in difficult listening situations
  d. Linear instruments were clearer

9. WHO stands for:
  a. Web for Hearing Organization
  b. World Health Organization
  c. It stands for nothing, it is like NOAH
  d. None of the above

10. In the WHO nomenclature, disability/activity dimension refers to:

a. Health problems in addition to hearing loss
b. Structured exercises developed by physical therapists
c. Person-level function and limitations in a patient's daily activities
d. None of the above

REFERENCES

Abrams, H. B., & Hnath-Chisolm, T. (in press). Outcome measures: The audiologic difference. In H. L. Hosford-Dunn, R. Roeser, & M. Valente (Eds.), *Audiology: Practice management*. New York: Thieme.

Bentler, R. A., & Dittberner, A. B. (1998). Outcome measures: Where should the focus be? *The Hearing Journal, 51*(11), 46–50.

Brooks, D. (1996). The time course of adaptation to hearing aid use. *British Journal of Audiology, 30*, 62.

Brooks, D. N. (1979). Counselling and its effect on hearing aid use. *Scandanavian Audiology, 8*, 101–117.

Brooks, D. N. (1981). Use of post-aural aids by national health service patients. *British Journal of Audiology, 15*, 79–86.

Cox, R. M. (1993). On the evaluation of a new generation of hearing aids. *Journal of Rehabilitation Research and Development, 30*(3), 297–304.

Cox, R. M. (1999). Personality and the subjective assessment of hearing aids. *Journal of the American Academy of Audiology, 10*(1), 1–13.

Cox, R. M., & Alexander, G. C. (1992). Maturation of hearing aid benefit: Objective and subjective measurements. *Ear and Hearing, 13*, 131–141.

Cox, R. M., & Alexander, G. C. (in press). Measuring satisfaction with amplification in daily life: The SADL scale. *Journal of the American Academy of Audiology*.

Dillon, H., Birtles, G., & Lovegrove, R. (1999). Measuring the outcomes of a national rehabilitation program: Normative data for the Client Oriented Scale of Improvement (COSI) and the Hearing Aid User's Questionnaire (HAUQ). *Journal of the American Academy of Audiology, 10*(2), 67–79.

Dillon, H., James, A., & Ginis, J. (1997). Client oriented scale of improvement (COSI) and its relationship to several other measures of benefit and satisfaction provided by hearing aids. *Journal of the American Academy of Audiology, 8*(1), 27–43.

Franks, J. R., & Beckmann, N. J. (1985). Rejection of hearing aids: Attitudes of a geriatric sample. *Ear and Hearing, 6*(3), 161–166.

Gatehouse, S. (1990). Determinants of self-reported disability in older subjects. *Ear and Hearing, 11*(Suppl.), 57S–65S.

Gatehouse, S. (1992). The time course and magnitude of perceptual acclimatization to frequency responses. Evidence from monaural fitting of hearing aids. *Journal of the Acoustical Society of America, 92*, 1258–1268.

Gerber, S. E., & Fisher, L. B. (1979). Prediction of hearing aid users' satisfaction. *Journal of the American Audiology Society, 5*(1), 35–40.

Gordon-Salant, S., Lantz, J., & Fitzgibbons, P. (1994). Age effects on measures of disability. *Ear and Hearing, 15*, 262–265.

Hall, C., & Norton, K. (1997). Clinical management and follow-up time for conventional, CIC and programmable instruments. *The Hearing Review, 4*(4), 36–41.

Hansen, V. (1998). Dealing with the psychological aspects of patient reluctance. *The Hearing Review, 5*(9), 8–14.

Horwitz, A. R., & Turner, C. W. (1997). The time course of hearing aid benefit. *Ear and Hearing, 18*, 1–11.

Hosford-Dunn, H., & Baxter, J. H. (1985). Prediction and validation of hearing aid wearer benefit: Preliminary findings. *Hearing Instruments, 36*(11).

Humes, L. E. (1999). Dimensions of hearing aid outcome. *Journal of the American Academy of Audiology, 10*, 26–39.

Iskowitz, M. (1998, September 7). Psychosocial issues. *Advance Magazine*, pp. 14–15.

Johnson, C. E., & Danhauer, J. (1997). The "Hearing aid effect" revisited: Can we achieve hearing solutions for cosmetically sensitive patients? In S. Kochkin, & K. E. Strom (Eds.), *High Performance Hearing Solutions, Vol I.* Supplement to *The Hearing Review*, pp. 37–44.

Kochkin, S. (1993). MarkeTrak III identifies key factors in determining customer satisfaction. *Hearing Journal, 46*(8), 39–44.

Kochkin, S. (1995). *Subjective measures of satisfaction and benefit: Establishing norms.* (Monograph). Collaborative Marketing Committee (CMC) Meeting (August 2, 1995).

Kochkin, S. (1996). MarkeTrak IV: 10-year trends in the hearing aid market—Has anything changed? *Hearing Journal, 49*(1), 1–6.

Kochkin, S. (1997). Customer satisfaction and subjective benefit with high performance hearing aids. In S. Kochkin & K. E. Strom, (Eds.), *High Performance Hearing Solutions, Vol 2.* Supplement to *The Hearing Review*, pp. 4–10.

Kochkin, S. (1999). MarketTrak V "Baby Boomers" spur growth in potential market, but penetration rate declines. *Hearing Journal, 52*(1), 33–48.

Martin, R. L. (1997). Nuts & bolts: Are you providing quality service? *Hearing Journal, 50*(8), 66.

Maurer, J., & Rupp, R. (1979). *Hearing and aging: Tactics for intervention.* New York: Grune & Stratton.

Morris, W. (Ed.). (1973). *The American Heritage dictionary of the English language.* New York: Houghton Mifflin.

Mueller, G. (1997). Outcome measures: The truth about your hearing aid fittings. *Hearing Journal, 50*(4), 21–32.

Naidoo, S. V., & Hawkins, D. B. (1997). Monaural/binaural preferences: Effect of hearing aid circuitry on speech intelligibility and sound quality. *Journal of the American Academy of Audiology, 8*(3), 188–202.

Noble, W. (1999). Nonuniformities in self-assessed outcomes of hearing aid use. *Journal of the American Academy of Audiology, 19*(2), 104–111.

Oja, G. L., & Schow, R. L. (1984). Hearing aid evaluation based on measures of benefit, use, and satisfaction. *Ear and Hearing, 5*(2), 77–86.

Palmer, C. V., Mueller, H. G., & Moriarty, M. (1999). Profile of aided loudness: A validation procedure. *The Hearing Journal, 52*(6), 34–42.

Purdy, J. K. (1999). Validation of hearing instruments. Part I: Patient questionnaires. *The Hearing Review, 6*(1), 16–22.

Resnick, S. (1998). Breakdown in the fitting process. In H. Tobin (Ed.), *Practical hearing aid selection and fitting.* Washington, DC: Department of Veterans Affairs.

Rupp, R. R. (1982, January). Predicting hearing aid use in maturing populations: The Feasibility Scale. *Hearing Aid Journal,* 10–15.

Rupp, R. R., Maurer, J., & Higgins, J. (1977). The feasibility scale for predicting hearing aid use (FSPHAU) with older individuals. *Journal of the Academy of Rehabilitation Audiology, 10*(1), 81–104.

Sandridge, S. A., & Newman, C. W. (1998, November). *Subjective satisfaction ratings for digital signal processing hearing aids.* Paper presented at the American Speech-Language-Hearing Association Annual Convention, San Antonio, TX.

Saunders, G. H., & Cienkowski, K. M. (1997). Acclimatization to hearing aids. *Ear and Hearing, 18*(2), 129–146.

Schow, R., Balsara, N., Smedley, T., & Whitcomb, C. (1993). Aural rehabilitation by ASHA audiologists: 1980–1990. *American Journal of Audiology, 3,* 28–38.

Schow, R. L., & Nerbonne, M. A. (1982). Communication screening profile: Use with elderly clients. *Ear and Hearing, 3*(3), 135–143.

Singer, J., Healey, J., & Preece, J. (1997). Hearing Instruments: A psychologic and behavioral perspective. In S. Kochkin, & K. E. Strom (Eds). *High Performance Hearing Solutions, Vol I.* Supplement to *The Hearing Review,* pp. 23–27.

Smedley, T. C. (1990). Self-assessed satisfaction levels in elderly hearing aid, eyeglass, and denture wearers. *Ear and Hearing, 11*(5), 41–47.

Strom, K. E. (1998). Rendezvous wrestles with the opportunities of new technology. *The Hearing Review, 5*(10), 46–48.

Surr, R. K., Schuchman, G. I., & Montgomery, A. A. (1978). Factors influencing use of hearing aids. *Archives of Otolaryngology, 104,* 732–736.

Traynor, R. M., & Buckles, K. M. (1997). Personality typing: Audiology's new crystal ball. In S. Kochkin, & K.E. Strom (Eds). *High Performance Hearing Solutions, Vol I.* Supplement to *The Hearing Review,* pp. 28–31.

Walden, B., Demorest, M., & Hepler, E. (1984). Self-report approach to assessing benefit derived from amplification. *Journal of Speech and Hearing Research, 27,* 49–56.

World Health Organization. (1980). *International classification of impairments, disabilities and handicaps—A manual of classification relating to the consequences of disease.* Geneva: Author.

World Health Organization. (1997). *Towards a common language for functioning and disablement: ICIDH-2 Betadraft for field trials.* Geneva: Author.

Yung, E. W., & Buckles, K. M. (1995). Discrimination of multichannel-compressed speech in noise: Long-term learning in hearing-impaired subjects. *Ear and Hearing, 16,* 417–427.

CHAPTER 16

Inventories of Self-Assessment Measurements of Hearing Aid Outcome

JUDY L. HUCH, M.S.
HOLLY HOSFORD-DUNN, PH.D.

OUTLINE

INTRODUCTION

This chapter reads like a books of lists. Its corpus is an inventory and commentary on available structured patient questionnaires that are designed to measure and validate hearing aid outcomes using a variety of separate and possibly related factors. The inventory is not exhaustive, but its length remains impressive. Readers may ask themselves why there are so many instruments and which one is best. The respective answers are:

- There are many instruments because there are a number of independent factors that influence different dimensions of hearing aid outcome in complex ways. As Humes (1999, p. 29) commented, "The development of separate measures of performance, benefit, satisfaction, and use reflect the clinical and research communities' belief that these are, in fact, independent aspects of outcome that must be measured separately."
- Until we understand enough about the multidimensionality of hearing aid outcome factors to develop a "complete" hearing aid outcome instrument, the "best" tool depends on what factor we want to measure.

The following scales and profiles are separated into four overlapping groups, according to application:

- I: Success Predictors
- II: Handicap Profiles
- III: Benefit Scales
- IV: Satisfaction Inventories

Benefit scales (Group III) are designed for pre- and postintervention administration, with measured difference indicating degree of aided improvement. Items in Group II can also be used after treatment intervention, but their original intent was to profile pretreatment handicap in order to determine appropriate intervention strategies. The Hearing Handicap Inventory for the Elderly (HHIE) is a good example of this. The original intent was to determine the emotional and social effects of a hearing loss on individuals, but many clinicians use it as a pre- and post-intervention tool to measure hearing aid benefit. Group IV scales measure satisfaction, which encompasses factors from the other three groups and also surveys that ask about the office environment directly. The latter factor is sometimes overlooked when clinicians evaluate satisfaction.

GROUP I: SUCCESS PREDICTORS

Feasibility Scale for Predicting Hearing Aid Use: FSPHAU

Development

In the 1970s, Rupp designed this scale for predicting success with hearing aid use (Rupp, 1982). The FSPHAU is shown in Table 16–1.

Description

The FSPHAU is designed to estimate or predict the probability of an older person with hearing impairment becoming a successful hearing aid user. The FSPHAU analyzes 11 factors:

1. **Motivation:** Refers to how the patient came to the professional's office. Did the patient self-refer for an acknowledged communication problem, or was the appointment instigated by friends or family who report a problem that the patient does not perceive? The individual's self-perceived listening needs are important to understand his or her motivation for obtaining hearing aids. Coming in for help on one's own, with a positive attitude, predicts future success with amplification.
2. **Self-evaluation:** Refers to how the patients view their receptive listening abilities, compared to the audiological information. Patients who report communication problems that agree with their audiologic data are reacting realistically to the handicapping effects of their hearing losses (Rupp, 1982). Individuals who report no communication difficulty in the presence of audiometric loss are in denial that hearing problems exist. In the FSPHAU, success is predicted based on the patient's perception of handicap. Congruence of self-evaluation and audiologic assessment predicts greater hearing aid success.
3. **Determination of cause:** Refers to how the person assigns fault for reduced listening ability. Some individuals report, "I keep asking people to repeat themselves," while others state, "I would understand people if they would just quit mumbling." Individuals who admit that the communication problems are theirs are more likely to succeed with hearing aids.
4. **Magnitude of loss:** Rupp suggests using aided and unaided measure of spondee threshold in the better ear and soundfield word recognition scores in quiet and noise. The higher the degree of improvement in these measurements, the more predictive of success.
5. **Commentary:** Examines the patient's informal comments relating to cosmetics, type of aid, manipulation, feedback, and so forth. Positive or negative comments are scored to determine the individual's attitude toward amplification on this factor.
6. **Audiologic estimates:** Refers to the clinician's judgment of the patient's general state of alertness, interaction, adaptabili-

Table 16–1. The Feasibility Scale for Predicting Hearing Aid Use (FSPHAU). (From "Predicting Hearing Aid Use in Maturing Populations: the Feasibility Scale," by R. R. Rupp, 1983, *Hearing Aid Journal, 13*, p. 12 Copyright 1983 by The Hearing Aid Journal. Reprinted with permission.)

1. Motivation/Referral	5. Completely on own behalf		
	4. Most on own behalf		
	3. Generally on own behalf		
	2. Half self, half others		
	1. Little self, mostly others		
	0. Totally at urging of others		
2. Self Assessment	5. Complete agreement		
	4. Strong agreement		
	3. General agreement		
	2. Some agreement		
	1. Little agreement		
	0. No agreement		
3. Verbalization as to "fault" of communicative difficulties	5. Clearly created by hearing loss		
	4. Usually created by loss		
	3. Created by loss and others		
	2. Created by environments and others		
	1. Created mostly by others		
	0. Others are totally at fault		
4. Magnitude of loss and results of amplification*		Understanding	
		in quiet at ___dB HTL	in noise at ___dBHTL
	ST shift		
	5. 30 + db	90%	70%
	4. 25	80-88%	60-68%
	3. 20	70-78%	50-58%
	2. 15	60-68%	40-48%
	1. 10	50-58%	30-38%
	0. 5	48%	28%
5. Informal verbalizations during hearing aid evaluation re: quality of sound, mold, size, weight, look	5. Completely positive		
	4. Generally positive		
	3. Somewhat positive		
	2. Guarded		
	1. Generally negative		
	0. Completely negative		
6. Flexibility and Adaptability:	5. 90th percentile		
A. Questionnaire and observation	4. 70		
B. Raven's Progressive Matrices	3. 50		
C. Face/Hand Sensory Test	2. 25		
	1. 10		
	0. 5-1		
7. Age	5. 65-69		
	4. 70-74		
	3. 75-79		
	2. 80-84		
	1. 85-89		
	0. 90+		

8. Manual/Hand Dexterity	5. Superior 4. Adequate 3. Slow but steady 2. Slow and shaky 1. "Arthritic"
9. Visual Ability (w/glasses)	5. Very good, no problems 4. Corrected, adequate 3. Adequate but safeguarded 2. Limited visibility 1. Very limited 0. Blind
10. Financial Resources	5. Unlimited resources 4. Generally unrestricted 3. Adequate 2. Adequate but close 1. Dipping into savings 0. Poverty level, on assistance
11. Significant Other Person	5. Always available 4. Often available 3. Sometimes available 2. Occasionally available 1. Seldom available 0. Never available

*Alternate scoring scheme for Factor 4 in cases where the ST shift was minimal due to loss in high frequencies only

Average threshold shift at 2 KHz and 3 KHz	5. 25+ dB	2. 11-15 dB
	4. 21-25 dB	1. 6-10 dB
	3. 16-24 dB	0. 0-5 dB

ty, and flexibility during the consultation. Is the individual willing or capable of modifying his or her behavior for the hearing aid? Rupp poses eight questions for the clinician to rate this estimation. Examples of the questions are: What kind of general orientation to the world does the client present? Is he or she generally positive in attitude toward life?

7. **Age:** Patient's age in the FSPHAU is a measure of whether the patient has waited too long for amplification. When Rupp (1982) developed the FSPHAU, he stated adjustment to amplification is poorer when the patient's age is beyond 60 or 70 years.
8. **Manual dexterity:** Judged by the clinician and used to decide hearing aid fit type, method of volume control adjustment, and battery size. Good manual dexterity predicts success on the FSPHAU.
9. **Visual capability:** Same as manual dexterity. The better the vision, the better success predictor on FSPHAU.
10. **Financial resources:** Resources may limit the type or sophistication of prescribed amplification. Limitations reduce FSPHAU predictions of success. A clinician may have some resources for the family to find help.
11. **Availability of a significant support person:** An important success predictor throughout all stages of aural rehabilitation. Communication strategy and appointment participation help the user become more successful with the hearing aid.

Application

This questionnaire is given to patients at the initial appointment (using stock hearing aid amplification) or at the time of the fitting (using custom amplification). The questionnaire is completed by the hearing aid provider.

Interpretation and Scoring

All 11 factors are scored on a scale of 1 through 5, where 5 is a "High" rating and 1 a "Low" rating for success. The factors are weighted according to prognostic importance, with Motivation receiving strongest weightings (20), and Determination or Cause, Magnitude of Loss, Commentary, and Visual Ability weighted lowest (5). Weighted values of all factors are summed and converted to a single percentage that is used to calculate success.

"Positive" (76% to 100%) is an ideal hearing aid candidate, "Equivocal" (61% to 75%) is a probable candidate, "Limited" (41% to 60%) is a doubtful candidate, and "Very Limited" (below 41%) is a noncandidate. Scoring, weighting, and success categories are shown on the form in Table 16–2.

Advantages and Disadvantages

Scoring the FSPHAU adds a few minutes to the evaluation or fitting appointment, but the process helps focus on factors that are helpful in counseling patients and planning intervention strategies. Hosford-Dunn and Baxter (1985), for example, found that Factors 1 (Motivation) and 4C (% discrimination in noise) were significant predictors of patient satisfaction with amplification after 3 months of use.

The FSPHAU has not been widely adopted for clinical use. The original format may not conform to some contemporary clinical protocols. Since this profile was developed in the 1970s, real ear measures have replaced sound field measures of functional gain in many clinics, and the validity of comparing aided versus unaided speech tests has been questioned (Thornton & Raffin, 1978). In Factor 4, for example, "Extent of Loss and Magnitude of Understanding Difficulties," the author outlined the process for function gain in a variety of situations and tests. It is not practical to do these tests before a fitting with either a stock aid or the patient's own amplification. Binaural testing is not specified in the test protocol, only "in the better ear" (Rupp, 1982).

A revised FSPHAU was proposed in 1988 by Chermak and Miller in which the magnitude of loss factor was deleted. The remaining factors were weighted the same as in the original. The authors found that the modified FSPHAU did not predict patient success with amplification.

Hearing Aid Needs Assessment: HANA

Development

In 1999, Schum developed the HANA as part of a self-report battery that examines the relationship between perceived communication needs/expectations and benefit achieved with new hearing aids. It is a companion scale to the Hearing Aid Performance Inventory (HAPI) and the shortened HAPI (described in section III). The HANA was administered to an unselected group of 82 patients. The HAPI was then administered after the hearing aid fittings to provide information on the relationship between expectations and results for the hearing aid fitting process (Schum, 1992).

Description

The HANA consists of 11 situational questions (Table 16–3) from the HAPI. The questions are grouped into four categories: Noise, Quiet, No Visual Cues, and Non Speech. Patients assign three ratings to each question that characterizes their unaided listening needs and hearing aid expectations. Patients who are previous hearing aid users answer the questions from their aided perspective. The ratings for the 11 situations are:

1. How often are you in this type of situation (hardly ever, occasionally, frequently)?
2. How much listening trouble do you have in situations like this one (very little, some, very much)?
3. How much help do you expect the hearing aid to provide (very little, some, very much)?

Table 16–2. Scoring FSPHAU. (From "Predicting Hearing Aid Use in Maturing Populations: the Feasibility Scale," by R. R. Rupp, 1983, *Hearing Aid Journal,* 13, p. 14 Copyright 1983 by The Hearing Aid Journal. Reprinted with permission.)

Prognostic Factors/Description (continuum, high to low)	*Assessment (5— high; 0—low)*	*Weight*	*Weighted Score Possible/ Actual*	
1. Motivation and referral (self...family)	5 4 3 2 1 0	X 4	(20)_____	1.
2. Self-assessment of listening difficulties (self…family)	5 4 3 2 1 0	X 2	(10)_____	2.
3. Verbalization as to "fault" of communication difficulties (self causes…projection)	5 4 3 2 1 0	X 1	(5)_____	3.
4. Magnitude of loss: HA results				4.
A. Shift in spondaic threshold:____	5 4 3 2 1 0	X 1	(5)_____	
B. Discrimination in quiet ____% at ____dB HTL	5 4 3 2 1 0	X 1	(5)_____	
C. Discrimination in noise: ____% at ____dB HTL	5 4 3 2 1 0	X 1	(5)_____	
5. Informal verbalizations during HAE re: quality of sound, mold, size (acceptable…awful)	5 4 3 2 1 0	X 1	(5)_____	5.
5. Flexibility and adaptability versus senility (relates outwardly…self)	5 4 3 2 1 0	X 1	(10)_____	6.
7. Age: 95 90 85 80 75 70 65 (0 0 1 2 3 4 5)	5 4 3 2 1 0	X 1.5	(7.5)_____	7.
8. Manual hand, finger dexterity, and general	5 4 3 2 1 0	X 1.5	(7.5)_____	8.
9. Visual ability (adequate with glasses...limited)	5 4 3 2 1 0	X 1	(5)_____	9.
10. Financial resources (adequate...very limited)	5 4 3 2 1 0	X 1.5	(7.5)_____	10.
11. Significant other person to assist individual (available…none)	5 4 3 2 1 0	X 1.5	(7.5)_____	11.
12. Other factors, please cite.	?	?	?	12.

Client_______________	FSPHAU: Very Limited	0 to 40%	TOTAL SCORE_____
Age_______________	Limited	41 to 60%	
Date_______________	Equivocal	61 to 60 %	
Audiologist_______________	Positive	76 to 100%	

Application

The HANA is intended for use at the evaluation appointment or when amplification is selected. The patient rates the 11 situations prior to hearing aid fitting.

The follow-up with the HAPI should be 2 to 3 months after fitting to give ample time for the patient to acclimatize to amplification. The HANA results are then compared to the HAPI to determine if prefit expectations match postfit benefit.

Interpretation and Scoring

The situations were scored on a 3-point system, "Hardly Ever" or "Very Little" equal to 1

Table 16–3. Hearing Aid Needs Assessment Questions. (From "Perceived Hearing Aid Benefit in Relation to Perceived Need," by D. J. Schum, 1999, *Journal of the American Academy of Audiology, 3.* Copyright 1999 by American Academy of Audiology. Reprinted with permission.

Question	***Categories***
1. Your are one of only a few customers inside your bank and are talking with a teller.	Quiet
2. You are at home reading the paper. Two family members are in another room talking quietly, and you want to listen in on their conversation.	No Visual Cues
3. You are in a quiet conversation with your family doctor in an examination room.	Quiet
4. You are driving your car with the windows down and are carrying on a conversation with others riding with you.	Noise
5. You are home in face-to-face conversation with one member of your family.	Quiet
6. You are at church listening to a sermon and sitting in the back pew.	No Visual Cues
7. You are at a large, noisy party and are engaged in conversation with one other person.	Noise
8. You are in your backyard gardening. Your neighbor is using a noisy power lawnmower and yells something to you.	Noise
9. Someone is trying to tell you something in a small quiet room while you have your back turned.	No Visual Cues
10. You are starting to cross a busy street, and a car horn sounds a warning.	Nonspeech
11. You are at home alone listening to your stereo system (instrumental music).	Nonspeech

point and "Frequently" or "Very Much" corresponding to 3 points. The higher the score, the more difficulty the patient is reporting. Each category (Quiet, No Visual Cues, etc.) is scored separately.

The scores from the HAPI are inverted to compare them to the HANA, as seen in Figure 16–1. Direct comparisons allow the clinician to evaluate the patient's expectations versus perceived benefit.

Schum (1999) found that most previous users' expectations are more realistic in noisy situations than those of new users. Both groups expected less benefit from amplification in noise than in quieter environments. The HANA can be used as a tool to identify unrealistic user expectations before they experience the situations. For example, if a new user answered the question, "You are driving your car with the windows down and are carrying on a conversation with others riding with you" with the statement "I expect the hearing aids to help very much," then counseling on signal to noise ratios in automobiles should be addressed immediately.

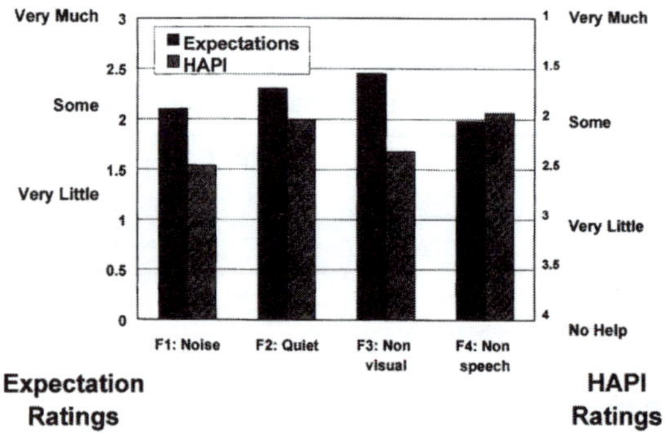

Figure 16–1. Average ratings for the HANA categories for the frequency of similar situations section. (Data from "Perceived Hearing Aid Benefit in Relation to Perceived Needs" by D. J. Schum, 1999, *Journal of the American Academy of Audiology, 3*, Figure 2. Copyright 1999 by American Academy of Audiology. Reprinted with permission.)

Advantages and Disadvantages

Schum (1999) reported that the HANA is a useful tool to evaluate patient expectations of hearing aid benefit. It is likely to be a reliable measure, because its items are derived from the HAPI, which has already been shown to be reliable (Walden, Demorest, & Helper, 1982). Nonetheless, the HANA had been tested only once at the time of writing (1999).

GROUP II: HANDICAP PROFILES

Communication Profile for the Hearing Impaired: CPHI

Development

The CPHI provides a systematic and comprehensive assessment of a broad range of communication problems (Erdman & Demorest, 1986). It was initially standardized on active duty service members at Walter Reed Army Medical Center. Later normative studies included older and wider ranges of clinical populations (Erdman et al., 1995; Garstecki & Erler, 1996; Hyde, Malizia, Riko, & Storms, 1992; Hyde, Malizia, Riko, & Storms, 1996).

The initial item pool was written to be relevant for the general population of individuals with hearing impairment. Two different but equivalent versions of the CPHI allow administration of a short (one form) or long (two forms) profile without the memory factor confounding results. The items, scales, and subscales of the CPHI have undergone rigorous statistical analyses to ensure their validity and reliability (Demorest & Erdman, 1987).

Description

The CPHI contains 145 items in five areas. For purposes of analysis, the areas are internally divided into 22 "scales." The five areas are described as follows:

The *Communication Performance Scales* assess ability to give and receive information or carry on a conversation. The authors recognize that individual communication in daily life is influenced by many factors depending on the patient's situations, expectations, and priorities. For this reason, the 18 items are designed to cover various types of situations and listening conditions. In contrast to other profiles developed around the same time (e.g., The Hearing Performance Inventory, HPI), the scales are not designed to provide detailed or specific information of the situation, listener, or speaker.

Through the development of *Communication Performance*, another area emerged. Communication Importance examines communication problems in different situations. The handicapping effects of a hearing loss may be less severe than if the same degree of difficulty is discovered in situations where communication is determined to be very important or essential (Demorest & Erdman, 1986). The 18 items of the Communication Performance scale have two response scales. The responses relating to Importance range from "Not Important" (1) to "Essential" (5).

The *Communication Environment Scales*, consisting of 31 items, assess the external environmental factors, strategies, and emotional adjustments the patient experiences in everyday life. Because the communication environment is the environment perceived by the patient, the possibility exists that the patient may incorrectly blame the environment and other persons for creating communication problems.

Communication Strategies Scales assess the person's verbal and nonverbal behaviors in 25 different situations. Behaviors are viewed as adaptive or maladaptive depending on their effects on communication. Maladaptive behavior items describe avoidance and other negative behaviors, such as ignoring others, dominating conversations, avoiding social interaction (Garstecki & Erler, 1996).

Personal Adjustment is composed of eight subscales, which assess the patient's acceptance of and adjustment to hearing loss and reaction to related communication problems. The subscales are as follows:

- Self-Acceptance: negative feelings toward self as a direct consequence of hearing loss
- Acceptance of Loss: the patient's ability to admit hearing impairment
- Anger: frustration from hearing loss and inability to communicate effectively
- Displacement of Responsibility: determines whether the patient places blame externally for communication difficulties
- Exaggeration of Responsibility: degree to which the patient blames external factors
- Discouragement: general feelings of discouragement or depression associated with communication difficulty or hearing loss
- Stress: the patient's reported discomfort, tension, nervousness, or anxiety in reaction to communication difficulties
- Withdrawal: the extent to which the patient removes himself/herself from communication situations or experiences feelings of isolation

The Denial scale is equivalent to the Problem Awareness scale. Its purpose is to identify patients' responses in the Personal Adjustment section that are inordinately positive given that they have a hearing loss. The items were designed to have the majority of the hearing impaired population agree with the statements. Most of the time these questions are qualified by the word "sometimes." The Denial section is not set as a main area, but intertwined in the Personal Adjustment section and given a separate score. The Denial scale reliability is reported to be very good (Demorest & Erdman, 1987).

Application

The CPHI is administered by the paper and pencil method before aural rehabilitation begins to define the patient's hearing profile and help plan appropriate intervention. The questionnaire generally takes less than 40 minutes to complete (Demorest & Erdman, 1987). The response scales range from 1 to 5 on a frequency ("almost never" to "almost always") or agree-disagree continuum.

Interpretation and Scoring

Because there are 25 individual scores on the CPHI, an automated database and scoring system are recommended. Responses can be entered in the computer by the clinician and a profile generated and printed within 2 minutes. Hand scoring is not recommended due to the number of items and the fact that some questions are reversed. Demorest and Erdman (1990) developed a database system and automated scoring system, which is available for a nominal fee.[1]

When interpreting the scores, a low score may suggest problems in a given area. Ineffective use of verbal communication strategies or a variable (ambient noise), for example, could contribute to communication difficulties. A high score that reflects effective communication may be due to appropriate use of compensatory strategies or indicate that the conditions described are not contributing to communication difficulty.

Advantages and Disadvantages

The scales give a wide range of clinical data that may be useful in creating an intervention plan. Perhaps the biggest advantage of the CPHI is that it is a demonstrably reliable and valid method to profile communication ability of patients with hearing loss.

The length of the CPHI and the cost of purchasing a database for scoring may discourage many offices from using this profile. Although there are norms for military and older populations, it is advisable to develop local norms where individual clients can be more appropriately compared (Erdman & Demorest, 1990). This may be too great a task for most offices to take on.

[1]Inquiries can be sent to CPHI Services, PO Box 444, Simpsonville, MD 21150-0444 or call/write the Hearing Rehabilitation Laboratory (HRL), Department of Psychology, University of Maryland Baltimore County, 1000 Hilltop Circle, Baltimore, MD 21250; (410) 455-3447.

Communication Scale for Older Adults: CSOA

Development

The CSOA is a self-assessment scale that evaluates the communication strategies and attitudes of independent, older patients (Kaplan, Bally, Brant, Busacco, & Pray, 1997). It was normed on 135 subjects with a mean age of 75 (60–88 years).

CSOA items were designed to "evaluate positive and negative communication strategies; perceived attitudes and behaviors of family, friends, and others; and interpersonal and emotional factors related to communication" (Kaplan et al., 1997, p. 204). The CSOA is based on the Hearing Performance Inventory (HPI) and the Communication Profile for the Hearing Impaired (CPHI), both described in this chapter. The CSOA has good internal consistency and high test-retest reliability (Kaplan et al., 1997).

Description

CSOA has two scales: Communication Strategies (41 items) and Communication Attitudes (31 items). The Communication Strategies scale measures actual or perceived communication breakdowns and strategies pertaining to each situation. The strategies may be positive or negative. An example of a positive strategy on this scale is when an individual with hearing loss asks someone to repeat a part of a sentence that he or she missed. Negative strategies include bluffing or avoidance behaviors on the part of the person with hearing loss.

The Communication Attitudes scale evaluates the patient's attitude toward his or her hearing loss and self perceptions as a hearing impaired individual. It is also touches on other people's perceptions of the hearing loss. Positive and negative perceptions of self and others are questioned.

Two response formats are available, a 3-point item response and a 5-point item response. The 3-point scale should be used when a complex format is too difficult for older adults who frequently only use the endpoints of scale responses (Kaplan, Feeley, & Brown, 1978). The five-point scale is designed for those older adults who desire more choices (Appendix 16A). On the 3-point scale, the responses are (1) Almost Always, (2) Sometimes, (3) Never. If the patient answers "never," he or she receives a score of 3. The higher the score, the more communication difficulty. Some items are answered in reverse, and "Almost Always" is 3.

The two scales are administered by the paper-and-pencil method and can be used independently of each other. The scores are computed separately by using the scale mean, and items that are not answered are not used in the mean score.

Application

The CSOA is used to help set up intervention. It is administered before and after treatment (which may or may not include amplification) to compare the change in communication. The initial COSA is given at the initial appointment and the final at 3 to 6 months postintervention. Aural rehabilitation and communication intervention can be used in situations of normal to mild hearing losses.

Interpretation and Scoring

An individual score on the Communication Strategies scale that exceeds 0.10 indicates benefit on the 3-point scale, and 0.04 or greater indicates benefit on the 5-point scale (Kaplan et al., 1997). For the Communication Attitude scale, a difference of 0.10 on the 3-point scale and of 0.11 on the 5-point indicates benefit (Kaplan et al., 1997).

One recommendation made in the original study is to compare scale results with the patient's case history and audiological testing results. A low score on the attitude scale with reported difficulty in the case history and aidable hearing loss could indicate denial of the hearing loss.

Advantages & Disadvantages

The ability to use a 3- or 5-point response is good when the clinician knows when a patient needs things a bit simpler. Another advantage of this scale is helping with planning intervention. The CSOA can be a tool to help the clinician customize intervention and decide whether amplification should be part of the rehabilitation process. This scale has not had other clinicians conduct test-retest studies on it and can be quite lengthy.

Denver Scales

The following four scales originated from the Denver Scale of Communication Function (Alpiner, Chervett, Glascoe, Mez, & Olsen, 1974) for purposes of estimating hearing handicap and effects of intervention on adults of different ages, abilities, and living situations.

Denver Scale of Communication Function: DSCF

The DSCF is a 25-item scale that queries adults with hearing impairment on the impact of hearing loss in a variety of experiential areas. The 25 statements are divided into four categories: family, self, social-vocational, general communication experience. The response scale is a seven-level semantic difference continuum from "agree" (1) to "disagree" (7). It is recommended that patients complete the scale with a 15-minute time limit to encourage first-impression responses.

Schow and Nerbonne (1980) quantified the scores of the DSSF and called it the Quantified Denver Scale (QDS). The scores are graphically represented on a profile form, with no handicap ranging from 0 to 15%, slight hearing handicap scores in the 16 to 30% range, and mild-moderate handicap scores 31% or greater. Degree of handicap increased with degree of hearing impairment based on puretone averages.

Denver Scale of Communication Function for Senior Citizens: DSCF-SC

This scale was one of the first designed for confined elderly patients. Zarnoch & Alpiner (1977) modified the original DSCF to allow older individuals to report their communication performance prior to and following rehabilitative intervention.

This scale is administered interview style because self-scoring scales are not always feasible with older confined persons. The questionnaire consists of seven key questions that cover the following topics:

- family
- emotions
- other persons
- general communication
- self-concept
- group situations
- rehabilitation.

Each question is followed by one "Probe Effect" and one "Exploration Effect" question, which examine the question further. The Probe Effect question isolates specific problem situations. The Exploration Effect determines how applicable the general question is to the individual. This area of the scale serves to eliminate questions that are irrelevant to the patient and therefore unnecessary in establishing intervention goals. The responses are "yes" or "no, " scored with pluses and minuses. A form for scoring is helpful when interpreting and comparing pre- and postintervention. This scale does not have scoring norms or group comparisons, but postintervention improvement is manifest by more plusses and fewer minuses than in the preintervention interview.

Denver Scale of Communication Function—Modified: DSCF-M

The modified version of the DSCF also was designed for use with older individuals living in retirement homes (Kaplan et al., 1978). DSCF was modified for this population, as follows:

- All items concerned with vocation were removed.
- The family category was changed to "peer and family attitudes" because many older people do not live with their families.
- The "self" and "socialization" categories were combined into one "socialization" category aimed at probing degrees and feelings of participation in social activities.
- A new category was added for "specific difficult listening situations."

In addition to these changes, an interview technique is used.

The DSCF-M consists of 34 items that are rated on a five-point "agree" to "disagree" continuum instead of the seven-point scale in the original. Each of the five points is defined for the patient on the form.

Advantages and Disadvantages

These scales offer different versions to cover a wide variety of populations. The scales can be given in either the interview format or the paper-and-pencil method according to clinician preference. When a clinician is setting up intervention, these scales help develop counseling strategies.

Except for the DSCF-M, these scales do not provide norms or group comparisons. Instead, they focus on the individual to provide an analysis of his or her communication performance. The DSCF-M is reliable when using group data but individual test-retest reliability is highly variable. For that reason, Kaplan et al. (1978) cautioned against using the scale as a pre- or postintervention evaluation tool.

Hearing Handicap Inventory for the Elderly: HHIE

Development

The HHIE was published by Ventry and Weinstein in 1982. The inventory assesses the perceived effects of hearing impairment on the emotional and social adjustment of elderly patients. Although originally the HHIE was designed to assess hearing impairment, it also is a reliable tool for measuring benefit (Newman & Weinstein, 1988). The HHIE has two areas interwoven throughout the profile, the Emotional Scale and the Social Scale. The Emotional Scale estimates the patient's attitudes and emotional responses to his or her hearing loss. The Social Scale measures the perceived effects of hearing loss in a variety of social situations.

Prototype testing was performed on 42 subjects with hearing loss who were over the age of 65. Internal consistency of the total scale was .82; reliability was .93 on the emotional subsection and .83 on the social/situational section (Ventry & Weinstein, 1982). A sensitivity section in the prototype was not included in the final inventory because of poor reliability (.24). The authors selected a three-point answering scale to simplify the response format for elderly patients.

The items used for the final version were selected on the basis of their strong correlation with pure-tone hearing sensitivity. The HHIE was administered to 100 subjects 65 years and older who had sensorineural hearing loss and no evidence of neurological or psychological problems. Results showed large standard deviations in the total score and both subscales, consistent with the prediction that patients respond differently to their hearing losses (Ventry & Weinstein, 1982). Weinstein, Spitzer, and Ventry (1986) subsequently evaluated reliability and found high test-retest correlations in the scores. They concluded that the HHIE is a highly reliable index of self-perceived hearing handicap in the elderly.

The HHIE-S (Appendix 16B) is a 10-item version, derived from the HHIE, that serves as a screening tool for profiling emotional and social aspects of hearing handicap. A companion inventory to the HHIE, called the HHIE-SP, is the spouse's version. It is identical to the HHIE except for small working changes in the questions (e.g., "your spouse" instead of "you"). The HHIE-SP supports using the spouse's judgments as an indicator of outcome of future rehabilitative intervention (Newman & Weinstein, 1988).

Description

The HHIE is composed of 25 questions in two subscales, Social (S) and Emotional (E) (Appendix 16C). All questions are labeled according to the scale to which they pertain. Administration time in the initial study was approximately 10 minutes (Ventry & Weinstein, 1982).

There is a three-point scale response system, "yes" (4 points), "sometimes" (2 points), "no"/not applicable (0 points). The maximum score is 100, and the minimum is 0.

Application

Self-perceived hearing handicap following a program of rehabilitation can be scrutinized using the interview format in the initial administration. Newman and Weinstein (1989) recommended that the HHIE be administered initially in a face-to-face interview format to reduce the "not applicable" answers.

If the HHIE is used as a benefit scale, the second application can be completed with the paper-and-pencil method by the patient. When the follow-up survey is given by paper and pencil, the results vary more than if it is given by face to face (Weinstein et al., 1986). If given face to face, there is a 95% confidence interval for detecting a change of 10 points, as opposed to 36 points from the paper-and-pencil administration.

Interpretation and Scoring

The higher the score, the greater the perceived hearing handicap. A "yes" response receives 4 points, "sometimes" receives 2 points, and "no" receives 0 points. Scores for the total scale range from 0 (no perceived handicap) to 100 (significant perceived hearing handicap) (Newman & Weinstein, 1989). A percentage change of 18% or greater is a significant change for each subscale when used as a benefit scale. One study reported a significant reduction in perceived emotional and social effects of hearing impairment following 1 year of hearing aid use (Newman & Weinstein, 1988).

Advantages and Disadvantages

This scale is easy for elderly patients to complete. It is straightforward to score and interpret. In addition, its reliability and validity are well documented for elderly persons with hearing loss. The screening version is a quick way to evaluate a patient's perceived hearing handicap. For these reasons, the HHIE and its variants have been widely used in the profession (Dancer & Gener, 1999).

Hearing Handicap Inventory for Adults: HHIA

Similar to the HHIE, the HHIA (Newman, Weinstein, Jacobson, & Hug, 1990) is a 25-item self-assessment scale composed of emotional and social/situation subscales that is scored in the same manner as the HHIE. This inventory is used to measure hearing handicap, as well as hearing aid benefit.

The HHIA was developed and normed on patients under the age of 65. Two questions differ from the HHIE, one social and one emotional. They focus on the occupational effects of hearing loss. A third item relates to leisure time activities. Table 16–4 shows the HHIE items that were omitted from the HHIA and the new items that were included. The HHIA has high internal reliability and excellent test-retest reliability (Newman, Weinstein, Jacobson, & Hug, 1991).

Hearing Handicap Scale: HHS

Development

The Hearing Handicap Scale, developed in 1964, was the first self-report questionnaire to assess hearing handicap (High, Fairbanks, and Glorig, 1964). Handicap in the HHS is defined as "any disadvantage in the activities

Table 16–4. Items omitted from HHIE and substituted in HHIA (Newman, et al, 1990).

HHIE	*HHIA*
E. Does a hearing problem cause you to feel "stupid" or "dumb?"	E. Does a hearing problem cause you to feel frustrated when talking to coworkers, clients, or customer?
S. Do you have difficulty hearing when someone speaks in a whisper?	S. Does a hearing problem cause you difficulty in the movies or theater?
S. Does a hearing problem cause you to attend religious services less often than you would like?	S. Does a hearing problem cause you difficulty hearing/understanding coworkers, clients, or customers?

of everyday living which derives from hearing impairment" (High et al., p. 215). In the original study, 40 items were given to 50 adults with hearing impairment along with a comprehensive audiological exam. The HHS is designed to estimate the effects of hearing loss on communication in various environments.

Description

The HHS has 40 questions on two equivalent forms (A and B) that have 20 questions each. The forms are used in pre- and post-testing. There are four content areas: *Speech Perception, Localization, Telephone Communication,* and *Noise Situations.* The 5-point responses range from "Almost Always," "Usually," "Sometimes," "Rarely," to "Almost Never."

Application

The HHS is given in a paper-and-pencil format at the initial appointment. The second form is given after intervention if it is used as a benefit scale.

Interpretation and Scoring

Schow and Tannahill (1977) suggested a categorical method for interpreting HHS results. Scores of 0 to 20% indicate no hearing handicap, 21 to 40% indicate a slight handicap, 41 to 70% indicate a mild-moderate hearing handicap, and 71 to 100% indicate severe handicap.

Advantages and Disadvantages

The two forms allow pre- and postrehabilitation assessment and can be used as a benefit scale as well (Schow & Tannahill, 1977). The HHS does not assess social or psychological impact of hearing loss, however.

Hearing Measurement Scale: HMS

Development

The Hearing Measurement Scale (HMS) was published in 1970. It assesses the degree of hearing handicap in patients with noise-induced hearing loss and relates handicap to audiological data (Nobel & Atherley, 1970). Four generations of the scale were tested on men engaged in trades that were noisy enough to cause chronic acoustic trauma.

The final version has 42 items and two identical forms, one for the subject (form A), the other for the subject's nearest relative (form B). Form B is used to check the reliability of the subjects' statements (Noble & Atherley, 1970).

Description

The HMS is a 42-item questionnaire of four sections (Table 16–5) divided into seven subsections:

Table 16–5. Number of Items and Maximum Possible Scores in Sections Combined According to Subject Matter. (From "The Hearing Measure Scale: A Questionnaire for the Assessment of Auditory Disability," by W. G. Noble and G. R. C. Atherley, 1970, *Journal of Auditory Research, 10,* pp. 229–250. Copyright 1970 by Journal of Auditory Research. Reprinted with permission.)

Sections	*Subject Matter*	*Number of Items*	*Maximum Score Possible*
1, 5	Speech Hearing	14	96
4, 6, 7	Hearing Handicap	13	74
2	Acuity	8	28
3	Localization	7	28

Sections

1. Speech hearing
2. Hearing handicap
3. Acuity
4. Localization

Subsections

1. Speech hearing
2. Acuity for nonspeech sound
3. Localization
4. Emotional response
5. Speech distortion
6. Tinnitus
7. Personal opinion

The seven subsections were weighted for importance by a panel of judges. The panel consisted of an otolaryngologist, a director of an audiology clinic, a psychologist, and a physician. The latter two were the authors of the HMS. Four main sections were developed grouping the original subsections with the corresponding weighting scale (Table 16–5).

The authors retested the same individuals 6 months later and found the test-retest scores were reliable over time. A 6-month interval was chosen to minimize noise and age effects on hearing while ensuring that subjects would not recall the test items.

Most answers are on a 5-point scale ranging from "Always" to "Never. " A few questions have answers that are designed specifically for the question (e.g., item 5 in Table 16–6). Several nonscoring questions are included (e.g., the nature of the tinnitus, information about lip-reading ability).

Application

The HMS is given at the initial appointment in paper-and-pencil form to the patient. It is best if used with a comprehensive audiogram in order to estimate expected and perceived handicap.

Interpretation and Scoring

Higher scores correlate with higher perceived handicap. In cases of denial, the perceived handicap does not correspond with the audiogram, and this discrepancy can be used during counseling. If the patient has a 50 dB hearing loss at 2000 Hz and reports no trouble in any situation, for example, denial is most likely present.

Advantages and Disadvantages

This scale is reliable for individuals with noise-induced hearing loss (Noble & Atherley, 1970). The authors are unsure of the validity in other populations. Scoring is not consistent and can be complicated. Not suprisingly, self-assessment of communication difficulties is consistent with audiological findings, but not highly correlated (Noble & Atherley, 1970).

Table 16–6. Hearing Measurement Scale nonscoring question. (From "The Hearing Measure Scale: A Questionnaire for the Assessment of Auditory Disability," by W. G. Noble and G. R. C. Atherley, 1970, *Journal of Auditory Research, 10,* p. 229–250. Copyright 1970 by Journal of Auditory Research. Reprinted with permission.)

5. Do you have difficulty in hearing when shopping or traveling in a car or bus?

All Most Half Occasionally Never

5. Modifier

Is this due to your hearing, due to background noise, or a bit of both?

Circle 1, 2, or 3

1. Due to hearing
2. Due to noise
3. A bit of both

Hearing Performance Inventory: HPI

Development

The HPI is designed to assess a patient's hearing performance in a variety of everyday listening situations to determine areas of communication breakdown (Giolas, Owens, Lamb, & Schuber, 1979). Later the HPI was used as a measure of benefit during and after intervention (Hosford-Dunn & Baxter, 1985; Owens & Fujikawa, 1980).

In the initial prototype, 500 items were narrowed to 289 items, which were administered to 190 patients with mild to severe hearing losses. Statistical analysis of these responses narrowed the selection to the 158 items that comprised the HPI in its final form.

Description

The HPI is divided into six sections. These sections address common listening situations that vary according to the speaker(s), communication situations, and noise environments. The six sections are as follows:

1. Understanding Speech Section: Patients judge how well they understand people whose voices are loud enough.
2. Intensity Section: Patients report their awareness of a particular sound in various situations (e.g., speech, doorbell, whistle).
3. Auditory Failure Section: Patients respond to how frequently they use particular behaviors in various situations (e.g., asking for repeats).
4. Social Section: Patients respond to selected items from Understanding Speech and Auditory Failure regarding situations in which a group of more than two people are gathered away from any occupational setting.
5. Personal Section: The patients report how they feel about the impairment and how it influences self-esteem and social interaction.
6. Occupational Section: Patients judge certain dimensions within an occupational context.

In 1983, Lamb, Owens, and Schubert revised the HPI to eliminate redundant items and shorten administration (Appendix 16D). The 90 items are arranged in the same six sections as the original.

Application

The HPI is administered by the clinician in an interview format in approximately 30 to 40 minutes (HPI-R about 20 minutes) at the initial visit. The 27 occupational items at the end of the profile can be omitted if the respondent is not employed. The spouse can fill an inventory out as well to highlight discrepancies that reflect the patient's denial of a hearing loss. If the HPI is used as a benefit scale, it is readministered face to face or in a paper-and-pencil format after intervention.

Interpretation and Scoring

The responses are answered in a 5-point scale. There are several questions in the Personal Section and Auditory Failure Section that are answered in reverse and need to be flagged before scoring is completed. To score, the numbers are added for all items answered, divided by the number of items answered, and multiplied by 20. (This does not apply to those not answered. They are counted as not attempted.) Scoring inventory can be conducted by individual sections individually as well. Templates have been used, as well as a computer program (Giolas et al., 1979).

Scores range from 20% (least amount of difficulty) to 100% (most difficulty). The more the scores between the spouse and the patient covary, the more likely the patient is realistic about communication difficulties. The greater the disparity of scores, the more likely that there is a lack of acknowledgment on the patient's part (Giolas et al., 1979).

The HPI-R authors found that the global inventory score was difficult to interpret due to poor correlation between audiometric hearing loss and individual patients' adjustment to the hearing loss. Rather, they recommend using individual section scores, with special emphasis on the Understanding Speech and the Intensity sections (Lamb et al., 1983).

Advantages and Disadvantages

An advantage to the HPI and HPI-R are the rigorous development studies with large numbers of subjects, which lead to good statistics and high reliability. The HPI-R inventory is also appropriate for those with profound hearing losses (Owens & Fujikawa, 1980).

At 90 items, it still takes 20 minutes to complete the HPI-R, but it is much shorter than the HPI. Either inventory can be mailed out before the initial visit. The authors of the HPI-R felt that further item reductions would sacrifice the integrity of the inventory (Lamb et al., 1983).

McCarthy-Alpiner Scale of Hearing Handicap: M-A Scale

Development

The McCarthy-Alpiner Scale of Hearing Handicap, developed in 1983, assesses the psychological, social, and vocational effects of hearing loss for an adult (McCarthy & Alpiner, 1983). The M-A Scale also has a parallel scale for a family member. Initially 100 items were given to a pilot group of 100 adults with acquired sensorineural hearing loss. Two weeks later a randomized form of the scale was readministered. Using a criteria of > 0.80 test-retest correlation, 34 items remained.

Sixty additional subjects and family members were given the 34-item scale to determine internal item consistency and correlation between subjects' scores and those of their family members on three subscales (Psychological, Social, and Vocational Effects). Results showed high correlations, high consistency, and good stability for the scales when administered to the subjects and their family members (McCarthy & Alpiner, 1983).

Description

The 34 items are divided into three categories:

- Psychological
- Social
- Vocational Effects

An example question is, "My hearing loss has affected my relationship with my spouse"

(McCarthy & Alpiner, 1983, p. 265). Response choices are on a 5-point scale ranging from "Always" to "Never." Audiometric results are also recorded for comparison to the reported perceived handicap.

Application

This scale is given prior to intervention and is used to design a rehabilitation program for the patient family members.

Interpretation and Scoring

Responses are weighted 1 to 5, with maximum handicap assigned a 5. Because the scale includes reversals, negative items are coded "N," and positive items are coded "P. " For "N" items, "Always" is 5 points, and "Never" is 1 point. For "P" items, "Always" is 1 point, and "Never" is 5 points. The higher the score, the greater the perceived handicap reported by the individual.

Attitudes and relationships of family members are compared to those of the patient and used for counseling. Several scenarios can emerge:

1. The patient does not accept, understand, or deal with the hearing problems, whereas the family member is keenly aware of the handicap.
2. The family member does not recognize, understand, or deal with the patient's hearing impairment.
3. The two people fail to agree on the impact of problem areas.
4. A combination of the above exists (McCarthy & Alpiner, 1983).

Advantages and Disadvantages

This scale is used to get family members involved in the patient's rehabilitation process. It is important to target and prioritize areas of counseling and this scale helps in this area of intervention.

Self-Assessment of Communication and the Significant Other Assessment of Communication: SAC and SOAC

Development

The Self-Assessment of Communication (SAC) and the Significant Other Assessment of Communication (SOAC) are two companion questionnaires developed by Schow and Nerbonne (1982) to screen primary communication difficulty and secondary emotional and social consequences of hearing impairment. The SAC and SOAC represent the nonaudiometric, subjective portion of Schow and Nerbonne's Communication Assess Profile (CAP).

In the initial phase of developing these scales, guidelines were developed through a Task Force. The CAP emerged from these guidelines.

There are two parts of the CAP, audiometric measures and nonaudiometric measures. The nonaudiometric section has two components:

1. Self-Assessment of Communication (SAC) —Personal attitudes of the patient regarding the hearing loss; and
2. Significant Other Assessment of Communication (SOAC)—Assessment of the hearing loss by a significant other. This component is useful in cases where a patient is either unaware of the extent of the hearing loss or attempts to minimize the severity (Show & Nerbonne, 1982).

The SAC and the SOAC have high test-retest reliability, 0.80 and 0.90, respectively (Schow & Nerbonne, 1982).

Description

The SAC is a 10-item screening test. Items 1 through 6 estimate communication in different environments. Items 7 and 8 look at the patient's overall feelings about the hearing handicap, and items 9 and 10 assess the patient's perception of other people's impression of the hearing loss. The SOAC contains the same questions but changes the pronouns in the questions to be appropriate for a family member.

Application

The authors suggested mailing the profiles and instructions prior to the initial appointment in order to save time.

Interpretation and Scoring

The responses are on a 5-point continuum from "Almost Never" (1) to "Practically Always" (5). The corresponding numerical responses are summed for a raw score. The raw score is converted to a percentage by multiplying by 2, subtracting 20, and multiplying by 1.25. For example, if the raw score is 43, the equation is: $43 \times 2 = 86 - 20 = 66 \times 1.25 = 82.5\%$.

The higher the percentage, the greater perceived hearing handicap of the patient. Percentage differences between the patient's and the family member's scores are taken into account to look for signs of denial on the patient's part.

Clinicians should develop their own norms over time to compare to individual patients (Schow & Nerbonne, 1982).

Advantages and Disadvantages

Using a quantifiable test battery helps set up guidelines for what constitutes normal overall communication functioning, to which individual patient responses can be compared. Even if clinicians do not complete their own norms, this test is quick and easy to administer, whether it is mailed out before hand or done in the office. Including the SOAC provides another perspective on the hearing impairment, which supports the patient's perceptions or serves as a counseling tool in cases of denial.

GROUP III: BENEFIT SCALES

Abbreviated Profile of Hearing Aid Benefit: APHAB

Development

The Abbreviated Profile of Hearing Aid Benefit, the APHAB, is a third-generation instrument whose precursors are the Profile of Hearing Aid Performance (PHAP) and the Profile of Hearing Aid Benefit (PHAB). All three instruments were developed at the University of Memphis, Hearing Aid Research Laboratory (HARL), by Dr. Robyn Cox and colleagues.

The PHAP was developed to measure hearing handicap in seven dimensions (Cox & Alexander, 1995). The PHAP is scored using three categories of speech communication and one environmental sound category: speech communication under relatively favorable conditions (SA), speech communication under unfavorable conditions that are not due primarily to background noise (SB), speech communication in noise (SC), and perception of environmental sounds (ES). Three of the categories or scales are further divided into subscales as seen in Table 16–7.

The PHAP was expanded to include responses to the items from the point of view of a listener in unaided and aided conditions. The differences between responses for "with my hearing aid" and "without my hearing aid" were compared to measure the user's subjective benefit from hearing aid use. Because it measures benefit as well as handicap, this expanded version of the PHAP was named the Profile of Hearing Aid Benefit (PHAB).

The PHAP and the PHAB both have 66 items and are too long for routine clinical use. As a result, 24 items were extracted from the PHAB and constructed into an Abbreviated PHAB (the APHAB). Item selection for the APHAB began by eliminating three of the PHAB subscales because of ceiling effects, and low internal consistency and test-retest corre-

Table 16–7. Scales and Respective Subscales for the PHAP.

Scales of PHAP	*Subscales of PHAP*
SA	FT: Familiar Talkers
	EC: Ease of Communication
SB	RV: Reverberation
	RC: Reduced Cues
SC	BN: Background Noise (referred to only)
ES	AV: Aversiveness
	DS: Distortion

lations (Cox & Rivera, 1992). The items for the APHAB were then selected based on an analysis of responses to the items in remaining four PHAB subscales: Ease of Communication (EC), Reverberation (RV), Background Noise (BC), and Aversiveness (AV).

Cox and Alexander (1995) established norms for the APHAB by administering it to three study groups that varied in their reported communication difficulties, hearing aid use, and age:

- Group I: established wearers of linear hearing aids
- Group II: elderly persons with few or no self-assessed hearing problems who do not wear amplification
- Group III: young normal hearing listeners

Cox and Alexander (1995) reported good item-total correlation, ranging from .54 to .66, for each of the subscales and also high internal reliability scores (.78 to .87).

Description

The APHAB is a three-page questionnaire with items arranged on the left and two response columns for "without my hearing aid" and "with my hearing aid" answers. The APHAB is composed of 24 items that are scored in four subscales, as described in the previous section and as seen in Appendix 16E. Each item belongs to one subscale. The items are statements that describe a specific situation (e.g., "I can understand my family at the dinner table."). Patients respond on a 7-point Likert scale by rating the frequency of the time that the statement is true in their experience. The responses range from "Always" (99%) to "Never" (0%).

The complete APHAB questionnaire is reproduced in Appendix 16E. The APHAB and associated scoring software are available through HARL's Web site (http://www.ausp.memphis.edu/harl) and are included in software fitting applications from several hearing aid manufacturers (e.g., Starkey PFS and Phonak).

Application

Probably the most common application of the APHAB is to evaluate benefit of new hearing aid fittings (Cox, 1997). In this case, the recommended procedure is to obtain the patient's "without my hearing aid" responses before the amplification device is fitted, and the "with my hearing aid" responses at least 2 weeks postfitting. The two sections can be completed at the same time, answering the "without my hearing aid" completely before starting "with my hearing aid."

To maximize the validity and reliability of the data, Cox suggested that patients be allowed to see their responses to the "without my hearing aid" portion while they are completing the "with my hearing aid" section.

She also suggested encouraging patients to review and even change the responses if they no longer agree with them (Cox, 1997).

The scale can be given in the office at initial appointment and follow-up or mailed out for completion after the fitting. If a patient fills out both "without" and "with" at the same time, instruct them to complete the "without" before starting the "with" column in order to minimize confusion and the possibility that data will be entered into the wrong column.

Patient responses are entered into the computer by the audiologist (see above for information on obtaining the scoring program). The program generates subscale scores and displays them graphically. The patterns of the graphs indicate areas of benefit and communication difficulty; they also help the audiologist determine whether the patient understood the APHAB and provided valid responses. This is because of the different types of items in the profile and the fact that some of them are presented in a reverse scoring paradigm (i.e., where "always" means fewer rather than more problems). As a result, it is likely that most of the response alternatives will be used at least once and the pattern of usage will not by systematic, as in Figure 16–2A. Patterns that do not vary, suggesting similar responses for all or most items, suggest that the patient does not understand the talk or did not read the instructions carefully (see Figure 16–2B).

Interpretation and Scoring

Interpretation is based on unaided versus aided subscore differences, as well as subscale patterns as in Figure 16–2A.

A difference of 22 points between unaided and aided scores is required to be certain of a significant difference between EC, RV, or BN conditions. Globally, the aided scores must exceed unaided scores on all three subscales by at least 10 points to establish true benefit accrues from hearing aid use (Cox, 1997).

The AV score is not well understood at present and more research is needed before

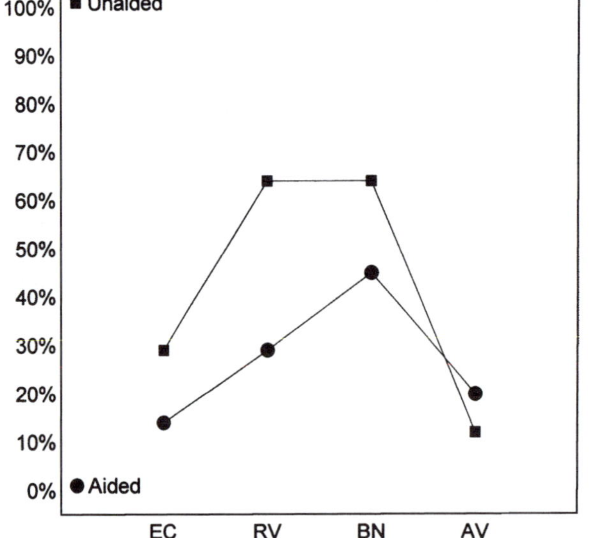

Figure 16–2. A. A patient's aided versus unaided scores and benefit on the four APHAB subscales.

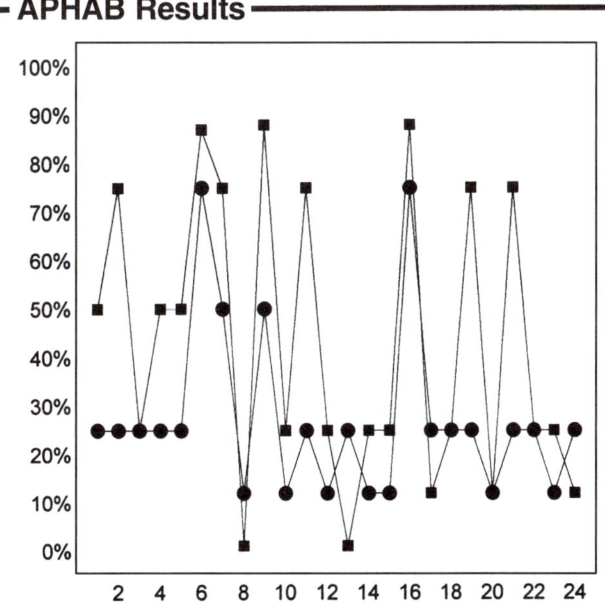

Figure 16–2. B. APHAB results pertaining to each question; square is unaided and circle is aided.

this score can be used in a scientific manner to improve hearing aid fittings (Cox, 1997). Therefore, it is not grouped with the other three subscales for interpretive purposes. Because the AV subscale focuses on perception of environmental sounds, answers on aided statements may give information about the appropriateness of an aid's maximum output level, and some clinicians have reported successfully using the AV scores as a basis for adjusting the SSPL 90 settings (Cox, 1997).

Advantages and Disadvantages

The APHAB is widely used due to its brevity and high internal reliability and because its software is readily available and automatically scored. The graphical representation of APHAB provides a quick way for the audiologist to understand the patient's communication needs and the effect of amplification on those needs. The graph is useful for explaining and discussing hearing handicap and aided benefit with a patient. It can also be printed and put in the patient's chart for future reference and comparison of hearing handicap status and aided benefit.

A recurring problem for most Group III questionnaires is that not all of the situationally specific items are relevant to all patients. The APHAB suffers from this problem and instructs patients to answer such items by estimating how they might respond, even if they are not likely to experience the situation. The APHAB was normed on patients who wore hearing aids with linear circuitry. More research is needed to determine whether normative data are different for patients who use higher performance instruments. Finally, the APHAB may be difficult for some patients to read and understand.

Abrams and Hnath-Chisolm (in press) note that patient or education questionnaires should not exceed a seventh to eighth grade reading level, but the APHAB's reading level is at or above the 11th-grade level.

Client Oriented Scale of Improvement: COSI

Development

The Client Oriented Scale of Improvement (COSI)[2] is an individually constructed statement of the patient's needs and the improvements resulting from the hearing rehabilitation process (Dillon, James, & Ginis, 1997). The COSI was developed by clinicians at the National Acoustic Laboratories (NAL) over several years in the early 1990s. In 1994, audiologists at different facilities were asked to use the COSI and five other outcome measures to estimate the benefits of the aural rehabilitation process and the value of the outcome measures. The audiologists reported a preference of the COSI over the others due to the simplicity, brevity, and the focus on the individual's particular situations (Dillon et al., 1997.

The COSI was normed on 98 Australian adults who were new hearing aid users. In that study, Dillon and colleagues (1997) reported on the scale's reliability, test-retest stability, validity, convenience of use, and capability to improve as well as measure rehabilitation outcomes. The first section of the COSI was completed at the initial appointment. The second section was administered 4 to 7 weeks after the hearing aid fitting and again at a 3 month check-up appointment. Test-retest scores show that the COSI is a reliable scale, with coefficients ranging from 0.73 to 0.84.

Description

In conference with the clinician, the patient identifies up to five situations in which he or she would like to hear better. These situations should be specific; for example, the patient should not state "I would like to hear better." The audiologist should help narrow this down to something like "I would like to understand conversational speech with a grocery store clerk."

After amplification is fitted, and after the patient has had a reasonable time to adapt to the aids (1 to 3 months), the patient rates how well the fitting has helped in the previously defined listening situations. There are two types of ratings to evaluate the COSI at this time which are recorded on the same sheet on which the situations were outlined:

1. Relative (degree of change): How much better do you hear in this situation (Worse, No Difference, Slightly Better, Better, Much Better)?
2. Absolute (final ability): How well do you do in this situation? I can hear: Hardly Ever, Occasionally, Half of the Time, Most of the Time, Almost Always.

Examples of the ratings are. "I hear my grandchildren on the phone" "slightly better," and I hear them "most of the time" or, "I hear the bids when playing bridge" "better," but I still only hear them "Half of the time."

Application

It is best to use the COSI at the initial appointment to individualize the patient's aural rehabilitation. The follow-up can be within the 30-day evaluation time or within a few months of the fitting, depending on acclimatization and other fitting factors.

Interpretation

The final assessment may highlight areas that require further improvement or counseling. Because the rehabilitation process is individualized according to patient needs and desires, the COSI helps clarify expectations, as well as remind the patient and clinician of original fitting goals. The COSI can also help define an endpoint for the fitting process.

Advantages and Disadvantages

This outcome measure is a quick, individualized tool that not only measures outcome, but also helps assess patient needs. For instance,

[2]A copy of the COSI can be obtained by contacting Dr. Harvey Dillon, National Acoustic Laboratories, 126 Greville St., Chatswood, 2067, Australia.

non-hearing-aid solutions can emerge from the assessment that solve needs that are not corrected by amplification.

As with many other hearing aid outcome measures, it is difficult to determine to what extent the patients' answers are related to how much they like their practitioners. The patients may overrate their responses if they admire the audiologist helping them (Dillon et al., 1997).

Glasgow Hearing Aid Benefit Profile: GHABP

Development

The Glasgow Hearing Aid Benefit Profile (GHABP) (Gatehouse, 1998) evaluates the effectiveness of rehabilitation services for adults with hearing impairment. It is based on data from the Hearing Disability and Aid Benefit Interview (HDABI) (Gatehouse, 1998). The HDABI contained 14 listening situations that were most likely to occur in everyday life. It was given to 943 subjects who were asked seven questions pertaining to each of the 14 listening situations. The seven follow-up questions are as follows:

1. How often does this happen?
2. Without your hearing aid, how much difficulty did you have in this situation?
3. Without your hearing aid, how much does any difficulty worry, annoy, or upset you in this situation?
4. In this situation, what proportion of the time do you wear your hearing aid?
5. In this situation, how much does your hearing aid help you?
6. In this situation with your hearing aid, how much difficulty do you have?
7. For this situation, how satisfied are you with your hearing aid?

After data collection, four of the most common situations were used to develop the GHABP, based on either maximum frequency of occurrence or maximum occurrence of hearing difficulty. Although test-retest reliability is high (0.86), the author suggested that this measure may be inflated because the scale is so short that subjects can recall the answers between test and retest.

Description

The GHABP has six scales:

1. Initial Disability
2. Handicap
3. Reported Hearing Aid Use
4. Reported Benefit
5. Satisfaction
6. Residual Disability

Information on these scales are obtained based on patient's answers to the seven questions of the HDABI, in each of the four specified listening circumstances. There are also up to four additional listening circumstances described by the patient (Appendix 16F).

Application

The author's goal is to use this profile during rehabilitation to help the patient and clinician focus on positive and negative aspects of amplification for the individual patient. It is best administered in an interview format.

Three questions are answered (Appendix 16F) at the visit when the decision to proceed with amplification is made:

1. Does this situation happen in your life? Yes (go to next question) No (stop)
2. How much difficulty do you have in this situation?
3. How much does any difficulty in this situation worry, annoy, or upset you?

Most patients give at least one (and as many as four) other examples in the subject-specified section, as seen in Appendix 16F and initially answer the two pertinent questions of difficulty (Gatehouse, 1999).

Interpretation

Questions are examined individually, but in each case the higher the number associated with the particular answer, the less difficulty.

Advantages and Disadvantages

The GHABP is just published as of this writing. It is a comprehensive profile that does not take much clinical time. Further testing is underway to evaluate self-completion by the patients and realistic use in clinical settings.

Hearing Aid Performance Inventory: HAPI

Development

The HAPI is a self-reported scale that measures success with amplification (Walden, Demorest, & Helper, 1984). The main question asked by the developers was: "Is perceived benefit from amplification relatively consistent across situations or is benefit too situation-specific to be assess with a single, global criterion measure?" (Walden et al., p. 49).

The HAPI was normed on 128 experienced hearing aid users (119 males, 9 females) who wore their aids an average of 10.8 hours per day and had a sloping sensorineural hearing loss. Subjects filled out the inventory at an appointment or mailed it and were instructed to answer based on the benefit received from the hearing aids and not based on the difficulty of the situation itself (Walden et al., 1984). Each situation had a "does not apply" option included in the answer format. The latter were not included in the statistical analysis.

The reliability of the HAPI is high (.96), even though there is high inter-subject variability. The reliability factor opened the door to shorter versions that were created later. Two different Shortened HAPI scales (both have been referred to as SHAPI) were modified by Schum (1992) and Dillon (1994) to decrease administration time but keep the reliability of the scale.

Description

The HAPI has 64 items organized into four subsections according to listening situations:

1. Noisy situations
2. Quiet situations with the speaker in proximity
3. Situations with reduced signal information
4. Situations with nonspeech stimuli

Common environments such as home and work are represented several times throughout the questionnaire. The items are broad in scope, applying to a variety of listening environments.

The patient chooses from a 5-item scale, as seen in Appendix 16G, ranging from "Very Helpful" (1) to "Hinders Performance" (5). In contrast to most other profiles, a low score is preferable.

Application

The original intent was to administer the HAPI when intervention is near completion by the paper-and-pencil method.

Interpretation and Scoring

The HAPI and its offspring were designed to report the amplification performance and the success of hearing aid use in daily life as one combined measure. The scores of all items are added together and averaged (leaving out the "not applicable" answers). The closer to "1" the averaged score is, the better the individuals feel they are doing.

Advantages and Disadvantages

Both the HAPI and Shortened HAPIs provide aided scores only. Although the scale is not designed for pre- and postintervention testing, some clinicians use it in this manner even though its reliability is not known for this application.

Because the items apply to a variety of listening environments, the HAPI may not be applicable to some elderly respondents (Newman & Weinstein, 1988). Schum (1992) and Dillon's (1994) Shortened HAPIs target the elderly population for ease of use. These scales do help clinicians reliably determine self-perceived benefit for those individuals who have been using amplification. The shortened forms reduce administration and scoring-time involvement.

Hearing Functioning Profile: HFP

Development

Singer, Healey, and Preece described The Hearing Functioning Profile (HFP) in 1997. This profile helps clinicians use rehabilitation tactics over and beyond amplification, such as communication strategies and closed captioning (Singer et al., 1997).

The HFP focuses on the psychological and behavioral changes that patients must go through in order to accept amplification. The profile is based on a psychological "transtheoretical approach" in which success and failure are related to "learned helplessness" (Singer et al., 1997). The HFP helps the clinician understand the patient's psychological profile based on learned helplessness and how different factors may influence the patient's function with hearing instruments. The HFP looks at the extent to which a patient is actively working to change his or her behaviors and whether his or her outlook is pessimistic or optimistic. The latter dictates whether an individual is at high risk for failure with amplification on this profile.

Description

The HFP examines three categories that encompass at least 10 hearing situations:

1. Alerting Category: telephone bell, doorbell, sound (e.g., baby), alarm clock, fire, and a section to add another alerting sound for that particular individual
2. Listening Category: television and phone conversation
3. Communication Category: planned (one to one), unplanned (one to one), group, and a fourth can be added to fit the needs of the individual

Application

The HFP was designed for postfitting management, but the authors did not feel it is limited to this intervention stage (Singer et al., 1997). The profile is conducted in an interview format with the clinician asking the patient about situations in each category and recording the responses. Each relevant situation is evaluated in terms of whether a problem is present in aided and unaided listening. If a problem exists, the patient is asked whether it is due to overall hearing, listening angle (e.g., if there is a "dead" ear or monaural fit), competing noise, distance, or visibility. Each situation has room for comments to elaborate on problems. If the patient has amplification, the final limitation that is examined is usage (i.e., is the individual a full-time or part-time user?)

Interpretation and Scoring

The HFP is not scored numerically. Rather, the clinician checks it on the form when a problem area is identified. A comments section is used for elaboration of the problem situation if needed. Evaluating the difficulties that patients report with amplification helps the clinician organize continuing rehabilitation for the patient. Treatment recommendations are based on "S.E.T." categories: Strategies, Environmental Manipulations, and Technology (Singer et al., 1997). *Strategies* include getting the individual's attention before speaking in an unplanned situation to optimize use of visual cues. *Environmental manipulations* can be as simple as turning the television down when conversation takes place or waiting for commercial breaks to converse. *Technology* refers to assistive listening devices of all types.

Advantages and Disadvantages

This profile encompasses many factors that are beneficial to the patient and clinician when searching for hearing solutions beyond amplification. As the authors pointed out, "The use of the Hearing Functioning Profile greatly enhances management of hearing loss. It benefits those fitted with hearing instruments, but should also be considered for individuals who do not use hearing instruments. The Profile forces the hearing health care professional to organize management around the numerous demands on a person in everyday life" (Singer et al., 1997, p. 26).

A few underlying issues are not clear on the form. For example, a limitation to communication is lack of hearing aid use, but daily (hourly) use is not queried on the form. The HFP might be easier to use if more question areas were on the form instead of relying on the clinician to think of unstated items when the profile is given to a patient.

Profile of Aided Loudness: PAL

Development

Mueller and Palmer developed the Profile of Aided Loudness (PAL) in 1998 to determine if loudness restoration is accomplished with amplification. In 1997, 53 subjects were fit binaurally with two-channel programmable CICs. The instruments had the capability of wide dynamic range compression (WDRC) or compression limiting (Mueller & Palmer, 1998). The authors found that the WDRC performance had better ratings for soft speech, but no difference was found in word understanding in noise using the speech perception in noise (SPIN) test. Mueller and Palmer reported a high consistency correlation of .70 or better on the PAL.

The pilot study normed loudness ratings for individuals without a hearing loss on 95 different sounds. This normative data is used when comparing answers of hearing aid users.

Description

There are 12 situations or noises in which the patient rates the loudness and the loudness satisfaction (see Appendix 16H). The loudness rating uses a 7-point scale as "cannot hear" (0) to "uncomfortably loud" (7). Each loudness (soft, medium, and loud) has four different examples to represent that situation.

The loudness rating is compared to the ratings of the normed (normal hearing) subjects. The target rating for each item is where 70% of the norm group selected that particular item. The acceptable rating is within ±1 standard deviation from the target, which establishes the loudness profile rating. Thus, soft speech goal is 2, ±1. For medium sounds, such as average speech, the target is 4, ±1.

Application

The original design is for administration after amplification is fit, but the PAL can also be executed prior to hearing aid fitting in order to establish baseline (Mueller & Palmer, 1998)

Interpretation and Scoring

There are four possible outcomes:

1. goal of normal aided loudness perception met, patient is satisfied
2. goal of normal aided loudness perception met, patient is dissatisfied
3. goal of normal aided loudness perception not met, patient is satisfied
4. goal of normal aided loudness perception not met, patient is not satisfied.

Each satisfaction rating is evaluated for each loudness level (soft, medium, and loud). The satisfaction profile is then compared to the loudness profile.

Advantages and Disadvantages

The PAL is easy to administer. It measures a specific component that affects wearer satisfaction and gives insight into the patient's fitting needs for loudness. This scale has only recently been published and remains to be tested in different dispensing environments.

GROUP IV: SATISFACTION INVENTORIES

Hearing Aid Users' Questionaire: HAUQ

Development

The Hearing Aid Users' Questionnaire (HAUQ) was developed and reported in Australia in

1988 (Dillon et al., 1997).[3] The HAUQ contains questions that relate to hearing aid use, difficulties, and other satisfaction-related issues. Little information is available on the HAUQ, and it is not widely known in the United States.

Description

This multi-item questionnaire looks at several different areas of hearing aid use. The primary goal is to detect problems that may affect the person's ability to use and benefit from the hearing aid (Dillon et al., 1999). Dillon described the questionnaire as:

- Questions 1 and 2 deal with usage of the hearing aid with the categories in question 2 scaled from 1-6
- Question 3 deals with benefits, with "not at all" scaled as a 1, "a little" scaled as a 2, and "a lot" scaled as a 3
- Question 4 deals with problems, with "no" scaled as 2 and "yes" scaled as 1
- Questions 5-7 deal with satisfaction, each scaled from 1 to 4. In all cases the larger the number the more favorable the outcome
- Question 8 attempts to find clients' assessment of whether they have problems that require another appointment
- Questions 9-11 are open-ended questions to determine what the clients likes and dislikes are of the services and instruments they have received (Dillon et al., p. 71).

Application

This questionnaire is given at some point post-intervention. Although no information is available on administration, it is lends itself to a paper-and-pencil format.

Interpretation and Scoring

This scale is useful when looking at the individual's satisfaction in several practical dimensions, but it is not appropriate to use it to rank patients according to satisfaction (Dillon et al., 1999). Dillon suggested looking at each question individually and using the data to identify those aspects of the hearing aid fitting that are less than satisfactory.

Advantages and Disadvantages

The scale is quick to administer and can be mailed to patients. Little is know of the HAUQ at this time. It is used by some professionals in Australia and has been reported on in the United States through the *Journal of the American Academy of Audiology*.

Satisfaction with Amplification in Daily Life: SADL

Development

The SADL examines the overall outcome of hearing aid fittings from the patient's point of view, using satisfaction rather than benefit as the measure of interest (Cox & Alexander, 1999). As the authors stated, "the focus on benefit as an outcome measure is in danger of becoming too narrow."

The investigator has hearing aid users rank a set of "Importance Factors." Those rankings showed that items of importance clustered into four factors: Benefit and Sound Quality, Physical and Psychological Comfort, Value, and Hearing Aid Stigma. Based on these four factors, a series of proposed satisfaction questions were developed and tested on older hearing aid users. The subjects wore conventional aids, half of which were dispensed in a VA setting. The results showed that satisfaction and importance were similar constructs but not identical. For example, a patient might be satisfied with one measure in an Importance Factor (e.g., phone use) but dissatisfied with another measure in the same factor (e.g., hearing in groups). Principle components analysis of the satisfaction data showed that items grouped into five Satisfaction Factors of varying importance to hearing aid users. Ultimately, this analysis and further testing produced a

[3]Information on the scale and scoring can be found at, URL: http://www.ausp.memphis. edu/harl.

15-item questionnaire with four subcategories corresponding to four dimensions of satisfaction.

Description

The SADL has 15 items that are scored into four subscales that correspond to these four satisfaction dimensions:

1. Positive Effect consists of 6 items associated with benefit and performance
2. Service and Cost consists of 3 items that address dispenser services and cost
3. Negative Features looks at 3 disparate areas of frustration with hearing aid use
4. Personal Image addresses hearing aid stigma and cosmetics in 3 items. The scale is shown in Appendix 16I.

The responses are in the form of a 7-point, equally spaced semantic scale, ranging from "Not at all" (A) to "Tremendously" (G).

There is a separate section that includes the experience, use, and hearing difficulty as recorded by the clinician. The SADL form has a back section for describing hearing aid information, which is also filled out by the clinician.

Application

The SADL is filled out by patients after they have become accustomed to their hearing aids. Responses can be compared to interim norms. The administration can be repeated at intervals (e.g., 3 months to 1 year) after the initial administration to track the patient's satisfaction over time.

The SADL requires less than 15 minutes. Some questions are reversed and may confuse a few patients. If a question is not applicable, patients are instructed to leave it unanswered. The scale can also be used to rate the difference in satisfaction between amplification devices.

The subscale scores allow more complete analysis of a patient's satisfaction status. If a patient is reporting global dissatisfaction, there is most likely an underlying cause that would show up in that particular subscale. Intervention in that area can be applied to improve satisfaction.

Interpretation and Scoring

The Global score is the mean of the scores for all of the completed items. Subscales are scored separately by averaging the item responses (e.g., if the three scores for Service and Cost are 6, 3, and 5 = 14, the score is (6 + 3 + 5/3 = 4.6). The higher the number, the more satisfied the patient is, whether it is on the individual subscale or the global scale.

Cox and Alexander reported that a critical difference (CD) calculated by test-retest scores, in global scores of 0.9, happens by chance only 10% of the time. Therefore, if the global scores differ by 0.9, there is a significant difference in satisfaction between the responses of one SADL and another for the same patient (Cox & Alexander, 1999).

As of this writing the scale is new and only interim norms from linear fittings are available.[3]

Advantages and Disadvantages

The SADL is short and does not take long to complete (about 10 minutes). It can be mailed to patients or filled out in the clinic.

One of the disadvantages of the APHAB that Cox also developed was the high reading level (Abrams & Hnath-Chisolm, in press) (the SADL is written at a seventh-grade reading level). The SADL is still in development. The subscales of Negative Features and Positive Image may not be reliable due to the small number of items and the diversity of content (Cox & Alexander, 1999). Four items (7, 11, 10, and 15) may be reworded due to clinical trials in progress.

Office Satisfaction Surveys

There are several surveys that relate to the user's overall satisfaction office and service delivery variables. An in-office adaptation of the ASHA survey (Appendix 16J) can be filled out by patients in the office, or it can be mailed. Another quality-of-service survey by Martin (1997) helps clinicians focus on quality issues in their own practices (Appendix 16K). It is important that clinicians remain aware of other services besides hearing aid delivery that influence patients' satisfaction. A remodeling project in the office, for instance, may interfere with mobility, patient flow, or scheduling. Any of these can reduce a patient's satisfaction with the overall hearing aid fitting process.

Industry Standards

Several surveys used by the hearing aid industry track hearing aid user satisfaction and other statistics. The MarkeTrack uses variations of the Knowles' Satisfaction and Benefit surveys (Kochkin, 1992, 1993, 1995). It is modified periodically to address changes in hearing aid technology and service delivery. The data are used by some audiologists to compare industry standards to the performance of individual offices or clinics. Some practices use this information to model incentive programs for their clinicians, using measures such as return-for-credit rate to reward employees whose rates are lower than the industry as a whole. *The Hearing Review* and *The Hearing Journal* also publish national hearing aid dispensing trends and statistics.

CONCLUSION

An exhaustive list of self-reported measures is beyond the scope of this book and would be incomplete by the time of publication. Another resource that describes profiles and scales is the *Handbook of Self-Assessment and Verification Measures of Communication Performance* (Geier, 1997) published by the Academy of Dispensing Audiologists (ADA) in the late 1990s.

When selecting and using outcome measures, it is important to first ask what factor needs to be measured. Is the goal to predict acceptance, to determine perceived benefit, or to measure satisfaction in one or more dimension? The clinician must evaluate the tools that best measure the desired factor(s). When the appropriate scale or scales are selected, clinicians must apply them consistently in their practices to realize improvement for their patients and their practices. In the long run, the tools only help if we use them.

REVIEW QUESTIONS

1. What is the main procedural difference between the "Benefit" scales and the other three types of profiles?
2. Name the four areas of scales in this chapter.
3. Name two examples for each group.
4. Which scales could be used on an elderly population to help design an aural rehabilitation program? Name two.
5. When would be an appropriate time to give a scale on satisfaction?

REFERENCES

Abrams, H. B. & Hnath-Chisolm, T. (2000, in press). Outcome measures: Audiologic difference.

Alpiner, J., Chevrett, W., Glascoe, O., Metz, M., & Olsen, B. (1974). *The Denver Scale of Communication Function*. Unpublished study, University of Denver, Colorado.

Chermak, G., & Miller, S. (1998). Shortcomings of a Revised Feasibility Scale for Predicting Hearing Aid Use with Older Adults. *British Journal of Audiology, 22*, 187–194.

Cox, R. M. (1997). Administration and application of the APHAB. *The Hearing Journal, 50*, 32–48.

Cox, R. M. & Alexander, G. C. (1995). The abbreviated profile of hearing aid benefit. *Ear and Hearing, 16*, 176–186.

Cox, R. M. & Alexander, G. C. (1997) Measuring satisfaction with amplification in daily life: The SADL scale. *Ear and Hearing, 10*, 306–320.

Cox, R. M. & Rivera, I. M. (1992). Predictability and reliability of hearing aid benefit measured using the PHAB. *Journal of the American Academy of Audiology, 3*, 242–254.

Dancer, J., & Gener, J. (1999). Survey on the use of adult hearing assessment scales. *The Hearing Review, 6*(1), 35.

Demorest, M. E., & Walden, B. E. (1984). Psychometric principles in the selection, interpretation, and evaluation of communication self-assessment inventories. *Journal of Speech and Hearing Disorders, 49*, 226–240.

Demorest, M. E. & Erdman, S. A. (1986). Scale composition and item analysis of the Communication Profile for the Hearing Impaired. *Journal of Speech and Hearing Research, 29*, 515–535.

Demorest, M. E., & Erdman, S. A. (1987). Development of the Communication Profile for the Hearing Impaired. *Journal of Speech and Hearing Disorders, 52*, 129–142.

Demorest, M. E., & Erdman, S. A. (1988). Retest stability of the Communication Profile for the Hearing Impaired. *Ear and Hearing, 9*, 237–242.

Demorest, M. E., & Erdman, S. A. (1989). Factor structure of the Communication Profile for the Hearing Impaired. *Journal of Speech and Hearing Disorders, 54*, 541–549.

Demorest, M. E. & Erdman, S. A. (1990). *User's guide to the CPHI database system* (2nd ed.). Simpsonville, MD: CPHI Services.

Dillon, H. (1994). Shortened Hearing Aid Profile Inventory for the Elderly. *Journal of Australian Audiology, 16*, 37–34.

Dillon, H., Birtles, G., Lovegrove, R. (1999). Measuring the outcomes of a national rehabilitation program: Normative data for the Client Oriented Scale of Improvement (COSI) and the Hearing Aid User's Questionnaire (HAUQ). *Journal of the American Academy of Audiology, 10*, 67–79.

Dillon, H., James, A., & Ginis, J. (1997). Client Oriented Scale of Improvement (COSI) and its relationship to several other measures of benefit and satisfaction provided by hearing aids. *Journal of the American Academy of Audiology, 8*, 27–43.

Erdman, S. A., Demorest, M. B., Wark, D. J., Skinner, M. W., Deming, J., Montano, J. J., & Madory, R. D. (1995). Psychosocial and behavioral adjustment to hearing impairment. *American Speech, Language and Hearing, 37*(10), 107.

Garstecki, D. C. & Erler, S. F. (1996). Older adult performance on the Communication Profile for the Hearing Impaired. *Journal of Speech and Hearing Research, 39*, 28–42.

Gatehouse, S. (1998). *The Glasgow Hearing Aid Benefit Profile: Derivation and validation of a client-centered outcome measure for hearing aid services.* Unpublished study, MRC Institute of Hearing Research (Scottish Section), Glasgow, Scotland.

Gatehouse, S. (1999). The Glasgow Hearing Aid Benefit Profile: Derivation and validation of a client-centered outcome measure for hearing aid services. *Journal of the American Academy of Audiology, 10*, 80–103.

Geier, K. (1997). *The handbook of self-assessment and verification measures of communication performance.* Columbia, SC: Academy of Dispensing Audiologists.

Giolas, T. G., Owens, B., Lamb, S. H., & Schuber, E. E. (1979). Hearing Performance Inventory. *Journal of Speech and Hearing Disorders, 44*, 169–195.

High, W. S., Fairbanks, G., & Glorig, A. (1964). Scale for self-assessment of hearing handicap. *Journal of Speech and Hearing Disorders, 29*, 215–230.

Hosford-Dunn, H., & Baxter, J. H. (1985). Prediction and validation of hearing aid wearer benefit: Preliminary findings. *Hearing Instruments, 36*, 35–41.

Humes, L. E. (1999). Dimensions of hearing aid outcome. *Journal of the American Academy of Audiology, 10*, 26–39.

Hyde, M. L., Malizia, K., Riko, K., & Storms, D. (1992). Evaluation of a self-assessment inventory for the hearing impaired. (*Project Rep. No. 66064122-45*). Toronto, Ontario, Canada: Mount Sinai Hospital, The Toronto Hospital, Otologic Function Unit.

Hyde, M. L., Malizia, K., Riko, K., & Storms, D. (1996, June). *CPHI results in a general clinical population.* Paper presented at the meeting of the Academy of Rehabilitative Audiology, Snowbird, UT.

Kaplan, H., Bally, S., Brandt, F., Busacco, D., & Pray, J. (1997). Communication Scale for Older Adults (CSOA). *Journal of the American Academy of Audiology, 8*, 203–217.

Kaplan, H., Feeley, J., & Brown, J. (1978). A Modified Denver Scale: Test-Retest Reliability. *Journal of the Academy of Rehabilitative Audiology, 11*, 15–32.

Kochkin, S. (1992). MarkeTrak III identifies key factors in determining consumer satisfaction. *The Hearing Journal, 45*, 39–44.

Kochkin, S. (1993, June). Customer satisfaction with hearing instruments in the united states. *The Marketing Edge.* Washington, DC: Hearing Industries Association.

Kochkin, S. (1995, August 2). Subjective measures of satisfaction and benefit: establishing Norms. Collaborative Marketing Committee (CMC).

Lamb, S. H., Owens, B., & Schubert, E. E. (1983). The revised form of the hearing performance inventory. *Ear and Hearing, 4*, 152–157.

McCarthy, P. A., & Alpiner, J. G. (1983). An assessment scale of hearing handicap for use in family counseling. *Journal of the Academy of Rehabilitative Audiology, 16*, 256–270.

Martin, R. L. (1997). Nuts and bolts; Are you providing quality service? *The Hearing Journal, 8*, 66.

Mueller, H. G., & Palmer, C. V. (1998). The profile of aided loudness: A new "PAL" for 98. *The Hearing Journal, 51*, 10–19.

Newman, C. W., & Weinstein, B. E. (1988). Test-retest reliability of the hearing handicap inventory for the elderly using two administration approaches. *Ear and Hearing, 10*, 90–191.

Newman, C. W., & Weinstein, B. E. (1989). The Hearing Handicap Inventory for the Elderly as a

Measure of Hearing Aid Benefit. *Ear and Hearing; 9*, 81–85.

Newman, C. W., Weinstein, B. E., Jacobson, G. P., & Hug, G. A. (1990). The Hearing Handicap Inventory for Adults: Psychometric adequacy and audiometric correlates. *Ear and Hearing, 11*, 430–433.

Newman, C. W., Weinstein, B. E., Jacobson, G. P., & Hug, G. A. (1991). Test-retest reliability of the hearing handicap inventory for adults. *Ear and Hearing, 12*, 355–357.

Noble, W. G., & Atherley, G. R. C. (1970). The Hearing Measure Scale: A questionnaire for the assessment of auditory disability. *Journal of Auditory Research, 10*, 229–250.

Owens, E., & Fujikawa, S. (1980). The Hearing Performance Inventory and hearing aid use in profound hearing loss. *Journal of Speech and Hearing Research, 23*, 470–479.

Rupp, R. R. (1982, January). Predicting hearing aid use in maturing populations: the Feasibility Scale. *Hearing Aid Journa*l, pp. 10–15.

Schow, R. L., & Nerbonne, M. A. (1980). Hearing Handicap and Denver Scales; Applications, categories, interpretation. *Journal of the Academy of Rehabilitative Audiology, 13*, 66–77.

Schow, R. L., & Nerbonne, M. A. (1982). Communication Screening Profile: Use with elderly clients. *Ear and Hearing, 3*, 135–147.

Schow, R., & Tannahill, C. (1977). Hearing handicap scores and categories for subjects with normal and impaired hearing sensitivity. *Journal of the American Auditory Society, 3*, 134–139.

Schum, D. J. (1992). Responses of elderly hearing aid users on the Hearing Aid Performance Inventory. *Journal of the American Academy of Audiology, 3*, 308–314.

Schum, D. J. (1999). Perceived hearing aid benefit in relation to perceived needs. *Journal of the American Academy of Audiology, 10*, 40–45.

Singer, J., Healey, J., & Preece, J. (1997). Hearing instruments: A psychologic and behavioral perspective. *High Performance Hearing Solutions, 1*, 23–27.

Tannahill, J. (1979). Hearing handicap scale as a measure of hearing aid benefit. *Journal of Speech and Hearing Disorders, 44*, 91–99.

Thornton, A. R., & Raffin, M. J. M. (1978). Speech discrimination scores modeled as a binomial variable. *Journal of Speech and Hearing Research, 21*, 507–518.

Ventry, I., & Weinstein, B. (1982). The Hearing Handicap Inventory for the Elderly: A new tool. *Ear and Hearing, 3*, 128–134.

Walden, B. E., Demorest, M. E., & Hepler, E. E. (1984). Self-report approach to assessment benefit derived from amplification. *Journal of Speech and Hearing Research, 27*, 49–56.

Weinstein, B., Spitzer J., & Ventry I. (1986). Test-retest reliability of the hearing handicap inventory for the elderly. *Ear and Hearing, 7*, 295–299.

Zarnoch, J. M., & Alpiner, J. G. (1977). The Denver Scale of Communication Function for Senior Citizens living in retirement centers. In *The Handbook of Adult Rehabilitative Audiology* (2nd ed.). Baltimore, MD: Williams and Wilkins.

APPENDIX 16A: COMMUNICATION SCALE FOR OLDER ADULTS

INSTRUCTIONS: Please read each situation. Decide if the situation is true: Please Respond to Each Question.

Communication Strategies

Please read each situation. Decide if the situation is true:
3-point: (1) Almost always, (2) Sometimes, or (3) Almost never
5-point: (1) Always, (2) Almost always, (3) Sometimes, (4) Almost never, or (5) Never
Please circle the appropriate answer. PLEASE RESPOND TO EACH QUESTION

1. You are talking with someone you do not know well. You do not understand. You ask her to repeat.
(1) Almost always (2) Sometimes (3) Almost never
(1) Always (2) Almost always (3) Sometimes (4) Almost never (5) Never

2. Your are talking with two people. You are not understanding. You change the topic so that you can control the conversation.
(1) Almost always (2) Sometimes (3) Almost never
(1) Always (2) Almost always (3) Sometimes (4) Almost never (5) Never

3. You ask a stranger for directions. You understand part of what he says. You tell him the part you understand and ask him to repeat the rest.
(1) Almost always (2) Sometimes (3) Almost never
(1) Always (2) Almost always (3) Sometimes (4) Almost never (5) Never

4. A friend introduces you to a new person. You do not understand the person's name. You ask the person to spell her name.
(1) Almost always (2) Sometimes (3) Almost never
(1) Always (2) Almost always (3) Sometimes (4) Almost never (5) Never

5. A stranger spells his name for you. You miss the first two letters. You ask him to say each letter and a word starting with that letter (A as in Apple, B as in Boy).
(1) Almost always (2) Sometimes (3) Almost never
(1) Always (2) Almost always (3) Sometimes (4) Almost never (5) Never

6. A person tells you his address. You do not understand. You ask him to repeat the street number, one number at a time.
(1) Almost always (2) Sometimes (3) Almost never
(1) Always (2) Almost always (3) Sometimes (4) Almost never (5) Never

7 You are talking with one person but are not understanding. You interrupt the person before he finishes to say what you think.

(1) Almost always (2) Sometimes (3) Almost never
(1) Always (2) Almost always (3) Sometimes (4) Almost never (5) Never

8. Your friend asks you to buy seven hamburgers. You do not understand how many he wants. You ask him to start counting from zero and stop at the correct number.
(1) Almost always (2) Sometimes (3) Almost never
(1) Always (2) Almost always (3) Sometimes (4) Almost never (5) Never

9. You are at a meeting. The speaker says something you do not understand. You pretend to understand and hope to get the information later.
(1) Almost always (2) Sometimes (3) Almost never
(1) Always (2) Almost always (3) Sometimes (4) Almost never (5) Never

10. Two people are talking. You do not understand the conversation. You ask them to tell you the topic.
(1) Almost always (2) Sometimes (3) Almost never
(1) Always (2) Almost always (3) Sometimes (4) Almost never (5) Never

11. You are talking with one person in a restaurant. His face is in the shadows. You know you could understand better if you changed seats with him. You ask to change seats.
(1) Almost always (2) Sometimes (3) Almost never
(1) Always (2) Almost always (3) Sometimes (4) Almost never (5) Never

12. You are visiting the doctor. He tells you what to do for your illness. You do not understand his speech. You ask him to write.
(1) Almost always (2) Sometimes (3) Almost never
(1) Always (2) Almost always (3) Sometimes (4) Almost never (5) Never

13. You are at a meeting. The speaker does not look at you when he talks. You feel angry but do nothing about it.
(1) Almost always (2) Sometimes (3) Almost never
(1) Always (2) Almost always (3) Sometimes (4) Almost never (5) Never

14. You are at a meeting. You realize you are too far from the speaker to understand him. There are empty seats in the front of the room. You change your seat.
(1) Almost always (2) Sometimes (3) Almost never
(1) Always (2) Almost always (3) Sometimes (4) Almost never (5) Never

15. You are at a meeting. You are the only hard of hearing person. You are afraid that you will not understand but you do not ask for help. You do the best you can.
(1) Almost always (2) Sometimes (3) Almost never
(1) Always (2) Almost always (3) Sometimes (4) Almost never (5) Never

16. You are talking to the dentist. He speaks very fast. You cannot lip-read him. You ask him to slow down.
(1) Almost always (2) Sometimes (3) Almost never
(1) Always (2) Almost always (3) Sometimes (4) Almost never (5) Never

17. You are taking a class. The teacher talks while she writes on the board. You talk to her after class. You explain that you need her to face you in order to speech read.
(1) Almost always (2) Sometimes (3) Almost never
(1) Always (2) Almost always (3) Sometimes (4) Almost never (5) Never

18. A speaker likes to move around the room while she lectures. You have problems reading her lips. You ask her after class to lecture from one place in the room.
(1) Almost always (2) Sometimes (3) Almost never
(1) Always (2) Almost always (3) Sometimes (4) Almost never (5) Never

19. You are going to a series of meetings or lectures. You ask the speaker to use slides, pictures, or the overhead projector whenever possible.
(1) Almost always (2) Sometimes (3) Almost never
(1) Always (2) Almost always (3) Sometimes (4) Almost never (5) Never

20. You are going to a series of meetings or lectures. You ask the speaker to find a person to take notes for you.
(1) Almost always (2) Sometimes (3) Almost never
(1) Always (2) Almost always (3) Sometimes (4) Almost never (5) Never

21. You are going to a series of meetings or lectures. You ask for an outline or a reading list.
(1) Almost always (2) Sometimes (3) Almost never
(1) Always (2) Almost always (3) Sometimes (4) Almost never (5) Never

22. You are going to a play. You read the play or reviews of the play before you see it.
(1) Almost always (2) Sometimes (3) Almost never
(1) Always (2) Almost always (3) Sometimes (4) Almost never (5) Never

23. You are talking with a clerk at the bank. A fire truck goes by. You ask him to stop talking until the noise stops.
(1) Almost always (2) Sometimes (3) Almost never
(1) Always (2) Almost always (3) Sometimes (4) Almost never (5) Never

24. You ask a person to repeat because you don't understand. He seems annoyed. You stop asking and pretend to understand.
(1) Almost always (2) Sometimes (3) Almost never
(1) Always (2) Almost always (3) Sometimes (4) Almost never (5) Never

25. You ask a stranger for directions to a place. You really want to understand his speech. You ask very specific questions like: "Is this place north or south of here?"
(1) Almost always (2) Sometimes (3) Almost never
(1) Always (2) Almost always (3) Sometimes (4) Almost never (5) Never

26. You need to ask directions. You avoid asking a stranger because you think you will have trouble understanding him.
(1) Almost always (2) Sometimes (3) Almost never
(1) Always (2) Almost always (3) Sometimes (4) Almost never (5) Never

27. You are at a store. You have trouble hearing the clerk because his voice is soft. You explain you are hearing impaired and ask him to talk louder.
(1) Almost always (2) Sometimes (3) Almost never
(1) Always (2) Almost always (3) Sometimes (4) Almost never (5) Never

28. You ask your family or friends to get your attention before they speak to you.
(1) Almost always (2) Sometimes (3) Almost never
(1) Always (2) Almost always (3) Sometimes (4) Almost never (5) Never

29. You are with five or six friends. You miss something important. You ask the person next to you what was said.
(1) Almost always (2) Sometimes (3) Almost never
(1) Always (2) Almost always (3) Sometimes (4) Almost never (5) Never

30. You have trouble understanding a man who is chewing gum. You explain that you need to speech read. You politely ask him to remove the gum when he talks.
(1) Almost always (2) Sometimes (3) Almost never
(1) Always (2) Almost always (3) Sometimes (4) Almost never (5) Never

31. You try to avoid people when you know you will have trouble understanding them.
(1) Almost always (2) Sometimes (3) Almost never
(1) Always (2) Almost always (3) Sometimes (4) Almost never (5) Never

32. You hate to bother other people with your hearing problem, so you pretend to understand.
(1) Almost always (2) Sometimes (3) Almost never
(1) Always (2) Almost always (3) Sometimes (4) Almost never (5) Never

33. You avoid wearing your hearing aid because it makes you feel different.
(1) Almost always (2) Sometimes (3) Almost never
(1) Always (2) Almost always (3) Sometimes (4) Almost never (5) Never

34. You are at a lecture on a subject of great interest. There is a microphone, but the speaker does not use it. You raise your hand and request that the speaker use the microphone.
(1) Almost always (2) Sometimes (3) Almost never
(1) Always (2) Almost always (3) Sometimes (4) Almost never (5) Never

35. You are at a lecture on a subject of great interest. There is a microphone, but it is not set loud enough for you to understand. You leave the meeting angry to complain to someone "in charge."
(1) Almost always (2) Sometimes (3) Almost never
(1) Always (2) Almost always (3) Sometimes (4) Almost never (5) Never

36. You are at a lecture on a subject of great interest. The speaker is talking too fast for you to understand. You leave the lecture because it has become a waste of time.
(1) Almost always (2) Sometimes (3) Almost never
(1) Always (2) Almost always (3) Sometimes (4) Almost never (5) Never

37. You are at a lecture on a subject of great interest. The speaker moves around so much that you have trouble understanding her. You complain to the organizers of the lecture after it is over.
(1) Almost always (2) Sometimes (3) Almost never
(1) Always (2) Almost always (3) Sometimes (4) Almost never (5) Never

38. You are at a holiday dinner. You can't understand the conversation because everyone is talking at once. You promise yourself you will not go back next year.
(1) Almost always (2) Sometimes (3) Almost never
(1) Always (2) Almost always (3) Sometimes (4) Almost never (5) Never

39. You are at a holiday dinner. You can't understand the conversation because everyone is talking at once. You ask for everyone's attention, explain the problem, and ask people to take turns so you can understand.
(1) Almost always (2) Sometimes (3) Almost never
(1) Always (2) Almost always (3) Sometimes (4) Almost never (5) Never

40. You are at a holiday dinner. You can't understand the conversation because everyone is talking at once. You explain the problem to the host so that he can handle the situation.
(1) Almost always (2) Sometimes (3) Almost never
(1) Always (2) Almost always (3) Sometimes (4) Almost never (5) Never

41. You are at a holiday dinner. You can't understand the conversation because everyone is talking at once. However, you don't say anything because you are glad to be at the party.
(1) Almost always (2) Sometimes (3) Almost never
(1) Always (2) Almost always (3) Sometimes (4) Almost never (5) Never

Attitudes

Please read each situation. Decide if the situation is true:
3-point: (1) Almost always, (2) Sometimes, or (3) Almost never
5-point: (1) Always, (2) Almost always, (3) Sometimes, (4) Almost never, or (5) Never
Please circle the appropriate answer. PLEASE RESPOND TO EACH QUESTION

1. I feel embarrassed when I don't understand someone.
(1) Almost always (2) Sometimes (3) Almost never
(1) Always (2) Almost always (3) Sometimes (4) Almost never (5) Never

2. I get upset when I can't follow a conversation.
(1) Almost always (2) Sometimes (3) Almost never
(1) Always (2) Almost always (3) Sometimes (4) Almost never (5) Never

3. I become angry when people do not speak clearly enough for me to understand.
(1) Almost always (2) Sometimes (3) Almost never
(1) Always (2) Almost always (3) Sometimes (4) Almost never (5) Never

4. I feel stupid when I misunderstand what a person is saying.

(1) Almost always (2) Sometimes (3) Almost never
(1) Always (2) Almost always (3) Sometimes (4) Almost never (5) Never

5. It's hard for me to ask someone to repeat things. I feel embarrassed.
(1) Almost always (2) Sometimes (3) Almost never
(1) Always (2) Almost always (3) Sometimes (4) Almost never (5) Never

6. Most people think I could understand better if I paid more attention.
(1) Almost always (2) Sometimes (3) Almost never
(1) Always (2) Almost always (3) Sometimes (4) Almost never (5) Never

7. I get angry when people speak too softly or too fast.
(1) Almost always (2) Sometimes (3) Almost never
(1) Always (2) Almost always (3) Sometimes (4) Almost never (5) Never

8. Sometimes I can't follow conversations at home. I still feel part of family life.
(1) Almost always (2) Sometimes (3) Almost never
(1) Always (2) Almost always (3) Sometimes (4) Almost never (5) Never

9. I feel frustrated when I try to communicate with people.
(1) Almost always (2) Sometimes (3) Almost never
(1) Always (2) Almost always (3) Sometimes (4) Almost never (5) Never

10. Most people do not understand what it is like to be hard of hearing. This makes me angry.
(1) Almost always (2) Sometimes (3) Almost never
(1) Always (2) Almost always (3) Sometimes (4) Almost never (5) Never

11. I am ashamed of being hearing impaired.
(1) Almost always (2) Sometimes (3) Almost never
(1) Always (2) Almost always (3) Sometimes (4) Almost never (5) Never

12. I get angry when someone speaks with his mouth covered or with his back to me.
(1) Almost always (2) Sometimes (3) Almost never
(1) Always (2) Almost always (3) Sometimes (4) Almost never (5) Never

13. I prefer to be alone most of the time.
(1) Almost always (2) Sometimes (3) Almost never
(1) Always (2) Almost always (3) Sometimes (4) Almost never (5) Never

14. My hearing loss makes me nervous.
(1) Almost always (2) Sometimes (3) Almost never
(1) Always (2) Almost always (3) Sometimes (4) Almost never (5) Never

15. My hearing loss makes me depressed.
(1) Almost always (2) Sometimes (3) Almost never
(1) Always (2) Almost always (3) Sometimes (4) Almost never (5) Never

16. My family does not understand my hearing loss.

(1) Almost always (2) Sometimes (3) Almost never
(1) Always (2) Almost always (3) Sometimes (4) Almost never (5) Never

17. I get annoyed when people shout at me because I have a hearing loss.
(1) Almost always (2) Sometimes (3) Almost never
(1) Always (2) Almost always (3) Sometimes (4) Almost never (5) Never

18. People treat me like a stupid person when I don't understand their speech.
(1) Almost always (2) Sometimes (3) Almost never
(1) Always (2) Almost always (3) Sometimes (4) Almost never (5) Never

19. Hard of hearing and hearing people often have difficulty communicating. It is only the responsibility of the hearing person to improve communication.
(1) Almost always (2) Sometimes (3) Almost never
(1) Always (2) Almost always (3) Sometimes (4) Almost never (5) Never

20. Hard of hearing and hearing people often have difficulty communicating. It is only the responsibility of the hard of hearing person to improve communication.
(1) Almost always (2) Sometimes (3) Almost never
(1) Always (2) Almost always (3) Sometimes (4) Almost never (5) Never

21. Members of my family get annoyed when I have trouble understanding them.
(1) Almost always (2) Sometimes (3) Almost never
(1) Always (2) Almost always (3) Sometimes (4) Almost never (5) Never

22. People who know I have a hearing loss think I can hear when I want to.
(1) Almost always (2) Sometimes (3) Almost never
(1) Always (2) Almost always (3) Sometimes (4) Almost never (5) Never

23. Members of my family leave me out of conversations.
(1) Almost always (2) Sometimes (3) Almost never
(1) Always (2) Almost always (3) Sometimes (4) Almost never (5) Never

24. Hearing aids don't always help people understand speech, but they can help in other ways.
(1) Almost always (2) Sometimes (3) Almost never
(1) Always (2) Almost always (3) Sometimes (4) Almost never (5) Never

25. I feel speech reading is helpful to me.
(1) Almost always (2) Sometimes (3) Almost never
(1) Always (2) Almost always (3) Sometimes (4) Almost never (5) Never

26. Even though people know I have a hearing loss, they don't help me by speaking clearly or repeating.
(1) Almost always (2) Sometimes (3) Almost never
(1) Always (2) Almost always (3) Sometimes (4) Almost never (5) Never

27. My family is willing to make telephone calls for me.

(1) Almost always (2) Sometimes (3) Almost never
(1) Always (2) Almost always (3) Sometimes (4) Almost never (5) Never

28. My family is willing to repeat as often as necessary when I don't understand them.
(1) Almost always (2) Sometimes (3) Almost never
(1) Always (2) Almost always (3) Sometimes (4) Almost never (5) Never

29. Hearing people get frustrated when I don't understand what they say.
(1) Almost always (2) Sometimes (3) Almost never
(1) Always (2) Almost always (3) Sometimes (4) Almost never (5) Never

30. Members of my family make it easy for me to speech read them.
(1) Almost always (2) Sometimes (3) Almost never
(1) Always (2) Almost always (3) Sometimes (4) Almost never (5) Never

31. Strangers make it easy for me to speech read them.
(1) Almost always (2) Sometimes (3) Almost never
(1) Always (2) Almost always (3) Sometimes (4) Almost never (5) Never

---

Source: From "Comunication Scale for Older Adults," by H. Kaplan, 1997. *Journal of the American Academy of Audiology, 8,* pp 203–217.

APPENDIX 16B: HEARING HANDICAP INVENTORY FOR THE ELDERLY-SCREENER

INSTRUCTIONS: The purpose of this questionnaire is to identify the problems your hearing loss may be causing you. Circle Yes, Sometimes, or No for each question. **DO NOT SKIP A QUESTION IF YOU AVOID A SITUATION BECAUSE OF A HEARING PROBLEM.**

E-1	Does your hearing problem cause you to feel embarrassed when meeting new people?	Yes Sometimes No
E-2	Does a hearing problem cause you to feel frustrated when talking to members of your family?	Yes Sometimes No
S-1	Do you have difficulty when someone speaks in a whisper?	Yes Sometimes No
E-3	Do you feel handicapped by a hearing problem?	Yes Sometimes No
S-2	Does a hearing problem cause you to visit friends, relatives, or neighbors less often than you would like?	Yes Sometimes No
S-3	Does a hearing problem cause you to attend religious services less often than you would like?	Yes Sometimes No
E-4	Does a hearing problem cause you to have arguments with family members?	Yes Sometimes No
S-4	Does a hearing problem cause you difficulty when listening to the TV or radio?	Yes Sometimes No
E-5	Do you feel that any difficulty with your hearing limits or hampers your personal or social life?	Yes Sometimes No
S-5	Does a hearing problem cause you difficulty when in a restaurant with relatives or friends?	Yes Sometimes No

Score E:

Score S:

Score T:

Source: Reprinted with permission of Barbara Weinstein.

APPENDIX 16C: HEARING HANDICAP INVENTORY FOR THE ELDERLY

INSTRUCTIONS: The purpose of this questionnaire is to identify the problems your hearing loss may be causing you. Circle Yes, Sometimes, or No for each question. **DO NOT SKIP A QUESTION IF YOU AVOID A SITUATION BECAUSE OF A HEARING PROBLEM.**

S-1	Does your hearing problem cause you to use the phone less often than you would like?	Yes Sometimes No
E-2	Does your hearing problem cause you to feel embarrassed when meeting new people?	Yes Sometimes No
S-3	Does your hearing problem cause you to avoid groups of people?	Yes Sometimes No
E-4	Does a hearing problem make you irritable?	Yes Sometimes No
E-5	Does a hearing problem cause you to feel frustrated when talking to members of your family?	Yes Sometimes No
S-6	Does a hearing problem cause you difficulty when attending a party?	Yes Sometimes No
E-7	Does a hearing problem cause you to feel "stupid" or "dumb"?	Yes Sometimes No
S-8	Do you have difficulty when someone speaks in a whisper?	Yes Sometimes No
E-9	Do you feel handicapped by a hearing problem?	Yes Sometimes No
E-10	Does a hearing problem cause you difficulty when visiting friends, relatives, or neighbors?	Yes Sometimes No
S-11	Does a hearing problem cause you to attend religious services less often than you would like?	Yes Sometimes No
E-12	Does a hearing problem cause you to be nervous?	Yes Sometimes No
S-13	Does a hearing problem cause you to visit friends, relatives, or neighbors less often than you would like?	Yes Sometimes No
S-14	Does a hearing problem cause you to have arguments with family members?	Yes Sometimes No
S-15	Does a hearing problem cause you difficulty when listening to the TV or radio?	Yes Sometimes No

S-16	Does a hearing problem cause you to go shopping less often than you would like?	Yes Sometimes No
E-17	Does any problem or difficulty with your hearing upset you at all?	Yes Sometimes No
E-18	Does a hearing problem cause you to want to be by yourself?	Yes Sometimes No
S-19	Does a hearing problem cause you to talk to family members less often than you would like?	Yes Sometimes No
E-20	Do you feel that any difficulty with your hearing limits or hampers your personal or social life?	Yes Sometimes No
S-21	Does a hearing problem cause you difficulty when in a restaurant with relatives or friends?	Yes Sometimes No
E-22	Does a hearing problem cause you to feel depressed?	Yes Sometimes No
S-23	Does a hearing problem cause you to listen to TV or radio less often than you would like?	Yes Sometimes No
E-24	Does a hearing problem cause you to feel uncomfortable when talking to friends?	Yes Sometimes No
E-25	Does a hearing problem cause you to feel left out when you are with a group of people?	Yes Sometimes No

Score E:

Score S:

Score T:

Source: Reprinted with permission of Barbara Weinstein.

APPENDIX 16D: HEARING PERFORMANCE INVENTORY REVISED*

Hearing Performance Inventory Revised

We are interested in knowing how your hearing problem has affected your daily living. Below you will find a series of questions that describe a variety of everyday listening situations and ask you to judge how much difficulty you would have hearing in these situations. Once we know which situations cause a person difficulty, we can begin to do something about them. Your answers will be confidential.

The questions cover many different listening situations. Some ask you to judge how well you can understand what people are saying when their voices are loud enough. The term *understand* means hearing the words a person is saying clearly enough to be able to participate in the conversation. Other questions ask whether you can hear enough of a particular sound (doorbell, speech, etc.) to be aware of its presence. Other questions concern occupational, social, or personal situations. Still others ask what you *do* when you miss something that was said.

To answer each question, you are asked to check the phrase that best describes how often you experience the situation being described:

Practically always	(or always)
Frequently	(about three-quarters of the time)
About half the time	
Occasionally	(about a quarter of the time)
Almost never	(or never)

For example, if you can understand what a person is saying on the telephone about 100% of the time, then you should check *practically always.* On the other hand, if you can understand almost nothing of what a person is saying on the telephone, then you should check *almost never.* If you can understand what a person is saying on the telephone about 50% of the time, then you should check *about half the time.*

Your answers to the questions should describe your hearing ability as it is now. If you wear a hearing aid in the situation described, answer the question accordingly. Please check one, and only one, phrase for each question. You should check *Does not apply* only if you have not experienced a particular situation or one similar to it.

There are also questions that appear identical but differ in at least one important detail. Please read each question carefully before checking the appropriate phrase.

We know that all people do not talk alike. Some mumble, others talk too fast, and others talk without moving their lips very much. Please answer the questions according to the way most people talk to you.

If the question does not specify whether the person speaking is male or female, answer according to which gender you have the most difficulty hearing.

1. You are watching your favorite news program on television. Can you understand the news reporter (female) when her voice is loud enough for you?
2. You are reading in a room with music or noise in the background. Can you hear a person calling you from another room?
3. You are with a male friend or family member in a fairly quiet room. Can you understand him when his voice is loud enough for you and you can see his face?
4. Can you hear an airplane in the sky when others around you can hear it?

5. You are watching a drama or movie on television. Can you understand what is being said when the speaker's voice is loud enough for you and there is music in the background?
6. Can you understand what a woman is saying on the telephone when her voice is loud enough for you?
7. You are at a restaurant and you hear only a portion of something the waitress/waiter said. Do you repeat the portion when asking him/her for a repetition?
8. You are with a child (6-10 years old) in a fairly quiet room. Can you understand the child when his/her voice is loud enough for you and you can see his/her face?
9. You are the driver in an automobile with several friends or family members. One or more of the windows are open. Can you understand the passenger behind you when his/her voice is loud enough for you?
10. You are at a restaurant and there is background noise such as music or a crowd of people. Can you understand the waiter/waitress when his/her voice is loud enough for you and you can see his/her face?
11. You are talking with a close friend. When you miss something important that was said, do you immediately adjust your hearing aid to help you hear better?
12. You are with five or six strangers at a gathering of more than 20 people and there is background noise such as music or a crowd of people. One person talks at a time. When you are aware of the subject, can you understand what is being said when the speaker's voice is loud enough for you and you can see his/her face?
13. You are at a play, movie, or are listening to a speech. When you miss something important that was said, do you ask the person with you?
14. You are with a child (6-10 years old) and several people are talking nearby. Can you understand the child when his/her voice is loud enough for you and you can see his/her face?
15. You are playing cards, Monopoly, or some similar game with several people and there is background noise such as music or a crowd of people. Can you understand what a friend or family member is saying to you when his/her voice is loud enough for you and you can see his/her face?
16. Does your hearing problem discourage you from attending lectures?
17. You are talking with five or six friends. When you miss something important that was said, do you ask the person talking to repeat it?
18. You are in an auditorium listening to a lecturer (female) who is using a microphone. Can you understand what she is saying when her voice is loud enough for you and you can see her face?
19. Can you hear water running in another room when others around you can hear it?
20. You are with a friend or family member and you hear only a portion of what was said. Do you repeat that portion before asking him/her for a repetition?
21. You are at a party or gathering of less than 10 people and the room is fairly quiet. Can you understand what a friend or family member is saying to you when his/her voice is loud enough for you, but you cannot see his/her face?
22. Does your hearing problem lower your self confidence?
23. You are in a fairly quiet room with five or six strangers. One person talks at a time. When you are aware of the subject, can you understand what is being said when the speaker's voice is loud enough for you, but you can not see his/her face?
24. You are with five or six friends or family members at a gathering of more than 20 people and several people are talking near by. One person talks at a time and the subject of conversation changes from time to time. Can you understand what is being said when the speaker's voice is loud enough for you and you can see his/her face?

25. When an announcement is given over a public address system in a bus station or airport, is it loud enough for you to hear?
26. You are talking with a stranger. When you miss something important that was said, do you ask for it to be repeated?
27. You are talking with a friend or family member. When you miss something important that was said do you pretend you understood?
28. You are at a fairly quiet restaurant. Can you understand the waiter/waitress when his/her voice is loud enough for you and you can see his/her face?
29. You are seated with five or six strangers around a table or in a living room. Often two persons are talking at once and one person frequently interrupts another. When you miss something important that was said, do you pretend you understood?
30. You are playing cards, Monopoly, or some similar game and the room is fairly quiet. The subject of conversation changes from time to time. Can you understand what is being said when the speaker's voice is loud enough for you, but you can his/her face?
31. You are at a party or gathering of less than 10 people and the room is fairly quiet. Can you understand what a friend or family member is saying to you when the speaker's voice is loud enough for you and you can see his/her face?
32. Does your hearing problem discourage you from going to concerts?
33. Do you find that children (6-10 years old) speak loudly enough for you?
34. When an announcement is given over a public address system in a bus station or airport, can you understand what is being said when the speaker's voice is loud enough for you?
35. You are seated with five or six strangers around a table or in a living room. Often two persons are talking at once and one person frequently interrupts another. Can you understand what is being said when the speaker's voice is loud enough for you and you can see his/her face?
36. You are seated with five or six friends around a table or in a living room. Often two persons are talking at once and one person frequently interrupts another. When you miss something that was said, do you ask the person talking to repeat it?
37. You are with a female stranger in a fairly quiet room. Can you understand her when her voice is loud enough for you and you can see her face?
38. You are with a stranger and there is background noise such as music or a crowd of people. Can you understand the person when his/her voice is loud enough for you, but you can not see his/her face?
39. Does your hearing problem tend to make you impatient?
40. You are talking with five or six strangers. When you miss something important that was said, do you let the person talking know you have a hearing problem?
41. You are at a party or gathering of less than 10 people and several people are talking near by. Can you understand what a friend or family member (female) is saying to you when her voice is loud enough for you and you can see her face?
42. Does your hearing problem discourage you from going to plays?
43. You are having dinner with five or six friends. When you miss something important that was said, do you ask the person talking to repeat it?
44. You are at a restaurant with a friend or family member and there is background noise such as music or a crowd of people. Can you understand the person when his/her voice is loud enough for you and you can see his/her face?
45. When you have difficulty understanding a person who speaks quite rapidly, do you ask him/her to speak more slowly?

46. You are talking to a woman sitting in a ticket or information booth and it is fairly noisy. She is giving directions or information. Can you understand her when her voice is loud enough for you and you can see her face?
47. You are having dinner with five or six friends. When you miss something important that was said, do you ask the person talking to repeat it?
48. When others are listening to speech on the radio or television, is it loud enough for you?
49. Does your hearing problem discourage you from going to the movies?
50. You are riding in an automobile with several friends or family members. One or more of the windows are open and you are sitting in the front seat. Can you understand the driver when his/her voice is loud enough for you and you can see his/her face?
51. You are at home watching television or listening to the radio. Can you hear the doorbell ring when it is located in the same room?
52. You are in a fairly quiet room talking with five or six strangers. One person talks at a time and the subject of conversation changes from time to time. Can you understand what is being said when the speaker's voice is loud enough for you and you can see his/her face?
53. You are seated with five or six friends or family members around a table or in a living room. Often two persons are talking at once and one person frequently interrupts another. When you miss something important that was said, do you remind the person talking that you have a hearing problem?
54. You are attending a stage play. Can you understand what the actors/actresses are saying when their voices are loud enough for you and you can see their faces?
55. You are with a friend or family member in a fairly quiet room, can you understand him/her when his/her voice is loud enough for you, but you cannot see his/her face?
56. A person is talking to you from a distance of no more than six feet with music or noise in the background. Would you be aware that he/she is talking if you did not see his/her face?
57. You are with five or six friends or family members and there is background noise such as music or a crowd of people. Can you understand what is being said when the speaker's voice is loud enough for you, but you cannot see his/her face?
58. When you have difficulty understanding a person with a pipe, toothpick, or similar object in his/her mouth, do you ask him/her to remove the object?
59. You are the driver in an automobile with several friends or family members. The windows are closed. Can you understand the passenger behind you when his/her voice is loud enough for you?
60. When you have difficulty understanding a person because he is holding his hand in front of his mouth, do you ask him to lower his hand?
61. You are at a party or gathering of more than 20 people and several people are talking near by. Can you understand what a stranger is saying to you when his voice is loud enough for you and you can see his face?
62. Do you feel that others cannot understand what it is to have a hearing problem?
63. You are at a movie. Can you understand what the actors/actresses are saying when their voices are loud enough for you and you can see their faces?
64. You are talking with five or six strangers. When you miss something important that was said, do you ask the person talking to repeat it?
65. You are at a party or gathering of less than 10 people and several people are talking nearby. Can you understand what a friend or family member (male) is saying to you when his voice is loud enough for you and you can see his face?
66. You are in a fairly quiet room. Can you carry on a conversation with a man in another room if his voice is loud enough for you?

67. You are with a male friend or family member and several people are talking nearby. Can you understand him when his voice is loud enough for you and you can see his face?
68. You are with five or six friends or family members. One person talks at a time. When you miss something important that was said, do you pretend you understood?
69. You are watching a drama or movie on television. Can you understand what is being said when the speaker's voice is loud enough for you and there is no music in the background?
70. You are with five or six friends or family members and there is background noise such as music or a crowd of people. One person talks at a time. When you are aware of the subject, can you understand what is being said when the speaker's voice is loud enough for you, but you cannot see his/her face?
71. You are at a lecture. If you have difficulty hearing what is being said, do you move to a place where you can hear better?
72. Does your hearing problem tend to make you nervous and tense?
73. You are with a female stranger and there is background noise such as traffic, music, or a crowd of people. Can you understand her when her voice is loud enough for you and you can see her face?
74. You are in a quiet place and the person seated on the side of your better ear whispers to you. Can you hear the whisper?
75. You are at a small social gathering. If you have difficulty hearing what is being said, do you move to a place where you can hear better?

Occupational Items

76. You are with a male coworker at work in a fairly quiet room. Can you understand him when his voice is loud enough for you and you can see his face?
77. You are with five or six coworkers at work. One person talks at a time. When you miss something important that was said, do you pretend you understood?
78. Does your hearing problem interfere with helping or instructing others on the job?
79. You are with a female coworker at work and there is background noise such as traffic, music, or a crowd of people. Can you understand her when her voice is loud enough for you and you can see her face?
80. You are with a coworker at work and you hear only a portion of what was said. Do you repeat that portion before asking the speaker for a repetition?
81. You are talking with a coworker at work. When you miss something important that was said, do you ask for it to be repeated?
82. You are talking with your employer (foreman, supervisor, etc.) and several people are nearby. Can you understand him/her when his/her voice is loud enough and you can see his/her face?
83. You are with a female coworker at work in a fairly quiet room. Can you understand her when her voice is loud enough for you and you can see his face?
84. You are talking with a coworker or employer. When you miss something important that was said, do you remind him/her that you have a hearing problem?
85. You are in a fairly quiet room at work with five or six coworkers. One person talks at a time and the subject of conversation changes from time to time. Can you understand what is being said when the speaker's voice is loud enough for you and you can see his/her face?
86. Does your hearing problem interfere with learning the duties of a new job easily?

87. You are seated with five or six coworkers around a table at work. Often two persons are talking at once and one person frequently interrupts another. Can you understand what is being said when the speaker's voice is loud enough and you can see his/her face?

88. You are talking with a coworker at work. When you miss something important that was said, do you pretend you understood?

89. You are with a male coworker at work and there is background noise such as traffic, music, or a crowd of people. Can you understand him when his voice is loud enough for you and you can see his face?

90. You are talking with a coworker at work. When you miss something important that was said, do you immediately adjust your hearing aid to help you hear better?

Note: Reprinted with permission from Stanford H. Lamb, Ph.D.

APPENDIX 16E: ABBREVIATED PROFILE OF HEARING AID BENEFIT*

INSTRUCTIONS: Please circle the answers that come closest to your everyday experience. Notice that each choice includes a percentage. You can use this to help you decide on your answer. For example, if a statement is true about 75% of the time, circle C for that item. If you have not experienced the situation we describe, try to think of a similar situation that you have been in and respond for that situation. If you have no ideas, leave that item blank.

A. Always (99%)
B. Almost Always (87%)
C. Generally (75%)
D. Half-the-time (50%)
E. Occasionally (25%)
F. Seldom (12%)
G. Never (1%)

	Without My Hearing Aid	With My Hearing Aid
1. When I am in a crowded grocery store, talking with the cashier, I can follow the conversation.	A B C D E F G	A B C D E F G
2. I miss a lot of information when I'm listening to a lecture.	A B C D E F G	A B C D E F G
3. Unexpected sounds, like a smoke detector or alarm bell, are uncomfortable.	A B C D E F G	A B C D E F G
4. I have difficulty hearing a conversation when I'm with one of my family at home.	A B C D E F G	A B C D E F G
5. I have trouble understanding dialogue in a movie or at the theater.	A B C D E F G	A B C D E F G
6. When I am listening to the news on the car radio, and family members are talking, I have trouble hearing the news.	A B C D E F G	A B C D E F G
7. When I am at the dinner table with several people and am trying to have a conversation with one person, understanding speech is difficult.	A B C D E F G	A B C D E F G
8. Traffic noises are too loud.	A B C D E F G	A B C D E F G
9. When I am talking with someone across a large empty room, I understand the words.	A B C D E F G	A B C D E F G

10. When I am in a small office, interviewing or answering questions, I have difficulty following the conversation.	A B C D E F G	A B C D E F G
11. When I am in a theater watching a movie or play, and the people around me are whispering and rustling paper wrappers, I can still make out the dialogue.	A B C D E F G	A B C D E F G
12. When I am having a quiet conversation with a friend, I have difficulty understanding.	A B C D E F G	A B C D E F G
13. The sounds of running water, such as a toilet or shower, are uncomfortably loud.	A B C D E F G	A B C D E F G
14. When a speaker is addressing a small group, and everyone is listening quietly, I have to strain to understand.	A B C D E F G	A B C D E F G
15. When I'm in a quiet conversation with my doctor in an examination room, it is hard to follow the conversation.	A B C D E F G	A B C D E F G
16. I can understand conversations even when several people are talking.	A B C D E F G	A B C D E F G
17. The sounds of construction work are uncomfortably loud.	A B C D E F G	A B C D E F G
18. It's hard for me to understand what is being said at lectures or church services.	A B C D E F G	A B C D E F G
19. I can communicate with others when we are in a crowd.	A B C D E F G	A B C D E F G
20. The sound of a fire engine siren close by is so loud that I need to cover my ears.	A B C D E F G	A B C D E F G
21. I can follow the words of a sermon when listening to a religious service.	A B C D E F G	A B C D E F G
22. The sound of screeching tires is uncomfortably loud.	A B C D E F G	A B C D E F G
23. I have to ask people to repeat themselves in one-on-one conversation in a quiet room.	A B C D E F G	A B C D E F G
24. I have trouble understanding others when an air conditioner or fan is on.	A B C D E F G	A B C D E F G

**Source:* Reprinted with permission of Robyn L. Cox.

APPENDIX 16F: GLASGOW HEARING AID BENEFIT PROFILE

Does this situation happen in your life?
0____No 1____Yes
Listening to the television with other family or friends when the volume is adjusted to suit other people.

How much difficulty do you have in this situation?	How much does any difficulty in this situation worry, annoy or upset you?	In this situation, what proportion of the time do you wear your hearing aid?	In this situation, how much does your hearing aid help you?	In this situation, with your hearing aid, how much difficulty do you now have?	For this situation, how satisfied are you with your hearing aid?
0__N/A	0__N/A	0__N/A	0_N/A	0_N/A	0_N/A
1__No Difficulty	1__Not at all	1__Never	1_Hgn aid no use	1_no difficulty	1_Not sat at all
2__Only sl diff	2__Only a little	2__about 1/4	2_Hng aid some help	2_Only slt diff	2_A little satis
3__Moder diff	3__A mod amt	3__about 1/2	3_Hng aid quite helpful	3_Mod diff	3_Reasonably
4__Great diff	4__Quite a lot	4__about 3/4	4_Hng aid is great help	4_Great diff	4_Very satisfied
5__Can't manag	5__Very much	5__All the time	5_Hng is perfect w/ aid	5_Can't manag	5_Delighted

Note: Reprinted with permission from Stuart Gatehouse.

APPENDIX 16G: HEARING AID PERFORMANCE INVENTORY

THE HEARING AID PERFORMANCE INVENTORY

INSTRUCTIONS: We are interested in knowing the extent to which your hearing aid helps you in your daily life. In this questionnaire you are asked to judge the helpfulness of your hearing aid in a variety of listening situations. You are asked to rate the benefit of your hearing aid in each situation and not the difficulty of the situation itself.

To answer each question, check the phrase that best describes how your hearing aid helps you in that situation.

——Very Helpful
——Helpful
——Very Little Help
——No Help
——Hinders Performance

There are items that appear similar but differ in at least one important detail. Therefore, read each item carefully before checking the appropriate phrase. We know that all people do not talk alike. Some mumble, others talk too fast, and others talk without moving their lips very much. Please answer the questions according to the way most people talk.

If you have never experienced the situation but can predict your hearing aid performance, respond to the item. A "Does Not Apply" response box is also provided. However, use the response "Does Not Apply" only if you do not know how helpful your hearing aid would be in the given situation.

Items

1. You are sitting alone at home watching the news on TV.
2. You are involved in an intimate conversation with your spouse.
3. You are watching TV and there are distracting noises such as others talking.
4. You are at home engaged in some activity and the telephone rings in another room.
5. You are at home in conversation with a member of your family who is in another room.
6. You are at a crowded outdoor auction bidding on an item.
7. You are listening to a speaker who is talking to a large group and you are seated toward the rear of the room. His back is partially turned as he makes notes on a blackboard.
8. You are starting to cross a busy street and a car horn sounds a warning.
9. You are riding on a crowded bus. You are in conversation with a friend seated next to you and you do not want others to overhear your conversation.
10. You are walking in the downtown section of a large city. There are the usual city noises and you are in conversation with a friend.
11. You are in a large office with the usual noise in the background (e.g., typewriters, air conditioners, fans, etc.). A coworker is telling you the latest gossip from close range in a soft voice.

12. You are riding in the back seat of a taxi. The window is down and the radio is on. The driver strikes up a conversation in a relatively soft voice.
13. You are driving your car and listening to a news broadcast on the radio. You are alone and the windows are closed.
14. You are in crowded grocery store checkout line and talking with the cashier.
15. You are alone in a small office with the door closed. People are talking quietly outside the door and you want to overhear their conversation.
16. You are at a crowded office picnic talking with a friend.
17. You are at home watching television and the doorbell rings.
18. You are with your family at a noisy amusement park and you are discussing which attraction to go to next.
19. You are taking an evening stroll with a friend through a quiet neighborhood park, there are the usual environmental sounds around (e.g., children playing, dogs barking).
20. You are at home alone listening to your stereo system (instrumental music).
21. You are listening to an orchestra in a large concert hall.
22. You are in whispered conversation with your spouse at an intimate restaurant.
23. You are in the kitchen in conversation with your spouse during the preparation of an evening meal.
24. You are at home in face to face conversation with a member of your family.
25. You are shopping at a large busy department store and talking with a salesclerk.
26. You are at church listening to the sermon and sitting in the front pew.
27. You are listening to a speaker who is talking to a large group and you are seated toward the rear of the room. There is an occasional noise in the room (e.g., whispering, rattling papers, etc.).
28. You are having a conversation in your home with a salesman and there is background noise (e.g., TV, people talking) in the room.
29. You are attending a business meeting where people are seated around a conference table. The boss is talking; everybody is listening quietly.
30. You are at church listening to the sermon and sitting in the back pew.
31. You are talking with a friend outdoors on a windy day.
32. You are driving your car with the windows up and carrying on a conversation with your spouse in the front seat.
33. You are in a small office interviewing for a job.
34. You are ordering food for the family at McDonald's.
35. You are at home reading the paper. Two family members are in another room talking quietly and you want to listen in on their conversation.
36. You are in a courtroom listening to the various speakers (witness, judge, lawyer).
37. You are talking with a teller at the drive-in window bank.
38. You are in a noisy business office talking with a stranger on the telephone.
39. You are in conversation with someone across a large room (such as an auditorium).
40. You are in conversation with a neighbor across the fence.
41. You are in a crowded reception room waiting for your name to be called.
42. You are in you backyard gardening. Your neighbor is using a noisy power lawnmower and yells something to you.
43. You are listening in a small quiet room to someone who speaks softly.
44. You are on an airplane and the stewardess is requiring a meal selection.
45. You are riding in a crowded bus and are in conversation with a stranger seated next to you.

46. You are alone driving your automobile and the cars around you are pulling to the side of the road. You begin to listen for what you anticipate is an emergency vehicle (firetruck, rescue squad, etc.).
47. Someone is trying to tell you something in a small quiet room while you have your back turned.
48. You are driving with your family and are listening to a news broadcast on the car radio. Your window is down and family members are talking.
49. You are driving your car with the windows down and are carrying on a conversation with others riding with you.
50. You are at an exciting sports activity (baseball, football game, etc.) and talk occasionally with those around you.
51. You are in a large business office talking with a clerk. There is the usual office noise (e.g., typing, talking , etc.).
52. You are in a quiet conversation with your family doctor in an examination room.
53. You are talking to a large group and someone from the back of the audience asks a question in a relatively soft voice. Audience is quiet as they listen to the question.
54. You are walking through a large crowded airport and are in conversation with a friend.
55. You are at a large noisy party and are engaged in conversation with one other person.
56. You are alone in the woods listening to the sounds of nature (e.g., birds, insects, small animals, etc.)
57. You are at the dinner table with your whole family and are in conversation with your spouse.
58. You are attending a business meeting where people are seated around a conference table. The discussion is heated as everyone attempts to make a point. The speakers are frequently interrupted.
59. You are one of only a few customers inside your bank and are talking with a teller.
60. You are at a theater watching a movie. There are occasional noises around you (e.g., whispering, wrappers rustling, etc.).
61. You are alone at home talking with a friend on the telephone.
62. You are downtown in a large city requesting directions from a pedestrian.
63. You are riding in a car with friends. The windows of the car are rolled down. You are in the back seat carrying on a conversation with them.
64. You are driving your car with the windows up and radio off and are carrying on a conversation with your spouse who is in the front seat.

APPENDIX 16H: PROFILE OF AIDED LOUDNESS

Profile of Aided Loudness (PAL)

Name ____ Date ____________________
Status: _______Unaided _______Previous Hearing Aids _______Current Hearing Aids

INSTRUCTIONS: Please rate the following items by both the level of loudness of the sound, and also by the level of satisfaction that you have for that loudness. For example, you might rate a particular sound as "Very Soft." If "Very Soft" is your preferred level for this sound, then you would rate your loudness satisfaction as "Just Right." If on the other hand, you would like the sound to be louder than "Very Soft," then your loudness satisfaction rating might be "Not Too Good" or "Not Good At All." The Loudness Satisfaction rating is not related to how "pleasing" the sound is to you, but rather, the appropriateness of the loudness. Here is an example:

The hum of a refrigerator motor:

Loudness Rating	*Loudness Satisfaction*
0 Cannot Hear	5 Just Right
1 Very Soft	4 Pretty Good
2 Soft	3 Okay
3 Comfortable, But Slightly Soft	2 Not Too Good
4. Comfortable	1 Not Good At All
5. Comfortable, But Slightly Loud	
6. Loud, But Okay	
7. Uncomfortably Loud	

In this example, the hearing aid user rated the loudness level of a refrigerator motor running as "Comfortable, But Slightly Soft" and rated his Loudness Satisfaction for this sound as "Just Right." This satisfaction rating indicates that this person believes that it is appropriate for a refrigerator motor to sound "Comfortable, But Slightly Soft."

Circle the responses that best describe your listening experiences. If you have not experienced one of the sounds listed (or a similar sound), simply leave that question blank.

Profile Of Aided Loudness (PAL)

1. An electric razor:

Loudness Rating	*Loudness Satisfaction*
0 Cannot Hear	5 Just Right
1 Very Soft	4 Pretty Good
2 Soft	3 Okay
3 Comfortable, But Slightly Soft	2 Not Too Good
4. Comfortable	1 Not Good At All

5. Comfortable, But Slightly Loud
6. Loud, But Okay
7. Uncomfortably Loud

2. A door slamming:

Loudness Rating
0 Cannot Hear
1 Very Soft
2 Soft
3 Comfortable, But Slightly Soft
4. Comfortable
5. Comfortable, But Slightly Loud
6. Loud, But Okay
7. Uncomfortably Loud

Loudness Satisfaction
5 Just Right
4 Pretty Good
3 Okay
2 Not Too Good
1 Not Good At All

3. Your own breathing:

Loudness Rating
0 Cannot Hear
1 Very Soft
2 Soft
3 Comfortable, But Slightly Soft
4. Comfortable
5. Comfortable, But Slightly Loud
6. Loud, But Okay
7. Uncomfortably Loud

Loudness Satisfaction
5 Just Right
4 Pretty Good
3 Okay
2 Not Too Good
1 Not Good At All

4. Water boiling on the stove:

Loudness Rating
0 Cannot Hear
1 Very Soft
2 Soft
3 Comfortable, But Slightly Soft
4. Comfortable
5. Comfortable, But Slightly Loud
6. Loud, But Okay
7. Uncomfortably Loud

Loudness Satisfaction
5 Just Right
4 Pretty Good
3 Okay
2 Not Too Good
1 Not Good At All

5. A car's turn signal:

Loudness Rating
0 Cannot Hear
1 Very Soft
2 Soft
3 Comfortable, But Slightly Soft
4. Comfortable
5. Comfortable, But Slightly Loud
6. Loud, But Okay
7. Uncomfortably Loud

Loudness Satisfaction
5 Just Right
4 Pretty Good
3 Okay
2 Not Too Good
1 Not Good At All

6. The religious leader during the sermon:

Loudness Rating
0 Cannot Hear
1 Very Soft
2 Soft
3 Comfortable, But Slightly Soft
4. Comfortable
5. Comfortable, But Slightly Loud
6. Loud, But Okay
7. Uncomfortably Loud

Loudness Satisfaction
5 Just Right
4 Pretty Good
3 Okay
2 Not Too Good
1 Not Good At All

7. The clothes dryer running:

Loudness Rating
0 Cannot Hear
1 Very Soft
2 Soft
3 Comfortable, But Slightly Soft
4. Comfortable
5. Comfortable, But Slightly Loud
6. Loud, But Okay
7. Uncomfortably Loud

Loudness Satisfaction
5 Just Right
4 Pretty Good
3 Okay
2 Not Too Good
1 Not Good At All

8. You chewing soft food:

Loudness Rating
0 Cannot Hear
1 Very Soft
2 Soft
3 Comfortable, But Slightly Soft
4. Comfortable
5. Comfortable, But Slightly Loud
6. Loud, But Okay
7. Uncomfortably Loud

Loudness Satisfaction
5 Just Right
4 Pretty Good
3 Okay
2 Not Too Good
1 Not Good At All

9. Listening to a marching band:

Loudness Rating
0 Cannot Hear
1 Very Soft
2 Soft
3 Comfortable, But Slightly Soft
4. Comfortable
5. Comfortable, But Slightly Loud
6. Loud, But Okay
7. Uncomfortably Loud

Loudness Satisfaction
5 Just Right
4 Pretty Good
3 Okay
2 Not Too Good
1 Not Good At All

10. A barking dog:

Loudness Rating
0 Cannot Hear
1 Very Soft

Loudness Satisfaction
5 Just Right
4 Pretty Good

2 Soft
3 Comfortable, But Slightly Soft
4. Comfortable
5. Comfortable, But Slightly Loud
6. Loud, But Okay
7. Uncomfortably Loud

3 Okay
2 Not Too Good
1 Not Good At All

11. A lawn mower:

Loudness Rating

0 Cannot Hear
1 Very Soft
2 Soft
3 Comfortable, But Slightly Soft
4. Comfortable
5. Comfortable, But Slightly Loud
6. Loud, But Okay
7. Uncomfortably Loud

Loudness Satisfaction

5 Just Right
4 Pretty Good
3 Okay
2 Not Too Good
1 Not Good At All

12. A microwave buzzer sounding:

Loudness Rating

0 Cannot Hear
1 Very Soft
2 Soft
3 Comfortable, But Slightly Soft
4. Comfortable
5. Comfortable, But Slightly Loud
6. Loud, But Okay
7. Uncomfortably Loud

Loudness Satisfaction

5 Just Right
4 Pretty Good
3 Okay
2 Not Too Good
1 Not Good At All

Source: Reprinted with permission of Catherine Palmer.

Normative Data
Profile of Aided Loudness (PAL)

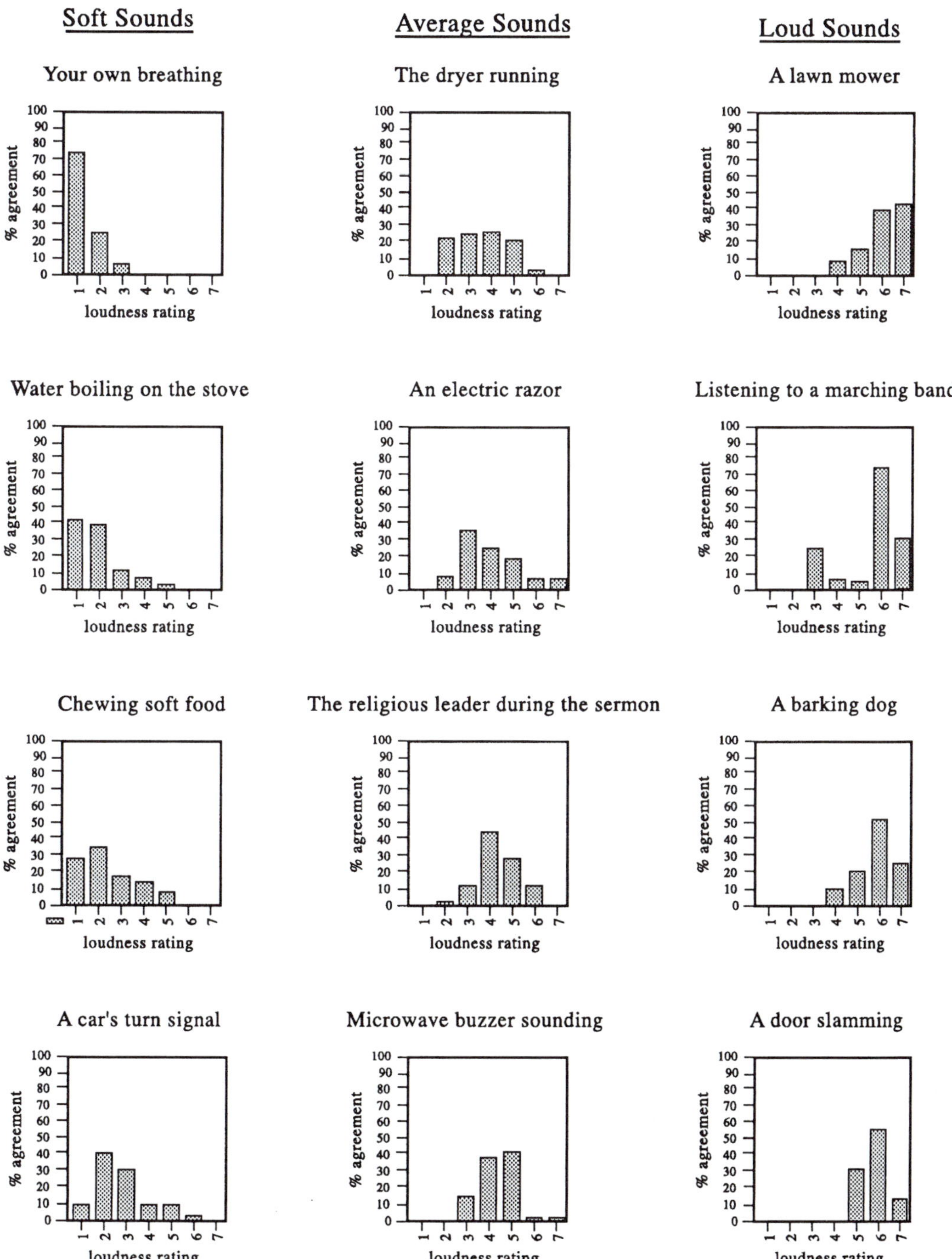

Note: Reprinted with permission from Catherine Palmer, Ph.D.

APPENDIX 16I: SATISFACTION WITH AMPLIFICATION IN EVERYDAY LIFE

Name ______________________________ D/O/B ____________ Today's Date ___________

INSTRUCTIONS: Listed below are questions about your experiences with obtaining and using your current hearing aid(s). For each question, please circle the letter that best corresponds to your opinion about your current hearing aid(s). Use the list of words below to determine your answer.

A: Not at all **B:** A little **C:** Somewhat **D:** Medium
E: Considerably **F:** Greatly **G:** Tremendously

Keep in mind that your answers should reflect your opinions about the hearing aids that *you are currently wearing or have most recently worn.*

While we would like you to answer every question, if you feel that a question cannot apply to your experiences, please write an "X" through the number in front of the question.

1. Compared to using no hearing aid at all, does your hearing aid(s) help you understand the people you speak with most frequently? A B C D E F G

2. Are you frustrated when your hearing aid(s) picks up sounds that keep you from hearing what you want to hear? A B C D E F G

3. Are you convinced that obtaining your hearing aid(s) was in your best interests? A B C D E F G

4. Do people notice your hearing loss more when you wear your hearing aid(s)? A B C D E F G

5. Does your hearing aid(s) reduce the number of times you have to ask people to repeat? A B C D E F G

6. Do you think your hearing aid(s) is worth the trouble? A B C D E F G

7. Are you bothered by an inability to turn your hearing aid(s) up loud enough without getting feedback (whistling)? A B C D E F G

8. How content are you with the appearance of your hearing aid(s)? A B C D E F G

9. Does wearing your hearing aid(s) improve your self-confidence? A B C D E F G

Experience with Current Hearing Aids:
❑ Less than 6 weeks
❑ 6 weeks to 11 months
❑ 1 to 10 years
❑ Over 10 years

Total Hearing Aid Experience
❑ Less than 6 weeks
❑ 6 weeks to 11 months
❑ 1 to 10 years
❑ Over 10 years

Daily Hearing Aid Use
Less than 1 hour
❑ 1 to 4 hours per day
❑ 4 to 8 hours per day
❑ 8 to 16 hours per day

Degree of Hearing Difficulties (without wearing a hearing aid)
❑ None
❑ Mild
❑ Moderate
❑ Severe

10. How natural is the sound from your hearing aid? A B C D E F G

11. How helpful is your hearing aid(s) on MOST telephones with NO amplifier or loudspeaker? A B C D E F G

12. How competent was the person who provided you with your hearing aid(s)? A B C D E F G

13. Do you think wearing your hearing aid(s) makes you seem less capable? A B C D E F G

14. Does the cost of your hearing aid(s) seem reasonable to you? A B C D E F G

15. How pleased are you with the dependability (how often it needs repairs) of your hearing aid(s)? A B C D E F G

Additional Comments: ____

____

____

____

____

____

____

Back of SADL

FOR AUDIOLOGIST'S USE ONLY

Hearing Aid Fitting Monaural Binaural

Right ear	Left ear
Make______________	Make______________
Model______________	Model______________
Ser. No.______________	Ser. No.______________
Fitting Date______________	Fitting Date______________

Hearing aid type	Hearing Aid Features (all that apply)		
CIC	Directional mic	Peak clipping	Multi-program
ITC	Output limiting	Multi-channel	K-amp
ITE	T-coil	WDRC	FM
BTE	Curvilinear	DAI	BILL
	Vent	Other______________	

Source: Reprinted with permission of Robyn L. Cox

APPENDIX 16J: ARE YOU PROVIDING QUALITY SERVICE?

Circle "Yes" or "No" for each question.

1. There is easy access for patients to my practice, including convenient parking, and they do not need to climb any stairs to get to my office.
☐ YES ☐ NO

2. I send maps or other written instructions to help new patients get to my office.
☐ YES ☐ NO

3. When a patient calls my office, there is someone knowledgeable available to help the person over the phone.
☐ YES ☐ NO

4. My office is a comfortable, well-lighted, climate-controlled facility with adequate working space. Amenities include coffee and other beverages, reading materials, information booklets, and comfortable chairs with arms.
☐ YES ☐ NO

5. Patients are not kept waiting if they arrive on time for their appointment.
☐ YES ☐ NO

6. When a patient has a problem, prompt help is available.
☐ YES ☐ NO

7. I use a "no pressure" sales approach.
☐ YES ☐ NO

8. The atmosphere in my office is friendly, and patience abounds. I always take a patient, unhurried approach to patients, no matter how busy I am.
☐ YES ☐ NO

9. For conducting hearing tests, I use a sound booth and a calibrated audiometer.
☐ YES ☐ NO

10. I give patients word-recognition tests at more than one level, as needed.
☐ YES ☐ NO

11. I use a fairly new, high-quality hearing aid test set.
☐ YES ☐ NO

12. I give clear, simple explanations, both orally and in writing, of all available hearing aids, including their price.
☐ YES ☐ NO

13. I have high-quality, informative, up-to-date booklets available for patients.
☐ YES ☐ NO

14. I have a functioning telephone amplifier device in my office that is demonstrated for every new patient; information on getting one is given to the patient.
☐ YES ☐ NO

15. There is an infrared TV system in my office that can be easily demonstrated to interested patients.

☐ YES ☐ NO

16. I follow a well thought out program for cerumen management, using written instructions and appropriate products and equipment, and I have received training from an accredited national association or some other formal instruction.

☐ YES ☐ NO

17. My practice has a facility for doing in-office minor repairs, including replacing broken battery doors, ear hooks, and tubing on earmolds (pre-bent tubing is mandatory), unplugging *deeply* impacted sound tubes, and using grinding/polishing equipment to adjust earmolds and shells.

☐ YES ☐ NO

18. I have a good supply of loaner BTE hearing aids (about 40) available for patients to use when their own hearing aids need to be sent in for service.

☐ YES ☐ NO

19. I have spare custom-made earmolds or high quality universal earmolds. (If you only have one or two boxes of 10-year-old universal earmolds, you don't get credit on this one.)

☐ YES ☐ NO

20. I provide batteries by mail.

☐ YES ☐ NO

Give yourself a point for every YES answer. If you scored 17 to 19, you did well.

Source: Reprinted with permission from "Nuts and Bolts: Are You Providing Quality Service, by R. Martin, 1997. *The Hearing Journal, 50*(8), 66.

APPENDIX 16K: ABC HEARING, INC. AUDIOLOGY SERVICES: EVALUATION AND/OR TREATMENT CONSUMER SATISFACTION MEASURE

READ each item carefully and **CIRCLE** the one answer that is best for you.

SA = Strongly Agree N = Neutral SD = Strongly Disagree A = Agree D = Disagree
NA = Not Applicable

1. Did we see you in a timely manner?

A. My appointment was scheduled in a reasonable period of time. SA A N D SD NA

B. I was seen on time for my scheduled appointment SA A N D SD NA

2. Did you benefit from Audiology Services?

A. I feel I gained valuable information from my visit. SA A N D SD NA

B. I feel I benefited from this appointment. SA A N D SD NA

3. Were you and your needs important to us?

A. The staff who serviced me were courteous and pleasant. SA A N D SD NA

B. Staff considered my special needs. SA A N D SD NA

C. Staff encourage participation by my family/friends/aides. SA A N D SD NA

4. Our staff are highly trained and qualified to serve you.

A. My clinician(s) were prepared and organized. SA A N D SD NA

B. My clinician(s) were experienced and knowledgeable. SA A N D SD NA

5. Was our office safe, acceptable, and accessible?

A. Health and safety precautions were taken when serving me. SA A N D SD NA

B. The environment was clean and pleasant. SA A N D SD NA

C. Test and consultation rooms were quiet and free of distractions. SA A N D SD NA

D. The office was easily accessible. SA A N D SD NA

6. Were your services and treatment efficient and comprehensive?

A. The purpose and nature of the procedures were explained clearly. SA A N D SD NA

B. My clinician(s) planned ahead and provided sufficient instruction. SA A N D SD NA

7. We respect and value your comments.

A. Overall, the program services were satisfactory. SA A N D SD NA

B. I would seek your services again if needed. SA A N D SD NA

C. I would recommend your services to others. SA A N D SD NA

My clinician(s) were: [ ] Ruth Smith [ ] Dan Owens [ ] Beverly Green [ ] Julie Carter

Comments:____

____

Thank you for your time. We will carefully review your comments to improve our practice!

Source: Reprinted with permission from ASHA Adaptation Office Survey, by American Speech-Language-Hearing Association.

CHAPTER 17

Psychology of Individuals with Hearing Impairment

ANDREW F. VALLA, M.S.
ROBERT W. SWEETOW, PH.D.

OUTLINE

Among the tools a successful hearing health care professional must possess is an understanding of the psychology of the individual with hearing impairment. As with any other group, individuals with hearing impairment possess a wide range of personalities, desires, and fears. By understanding the factors exerting influence on the thoughts and emotions of these patients, we will be better equipped to meet their amplification needs.

In this chapter, we will analyze the psychology of listeners with hearing impairment, how their behaviors and thoughts are shaped and developed by both internal and external factors and events, and how the hearing health care professional must utilize this knowledge in order to serve this population.

TERMINOLOGY

There may be confusion when discussing certain terms related to persons with hearing impairment. While there is some degree of overlap in these terms, we will use the following definitions as our discussion continues in this chapter:

A. *Hard of hearing*: disabled to an extent that makes difficult, but does not preclude, the understanding of speech through audition alone, with or without hearing aids
B. *Deafness*: disability that precludes understanding speech through the auditory channel alone, with or without the use of hearing aids
C. *Degree of loss*: generally categorized as mild, moderate, severe, or profound
D. *Disorder*: disease process or malformation of a physical system
E. *Impairment*: loss or abnormality of psychological, physiological, or anatomical structure or function.
F. *Disability*: restriction or lack of ability (resulting from an impairment) to perform an activity in a manner that is considered within the range of normal for a human being
G. *Handicap*: disadvantage for a given individual, resulting from an impairment or a disability, that limits or prevents the fulfillment of a normal role (depending on age, sex, social, and cultural factors)
H. *Benefit*: decrease in the amount and degree of handicap for an individual
I. *Satisfaction*: personal gratification comprised of a complex combination of benefit, communication needs, and personality traits

PSYCHOLOGICAL LEVELS OF HEARING

Ramsdell (1978) proposed that people function in an auditory sense at three different levels: primitive, warning, and symbolic. Each level has a distinct importance and therefore will be discussed separately.

Primitive Level of Hearing

A major boost in the interest of the psychology and rehabilitation of individuals with hearing impairment occurred following World War II when army veterans returning home complained of changes in their perception of the auditory world. Ramsdell hypothesized it was not simply the loss of the ability to understanding speech that so adversely affected these veterans but the loss of background environmental sounds that are heard subconsciously and taken for granted that were sorely missed. Hull (1992) stated that at the primitive level, sound functions as an auditory coupling to the world. People react to the changing background sounds around them without being aware of it. It is this level of hearing that connects us to our environment. A loss of hearing at the primitive level can cause disorientation and even result in an acute state of depression. Because this level of hearing is not at the conscious level, it may be difficult to identify it as the source of depression. Prominent audiologist Dr. Mark Ross recently noted a practical example of the effect of a loss of hearing at the primitive level. Ross (1999), who has a longstanding profound hearing loss, contracted an external ear infection and was unable to wear his hearing aids. As a result, sounds and noises that were otherwise taken for granted while wearing his hearing aids were no longer audible and left him "with a feeling of being cut off from the world."

Signs and Warning Level of Hearing

The next level of hearing goes beyond the realm of background sounds and interprets sounds that serve as warning signals and as signs conveying information. The warning level of hearing provides the listener with essential information about the environment. It is critical because audition can notify us of events that occur outside of the range of the other senses. Alerting sounds have a direct meaning attached to them and require an immediate response. Some examples of alerting sounds include a siren or a smoke alarm. At this level of hearing, not all sounds signal danger, however. Sounds also convey information about objects or events. Examples include a knock at the door or the ring of the telephone. The sound of an alarm clock informs us that it is time to wake up. When hearing is lost at this level, the individual's safety and connection with nonlanguage bearing information is altered. This can lead to feelings of insecurity. Because signal warning hearing and the associated meanings attached to these auditory symbols occur at the conscious level, compensatory strategies can and should be developed. It is also at this level that people utilize hearing as a tool to determine the location of sound (which can provide both warning information and information that will provide cues regarding how to position oneself so that the signal can be most efficiently received). Additionally, we utilize this stage of hearing to enhance our aesthetic pleasure, for example, when listening to music.

Symbolic Level of Hearing

The highest psychological stage of hearing occurs at the symbolic level. It is here that sound forms the major component of communication and becomes the foundation for language. A loss of hearing at the symbolic level may cause an individual who is hard of hearing to misunderstand certain key words in sentences. Even the emotional content of the spoken message can be lost if linguistic cues inherent in the sentence and prosodic cues bearing information about stress cannot be heard. Loss of hearing at this most identifiable level (communication) with other individuals can cause depression, withdrawal, and isolation.

HEARING LOSS CHARACTERISTICS

The psychological influence and the effect on personality that hearing loss bears on an individual may vary depending on 1) the degree of the impairment, 2) the time at which the loss occurred in the individual's life, and 3) the amount of handicap produced by the disability. These factors will influence the choices that the individual will make with regard to the effect the hearing impairment will exert on his or her life.

Degree of Hearing Loss

Individuals who have little or no usable hearing are likely to have a different perspective than individuals who have partial hearing and are able to utilize audition as the primary channel of receptive communication. For individuals with deafness, the realization that they must employ a sensory shift is apparent. For people who are hard of hearing, the propensity to "hold on" to what they have may lead to denial of the problem.

Recognizing inevitable individual variations, certain general statements can be posed regarding the difference in the manner in which individuals with deafness versus those with lesser degrees of hearing loss have historically been viewed and treated by society. As a consequence of this treatment, people with both degrees of hearing loss often face separate struggles and choices revolving around their hearing handicap.

Deafness

Individuals with deafness, as a group, have suffered the indignities of being treated as outsiders or even as people of inferior intellect. Such treatment rose from the historical concept that thinking could not develop without language, language could not develop without speech, and speech could not develop without hearing, hence the term "deaf mute." It therefore was concluded that those who could not hear could not think. Even Aristotle surmised that those born deaf were also dumb, hence the term deaf and dumb. Early Greek translators often interchanged the words for speechless and senseless. In the Roman Empire, individuals with hearing impairment who could not speak were stripped of all legal rights. Christians from St. Augustine's era believed that, unlike those with normal hearing, the deaf could not achieve immortality because they could not speak the sacraments. Legal statutes from the 19th century United States continued to impede the rights of the deaf. In New York, for example, deaf individuals were not allowed to vote. Ship owners arriving in the United States were required to report the names of all deaf persons on board and were obligated to pay exorbitant taxes (Higgins, 1980).

Today it is the unfortunate reality that individuals with greater degrees of hearing loss continue to be frequently excluded from or avoided by normal-hearing society. This prejudiced attitude is likely an outcome of the lack of education about deafness. The normal-hearing person watching people living with deafness sign or who hear their speech may, in fact, be fearful of his or her own inappropriate response to the situation. Ignorance breeds fear. This is not to imply that the struggles and choices made by a given deaf individual are created only by the reactions of the normal-hearing society. Individuals with deafness do have options. One of the most fundamental choices they can make is whether to attempt to assimilate completely into normal-hearing society with the help of hearing aids or cochlear implants or to assume their role as a member of the "deaf culture." One might argue that selection of the first choice affords a greater number of opportunities, both social and vocational. To do this, however, individuals must be willing to face both intentional and unintentional ridicule, to develop compensation strategies for enhanced communication, and to take chances.

The alternative choice persons living with deafness can make is to separate themselves from the normal-hearing world and enter into a lifestyle often termed "Deaf Culture." One could presume that deaf culture might be selected because the person's role in society might not be accepted by those with normal hearing. In other words, the person with deafness could be considered an outsider due largely to the cultural norms created and controlled by normal-hearing society. On the other hand, a person with deafness who desires to associate primarily with others who share similar struggles and life situations is no different, for example, than people who choose to befriend others who share an interest in art. If individuals desire acceptance into certain deaf cultures, they may be required to accept their values, particularly the use of American Sign Language (ASL), associate and identify primarily with other people who have significant degrees of hearing loss (Padden, 1980), and, relevant to this chapter, reject the use of amplification. Conversely, the benefits of this choice of lifestyle are that some of the struggles facing the individual who attempts to fully integrate into "normal-hearing" society may be minimized or eliminated. This individual may be rewarded with the luxury of "letting his or her guard down" and not feeling the need to hide the hearing disability.

Hard of Hearing

A major difference between the person who is hard of hearing and the person with deafness is that the hearing disability may not be as apparent to the rest of society. Therefore, the struggles and choices facing the person with a lesser hearing loss are often quite different than those for the deaf population. Because of learned reactions to disabilities, persons with lesser degrees of hearing loss must contend not only with society's reactions to their disabilities, but also with the internal psychological battle of acceptance of a loss. The choices they make regarding these struggles also will affect their quality and outlook on life.

Similar to people with deafness, persons who are hard of hearing must face the reaction of the normal-hearing society. Society's reactions to disabilities are strange and confusing. Traditionally, people with disabilities have been viewed in a negative and unsympathetic manner in many cultures and are often avoided (Ross, 1999). Frequently, there are behavioral changes that occur when normal-hearing persons first become aware that the individual they are engaged in a conversation with has a hearing loss. Why does this occur? Were they surprised by the individual's disability, did they feel like they were tricked in some way or taken advantage of? These reactions, no matter how inappropriate they may seem, are learned and practiced on almost a daily basis because this is how societal norms are structured. Conversely, when individuals who were once a part of this learned lifestyle recognize they have a hearing loss, they may withdraw or isolate themselves from society in an effort to protect themselves from being discovered. Danhauer, Johnson, Kasten, and Brimacombe (1985) identified the negative attitudes that normal-hearing individuals have when viewing people wearing hearing aids. They defined this as the "hearing aid effect." This effect is likely a contributing factor in the decision by many persons with lesser degrees of hearing loss not to pursue the use of hearing aids. These individuals thus must face a tough choice: to deny their hearing loss or to accept and recognize their disability and seek professional advise.

Time of Onset

The individual who acquires hearing loss after developing language may view hearing loss from a different perspective than an individual who has had hearing impairment since birth. To congenitally impaired listeners, their auditory status is their personal norm. Life without hearing has shaped the core of their lives; they only have the life experience of *not* being able to draw information about their environment from their sense of hearing. People who have a congenital hearing loss must face the challenge of learning language via channels that are not the primary route and gathering information about their environment through other means.

For individuals who lose their hearing following the acquisition of language, however, a different set of attitudes occurs. People who had normal hearing may have difficulty reconciling the prejudices and attitudes they developed at an earlier stage of life with their present hearing status. As their hearing loss becomes more conspicuous, this realization can create psychological strife because it becomes evident that they have a disability that will cause modifications to their daily life. As a result, insecurities may develop because of previously learned attitudes regarding hearing disabilities. Individuals who are hard of hearing may suffer from a lack of internal reference. For instance, they may face uncertainty regarding whether the messages being received from improperly functioning sensory organs are being interpreted accurately. They may be concerned that they are violating social rules by speaking at inappropriate loudness levels, asking others to repeat too often, and so forth (Hetu, Jones, & Getty, 1993). The hard of hearing may worry about misunderstandings that occur when they truly do not hear compared to when others incorrectly assume they are engaging in "selective listening." Their initial reaction may be to deny a hearing loss in order to justify remaining an active member of a normal-hearing society and to maintain a certain component of illusion that they do not have a hearing loss. It may be easier, or psychologically less painful, to deny the presence of a hearing loss and the necessity for hearing aids because these issues do not calculate into their perception of self–image (Orlans, 1985). In addition, the longer persons with hearing impairment deny their hearing loss and the longer they live with it, the more they may withdraw socially and develop other compensatory behaviors that may become difficult to break at a later time.

Handicap Produced by the Disability

Identical audiograms produced by similar impairments do not necessarily create comparable handicaps. Recall that handicap can be defined as a disadvantage for a given individual, resulting from an impairment or a disability, that limits or prevents the fulfillment of a normal role (depending on age, sex, and social and cultural factors). Thus, the handicapping effects of a hearing impairment are the combined result of the following elements:

- disorders
- impairments
- disabilities
- resources
- beliefs
- perceptions
- attitudes
- aptitudes
- lifestyles
- behaviors

Therefore, it is critical to recognize that it is the handicaps that become the critical issue to address in rehabilitation rather than the disability. Furthermore, not only does each individual present distinct sets of handicaps, but these handicaps are constantly changing throughout the course of the psychological adjustment to the hearing loss, as well as the rehabilitation process itself.

PSYCHOLOGICAL ADJUSTMENT TO HEARING LOSS

Kyle, Jones, and Wood (1985) described three phases (awareness, acceptance, and adjustment) that persons with hearing loss must transverse in order to come to terms with their disability. The length of time a person remains affixed in each stage depends on psychological state, family support, and expectations regarding the hearing impairment.

Awareness Phase

This first phase can last just a few days or as long as a lifetime. Recognition of a hearing loss during the awareness phase may actually begin as an unconscious event. An individual with a gradually progressing mild hearing loss may not even be aware of the deficit because the body and brain may be making the necessary calibration adjustments to compensate. As the hearing loss progresses, it reaches a point at which the individual becomes aware of a change in function. Consequently, compensation strategies are consciously or subconsciously developed to adjust for the change. Eventually, the disability becomes sufficient so that the person can no longer deny or hide its existence. When this occurs, the need for remedial help (hearing aids, aural rehabilitation, or both) may be recognized, though not necessarily accepted. As this awareness grows, so does the person's observation of other people's ears and the presence of hearing aids. This increasing awareness is analogous to that one encounters after buying a new car and realizing just how many other drivers own the same model. It occurs because the novelty of the car is in the forefront of the new owner's mind, and it is common to check out who else is driving the same automobile. As the newness wears off, the owner tends to notice the same car less and less because the interest wanes. Similarly, people with hearing loss in the awareness phase may turn their attention to other people's ears to view others wearing hearing aids, the style of device, and so forth. Prior to becoming aware of their own hearing loss, they paid no attention to people's ears, and if they did see someone wearing hearing aids, it was probably by accident. Once awareness of a personal hearing loss is reached, persons with hearing impairment may wish to discover which hearing aids are the most popular and least conspicuous so that they might continue to fit into a normal-hearing society in some capacity. Other individuals may become aware of their hearing loss via external channels. In other words, it may be the frequent remarks of others that will alert an individual that something is awry. Either way, it is necessary to first be aware of the loss before moving to the second stage, acceptance.

Acceptance Phase

The acceptance phase typically lasts a few months following awareness (Kyle, Jones, & Wood, 1985). When individuals come to terms with the fact that they have a hearing loss and are now willing to seek professional advice. This is a challenging time for both the hearing health care professional and the patient, as each may have separate goals and objectives they want to address. The hearing health care professional must not dismiss the person's fears of having a hearing loss. We will go into greater detail later in this chapter about the clinician's psychological influences in rehabilitation. Kyle et al. stated, "The diagnosis of decreasing hearing presents a wide range of unpleasant prospects; loss of all hearing, loss of job, independence, and control of social situations; rejection by family and friends; and fear of perceived stigma" (p. 124). It is the responsibility of the clinician to address these fears and gain the trust of patients. Only when this trust is established will patients be willing to accept hearing treatment options, such as amplification or aural rehabilitation.

Acknowledgement is the simple but crucial first step in successfully coping with a hearing loss (Ross, 1999). The first stage of an effective rehabilitation solution is an admission on the part of the individual that he or she has a hearing loss. It is crucial that the person recognize a hearing loss and begin to explore how this loss will affect his or her life and the lives of significant others.

Adjustment Phase

It is difficult to place an average length of time that individuals will spend in the adjustment phase because they are in a constant evolution of change and adjustment to their hearing loss. Adjustment involves establishing control over their disability and having the power to conform their environment to enhance speech understanding. A loss of power or control can result in an increased awareness of the disability, which can subsequently be transformed into increased handicap. It is believed that a person's power/powerlessness and ability to control situations is instilled during childhood and reinforced in adulthood (Lerner, 1979). We will return to the topic of power and powerlessness later in this chapter in the section discussing the effects of hearing loss on personality. The use of amplification and aural rehabilitation strategies, therefore, can provide the necessary assistance and information in order to institute increased control over personal listening situations.

EFFECTS OF HEARING LOSS ON PERSONALITY

Hearing loss can wield profound effects on aspects of an individual's personality. Three of the most important factors constituting a person's nature are emotions, behaviors, and relationships. These factors influence each other in a type of closed-circle manner. Emotions shape behaviors, behaviors alter relationships, relationships induce emotions, and so on.

Emotions

Negative emotions such as anger, anxiety, guilt, paranoia, embarrassment, frustration, and sadness are not confined to people with hearing loss, but the presence of an impairment certainly can fuel these feelings. People who have difficulty hearing at a cocktail party, for example, may experience a heightened sense of anxiety because they are concerned about responding inappropriately, ignoring someone speaking outside of their visual range, worried about statements others may be making "behind their backs," and so forth. These worries can produce tension, nervousness, irritability, and uncertainty. As stress and anxiety rise, understanding of speech can diminish as the listener tries too hard to distinguish every word and the probability of failure increases. The listener may become frustrated, guilty, or even angry, wondering why he or she has to be in this position. Alternatively, the listener may choose to deflect the blame on to others and suggest it is they who have the "mumbling" problem. In the extreme case, the listener with hearing impairment may develop serious depression (Meadow-Orlans, 1985).

Another force exerting an effect on emotions is the presence of fatigue. Normal-hearing individuals do not typically have to expend significant energy to hear in most environments. The impaired listener, on the other hand, may (even without recognizing the effort) need to physically strain to hear during much of the day. Increases in stress and fatigue produce physical changes, such as release of certain hormones and neurotransmitters that can diminish control over emotions. Thus, individuals with hearing impairment may recognize the heightened level of anxiety they experience in adverse listening situations and choose to withdraw and isolate themselves from that environment.

Behaviors

When a person experiences the negative emotions described above, a reaction—likely to take the form of a behavior—is soon to follow. As stated above, anxious, frustrated persons may decide that pain and embarrassment can be minimized or even eliminated by simply removing themselves from anxiety-producing situations. Isolation and withdrawal from social situations is indeed a common defense mechanism. Weiss (1973) describes two types of isolation. Social isolation results from being detached from a social network or community; emotional isolation stems from the loss or absence of an attachment figure. As a person withdraws more from society and social situations, important attachment figures also begin to withdraw from the individual with hearing impairment. Just as it may be easier psychologically for persons with hearing loss to avoid adverse situations and remain at home where they can regulate their listening environment, it may be easier for the normal-hearing person to avoid potentially difficult situations and the negative emotions carried by the anxious or unpleasant associate with hearing impairment. An individual with hearing loss can experience social isolation and emotional isolation simultaneously or separately. These behaviors are typically the result of past experiences and individual reactions toward hearing loss (Surr and Hawkins, 1988). In cases of withdrawal and isolation, persons with hearing losses may develop a certain amount of loneliness. Loneliness is often associated with other emotionally debilitating conditions, such as depression, grief, and anxiety (Dugan & Kivett, 1994).

As discussed earlier, another common behavior associated with psychological adjustment to hearing loss is denial. Kyle et al. (1985) stated that "denial of hearing loss is rational in terms of preserving a self-image, but dysfunctional from a control point of view and will almost certainly lead to rejection of situations that produce the dilemma" (p. 133). Individuals exhibiting this behavior mode are not ready to accept or deal with the effects of hearing loss and tend to make excuses for missed speech information (i.e., "everyone mumbles"). A time will be reached, however, when one's denial of a hearing loss may become intolerable to others who recognize the handicapping nature of the hearing impairment. One of the reasons this occurs is that even though behaviors develop as a consequence of experiences with a hearing disability, it may be difficult for those without disabilities to recognize these behaviors as a normal progression, and they may instead view them as an annoyance. This aspect of how an individual's hearing impairment affects others will be discussed shortly.

Individuals with hearing impairment can exert a certain amount of power and control over life's situations to keep themselves feeling secure and unthreatened by society. When listening in background noise, for example, it helps to be familiar with the topic being discussed, the talker's speaking pattern, and to be able to control the environment to increase understanding. Such controls include moving closer to the speaker, moving to a quieter area, positioning the speaker toward the better ear and away from the noise source, and so forth. Every individual's level of power varies based in part on personality, learned strategies, and the effort one will make to manipulate the environment. The person with a hearing loss often finds, however, that with the progression of a hearing disability, the strategies that had once worked so effectively no longer succeed. If the individual's sense of power to control situations becomes unreliable, a sense of powerlessness or learned helplessness develops. The individual's personality may influence how successful the adaptations will become. It is here that people make decisions that ultimately determine the degree to which the disability becomes a handicap.

There are many ways personality can be classified. A classification that has been shown to be particularly pertinent to hearing impairment is introversion versus extraversion. Persons who are introverted tend to direct their actions or events toward the self, in contrast to extroverted persons who direct actions or events toward the environment (Cox, Alexander, & Gray, 1999). Introverts dealing with the effects of a hearing disability may allow the loss to overtake their lifestyles and could become more withdrawn and isolated. Introverts may find it easier to avoid conflicts related to hearing disability rather than to experience the stress involved in trying to communicate with others. Introverts initially may not be prepared or confident enough to take on the issue of hearing loss by themselves.

Extroverts, on the other hand, use compensation strategies for listening but are not afraid to disclose their disability to a stranger. Extroverts do not easily allow themselves to be dismissed from society; they will do what is necessary to remain active members of the normal-hearing world. This characteristic may include the use of hearing aids to address their hearing disability.

Cox et al. (1999) reported that individuals' personalities influence their benefits from hearing aids. This research suggests that personality type is correlated with subjects' responses on the subjective Abbreviated Profile of Hearing Aid Benefit (APHAB). "Of the personality variables assessed, the introversion-extroversion dimension was clearly the most salient predictor of hearing aid benefit" (Cox et al., p. 10). The authors attributed this finding to the extrovert's external locus of control. It is recommended that since personality can be a possible predictor to successful use of a hearing aid, it should be assessed by the hearing health care professional.

It is also important to keep in mind that benefit from hearing aids does not equate to satisfaction with hearing aids. Cox (1997) estimated that satisfaction is comprised of 40% benefit (both psychosocial and acoustic), 25% personal image, 19% service and cost, and 16% negative features. In other words, a person may achieve significant benefit from hearing aid use, in terms of reducing handicap, but may still fail to be satisfied. Here too, personality and attitude play a major role in the final outcome.

Relationships

The effects of a hearing disability and the ensuing psychological adjustment can have damaging effects on interpersonal and family functions. All involved individuals experience separate and distinct issues regarding the hearing loss. "The impaired person experiences the disabilities (and the resulting handicaps) while the unimpaired person experiences the consequences as well as the effects of trying to adjust to these disabilities" (Hetu et al., 1993, p. 364). Embarrassment associated with the inability to understand spoken messages, fatigue from straining to hear, increased irritability and tension, social avoidance and withdrawal, rejection, negativism, and depression can have devastating effects on family relationships (Oyer and Oyer, 1985). It is for this reason that involvement of significant family members or friends is critical to the rehabilitation process. If only the person with hearing loss is involved, the burden of adjustment rests solely on his or her shoulders. The active participation of members in the support structure will provide the necessary information and education about hearing loss, as well as an understanding of the various psycho logical emotions and behaviors associated with a hearing disability. This knowledge will allow the persons without impairment to experience the consequences of the hearing loss as well as the effects of trying to adjust to disabilities (Hetu et al.). To illustrate this process, let's use a hypothetical example of a couple that has been living together for many years. As one of the members begins to lose hearing, the couple's comfortable and compatible lifestyle begins to change. Communication habits that had worked in the past may no longer be acceptable. Among the difficulties they may experience are understanding each other from separate rooms, carrying on conversations over the telephone, and even conducting discussions at the dinner table. In addition, the need to increase the volume of the television set can lead the couple to move to separate rooms when watching their favorite shows. This may reduce the shared experiences they would normally enjoy discussing together. Also, social situations may become a burden to the couple. Restaurants may seem too loud, and movie or theatre dialogue may be difficult to understand. The partner without hearing impairment may find a reduction in the activities he or she can participate in because of the spouse. Frustration may ensue because the normal-hearing spouse has to act as an interpreter and constantly fill in missed information. A modification in communication habits is thus required. If the adjustment process is going to be successful, both parties need to be involved. Each needs to take an active membership in the rehabilitation process in order for healthy adaptation to occur.

The personality characteristics of normal hearing partners can be a significant factor in their reaction to the onset of a hearing disability. The make-up of one's personality is molded and shaped throughout childhood. Personalities are shaped from observations, reactions to various issues, situations, and conversations of parents and family members. Personalities are refined and manipulated through interactions with the world through trial and error.

CULTURAL INFLUENCES OF AGE, DISABILITY, AND HEARING LOSS

The hearing health care professional needs to be sensitive not only to the auditory disabilities of individuals with hearing loss, but must also acknowledge and recognize the effect of cultural background and expectations on psychological impact and subsequent behaviors. Various cultures perceive disabilities in diverse manners. Hearing loss may be perceived as a weakness and, as dubious as the logic may be, an indication of aging. Psychological reaction to aging is also quite diverse and is dictated by many factors including individual feelings, familial expectations, and society's view of the elderly.

Some cultures rely heavily on the elderly for their guidance, experience, and knowledge. The aging process is embraced and valued. Younger individuals in these types of cultures learn the norms of society through the direction and observation of their elders. Other cultures, including our own Western culture, focus more on "the negative, the loss of self-esteem, the weakness, and increasing threats to security" (Busse, 1965, p. 81). Rather than embracing and living out this unique period of life, many people view aging as an inconvenience or a period leading to disability. The elderly in our culture frequently do not share their experiences because they are left out and because this culture focuses on the value of youth and youthful appearance. As a result, efforts are often made to curb or hide the aging process and the many physical and emotional challenges aging presents. People may try to hide the outward signs of growing old by having plastic surgery or dying their hair. Others may withdraw from social situations that highlight their growing physical limitations. Efforts to hide or delay the aging process may include a denial of health-related issues. The presence of a hearing impairment and the need for amplification may be summarily rejected simply because it is associated with aging and the underlining cultural message that the person is becoming weak and a burden on society. Steps need to be taken by the hearing health care professional to address not only the physical but also the psychological needs of the individual with hearing loss. It is the responsibility of the hearing health care professional to address healthy treatment options and strategies for managing the aging process and the person's hearing disability.

Just as cultural and social criteria affect reaction to a disability, they also may influence the way disabilities are addressed and dealt with. For instance, certain cultures may view disabilities as a sign of weakness that reflects a negative image on the entire family. This can lead to an additional emotional challenge for the impaired individual as that person begins to address physical needs through rehabilitation solutions. Thus, these individuals may be torn between their desire to achieve personal goals through rehabilitation at the same time be reluctant to seek help and show outward displays of physical needs (i.e. wearing hearing aids) because of the perceived impact their disability has on the family. It is interesting that some of the cultures that show the greatest respect for the elderly also have difficulty accepting the disabilities of the young. Therefore, the key for the hearing health care professional is to acknowledge and understand how the patient's culture may impact the acknowledgement and treatment of a disability. It is important to work with persons with hearing impairment to explore how their cultural norms and expectations will impact the treatment of their hearing disability.

THE CLINICIAN'S PSYCHOLOGICAL INFLUENCES ON REHABILITATION

Successful rehabilitation requires the collaboration of both the individual with the hearing impairment and the hearing health care professional. Persons with hearing loss are vital to the rehabilitation process in that they must be able to operationally articulate the various barriers and handicaps their hearing disorders are creating in their daily lives. Thus, they must not only recognize the various limitations of their hearing loss, but they must become active participants in the rehabilitation process. Concurrently, the hearing health care professional must be able to utilize counseling skills to break down emotional barriers producing denial, to motivate and to understand the individual's needs, and to convey information in a constructive manner (Sweetow, 1999a). This must be done not only for the patient, but for the family and critical members of the support structure as well.

A primary objective of the clinician in the rehabilitation process is to gain the patient's trust. This is a process that begins at the initial meeting and continues to develop over the course of the professional relationship. While hearing health care professionals focus on the assessment of their patients' hearing needs relevant to their lifestyle and medical background, their patients are developing opinions about the clinician's competence to provide the appropriate treatment and direction for their disability.

Sweetow (1999b) stated that there are three things patients with hearing impairment need to confirm about the hearing health care professional: (1) The professional knows what s/he is talking about, (2) the professional cares about the patient as a person, and (3) the professional has the patient's best interest at heart.

He goes on to say that clinicians must establish themselves as having the knowledge, the desire, and the ability to help the patient effect a desired change. Before advice can be offered that is regarded as having great value, the patient must be convinced of the professional's desire to be part of the solution. The patient must believe that the professional not only can help provide the answer to his or her hearing problem, but that the professional is emotionally vested in providing it. In short, the patient must feel that the professional cares.

One of the most effective methods of obtaining trust is through deep listening, creating an atmosphere of security, and identifying and understanding an individual's "salient event" (Hansen, 1998). A "salient event" is what brought the person into the clinic: the individual's own awareness of hearing difficulties or pressures from family or friends. "Salient events" provide the hearing health care professional with a base to understand individuals with hearing impairment and with insight into their emotional needs.

There are three facilitative conditions that must be present if a clinician is to be successful in the rehabilitation process: (1) empathy, (2) respect for the view and feelings of the individual, and (3) a relaxed, friendly attitude toward the person, coupled with an ability to accept criticism and communicate in an understandable manner (Kaplan, 1992). These conditions underscore the fact that each person is different and presents distinctive reactions to hearing impairment. The challenge for the hearing health care professional is to recognize these individual characteristics and stages of hearing loss acceptance and to provide the necessary counseling and treatment. Hearing health care professionals should foster the understanding that patients are not alone in their endeavor. The clinician needs to guide patients to view their hearing loss with hope and confidence so they can address their disability and reduce their handicap.

SUMMARY

- Among the tools a successful hearing health care professional must possess is an understanding of the psychology of the individual with hearing impairment. As with any other group, a wide range of personalities, desires, and fears characterize people with hearing impairment. By understanding the factors exerting influence on the thoughts and emotions of our patients, the professional will be better equipped to meet their amplification needs.
- Humans utilize their auditory sense at three different levels: primitive, warning, and symbolic. Hearing at the primitive

level occurs at an unconscious level and produces a connection to the environment; warning conveys information; and symbolic forms the major component of communication and becomes the foundation for language.

- The psychological influence and the effect on personality that hearing loss bears on an individual may vary depending on the degree of the impairment, how it affects the level of disability, the time at which the loss occurred, and the handicapping situations that result.
- There are three phases of psychological adjustment to hearing loss. The awareness phase is the time during which individuals recognize they have a hearing loss. The acceptance phase occurs when individuals come to terms with the fact that they have a hearing loss. The adjustment phase involves establishing control over their impairment and having the power to modify their environment to enhance speech understanding.
- Hearing loss can exert profound effects on aspects of an individual's personality. Three of the most important factors constituting a person's nature are emotions, behaviors, and relationships. These factors influence each other in a type of closed-circle manner. Specifically, emotions shape behaviors, behaviors alter relationships, relationships induce emotions, and so on.
- The clinician's directives in the rehabilitation process include not only the patient with hearing loss, but also their significant other. A key role the hearing health care professional plays is to develop an atmosphere that allows patients to accept their hearing loss and gives them the confidence to address their needs.

REVIEW QUESTIONS

1. What are the three different levels of hearing?
2. What society-based struggles do people with hearing impairments face?
3. What choices can people with hearing impairments make with regard to their hearing loss?
4. List the three psychological phases to hearing loss adjustment and identify one important factor that was discussed for each of the phase.
5. During the acceptance phase to psychological adjustment to hearing loss, what is the role of the hearing health care professional?
6. List some of the emotions and behaviors a person with hearing loss might exhibit.
7. What are some of the effects a hearing loss can have on significant others and/or family members?
8. Discuss the importance of personality traits of the individual with hearing impairment and how they apply to the prognosis success with hearing aids.
9. What is the significance of cultural influences on one's reaction to disabilities?
10. Name three facilitative conditions to successful rehabilitation.

REFERENCES

Busse, E. W. (1965). Research on aging: Some methods and findings. In M. A. Barezin & S. H. Cath (Eds.), *Geriatric psychiatry*. New York, NY: International Universities Press.

Cox, R. M., Alexander, G. C., & Gray, G. (1999). Personality and the subjective assessment of hearing aids. *Journal of the American Academy of Audiology, 10*, 1–13.

Cox, R. (1997). *Satisfaction from Amplification for Daily Living (SADL)*. Paper presented at the University of California, San Francisco/International Hearing Aid Seminars Audiology/Amplification Update III, San Francisco, CA.

Danhauer, J. L., Johnson, C. E., Kasten, R. N., Brimacombe, J. A. (1985). The hearing aid effect—summary, conclusions and recommendations. *Hearing Journal, 38*, 12–23.

Dugan, E., & Kivett, V. R. (1994). The importance of emotional and social isolation to loneliness among very old rural adults. *The Gerontologist, 34*, 340–346.

Hansen, V. (1998). Dealing with the psychological aspects of patient reluctance. *The Hearing Review, 5*, 8–14.

Hetu, R., Jones, L., & Getty, L. (1993). The impact of acquired hearing impairment on intimate relationships: Implications for rehabilitation. *Audiology, 32*, 363–381.

Higgins, P. C. (1980). *Outsiders in a hearing world*. Beverly Hills, CA: Sage Publications.

Hull, R. H. (1992). The impact of hearing loss on older persons: A dialogue. In R. H. Hull (Ed.), *Aural rehabilitation* (2nd ed., pp. 247–256). San Diego, CA: Singular Publishing Group.

Kaplan, H. F. (1992). The impact of hearing impairment and counseling adults who are deaf or hard of hearing. In R. H. Hull (Ed.), *Aural rehabilitation* (2nd ed., pp. 135–148). San Diego, CA: Singular Publishing Group.

Kyle, J. G., Jones, L. G., & Wood, P. L. (1985). Adjustment to acquired hearing loss: A working model. In H. Orlans (Ed.), *Adjustment to adult hearing loss* (pp. 119–138). San Diego, CA: College-Hill Press.

Lerner, M. (1979). Surplus powerlessness. *Social policy, 9*, 11–27.

Meadow-Orlans, K. P. (1985). Social and psychological effects of hearing loss in adulthood: A literature review. In H. Orlans (Ed.), *Adjustment to adult hearing loss* (pp. 35–57). San Diego, CA: College-Hill Press.

Orlans, H. (1985). Reflections on adult hearing loss. In H. Orlans (Ed.), *Adjustment to adult hearing loss* (pp. 179–194). San Diego, CA: College-Hill Press.

Oyer, H. J., & Oyer, E. J. (1985). Adult hearing loss and the family. In H. Orlans (Ed.), *Adjustment to adult hearing loss* (pp. 139–154). San Diego, CA: College-Hill Press.

Padden, C. (1980). The deaf community and the culture of deaf people. In C. Baker & R. Battison, (Eds.), *Sign language and the deaf community: Essays in honor of William C. Stokoe*. Silver Spring, MD: Aspen.

Ramsdell, D. A. (1978). The psychology of the hard of hearing and the deafened adult. In H. Davis & S. R. Silverman (Eds.). *Hearing and deafness* (4th ed., pp. 499–510). New York: Holt, Rinehart and Winston.

Ross, M. (1999a). *My "near deaf" experience*. Unpublished manuscript.

Ross, M. (1999b). *Why people won't wear hearing aids*. Unpublished manuscript.

Surr, R. K., & Hawkins, D. B. (1988). New hearing aid users' perception of the "hearing aid effect." *Ear and Hearing, 9*, 113–118.

Sweetow, R. W. (1999a). Counseling: It's the key to successful hearing aid fittings. *The Hearing Journal, 52*, 10–17.

Sweetow, R. (1999b). Counseling: The secret to successful hearing aid fittings. In R. Sweetow (Ed.), *Counseling for hearing aid fittings* (pp. 1–20). San Diego, CA: Singular Publishing Group.

Weiss, R. S. (1973). *Loneliness: The experience of emotional and social isolation*. Cambridge, MA: MIT Press.

CHAPTER 18

Considerations for Selecting and Fitting of Amplification for Geriatric Adults

ROBERT E. NOVAK, PH.D.

OUTLINE

(In 1988, when the first edition of the *Handbook of Hearing Aid Amplification* was published, the combined efforts of Drs. Glorig and Novak resulted in an excellent treatise on hearing problems among the geriatric population. Dr. Glorig was especially instrumental in describing some of the neurophysiological changing associated with the aging process. With the recent death of Dr. Glorig, the task of revising the chapter fell on the ample shoulders of Dr. Novak. Every attempt has been made to maintain the significant contributions of Dr. Glorig, yet offer needed revisions to be consistent with more recent knowlege relating to the aging patient and hearing aid use. One feels certain that Dr. Glorig would approve of the revisions.)

The number of persons age 65 years and older with hearing loss significant enough to interfere with communication is growing rapidly. It is estimated that 75 of 1,000 persons aged 65–74 years cannot hear and understand normal conversational levels of speech, with this number growing to 150 out of 1,000 (15%) of persons age 75 years and older (Ries, 1994). Others report that, by age 65 years, one third of the U.S. population develop a hearing loss serious enough to interfere with daily communication (National Ear Care Plan, 1999). As many as 48% or more of older residents of skilled nursing facilities also have hearing thresholds for the speech frequencies (500 Hz-4 KHz) in excess of 40 dB Hearing Level (HL), (re: ANSI, 1989) (Schow & Nerbonne, 1980). Currently, 12.5% of the United States population is 65 years of age and older. The population of 31 million persons over the age of 65 years in 1990 is predicted to increase to 65 million by the year 2030. It is predicted that 1 in 12 U.S. citizens will be 80 years or older by the year 2050 (Taeuber, 1992). Americans are living longer and generally healthier lives.

The geriatric population is marked by significant heterogeneity as it includes the "young old," for the purposes of this chapter defined as 65–75 years, the old, 76–85 years, and the old-old, 86 years and older. Within each of these groups again are a remarkably diverse cohort of people, with great variability in education, socio-economic status, family support, psychological and physical health, community avocational and ongoing vocational involvement. The over-65 group is also rich in its ethnic and cultural diversity, which affects how they view the need for aural rehabilitation and participate in the rehabilitation process. The majority of the population of persons over age 65 years with hearing impairment still do not seek help for their hearing loss. Seven million cannot afford hearing aids, and nearly 15 million experience prejudice and embarrassment about hearing loss that prevents them from seeking help (Better Hearing Institute, 1999). However, those who do seek amplification share many clinical issues and desired outcomes. The purpose of this chapter is to present a framework for audiologic intervention that emphasizes the desired clinical outcomes shared by the majority of geriatric patients, and to present information that should be considered when designing an amplification system and aural rehabilition program to achieve these goals.

The process of aging can be divided into three related fields: biologic aging, the physiologic changes that occur at all levels of the individual organism and in all of its functions; psychologic aging, the age-related changes that occur in the behavior of the individual (i.e., perceiving, feeling, thinking, acting, and reacting); and social aging, the changing roles of the individual in society as a result of age-related biologic and psychologic changes.

The first part of this chapter is concerned in part with the aging process in the auditory system. Technically, this is defined as hearing loss due to biologic and physiologic changes that are strictly a function of the cell and its organisms. It is impossible to extract age-related cellular changes from changes facilitated by the addition of environmental stressors (e.g., noise, disease, iatrogenesis). The fact that one ages physiologically and biologically also means that there are effects of changing environments over the aging period. Any study of aging and its effects must assume that the effects that are found are a combination of intrinsic biologic factors and extrinsic environmental factors. At best, the selection of amplification systems is not a simple task, and the probable effects of aging in the selection process should be evaluated. Subsequent portions of the chapter deal with various aspects of the application of hearing aids to the geriatric population with hearing impairment.

PRESBYCUSIS

Physiological Considerations

High-frequency hearing loss associated with aging was first described in 1891, as was the term presbycusis (Zwaardemaker, 1891). The original spelling was presbyacusis; however, presbycusis has become the preferred spelling. Pathologic studies have failed to identify anything pathognomonic of presbycusis. It appears to be a collection of different entities that occur in various combinations and affect the entire auditory system from the middle ear up to and including the central nervous system. There are predictable changes in function and such changes require special consideration in the evaluation, selection, and fitting of hearing aid devices.

If one looks at the external ear in the aged, one finds that it has become flabby, the earlobe has become larger and loose, and the ear canal has become quite flexible and sometimes has partially collapsed. These changes are due to changes in the elasticity of the skin as well as in the cartilaginous framework. Cartilaginous changes introduce a special concern when fabricating the earmold impression. The obvious problem presented is that, to make an acceptable impression, one must manipulate the ear in a manner that permits a canal opening adequate to allow the finished earmold, in-the-ear aid (ITE), or canal or CIC aid to pass amplified sound from the hearing aid earphone through the canal bore of the earmold, ITE, or canal hearing aid and, subsequently, to the eardrum.

Insertion of the earmold or hearing aid device into the external canal may produce soreness or irritation at the canal opening due to the sensitivity of the canal tissue when pressure is applied by the physical presence of the earmold or the canal portion of a hearing aid. These cartilaginous changes are so pronounced for some geriatric patients that the entrance to the canal is extremely narrow.

When the earmold impression is taken, the opening to the canal must be of sufficient size to permit effective use of the earmold. While taking the impression of the external ear canal, the pinna must be manipulated so that the narrow entrance to the canal opening is expanded to permit the impression material to be introduced and a usable ear impression to be taken. Sometimes, in an effort to make the opening as favorable as possible in the ear impression process, too much pressure is exerted against the canal wall when the finished product is inserted. It is this constant pressure that creates soreness or irritation and subsequent rejection of the device if early resolution is not provided. The impression gun technique, which mixes the agents of the impression material as it is inserted into the ear, is preferred for persons with collapsed canals. The impression material has a liquid consistency as it exits the gun that applies minimal pressure to the canal walls as the impression is being taken. Also, patients with extremely narrow canals are not good candidates for ITE aids and should be provided with BTE aids allowing for the use of earmolds that better accommodate the true architecture of the external ear canal.

Similar changes may occur in the structures of the middle ear, with associated changes in the sound transmission characteristics of the ossicles. This was demonstrated by Nixon and Glorig (1962) in a study of air- and bone-conduction thresholds as a function of age. They found an air-bone gap at 4000 Hz in many individuals age 55 years and older. Air-bone gaps also were discovered by Rosen, Bergman, Plester, El Mofty, and Sotti (1962) in their study of elderly members of the Mabaan tribe in rural Sudan.

Glorig and Davis (1961) reported that they believed that an air-bone gap of this kind could be caused by an inner ear conductive hearing loss as the result of changes in the basilar partition of the inner ear. These changes, which include the lessening of elastic tissue and the stiffening of the remaining components, have been identified via microscopic analysis. It is unclear what, if any, role these air-bone gap phenomena play in the determination of the recommended frequency-intensity response characteristics of the hearing aid. Their presence may account for a higher-than-expected Most Comfortable Listening level (MCL) at frequencies at which air-bone gaps occur. Higher MCLs may translate into higher gain prescriptions for older adults who have these air-bone gaps compared to other older and younger patients who have similar air-conduction thresholds but an absence of high-frequency air-bone gaps.

Schuknecht (1974) described four types of inner ear loss in presbycusis: sensoripresbycusis, neuropresbycusis, striapresbycuis, and inner ear conductive presbycusis. Glorig and Davis (1961) suggested a similar classification based on their own theoretical constructs.

Sensoripresbycusis is characterized by slowly progressive, bilaterally symmetrical high-frequency sensorineural hearing loss, with good single-syllable word identificaion. The primary histopathologic finding is an absence or reduction of hair cells, primarily in the basilar portion of the cochlea.

Neuropresbycusis is characterized by high-frequency sensorineural hearing loss with poor single-syllable word identification. Atrophy of the spiral ganglion and nerves of the osseous spiral lamina, mainly in the basal corridor, are the most consistent histopathologic finding with this type of presbycusis.

Striapresbycusis, or metabolic presbycusis, is characterized by a slowly progressive, flat, bilaterally symmetrical sensorineural hearing loss starting in the third through sixth decades of life. Single-syllable word identification is good, and there is usually no recruitment. The pathophysiology of striapresbycusis is related to the atrophy of the stria vascularis and a general reduction in sensitivity of all hair cells due to the metabolic changes of the endolymph.

Inner ear conductive presbycusis has been suggested by several authors (Glorig & Davis, 1961; Mayer, 1970; Schuknecht, 1974). Schuknecht (1974) described changes in the cochlear ducts that cause changes in the mass, stiffness, and friction of the moving membranes, thus affecting the transmission of acoustic energy. Mayer (1970) described thickening and hyalinization of the basilar membrane and calcium deposits located mainly in the basal coil. He suggested that the aging process of the basilar membrane causes stiffness and decreased mobility. The hypothesis of hearing loss due to increased stiffness of the basilar membrane correlates with its anatomical shape. The basilar membrane is narrow and thin at the basal coil and wide and relatively thick at the apical turn. The basal portion of the basilar membrane is more prone to loss of elastic properties due to aging, thus accentuating hearing loss in the high frequencies.

Figures 18–1 through 18–6 are diagrammatic representations of pathology found in microscopic studies of the temporal bones in individuals over 65 years of age. They are accompanied by pure-tone air conduction audiograms and word identification scores obtained by using phonetically balanced (PB) words. The diagrammatic cochlea shows hair cell rows. Open circles indicate cells that are pathologic. Note the correlation with the dark areas in the organ of Corti shown in the rectangles. Figures 18–1 and 18–2 show findings in patients with primarily cochlear pathology like that found with sensoripresbycusis. Figure 18–3 shows a patient with basal cochlear pathology and significant damage to the spiral ganglion. Note that, although pure-tone thresholds are normal through 2000 Hz, the PB score in quiet is only 82%.

Figure 18–4 shows more diffuse hair cell loss with spiral ganglion damage throughout the cochlea. These findings are consistent with the neuropresbycusis classification. Note the very poor (55%) PB-word identification score and compare it to the relatively good identification score of 80% in Figure 18–2, which depicts similar pure-tone threshold results but minimal spiral ganglion damage (sensoripresbycusis). The loss of central auditory nerve cells also may be related to a loss of synchrony in the central auditory pathways. Such a loss can be detected electrophysiologically by the decreased phase coherence of the middle latency response (MLR) in elderly adults exhibiting central auditory processing disorders (CAPD) (Musiek & Rintelmann, 1999). Audiometrically measured CAPD in the geriatric population is independent of peripheral loss of hearing sensitivity (Jerger, Jerger, Oliver, & Priozzolo, 1993), but the decreased speed of information processing created by CAPD can reduce speech discrimination sig-

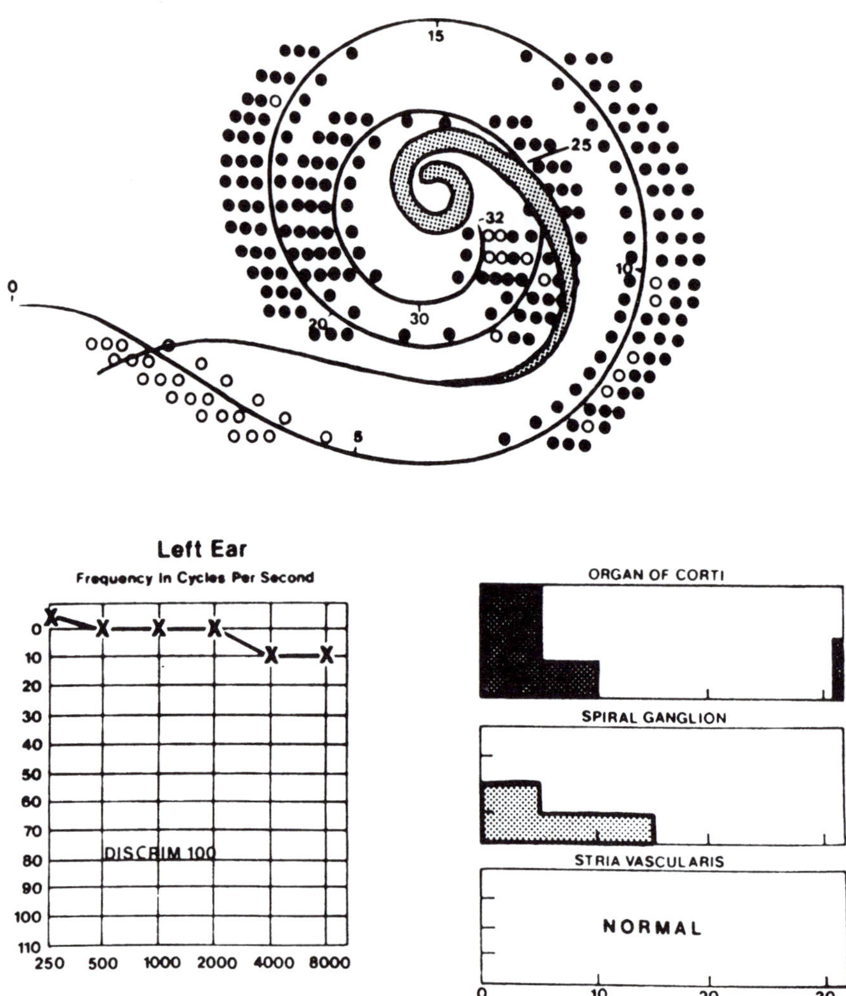

Figure 18–1. Pathology evident in a patient with primarily cochlear hair cell loss. Some damage also is evident in the spiral ganglia. Open circles indicate areas of hair cell loss.

nificantly. Jerger et al. (1993) found that CAPD can exist independently of cognitive dysfunction in the elderly. This is the case for most elderly patients who report that reduced conversational rate serves to enhance understanding of what was said.

Figure 18–5 depicts results consistent with the classification of striapresbycusis or metabolic presbycusis: minimum hair cell damage and spiral ganglion pathology but diffuse striavascularis abnormality. Note the excellent PB score (100%), which is consistent with this diagnostic classification.

Figure 18–6 depicts the results obtained from a patient with diffuse damage of the organ of Corti, spiral ganglia, and stria vascularis (a combination of types of presbycusis). Note the very poor word identification score. Of all the patients described, certainly this individual would have the poorest prognosis for benefit from the use of hearing aid amplification.

Of significance, when one reviews Figures 18–1 through 18–6, is that conventional pure-

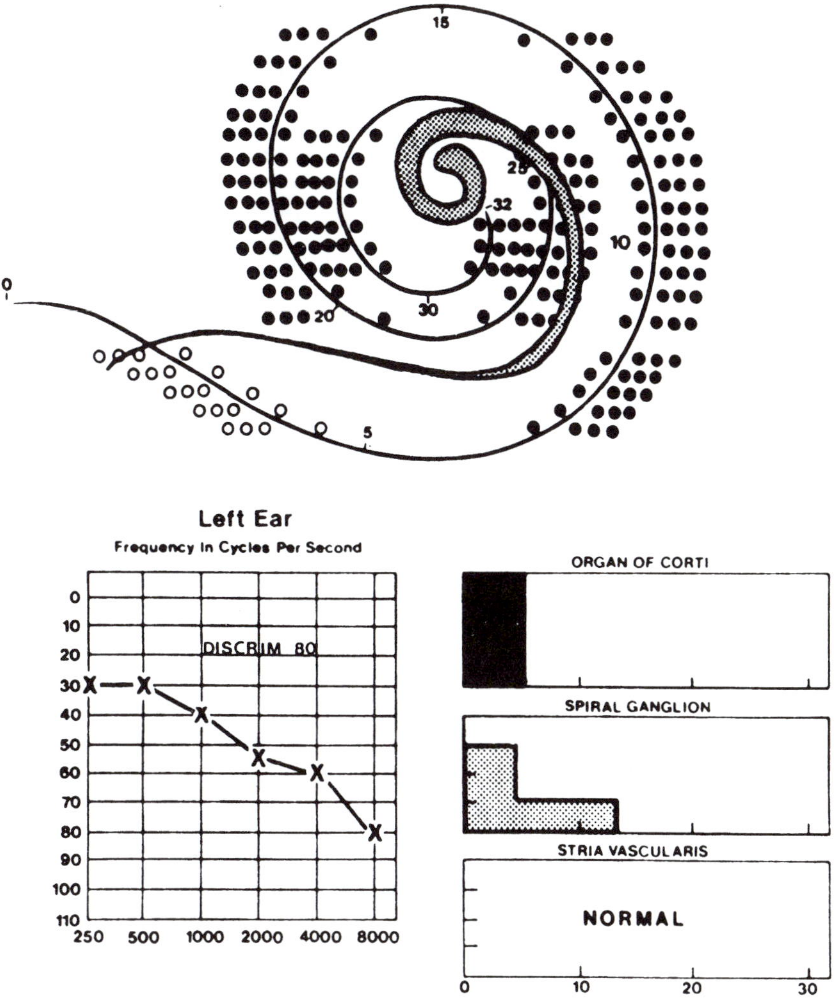

Figure 18–2. Pathology consistent with sensoripresbycusis. Open circles indicate areas of damage in the cochlea.

tone audiometry, in terms of signal detection, MCL, and tolerance discomfort thresholds, may not provide enough information to predict the benefit to be expected in understanding intended verbal messages when hearing aid amplification is provided. Although conventional word identification tests are suspect in ferreting out the best hearing aid device from among several choices, it is readily apparent that some form of speech or speech-like assessment is critical to the successful management of the aging patient. For example, the relatively low identification score shown in Figure 18–4 may suggest that appreciable improvement in speech understanding over time will not differ greatly from the measures obtained initially. Such an observation would have a profound effect on the counseling strategy devised to deal effectively with this patient as a result of the limitations imposed not only by the hearing aid but also by the auditory system itself.

Vasodilation is a common medical treatment for various inner ear diseases, including

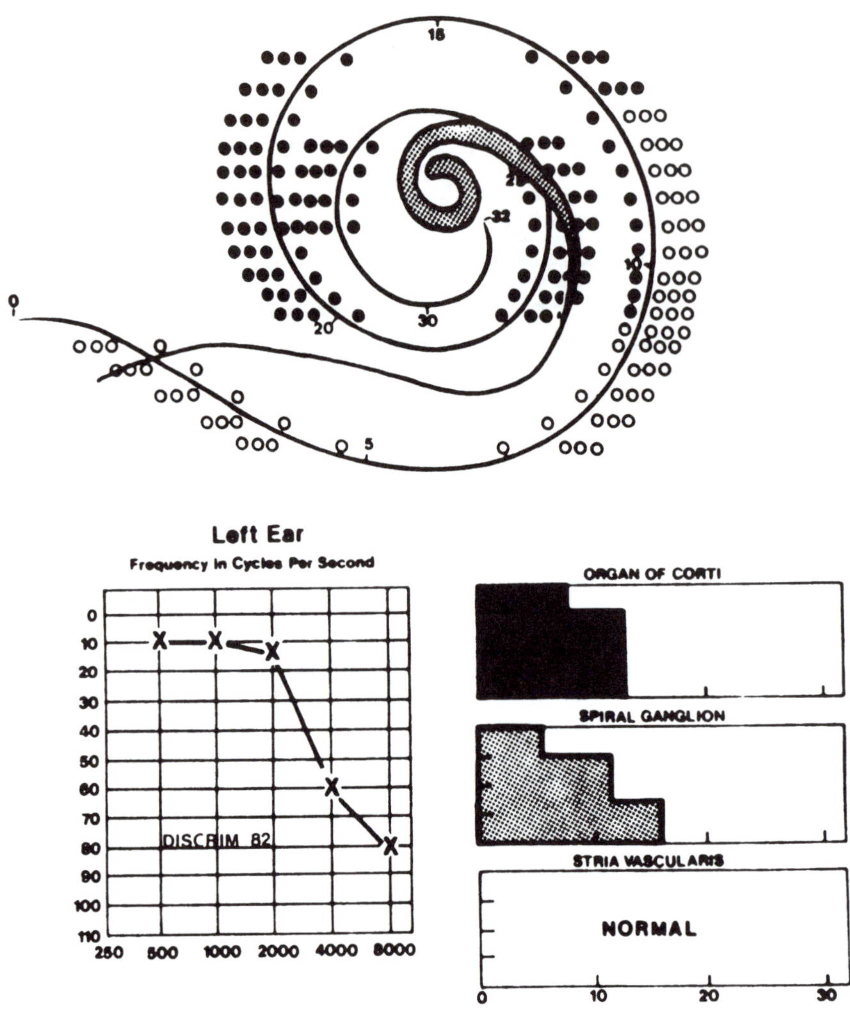

Figure 18–3. Pathology found in a patient with basal cochlear damage and marked changes in the spiral ganglion. Open circles show areas of cochlear damage.

Ménière's, sudden hearing loss, tinnitus, and presbycusis. The dependence of the inner ear on a single-ended artery without cross-circulation has led to speculation that vascular insufficiency may, in part, be the cause of these inner ear disorders.

Further understanding of pathologic processes in the internal auditory canal that are responsible for inner ear vascular degeneration and neural loss was contributed by the excellent observations of Krmpotic-Nemanic (1971). She studied 2600 temporal bones of all ages and demonstrated an apposition of fibrous osteoid and bony material in the fundus of the internal auditory canal in the region of the spiral tract, beginning at the basal coil. This process reduced the diameter of the hole in the spiral tract through which nerve bundles cross from the inner ear to the internal auditory canal. Hawkins and Johnsson (1985), citing similar findings, called this Hyperstotic Presbycusis. For patients who exhibit severe cochlear-vascular changes, the hearing health care professional should be aware of the pronounced limitations imposed on the probable contributions of the hearing aid.

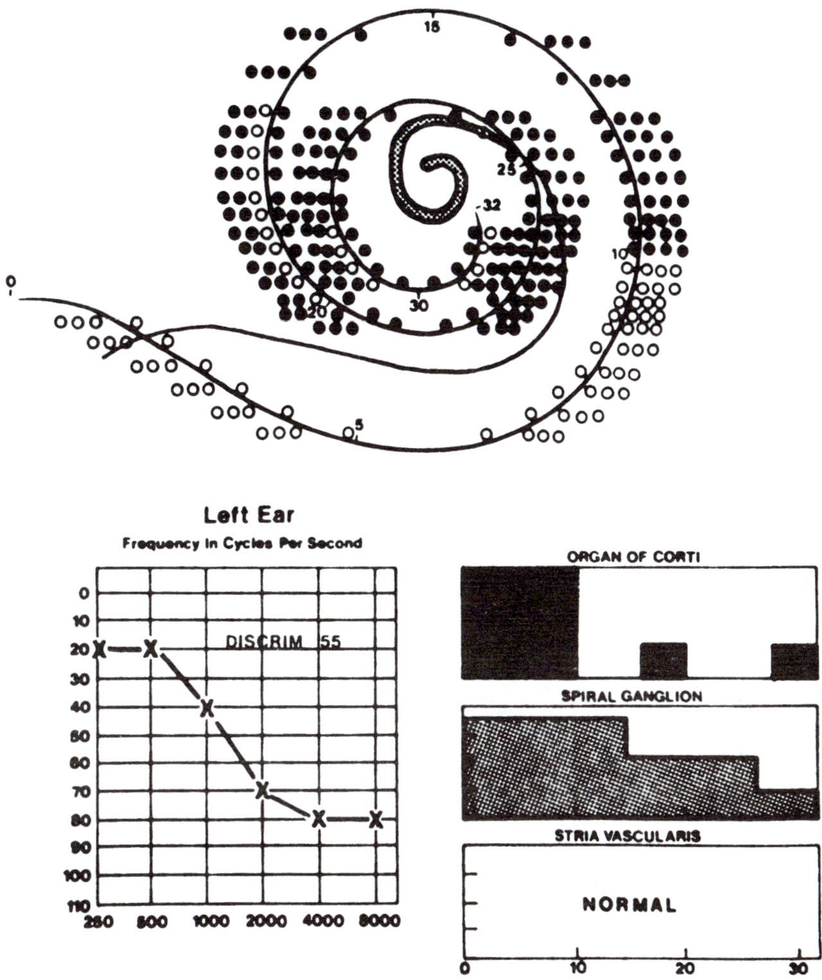

Figure 18–4. Pathologic findings for the patient shown indicate significant hair cell loss as well as spiral ganglion damage. Such findings are consistent with neuropresbycusis. Open circles indicate areas of damage in the cochlea.

Extrinsic Etiologic Factors

Hearing loss in the aging ear is believed to be the end result of the cumulative effects of various extrinsic factors in addition to genetically determined patterns of aging. There is a growing interest in environmental factors known to cause hearing loss that can be attenuated or eliminated as part of the overall efforts of hearing conservation.

Glorig and Nixon (1962) used the term socioacusis to describe the inevitable effects of daily, nonoccupational noise exposure. The hearing loss of aging, therefore, is the combined result of presbycusis (physiologic aging), socioacusis, and occupational noise.

Relation to Amplification

The end result of the many factors that cause hearing loss in the aged individual is multifaceted and highly complex. Some of these factors affect the application of amplification

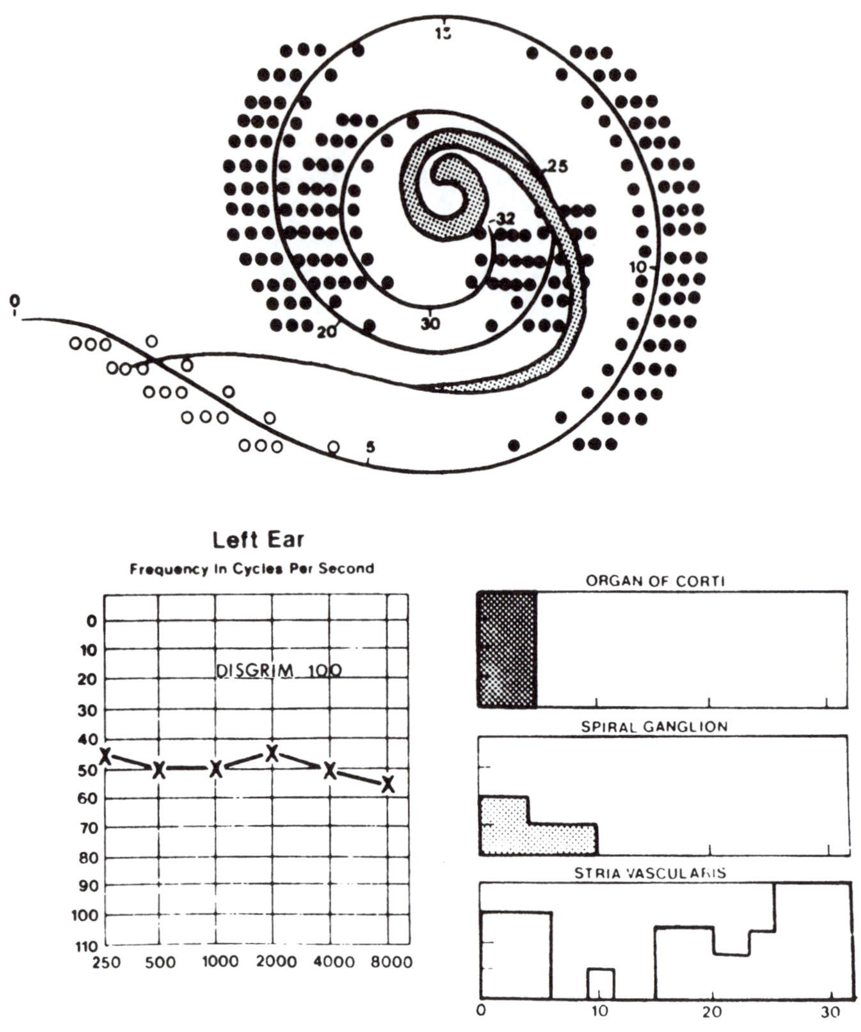

Figure 18–5. Hair cell loss consistent with striapresbycusis or metabolic presbycusis. Note the excellent word identification score. Open circles indicate areas of damage in the cochlea.

more than others. The primary biologic factor that limits adapting amplification to the aged ear is related to the pathology in the inner ear. Pathology that affects the spiral ganglion causes the most difficulty in applying successful amplification. In general, in the absence of causes directly affecting the hair cells, such as noise and ototoxicity, the pathology of aging lies principally in the changes in the spiral ganglion and the neural elements that leave the calyces of the hair cells and proceed through the auditory nerve to the various stations in the midbrain and cortex.

The cochlea serves as: (1) a coding mechanism in which the hair cells are the center of the coding system and (2) a processor of information, which is garnered by the hair cells and then transferred to the central nervous system by way of the neural elements.

In the case of abnormal first-order auditory neurons, the neural elements leaving the

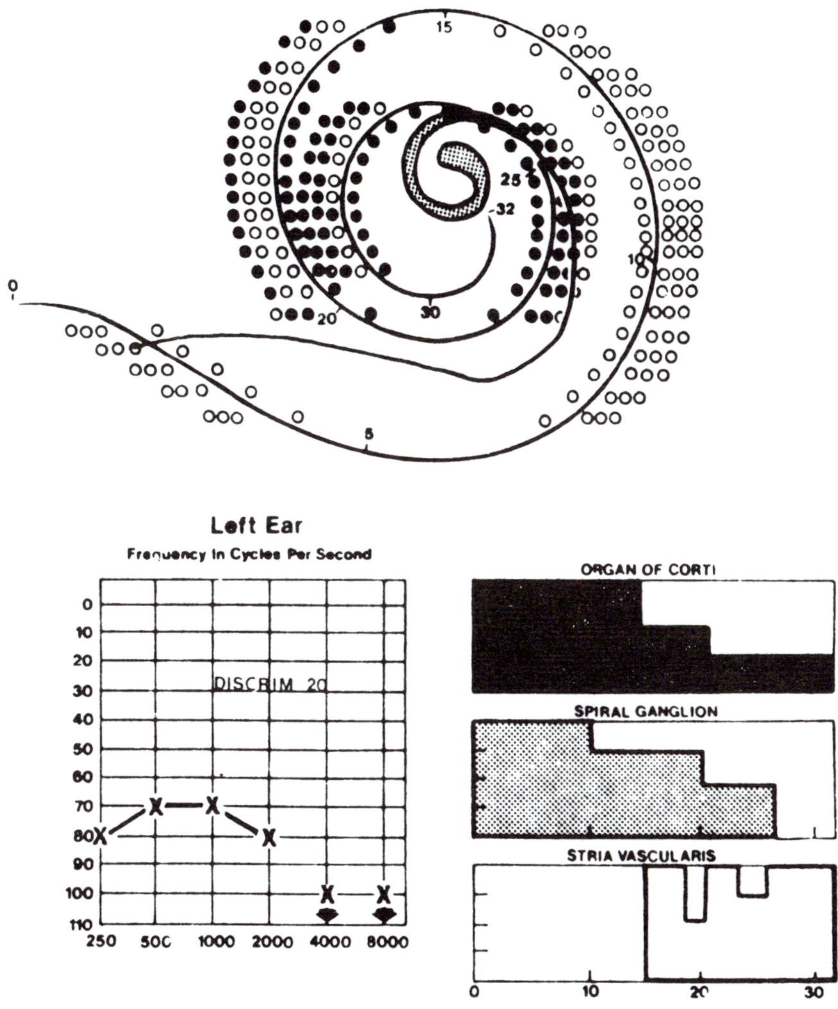

Figure 18–6. Pathology found in a patient with widely diffused damage of the organ of Corti, spiral ganglion, and stria vascularis. Note the poor word identification score for this patient. Cochlear hair cell loss is indicated by the open circles.

cochlea are reduced in their ability to process information. The decoding system, the central nervous system, thus receives sparse, poorly coded auditory information. In other words, the principal site of auditory processing is the neural system of the cochlea. If this is faulty, it is difficult to build an extrinsic signal processor (hearing aid device) to correct it. The success of extrinsic signal processing is highly dependent on the degree of pathology in the spiral ganglion and the neural elements that transmit auditory information to the cortex. Differences in amplification results found in patients with similar test data may be explained by differences in cochlear pathology that are not apparent in the test data. In these cases, amplification can be compared to trying to use a public address system with a defective microphone by tailoring the input to the microphone so that the output of the system will be understandable. This has never been done successfully. Good public address systems depend on good microphones or transducers. Successful use of traditional hearing aids depends on a functioning cochlea, which is present in varying degrees in persons with various types of presbycusis.

Independent of the presence of hearing loss and type of presbycusis when hearing loss exists, it has been reported that understanding of speech in noise is more difficult for geriatric patients than for their younger counterparts. The more difficult the speech material becomes, the more favorable the signal to noise ratio must be for older listeners to achieve the same listening performance as younger listeners. This is true even for older listeners with normal pure-tone sensitivity. (Dubno, Dirks, & Morgan, 1984; Schum, 1991). Difficulty understanding speech in noise is a universal complaint of geriatric patients with hearing impairment and presents a consistent challenge to the design of signal processing algorithms in hearing aids and the matching of these algorithms to the unique needs of each patient with hearing impairment.

In spite of the limitations of the geriatric auditory system, hearing health professionals should not give up trying to apply amplification to older persons with hearing losses because, to date, there is no other alternative. Minimal improvement in speech understanding skills is better than no improvement. The challenge for clinicians is to develop assessment procedures that allow the most specific application of amplification to each older hearing-impaired patient and follow-up protocols that maximize acceptance and successful use. To fully appreciate the factors related to hearing aid use in the geriatric population, practitioners also should be aware of the sociological and psychological factors presented by this population of individuals.

PSYCHOLOGICAL AND SOCIOLOGICAL PERSPECTIVES

In addition to changes in sensory and neural auditory processes, aging may be accompanied by modifications in adjustment strategies, problem-solving capacities and stress-coping responses, emotional states, perception, and memory (Mauldin, 1976). These changes are not consistent across the elderly population with hearing impairments and also may vary as a function of race and culture. The focus of this portion of the chapter is on the relationship these modifications have to the rehabilitation of hearing loss and specifically to the successful fitting of amplification devices in elderly populations.

As with their younger clinical counterparts, successful utilization of amplification by the geriatric population certainly is dependent on the critical audiometric factors of magnitude of loss in threshold sensitivity, reduced tolerance for loud sounds, and the related reduction in speech understanding skills. Although all hearing aid candidates have these problems, many hearing health professionals are not fully aware of other age-related factors that contribute to acceptance and use of amplification systems. Therefore, some of the behaviors manifested by the elderly are reviewed here and their importance in the consideration of hearing aid use is assessed.

Cultural influences, coupled with the aging process and the changes that accompany it, are often major determinants of the elderly adult's behavior. Social, physical, and economic conditions also may affect attitudes, assessment of need, and ability to afford hearing aid use and care in the face of other, sometimes more pressing, economic realities. The need for hearing amplification is a physical reality. The use and acceptance of any amplification system, however, is tempered by a number of other concerns.

The stereotype of the elderly as physically feeble, severely hearing impaired, partially sighted, and demented fits less than three percent of the aged population. This stereotype would be true if survival to the maximum life span of 110 years was typical (Eisenberg, 1985). Aging can be viewed as both positive and negative, as growth and decline; however, compared to years past, tomorrow's elderly adults will be living longer and healthier lives. The reality also is that the majority of them will be doing it with significant hearing loss requiring the need for amplification and aural rehabilitation.

Psychology of Adult Onset Hearing Loss

It has been documented recently that untreated hearing loss in older people can lead to a variety of problems including depression, anxiety, and social isolation (National Council on the Aging Survey, 1999). In a comparison of hearing aid using and non-using groups of hearing impaired older people matched for age, gender, and income, the study found hearing-impaired people who do not use hearing aids are more likely to report sadness, depression, worry and anxiety, paranoia, reduced social activity, and emotional turmoil and insecurity. For example, chronic sadness or depression was reported by 14% of hearing aid users versus 23% of non-users with mild hearing loss. Hearing aid users report improvements in many aspects of their lives, including their family relationships, sense of independence, and sex life. More than 2,000 family members or close friends of the hearing-impaired respondents asked a parallel set of questions also noticed the same improvement in the lives of the hearing-aid users.

Preference for nonuse of hearing aids by the elderly who are candidates for the use of amplification is related to a variety of variables. Popelka, Cruickshanks, Wiley, Tweed, and Klein (1998) found that the prevalence of hearing aid use among those with a pure-tone average greater than 25 dB HL (average of 500 Hz, 1 KHz, 2 KHz, and 4 KHz) in the poorer ear was 14.6%. The prevalence in a subset of the most severely affected subjects was 55%. Their analysis reveals that current hearing aid use was inversely correlated with word recognition scores, and directly correlated with age, education, severity of loss, self-reported hearing loss, self-perceived hearing handicap, and history of noise exposure. Garstecki and Erler (1998) found that non-use of hearing aids by those who have been advised to use them by hearing professionals is related to a variety of factors. Female users of hearing aids demonstrated greater hearing loss and poorer word recognition ability, but less hearing handicap, higher internal locus of control, higher ego strength, and fewer depressive tendencies than females who have not obtained recommended hearing aids. Female hearing aid users also assumed responsibility for effective communication. Male users of hearing aids were more accepting of their hearing losses, took responsibility for communication problems, and found hearing aids less stigmatizing than their male non-hearing aid using counterparts.

Seeking help for hearing loss is influenced by economic constraints. Maulding (1976) observed that certain consequences of aging present problems because they directly impact the older person's consumer needs. Digestive and metabolic changes may require changed diets. Changes in sensory processes, such as eyesight and hearing, may require eyeglasses and hearing aids; physical disabilities may require medical services, medical products, and institutionalization. The hearing health care professional must determine whether the hearing loss is considered a problem by the aged individual and, if it is a problem, where the remediation of hearing loss fits into the older person's priorities of consumer needs.

Cultural Considerations

In American culture, if one can generalize, the aged often have not been given, or allowed to assume, the esteemed role given to elders in some other societies (e.g., China). Rather, they often are treated with impatience and patronization. Approximately 6% reside in extended care facilities. For a significant subset of the older Americans, as their life expectancy increases, they are given less reason to live (Parenti, 1978). Chinese psychiatrist Wer Chen-1 contended that depression in the elderly is found more often in western cultures because "the west extrudes older citizens, they lose place in the family, industry, community, their sphere of influence collapses as does their morale, leaving them vulnerable to disability and disease" (Greenblat & Chien, 1983). When hearing loss exists in the older American patient, great potential for depression and low morale must be assessed as possible etiologies of a lack of desire to communicate and to pursue use of amplification and aural rehabilitation.

It is very difficult to make generalizations about older Americans due to the ethnic diversity of the population in the United States and the existence of relatively pure ethnic and cultural subgroups, such as Asians, native Americans, and "neighborhood" Hispanics and blacks. The sociological ramifications of group membership, sexual differences, and educational and economic levels in each of these subcultures relative to hearing help-seeking behaviors of their older members are complex and should be assessed. Although a thorough review of the help-seeking practices of all cultures represented among American elderly is beyond the scope of this chapter, the following is a fairly detailed account of how cultural differences among the Asian elderly may affect hearing aid use.

Cheng (1988, interview) described three subgroups of Asians in America: new immigrants; refugees, including those from Indochina, Vietnam, Laos, and Cambodia; and second-generation Asian-Americans. New immigrants are defined as people who came to the United States as young people after 1950. If they have hearing problems, they are the most likely to seek help. Refugees may rely on remedies from nontraditional health care providers for various ailments, including hearing loss. There are many sheltered, protected, and isolated older people in the refugee subgroup who do not speak English and who live with their extended families. Barriers to the pursuit of hearing health care and hearing aid use in this group include:

- fear of American culture
- illiteracy in their own language and lack of knowledge of English
- lack of knowledge of available help
- psychological maladjustment to life in the United States

The third subgroup is American-born Asians. Cheng described two subgroups within this group. The "Chinatown ghetto" group in which members are born, raised, and never leave the Chinatown area is limited in its understanding of hearing problems and access to audiologic services. On the other hand, individuals who left Chinatown early and established their own lifestyles typically have their own English-speaking physicians and may seek help if they have a hearing problem.

For all groups, Asian cultural themes affect behavior in response to significant hearing loss. A general Asian belief that aging is a natural process that does not require intervention is common. In Asian cultures, for example, the young show respect for adults with hearing impairment either by speaking loudly or nodding to the elder during conversation, even when they cannot hear or understand the speech. In this case, the elders may not feel a need to improve communication because they consistently are acknowledged during family conversations. If they purchase a hearing aid and it does not work satisfactorily, they will simply not wear it rather than seek confrontation. When asked if a problem exists, they will deny it ("How can the audiologist or the dispenser be wrong? It must be me.") Cheng (1988) asserted that these problems will not subside through acculturation in the forseeable future because increasing numbers of immigrants from Hong Kong and mainland China are expected in the coming years.

Culturally specific issues related to hearing help-seeking behaviors and application of amplification devices in all ethnic subgroups of the American population demand further investigation. The reader is referred to Spector (1996), Purnell & Paulanka (1998), and Geissler (1994) for more detailed information on transcultural issues as they relate to health, illness, and health care, all of which have direct application to the delivery of aural rehabilitative services to elderly members of other cultures.

Sociologic Considerations: The Nursing Home Population

Of elderly individuals living in the United States at any one time, only 5% to 6% live in intermediate and skilled convalescent care facilities (nursing homes). This aged subpopulation consists of four subgroups:

1. Residents who are in nursing homes for rehabilitation with the realistic expectation of again living independently in the community, depending to various degrees on community-based services and their own resources,
2. Residents who have physical limitations that prevent them from living independently but otherwise are mentally intact,
3. Residents who, like group 2, are limited physically and are also mentally impaired, and
4. Residents who are critically and terminally ill.

Nursing home residents, like all older people, have an increased desire for privacy. The paradox, however, is that institutional living reduces the ability to maintain privacy. For a significant subset of hearing-impaired adults, long-term nursing home residents, hearing loss may be their source of privacy, their insulation from the ever-present intrusions on their personal space. Ulatowska (1985) cited gestures, degree of eye contact, gaze, and orientation of body parts as methods used by nonambulatory nursing home residents to declare their territory and desire for solitude. Even a slight movement of the body or chair away from a fellow resident or staff member can indicate the termination of a conversation (Lipman, 1968). With this in mind, the hearing health care professional must ask what maintenance-of-privacy function the hearing loss serves for each of the subgroups of residents, and how truly motivated each group is to improve hearing for purposes of communication.

Specific hearing aid related services that the hearing health care professional might provide for each of these subgroups include the following:

Group One

For rehabilitation patients bound to return to their homes, the goal is to maximize the electroacoustic function of existing hearing aids and assure proper use and application of the hearing aids by the patient and nursing home staff, respectively. Electroacoustically appropriate loaner hearing aids or new hearing aids should be provided in cases in which patients need amplification and do not have their own hearing aids.

Maximum use of residual hearing by members of this group is of paramount importance if they are to have optimum receptive and expressive communication during the rehabilitation process.

Group Two

For permanent residents with good mentation, the goal is to maximize long-term life quality in the nursing home by allowing the hearing-impaired resident the option of using appropriate amplification when they desire to communicate. The ability to succeed in communicating when they desire to and when others must get through is imperative to the quality of life for this population of nursing home residents. The hearing health care professional, therefore, must ensure that:

- Residents have access to functional and appropriate amplification,
- Staff participate in regular staff inservice instruction in the use of amplification systems including personal hearing aids and assistive listening devices,
- They have regular (monthly) follow-up with residents using hearing aids on site,
- Hearing aid assessment and fitting procedures ensure valid application of amplification (the use of portable hearing aid test box/real-ear equipment is required if the hearing professional is to be able to deliver valid hearing aid services on-site),
- An in-house loaner hearing aid bank exists to ensure access to amplification for new and experienced hearing aid users (hearing aids in the loaner bank can be do-

nated by former residents, their families, and staff members, and electroacoustically analyzed and catalogued for appropriate use. Supportive aural rehabilitation programs and the availability of trained resident peer support and hearing-impaired patient advocate groups also are important for the optimum use of hearing aids by this subgroup), and

- Assistive devices (e.g., infra-red television listening systems, one-on-one communication systems such as the Pocket Talker, telephone amplifiers, etc.) are available either to augment the residents' hearing aids or to serve as the primary amplifier if personal hearing aids are not used or available.

Group Three

For the cognitively impaired long-term resident with hearing loss, the goal is to maximize functional mentation through the enhancement of meaningful sensory stimulation. The questions that the hearing health care professional must answer for this group include:

- To what degree is inadequate and inconsistent sensory input responsible for the resident's impaired mental health?
- Are the symptoms displayed by this subgroup indicative of true chronic brain degeneration (dementia) or can the symptoms, in part, be described as signs of pseudodementia with the etiology of those symptoms being reduced meaning of sensory input (e.g., remediable auditory dysfunction)?

To the extent that the latter is true, the hearing health professional is challenged to fit appropriate amplification and optimize successful use through effective staff involvement and support. The availability of portable auditory brainstem evoked potential equipment and distortion product otoacoustic emission equipment for assessing hearing loss and real-ear probe tube microphone systems for assessing the insertion gain provided by hearing aids and assistive devices can be very helpful in working with this subgroup. For this group, the use of one-on-one amplification devices such as the Pocket Talker under supervision when communication is desired may be preferable to the full-time attempted use of personal hearing aids.

Group Four

For the terminally-ill or dying resident, the goal is to support receptive and expressive communication through the final stages of the terminally ill resident's life. The hearing health care professional may be critical in facilitating meaningful communication of the terminally hearing impaired resident with his or her family physician, clergy, nursing staff, and friends. If hearing-impaired members of this subgroup are not currently hearing aid users, they are logical candidates for use of hearing aids provided from the facility's loaner hearing aid bank or use of institutionally owned assistive listening devices.

The hearing health care professional often must act as a vocal advocate for access of this patient subgroup to hearing aids and assistive listening devices. The Americans With Disabilities Act of 1992 certainly provides legislation to support equal access of residents with hearing impairment in public or corporately owned nursing home facilities. Access by the hearing professional to the hearing-impaired nursing home resident, in most cases, is determined by requests for services by the patient, nursing home staff, patient's physician, or family. Extended care facilities should have nonexclusive contracts with appropriate health care professionals to whom referrals for medical and audiologic intervention can be made. In most states, however, it is only with the consent of the resident's physician that these referrals can be consummated. Therefore, it is imperative for the nursing staff and personal physicians of extended care facility residents to be educated regarding the symptoms that indicate the need for and the potential benefit of appropriate intervention (e.g., hearing aids, assistive listening devices, aural rehabilitation therapy, otologic medical and surgical treatment) by hearing health care professionals.

Sociological Considerations: Physically Impaired Adults Living at Home

Ten percent of the elderly individuals who live at home are as functionally impaired as individuals who live in nursing homes. Mutual access of this subgroup of the aged population to the variety of hearing health care services is limited by the individual's motivation to seek help for hearing problems either because of low priority in the list of more fundamental human needs or because of minimal demands for communicative efficacy (i.e., few visitors, no televison or radio, no telephone use, or use of communication devices at high volume to compensate for the individual's hearing loss). Access is also limited by the person's ability to get hearing health care services for initial and necessary follow-up appointments. The logistical problems of follow-up may be so overwhelming to the individual that it may seem impossible to overcome them; therefore, the person does not try. If services are to be provided to this group, they must be more accessible to them than they typically are to the more flexible ambulatory consumer with hearing impairment.

Sociological Considerations: Independent Ambulatory Older Adults

Eighty-five percent of the older population live independently in varying stages of wellness and well-being. This group by far contains the majority of aged persons with hearing impairment. The total population of aged individuals with hearing impairment constitutes 55% of adults with hearing losses severe enough to interfere with receptive communication (Berkowitz, 1975). Of this population, Maurer and Rupp (1979) asserted that four out of five individuals are probably experiencing some communication problems in listening. Less than 25% of the persons over age 65 with hearing impairment who need and could benefit from amplification, however, have purchased hearing aids (Skafte, 1986). The reasons for this, surmised from clinical experience, include:

- Lack of acknowledgment of hearing loss as a problem,
- Lack of desire to rehabilitate acknowledged hearing loss,
- Lack of knowledge of available services and technology,
- Lack of appropriate support system and ability to manage use of hearing aids,
- Financial inability to purchase hearing aids,
- Erroneous understanding of what hearing aids can do and dissatisfied testimony from other hearing aid users or their own dissatisfaction with previous hearing aid use,
- Inadequate audiometric and psychosocial assessment of the residual auditory function and communication needs of the aged individual with hearing impairment,
- Amplification that was inappropriately applied because of electroacoustic and personal style preference inappropriateness, and
- Lack of or poor supportive aural rehabilitation services for the first-time hearing aid user.

Adjustment to Adult Onset Hearing Loss

Kyle, Jones, and Wood (1985) presented a model that described the phases of acquisition and adjustment to adventitious hearing loss in adults. It is important to assess which stage an individual is in when hearing aid assessment and fitting is being attempted. Phase 1, Acquisition of Hearing Loss, is described as the period when the loss is not acknowledged. It may last less than 1 month or go on for 20 years or more. It is the time period between initial onset of loss and the first visit to a hearing health care provider. Up to 75% of the population with acquired hearing loss may be in this phase at any time (Medical Research Council, 1981). During this phase, the unaided person receives feedback from the environment that he or she is talking too loud, the television or radio is too loud, he or she has misheard important information, and so on. During the initial stages of this phase, the person with hearing impairment ascribes the inability to hear to the faulty speech of others and other problems external to him- or herself. The initial visit to a hearing health care professional for evaluation may be made only in acquiescence to the demands of family members. Since realization of the existence of the loss is fundamental to initiation of help-seeking behavior, Kyle and colleagues suggested that when persons are forced to be in situations where they cannot control the volume of speech (e.g., lectures, church), they are apt to more quickly realize the extent of their impairment than if their time is spent in listening activities in which they can control the volume of speech (e.g., watching television) or ascribe their inability to understand to faulty connections (e.g., using the telephone) may be important. The use of self-assessment scales or hearing handicap inventories at the initial evaluation can help to shorten the duration of Phase 2 by focusing the individual on communication, social, and emotional problems they may be having that are related to their newly identified hearing loss.

Phase 2 is described as the time between first contact with a professional and diagnosis of permanent hearing loss and the receipt of a hearing aid. Kyle and colleagues found that, in England, where hearing aids are provided at no charge, this phase lasted a few months. In the United States, where the cost of hearing aids represents a significant financial investment, this phase may last a year or more. It is marked by uncertainty as to the ramifications of the newly identified hearing loss, and the resolution of this phase in large part is dependent on the accommodation and support of the person's family and friends. The resolution of this phase also is dependent on the person's willingness to accept responsibility for his or her own successful use of assertive communication techniques and speechreading skills taught in supportive aural rehabilitation sessions.

Phase 3 is the period of subsequent accommodation to the hearing loss. This phase is characterized by the individual's realization of the level of control he or she can expect to have in various communication settings. The ultimate goal of hearing aid fitting and supportive rehabilitation is to maximize the independence and control of the hearing-impaired individual in all desired communication environments. Kyle and colleagues cited maladaptive behaviors in this phase as behavioral changes resulting in: (1) excessive introversion and control of conversations with minimal listening, and (2) withdrawal from communication situations that threaten control and independence.

An acceptable resolution of Phase 3 is dependent on how the individual adjusts to the use of the hearing aid in various personal and social situations, vocational and avocational demands, and the dynamics of family life. It also depends on an optimum match between how much control an individual believes they have over the rehabilitation of his or her hearing loss (internal versus external locus of control) versus how much control truly exists. Also fundamental to adjustment to the hearing aid are acceptance of its physical appearance, optimum electroacoustic compatibility with and compensation for the hearing loss, independence in the use of the amplification system, acknowledgment of the use of a less than perfect amplification system to others with whom communication is initiated, and realistic expectations of others regarding the aided benefit the new hearing aid user can derive in a variety of listening environments.

Kyle and Wood (1983) found that, although 89% of their aided respondents had difficulty with street conversations, 79% would not tell people that they had a hearing problem. This also is typical of the reactions of new hearing aid users in the United States. If audiologists and dispensers were able to match perfectly the hearing aid configuration to the psychophysical needs of the patient, there would be no need for public acknowledgment of the loss and the use of hearing aids. However, given the fact that current hearing aids do not fully restore normal hearing function in the damaged cochlea and central auditory pathways, acknowledgment of the hearing loss and use of hearing aids remain critical to the successful resolution of the aural rehabilitation process.

The remainder of this chapter deals with assessment and intervention strategies.

AUDITORY ASSESSMENT FINDINGS IN THE AGED POPULATION

This section concentrates on threshold and suprathreshold auditory function in the aged listener. This information is, of course, most important when considering appropriate assessment and intervention strategies to amplify the older patient with hearing impairment.

Marshall (1981) suggested the following hypotheses in the clinical evaluation of the older hearing-impaired listener: (1) Aging listeners are no different than young listeners with equal degrees of hearing loss and (2) aging listeners will show auditory function problems in addition to those shown by younger listeners with similar hearing losses, possibly due to peripheral problems associated with presbycusis, which are not adequately assessed by the pure-tone audiogram, central auditory nervous system degeneration, cognitive differences, or a combination of all of the above.

Assessment Problems Related to Age

The incidence of excessive impacted cerumen is higher in the older versus younger population (Fisch, 1978; Schow, Christensen, Hutchinson, & Nerbonne, 1978). Otoscopy must be performed prior to auditory and hearing aid evaluation.

Collapsing ear canals with the application of earphones also has been found to occur more frequently in older listeners (Schow & Goldbaum, 1980; Zucker & Williams, 1977) and may explain the high incidence of conductive loss cited in several studies (Rosen, Plester, El Mofty, & Rosen, 1964). The implication is to assess the anteroposterior relationship of the tragus to the cavum of the concha and the relative collapsibility of the tragus and cartilaginous portion of the external auditory meatus. Calibrated insert earphones should be used to eliminate this problem. As described earlier, collapsing ear canals also present a challenge for the fabrication of earmolds and ITE hearing aids.

It has been suggested that aged listeners are more conservative in their threshold criterion than younger listeners when they are asked to respond yes or no to the presence of an auditory signal (Rees & Botwinick, 1979; Potash & Jones, 1977). Clinical observations indicate that aged listeners may be less willing to guess in their discrimination of suprathreshold auditory signals if only a portion of the signal is heard (as with a suprathreshold single-word identification task). This symptom may be representative of older listeners or it may be endemic only to the current aged population as a consequence of low self-esteem and the low value generally placed on the aged by our society. In either case, the implication for the hearing health care professional is to reduce auditory test anxiety and re-instruct the older patient regarding the clinician's expectation that errors in signal identification are expected, and in fact necessary, if an accurate evaluation is to be obtained. Implications for the test procedures include changing the threshold response to a two-interval forced choice task (eliminating the possibility of a nonresponse) and using closed-set, forced choice suprathreshold speech identification tests, such as a Modified Rhyme type test, the Synthetic Sentence Identification Index, or a comparison of closed set (high redundancy) to open-set (low-redundancy) word identification performance using a tool such as the Speech in Noise test (SPIN).

Loudness and Adaptation

"Other than using uncomfortable loudness thresholds as a recruitment measure, there is currently no behavioral test of recruitment for elderly listeners" (Marshall, 1981). Loudness recruitment in the elderly listener with sensorineural hearing loss does exist and is demonstrated by the elevation in hearing thresholds with perceptions of loud sounds that either are similar to or are reduced relative to those for normal hearing listeners. It has been suggested by clinical audiologists that uncomfortable loudness measures using speech and pure tones lack validity as representations of the levels of sound a person will truly accommodate when they are motivated to do so (i.e., in social or vocational situations).

In spite of this perception, it is important to assess frequency-specific tolerance limits, known by various names such as Uncomfortable Loudness Levels (UCLs), Upper Limits of Comfortable Loudness (ULCL), and Loudness Discomfort Levels (LDLs), in each ear for each subject to make the most appropriate initial decisions regarding the appropriate frequency-specific Saturation Sound Pressure level (SSPL) characteristics of hearing aids.

Adaptation, or reduction in the loudness percept of suprathreshold continuous pure tones, has been assessed in older individuals using Békésy and conventional tone decay tests. Békésy tracings usually are consistent with normal hearing or a cochlear site of lesion (type I or II tracings, respectively) (Jerger, 1960; Harbert, Young, & Menduke, 1966), and tone decay is typically less than 30 dB, also consistent with cochlear site of lesion (Olsen & Noffisinger, 1974; Ganz, 1976).

Implications for Amplification

The primary behavioral assessment of recruitment for the aging listener is loudness tolerance for pure-tones, warble tones, or speech. The dynamic range from threshold to these levels is reduced in persons with sensorineural hearing loss. Although the usable auditory dynamic range is not reduced inordinately for aged listeners with hearing impairment as compared to younger listeners with similar hearing loss, they often have a decreased ability to ignore the presence of loud environmental noise. This interferes with their understanding of important auditory input to a greater degree than that experienced by their younger counterparts.

The aided listener with sensorineural hearing loss requires a comparatively wide range of input signal intensities to be amplified to suprathreshold levels and maintained within the compressed suprathreshold dynamic range of the individual. These findings suggest that, if maximum hearing aid benefit is to be achieved for the elderly and all persons with sensorineural hearing loss, SSPL90 values that closely correspond to obtained frequency-specific UCLs must be utilized, while at the same time providing enough gain to boost important auditory stimuli to the person's Most Comfortable Levels (MCLs). Depending on the separation in dB between the person's MCL and UCL at each frequency, these criteria may be met with the use of a linear amplifier with high-level compression limiting to minimize distortion of high-level inputs and accommodate UCLs. However, as MCLs approach the levels of the UCLs, reducing the dynamic range, it may be possible only to provide adequate gain for lower level input signals to keep all amplified signals below the UCLs. This situation would necessitate the use of a wide dynamic range compression circuit with a low knee-point of compression. Current compression circuits employ the concepts of expansion, compression, unity gain, and high-level output compression limiting. Compression amplifiers that incorporate each of these may have three knee points, defined as: (1) the input level at which the aid stops increasing in gain for progressively louder soft sounds (expansion) and goes into compression (or gain reduction for successively louder inputs), (2) the input level at which the aid no longer compresses the signal but gives no gain (unity gain) with the output being equal to the input, and (3) output limiting, which is the input level beyond which there is no further increase in output regardless of the change in input.

Multichannel compression circuits give the flexibility to fit a hearing aid that has unique input/output functions for two or more frequency bands. This allows the aid to be programmed to accommodate the unique loudness growth characteristics for each individual in the various frequency bands accommodated by the hearing aid. Although there are aids with as little as two channels and as many as nine channels or more, it is not clear how many channels are minimally necessary and optimal. The audiologist or the dispenser who uses frequency-specific stimuli to determine MCLs and UCLs also should evaluate whether MCLs and UCLs for more complex signals (e.g., speech and environmental noise) might be somewhat lower due to loudness summation resulting from the simultaneous presentation of the multiple frequency components contained in these stimuli. If this is true, the overall gain of the instrument may need to be reduced once the independent channels have been set to accommodate the loudness of sounds with complex spectra.

The Independent Hearing Aid Fitting Forum (IHAFF, 1994) proposed a method for assessing loudness growth in a low- and high-frequency band from threshold to perceived uncomfortable loudness. Using the first seven of the loudness levels recommended by Hawkins, Walden, Montgomery, and Prosek (1987), the patient rates the audibility of presented pure-tones at increasing loudness levels typically at 500 Hz and 3000 Hz (the peak of the frequency response for most Class-D amplifiers). With current digitally programmable and programmable true digital signal processing hearing aids, it probably is adequate to assess only threshold and the UCL at each of these frequencies to define the dynamic range accurately. The hearing aid simply will interpolate the appropriate input/output function with associated compression knee points and ratios based on these two end points of the loudness function. In hearing aids with three or more channels, loudness growth using this procedure should be assessed using a frequency at the center of each frequency band included in each channel.

Frequency Discrimination

Reduced frequency selectivity in persons with sensorineural hearing loss has been shown using difference limens for frequency (DLF) (Zurek & Formby, 1979). DLFs have been shown to increase with increased magnitude of loss and for low frequencies as well as high frequencies in persons with only high-frequency loss. It has not been established whether aged hearing-impaired listeners have inordinately greater DLFs than their younger counterparts when learning effects and potential age-related criterion effects are controlled (Marshall, 1981).

Psychophysical tuning curves for listeners with sensorineural hearing loss, obtained by fixing the level and frequency of a probe tone and measuring the level of a second tone at various frequencies required to mask the probe, have shown abnormal broadening, abnormal shape, and loss of the tip in regions of hearing loss (Zwicker & Shorn, 1978; Tyler, Fernandes, & Wood, 1984) and abnormality in regions of normal hearing sensitivity (Mills, Gilbert, & Adkins, 1979), especially in the presence of significant high-frequency loss (Nelson, 1979). It is not clear whether these results differ in older versus younger persons with similar audiograms (Marshall, 1981).

It has been suggested that each frequency is surrounded by its own critical bandwidth of frequencies and that all frequencies within the critical band of a probe frequency are processed equally. Thus, formants in the speech signal that are separated by a critical bandwidth are perceived as different frequencies; however, environmental noise located within the critical band of each formant frequency is processed along with the speech signal. A widening of critical bandwidths, or loss of frequency selectivity, has been found with the advent of sensorineural hearing loss (deBoer & Bowmeester, 1974, 1976). The widening of critical bands may be due to cochlear changes (efferent olivocochlear neuron degeneration) not related to afferent input, and frequency discrimination may be independent of loss of pure-tone hearing sensitivity (Bienvenue & Michael, 1979). It has not been shown definitively, however, that the widening of critical bandwidths in aged listeners with sensorineural loss is in excess of that for young hearing-impaired listeners. Bienvenue and Michael (1979) listed four functions of critical bands: (1) to band-limit the effect of background noise on the target signal serving to enhance the signal-to-noise ratio, (2) to determine ability to perceive harmonic content and formant content (in the case of speech) of complex signals, (3) to determine ability to perceive phase relationships among tone complexes, and (4) to sharpen frequency discrimination beyond that which can be described by basilar membrane mechanics.

Critical ratios (signal-to-noise ratio at masked threshold) and upward spread of masking have been assessed in aged listeners and are a reflection of critical bandwidth. Critical ratios have been demonstrated to increase for higher frequencies in both normal hearing listeners (Reed & Bilger, 1973) and listeners with high-frequency noise-induced listeners with hearing impairment (Tyler, Fernandes, & Wood, 1984). Margolis and Goldberg (1980) concluded that critical ratios are not a simple reflection of auditory filter bandwidth in aged listeners. Upward spread of masking in aged listeners with hearing impairment has not been shown to be any greater than for younger cochlear hearing-impaired counterparts. Although upward spread of masking has been found to be detrimental to speech discrimination of normal hearing listeners at high signal intensities (95-100 dB SPL) (Danaher, Osberger, & Pickett, 1973), it has not been shown to be abnormally broad in all listeners with sensorineural hearing loss (Jerger et al., 1960; Leshowitz & Lindstrom, 1979).

Implications for Amplification

It is quite possible that peripheral deterioration of the frequency selectivity of the cochlea accounts in large part for the reduced understanding of speech in noise in the aged listener with hearing impairment. It is also possible that aged persons with different audiometric configurations and etiologies of hearing loss have varying degrees of alteration in critical bandwidths and cochlear-based frequency specificity.

Once a reliable data base is established regarding the frequency discrimination of older versus younger hearing-impaired listeners with controls for loss configuration, etiology, and task-response criterion effects, it seems imperative that tasks that assess frequency discrimination be included in the hearing aid assessment process. The information obtained would make it possible to severely band limit the amplified signal, based not only on the audiometric configuration of the pure-tone loss, but also on the extent of abnormality of frequency selectivity across the frequency range, even in the presence of what appear to be normal pure-tone thresholds. This information then could be used to help determine the optimum crossover frequencies in multichannel hearing aids with the steep skirts of digital filters controlling interaction between adjacent frequency bands. This is quite possible with current digital signal-processing technology.

Speech Discrimination

From the previous discussion of the importance of peripheral frequency selectivity to the discrimination of complex signals (speech) in noise, it can be argued that, if population-specific information was available, much of the responsibility for reduction in speech discrimination in noise demonstrated by significant numbers of aged hearing-impaired listeners could be described on the basis of impaired frequency selectivity at the level of the cochlea. If this were true, particularly with the advent of digital-processing technology, algorithms could be designed into the hearing aid to compensate specifically for abnormal cochlear function. An additional portion of the reduction in speech understanding in aged listeners can be explained solely on the basis of inadequate sensation levels, particularly of high-frequency speech sounds and higher formants (F1, F2, and F3) and their transitional cues.

To determine age-only related changes in auditory temporal processing, Blackington, Novak, and Kramer (1988) examined NU-6 word identification in normal-hearing young and elderly subjects with 0% and 60% temporal compression of the speech signals. The authors compared these data to forward masking threshold results using 500 and 2000 Hz as the target stimuli with wide-band noise as the masker. The older subjects, ages 60 to 79 years, obtained 70% correct identification on the compressed speech presented at 40 dB HL compared to 82% correct identification for the young controls. There was no difference in word identification scores between the two groups for non-compressed speech stimuli (97 to 99% for all subjects). Blackington, Novak, and Kramer also found that, for separations between the masker and target stimuli of 0 to 250 ms, the older subjects required higher tone sensation levels in order to achieve the same 70% correct detection level as their younger counterparts. This was particularly true for the 2000 Hz stimuli.

Implications for Amplification and Aural Rehabilitation

A common clinical observation from aged hearing-impaired listeners is that their understanding of speech improves with a mildly reduced rate of speech. The results of many of the altered speech studies have shown excessively reduced performance in aged hearing-impaired listeners. The results of Blackington, Novak, and Kramer (1988), which showed the same reduction of performance in normal-hearing aged listeners, suggest that the critical causal factors are age-related central factors that are not dependent on changes in pure-tone sensitivity. This has been confirmed more recently by Gordon-Salant and Fitzgibbons (1999). They found that age-related problems for recognition of time-compressed speech are independent of attenuation imposed by hearing loss. This supports the contention that aging, in and of itself, imposes a limitation on the ability to process rapid speech segments. These limitations are believed to be central in nature and most likely associated with deterioration of central timing mechanisms. Although possible, current digital hearing aids are not able to slow the rate of speech being processed in real time. As a result, it is imperative for older listeners to realize that difficulty understanding rapid speech is a common problem of the elderly that is not significantly helped with amplification and that can be reduced simply by asking speakers to slow their rate of speech. The temporal characteristics (attack and release times) of compression circuits also can be a signficant factor in reducing the use of temporal and frequency cues in speech. The attack times must be rapid enough to accommodate the loudness of the offending loud sounds while, at the same time, the release times must allow recovery quickly enough to allow for the audibility of the subsequent temporal and frequency cues carried by the softer speech sounds. The selection of appropriate release times is particularly important for the elderly hearing aid user and is deserving of further research.

Binaural Integration

Binaural auditory fusion and release from masking tasks have been used to assess central auditory nervous system integrity. Binaural auditory fusion compares word identification when high- and low-frequency information is presented monaurally versus when high-pass filtered speech is presented to one ear and low-pass filtered speech to the other. Breakdown in the former task can be attributed solely to abnormal cochlear filter effects, whereas breakdown in the dichotic high pass-low pass task can be impaired also by brainstem pathology and bilateral and diffuse cerebral pathology (Lynn & Gilroy, 1976). Investigators have found that the aged listener's binaural fusion ability is not significantly poorer than younger listeners with similar pure-tone thresholds (Harbert et al., 1966; Palva & Jokenen, 1970). In fact, older listeners often perform more poorly on the monaural task than on the dichotic speech fusion task, which is consistent with peripheral auditory system pathology. Franklin (1975) also found this to be true with young (13–23 years) listeners with sensorineural hearing loss.

The binaural Masking Level Difference (MLD) is a psychophysical task that also relies on intact lower brainstem function for maximum MLD results. Many studies that have reported MLD results for presbycusic listeners have concluded that MLDs are generally smaller for the presbycusic population (Olsen, Noffsinger, & Carhart, 1976; Warren, Wagener, & Herman, 1978) in spite of considerable overlap of MLD values between young normal hearing and older hearing-impaired groups. Novak and Anderson (1982) were the first to attempt to systematically control for age, degree of hearing loss, bilateral symmetry of loss, shape of loss, and central auditory integrity in the evaluation of the MLD in older hearing-impaired listeners. They found that, for older listeners, MLD magnitudes for 500 Hz were significantly reduced only for the neural presbycusic (Schuknecht, 1964, 1974) group. The authors concluded that central auditory system function as measured by the MLD task was significantly different only for the neural presbycusic group with high-frequency sloping sensorineural hearing loss and single-word identification scores less than 70%. These binaural speech fusion and MLD studies support the contention that binaural integration is intact for many aged hearing-impaired listeners.

Despite these findings, a small percentage of elderly hearing aid users will perform better with monaural than with binaural amplification. Chmiel, Jerger, Murphy, Pirozzolo, and Tooley-Young (1997) studied this phenomenon extensively in one such elderly listener. Their results suggest that age-related changes in interhemispheric transfer of auditory input via corpus callosum may underlie the preference for monaural amplification. These results support the inclusion of behavioral and electrophysiologic dichotic speech perception tests for older hearing aid candidates who are not successful with binaural amplification.

Implications for Amplification

From the results of the studies cited in the previous two sections, it must be concluded that, although problems of speech understanding in the aged hearing-impaired listener can be attributed in large part to cochlear filtering effects due to pathology at the level of the cochlea, even older normal-hearing listeners show poorer performance than their younger counterparts on temporal masking tasks (compressed speech identification, forward masking signal detection). In this case, age appears to be a critical factor in determining the ability to understand rapid speech. On the basis of the forward-masking data of Blackington, Novak, and Kramer (1988), even normal-hearing older listeners may benefit from mild high-frequency emphasis amplification to improve their detection and processing of rapidly presented auditory information.

In the case of bilaterally symmetrical hearing loss and PB word discrimination scores in excess of 80%, binaural fitting of aids must not be ruled out solely on the basis of concern for inability to binaurally integrate dichotically presented information (typical sound-field listening). Age, in and of itself, does not appear to be a significant factor in reduction of binaural auditory integration or binaural release from masking abilities in the majority of older persons with cochlear-based hearing loss; however, in a small subgroup of hearing aid candidates, monaural speech processing may be better than that achieved with binaural amplification and probably due to higher-level central processing problems. For these reasons, the inclusion of central auditory processing tasks such as compressed speech or dichotic listening tasks could allow for better evaluation of hearing aid candidacy and potential hearing aid benefit (Givens, Arnold, & Hume, 1998). These assessment tools could help identify those patients who are going to need more rehabilitative support because of the poor prognosis for successful use of hearing aids in difficult listening situations.

The implications of all of the psychoacoustic findings with aged hearing-impaired listeners are that:

- The population is indeed composed of subgroups as defined by different peripheral and central auditory system function.
- The pure-tone audiogram, in and of itself, is not an adequate descriptor of important auditory psychophysical abilities.
- The onus is on the audiologist to develop a valid, reliable, and efficient test battery that will delineate cochlear versus retrocochlear function as it relates specifically to the specification of hearing-aid parameters. This test battery must differentiate between improved auditory function that can be expected based solely on differential hearing aid design and benefits from "appropriate" amplification predicted on the basis of psychosocial motivational parameters unique to each aged listener.

APPLYING HEARING AIDS TO OLDER PATIENTS

The audiologist must apply hearing aids that: (1) have the electroacoustic characteristics most appropriate for the patient's residual auditory function and (2) are acceptable to the patient. Satisfaction of the first requirement does not always ensure satisfaction of the second. Barford (1979) stated that user satisfaction across patients, as measured by speech perception ability, can be high or low with similar sudden significant changes in aided versus unaided auditory sensitivity. High satisfaction results if the additional frequency information provided to the "recognition device" is indeed meaningful and useful. Low satisfaction results when enhanced aided sensitivity for high frequencies relative to low frequencies causes a "mismatch of the recognition device and the input code." A degradation in speech perception ability at the time of initial hearing aid use will result if the latter effect dominates. Barford suggested that, "This mismatch will gradually decrease as a result of adaptation, if adaptation is possible." However, the length of the adaptation is not easily predicted (re: age of patient, type of loss, and a variety of psychosocial variables) for each individual patient and may last from a few days to 6 months or longer. Surr and Wladen (1998) examined long-term versus short-term hearing aid benefit. This study compared hearing aid benefit obtained 6 weeks and a minimum of 1 year after fitting to determine if changes occurred over time. Fifteen patients were fitted binaurally with a programmable two-channel aid with wide dynamic range compression. The manufacturer's recommended loudness growth in octave bands, and audiogram programming algorithm and fitting procedures were used. Following an initial 6-week period and again following a minimum of one year of use, the Profile of Hearing Aid Benefit (PHAB) was administered. Speech recognition performance was tested using the Connected Speech Test (CST) in six-talker speech babble at 50 dBA, +10 dB signal-to-noise ratio, 60dBA, +5 dB signal to noise ratio, 70 dBA, +2 dB signal-to-noise ratio, and in quiet with a reverberation time of 0.78 second. Significant aided benefit was shown. A comparison of short term versus one year PHAB and CST results showed no significant differences in hearing aid benefit with long-term use. This suggests that the 6-week acclimatization period evaluated in this investigation is sufficiently long for clinical trials of this type of Wide Dynamic Range amplification. The question remains as to whether the typical 30-day trial period can be sufficiently long enough as well.

Needs and Expectations of the Older Patient

Today, audiologists have the option of recommending traditional screw-adjusted potentiometer analogue hearing aids, digitally programmable analogue hearing aids, and digitally programmable true digital signal processing hearing aids to their geriatric patients. The technology selected will be chosen on the basis of patient auditory measurments, the demands of the patients' listening environments and the importance of functioning in these environments, the patients' desire for state-of-the art technology, the patients' cosmetic demands, desire for more or less automatic function, and the patients' financial resources. More and more of the older patients seeking help for their hearing loss have the financial resources to purchase state-of-the art technology. Many want the best of what is available and expect that, if they pay the higher price, the hearing aid will allow them to hear well in all listening environments, with minimal adjustment or maintenance on their part. In reality, the expectations of older patients and their families may be unrealistic. However in light of the high price tag (possible $3,000–$4,000 per aid) on today's most sophisticated hearing aids, it is understandable that the patients and their families may have unrealistic expectations of hearing aid benefit. As audiologists help their older patients decide between the various types of technology, it must be determined if the demands of their typical listening situations warrant the expense of the most sophisticated digital signal processing (DSP) technology. Manufacturers claim to be building algorithms into their true DSP aids that attempt to optimize the understanding of speech in noise either by "recognizing" speech as different from noise and enhancing the amplification of it, minimizing the amplification of noise-like signals, or both. Although objective and subjective reports are demonstrating benefits of true DSP technology over other types of amplification, the research data indicating the significant advantage of these DSP algorithms over multi-channel compression high-quality digitally programmable analogue aids for geriatric patients in their variety of listening environments has yet to be completed. Therefore, at this point in the evolution of hearing aid technology, it cannot be said definitively that DSP truly is better for all geriatric patients and warrants the high cost. In the absence of this research data, audiologists are prone to encourage their geriatric patients to purchase the high-end DSP products because they must be better than the analogue alternatives, particularly for the more challenged auditory processing system of the geriatric patient. Although older, experienced hearing aid patients often describe a preference for true DSP technology over analogue alternatives, this could be a function of the amount of money that they have paid for the DSP product and the "digital" halo effect which may elevate the benefit they perceive they are receiving from the DSP aids. The high cost of DSP technology also encourages the older patient to have unrealistic expectations of the benefit they should be receiving from their aids in all difficult listening environments. Also, to the extent that the more sophisticated technology may require greater understanding of its use and dexterity in its adjustment, there will be a greater opportunity for failure of the older patient to use it successfully. Given these issues and the fact that the older patient often requires more time for all aspects of hearing assessment, hearing aid fitting, counseling, and adjustment to hearing aid use, time and attention are critical variables in the design of an effective hearing aid intervention program for the elderly patient.

Steps in the geriatric hearing aid evaluation and orientation process include:

- Selection of electroacoustic parameters of the hearing aid based on the audiometric evaluation,
- Assessment of self-perceived handicap imposed by the hearing loss and prediction of hearing aid benefit,
- Selection of the technology to be used and verification of hearing aid benefit,

- Fine tuning,
- Validation of self-perceived hearing aid benefit, and
- Participation in a group aural-rehabilitation program (ReACT) during the 30-day trial period.

Selection of Electroacoustic Parameters of Hearing Aids

Auditory Evaluation

It is recommended that, at a minimum, the following parameters should be assessed:

1. Pure-tone thresholds and UCLs under earphones should be obtained to specify general frequency response characteristics and absolute gain and output requirements. Some digitally programmable and true digital signal processing hearing aid products allow for determination of thresholds and UCLs using the aid in the ear as the transducer. For many years, prescriptive methods like POGO II, NAL-R, and DSL 3.0 have been considered the standard approach to identifying target hearing aid insertion or functional gain. (Hawkins, 1992; Mueller, 1997). These approaches used threshold data to calculate hearing instrument gain as a function of frequency. Some also calculated a recommended maximum output level of the hearing aid assuming an input of 60-65 dB SPL. As these procedures have no way of determining gain appropriate for softer and louder signal input levels they are not adequate to define the input/output (I/O)gain functions of non-linear compression aids. The Desired Sensation Level (DSL) I/O algorithm was developed later as an approach for fitting non-linear compression instruments (Seewald, Moodie, Sinclair, & Cornelisse, 1997). To achieve loudness equalization, DSL I/O recommends target output levels for different sound input levels (40, 65, and 95 dB) as a function of frequency. These target output levels are based on the listener's measured thresholds and UCLs. If loudness judgements are not available, DSL I/O will default to predicted data for UCLs which are about one standard deviation below the mean loudness discomfort levels reported by Pascoe (1988). Loudness equalization should enable the listener to perceive soft sounds as soft, but audible, average conversational sounds should be perceived as comfortable, and loud sounds should be perceived as loud but not uncomfortably loud. This approach is used by a variety of hearing aid manufacturers in their gain and output determination algorithms and is available in several real-ear probe microphone measurement systems. It is appropriate for the fitting of current hearing aid technology in geriatric patients.
2. In applying audiometric data to determinations of frequency response requirements and preselection of specific hearing aids, it is important to realize that 2 cc coupler values indicated on manufacturers' specification sheets may over-represent desired functional gain (aided versus unaided thresholds for warble tones or narrow band noise) or insertion gain (aided versus unaided ear canal sound pressure levels) (Hawkins & Schum,1984). This difference will be greater for BTE than for ITE hearing aids, particularly for frequencies above 1000 Hz. Lower insertion and functional gain also will be seen in persons with large ear canal volumes medial to the tip of the hearing aid on the earmold and with very flaccid middle ear systems. This is not so much of a problem when using highly flexible, multi-channel digitally programmable aids and real-ear probe tube measurements to assess changes in insertion gain as gain and output parameters of the hearing aid are manipulated to achieve DSL I/O targets
3. Real-ear unaided response measurements indicating the location and amplitude of the ear canal resonance frequency are helpful in predicting the amount of gain

that will be necessary to achieve targets. They should be used to determine if the selected hearing aid has the flexibility to accommodate the gain requirements necessitated by the ear canal resonance values and the target values.

4. Frequency-specific LDLs or UCLs for those frequencies for which amplification is desired should be obtained to specify SSPL90 values to which the aid should be adjusted first. Etymotic insert earphones, available through the Etymotic Research Lab, calibrated in the 2 cc coupler are an appropriate transducer for these measurements. LDLs should be obtained for both frequency-specific and broad-band stimuli (speech or speech noise) to determine the extent to which loudness summation may necessitate the lowering of the gain and SSPL90 requirements.
5. Dichotic assessment using the Dichotic Digits Test, a test of discrimination of temporally compressed speech, and a test of the discrimination of speech in noise (e.g., high predictability versus low predictability speech-in-noise test; SPIN) should be completed to assess the prognosis for successful use of binaural amplification and the need for additional counseling based on unusual difficulty processing rapid speech and speech in noise.
6. Standard single syllable word identification tests should be completed under phones at the patient's MCLs for speech to determine symmetry between ears. Low discrimination scores for this test should not be a reason for not considering amplification for the geriatric patient. Low discrimination scores in this test condition, particularly for persons with sloping high-frequency losses, are probably a result of inadequate sensation level for high-frequency speech sounds and upward spread of masking of louder low-frequency components in the speech spectrum. If scores are asymmetrical in the presence of symmetrical hearing loss, this should be assessed further to rule out active retrocochlear pathology. Unaided speech discrimination scores also should be obtained in the sound field at 50 dB HL to determine the effect of increased audibility of speech sounds provided by the hearing aid on the aided versus unaided difference score.

In a less than optimal testing environment, the effects of background noise are reduced for persons with thresholds of 40 dB HL at or above 500 Hz. Methods utilized include assessment of pure-tone thresholds and UCLs under earphones using a portable audiometer, and identification of recorded words under earphones using recorded speech and an audiometer with speech presentation capabilities. Probe microphone measures are invaluable in allowing a quick and reliable comparison of aided versus unaided ear canal sound pressure levels (insertion gain) to assess adequacy of hearing aid gain without requiring subjective judgments from the patient. Aided versus unaided speech identification can be assessed in the sound field at a pragmatic distance of three feet with the clinician's speech being monitored at 55 to 60 dBA at the patient's location using a sound level meter. The speech stimuli used will vary with the abilities of the patient (standard word lists for more intact patients or abbreviated word lists emphasizing high-frequency words, the Ling 5 sounds test incorporated into real words [e.g., shaw, she, shoe, saw, see, sue], and more meaningful questions about the patient and his or her environment for less intact patients). Speech testing, aided versus unaided, also should be done with and without the use of lip cues to show the older patient the importance of enhancing hearing aid use by watching the speaker's face.

Assessment of Self-Perceived Handicap Imposed by the Hearing Loss

There are a variety of self-assessment inventories designed to allow patients to rate the psychological, social, vocational, and emotional handicaps imposed by their hearing losses.

Use of the Hearing Handicap for the Elderly (Weinstein & Ventry, 1983; Ventry and Weinstein, 1982) is recommended because it has been used and validated with hearing-impaired older persons typically seen in speech and hearing clinics. It is relatively short and assesses the critical concerns of the emotional, social, and situational effects of the hearing loss. Weinstein and Ventry found that older patients with pure-tone averages of 0 to 25 dB HL (500, 1000, 2000 Hz) almost never described their hearing losses as handicapping. Half of the patients with pure-tone averages of 26 to 40 dB HL perceived the hearing loss as a handicap and half did not. Older patients with hearing losses greater than 41 dB HL very often (88–92%) perceived their hearing loss as handicapping. There was, however, considerable variability even for the greater-than-40-dB loss group in the degree (mild to significant) of perceived handicap. Results for older persons were very similar to the results for younger persons, and audiometric data (e.g., pure-tone averages, speech reception thresholds, and speech discrimination scores) accounted for less than 50% of the variance in self-assessed hearing handicap. These results are consistent with the recommendation that, although pure-tone thresholds are important for the description of the desired hearing aid electroacoustic parameters, they do not adequately describe the functional deficits imposed by a given hearing loss, particularly for losses less than 40 dB HL for the three-frequency pure-tone average.

Most aged patients who admit that they are having communication difficulties secondary to hearing loss complain that, with previous hearing aids, sounds were often too loud and speech was difficult to understand when background noise was present (e.g., during informal group gatherings). If bilaterally impaired, sounds originating on the unaided ear were often difficult to detect initially and process if relocation was not easy (e.g., when seated in a car). Mueller, Hawkins, and Sedge (1984) suggested that, for the majority of the hearing-impaired population who have potential for bilateral amplification, it is preferable to use compression, directional microphones and binaural fitting. If the patient is over 70 years of age and a first-time hearing aid user, the recommendation for binaural fitting might be qualified, based on the person's ability to physically and mentally cope with, at first, just one new hearing aid and then, at a later time, possibily a second hearing aid.

Prediction of Ability to Successfully Use Amplification

The Rupp Feasibility Scale for Predicting Hearing Aid Use (Rupp, Higgins, & Maurer, 1977) differentially weights factors of motivation, fault, initial impression, age, vision, significant others, self assessment, functional gain for speech, adaptability, manual dexterity, and financial resources and, accordingly, allows for scoring of each patient from poor (0) to excellent (100) prognosis for successful use of hearing aids. Hosford-Dunn and Baxter (1985) found that, in a group of 95 patients (mean age, 65 years) with mild to severe hearing losses at 1000 to 4000 Hz, clinician-assessed "motivation" and "initial subjective impressions of amplification" to be the two best predictors of long-term (first 3 months of aid use) satisfaction. As Hosford-Dunn and Baxter suggested, for patients older than 70 years of age, other factors of this instrument may have predictive value as well and should not be eliminated for that population. Hosford-Dunn and Baxter also examined the predictive value of standard audiometric measures relative to the successful use of amplification. Only aided versus unaided single syllable word identification scores in quiet were found to be of predictive value.

Verification of Hearing Aid Benefit

Whether the prescriptive approach is used with a presetting of the hearing instrument, or whether the instrument is adjusted to match prescribed amplification targets, it is important to remember that achievement of the targets cannot be assumed and must be measured. Two verification methods are recommended: (1) probe-microphone measurements, and (2) aided loudness scaling.

Some probe microphone measurements display the DSL I/O targets. Real-ear insertion gain measurements then can be taken to determine closeness of fit of the actual hearing aid real ear insertion gain measures to the DSL I/O targets. The aid then can be adjusted while the signal is present to bring the output levels within target values for the various input levels of 40 dB, 65 dB, and 90 dB. Probe microphone measurements can be obtained with both analogue and digital signal processing aids and can be useful in assessing the effect of noise reduction algorithms when they are engaged. Probe microphone measures also are comforting to the older patient in that their use builds trust with the dispenser. The patient is able to see targets for amplification represented on the equipment screen, the closeness of fit of the obtained real-ear data, and the relationship between changes in measures of real-ear insertion gain on the screen and changes in their perception of speech and other environmental sounds.

Aided loudness scaling can be used to verify that desired gain is delivered across a wide range of input levels. Narrow-band signals for three or more different frequencies can be used to assure that loudness is restored across frequencies for different inputs. With multi-channel instruments, it is recommended that at least one frequency lies within each channel. Some hearing care professionals use a modified scaling technique for the aided speech testing modeled after the Independent Hearing Aid Fitting Forum (IHAFF) verification guidelines (Valente & Van Vliet, 1997). Speech inputs at three different levels (45, 65, and 85 dB SPL) are presented and the patient is required to rate these speech inputs as "soft," "comfortable," and "loud but okay" (Zelisko, Wolf & Burton, 1999). Other time-honored methods of loudness assessment include tolerance for clapping, sudden loud sounds such as keys dropping on a table top, a door slamming, and live-voice loud-speech at a six-foot distance from the speaker.

Fine Tuning

Following verification of the performance of the hearing aids on each ear, the patient then can participate in the fine tuning of the hearing aid(s). Real-ear probe tube measurements using a composite signal provide the best method for real time assessment of the effects of changes in such parameters as gain for soft, medium, and loud sounds in each channel, and channel specific compression thresholds and ratios. Some dispensers avoid using real-ear measurements because they believe they take too much time. They are certainly less time-consuming than sound field functional gain measures, provide much more information, give the patient a means to monitor the effects of changes in hearing aid settings, and minimize the need for fine tuning beyond the weekly monitoring conducted during the 30-day trial period.

Validation Through Self-Assessment Inventories

On completion of the verification measures and fine-tuning adjustments, subjective validation of the effectiveness of the fitting is an essential component to the fitting and follow-up protocol. There are a variety of scales that can be used for this purpose. It is best to have the patient complete the scale at least twice, once prior to the fitting of the instrument(s) and at the completion of the trial period. Regardless of the instruments used, it is important that they be completed under the supervision of the clinician with the audiologist presenting each scale item in an interview context. The older patients often appreciate ongoing explanation of the rating scale and interpretation of the questions to minimize the chance for confusion during the completion of the inventory. Although there are many outcome scales available, the following are ones that have good utility with senior patients:

Hearing Handicap Inventory for the Elderly-Screening Version (HHIE-S) (Ventry and Weinstein,1982). This 10-item tool assesses both social and emotional handicap that is created by the hearing loss and the reduction of the handicap as a result of utilization of the hearing aid(s).

Client Oriented Scale of Improvement (COSI) (Dillon & Ginis, 1997). The COSI is a self-assessment scale in which, prior to hearing aid fitting, the patient selects and rank orders up to five communication settings/goals that are important to him/her. The scale then is readministered during the 30-day trial and rehabilitation program, and at each visit, allows the patient to indicate the degree of change on a 5-item scale from "worse" to "much better." This scale focuses the patients on their most important amplification goals and allows them to reassess the importance of these goals throughout the trial period.

Profile of Aided Loudness (PAL) (Mueller & Palmer, 1998). The PAL is designed to assess if normal loudness restoration has been establish. Patients rate their loudness perceptions for 12 real-world sounds (e.g., a door slamming, an electric razor, their own breathing, etc.) and also rate their satisfaction with the loudness levels of each ("just right" to "not good at all"). The results are compared to similar loudness ratings provided by normal-hearing listeners. This can be completed also by the normal-hearing spouse as a second assessment for the actual noises being rated by this patient in his or her environment (e.g., a barking dog, a clothes dryer that may be unusually loud in a given environment and not "typical").

Abbreviated Profile of Hearing Aid Benefit (APHAB) (Cox, 1997; Cox & Alexander, 1995). This is a 24-item survey designed to measure disability and benefit from amplification. The 24 items are divided into 4 subscales that include listening in quiet, noise, and reverberation, and aversiveness for sounds. Each item is ranked on a 7-item scale ("never" to "always"). It is best used as a pre- and post-rehabilitation program assessment and must be given to the elderly patient in an interview format with the clinician presenting each item and reminding the patient of how the scale relates to the question. Without this support, the elderly patient often is confused by the questionnaire.

As appropriate, the patient and his or her spouse should complete these questionnaires to triangulate what the patient is saying, what the clinician is observing, and what a third party living in the patient's environment also is observing.

Participation in a Group Aural Rehabilitation Program (ReACT) During the Trial Period

It is essentially unethical to dispense amplification to elderly patients without the benefit of a structured aural rehabilitation program during the trial period with their new hearing aid(s). This is true of both new and experienced users, as experienced users typically are graduating to more sophisticated technology and can benefit from the technical support, the ongoing audiological assessment, and the social support of their peers. Novak has titled his program Rehabilitating Auditory Communication Techniques (ReACT). It is helpful to have a meaningful acronym for the rehab program so that it can be referred to easily both in advertisement and discussion with the patient. This program is dispensed with the hearing aid and the cost is bundled into the cost of the aid(s). It includes the attendance of the spouse, friend, or significant other of the person receiving the aids and typically is limited to about eight people per session. ReACT is a 4-week, 2-hour per week family-centered program. The ultimate goal is to enable successful adjustment to and use of hearing amplification and reduce the hearing loss from the status of a handicapping condition to an inconvenience fully managed by the elderly patient and his or her family. Components of ReACT include:

- Education of the patient regarding his or her hearing loss, the probable etiology, and other hearing disorders common to the elderly population,
- Development of educated consumers regarding effective use of their new hearing aids and other assistive listening devices,
- Development of new assertive communication skills, speechreading skills, and an understanding of the commonality of communication, social, and emotional issues shared by seniors with hearing loss,
- Use of the group process to seek solutions to hearing loss-related problems and, as a laboratory, to practice assertive communication techniques and communication repair strategies,
- Ongoing electroacoustic fine tuning of the hearing aids using real-ear probe microphone measurments and modification of the physical characteristics of the earmold or ITE aids as needed according to the feedback from each patient, and
- Gradual adjustment of the hearing aid electroacoustic parameters of the hearing aids to achieve ultimate target goals as tolerated by the patient during the trial period.

The best schedule for ReACT for the elderly patient population is typically late morning or early afternoon. Saturday clinics are also an option. The majority of older patients do not want to drive at night and do not like early morning appointments or appointments that require driving in "rush hour" traffic or that interfere with traditional meal times.

SUMMARY

The aged hearing-impaired population presents infinitely complex diagnostic and rehabilitative challenges to hearing health care professionals. Older hearing aid candidates may have a variety of physical changes in addition to hearing loss that provide a complicated backdrop to problems created by hearing loss, or hearing loss may be their only significant disorder. Aged patients may present themselves alone with no one to assist in the aural rehabilitation process, or they may be warmly supported by a child, a spouse, or a friend in their adaptation to the use of hearing aids and new assertive communication skills. They may have predominantly cochlear-based sensorineural hearing loss and seem no different than their younger counterparts, or they may have more difficulty understanding aided speech than would be predicted on the basis of their pure-tone audiograms. They may present themselves at hearing aid clinics because they truly realize the extent of their disability and desire rehabilitation or may come only to appease a significant other with no acknowledgment of responsibility for the communication problems they are having.

Knowledge of appropriate psychophysical data necessary to describe discretely the auditory function of presbycusic subgroups is incomplete. Our ability to model "normal" auditory function in each aged hearing-impaired patient with uniquely appropriate amplification is, therefore, also imperfect. The procedures that are used in the assessment of the aged patient for use of amplification should specifically define unique cochlear versus central auditory function in presbycusic subgroups. The resultant data should be adaptable to a prescriptive approach for the recommendation of state-of-the art hearing aids or more traditional analogue technology in a way that minimizes the time spent in hearing aid evaluation and fitting and maximizes time spent in counseling and family-centered aural rehabilitation.

In the final analysis, the clinician is best advised to listen to elderly patients and to understand, as much as possible, the orientation (cultural, social, psychological) of the patient with respect to the hearing aid and aural rehabilitation process. Successful aural rehabilitation of the older patient is possible only if there is mutual respect and honesty between the patient and the hearing health care professional. The onus is on the individual professional to recommend the most appropriate hearing aid or aids, to provide supportive family-centered aural rehabilitation counseling to the aged patient, and to involve the patient in a manner that will maximize independent use of all of the equipment and communication strategies offered.

REVIEW QUESTIONS

1. What are the various types of presbycusis, the bases for their classification, and the audiometric patterns unique to each?

2. What audiometric data is recommended to provide the basis for hearing aid selection for elderly patients?

3. Why are cultural considerations important when attempting to provide hearing aids to older patients whose culture identity is other than American.

4. How would you uniquely approach Asian Elders from the various subgroups described in this chapter?

5. Are two hearing aids always better than one for geriatric patients? How would you determine this in your patients, particularly when low communication demands and economics encourage consideration of monaural amplification?

6. Do we know that Digital Signal Processing technology offers the same benefits to the elderly as to younger adult patients?

7. How would you take into consideration the concepts discussed in this chapter in counseling your geriatric patients about selecting from the array of hearing aid and assistive device technology that exists and that are described in greater detail elsewhere in this text?

8. Is there a relationship between the cost of the hearing aid and the expectations for success of the elderly hearing aid user?

9. Do the elderly have greater needs for support services than younger adult patients?

10. What methods would you propose to assess the patient's ability to manipulate the hearing aid that you are recommending?

11. What are the recommended steps in the Geriatric Hearing Aid Evaluation and Orientation Process?

12. Should hearing aids ever be delivered to first-time geriatric hearing aid users without the support of a group aural rehabilitation program during the trial period?

REFERENCES

Alpiner, J. G. (1992). *Handbook of adult rehabilitative audiology*. Baltimore, MD: Williams & Wilkins.

Barford, J. (1979). Speech perception processes and fitting of hearing aids. *Audiology, 18*, 430–441.

Becker, G. (1980). *Growing old in silence*. Berkeley: University of California Press.

Berkowitz, A. (1975). Audiologic rehabilitation of the geriatric patient. *Hearing Aid Journal, 8*, 30–34.

Better Hearing Institute. (1999, June). Available at http://www.betterhearing.org/demograp.htm.

Bienvenue, G., & Michael, P. (1979). Digital processing techniques in speech discrimination testing (critical bandwidth measurements for use in hearing aid testing). In P. Yaneck (Ed.), *Rehabilitative strategies for sensorineural hearing loss*. New York, NY: Grune & Stratton.

Blackington, B., Novak, R. E., & Kramer, S. A. (1988). Temporal masking effects for speech and puretone stimuli in normal hearing aged subjects. Unpublished master's thesis, San Diego State University, San Diego, CA.

Cheng, L. R. (1988). Personal interview with R. E Novak. San Diego, CA.

Corso, T. F. (1963). Age and sex differences in puretone thresholds. *Archives of Otolaryngology, 77,* 53–73.

Cox, R. M. (1997). Administration and application of the APHAB. *Hearing Journal, 50,* 42–48.

Cox, R. M., & Alexander, G. C. (1995). The abbreviated profile of hearing aid benefit. *Ear and Hearing, 16,* 176–186.

Crowe, S. J., & Guild, S. R. (1934). Observation of the pathology of high tone deafness. *Johns Hopkins Hospital Bulletin, 54,* 315–380.

Danaher, E. N., Osberger, M., & Pickett, J. (1973). Discrimination of formant frequency transitions in synthetic vowels. *Journal of Speech and Hearing Research, 16,* 439–451.

deBoer, E., & Bowmeester, J. (1974). Critical bands and sensorineural hearing loss. *Audiology, 13,* 236–259.

deBoer, E., & Bowmeester, J. (1975). Clinical psychophysics. *Audiology, 14,* 274–299.

Dillon, H. J., & Ginis, J. (1997). Patient oriented scale of improvement (COSI) and its relationship to other means of benefit and satisfaction provided by hearing aids. *Journal of the American Academy of Audiology, 8,* 27–43.

Dubno, J. R., Dirks, D. D., & Morgan, D. E. (1984). Effects of age and mild hearing loss on speech recognition in noise. *Journal of the Acoustical Society of America, 76,* 87–96.

Eisenberg, S. (1985). Communication with elderly patients: The effects of illness and medication on mentation, memory, and communication. In H. K. Ulatowska (Ed.), *The aging brain and communication in the elderly.* Boston. MA: College-Hill Press.

Fabini, G. (1931). Regarding morphological and functional changes in the internal ear arteriosclerosis. *Laryngoscope, 4,* 663–670.

Feller, B. (1981). *Prevalence of selected impairments.* United States, 1977 (Series 10, No. 134) National Center for Health Statistics. Washington, DC: U.S. Government Printing Office.

Fisch, L. (1978). Special senses: The aging auditory system. In J. C. Brocklehurst (Ed.), *Textbook of geriatric medicine and gerontology.* New York: Churchill Livingstone.

Fisch, U. (1972). Degenerative changes of the arterial vessels of the internal auditory meatus during the process of aging. *Acta Otolaryngologica, 73,* 259–260.

Franklin, B. (1975). The effects of combining low- and high-frequency pass bands on consonant recognition in the hearing impaired. *Journal of Speech and Hearing Research, 18,* 719–727.

Ganz, R. P. (1976). The effects of aging on the diagnostic utility of the rollover phenomenon. *Journal of Speech and Hearing Disorders, 41,* 63–69.

Garstecki, D. C., & Erler, S. F. (1998). Hearing loss, control and demographic factors influencing hearing aid use among older adults. *Journal of Speech, Language and Hearing Research, 41,* 527–537

Gelfand, D. (1982). *Aging—The ethnic factor*: Boston, MA: Little, Brown.

Geissler, E. M. (1994). *Pocket guide to cultural assessment.* St. Louis, MO: Mosby.

Gentile, A. (1971). Persons with impaired hearing. United States, 1971 (Series 10, No. 134). Washington, DC: U.S. Government Printing Office.

Givens, G. D., Arnold, T., & Hume, W. G. (1998). Auditory processing skills and hearing aid satisfaction in a sample of older adults. *Perceptual and Motor Skills, 86,* 795–801.

Glorig, A., & Davis, H. (1961). Age, noise and hearing loss. *Annals of Otology, 70,* 556–571.

Glorig, A., & Nixon. H. L. (1962). Hearing loss as a function of age. *Laryngoscope, 27,* 1596–1610.

Goldman, R. (1971). Decline in organ function with aging. In L. Rossman (Ed.*), Clinical geriatrics.* Philadelphia, PA: Lippincott.

Gordon-Salant, S., & Fitzgibbons, P. J. (1999). Profile of auditory temporal processing in older listeners. *Journal of Speech Language Hearing Research, 42* 300–311.

Greenblatt, N., & Chien, C. (1983). Depression in the elderly. In L. Breslau & M. Haug (Eds.), *Depression and aging—Causes, care and consequences.* New York: Springer-Verlag.

Harbert, R., Young, J., & Menduke, H. (1966). Audiological findings in presbycusis. *Journal of Auditory Research, 6,* 297–312.

Hawkins, D. B. (1992). Prescriptive approaches to selection of gain and frequency response. In H. G. Mueller, D. B. Hawkins, & J. L. Northern (Eds.), *Probe microphone measurements.* San Diego, CA: Singular Publishing Group.

Hawkins, D. B. (1984). Selection of a critical electroacoustic characteristic: SSPL-90. *Hearing Instruments, 35,* 28–32.

Hawkins, D. B. (1985). Reflections of amplification: Validation of performance. *Journal of the Academy of Rehabilitative Audiology, 17,* 87–96.

Hawkins, D. B., & Schum, D. J. (1984). Relationship among various measures of hearing aid gain. *Journal of Speech and Hearing Disorders, 49,* 94–97.

Hawkins, D. B., Walden, B., Montgomery, A., & Prosek, R. (1987). Description and validation of an LDL procedure designed to select SSPL90. *Ear and Hearing, 8,* 162–169.

Hosford-Dunn, H., & Baxter, J. H. (1985). Prediction and validation of hearing aid wearer benefit: Preliminary findings. *Hearing Instruments, 36,* 34–41.

IHAFF unveils fitting protocol at Jackson Hole Rendezvous. (1994). *The Hearing Review, 9.*

Iler, K., Danhauer, J. L., & Mulac, A. (1982). Peer perceptions of geriatrics wearing hearing aids. *Journal of Speech and Hearing Disorders, 47*, 433–438.

Jerger, J. (1960). Békésy audiometry in analysis of auditory disorders. *Journal of Speech and Hearing Research, 3*, 275–287.

Jerger, J., Jerger, S., Oliver, T., & Pirozzolo, F. (1993). Speech understanding in the elderly. In B. R. Alford & S. Jerger (Eds.), *Clinical audiology: The Jerger perspective*. San Diego, CA: Singular Publishing Group.

Krmpotic-Nemanic, J. (1971). A new concept of the pathogenesis of presbycusis. *Archives of Otolaryngology, 93*, 161–166.

Kyle, J. G., Jones, L. G., & Wood, P. L. (1985). Adjustment to acquired hearing loss: A working model. In H. Orlans (Ed.), *Adjustment to adult hearing loss*. Boston, MA: College-Hill Press.

Kyle, J. G., & Wood, P. L. (1983). Social and vocational aspects of acquired hearing loss. Final report to MSC School of Education, Bristol. (Reported in Kyle, J. G., Jones, L. G., & Wood, P. L. [1985]). Adjustment to acquired hearing loss: A working model. In H. Orlans [Ed.], *Adjustment to adult hearing loss*. Boston, MA: College-Hill Press.)

Lipman, A. (1968). A socio-architectural view of life in three homes for older people. *Gerontologica Clinica, 10*, 88–101.

Lynn, G. E., & Gilroy, J. (1976). Central aspects of audition. In J. Northern (Ed.), *Hearing disorders*. Boston, MA: Little, Brown.

Margolis, R., & Goldberg, S. (1980). Auditory frequency selectivity in normal and presbycusic subjects. *Journal of Speech and Hearing Research, 23*, 603–613.

Marshall, L. (1981). Auditory processing in aging listeners. *Journal of Speech and Hearing Disorders, 46*, 226–236.

Mauldin, C. R. (1976). Communication and the aging consumer. In H. J. Oyer & E. J. Oyer (Eds.), *Aging and communication*. Baltimore, MD: University Park Press.

Maurer, J. F., & Rupp, R. R. (1979). *Hearing and aging—tactics for intervention*. New York: Grune & Stratton.

Mayer, O. (1970). Das anatomische Substrat der Altersschwerhörigkeit. *Archiv Ohren-Nasen-und Kehlkopf Heilkunde, 105*, 1313.

McCartney, J. (1977, November/December). A look at hearing loss. *Perspectives on Aging*, 10–11.

Meadow-Orlans, K. P. (1985). Social and psychological effects of hearing loss in adulthood: A literature review. In H. Orlans (Ed.), *Adjustment to adult hearing loss*. Boston, MA: College-Hill Press.

Medical Research Council Institute of Hearing Research. (1981). Population study of hearing disorders in adults. *Journal of the Royal Society of Medicine, 74*, 819–827.

Merluzzi, F., & Hinchcliffe, R. (1973). Threshold of subjective auditory handicap. *Audiology, 12*, 65–69.

Mills, J. H., Gilbert, R. M., & Adkins, W. V. (1979, February). *Some effects of noise on auditory sensitivity, temporal integration and psychophysical tuning curves*. Paper presented at Second Midwinter Research Meeting of the Association for Research in Otolaryngology, St. Petersburg, FL.

Mueller, H. G. (1997). Prescriptive fitting methods: The next generation. *Hearing Journal, 50*, 10–16.

Mueller, H. G., & Palmer, C. V (1998). The profile of aided loudness: A new "PAL" for '98. *Hearing Journal, 51*, 10–16.

Mueller, H. G., Hawkins, D., & Sedge, R. K. (1984). Three important variables in hearing aid selection. *Hearing Instruments, 35*.

Musiek F., & Rintelmann, W. (1999). *Contemporary perspectives in hearing assessment*. Boston, MA: Allyn and Bacon.

National Ear Care Plan. (1999, June). Available at http://www.necp.com/hrstats.htm.

National Council on the Aging. (1999). Survey of hard of hearing hearing aid users and non-users and their families. Washington, DC: Author.

Nelson, D. A. (1979, February). *Frequency selectivity in listeners with sensori-neural hearing loss*. Paper presented at Second Midwinter Research Meeting of the Association for Research in Otolaryngology, St. Petersburg, FL.

Nixon, J. C., & Glorig, A. (1962). Changes in air and bone conduction thresholds as a function of age. *Journal of Laryngology, 76*, 288–292.

Novak, R. E., & Anderson, C. V. (1982). The differentiation of types of presbycusis using the masking level difference. *Journal of Speech and Hearing Research, 25*, 504–508.

Olsen, W. O., & Noffsinger, D. (1974). Comparison of one new and three old tests of auditory adaptation. *Archives of Otolaryngology, 99*, 94.

Olsen, W., Noffsinger, D., & Carhart, R. (1976). Masking level difference encountered in clinical populations. *Audiology, 15*, 287–301.

Oyer, H. J., & Oyer, E. J. (1979). Social consequences of hearing loss for the elderly. *Allied Health and Behavioral Sciences, 2*, 123–137.

Palva, A., & Jokenen, H. (1970). Presbycusis v. filtered speech test. *Acta Otolaryngologica, 70*, 232–241.

Parenti, M. (1978). *Power and powerlessness*. New York, NY: St. Martin's Press.

Pascoe, D. (1988). Clinical measurements of the auditory dynamic range and their relation to formulas for hearing aid gain. In J. H. Jensen (Ed.), *Hearing aid fitting: Theoretical and practical views*. Copenhagen: Stougaard/Jensen.

Popelka, M. M., Cruickshanks, K. J., Wiley, T. L., Tweed, T. S., Klein, B. E., Klein, R. (1998). Low prevalence of hearing aid use among older adults with hearing loss: the Epidemiology of hearing loss study. *Journal of the American Geriatric Society, 46*, 1075–1078.

Potash, M., & Jones, B. (1977). Aging and decision criteria for the detection of tones in noise. *Journal of Gerontology, 32*, 436–440.

Purnell, L. D., & Paulanka, B. J. (1998). *Transcultural health care: A culturally competent approach.* Philadelphia, PA: F.A. Davis Company.

Reed, C. M., & Bilger, R. C. (1973). A comparative study of S/NO and E/NO. *Journal of the Acoustical Society of America, 53*, 1039–1044.

Rees, J. N., & Botwinick, J. (1971). Detection and decision factors in auditory behavior of the elderly. *Journal of Gerontology, 26*, 133–136.

Ries, P. W. (1982). *Hearing ability of persons by sociodemographic and health characteristics.* United States (Series No. 10, No. 140). National Center for Health Statistics. Washington, DC: Government Printing Office.

Ries, P. W. (1994). *Prevalence and characteristics of persons with hearing trouble: United States, 1990–91.* National Center for Health Statistics. Vital Health Statistics, 10 (188).

Rosen, S., Bergman, M., Plester, D., El Mofty, A., & Sotti, M. (1962). Presbycuses study of a relatively noise free population in the Sudan. *Annals of Otolaryngology, 71*, 727–743.

Rosen, S., Plester, D., El Mofty, A., & Rosen, H. (1970). High-frequency audiometry in presbycusis. *Annals of Otolaryngology, 79*, 18–32.

Rupp, R., Higgins, J., & Maurer, J. F. (1977). A feasibility scale for predicting hearing aid use (FSPHAU) with older individuals. *Journal of the Auditory Rehabilitation Association, 10*, 81–194.

Schow, R. L., Christensen, J. M., Hutchinson, J. M., & Nerbonne, M. A. (1978). *Communicative disorders of the aged.* Baltimore, MD: University Park Press.

Schow, R. L., & Goldbaum, D. E. (1980). Collapsed ear canals in the elderly nursing home population. *Journal of Speech and Hearing Disorders, 45*, 259–267.

Schow, R.L., & Nerbonne, M.A. (1980). Hearing levels among elderly nursing home residents. *Journal of Speech and Hearing Disorders, 45*, 124–132.

Schuknecht, H. F. (1951). Lesions of the organ Corti. *Transactions of the American Academy of Ophthalmology and Otolaryngology, 57*, 366.

Schuknecht. H. F. (1955). Presbycusis. *Laryngoscope, 65*, 42.

Schuknecht, H. F. (1964). Further observations on the pathology of presbycusis. *Archives of Otolaryngology, 80*, 369–382.

Schuknecht, H. F. (1974). *Pathology of the ear.* Cambridge, MA: Harvard University Press.

Schum, E., Matthews, L., & Lee, F. (1991). Actual and predicted word-recognition performance of elderly hearing-impaired listeners. *Journal of Speech and Hearing Research, 34*, 636–642.

Seewald, R. C., Cornelisse, L. E., Ramji, K.V., Sinclair, S.T., Moodie, K.S., & Jamieson, D. G. (1997). *DSL v 4 1a for Windows. A software implementation of the desired sensation level* DSL i/o method for fitting linear gain and wide dynamic range compression hearing instruments. London, ON: Univ of Western Ontario.

Skafte, M. (1986). Communicate for a longer life. *Hearing Instruments, 37*, 4.

Spector, R. E. (1996). *Cultural diversity in health and illness.* Stamford, CT: Appleton & Lange.

Thomas, A., & Gilhome-Herbst, K. (1980). Social or psychological implications of acquired deafness for adults of employment age. *British Journal of Audiology, 14*, 76–85.

Taeuber, C. (1992). *Sixty-five plus in America.* Washington, DC: U.S. Department of Commerce, Economics and Statistics Administration. Bureau of the Census.

Tyler, R. S., Fernandes, M., & Wood, E. J. (1984). Masking temporal integration and speech intelligibility in individuals with noise induced hearing loss. In G. Taylor (Ed.), *Disorders of auditory function III.* New York, NY: Academic Press.

Ulatowska, H. K. (1985). *The aging brain: Communication in the elderly.* Boston, MA: College-Hill Press.

Valente, M., & Van Vliet, D. 1997. The IHAFF protocol. *Trends in Amplification, 2.*

Ventry, L. M., & Weinstein, B. E. (1982). The hearing handicap inventory for the elderly: A new tool. *Ear and Hearing, 3*, 128–134.

Warren, L. R., Wagener, J., & Herman, G. (1978). Binaural analysis in the aging auditory system. *Journal of Gerontology, 33*, 731–736.

Weinstein, B. E., & Ventry, L. M. (1983). Audiometric correlates of the hearing handicap inventory for the elderly. *Journal of Speech and Hearing Disorders, 84*, 379–383.

Zelisko, D., Wolf, R., & Burton, P. (1999). Matching new technology to patient's needs. *The Hearing Review, 6.*

Zucker, K., & Williams, P. S. (1977, November). *Audiological services in extended care facilities.* Paper presented at the American Speech and Hearing Convention, Chicago, IL.

Zurek, P., & Formby, C. (1977). *Frequency discriminability of sensorineural listeners.* Paper presented at the Second Midwinter Research Meeting of the American Speech and Hearing Association, Chicago, IL.

Zwaardemaker, H. (1981). Der verlust an horen tonen mit zunehemendum alter: ein neues gesetz. *Arch Ohr Nas-Kehlk-Heilk, 32*, 53.

Zwicker, E., & Shorn, K. (1978). Psychoacoustical tuning curves in audiology. *Audiology, 17*, 120–140.

CHAPTER 19

Hearing Aid Amplification and Central Auditory Disorders

BRAD A. STACH, PH.D.

OUTLINE

(continued)

The central auditory nervous system is a highly complex network that analyzes and processes neural information from both ears and transmits it to the auditory cortex and other areas within the nervous system. Auditory processing ability is usually defined as the capacity with which the central auditory nervous system transfers information from the VIIIth nerve to the auditory cortex. Central auditory processing disorders (CAPDs) are impairments in this function of the central auditory nervous system.

The central auditory nervous system plays an important role in comparing sound at the two ears for the purpose of sound localization. It also plays a major role in extracting a signal of interest from a background of noise. While signals at the cochlea are analyzed exquisitely in the frequency, amplitude, and temporal domains, it is in the central auditory nervous system where those fundamental analyses are eventually perceived as speech or some other meaningful non-speech sound.

The ability of the central auditory nervous system to process sound was evaluated historically for diagnostic purposes to identify specific lesions or disease processes of the nervous system. Numerous measures of auditory nervous system function were scrutinized for what they could reveal about the presence of such neurologic disorders and form a basis for the assessment of central auditory disorders today, which is much more focused on describing communication disorder than on diagnosing specific neurologic disorders. Results of such an assessment provide an estimate of central auditory processing ability and a more complete profile of a patient's auditory abilities and handicap (Chmiel and Jerger, 1996; Jerger, Oliver, & Pirozzolo, 1990). Such information is often useful in providing guidance regarding appropriate amplification strategies or other rehabilitation approaches (Chmiel, Jerger, Murphy, Pirozzolo, & Tooley-Young, 1997; Stach, Jerger, & Fleming, 1985; Stach, Loiselle, & Jerger, 1991).

Although conventional hearing aid amplification can be used to effectively treat hearing sensitivity loss, its effectiveness may be reduced by concomitant central auditory disorder. Elderly patients, who constitute the largest number of hearing aid users, often have hearing problems characterized by both hearing sensitivity loss and central auditory disorder (Hayes, 1980; Jerger, 1973; Jerger & Hayes, 1977; Otto & McCandless, 1982; Pestalozza & Shore, 1955; Schuknecht & Igarashi, 1964; Welsh, Welsh, & Healy, 1985). The impact of such deficits on amplification solutions for these older patients, as well as for children with specifically-auditory central processing disorder, warrants careful attention.

Perhaps an even greater challenge than delineating the relationship between hearing aid use and central auditory disorder is developing beneficial amplification strategies. Merely amplifying sound to overcome a peripheral hearing loss may provide little, if any, advantage to a young or aging auditory system that requires an enhanced signal-to-noise ratio

(SNR) because of central auditory disorder. Remote and directional microphones, as well as better noise reduction circuitry in conventional hearing aids, hold promise as effective intervention strategies for those with central auditory disorder.

THE NATURE OF CAPD IN ADULTS

Although there is a tendency to think of hearing impairment as the sensitivity loss that can be measured on an audiogram, there are other types of hearing impairment that may or may not be accompanied by sensitivity loss. These other impairments result from disease, damage, or degradation of the central auditory nervous system in adults or delayed or disordered auditory nervous system development in children.

A disordered auditory nervous system, regardless of cause, can have functional consequences that range from subclinical to substantial. Auditory nervous system impairments tend to be divided into two groups, depending on the nature of the underlying disorder, even though the functional consequences may be similar. When an impairment is caused by active, measurable disease process, such as a tumor or other space-occupying lesion, or from damage due to trauma or stroke, it is often referred to as a retrocochlear disorder. That is, retrocochlear disorders result from structural lesions of the nervous system. When an impairment is due to developmental disorder or delay or from diffuse changes such as the aging process, it is often referred to as a central auditory processing disorder. That is, central auditory processing disorders result from "functional lesions" of the nervous system. The term central auditory processing disorder is also used to describe the functional consequence of a retrocochlear disorder.

Retrocochlear disorders are those that are often addressed first by medical management. Residual communication disorder is often a secondary consideration because of the immediate health threat of retrocochlear disease. Central auditory processing disorders often present as communication disorders and are either the residual consequence of a retrocochlear disorder or are the consequence of diffuse changes or disorders that are not amenable to medical management. That both types of disorder may present similar audiologic findings can be challenging clinically, but their treatment as a communication disorder is not likely to differ, because the functional deficit to the patient will be similar despite the underlying cause.

Causes and Effects of CAPD

There are two primary causes of central auditory processing disorders. One is neuropathology of the peripheral and central auditory nervous systems, resulting from tumors, other space-occupying lesions, or damage due to trauma or stroke. The other is from diffuse changes in brain function or developmental delays or disorders.

Disorders Secondary to Neuropathology

A retrocochlear disorder is caused by a change in neural structure of some component of the peripheral or central auditory nervous system. The influence that this structural change will have on function depends primarily on lesion size, location, and impact. For example, a retrocochlear lesion may or may not affect auditory sensitivity. A tumor on the VIIIth cranial nerve can cause a substantial sensorineural hearing loss, depending on how much pressure it places on the nerve, the damage that it causes to the nerve, or the extent to which it interrupts blood supply to the cochlea. A tumor in the temporal lobe, however, is quite unlikely to result in any change in hearing sensitivity, although it may result in a more subtle hearing disorder as noted in measures of suprathreshold function such as speech recognition ability.

VIIIth Nerve Disorder

Retrocochlear neuropathology can occur at any level in the peripheral and central auditory nervous system pathway. The most peripheral of retrocochlear disorders result from lesions of the VIIIth cranial nerve. The most common neoplastic growth affecting the auditory nerve is called a cochleovestibular schwannoma, which is a benign, encapsulated tumor composed of Schwann cells that arises from the VIIIth cranial nerve. Acoustic tumors are unilateral and most often arise from the vestibular branch of the VIIIth nerve. In addition to cochleovestibular schwannoma, a number of other types of tumors, cysts, and aneurysms can affect the VIIIth nerve and the cerebellopontine angle, where the VIIIth nerve enters the brain stem. In addition, not unlike any cranial nerve, the VIIIth nerve can develop neuritis, or inflammation of the nerve. Although rare, acute cochlear neuritis can occur as a result of a direct viral attack on the cochlear portion of the nerve.

Among the most common symptoms of cochleovestibular schwannoma and other acoustic tumors are unilateral tinnitus and unilateral hearing loss. The hearing disorder varies in degree depending on the location and size of the tumor. Hearing sensitivity can range from normal to a profound hearing loss. Speech recognition ability typically is disproportionately poor for the degree of hearing loss. If the tumor is affecting function of the VIIIth nerve, its effects are unlikely to be subtle.

Brain Stem Disorders

Brain stem disorders that affect the auditory system include infarcts, gliomas, and multiple sclerosis. Brain stem infarcts are localized areas of ischemia produced by interruption of the blood supply. Gliomas are tumors composed of neuroglia, or supporting cells of the brain. They develop in various forms, depending on the types of cells involved. Multiple sclerosis is a demyelinating disease. It is caused by an autoimmune reaction of the nervous system that results in small scattered areas of demyelination and the development of demyelinated plaques.

Central auditory processing disorders associated with brain stem lesions will vary depending on level at which they occur in the brain stem as well as the extent of the lesion's influence. Generally, the higher in the brain stem, the more subtle are the effects of the lesion. In lower brain stem lesions, performance on difficult monotic tasks is typically poor in the ear ipsilateral to the disorder. In addition, abnormalities are often found in measures of binaural release from masking. In higher brain stem lesions, performance on difficult monotic tasks can be abnormal in both the ipsilateral and contralateral ear. Brain stem lesions have also been associated with reduction in localization, lateralization, and temporal processing abilities.

Cortical Disorders

One of the more common cortical pathologies is caused by cerebrovascular accident, or stroke, which results from an interruption of blood supply to the brain due to aneurysm, embolism, or clot. This in turn causes a sudden loss of function related to the affected portion of the brain. Any other disease processes, lesions, or trauma that affect the central nervous system can affect the central auditory nervous system as well. When the temporal lobe is involved, audition may be affected, although more typically, receptive language processing is affected while hearing perception is relatively spared.

Central auditory processing disorders associated with temporal lobe lesions include poor dichotic performance, some reduction in performance on difficult monotic tasks typically in the ear opposite to the lesion, impaired localization ability, and reduced temporal processing ability. In cases of bilateral temporal lobe lesions, "cortical deafness" can occur, resulting in symptoms that resemble auditory agnosia or profound hearing sensitivity loss (Hood, Berlin, & Allen, 1994; Jerger, Lovering, & Wertz, 1972; Jerger, Weikers, Sharbrough, & Jerger, 1969).

Central Disorders of Aging

Changes in structure and function occur throughout the peripheral and central auditory nervous systems as a result of the aging process. Structural degeneration occurs in the cochlea and in the central auditory nervous system pathways. Histopathologic and morphologic studies have documented structural degeneration in the auditory nerve (Krmpotic-Nemanic, 1971; Schuknecht, 1964) and at the level of the auditory brain stem and cortex (Brody, 1955; Corso, 1976; Hansen & Reske-Nielsen, 1965; Hinchcliffe, 1962; Kirikae, Sato, & Shitara, 1964).

Anatomic and physiologic aging of the auditory system results from at least two processes (Willott, 1996). One is the central effects of peripheral pathology, or those that are secondary to the deprivational effects of cochlear hearing loss. The other is the central effects of biologic aging of the nervous system structures themselves. As with all other structures of the body, the brain undergoes changes related to the aging process. These central effects of biologic aging include a loss of neuronal tissue; loss of dendritic branches, reducing the number of synaptic contacts; changes in excitatory and inhibitory neurotransmitter systems; and other degenerative changes.

Because age related changes can occur throughout the auditory system, many patients with presbyacusis will demonstrate behavior suggestive of both peripheral and central auditory disorder. The effect of structural changes in the auditory periphery is to attenuate incoming sound. For the most part, speech understanding deficits can be explained by the degree of loss and shape of the audiometric contour (Goetzinger, Proud, Dirks, & Embrey, 1961; Jerger & Hayes, 1977; Mills, 1978). In contrast, the major effect of structural changes in the central auditory pathways is one of degradation of suprathreshold speech perception (Antonelli, 1970; Arnst, 1982; Bergman, 1971; Bergman et al., 1976; Bosatra & Russolo, 1982; Hinchcliffe, 1962; Konkle, Beasley, & Bess, 1977; Lutterman, Welsh, & Melrose, 1966; Orchik & Burgess, 1977; Sticht & Gray, 1969). Aging patients have been shown to perform more poorly than would be predicted on the basis of the audiogram alone on tests that incorporate frequency- and time-altered speech materials or speech presented in a background of noise (Bocca, 1958; Goetzinger et al., 1961; Hayes, 1984; Helfer and Wilber, 1990; Jerger, 1973; Jerger & Hayes, 1977; Konig, 1969; Letowski and Poch, 1996; Pestalozza & Shore, 1955; Price and Simon, 1984; Shirinian & Arnst, 1982; Wiley et al., 1998).

The number of elderly adults with central auditory disorder may be substantial. After degree of hearing loss is accounted for, as many as 80 percent of clinical patients ranging in age from 75-79 years have some degree of central disorder (Stach, Spretnjak, & Jerger, 1990). As many as 25% of older patients have some degree of dichotic deficit (Jerger, Stach, Johnson, Loiselle, & Jerger, 1990). The prevalence is significantly lower in the non-clinical elderly population (Cooper & Gates, 1991).

The question of whether central auditory disorder exists as a result of the aging process has not been without controversy over the years. Clinical measurement of central processing ability is based primarily on speech audiometric techniques, many of which have been validated on patients with neurologic disorders (Lynn, Benitez, Eisenbrey, Gilroy, & Wilner, 1972; Jerger & Jerger, 1975; Musiek & Baran, 1987). By inference, then, a patient whose poor performance on speech audiometric tasks resembles that of a neurologically impaired patient is said to have a processing disorder at the level of the central auditory nervous system, or CAPD.

Because the diagnosis of CAPD has been so dependent on behavioral, speech-based techniques, its very existence has been questioned. In the elderly, decline in memory, speed-of-information processing, and peripheral hearing sensitivity have all been implicated as the cause of reduced speech understanding (Humes, Christopherson, & Cokely, 1992; Working Group on Speech Understanding and Aging, 1988). Recent evidence suggests that neither cognitive decline, language deficit, nor peripheral hearing loss can be invoked as the simple explanation for the decline in speech processing that characterizes CAPD, however. Indeed, auditory processing disorders that cannot be explained on the basis of these nonauditory factors have been isolated in aging patients (Jerger, Jerger, Oliver, & Pirozzolo, 1989; Jerger, Mahurin, & Pirozzolo, 1990; Jerger, Stach, Pruitt, Harper, & Kirby, 1989).

Central auditory processing ability has been measured in a number of ways. Although the strategies used have been found to be more or less sensitive as measures of central auditory ability, problems in interpretation of many of them can occur if a peripheral hearing loss, a language disorder, or a cognitive deficit is present. That is, performance on such tests can be affected by other auditory and nonauditory factors, and differentiation of peripheral or cognitive components from central components can be difficult. These confounding variables either need to be controlled during the test session or their influence on test results must be quantified.

Symptoms and Signs

Disorders of central auditory processing have two fundamental characteristics. First, auditory sensitivity loss rarely results from CAPD. Pure-tone thresholds, in the absence of other deleterious factors, are usually normal in patients with CAPD. Second, the most pervasive characteristic of central auditory disorder is poor speech understanding. Although performance is typically normal on tests in which unaltered speech materials are presented in quiet, performance is reduced on complex speech tasks that stress the central processing of auditory information.

Symptoms

Some individuals with central auditory processing disorders will have normal hearing sensitivity. Others, especially those who are elderly, will have some degree of peripheral hearing sensitivity loss upon which the central auditory disorder is imposed. In the former group, the most common symptom is that of a hearing disorder in the presence of normal hearing sensitivity. Such patients will describe difficulty hearing in certain listening situations despite their ability to detect faint sounds. In the latter group, the most common symptom will be a hearing disorder that seems to be disproportionate to the degree of hearing sensitivity loss. Regardless of category, those with central auditory processing disorders share common difficulties along a continuum of severity.

The most common symptom of central auditory processing disorder is difficulty extracting a signal of interest from a background of noise. Patients with central auditory disorders will simply have difficulty hearing in noise. Another common symptom is difficulty spatially locating a sound source, especially in the presence of background noise. Perhaps as a consequence of these symptoms, patients and their families are also likely to describe behaviors such as inattentiveness and distractibility.

These symptoms, of course, are not necessarily unlike those of patients with peripheral hearing sensitivity loss. It should be no surprise that an auditory disorder, regardless of its locus, would result in similar perceived difficulties. Perhaps the distinguishing feature for patients with central auditory processing disorder is the inability to extract sounds of interest in noisy environments despite an ability to perceive the sounds with adequate loudness.

Signs

Not surprisingly, clinical findings in patients with central auditory processing disorders reflect impairments in those functions attributable to the central auditory nervous system. Although the clinical signs attributable to a central disorder may provide insight into the basis and locus of the underlying disorder, the symptoms related to the various signs seem to be reasonably similar across patients. That is, whether a disorder is identified as a problem in temporal processing, dichotic listening, or localization, the functional consequence to the patient tends to be difficulty hearing in adverse listening environments.

Subtlety and Bottleneck Principles

As a general rule, the more peripheral a lesion, the greater its impact will be on auditory function (the bottleneck principle). Conversely, the more central the lesion, the more subtle its impact will be (the subtlety principle). A well placed lesion on the auditory nerve can substantially impact hearing, whereas a lesion in the midbrain is likely to have more subtle effects.

Perhaps the best illustration of the bottleneck principle comes from reports of cases with lesions that effectively disconnect the cochlea from the brain stem. These cases demonstrate the presence of severe or profound hearing loss and very poor speech recognition despite normal cochlear function, as indicated by normal otoacoustic emissions or VIIIth nerve action potentials. In cases involving lesions of the cerebellopontine angle secondary to tumor (Cacace, Parnes, Lovely, & Kalathia, 1994), multiple sclerosis (Stach & Delgado-Vilches, 1993), and miliary tuberculosis (Stach, Westerberg, & Roberson, 1998), results have shown how a strategically placed lesion at the bottleneck can substantially affect hearing ability. The bottleneck in the case of the auditory system is, of course, the VIIIth nerve as it enters the auditory brain stem.

One specific type of auditory nervous system disorder identified recently is auditory neuropathy (Starr, Picton, Sininger, Hood, & Berlin, 1996; Starr, et al., 1998), a term used to describe a condition in which cochlear function is normal and VIIIth nerve function is abnormal. It is distinguishable from disorders due to space-occupying lesions in that imaging results of the nerve and brain stem are normal. Nevertheless, auditory neuropathy is a disorder that exemplifies the consequences of a disorder at the level of the bottleneck.

If the bottleneck is unaffected, then lesions at higher levels will have effects on auditory processing ability that are more subtle. These effects tend to become increasingly subtle as the lesions are located more centrally in the system. For example, whereas a lesion at the bottleneck can cause a substantial hearing sensitivity loss, a brain stem lesion often results in only a mild low-frequency sensitivity loss (Jerger & Jerger, 1980), and a temporal lobe lesion is unlikely to affect hearing sensitivity at all. Similarly speech recognition of words presented in quiet can be very poor in the case of a lesion at the periphery but will be unaffected by a lesion at the level of the temporal lobe.

Reduced Speech Recognition

One hallmark sign of central auditory processing disorder is a reduction in recognition of speech materials that have been altered in some way, such as by limiting the frequency content of the signal. It has been known for over 40 years that reducing the informational content, or redundancy, of speech targets by low-pass filtering creates a challenge to an impaired auditory nervous system that is not present in an intact system (Boca, Calearo, & Cassinari, 1954). As a result, patients with auditory processing disorder are likely to perform more poorly on a low-pass filtered speech test than those with normal hearing ability.

Another sign of central auditory disorder is an inability to extract signals of interest, usually speech, from a competing background. In general, the more meaningful or speech-like the competition, the more interfering will be its influence on perception (Sperry, Wiley, & Chial, 1997; Stuart & Phillips, 1996).

In cases of normal auditory processing ability, speech recognition performance increases systematically as speech intensity is increased, to an asymptotic level representing the best speech understanding that can be achieved in that ear. In some cases, however, there is a paradoxical *rollover* effect, in which performance declines substantially as speech intensity increases beyond the level producing the maximal performance score. In other words, as speech intensity increases, performance rises to a maximum level, then declines or "rolls over" sharply as intensity continues to increase. This rollover effect is commonly observed when the site of the hearing loss is retrocochlear, in the auditory nerve or the auditory pathways in the brain stem (Dirks, Kamm, Bower, & Betsworth, 1977; Jerger & Jerger, 1971).

Impairment in processing in the time domain is also a common sign in central auditory disorders. Temporal processing deficits have been identified based on a number of measures, including time compression of speech, duration pattern discrimination, duration difference limens, gap detection, and so on. Some researchers believe that deficits in temporal processing are the underlying cause of and primary contributors to many of the other measurable deficits associated with central auditory processing disorders.

Binaural Disorders

The ability to localize acoustic stimuli generally requires auditory system integration of sound from both ears. Some patients with central auditory disorders have difficulty locating the directional source of a sound in a soundfield or lateralizing the perception of a sound within the head.

Most people with intact auditory nervous systems are able to identify different signals presented simultaneously to both ears. If the signals are linguistic in nature, most individuals will experience a slight right ear advantage in dichotic listening ability. Central auditory processing disorder, particularly due to impairment of the corpus callosum and auditory cortex, often results in dichotic deficits characterized by substantial reduction in performance in one or both ears.

The binaural auditory system is an exquisite detector of differences in timing of sound reaching the two ears. This helps in spatial location of low frequency sounds, which reach the ears at different points in time. Abnormal ability in processing these timing cues is a common sign of auditory disorder that occurs as a result of impairment in the lower auditory brain stem.

A different kind of deficit in binaural processing is referred to as *binaural interference*. Under normal circumstances, binaural hearing provides an advantage over monaural hearing. This so-called binaural advantage has been noted in loudness judgements, speech recognition, and evoked potential amplitudes. In contrast, in cases of binaural interference, binaural performance is actually poorer than the best monaural performance. In such cases, performance on a perceptual task with both ears can actually be poorer than performance on the better ear in cases of asymmetric perceptual ability. It appears that the poorer ear actually reduces binaural performance below the better monaural performance.

AMPLIFICATION AND CAPD IN ADULTS

Conventional hearing aid amplification is designed to amplify sound as a means of overcoming hearing sensitivity loss. Improvements in modern hearing aids permit the adjustment of gain across frequencies in a manner that packages amplified sound within the range of a patient's hearing sensitivity and loudness discomfort levels. These efforts to make speech audible, although sufficient in many cases of peripheral sensitivity loss, do not necessarily address the problems in hearing caused by central auditory disorders.

The issue of amplification and central auditory disorders in adults is primarily related to those with central auditory disorder resulting from the aging process. In other patients, those with documented neuropathology, the answer to the question of amplification is ordinarily clear. In cases where the pathology causes a change in hearing sensitivity, the disorder is usually unilateral and results in sufficient distortion of the signal to preclude conventional hearing aid use. In cases where the pathology does not cause a change in sensitivity, conventional hearing aids are not ordinarily considered, and any amplification that might be used is usually some form of remote-microphone system. In the case of aging, however, the challenge is greater. In most cases, patients with central auditory aging also have a peripheral hearing sensitivity loss, either causing or coincident with a central processing deficit. In these cases, conventional hearing aids are indicated for the sensitivity loss. Whether their use is beneficial for the central disorder or whether the central disorder detrimentally influences their use can be an important factor in successful implementation.

For purposes of reviewing the known influences of central auditory disorder on success with conventional hearing aid amplification, they will be categorized into one of five types of deficits, those of temporal processing, SNR loss, acquired suprathreshold asymmetry, dichotic listening, and binaural processing.

Temporal Processing Disorders

Nature of the Disorder

One consequence of central auditory disorder, particularly notable in auditory aging, is the presence of temporal processing deficits (Fitzgibbons & Gordon-Salant, 1996; Gordon-Salant & Fitzgibbons, 1999; Grose, 1996), or a reduction in the ability to perceive or discriminate short duration acoustic signals or changes. Temporal processing deficits have been identified in aging subjects based on a number of measures, including time compressed speech (Konkle, Beasley, & Bess, 1977; Letowski and Poch, 1996; Sticht and Gray, 1969), duration pattern discrimination (Abel, Krever, & Alberti, 1990; Phillips, Gordon-Salant, Fitzgibbons, & Yeni-Komshian, 1994), duration difference limen (Fitzgibbons and Gordon-Salant, 1996), gap detection (Lutman, 1991; Moore, Peters, & Glasberg, 1992; Schneider, Pichora-Fuller, Kowalchuk, & Lamb, 1994), and the precedence effect (Cranford and Romereim, 1992).

Deficits in temporal processing may be the underlying cause of and primary contributors to many of the other measurable deficits associated with central auditory processing disorders. This may be intuitively appealing in explaining some of the difficulty that older patients have hearing speech in the presence of background competition. Performance of aging patients in the identification of speech in the presence of a constant background of white noise is not greatly different from performance of younger patients, once hearing loss is controlled. However, if the competition is that of a single talker, for example, younger listeners can perceive speech through the acoustic gaps that occur in the competition. Older listeners appear to be relatively less able to make use of these temporal windows and often have considerable difficulty with such a task. It is conceivable, then, that underlying fundamental changes in the ability to process temporally can have broad implications in the hearing ability of patients with central auditory disorders.

Given that older individuals do not perceive rapid or time-compressed speech as well as younger ones, it stands to reason that if the temporal characteristics of speech could be reduced to effectively slow the rate, then the older group should show improved speech perception. Nakamura and colleagues (1994) described results of a study in which they temporally altered speech in real time to slow the rate of initial portions of speech phrases. Results of the study showed that speech intelligibility was enhanced substantially in older individuals by slowing speech rate. These results may have implications for signal processing algorithms in digital hearing aids in the future.

Influence of the Disorder on Amplification

Except as these temporal processing disorders are reflected in other consequences of central auditory disorder such as SNR deficits, there have been few, if any, studies that clarify the relationship of temporal disorders to success with hearing aid amplification.

In one pertinent study, Wingfield, Poon, Lombardi, and Lowe (1985) showed that rate of speech had an adverse influence on speech perception in older subjects for random strings of words, but relatively less influence as sentences became more meaningful. These results suggest an interaction of rate and semantic content, so that the less meaningful the speech signal, the more detrimental will be the effect of rate. Conversely, the more meaningful the speech, the less likely that rate will be an influence in perception by the elderly. The obvious implication is that higher fidelity amplification of speech by hearing aids, permitting better audibility for semantic processing, will reduce some of the detrimental influences of rate on speech perception.

Signal-to-Noise Ratio Deficits

Nature of the Disorder

One of the most important consequences of central auditory processing disorder is an inability to identify speech in the presence of competition. Much of the early work in this area focused on monaural perception of speech targets in a background of competition presented to the same ear. Results showed that aging listeners do not perform as well as younger listeners on tasks that involve the understanding of speech in the presence of background noise (Goetzinger et al, 1961; Helfer & Wilber, 1990; Jerger, 1973; Jerger & Hayes, 1977; Konig, 1969; Orchik & Burgess, 1977; Pestalozza & Shore, 1955; Shirinian & Arnst, 1982; Wiley et al., 1998). Other results have shown deficits in patients with central auditory disorders when competition is presented to the opposite ear or when both targets and competition are presented to both ears in a soundfield (Jerger & Jordon, 1992; Jerger, Johnson, et al., 1991).

Influence of the Disorder on Amplification

However well substantiated the phenomenon of central auditory aging appears to be, the question of its effect on hearing aid use is not altogether clear. Some studies have suggested that elderly patients are generally less satisfied with amplification than younger patients (Berger & Hagberg, 1982; Jerger & Hayes, 1976;), but it is not clear whether this dissatisfaction is related to nonauditory aging problems or central auditory aging. Two areas of research have addressed this question. The first is the relationship between central auditory disorder and clinical performance with amplification, and the second is the relationship between central auditory disorder and satisfaction with or benefit from hearing aid use.

Central Presbyacusis and Hearing Aid Performance

If central processing disorder affects hearing aid use, then the elderly patient with central auditory disorder should perform more poorly during hearing aid evaluations. Hayes and Jerger (1979) studied performance with hearing aids of 154 patients aged 60 years or older. They divided the patients into three groups based on speech recognition ability. Figure 19–1 shows the results of aided performance for the three groups. The group with central disorder, characterized by reduced SNR ability, performed more poorly than the other groups at all message-to-competition ratios (MCRs). A systematic decline in performance also occurred as the central component increased. The authors further divided the groups to match for age and degree of sensitivity loss in an attempt to rule out any possible contribution of these factors to the performance differences. Even with age and degree of hearing loss accounted for, the group with central auditory disorder performed more poorly. The authors concluded that central processing disorder has a detrimental effect on performance with hearing aids in the clinical setting.

Pruitt, Loiselle, Jerger, and Stach (1990) studied the effects of aging and hearing loss on binaural hearing aid advantage. Results were from 72 patients matched for better-ear aided performance, 35 of whom had central auditory disorder. Aided speech recognition performance showed a larger binaural advantage in patients with central auditory disorder. Interestingly, absolute binaural performance was equivalent between groups, suggesting that the CAPD group exhibited more of a monaural disadvantage than the non-CAPD group. Results also showed that age, per se, was not a factor, except as it covaried with hearing loss and central auditory processing ability.

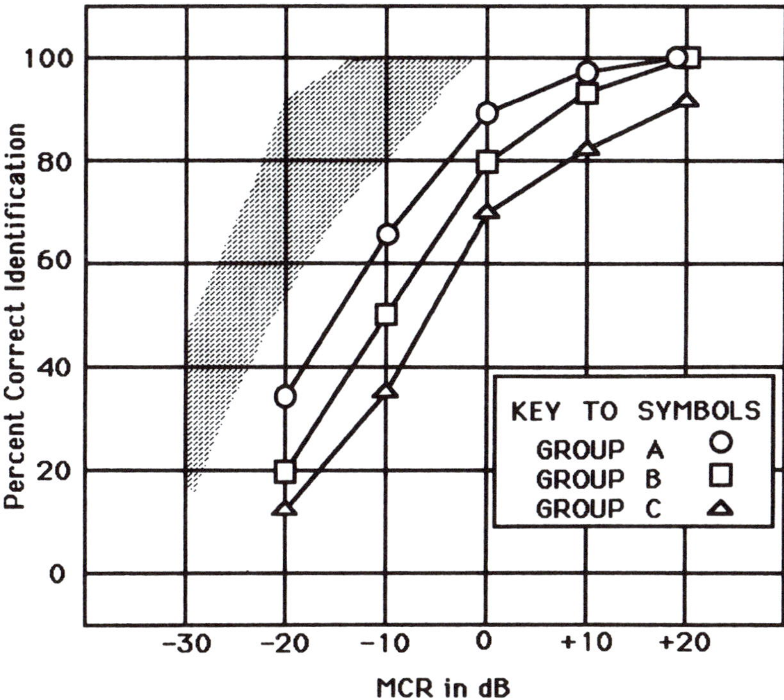

Figure 19–1. Aided performance in the sound field for three groups of elderly subjects: Group A = peripheral, Group B = intermediate, Group C = central, MCR = message-to-competition ratio. *Note:* From "Aging and the Use of Hearing Aids," by D. Hayes and J. Jerger, 1979. *Scandinavian Audiology, 8*, 33–40. Copyright 1979. Reprinted with permission.

Central Presbyacusis and Hearing Aid Satisfaction

Several studies have reported on the relationship between central presbyacusis, as measured by SNR ability, and hearing aid user satisfaction. Jerger and Hayes (1976) sent questionnaires to patients who received hearing aid evaluations, asking them to rate their hearing aid use as satisfactory, sometimes helpful, or unsatisfactory. Of 47 respondents who had purchased hearing aids, 72% rated the aid as satisfactory, 15% as sometimes helpful, and 13% as unsatisfactory. Noting an inverse relationship between satisfaction and age, they studied aided sound field performance. Results showed little difference in performance between groups at an easy MCR (+10 dB), but a progressive separation of groups as the listening condition became more difficult. At a difficult listening condition (−10 dB), aided performance for the unsatisfactory group was substantially poorer than aided performance for the satisfactory group.

McCandless and Parkin (1979) classified 140 hearing aid users into site of lesion categories based on 12 audiological measures. Criterion for successful hearing aid use was total daily wearing time. Of all hearing aid users with central site of lesion, only 11% were classified as successful users, and 89% rejected hearing aid use. In contrast, 84% of those with middle ear site and 71% of those with cochlear site were considered successful.

In another study relating hearing aid performance to hearing aid user satisfaction, Hayes, Jerger, Taff, and Barber (1983) surveyed 78 hearing aid users who were asked to judge their satisfaction. Aided results in a difficult listening condition (−10 MCR) were 30% poorer for those in the "unsatisfactory" and "sometimes helpful" category than for those in the "very helpful" category. It appears that hearing aid users who have central processing difficulty are generally less satisfied with hearing aid use than those with more peripheral losses (see however, Kricos, Lesner, Sandridge, & Yanke, 1985; 1987).

Central Presbyacusis and Hearing Aid Benefit

Stach, Jerger, & Smith (1986) evaluated the question of hearing aid benefit in patients with CAPD by using an interviewing technique in an attempt to circumvent some of the problems associated with patients' definitions of satisfaction. Two groups of patients with hearing loss matched on the basis of age and degree of peripheral sensitivity loss, one with speech audiometric patterns suggesting peripheral disorder and the other with patterns suggesting mixed peripheral and central disorder, were formed. Benefit from hearing aid use was then determined by telephone interview and judged on a 5-point scale from very helpful (rating of 5) to no benefit (rating of 1).

Benefit ratings assigned to the central group were poorer than those assigned to the peripheral group. The mean rating for the central group was 3.0, and the mean rating for the peripheral group was 4.0. While the mean difference was small, the distribution of ratings for the two groups was strikingly different. Figure 19–2 shows these distributions. Ratings for the peripheral group were distributed in a manner that was not unexpected. Most of the patients reported hearing aid use that was rated by the examiner as either very helpful or often helpful. None of the patients in the peripheral group reported usage consistent with no benefit. Ratings from the central group, however, were fairly evenly distributed across the rating range. While some reported usage consistent with a very helpful rating and most reported usage consistent with a helpful rating, 33% of the patients reported usage consistent with no benefit from hearing aid use.

These results are challenging from a clinical perspective. In general, patients with central auditory disorder were not judged to be receiv-

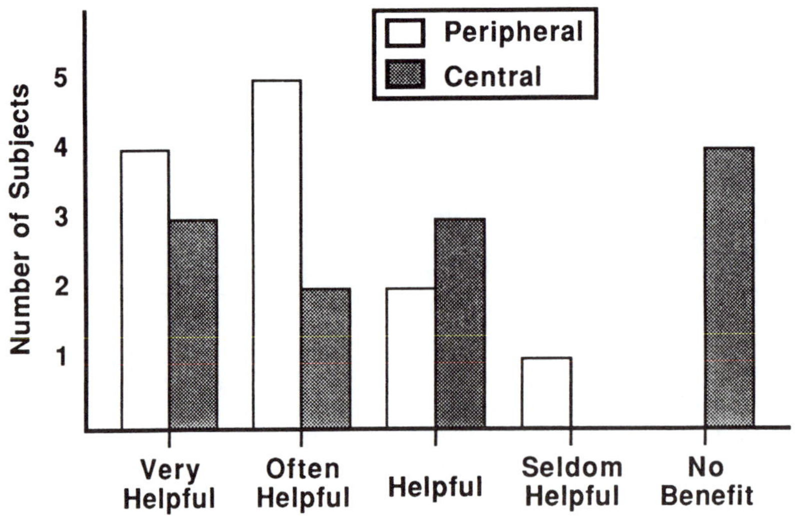

Figure 19–2. Distribution of ratings of hearing aid benefit for two groups, one with central auditory disorder (central) and one with normal auditory processing ability (peripheral).

ing as much benefit from hearing aid use as patients with peripheral hearing loss. They also did not perform as well as a group on aided measures of speech understanding in difficult listening situations. Of even greater interest was the finding of a large disparity among individual benefit ratings within the central group. It appears that, while central processing disorder does not necessarily contraindicate hearing aid use in an individual patient, there is a reasonably high probability that a patient with central disorder will not receive optimal amplification benefit.

Illustrative Case

Central processing disorder can result from aging. These senescent changes in central ability are quite likely to progress with increasing age. Considering the relationship between dissatisfaction with hearing aid use and central presbyacusis, it seems likely that a satisfied hearing aid user could become dissatisfied as the pattern of auditory aging changed over time from peripheral to central. If there truly is a relationship between central processing ability and hearing aid benefit, then the insidious progression of central auditory aging might result in a progressive decline in ability to use amplification successfully.

Stach, Jerger, & Fleming (1985) reported audiological findings in an elderly patient over a 9-year period. The patient was first seen at the age of 70. Results of pure-tone audiometry revealed a hearing-sensitivity loss that was mildly sloping and symmetrical. Speech audiometry was slightly asymmetrical. The right ear was characterized by a small word-sentence discrepancy and slight rollover of the sentence function. In this case, sentences were from the Synthetic Sentence Identification (SSI) test (Jerger, Speaks, & Trammel, 1968), presented with ipsilateral competition at an MCR of 0 dB. At the time, the patient noted significant communication difficulty but did not feel that it warranted the use of amplification.

The patient returned at the age of 75 with increased communication complaints. Pure-tone sensitivity and word-recognition scores were essentially unchanged, but results from the SSI showed a decrease in the maximum score and significant rollover on both ears. He was fitted with a hearing aid on the right ear at that time. Over the next four years, he reported successful hearing aid use in quiet listening conditions, but increasing difficulty understanding speech in noisy situations.

At the age of 79, the patient returned to the clinic because he felt that his hearing aid was no longer working appropriately. He reported the aid to be increasingly less useful and finally quit wearing it altogether. One day when he tried it again, he was convinced that it had ceased functioning. He reported that it still seemed to amplify sound but that the clarity was very poor. A routine electroacoustic analysis of the hearing aid showed it to be functioning within manufacturer's specifications and unchanged from the original analysis.

On the assumption that his peripheral sensitivity must have changed during the intervening years, the patient was re-tested during that visit. Pure-tone sensitivity was relatively unchanged, as were maximum word-recognition scores. Performance on the SSI, however, had decreased dramatically. Figure 19–3 shows pure-tone sensitivity, maximum word-recognition scores, and maximum SSI scores on four occasions over the 9-year period. While sensitivity and ability to understand speech in quiet had changed little, understanding of speech presented in competition showed a progressive and substantial decline.

The decline in central auditory function, apparently quite independent of any peripheral changes, resulted in a parallel decline in benefit from hearing aid use. There was no evidence of significant general cognitive decline or any other intervening factors to explain the progression away from satisfactory use of amplification.

Acquired Suprathreshold Asymmetry

Nature of the Disorder

The brain has ample plasticity to adjust to long-term changes in auditory input. For example, evidence suggests that the auditory cortex and

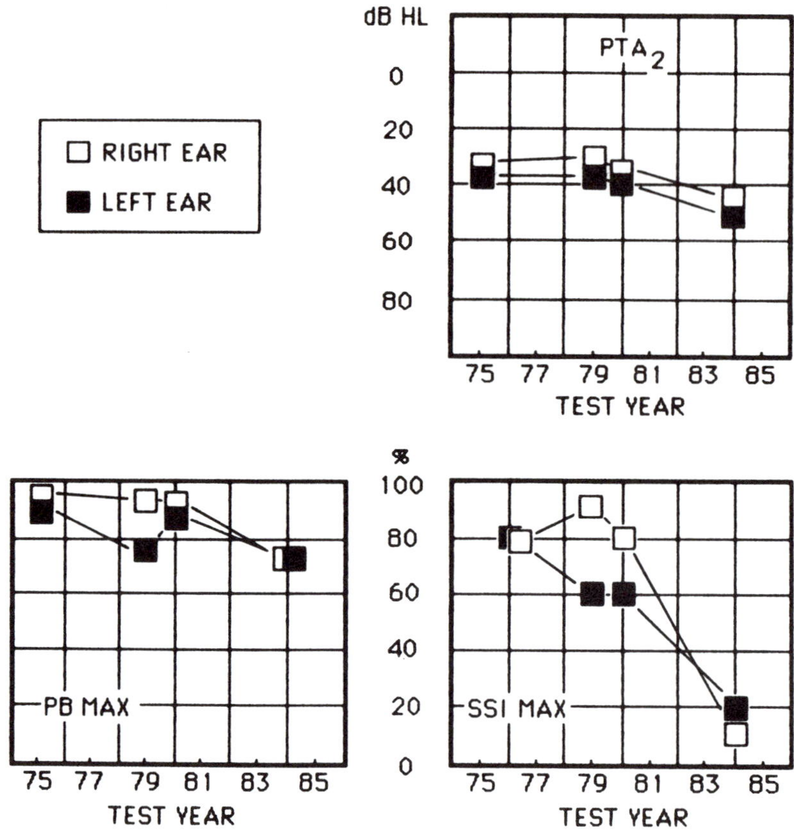

Figure 19–3. Changes in pure-tone and speech-audiometric scores in a single patient over a 9-year period. PTA_2 = average of hearing threshold levels at 1000, 2000, and 4000 Hz. PB MAX = maximum word recognition score on phonetically-balanced (PB) word lists. SSI MAX = maximum score on the synthetic sentence identification test. *Note:* From "Central Presbyacusis: A Longitudinal Case Study," by B. A. Stach, J. F. Jerger, and K. A. Fleming, 1985, *Ear and Hearing, 6,* 304–306. Copyright 1985. Reprinted with permission.

other nervous system structures can undergo extensive organizational changes as a result of some form of interruption to or deprivation of auditory input (Harrison, Nagasawa, Smith, Stanton, & Mount, 1991; Harrison, Stanton, Ibrahim, Nagasawa, & Mount, 1993; Robertson & Irvine, 1989). As another example, it is quite common for patients who wear hearing aids or use cochlear implants to undergo a significant adjustment period when they obtain new hearing aids or get a new map on their processor. One of the more intriguing findings in this area is that substantive changes are noted in auditory nervous system structures in cases of unilateral or asymmetric deprivation that are not apparent in bilateral, symmetric deprivation (Coleman & O'Connor, 1979).

In 1984, Silman, Gelfand, and Silverman described what they termed "late-onset auditory deprivation," an acquired asymmetry in suprathreshold speech recognition that appeared to result from the relative deprivation of one ear by the fitting of hearing aid amplification to the other. In 40% of individuals wearing monaural hearing aids, word-recognition scores declined after a period of asymmetrical stimulation.

Emerging from these fascinating data is the notion that asymmetry in peripheral hearing sensitivity can adversely effect suprathreshold speech perception on the poorer hearing, or deprived ear. Results are intriguing in that they point to changes in central auditory function as a consequence of the asymmetry. Progressive suprathreshold asymmetry can occur naturally as a result of greater cochlear disorder in one ear than the other. In such cases, evidence is mounting that processing by the poorer ear is adversely affected beyond that which might be expected if the loss was symmetric (Moore, Vickers, Glasberg, & Baer, 1997; Silverman and Emmer, 1993).

Suprathreshold asymmetry can also occur by fitting a hearing aid on one ear only, as discovered by Silman et al. (1984). These findings have since been verified in a number of studies and case reports (Dieroff, 1993; Gelfand & Silman, 1993; Gelfand, Silman, & Ross, 1987; Hattori, 1993; Neuman, 1996; Silman, Silverman, Emmer, & Gelfand, 1992; Silverman and Silman, 1990). In a patient fitted with one hearing aid, speech recognition ability in that ear remains constant over time, while the same ability in the unaided ear begins to show signs of deterioration. So long as hearing is symmetric in both ears, this decline is not apparent. However, once a hearing aid is fitted in one ear, resulting in asymmetric hearing, ability appears to decline in the disadvantaged ear.

Influence of the Disorder on Amplification

Acquired suprathreshold asymmetry may be reversible if the unaided ear is aided within a reasonable time frame (Boothroyd, 1993; Hurley, 1993; Silverman & Silman, 1990). In some patients, however, the decline in speech recognition in the unaided ear may not recover (Silverman & Silman; Hurley, 1993; Gelfand, 1995) and may actually preclude the successful use of binaural amplification.

Gelfand (1995) described six cases of acquired suprathreshold asymmetry. In two cases, the unaided ear showed a decline in word-recognition scores following the fitting of a hearing aid on the opposite ear. Once the binaural fit was completed, the word-recognition scores returned to premorbid baselines. In two other cases, the completion of a binaural fit resulted in improvement in the formerly unaided ear, but the improvement never quite reached the original baseline or performance of the originally aided ear. The final cases showed a decline in word-recognition ability in the unaided ear that did not recover following the addition of a hearing aid. These cases suggest that acquired asymmetry may be reversible if the unaided ear is aided within a reasonable time frame, although the critical duration of the deprivation is not known. Clearly in some patients the decline in speech recognition does not recover. It has been hypothesized that, as a result, a binaural interference phenomenon may occur, wherein binaural ability is actually poorer than the better monaural ability.

Dichotic Deficits

Nature of the Disorder

Dichotic listening ability has been found to be adversely affected by aging (Arnst, 1982; Fifer, Jerger, Berlin, Tobey, & Campbell, 1983; Gelfand, Hoffman, Waltzman, & Piper, 1980; Jerger, Chmiel, Allen, & Wilson, 1994; Jerger, Stach, Johnson, Loiselle, & Jerger, 1990; Wilson & Jaffe, 1996). Jerger, Stach, and colleagues (1990) studied dichotic listening ability in 172 elderly patients with varying degrees of sensorineural hearing loss. After controlling for the influences of task-related factors such as memory and other non-auditory influences, results showed that 23% of these older patients showed some degree of dichotic deficit. In another study, Chmiel and Jerger (1996) described results from 115 elderly subjects, 33 (29%) of whom exhibited dichotic deficits. Interestingly, the pattern of dichotic listening deficits found in some aging patients was similar to that found in patients with lesions of the corpus callosum, implicating a loss in the efficiency of interhemispheric transfer of auditory information (Jerger, Alford, Lew, Rivera, & Chmiel, 1995).

Influence of the Disorder on Amplification

The influence of dichotic deficits on successful use of hearing aid amplification is not altogether clear, although studies of aging patients with dichotic processing difficulty suggest the possibility of an adverse effect. Chmiel and Jerger (1996) evaluated self-reported handicap in elderly subjects before and 6 weeks after first-time hearing aid use. Results showed that self-assessment of handicap was equivalent for both a normal-dichotic subgroup and an abnormal-dichotic subgroup prior to hearing aid use. After 6 weeks of use, self-reported handicap improved significantly, but only in the normal-dichotic group. It appears that the presence of a central auditory disorder, in this case a dichotic deficit, can prevent an older patient from realizing the full potential of hearing aid use.

Stach, Wilson, and Gilbert (unpublished report) studied the effect of dichotic listening ability on performance with hearing aids in 74 subjects with symmetric hearing sensitivity and word-recognition ability, 25 of whom had abnormal dichotic performance. Aided sentence-recognition testing showed no difference between right and left ears of either group. However, aided binaural performance of the normal-dichotic group was, on the average, approximately 10% better than that of the dichotic-deficit group. To assess the question of binaural versus monaural performance more directly, binaural performance was compared to best-monaural performance, regardless of whether best performance was on the right or left ear. The mean binaural-monaural difference for the dichotic-deficit group was –3.6%, and the mean difference for the normal-dichotic group was 7.3%. In terms of individual results, there was substantial overlap of subjects between groups. Fifty-five percent of the normal-dichotic group, and 28% of the dichotic-deficit group, had better binaural scores than monaural scores, whereas 45% of the normal-dichotic group, and 72% of the dichotic-deficit group, had equal scores or better monaural than binaural scores. With such overlap in individual performances, it would be precarious to apply these results on an individual basis. That is, although the presence of a dichotic deficit appears to place a patient at risk for reduced binaural benefit, it does not preclude the use of binaural hearing aids. Nevertheless, a patient with a dichotic deficit appears less likely to enjoy the benefits of binaural amplification to the extent that those with normal dichotic ability might.

An extreme example of this effect was reported by Chmiel, Jerger, Murphy, Pirozzolo, and Tooley-Young (1997). They described clinical results from a 90-year old patient who preferred and performed better with monaural versus binaural amplification. Clinical results showed symmetric hearing sensitivity and slightly asymmetric monaural speech recognition ability. However, on dichotic measures, the patient showed a significant left ear deficit both behaviorally and electrophysiologically. Performance with hearing aids was similarly affected. Soundfield speech recognition was superior with a hearing aid in the right ear only and was poorest with a hearing aid in the left ear only. Binaural performance was better than left ear performance but significantly poorer than right ear performance.

Illustrative Case

A 78-year-old woman with bilateral sensorineural hearing loss reported that her hearing impairment progressed slowly over a 15-year period. She had worn hearing aids for the past 10 years and had an annual audiologic re-evaluation each year. Her major complaints were in communicating with her grandchildren and trying to hear in noisy restaurants. Although her hearing aids worked well for her at the beginning, she was not receiving the benefit from them that she had 10 years before.

At the time of her most recent evaluation, immittance audiometry was consistent with normal middle ear function, characterized by a Type A tympanogram, normal static immittance, and normal crossed and uncrossed reflex thresholds bilaterally. Pure-tone and speech audiometric results are shown in Figure 19–4A.

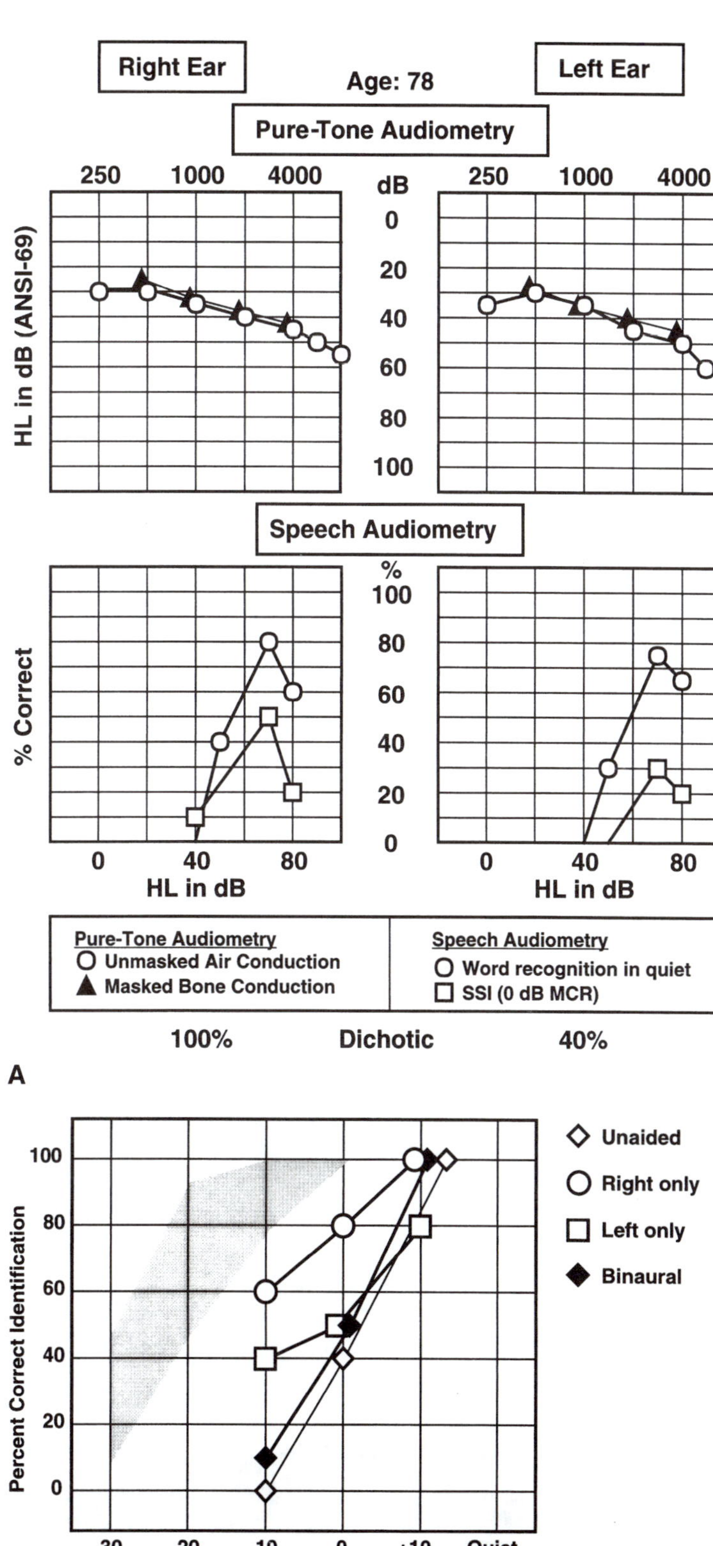

Figure 19–4. Audiometric results **(A)** in a 78-year-old woman with long-standing, progressive hearing loss. Pure-tone audiometric results show bilateral, symmetric, moderate, sensorineural hearing loss. Speech audiometric results show symmetric word recognition in quiet, consistent with the degree and configuration of cochlear hearing loss, symmetric sentence recognition in competition that is substantially reduced, and a dichotic performance deficit on the left. Aided speech recognition performance **(B)** shows the influence of the dichotic deficit, reducing left-ear and binaural scores.

The patient had a moderate, bilateral, symmetric, sensorineural hearing loss. Hearing sensitivity was slightly better in the low frequencies than in the high frequencies.

Speech audiometric results were consistent with those found in older patients. Word-recognition scores were reduced symmetrically, but not below a level predictable from the degree of hearing sensitivity loss. Speech recognition in the presence of competition was substantially reduced bilaterally, consistent with the patient's age. Despite symmetric reduction in monotic performance, however, results show evidence of a dichotic deficit, with reduced performance in the left ear. Aided performance is shown in Figure 19–4B. Right ear performance was superior to left-ear and binaural performance at all MCRs, reflecting the influence of the central auditory disorder in dichotic listening.

Results of a hearing handicap assessment show that she has communication problems a significant proportion of the time in most listening environments, especially those involving background noise. These results are not uncommon in many aging patients with hearing disorders. Word recognition in quiet is consistent with the degree of hearing loss. Speech perception in the presence of competition is reduced beyond what might be expected from the hearing sensitivity loss.

Other Binaural Deficits

Some patients with central auditory disorders have difficulty locating the directional source of a sound. Disorders of the central auditory nervous system have been associated with deficits in ability to localize the source of a sound in a soundfield or to lateralize the perception of a sound within the head. These deficits are probably related to difficulties in spatial location of sound in noisy and reverberant environments. Older subjects often have difficulty perceiving speech in backgrounds of competition, particularly when the source location is on the left side (Jerger & Jordan, 1992). The inability to spatially locate sounds adds to the difficulty in understanding speech in noisy environments.

Difficulties in spatial location are most likely exacerbated by the use of conventional hearing aids. Monaural hearing aid fittings can substantially diminish the advantage in sound localization afforded by binaural hearing. Even when binaural amplification is used, behind-the-ear and in-the-ear devices have microphone locations that reduce the natural spectral contributions of the pinna, concha, and ear canal critical for separating signal sources.

Another type of deficit in binaural processing is referred to as binaural interference, in which performance on a perceptual task with both ears is actually poorer than performance on the better ear in cases of asymmetric auditory ability. It appears that the poorer ear actually reduces binaural performance below the better monaural performance. Binaural interference has been reported in elderly individuals (Jerger, Silman, Lew, & Chmiel, 1993) and in patients with multiple sclerosis (Silman, 1995).

The functional consequence of binaural interference may be to reduce the potential benefit of binaural hearing aids when hearing with both ears is poorer than hearing with one ear. Not unlike the case of a substantial dichotic deficit, when auditory processing is significantly asymmetric, hearing aid use may be precluded in the poorer-hearing ear. Jerger, Silman, et al. (1993) describe aided performance by a patient who demonstrated binaural interference on electrophysiological and behavioral measures. Aided responses were best for the better monaural ear. Interestingly, on one aided condition, binaural performance was actually poorer than either the better- or poorer-ear monaural performance. It appears that in cases of binaural interference, binaural hearing aid use may be contraindicated.

SUCCESSFUL AMPLIFICATION STRATEGIES IN ADULT CAPD

Evidence of decreased hearing aid performance resulting from central auditory disorder is interesting and certainly helps guide the professional in terms of patient counseling about reasonable expectations and optimal listening conditions and strategies. Approaches to conventional amplification that can be taken to help ameliorate the communication difficulty resulting from central auditory disorder are directed toward enhancing SNR and restoring spatial location to the extent possible. The other approach that has proven successful is the use of remote microphone technology.

Conventional Hearing Aid Amplification

One important aspect of conventional hearing aid fitting is the use of techniques to enhance the SNR. Although the techniques for doing so are no different for those with central auditory problems than for those with purely peripheral hearing loss, their application is probably more important. Enhancement of SNR can be achieved in three ways in conventional ear-level hearing devices, through electroacoustic alteration, fitting of binaural hearing aids, and use of directional microphones. Binaural hearing aids also present an opportunity to preserve or restore spatial hearing to a certain extent.

Electroacoustic Alteration of Conventional Hearing Aids

If patients with CAPD are to be successful with hearing aid use, alterations that reduce background noise and enhance SNR are critical. The presence of background noise is probably more detrimental to patients with CAPD than to any other group of hearing aid users. It is even quite likely that hearing aid amplification of background noise makes hearing aid use counterproductive for some of these patients. The same electroacoustic modification strategies that are used to reduce noise for patients with peripheral hearing loss are even more critical for those with central disorder. Recent technology advances have created better amplifiers with wide bandwidth, smooth frequency response, variable-recovery time compression, and improved fitting targets (Killion, 1997), all of which can enhance the SNR to an extent. Although experimental data are not available, recent clinical experience suggests that the consequent amplification benefit for those with central auditory disorder has improved accordingly.

Binaural Hearing Aids

Except in cases of binaural interference or substantial dichotic deficits, binaural amplification is indicated for patients with central auditory disorder as a means for enhancing speech understanding in noise and for enhancing spatial localization. There is some evidence that microphone location may impact on the benefits of binaural amplification. Completely-in-the-canal hearing aids tend to preserve the natural influences of the pinna and concha, which provide important spectral shaping for sound localization. BTE and ITE hearing aids eliminate these influences and can reduce localization ability. In cases where low frequency hearing is good, open earmolds for BTE fittings enhance the potential for appropriate localization ability (Byrne & Noble, 1998).

Directional Microphones

Most conventional hearing devices use omnidirectional microphones that provide wide-angle reception of acoustic signals. Although useful for monitoring the environment, the hearing aid user is often challenged by difficulty in localizing the source of a sound and separating a desired signal from a background of noise. The problem is worsened by placing the microphone over the ear on a behind-the-ear hearing aid, thereby eliminating the natural effects of the pinna for gathering sound.

One alternative is a directional microphone, which has a more focused field. Although directional microphones have been available for many years, they have only recently achieved a level of directivity necessary to sufficiently benefit patients with SNR loss. Recently, microphone systems have been developed that provide the capability of both directional and omnidirectional reception in the same hearing device. Multi-microphone systems are currently available for both behind-the-ear and in-the-ear hearing aids. Some systems have both omnidirectional and directional settings that can be switched via remote control from one to the other. Studies have confirmed that directional microphones can provide a significant enhancement in signal-to-noise ratio over omnidirectional microphones (Killion, et al., 1998; Lurquin & Rafhay, 1996; Valente, Fabry, & Potts, 1995). In addition there is evidence of improved consumer satisfaction ratings for hearing aids with directional microphones (Kochkin, 1996).

It can be expected that directional microphones will be superior to omnidirectional microphones for hearing in noise. However, such improvements may be gained at the expense of spatial locating capability. It is not yet clear whether the relative advantage of this sophisticated microphone technology for improving SNR is superior to the advantage in spatial location and SNR realized with deep-canal hearing aid fittings. Regardless, SNR enhancements gained by the added directivity of these microphones are likely to provide added benefit to patients with central auditory disorders.

Remote Microphone Technology

Hearing in the presence of background noise is a significant problem for individuals with central auditory disorders and particularly for those who wear conventional hearing devices. Despite technical advances made over the past few years that address this issue, some patients need additional assistance with hearing in unfavorable SNRs. In these patients, use of remote-microphone technology can provide substantial assistance.

Conventionally, a remote-microphone system is an FM system or similar device consisting of a microphone/transmitter that the talker uses and a receiver/amplifier that the listener uses. Signals are sent via FM radio waves from the talker to the listener, thereby reducing background noise and enhancing the SNR.

Personal FM systems have been used successfully in adults with central auditory disorders (Stach, Loiselle, Jerger, Mintz, & Taylor, 1987). In cases where a conventional FM system is used, the speaker wears a microphone that is attached to an FM transmitter. The listener wears an FM receiver tuned to the transmitter frequency, and the signal is delivered to the ear in one of two ways. For cases in which the hearing loss has both a peripheral and central component, hearing aids are used to overcome the peripheral loss in conjunction with FM systems for the central disorder. Transduction of signals is typically done through the hearing aid telecoil via a neckloop. In other cases in which the disorder is primarily central, the FM system alone is recommended, and the signal is transduced via an insert receiver or lightweight headphones.

Recent advances in both transmitter and receiver technology are bringing remote-microphone fittings into the mainstream. Transmitters have been introduced that have sophisticated array microphones, designed for directionality. The transmitter can be enclosed in a case the size of a large pen and can be directed at a sound source or handed to a speaker during communication in a noisy environment. FM transmitters are also included in the remote controls of some programmable hearing instruments. Similar advances have been made on the receiver portion of the FM system. Receivers have been developed that contain the entire FM reception system in a conventional ear-level hearing device or in a behind-the-ear hearing aid "boot." As the transmitters and receivers become more practical and advanced, the use of remote-microphone technology is likely to become a more common option.

Illustrative Case

The following case serves as an illustrative example of the success that can be experienced with the application of FM assistive devices to patients with central auditory disorder.

A 75-year-old man had a long history of progressive hearing loss and hearing aid use. While he still found his hearing aids to be beneficial in quiet situations, he complained of increasing difficulty at his weekly lunch meetings and other social occasions. His wife reported that he was becoming increasingly withdrawn socially because he was no longer able to communicate effectively with his friends.

Figure 19–5A shows results of the audiological evaluation. The hearing loss was sensorineural and moderate-to-severe in degree. Understanding of words presented in quiet was depressed, consistent with the configuration of the peripheral hearing loss. SSI results were disproportionately depressed, consistent with CAPD.

Figure 19–5B shows results of the hearing aid evaluation. Despite all efforts, a hearing aid could not be found that outperformed his own, nor could a binaural advantage be shown. Yet even his best aided performance was relatively depressed in difficult listening situations. When an FM system was used in conjunction with his own hearing aid, performance increased dramatically.

At his follow-up visit, his wife described what she considered to be a rebirth in his social activity level since using the FM system. In this case, the amplification arrangement necessary for benefit was one that both overcame the attenuation deficit resulting from a peripheral sensitivity loss and provided the needed SNR advantage that had been reduced by central presbyacusis.

THE NATURE OF CAPD IN CHILDREN

Not unlike in adults, childhood CAPD can be thought of as an auditory disorder that occurs as a result of dysfunction in the manipulation and utilization of acoustic signals by the central auditory nervous system. It is broadly defined as an impaired ability to process acoustic information that cannot be attributed to impaired hearing sensitivity, impaired language, or impaired intellectual function.

Central auditory processing disorders have been characterized based on models of deficits in children and adults with acquired lesions of the central auditory nervous system (Jerger, Johnson, & Loiselle, 1988). Such deficits include reduced ability to understand in background noise, to understand speech of reduced redundancy, to localize and lateralize sound, to separate dichotic stimuli, and to process normal or altered temporal cues. Children with CAPD exhibit deficits similar to those with acquired lesions, although they may be less pronounced in severity and are more likely to be generalized than ear-specific.

Although some children may be genetically predisposed to CAPD, it is more likely to be a developmental delay or disorder, resulting from inconsistent or degraded auditory input during the critical period for auditory perceptual development. CAPD is symptomatic in nature and is often confused with an impairment of hearing sensitivity. It can be an isolated disorder, or it can co-exist with attention deficit disorders, learning disabilities, and language disorders. Clinically, CAPD is operationally defined most often on the basis of speech audiometric results. Recent advances in speech audiometry and recent studies of auditory evoked potentials hold promise for refinement in the diagnosis.

Functionally, children with CAPD act as if they have hearing-sensitivity deficits, although they are usually capable of hearing faint sounds. In particular, they exhibit difficulty in perceiving spoken language or other sounds in hostile acoustic environments. Thus, a common age of identification is early in the children's academic lives, when they enter a conventional classroom situation and are unable to understand instructions from the teacher.

Many children with language and learning deficits have been found to have auditory

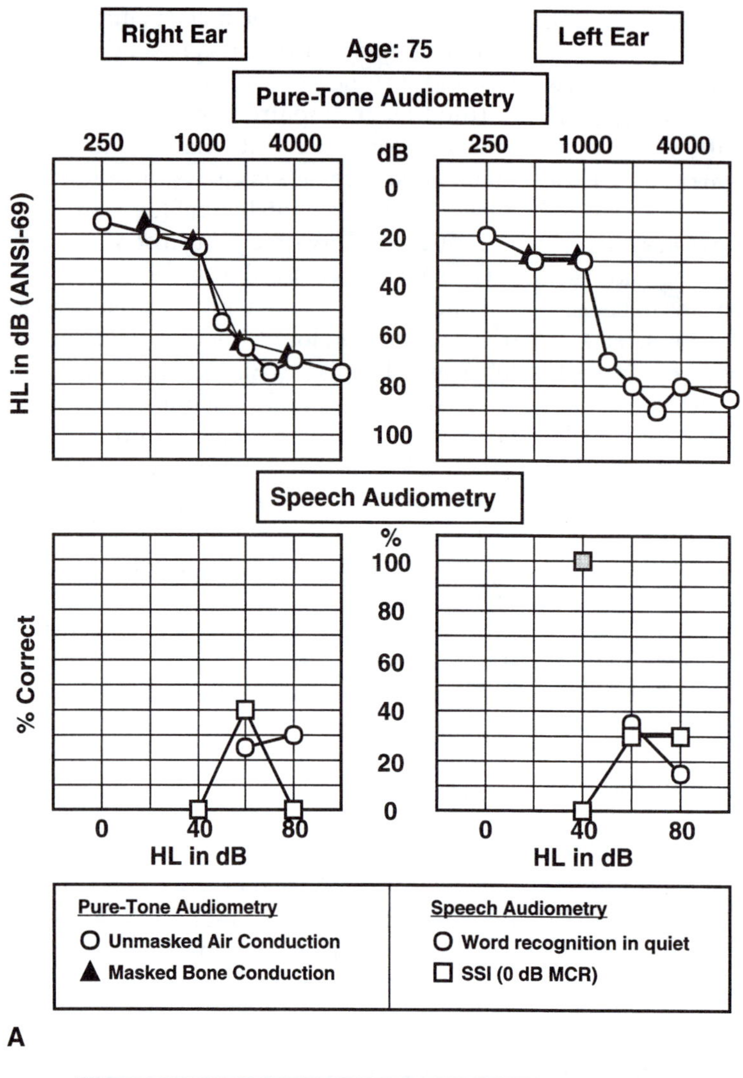

A

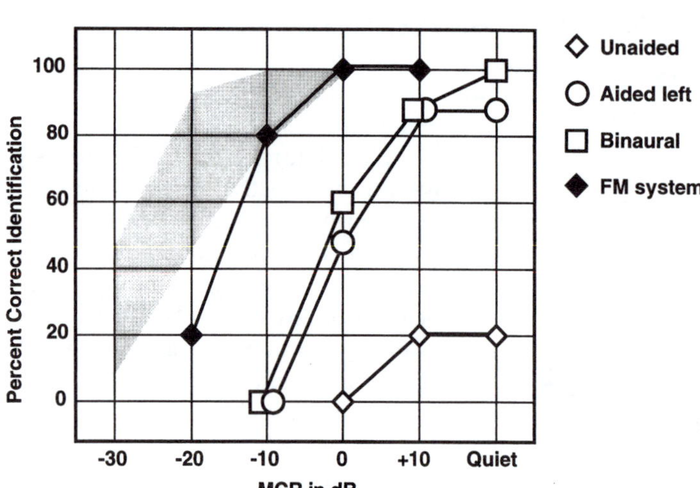

B

Figure 19–5. Pure-tone and speech-audiometric results **(A)** in a 75-year-old patient with hearing sensitivity loss and central auditory disorder. Speech audiometric results are for word-recognition in quiet and the SSI at 0 dB MCR. Soundfield speech recognition performance **(B)** without hearing aids, with an aid on the left ear, on both ears, and with an FM system.

perceptual impairment (Farrer & Keith, 1981; Freeman & Beasley, 1978; Johnson, Enfield, & Sherman, 1981; Lubert, 1981; Pinheiro, 1977; Willeford, 1977; Willeford & Billger, 1978). However, because of a wide range of tests designed to measure auditory perception, a large number of classification schemes for children with disorders of this nature, varied educational strategies used for intervention, philosophical differences among professionals involved, and the tendency toward multimodality deficits in these children, the nature and scope of central auditory processing disorder has not been altogether clear. Despite this confusion, evidence continues to accumulate, from both clinical and research settings, attesting to the reality of what so many clinicians have for so long suspected: that some children may have a problem as a result of a specific deficit in auditory processing and that such deficits may co-exist with peripheral hearing loss or may exist independently of any actual sensitivity deficit.

Clinical experience with children has convinced many of the reality of the concept of CAPD and the need to take seriously the implications of its impact on communication. For example, there is increasing evidence of a population of children with isolated CAPD. In almost a syndrome-like manner, these children have a history of chronic otitis media and parental and teacher complaints of inattentiveness, distractibility, and difficulty hearing in the presence of background noise. Clinical manifestations include normal hearing sensitivity, normal performance on single-syllable word recognition tests presented in quiet, and an assortment of deficits on tests of central auditory processing.

Causes of Childhood CAPD

Childhood central auditory disorders can be classified into two groups, those associated with identifiable neuropathology and those of idiopathic origin that present as communication disorders. Central auditory disorders related to neuropathologic conditions are rare. When neoplasms affect the auditory nervous system, they are usually diagnosed with radiographic techniques and on the basis of associated medical problems. Treatment strategies for such disorders are often similar to those that would be appropriate in adults with similar pathology.

There are relatively few reports of central auditory disorder in children with central nervous system lesions due, in part, to the rarity of the lesions and, presumably, because hearing disorders tend to be a relatively minor aspect of the generally deteriorated health of such children. Jerger (1987) summarized results of an audiometric battery in 21 children with documented central nervous system lesions. Results showed patterns of abnormality consistent with those found in adults with similar lesions. Specifically, those children with extra- and intra-axial gliomas had abnormal, degraded monotic speech perception, and those with temporal lobe lesions had abnormal dichotic speech perception. Most other reports corroborate these findings that children and adults tend to exhibit similar patterns of abnormality (Bergman, Costeff, Koren, Koifman, & Reshef, 1984; Goodglass, 1967), although some have suggested that auditory deficits in children with central nervous system lesions may be more generalized and less severe than in adults with similar lesions (Woods, 1984). Regardless, the probability of encountering such children in a clinical setting is low, and auditory disorders are likely to be a minor component of care, except in such extreme cases as bilateral acoustic tumors.

The vast majority of childhood central auditory disorders do not result from documented neuropathologic conditions. Rather, they present as communication disorder that resembles hearing impairment. The specific hearing impairment is related to an idiopathic dysfunction of the central auditory nervous system and is commonly referred to as central auditory processing disorder. Although the auditory symptoms and clinical findings in children with CAPD may mimic those of children with auditory disorders due to discrete pathology in the central auditory nervous system, they result from no obvious pathological condition that requires medical intervention.

The etiology of CAPD is not known. There have been anecdotal reports of families with CAPD, including parents and siblings. In addition, in larger series of children with CAPD, there is an indication of a high prevalence of chronic otitis media. Until further evidence can be gathered, it remains only a conjecture that children who have aperiodic disruption in auditory input during the critical period for auditory development may be at risk for developing central auditory processing disorder. However, several reports have shown convincing delays in auditory processing ability in children with a history of chronic otitis media (Brown, 1994; Hall, Grose, & Pillsbury, 1995; Jerger, Jerger, Alford, & Abrams, 1983; Schilder, Snik, Straatman, & van den Broek, 1994).

Consequences of Childhood CAPD

In general, children with CAPD will act as if they have a hearing sensitivity loss, even though most will have normal audiograms. They will ask for repetition, fail to follow instructions, and so on, particularly in the presence of background noise or other factors that reduce the redundancy of the acoustic signal (Chermak, Somers, & Seikel, 1998). To the extent that such difficulties result in frustration, secondary problems may develop related to their behavior and motivation in the classroom. Some children with CAPD will have concomitant speech and language deficits, learning disabilities, and attention deficit disorders (Keller, 1992). Thus, CAPD may be accompanied by distractibility, attention problems, memory deficits, language comprehension deficits, restricted vocabulary, and reading and spelling problems.

Consequences of CAPD can range from mild difficulty understanding a teacher in a noisy classroom to substantial difficulty understanding speech in everyday listening situations at home and school. One of the most important deficits in children with CAPD is difficulty understanding in background noise. In an acoustic environment that would be adequate for other children, a child with CAPD may have substantial difficulty understanding what is being said. Thus, parents will often complain that the child cannot understand them while the television is on, while riding in the car, or while the parents are speaking from another room. The teacher will complain of the child's inability to follow directions, distractibility, and general unruliness. In effect, the complaints will be similar to those expressed by parents or teachers of children with impairments of hearing sensitivity. In a quiet environment, with one-on-one instruction, a child with CAPD may thrive in a manner consistent with academic potential. In a more adverse acoustical environment, a child with CAPD will struggle.

It seems likely that the presence of CAPD in a child will have an adverse impact on speech and language development. Some even argue that it is unlikely that a child could have CAPD and not have some consequent language disorder. Evidence suggests that CAPD is prevalent in groups of children with speech and language disorders. A causal relationship, while implied, has not been confirmed. Evidence also suggests that CAPD can occur in isolation, suggesting that CAPD and language disorder are not necessarily consequential (Jerger, Martin, & Jerger, 1987).

AMPLIFICATION AND CAPD IN CHILDREN

Although benefit from hearing aid use in children with both hearing loss and central disorder has eluded careful study, attempts have been made to use amplification systems with educationally handicapped children who have normal hearing or mild hearing loss and who are not considered by traditional criteria to be candidates for hearing aids. The underlying assumption of these studies is that educational deficits are often related to auditory deficits. Alteration of auditory information with amplification, therefore, should enhance auditory processing and have a positive effect on educational intervention.

Early studies of classroom amplification provided encouragement for generalized solutions to hearing problems in schools. Sarff (1981) and Sarff, Ray, and Bagwell (1981) described a program entitled Mainstream Amplification Resource Room Study (MARRS) in which 110 children from grades 4, 5, and 6 were selected for study. Each child in the group had an academic deficit and auditory thresholds of no better than 15 dB HL and no poorer than 35 dB HL. Although central processing ability was not measured directly, the educational difficulties of these children were presumed to relate directly to auditory deficits resulting from minimal hearing loss.

Students from the MARRS study were assigned to one of two groups. The intervention procedure for one group was in the form of special help in a learning disabilities resource room as an adjunct to the traditional classroom setting. The other group had no special resource room. Instead, the students were confined to a standard classroom in which amplification equipment was installed. The teacher wore a microphone and wireless transmitter coupled to two loudspeakers. The teacher's lectures and instructions were thus amplified before being presented to the students.

Preceding and following these intervention strategies, student competency in various academic areas was measured. Results showed increased academic achievement for both groups and a tendency for greater achievement by students in the amplified classroom. Apparently, the enhancement of SNR by amplification intervention altered the classroom listening environment enough to reduce the negative educational effect of auditory deficits.

These positive results may well have resulted simply from overcoming the mild peripheral hearing loss present in these children. An alternative explanation is that many of these children with minimal hearing loss and educational deficits had CAPD, although auditory processing ability was not measured directly. If so, then it would follow, based on the MARRS study, that amplification intervention on a group or an individual basis might prove to be a beneficial strategy for children with such an auditory disorder. Regardless, these findings are intriguing in terms of the potential for benefit from classroom amplification in children with educational problems.

Children with central processing disorders may or may not have concomitant peripheral hearing loss. Similarly, children with peripheral hearing loss may or may not have central processing disorder. As a result, few children with central disorder are fitted with amplification. Consequently, the effect of amplification on central disorder in this population is not well known.

SUCCESSFUL AMPLIFICATION STRATEGIES IN CHILDREN

Childhood CAPD can be thought of as an auditory disorder that has as one of its main components the difficulty in understanding speech in background noise. Treatment strategies that focus on this component are often effective in forestalling or changing the expected outcome related to the presence of CAPD.

Enhancing the SNR

Intervention strategies directed toward enhancement of signal-to-noise ratio have proven successful in the treatment of children with CAPD (Stach et al., 1987; Stach, 1990). There are at least two approaches to this type of intervention. The first approach is to alter the acoustic environment in order to enhance the SNR. Environmental alterations include such practical approaches as preferential seating in the classroom and manipulation of the home environment so that the child is placed in more favorable listening situations. Alterations may also include equipping the classroom with sound field speakers to provide amplification of the teacher's speech.

It is not uncommon in children with CAPD for the diagnosis itself to serve as the treatment. That is, once parents and teachers become aware of the nature of the child's problem and that the solution is one of enhancement of SNR, they manipulate the environment in such a manner that the problem situations are eliminated, and the child's auditory processing difficulties become inconsequential.

In other cases, however, when severity of the auditory processing disorder is greater, the use of remote microphone technology may be indicated. Personal FM systems, which use remote microphones for SNR enhancement, have been used to assist these children in overcoming their deficit in understanding speech in background noise. In 1987, some of my colleagues and I summarized our experience at the Neurosensory Center of Houston with intervention in children with CAPD (Stach et al., 1987). Of those children who were considered to have CAPD, 30 were successfully treated by enhancing the awareness of parents and teachers to the need for environmental alteration to reduce background noise. In 11 others, however, the more aggressive approach of personal FM-system use was taken. These were relatively young children whose average age was 7 years. Although some of the children had slight, low-frequency hearing loss, all had pure-tone averages that were within normal limits. The majority (72%) also had a history of chronic otitis media. Evidence of improvement in 9 of the children using FM systems was gathered from interviews with parents and teachers. In 8 of the 9 children, improved grades and improved behavior were reported anecdotally by the teacher and parents. In addition, 2 of the children were reported to have improved speech and language abilities, 2 had improved attention, and, in 2, there was a school placement change from a special-education classroom to a regular classroom.

Children with CAPD may also benefit from auditory-training therapy, directed toward enhancement of the ability to process auditory information (Schneider, 1992) and to development of compensatory skills (Chermak & Musiek, 1992). While it may seem counterintuitive to try to train away a sensory deficit, there is convincing evidence of functional plasticity of the maturing central auditory nervous system (Aoki & Siekevitz, 1988). It seems likely that stimulation of the auditory system through therapy could exploit such neural plasticity.

Sequelae of CAPD in younger children are related to appropriate speech and language development. Although data on outcomes are limited, anecdotal evidence suggests that early detection results in early referral for speech and language evaluation and monitoring. Sequelae of CAPD in older children are related mostly to the extent to which the auditory problem affects hearing in the classroom. Successful intervention is expected to reduce achievement problems, while undetected or unmanaged problems are likely to result in academic underachievement.

Illustrative Cases

The first illustrative case had a history of chronic otitis media that lasted until he was 4 years of age. At age 6 years, he was exposed to a gun-shot that reportedly left him with a hearing loss for approximately 48 hours. Audiological testing at that time showed a mild sensorineural hearing loss with a notch at 4000 Hz. When he was 11 years old, his parents again sought audiological consultation for behaviors that included the inability to simultaneously write and listen and a propensity for turning up the television volume control. By this time he was in the fifth grade, and although results of educational testing had always placed him in the above average categories, he was diagnosed as having auditory retention and recall difficulties. His teachers assigned him preferential seating in the classroom because of what they described as an inability to pay attention and a mild degree of recalcitrance. He was seen by another audiology facility one month earlier and was fitted with hearing aids. Because of his complaints about increased listening difficulty while wearing the aids, the parents came to us for a second opinion.

Figure 19–6A shows results from our audiological evaluation. The patient had a peripheral, mild- to-moderate, sensorineural hearing

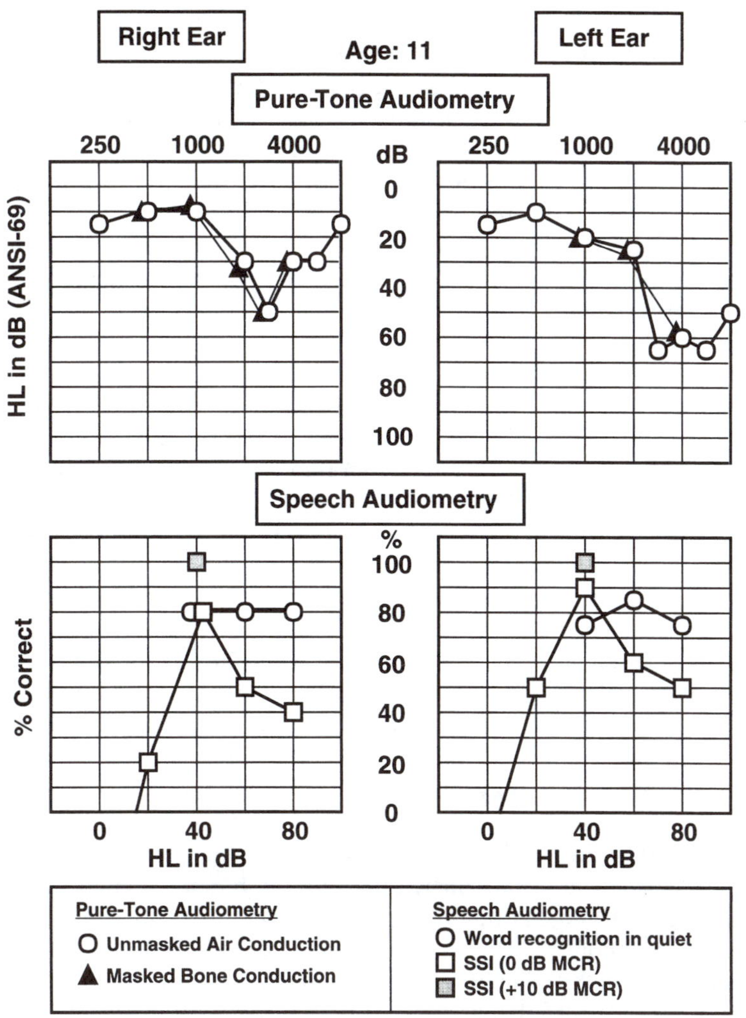

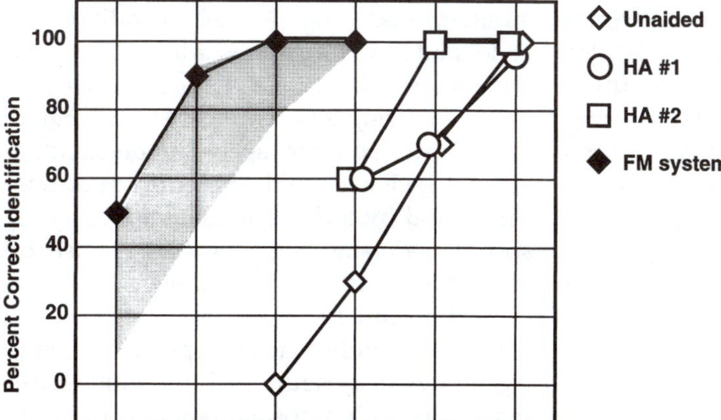

Figure 19–6. Pure-tone and speech-audiometric results **(A)** in an 11-year-old patient with a hearing sensitivity loss and central auditory disorder. Speech audiometric results are for word-recognition in quiet, SSI at 0 dB MCR, and SSI at +10 dB MCR. Soundfield speech recognition performance **(B)** without hearing aids, with two different hearing aids, and with an FM system.

loss and normal middle ear function. Results of speech audiometry were characterized by a word-sentence discrepancy that could not be explained by the configuration of the sensitivity loss. Further, the SSI function showed significant rollover. These speech results suggested to us that he had a concomitant central auditory disorder and that the disorder was exacerbated at higher intensities. Auditory evoked potential measures were also abnormal. The auditory brainstem response was well-formed, with peak latencies and interpeak intervals within normal limits. Late latency responses were also present and well-formed. Middle latency responses, however, were abnormal bilaterally.

It is likely that the patient's problems with traditional amplification resulted from an increased difficulty understanding speech in competition when the hearing aids amplified sound to these higher levels. Figure 19–6B shows results of the hearing aid evaluation. Speech understanding of synthetic sentences was measured at several MCRs with no hearing aid, with his own hearing aid (Hearing Aid 1), with an aid that we predicted might be more appropriate for his sensitivity loss (Hearing Aid 2), and with a personal FM system. Results showed very minor aided improvement and only in easy and average listening conditions. However, he showed substantial improvement in performance, especially in difficult listening conditions, when the SNR ratio was made more favorable by use of an ALD.

The patient wore the FM system at all times in the classroom for several years. He also found it particularly useful at home during conversations at dinner and while watching television. Anecdotal parent and teacher reports were extremely positive, and his grades in school improved substantially.

The second case illustrates a similar approach to treatment of CAPD in a younger child with normal hearing sensitivity. Results are from a 5-year old female with a speech and language disorder who also had symptoms of hearing impairment (Stach & Loiselle, 1993). Results revealed a deficit in speech understanding in the presence of background competition and abnormal late-latency auditory evoked potentials. In both speech treatment sessions and in the classroom, the child used a personal FM amplification system as a means of enhancing the SNR. Anecdotal reports suggested that the device was of benefit in her learning environments.

The child was 5 years, 2 months old when her hearing was first evaluated. Her mother had been concerned about her speech for over two years. Her perinatal history was unremarkable. During early childhood, she had numerous bouts of rhinitis. Her medical history was otherwise unremarkable. Although her mother reported normal language milestones, she also reported that she was the only one who could understand the child because of her poor articulation.

A speech/language evaluation indicated that the patient had moderate dysarthria and possible apraxia that resulted in a moderate-to-severe articulation disorder, with limited speech intelligibility related to deficiencies in oral-motor timing and range of motion. She may also have had a mild expressive language disorder with deficits noted in morphologic (plurals) and syntactic (grammatical) structures, although such deficits are difficult to separate from the influence of an articulation disorder. In addition, receptive language skills were within normal limits for her age.

The overall pattern of results from the audiologic test battery was consistent with central auditory processing disorder. In addition, the child had middle ear disorder on the left, accompanied by a mild, low-frequency conductive hearing loss. The CAPD was characterized by depressed speech understanding of single-syllable words presented in competition, and by a dichotic deficit. Depressed speech understanding was accompanied by abnormality in the late-latency auditory evoked potentials.

Results of pure-tone and speech audiometry are shown in Figure 19–7. Pure-tone sensitivity was within normal limits in the right ear. The left ear showed a mild, low frequency conductive hearing loss.

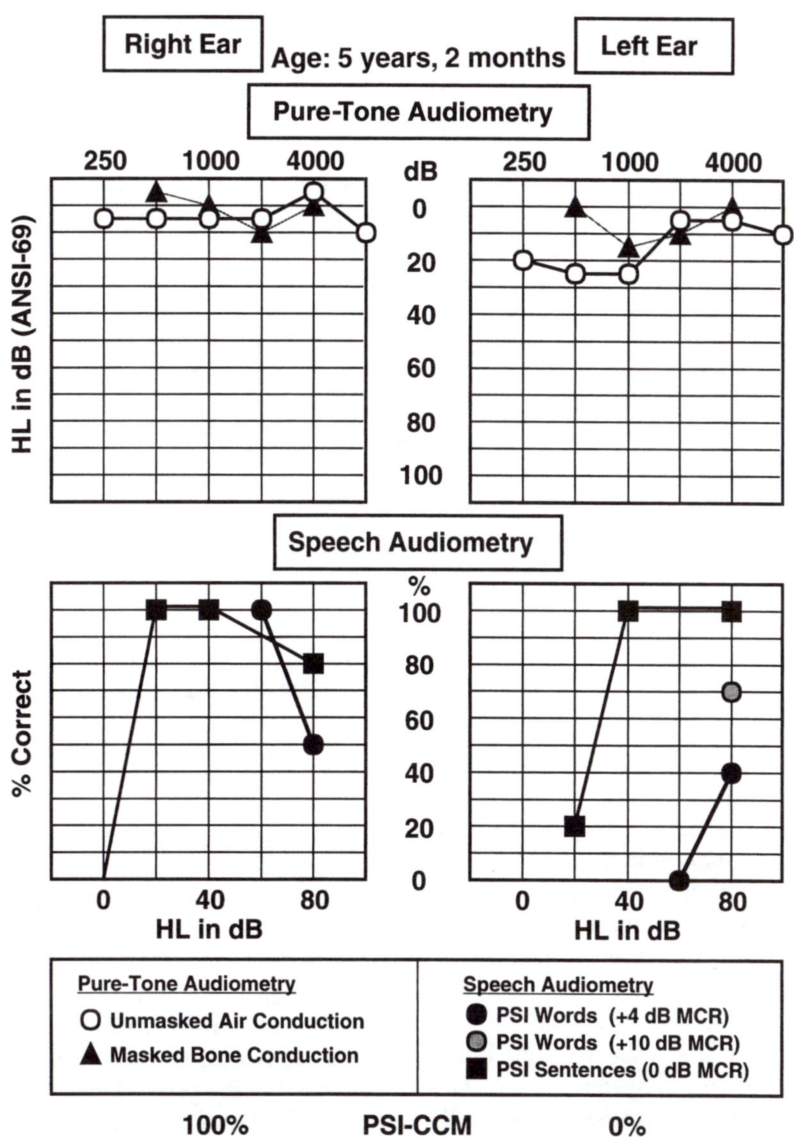

Figure 19–7. Pure-tone and speech-audiometric results in a 5-year-old child with a central auditory processing disorder. Speech audiometric results on PSI test are for word-recognition at +4 and +10 dB MCR and for sentence recognition at 0 dB MCR. Dichotic performance was assessed with the PSI sentence materials with contralateral competing message (CCM).

The Pediatric Speech Intelligibility (PSI) test (Jerger, Lewis, Hawkins, & Jerger, 1980) was used to assess auditory processing ability. Performance-intensity functions were obtained for both words and sentences in the presence of ipsilateral competition at 4 and 0 dB MCR, respectively. Initial practice was carried out at a 10 dB more favorable MCR to assure that the patient was capable of performing the task. Performance on the PSI sentence task was also measured with a contralateral competing message over a range of 0 to −20 dB MCR.

Results were abnormal in both ears. Although her ability to identify sentences in the presence of competition was within normal limits, her ability to identify words in competition was abnormal for both ears. The right ear performance-intensity function showed rollover. For the left ear, the absolute score at the point of maximum performance was abnormally depressed. In addition, for the dichotic listening task, wherein sentences are presented with a contralateral competing message, performance was markedly abnormal, with a score of 0% in the left ear and 100% in the right ear.

Results of an auditory evoked potential assessment showed that both the middle-latency responses and auditory brain stem responses were well formed and had peaks at appropriate and symmetric latencies. Late-latency responses were not identifiable for either ear, however.

Because the patient demonstrated difficulty in understanding speech in the presence of background competition, the clinical goal was to determine the extent to which she could benefit from an enhancement in SNR.

She reported having difficulty understanding the teacher when she wrote on the board and that she could not listen to her teacher and write at the same time. Coupled with parental and teacher concerns over progress in school, the decision was made to implement trial use of an FM system in the classroom. The patient was enthusiastic about the trial and began using the device at school on a regular basis.

After wearing the device for a month, reports from the teacher and parents suggested that its use was having a noticeable impact. Evidence of FM system benefit included: (1) a reduction in the number of emotional outbursts in the classroom; (2) an improvement in the care in which her assignments were carried out; and (3) improvement in the quality of her overall classroom performance.

For the next 2 years, she continued FM-system use and speech treatment. Continual progress was noted in her motor speech ability, and her academic achievement flourished. Hearing sensitivity was monitored and showed no significant change.

This patient was not unlike many children who are referred for audiological assessment to rule out central auditory processing disorder. While some have no apparent speech and language deficits, others have language deficits that are considerably more severe. Her audiologic profile and the course of her treatment and progress serve to illustrate that intervention strategies directed toward enhancement of signal-to-noise ratio can be effective in the treatment of children with CAPD. In this case, due to the severity of the auditory processing disorder, the use of remote-microphone technology was indicated and proved to be effective in overcoming her deficit in understanding speech in background noise in the classroom.

SUMMARY

For many patients with central auditory disorders, conventional hearing aid amplification may not provide adequate benefit or may even be contraindicated. It is also quite possible that a previously satisfied hearing aid user can become progressively dissatisfied as central disorder progresses.

For both children and adults with central auditory disorders, prosthetic devices that go beyond mere amplification of sound may be needed to overcome communication disorder associated with poor speech understanding ability. The use of directional microphones and remote-microphone assistive listening devices can be effective amplification solutions for these populations.

REVIEW QUESTIONS

1. Define auditory processing.

2. What is the primary function of the central auditory nervous system?

3. Define central auditory processing disorders.

4. Is it possible to have normal hearing and a CAPD? If your answer is YES, what is your rationale for answering in the affirmative?

5. What are the two primary causes of CAPD in adults?

6. How does a retrocochlear disorder differ from disorders causing CAPD?

7. True or False: In lower brain stem lesions, performance on difficult monotic tasks is typically poor in the ear *ipsilateral* to the disorder.

8. True or False: Central auditory processing disorders associated with temporal lobe lesions include poor dichotic performance.

9. Why is one of the most pervasive characteristics of central auditory disorder poor speech understanding?

10. Relative to site of lesion, what is meant by the "bottleneck principle"?

11. Relative to those with CAPD, what is the significance of increasing the SNR in difficult listening environments?

12. Does suprathreshold asymmetry *always* present a significant problem to the hard of hearing CAPD patient? Why or why not?

13. Is it true or false that children having a history of otitis media may be prone to developing CAPD?

14. Briefly discuss the advantages of FM systems for those children having diagnosed CAPD.

15. Compared to the normal hearing person, why is it that children and adults with CAPD have difficulty in localizing sound in space and comprehending the spoken word in a background of noise?

REFERENCES

Abel, S., Krever, E., & Alberti, P. W. (1990). Auditory detection, discrimination and speech processing in aging, noise-sensitive and hearing-impaired listeners. *Scandinavian Audiology, 19*, 43–54.

Antonelli, A. (1970). Sensitized speech tests in aged people. In C. Rojskjaer (Ed.), *Speech audiometry. Second Danavox Symposium*. Odense, Denmark: Danavox.

Aoki, C., & Siekevitz, P. (1988). Plasticity in brain development. *Scientific American, 259*, 56–64.

Arnst, D. (1982). Staggered spondaic word test performance in a group of older adults. A preliminary report. *Ear and Hearing, 3*, 118–123.

Berger, K.W., & Hagberg, E.N. (1982). Hearing aid users' attitudes and hearing aid usage. *Monographs in Contemporary Audiology, 3*(4).

Bergman, M. (1971). Hearing and aging. *Audiology, 10*, 164–171.

Bergman, M., Blumfield, B., Cascardo, D., Dash, B., Levitt, H., & Marguiles, M. (1976). Age-related decrement in hearing for speech: Sampling and longitudinal studies. *Journal of Gerontology, 31*, 533–538.

Bergman, M., Costeff, H., Koren, V., Koifman, N., & Reshef, A. (1984). Auditory perception in early lateralized brain damage. *Cortex, 20*, 233–242.

Bocca, E. (1958). Clinical aspects of cortical deafness. *Laryngoscope*, 68, 301–309.

Bocca, E., Calearo, C., & Cassinari, V. (1954). A new method for testing hearing in temporal lobe tumours. *Acta Otolaryngologica, 44*, 219–221.

Boothroyd, A. (1993). Recovery of speech perception performance after prolonged auditory deprivation: Case study. *Journal of the American Academy of Audiology, 4*, 331–336.

Bosatra, A, & Russolo, M. (1982). Comparison between central tonal tests and central speech tests in elderly subjects. *Audiology, 21*, 334–341.

Brody, H. (1955). Organization of the cerebral cortex, III: A study of aging in human cerebral cortex. *Journal of Comparative Neurology, 102*, 511–556.

Brown, D. P. (1994). Speech recognition in recurrent otitis media: Results in a set of identical twins. *Journal of the American Academy of Audiology, 5*, 1–6.

Byrne, D., & Noble, W. (1998). Optimizing sound localization with hearing aids. *Trends in Amplification, 3*, 51–73.

Cacace, A.T., Parnes, S.M., Lovely, T.J., & Kalathia, A. (1994). The disconnected ear: phenomenological effects of a large acoustic tumor. *Ear and Hearing, 15*, 287–298.

Chermak, G.D., & Musiek, F.E. (1992). Managing central auditory processing disorders in children and youth. *American Journal of Audiology, 1*(3), 61–65.

Chermak, G.D., Somers, E.K., & Seikel, J.A. (1998). Behavioral signs of central auditory processing disorder and attention deficit hyperactivity disorder. *Journal of the American Academy of Audiology, 9*, 78–84.

Chmiel, R., & Jerger, J. (1996). Hearing aid use, central auditory disorder, and hearing handicap in elderly persons. *Journal of the American Academy of Audiology, 7*, 190–202.

Chmiel, R., Jerger, J., Murphy, E., Pirozzolo, F., & Tooley-Young, C. (1997). Unsuccessful use of binaural amplification by an elderly person. *Journal of the American Academy of Audiology, 8*, 1–10.

Coleman, J. R., & O'Connor, P. (1979). Effects of monaural and binaural sound deprivation on cell development in the anteroventral cochlear nucleus of rats. *Experimental Neurology, 64*, 553–566.

Cooper, J. C., & Gates, G. A. (1991). Hearing in the elderly – The Framingham cohort, 1983–1985: Part II. Prevalence of central auditory processing disorders. *Ear and Hearing, 12*, 304–311.

Corso, J. (1976). Presbyacusis in noise-induced hearing loss. In D. Henderson, R.P. Hamernik, D.S. Dosanjh, & J.H. Mills (Eds.), *Effects of noise on hearing* (pp. 497–524). New York: Raven Press.

Cranford, J. L., & Romereim, B. (1992). Precedence effect and speech understanding in elderly listeners. *Journal of the American Academy of Audiology, 3*, 405–409.

Dieroff, H. (1993). Late-onset auditory inactivity (deprivation) in persons with bilateral essentially symmetric and conductive hearing impairment. *Journal of the American Academy of Audiology, 4*, 347–350.

Dirks, D. D., Kamm, C., Bower, D., & Betsworth, A. (1977). Use of performance-intensity functions for diagnosis. *Journal of Speech and Hearing Disorders, 42*, 408–41 5.

Farrer, S. M., & Keith, R. W. (1981). Filtered word testing in the assessment of children's central auditory abilities. *Ear and Hearing, 2*, 267–269.

Fifer, R. C., Jerger, J. F., Berlin, C. I., Tobey, E. A., & Campbell, J. C. (1983). Development of a dichotic sentence identification test for hearing-impaired adults. *Ear and Hearing, 4*, 300–305.

Fitzgibbons, P. J., & Gordon-Salant, S. (1996). Auditory temporal processing in elderly listeners. *Journal of the American Academy of Audiology, 7*, 183–189.

Freeman, B. A., & Beasley, D. S. (1978). Discrimination of time-altered sentential approximations and monosyllables by children with reading problems. *Journal of Speech and Hearing Research, 21*, 497–506.

Gelfand, S. A. (1995). Long-term recovery and no recovery from the auditory deprivation effect with binaural amplification: Six cases. *Journal of the American Academy of Audiology, 6*, 141–149.

Gelfand, S. A., Hoffman, S., Waltzman, S. B., & Piper, N. (1980). Dichotic CV recognition at various interaural temporal onset asynchronies: effect of age. *Journal of the Acoustical Society of America, 68*, 1258–1261.

Gelfand, S. A., & Silman, S. (1993). Apparent auditory deprivation in children: Implications of monaural versus binaural amplification. *Journal of the American Academy of Audiology, 4*, 313–318.

Gelfand, S. A., Silman, S., & Ross, L. (1987). Long-term effects of monaural, binaural and no amplification in subjects with bilateral hearing loss. *Scandinavian Audiology, 16*, 201–207.

Goetzinger, C., Proud, G., Dirks, D., & Embrey, J. (1961). A study of hearing in advanced age. *Archives of Otolaryngology, 73*, 662–674.

Goodglass, H. (1967). Binaural digit presentation and early lateral brain damage. *Cortex, 3*, 295–306.

Gordon-Salant, S., & Fitzgibbons, P. J. (1999). Profile of auditory temporal processing in older listeners. *Journal of Speech, Language, and Hearing Research, 42*, 300–311.

Grose, J. H. (1996). Binaural performance and aging. *Journal of the American Academy of Audiology, 7*, 168–174.

Hall, J. W., Grose, J. H., & Pillsbury, H. C. (1995). Long-term effects of chronic otitis media on binaural hearing in children. *Archives of Otolaryngology, 121*, 847–852.

Hansen, C., & Reske-Nielsen, E. (1965). Pathological studies in presbyacusis: Cochlear and central findings in 12 aged patients. *Archives of Otolaryngology, 82*, 115–132.

Harrison, R. V., Nagasawa, A., Smith, D. W., Stanton, S., & Mount, R. J. (1991). Reorganization of auditory cortex after neonatal high frequency cochlear hearing loss. *Hearing Research, 54*, 11–19.

Harrison, R. V., Stanton, S. G., Ibrahim, D., Nagasawa, A., & Mount, R.J. (1993). Neonatal cochlear hearing loss results in developmental abnormalities of the central auditory pathways. *Acta Otolaryngologica, 113*, 296–302.

Hattori, H. (1993). Ear dominance for nonsense-syllable recognition ability in sensorineural hearing-impaired children: Monaural versus binaural amplification. *Journal of the American Academy of Audiology, 4*, 319–330.

Hayes, D. (1980). Central auditory problems and the aging process. In D.S. Beasley & G.A. Davis (Eds.), *Aging communication processes and disorders* (pp. 257–266). New York: Grune and Stratton.

Hayes, D. (1984). Hearing problems of aging. In J. Jerger (Ed.), *Hearing disorders in adults* (pp. 311–337). Boston: College-Hill Press.

Hayes, D., & Jerger, J. (1979). Aging and the use of hearing aids. *Scandinavian Audiology, 8*, 33–40.

Hayes, D., Jerger, J., Taff, J., & Barber, B. (1983). Relation between aided synthetic sentence identification scores and hearing aid user satisfaction. *Ear and Hearing, 4*, 158–161.

Helfer, K. S., & Wilber, L. A. (1990). Hearing loss, aging, and speech perception in reverberation and noise. *Journal of Speech and Hearing Research, 33*, 149–155.

Hinchcliffe, R. (1962). The anatomical locus of presbycusis. *Journal of Speech and Hearing Disorders, 27*, 301–310.

Hood, L. J., Berlin, C. I., & Allen, P. (1994). Cortical deafness: a longitudinal study. *Journal of the American Academy of Audiology, 5,* 330–342.

Humes, L., Christopherson, L., & Cokely, C. (1992). Central auditory processing disorders in the elderly: Fact or fiction? In J. Katz, *Central auditory processing: A transdisciplinary view* (pp.141–150). St. Louis, MO: Mosby Year Book.

Hurley, R. M. (1993). Monaural ear effect: case presentations. *Journal of the American Academy of Audiology, 4,* 285–295.

Jerger, J. (1973). Audiological findings in aging. *Advances in Oto-Rhino-Laryngology, 20,* 115–124.

Jerger, J., Alford, B., Lew, H., Rivera, V., & Chmiel, R. (1995). Dichotic listening, event-related potentials, and interhemispheric transfer in the elderly. *Ear and Hearing, 16,* 482–498.

Jerger, J., Chmiel, R., Allen, J., & Wilson, A. (1994). Effects of age and gender on dichotic sentence identification. *Ear and Hearing, 15,* 274–286.

Jerger, J., & Hayes, D. (1976). Hearing aid evaluation: Clinical experience with a new philosophy. *Archives of Otolaryngology, 102,* 214–225.

Jerger, J., & Hayes, D. (1977). Diagnostic speech audiometry. *Archives of Otolaryngology, 103,* 216–222.

Jerger, J., & Jerger, S. (1971). Diagnostic significance of PB word functions. *Archives of Otolaryngology, 93,* 573–580.

Jerger, J., & Jerger, S. (1975). Clinical validity of central auditory tests. *Scandinavian Audiology, 4,* 147–163.

Jerger, J., Jerger, S., Oliver, T., & Pirozzolo, F. (1989). Speech understanding in the elderly. *Ear and Hearing, 10,* 79–89.

Jerger, J., Johnson, K., Jerger, S., Coker, N., Pirozzolo, F., & Gray, L. (1991). Central auditory processing disorder: A case study. *Journal of the American Academy of Audiology, 2,* 36–54.

Jerger, J., & Jordan, C. (1992). Age-related asymmetry on a cued-listening task. *Ear and Hearing, 4,* 272–277.

Jerger, J., Lovering, L., & Wertz, M. (1972). Auditory disorder following bilateral temporal lobe insult: report of a case. *Journal of Speech and Hearing Disorders, 37,* 523–535.

Jerger, J., Mahurin, R., & Pirozzolo, F. (1990). The separability of central auditory and cognitive deficits: implications for the elderly. *Journal of the American Academy of Audiology, 1,* 116–119.

Jerger, J., Oliver, T. A., & Pirozzolo, F. (1990). Impact of central auditory processing disorder and cognitive deficit on the self-assessment of hearing handicap in the elderly. *Journal of the American Academy of Audiology, 1,* 75–80.

Jerger, J., Silman, S., Lew, H. L., & Chmiel, R. (1993). Case studies in binaural interference: converging evidence from behavioral and electrophysiologic measures. *Journal of the American Academy of Audiology, 4,* 122–131.

Jerger, J., Speaks, C., & Trammel, J. (1968). A new approach to speech audiometry. *Journal of Speech and Hearing Disorders, 33,* 318–327.

Jerger, J., Stach, B., Pruitt, J., Harper, R., & Kirby, H. (1989). Comments on "Speech understanding and aging." *Journal of the Acoustical Society of America, 85,* 1352–1354.

Jerger, J., Stach, B. A., Johnson, K., Loiselle, L. H., & Jerger, S. (1990). Patterns of abnormality in dichotic listening in the elderly. In J.H. Jensen (Ed.), *Proceedings of the 14th Danavox Symposium on Presbyacusis and Other Age Related Aspects* (pp. 143–150). Odense, Denmark: Danavox.

Jerger, J., Weikers, N., Sharbrough, F., & Jerger, S. (1969). Bilateral lesions of the temporal lobe: A case study. *Acta Otolaryngologica,* Suppl. 258.

Jerger, S. (1987). Validation of the pediatric speech intelligibility test in children with central nervous system lesions. *Audiology, 26,* 298–311.

Jerger, S., & Jerger, J. (1980). Low frequency hearing loss in central auditory disorders. *American Journal of Otology, 2,* 1–4.

Jerger, S., Jerger, J., Alford, B. R., & Abrams, S. (1983). Development of speech intelligibility in children with recurrent otitis media. *Ear and Hearing, 4,* 138–145.

Jerger, S., Johnson, K., & Loiselle, L. (1988). Pediatric central auditory dysfunction: comparison of children with confirmed lesions versus suspected processing disorders. *American Journal of Otology Supplement, 9,* 63–71.

Jerger, S., Lewis, S., Hawkins, J., & Jerger, J. (1980). Pediatric speech intelligibility test. I. Generation of test materials. *International Journal of Pediatric Otorhinolaryngology, 2,* 217–230.

Jerger, S., Martin, R. C., & Jerger, J. (1987). Specific auditory perceptual dysfunction in a learning disabled child. *Ear and Hearing, 8,* 78–86.

Johnson, D. W., Enfield, M. L., & Sherman, R. E. (1981). The use of staggered spondaic word and the competing environmental sounds test in the evaluation of central auditory function of learning disabled children. *Ear and Hearing, 2,* 70–77.

Keller, W. D. (1992). Auditory processing disorder or attention-deficit disorder? In J. Katz, N. Stecker, & D. Henderson (Eds.), *Central auditory processing: A transdisciplinary view* (pp. 107–114). St Louis, MO: Mosby Year Book.

Killion, M. C. (1997). Hearing aids: Past, present, future: Moving toward normal conversations in noise. *British Journal of Audiology, 31,* 141–148.

Killion, M., Schulein, R., Christensen, L., Fabry, D., Revit, L., Niquette, P., & Chung, K. (1998). Real-world performance of an ITE directional microphone. *The Hearing Journal, 51*(4), 1–6

Kirikae, I., Sato, T., & Shitaro, T. (1964). Study of hearing in advanced age. *Laryngoscope, 74,* 205–221.

Kochkin, S. (1996). Customer satisfaction and subjective benefit with high-performance hearing aids. *The Hearing Review, 3*(12), 16–26.

Konig, E. (1969). Audiological tests in presbycusis. *International Audiology, 8,* 240–259.

Konkle, D., Beasley, D., & Bess, F. (1977). Intelligibility of time-altered speech in relation to chronological aging. *Journal of Speech and Hearing Research, 20*, 108–115.

Kricos, P. B., Lesner, S. A., Sandridge, S. A., & Yanke, R. B. (1985). Influence of central auditory function on perceived amplification benefits in the elderly: Case reports. *Journal of the Academy of Rehabilitative Audiology, 18*, 871–875.

Kricos, P. B., Lesner, S. A., Sandridge, S. A., & Yanke, R. B. (1987). Perceived benefits of amplification as a function of central auditory status in the elderly. *Ear and Hearing, 8*, 337–342.

Krmpotic-Nemanic, J. (1971). A new concept of the pathogenesis of presbycusis. *Archives of Otolaryngology, 93*, 161–166.

Letowski, T., & Poch, N. (1996). Comprehension of time-compressed speech: effects of age and speech complexity. *Journal of the American Academy of Audiology, 7*, 447–457.

Lubert, N. (1981). Auditory perceptual impairments in children with specific language disorders: A review of the literature. *Journal of Speech and Hearing Disorders, 46*, 3–9.

Lurquin, P., & Rafhay, S. (1996). Intelligibility in noise using multimicrophone hearing aids. *Acta Otorhino-laryngologica, 50*, 103–109.

Lutman, M.E. (1991). Degradations in frequency and temporal resolution with age and their impact on speech identification. *Acta Otolaryngologica*, Suppl. *476*, 120–126.

Lutterman, D., Welsh, O., & Melrose, J. (1966). Responses of aged males to time altered speech stimuli. *Journal of Speech and Hearing Research, 9*, 226–230.

Lynne, G., Benitez, J., Eisenbrey, A., Gilroy, J., & Wilner, H. (1972). Neuroaudiological correlates in cerebral hemisphere lesions. *Audiology, 11*, 115–134.

McCandless, G. A., & Parkin, J. L. (1979). Hearing aid performance relative to site of lesion. *Otolaryngology Head—Neck Surgery, 87*, 871–875.

McCroskey, R., & Kasten, R. (1982). Temporal factors and the aging auditory system. *Ear and Hearing, 3*, 124–127.

Mills, J. H. (1978). Effects of noise on young and old people. In D. Lipscomb (Ed.), *Noise and audiology* (pp. 229–241). Baltimore: University Park Press.

Moore, B. C. J., Peters, R. W., & Glasberg, B. R. (1992). Detection of temporal gaps in sinusoids by elderly subjects with and without hearing loss. *Journal of the Acoustical Society of America, 92*, 1923–1932.

Moore, B. C. J., Vickers, D. A., Glasberg, B. R., & Baer, T. (1997). Comparison of real and simulated hearing impairment in subjects with unilateral and bilateral cochlear hearing loss. *British Journal of Audiology, 31*, 227–245.

Musiek, F. E., & Baran, J. A. (1987). Central auditory assessment: Thirty years of challenge and change. *Ear and Hearing, 8*, 22S–35S.

Nakamura, A., Seiyama, N., Imai, A., Takagi, T., & Miyasaka, E. (1994). A new approach to compensate degeneration of speech intelligibility for elderly listeners. ICSLP94, Yokohama, 2115–2118.

Neuman, A. C. (1996). Late-onset auditory deprivation: a review of past research and an assessment of future research needs. *Ear and Hearing Supplement, 17*, 3S–13S.

Orchik, D., & Burgess, J. (1977). Synthetic sentence identification as a function of age of the listener. *Journal of the American Audiology Society, 3*, 42–46.

Otto, W. C., & McCandless, G. A. (1982). Aging and auditory site of lesion. *Ear and Hearing, 3*, 110–117.

Pestalozza, G., & Shore, I. (1955). Clinical evaluation of presbycusis on the basis of different tests of auditory function. *Laryngoscope, 65*, 1136–1163.

Phillips, S. L., Gordon-Salant, S., Fitzgibbons, P. J., & Yeni-Komshian, G. H. (1994). Auditory duration discrimination in young and elderly listeners with normal hearing. *Journal of the American Academy of Audiology, 5*, 210–215.

Pinheiro, M. L. (1977). Tests of central auditory function in children with learning disabilities. In R. W. Keith (Ed.), *Central auditory dysfunction* (pp. 223–256). New York, Grune & Stratton.

Price, P. J., & Simon, H. J. (1984). Perception of temporal differences in speech by "normal-hearing" adults: Effect of age and intensity. *Journal of the Acoustical Society of America, 76*, 405–410.

Pruitt, J. R., Loiselle, L. H., Jerger, J. F., Stach, B. A., & Stoner, W. R. (1990). Effects of aging and hearing loss on binaural hearing aid advantage. *Asha, 32* (10), 156 (abstract).

Robertson, D., & Irvine, D. R. F. (1989). Plasticity of frequency organization in auditory cortex of guinea pigs with partial unilateral deafness. *Journal of Comparative Neurology, 282*, 456–471.

Sarff, L. S. (1981). An innovative use of free field amplification in regular classrooms. In R. J. Roeser & M. P. Downs (Eds.), *Auditory disorders in school children* (pp. 263–272). New York: Thieme-Stratton.

Sarff, L. S., Ray, H. R., & Bagwell, C. L. (1981). Why not amplification in every classroom? *Hearing Aid Journal, 34*, 11.

Schilder, A. G. M., Snik, A. F. M., Straatman, H., & van den Broek, P. (1994). The effect of otitis media with effusion at preschool age on some aspects of auditory perception at school age. *Ear and Hearing, 15*, 224–231.

Schneider, D. (1992). Audiologic management of central auditory processing disorders. In J. Katz, N. Stecker, & D. Henderson (Eds.), *Central auditory processing: A transdisciplinary view* (pp. 161–168). St Louis, MO: Mosby Year Book.

Schneider, B. A., Pichora-Fuller, M. K., Kowalchuk, D., & Lamb, M. (1994). Gap detection and the precedence effect in young and old adults. *Journal of the Acoustical Society of America, 95*, 980–991.

Schuknecht, H. (1964). Further observation on the pathology of presbycusis. *Archives of Otolaryngology, 80*, 369–382.

Schuknecht, H., & Igarashi, M. (1964). Pathology of slowly progressive sensorineural deafness. *Transactions of the American Academy of Ophthalmology and Otolaryngology, 68*, 222–242.

Shirinian, M., & Arnst, D. (1982). Patterns in performance intensity functions for phonetically balanced word lists and synthetic sentences in aged listeners. *Archives of Otolaryngology, 108*, 15–20.

Silman, S. (1995). Binaural interference in multiple sclerosis: case study. *Journal of the American Academy of Audiology, 6*, 193–196

Silman, S., Gelfand, S. A., & Silverman, C. A. (1984). Effects of monaural versus binaural hearing aids. *Journal of the Acoustical Society of America, 76*, 1357–1362.

Silman, S., Silverman, C. A., Emmer, M. B., & Gelfand, S. A. (1992). Adult-onset auditory deprivation. *Journal of the American Academy of Audiology, 3*, 390–396.

Silverman, C. A., & Emmer, M. B. (1993). Auditory deprivation from and recovery in adults with asymmetric sensorineural hearing impairments. *Journal of the American Academy of Audiology, 4*, 338–346.

Silverman, C. A., & Silman, S. (1990). Apparent auditory deprivation from monaural amplification and recovery with binaural amplification: two case studies. *Journal of the American Academy of Audiology, 1*, 175–180.

Sperry, J. L., Wiley, T. L., & Chial, M. R. (1997). Word recognition performance in various background competitors. *Journal of the American Academy of Audiology, 8*, 71–80.

Stach, B. A. (1990). Hearing aid amplification and central processing disorders. In R. E. Sandlin (Ed.), *Handbook of hearing aid amplification, Volume II: Clinical considerations and fitting practices* (pp. 87–111). Boston: College-Hill Press.

Stach, B. A., & Delgado-Vilches, G. (1993). Sudden hearing loss in multiple sclerosis: Case report. *Journal of the American Academy of Audiology, 4*, 370–375.

Stach, B. A., Jerger, J. F., & Fleming, K. A. (1985). Central presbyacusis: a longitudinal case study. *Ear and Hearing, 6*, 304–306.

Stach, B. A., Jerger, J. F., & Smith, S. L. (1986). Central auditory disorder and hearing aid satisfaction. *Asha, 28*(10), 69 (abstract).

Stach, B. A., & Loiselle, L. H. (1993). Central auditory processing disorder: Diagnosis and management in a young child. *Seminars in Hearing, 14*, 288–295.

Stach, B. A., Loiselle, L. H., & Jerger, J. F. (1991). Special hearing aid considerations in elderly patients with auditory processing disorders. *Ear and Hearing Supplement, 12*, 131S–138S.

Stach, B. A., Loiselle, L. H., Jerger, J. F., Mintz, S. L., & Taylor, C. D. (1987). Clinical experience with personal FM assistive listening devices. *The Hearing Journal, 40*(5), 24–30.

Stach, B. A., Spretnjak, M. L., & Jerger, J. (1990). The prevalence of central presbyacusis in a clinical population. *Journal of the American Academy of Audiology , 1*, 109–115.

Stach, B. A., Westerberg, B. D., & Roberson, J. B. (1998). Auditory disorder in central nervous system miliary tuberculosis: A case report. *Journal of the American Academy of Audiology , 9*, 305–310.

Starr, A., Picton, T. W., Sininger, Y., Hood, L. J., & Berlin, C. I. (1996). Auditory neuropathy. *Brain, 119*, 741–753.

Starr, A., Sininger, Y., Winter, M., Derebery, M.J., Oba, S., & Michalewski, H. J. (1998). Transient deafness due to temperature-sensitive auditory neuropathy. *Ear and Hearing, 19*, 169–179.

Sticht, T., & Gray, B. (1969). The intelligibility of time-compressed words as a function of age and hearing loss. *Journal of Speech and Hearing Research, 12*, 443–448.

Stuart, A., & Phillips, D. P. (1996). Word recognition in continuous and interrupted broadband noise by young normal-hearing, older normal-hearing, and presbyacusic listeners. *Ear and Hearing, 17*, 478–489.

Valente, M., Fabry, D., & Potts, L. (1995). Recognition of speech in noise with hearing aids using dual microphones. *Journal of the American Academy of Audiology, 6*, 440–449.

Welsh, L. W., Welsh, J. J., & Healy, M. P. (1985). Central Presbyacusis. *Laryngoscope, 95*, 128–136.

Wiley, T. L., Cruickshanks, K. J., Nondahl, D. M., Tweed, T. S., Klein, R., & Klein, B. E. K. (1998). Aging and word recognition in competing message. *Journal of the American Academy of Audiology, 9*, 191–198.

Willeford, J. (1977). Assessing central auditory behavior in children: A test battery approach. In R. Keith (Ed.), *Central auditory dysfunction* (pp. 43–72). New York, Grune and Stratton.

Willeford, J. A., & Billger, J. M. (1978). Auditory perception in children with learning disabilities. In J. Katz (Ed.), *Handbook of clinical audiology* (2nd ed., pp. 410–425). Baltimore: Williams & Wilkins.

Willott, J. F. (1996). Anatomic and physiologic aging: A behavioral neuroscience perspective. *Journal of the American Academy of Audiology, 7*, 141–151.

Wilson, R. H., & Jaffe, M. S. (1996). Interactions of age, ear, and stimulus complexity on dichotic digit recognition. *Journal of the American Academy of Audiology, 7*, 358–364.

Wingfield, A., Poon, L. W., Lombardi, L, & Lowe, D. (1985). Speed of processing in normal aging: Effects of speech rate, linguistic structure, and processing time. *Journal of Gerontology, 40*, 579–585.

Woods, B. (1984). Dichotic listening ear preference after childhood cerebral lesions. *Neuropsychologia, 22*, 303–310.

Working Group on Speech Understanding and Aging. (1988). Speech understanding and aging. *Journal of the Acoustical Society of America, 83*, 859–894.

CHAPTER 20

Assistive Technologies for the Hearing Impaired

CARL C. CRANDELL, PH.D.
JOSEPH J. SMALDINO, PH.D.

OUTLINE

(continued)

It is well recognized that the major complaint of individuals with sensorineural hearing loss (SNHL) is communicative difficulty, particularly in noisy and reverberant listening environments (Cooper & Cutts, 1971; Crandell, 1991; Crandell, Henoch, & Dunkerson, 1991b; Crandell & Smaldino, 1996a, 1996b; Crum, 1974; Dirks, Morgan, & Dubno, 1982; Duquesnoy & Plomp, 1983; Finitzo-Hieber & Tillman, 1978; Humes, 1991; Nabelek, 1982; Nabelek & Pickett, 1974a, 1974b; Needleman & Crandell, 1996a, 1996b; Plomp, 1978, 1986; Ross, 1978; Suter, 1985). Due to the deleterious effects of SNHL on communication, additional research has indicated that hearing loss may detrimentally affect both psychosocial and physical health status (see Crandell, 1998, for a review of these studies). Unfortunately, many forms of hearing aid technology have been shown to offer minimal speech-recognition benefit to listeners with hearing impairment in adverse listening environments (Boothroyd, 1991; Crandell, 1991a, 1991b; Crandell & Smaldino, 1999a, 1999b; Crandell, Smaldino, & Flexer, 1995; Festen & Plomp, 1983; Moore, 1997; Plomp, 1978, 1986; Van Tassell, 1993). Plomp (1986), for example, reported that hearing aids offered limited improvements in speech recognition when background noise levels exceeded 50 dB(A), a noise level commonly encountered in everyday listening environments. With these considerations in mind, this chapter will examine various rehabilitative technologies for improving communicative efficiency within commonly used noisy and reverberant listening environments. The terms rehabilitative technology or assistive technology will be used to describe these technologies. These terms were selected over the more commonly used assistive listening devices (ALDs), as many of these technologies are not limited to simply improved listening ability.

EFFECTS OF REVERBERATION, NOISE, AND DISTANCE ON SPEECH RECOGNITION

The accurate transmission of speech in a room can be affected by the acoustic characteristics of the room, including reverberation time (RT), the intensity of ambient noise in comparison to the intensity of the desired signal, and the distance from the speaker to the listener. Prior to examining rehabilitative technologies that can improve speech recognition in adverse listening environments, it is first imperative to summarize some of the general effects of these variables on speech recognition. For more detailed information on the effects of noise, reverberation, and distance on speech recognition, the reader is directed to Crandell and Smaldino (1994, 1995, 1996a, 1996b, 1999a, 1999b) and Siebein (1994).

Reverberation time refers to the amount of time it takes for a steady-state sound to decrease 60 dB from its peak amplitude. In a reverberant room, the reflected speech from the room surfaces reaches the ear of the listener temporally delayed and overlaps with the direct speech signal (the signal not reflected before reaching the listener's ear), which masks certain acoustic speech components (Bolt & MacDonald, 1949; Lochner & Burger, 1964; Siebein, Crandell, & Gold, 1997). Because vowels are more intense than consonants, reverberation tends to produce a prolongation of the spectral energy of vowel phonemes, which reduces consonant recognition. A reduction of consonant information can have a significant effect on speech recognition because the vast majority of the acoustic information that is important for speech recognition is provided by consonants (French & Steinberg, 1947; Licklider & Miller, 1951; Wang, Reed, & Bilger, 1978). Speech recognition tends to decrease with increases in RT. Speech recognition in adults with normal hearing is not significantly degraded until the RT exceeds approximately 1 second (Crum, 1974; Gelfand & Silman, 1979; Houtgast, 1981; Nabelek & Pickett, 1974a, 1974b; Moncur & Dirks, 1967). Listeners with SNHL, however, need considerably shorter RTs (0.4 to 0.5 second) for optimal communication (ASHA, 1995; Crandell, 1991b; 1992a; Crandell & Smaldino, 1994, 1995, 1996a, 1996b, 1999a, 1999b; Crandell et al., 1995; Finitzo-Hieber, 1988; Finitzo-Hieber & Tillman, 1978; Gengel, 1971; Neimoeller, 1968; Olsen, 1981, 1988). In addition to listeners with SNHL, there are a number of populations of individuals (primarily children) with "normal hearing" sensitivity that exhibit greater perceptual difficulties in reverberation (and noise) than young adults with normal hearing (Berg, 1993; Bess, 1985; Bess & Tharpe, 1986; Boney & Bess, 1984; Crandell, 1991b, 1992a; 1993; Crandell & Bess, 1986; Crandell & Smaldino, 1992; 1994; Flexer, 1992; Nabelek & Nabelek, 1994; Crandell et al., 1995; Crandell & Smaldino, 1995; 1996a, 1996b). A list of these "normal hearing" listeners is presented in Table 20-1. Due to this increased difficulty listening in noise, acoustical guidelines for hearing impaired and "normal-hearing" populations suggest that RTs should not exceed 0.4 to 0.5 second in communication environments frequented by these individuals.

Background noise in a room also reduces speech recognition by masking the acoustic/linguistic cues in the message. As with reverberation, background noise in a room tends to mask the weaker consonant phonemes significantly greater than the more intense vowel phonemes. The most important factor for accurate speech recognition is often the ratio of the intensity of the desired signal compared to the intensity of the undesired signal or noise. This ratio is referred to as the signal-to-noise ratio (SNR) and is reported as the decibel difference between the two intensities. Speech recognition is generally highest at advantageous SNRs and decreases as the SNR of the

Table 20–1. Populations of listeners with "normal hearing" who may be affected by poor room acoustics.

- Elderly listeners with normal hearing sensitivity
- Young children (less than 15 years)
- Conductive hearing loss
- History of otitis media
- Articulation and/or language disorders
- Learning disabled
- Non-native English
- Central auditory processing deficits
- Minimal or borderline degrees of SNHL (16–25 dB HL)
- Unilateral hearing loss
- Developmental delays
- Attentional deficits
- Reading deficits (dyslexia)

environment is reduced (Cooper & Cutts, 1971; Crum, 1974; Finitzo-Hieber & Tillman, 1978; Miller, 1974; Nabelek & Pickett, 1974a, 1974b). Speech-recognition ability in adults with normal hearing is not significantly reduced until the SNR is reduced below 0 dB. To obtain recognition scores equal to those of normal hearers, listeners with SNHL require the SNR to be improved by 4 to 12 dB (Crandell et al., 1995; Moore, 1997; Plomp, 1986) and by an additional 3 to 6 dB in rooms with moderate levels of reverberation (Hawkins & Yacullo, 1984). Based on these data, acoustical guidelines for hearing-impaired populations (and "normal hearers") suggest that SNRs should exceed +15 dB for peak speech recognition.

The acoustics of a speaker's voice also vary as a function of the distance to the listener. When the listener is relatively near to the speaker, the direct sound field dominates and the listener receives the sound directly from the speaker unaffected by reflections from surfaces within the room. Direct sound pressure decreases 6 dB for every doubling of distance from the sound source, a phenomena referred to as the inverse square law. As speaker-listener distance increases, there is a point at which the direct sound energy and the intensity of sound reflected off room surfaces (reverberation) is equal. This point is called the critical distance of the room. Beyond the critical distance, the direct sound from the speaker arrives at the listener first (but at a decreased intensity) and is quickly followed by reflections of the direct sound from the walls, floor, and ceiling. Because there is a decease in sound intensity with distance and because some frequencies will be absorbed more than others by the absorptive elements in the room (including the occupants), the reflected sound reaching the listener will have a different acoustic signature in the intensity, frequency, and temporal domains. Speech recognition tends to decrease until the critical distance (the point at which the direct and reverberant sound energy is equal) of the room is reached. The critical distance in most small rooms (such as classrooms) is approximately 3 to 6 feet from the speaker. Beyond the critical distance, recognition ability tends to remain essentially constant unless the room is very large (such as an auditorium). In larger rooms, speech recognition may continue to decrease as a function of increased distance. These findings suggest that speech recognition can only be improved by decreasing the distance between a speaker and listener within the critical distance of the room. Stated another way, the simple recommendation of preferential seating for a listener with hearing loss is often not adequate to ensure optimal communication.

Reverberation, background noise, and distance from the speaker synergistically interact in a room. That is, when each factor is combined (which is the case in virtually all real world listening environments), they affect speech recognition more than any one of the factors alone. Finitzo-Hieber and Tillman (1978), for example, demonstrated that children with SNHL obtained speech-recognition scores of only 29% in typical classroom learning environments (RT = 0.4 second; SNR = dB; distance of 12 feet). Leavitt and Flexer (1991), using the Rapid Speech Transmission Index (RASTI), demonstrated that 83% of the speech energy was available to the listener in the front row of a typical classroom-sized environment. In the back row of the classroom, however, only approximately 50% of the speech energy was available. Even less of the signal would be available if the listener has a hearing loss, attentional difficulties, or reduced auditory/language processing. That is, add the loss of the speech signal due to the acoustical environment to the distortion imposed by a damaged auditory or linguistic system and it becomes apparent why simply turning up the gain of a hearing aid is frequently not a satisfactory communicative solution.

HEARING ASSISTIVE DEVICES

Whether the goal is group communication or one-to-one communication, the initial approach for improving speech recognition in a room is modification of the acoustics within that environment. For a detailed review of acoustical modifications, the reader is directed to Crandell and Smaldino (1999a). Unfortunately, due to cost factors, appropriate acoustical conditions for the hearing impaired are infrequently met with physical acoustical modification of the room. Consequently, assistive technologies must often be implemented. One well-recognized strategy for improving speech recognition in rooms is the utilization of group or personal room amplification systems. Often, these devices are called hearing assistive devices. As seen in Table 20–2, possible hearing assistive devices include hard wired, personal Frequency Modulation (FM), sound field FM, induction loop, and infrared systems. The goals of assistive systems are depicted in Table 20–3.

Hard Wired Systems

With hard-wired systems, a wire connects the microphone of the speaker to the amplifier and the amplifier to the receiver used by the listener. Thus, with hard-wired systems, there is a direct physical connection between the sound source and the individual. Due to the "hard wiring" involved in such systems, and consequently the reduced mobility for both the speaker and the listener, they are generally not recommended for most listening environments. It should be noted, however, that several investigators have reported that some small, inexpensive hard-wired systems may be beneficial for individuals who can not manage a hearing aid due to conditions such as dementia or severe manual dexterity difficulties (Crandell & Smaldino, 1999a, 1999b; Weinstein & Amsel, 1986). A summary of the advantages and disadvantages of hard-wired systems are shown in Table 20–4.

Table 20–2. Various types of hearing assistive devices.

- Hard wired
- Personal FM
- Sound field FM
- Induction loop
- Infrared

Table 20–3. The primary goals of hearing assistive devices.

- Maintain favorable SNR with minimal reverberation at the listener's ears
- Allow the acoustic signal to be modified to meet the hearing needs of the individual
- Provide wide frequency amplification with a minimal degree of distortion
- Allow mobility for both speaker and listener
- Allow the listener to not only hear the primary speaker, but also other speakers in the room and their own voice
- Accept auditory inputs such as compact disks, tape recorders, and televisions

Source: Adapted from *Management of Hearing Handicap: Infants to Elderly*, by D. Sanders, 1993. Englewood Cliffs, NJ: Prentice Hall

Table 20–4. Potential advantages and disadvantages of hard-wired systems.

Advantages

- Inexpensive
- May be useful in some patients with hearing impairment who may not be able to use conventional amplification (cognitive declines, physical disabilities and/or severe manual dexterity difficulties)
- Installation of such systems tends to be relatively easy
- Not susceptible to electromagnetic interference

Disadvantages

- Hard-wired systems are not specified as medical devices by the Food and Drug Administration (FDA); therefore, there are no standards for the electroacoustic characteristics (gain, frequency response, SSPL90, harmonic distortion) of such devices
- Limited mobility for the speaker and/or listener
- Installation costs can be high, particularly in already-constructed buildings

Personal Frequency Modulation (FM) Amplification

With a personal FM system (often called an Auditory Trainer), the speaker's voice is picked up via an FM wireless microphone located 3 to 4 inches from the speaker's mouth (where the detrimental effects of reverberation and noise are minimal). The acoustic signal is converted to an electrical waveform and transmitted via an FM radio signal to a receiver (see Figure 20–1). The electrical signal is then amplified, converted back to an acoustical waveform, and conveyed to one or more listeners in the room.

Often, FM systems can improve the SNR of the listening environment by 20 to 30 dB. The Federal Communication Commission (FCC) has allocated the frequency region of 72 to 76 MHZ (and recently 216 to 217 MHZ) for FM devices utilized for the hearing impaired.

As noted in Table 20–5, there are several ways of coupling an FM system to the user. For a discussion of the advantages and disadvantages of various coupling strategies the reader is directed to Crandell and Smaldino (1999b) and Lewis (1998). For listeners with hearing loss, the FM signal can be presented through headphones, earbuds coupled directly to the ear via a button or behind-the-ear transducer, or directly to hearing aids via in-

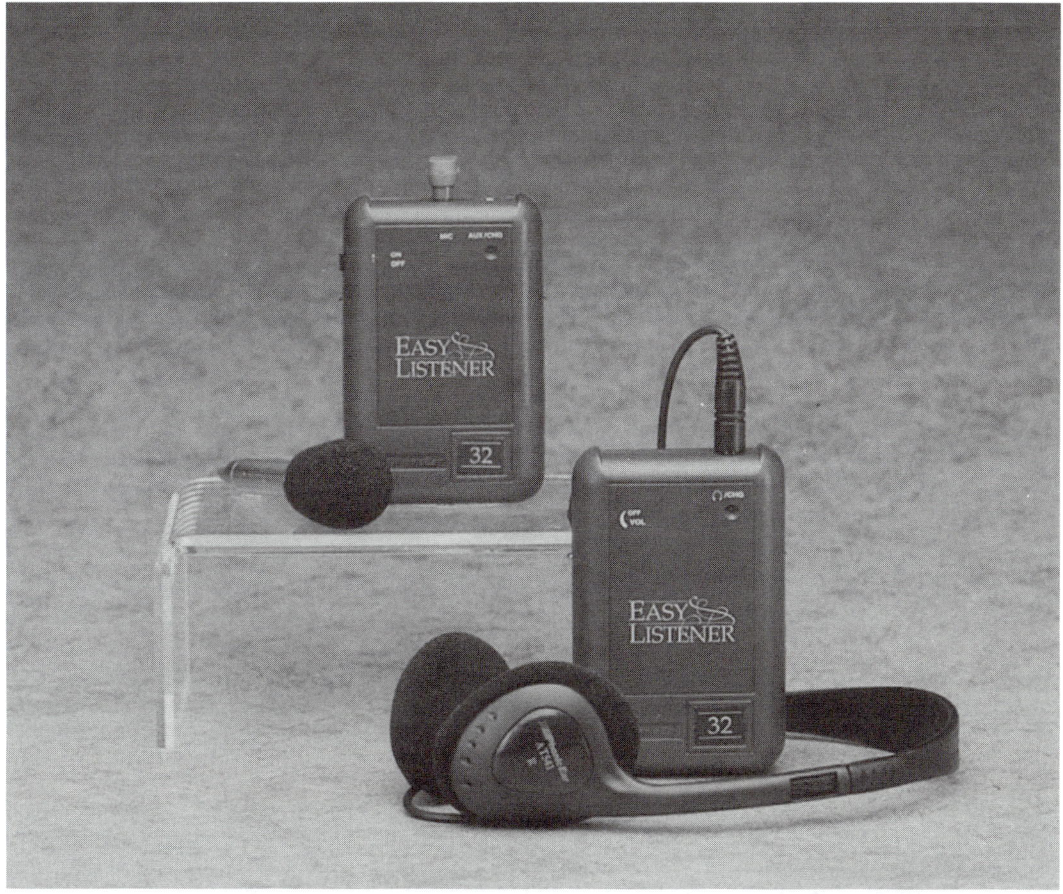

Figure 20–1. An example of a frequency modulation (FM) system. (Photo courtesy of Phonic Ear.)

Table 20–5. FM coupling strategies for listeners with hearing loss and "normal hearing."

Individuals with Hearing Loss

- Headphones
- Earbuds
- Direct to the ear via a button/behind-the-ear transducer
- Direct to hearing aids via induction loop/Direct Auditory Input (DAI).
- Ear level (audio boot or behind-the-ear style device with hearing aid + FM system integrated)
- Bone conduction transducer

Individuals with "Normal Hearing"

- Headphones
- Earbuds
- Ear level (behind-the-ear style device with FM system integrated)

duction loop or Direct Audio Input (DAI) (see Figure 20–2). For individuals with conductive or mixed hearing losses, the FM system can be coupled to a bone conduction transducer. For "normal-hearing" individuals, the signal can be presented through earbuds or Walkman-style earphones. Recently, personal FM systems have become available for both individuals with SNHL and "normal hearing" in ear-level models. For listeners with SNHL, this type of FM system provides the user with a combination of *both* a hearing aid and an FM system in the same ear-level device. For individuals with "normal hearing," the FM system is simply located in a behind-the-ear configuration. In both cases, these types of systems allow the user the freedom of not having to use the body-worn receivers required with traditional FM systems. Another current advancement in FM technology allows a personal FM receiver to be coupled to a hearing aid via an "audio boot" (see Figure 20–3). This

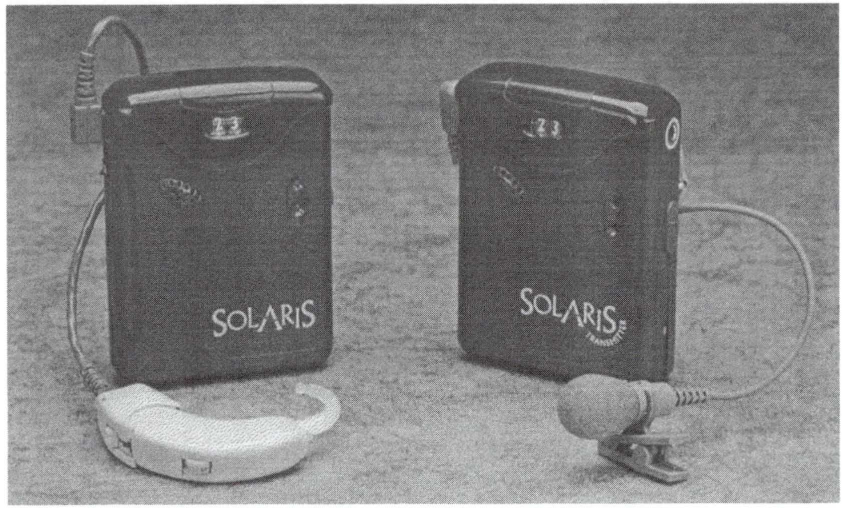

Figure 20–2. Frequency modulation (FM) system coupled to a hearing aid via direct audio input (DAI). (Photo courtesy of Phonic Ear.)

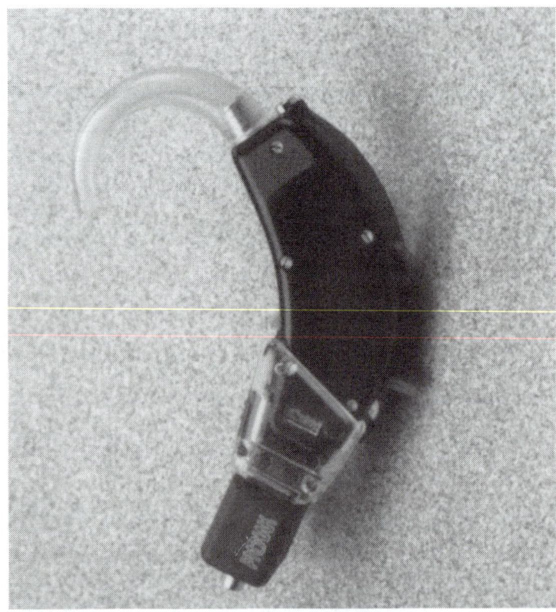

Figure 20–3. Frequency modulation (FM) system coupled to a hearing aid via a wireless "audio boot." (Photo courtesy of Phonak.)

technology allows the user to convert his or her personal hearing aid into an FM system simply by attaching the audio boot. These FM systems may be particularly useful for individuals who may not want to utilize personal FM systems due to the potential negative stigma that may be associated with such devices.

Finally, prior to concluding this section, it should be noted that although FM systems are the most popular room amplification used in theaters, classroom, and therapy-room settings, they also can be beneficial in other settings. For example, FM systems can be used to provide important early auditory input to infants with hearing impairment, particularly when limited auditory information is available (Crandell & Smaldino, 1999a, 1999b). Advantages and disadvantages of personal FM systems are found in Table 20–6.

Sound Field FM Amplification

A sound field FM system is similar to a personal FM system, but with sound field FM amplification, the speaker's voice is conveyed to all listeners in the room via one or more strategically placed loudspeakers (see Figure 20–4). Sound field FM systems are generally used to assist "normal-hearing" individuals, such as children in a classroom setting. The objectives when placing a sound field FM system in a classroom are to: (1) amplify the speaker's voice by approximately 8 to 10 dB, thus improving the SNR of the listening environment and (2) provide amplification uniformly throughout the classroom regardless of teacher or student position. Sound field systems vary from compact, portable, battery-powered single-speaker units to more permanently placed, alternating-current (AC) powered speaker systems that utilize multiple (usually four) loudspeakers. Loudspeakers are generally placed on stands and strategically placed within the classroom. Several companies now sell loudspeakers that can be placed in the ceiling (see Figure 20–5). A number of studies have demonstrated that when sound field amplification systems are correctly placed within learning settings (such as classrooms and lecture halls) speech recognition, psychoeducational, and psychosocial improvements occur for listeners

Table 20–6. Potential advantages and disadvantages of personal FM systems.

Advantages

- High degree of portability
- Simple installation
- FM systems can be used in many communication situations (large rooms, small rooms, indoor, outdoors, field trips, broadcast media) that may not be practical for other forms of room amplification
- High degree of electroacoustic flexibility
- Buildings can have many rooms using FM systems as long as the transmission channels are selected to not interfere with one another
- High mobility for speaker and listener
- Not susceptible to electromagnetic interference

Disadvantages

- User often has to wear a body-worn receiver
- May be susceptible to FM interference from other sources
- Relatively high unit cost
- Learning curve for use and maintenance

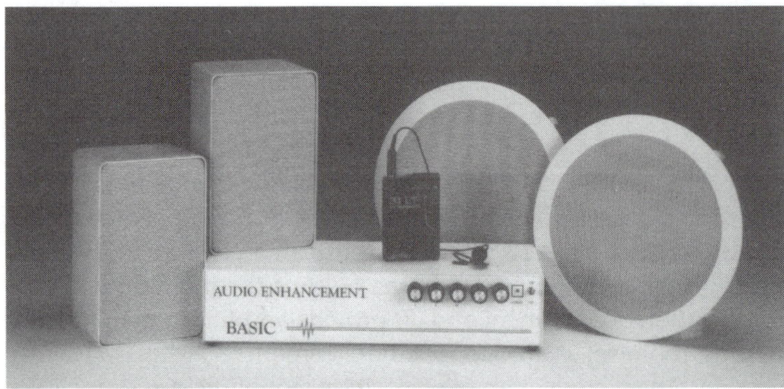

Figure 20–4. Components of a frequency modulation (FM) sound field system with varying loudspeaker arrays, floor and ceiling mounted. (Photo courtesy of Audio Enhancement.)

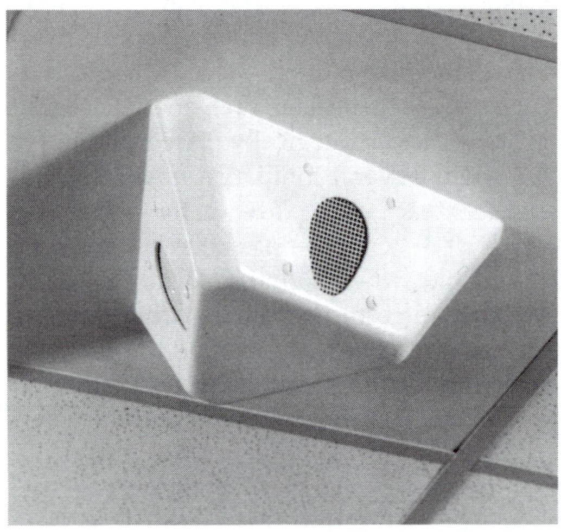

Figure 20–5. A frequency modulation (FM) sound field system loudspeaker located in the ceiling. (Photo courtesy of Lightspeed.)

with "normal hearing" (see Berg, 1993, Crandell et al., 1995; Crandell & Smaldino, 1996b for a review of these studies). At present, there remains limited data concerning the effects of sound field FM systems on individuals with moderate to severe degrees of SNHL. Advantages and disadvantages of sound field FM systems are found in Table 20–7.

Infrared Light Wave Systems

Infrared systems consist of a wireless microphone, infrared converter, and infrared receiver. The microphone converts the acoustical signal to an electrical signal, which is then transmitted to the converter. The converter transduces the electrical signal to an invisible infrared signal and transmits it to a receiver worn by the listener. The receiver (which often also has an amplifier) contains photo-detector diodes that pick up the infrared signal to transduce the infrared signal back into electrical energy. The electrical signal is then changed into acoustical energy and routed to the listener via an induction loop and hearing aid telecoil setup, through headphones or insert earphones or DAI. The majority of infrared systems designed for individuals with SNHL use a carrier frequency of 95 kHz. Infrared systems are often used in larger room settings, such as auditoriums, conference halls, theaters, and churches. For large rooms, such as theaters and auditoriums, arrays of transmitters must be utilized to ensure that all listeners are appropriately placed with the infrared light beam. In the clinical setting, infrared systems are often recommended for television and radio communication. An example of one such device is found in Figure 20–6. A summary of the advantages and disadvantages of infrared systems are found in Table 20–8.

Large Area Electromagnetic Induction Loop Systems

A large area induction loop system consists of a microphone connected via a hardwire or an FM transmitter to an amplifier. A length of wire, which is wound around a magnetic core

Table 20–7. Potential advantages and disadvantages of sound field FM systems.

Advantages

- Provides benefit to all "normal hearing" listeners in the room
- Can provide benefit to children with SNHL while malfunctioning hearing aids or auditory trainers are being repaired
- Often the most inexpensive procedure of improving classroom acoustics
- Sound field system does not stigmatize certain listeners
- Speakers/teachers overwhelmingly accept sound field amplification system once they receive an in-service on the instrumentation or utilize the equipment
- Speakers/teachers report lessened stress and vocal strain during teaching activities
- Parents and students overwhelmingly accept sound field amplification systems
- Sound field systems can be used to enhance the auditory signal from other instructional equipment (e.g., television, cassette tape/compact disk players)
- High mobility for speaker and listener
- Not susceptible to electromagnetic interference

Disadvantages

- May not provide adequate benefits in excessively noisy or reverberant listening environments
- Primarily used only for "normal hearers" and listeners with milder degrees of SNHL
- Loudspeaker arrangement and/or number of loudspeakers(s) must be appropriate
- May not be feasible in smaller rooms due to feedback problems associated with the interactive effects of reflective surfaces and speaker closeness
- May not benefit children with severe recruitment or hypersensitive hearing
- Sound field systems may not be portable (unless desktop units are used)

under its installation, extends from the amplifier. This wire is placed either around the head of an individual (neckloop) or around a designated area, such as a classroom or theater (see Figure 20–7). When an electrical current flows through the wire loop, it creates a magnetic field, which can be picked up by any device utilizing telecoil technology (such as a hearing aid). Advantages and disadvantages of large area induction loop systems are presented in Table 20–9.

To avoid many of the difficulties associated with traditional induction loop systems, Hendricks and Lederman (1991) developed a three-dimensional (3D) induction loop system. In the 3D induction loop system, a wireless microphone transmits the speaker's voice to an audio mixer, signal processor, and power amplifier. The amplified signal is then transmitted to specially designed induction loops that are placed within a floor mat that is placed under the room's carpet. Advantages of such systems over traditional induction loop systems include that "spillover" is significantly reduced and that the signal tends to be more uniform, thus aiding more listeners in the room.

IMPROVING TELEPHONE COMMUNICATION WITH REHABILITATIVE TECHNOLOGIES

In addition to communicative difficulties in rooms, another common complaint of indi-

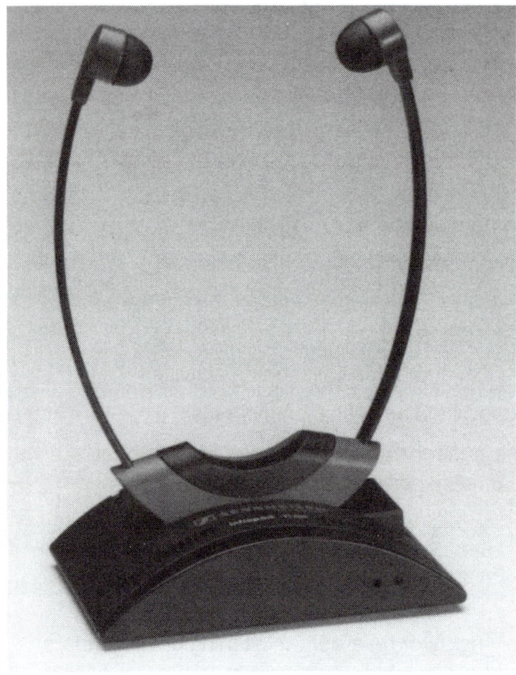

Figure 20–6. A personal infrared device commonly used for improving television communication. (Photo courtesy of Sennheiser.)

Table 20–8. Potential advantages and disadvantages of infrared systems.

Advantages

- Worldwide use is high
- Not susceptible to electromagnetic interference
- Relatively Inexpensive

Disadvantages

- Because the infrared cannot penetrate solid barriers, listener must be in a direct line of sight with the transmitter
- Cannot be used outside, or in highly lit rooms, because infrared is susceptible to interference from sunlight

viduals with SNHL is speech-recognition difficulties when communicating via the telephone. The present section examines various strategies for improving communication over the telephone.

Hearing Aid Telecoils and Telephone Use

A common procedure to improve telephone communication is through a hearing aid telephone induction pickup coil, or telecoil. A hearing aid telecoil picks up the electromagnetic leakage from the telephone receiver. The signal is then amplified, transduced into acoustical information, and delivered to the individual's ear. Improved telephone communication is obtained because (1) the hearing microphone is turned off, reducing the level of the background noise and reverberation and (2) the frequency response of most telecoils tends to be smoother than when the hearing aid is acoustically coupled to the tele-

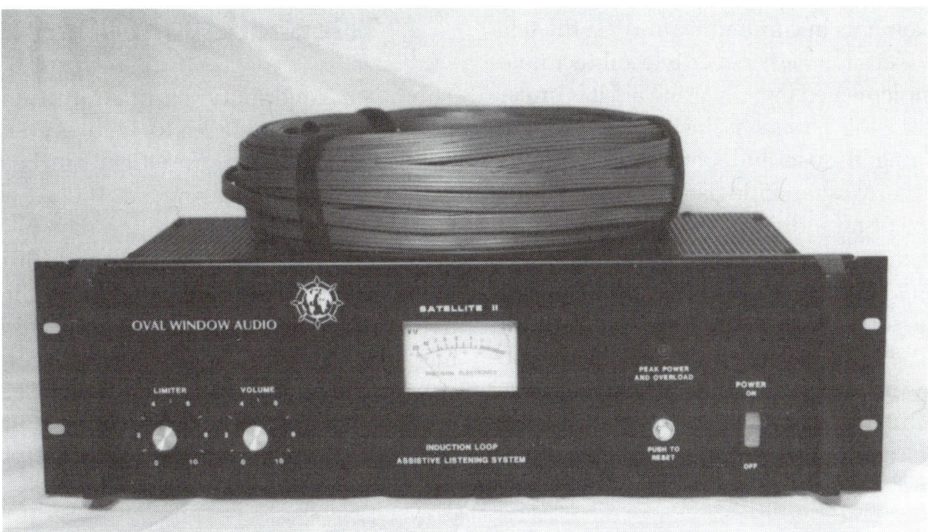

Figure 20–7. Components of a large area induction loop system. (Photo courtesy of Oval Window Audio.)

Table 20–9. Potential advantages and disadvantages of large area induction loop systems.

Advantages

- Often least costly of the room amplification systems
- Installation, portability, troubleshooting, and maintenance of such systems tend to be relatively easy
- Hearing aid users already have receiver if their hearing aid contains a telecoil
- High degree of electroacoustic flexibility (due to hearing aid telecoil)

Disadvantages

- Require functional telecoil that is sensitive enough to pick up the magnetic field throughout the room and/or incorporate a preamplifier
- Require hearing aids (or some device with telecoil) that limits use for "normal hearers"
- Require hearing aids that contain telecoil option
- Signal quality may decrease as the listener moves away from the induction loop
- Reduced portability; for example, it is not practical to move such systems to accommodate outdoor activities
- Number of rooms in a building that can be equipped with such technology may be limited, because "spillover" can occur across systems
- Signal quality may be reduced by additional devices in the room that produce electromagnetic fields (and 60 Hz hum), such as fluorescent lighting and electric power lines

phone. Unfortunately, due to the miniaturization of hearing aids, many hearing aids are not equipped with telecoils or are equipped with telecoils that produce inappropriate amounts of amplification. Often amplified telecoils must be ordered to provide significant improvements in communication via the telephone. Certainly, whenever telecoil technology is implemented into a hearing aid it is imperative that the patient is instructed properly concerning its use and placement with the telephone. Most audiologists have had the experience of an individual with a hearing aid attempting (with no success) to place the telephone receiver over his or her ear instead of near the telecoil. Moreover, patients should be warned that hearing aid telecoil technology may not be particularly beneficial within environments where electromagnetic interference (computers, fluorescent lights) may be high.

Rehabilitative Technologies and Telephone Use

A number of individual rehabilitative technologies can also be used with the telephone to improve communication for the individual with hearing loss. One device, for example, consists of a disk-shaped microphone that attaches to the telephone handset. The signal is then routed into the listener's personal hearing aid via DAI. Often, the use of an individual personal rehabilitative technology, particularly DAI, can be beneficial in environments where electromagnetic interference is high.

Acoustic Couplers

Acoustic couplers are foam or plastic cushions that fit on the receiver of the telephone handset. Such cushions come in both square or round shapes to fit ear- and mouthpieces. In addition to providing comfort, these cushions allow the hearing aid user to acoustically utilize the telephone with reduced feedback, particularly when the telephone is equipped with amplification. Acoustic telepads may be particularly useful for those individuals with hearing aids that are too small to adequately incorporate telecoil circuitry.

Telephone Amplifiers

There are several types of amplifiers for telephones (see Table 20–10, Figures 20–8 and 20–9). Each of these amplifiers can be used with or without a hearing aid. If used with a hearing aid, such amplification systems may be used through acoustic coupling (through the microphone of the hearing aid) or inductive coupling (through the telecoil of the hearing aid).

Amplified telephones often provide adjustable gain characteristics, tone controls, and an enhanced dynamic range. Amplified telephones

Table 20–10. Various types of amplifiers for telephones.

- Amplified telephones
- Amplified telephone handsets
- In-line amplifiers
- Portable telephone amplifiers
- Acoustic-induction loop amplifiers

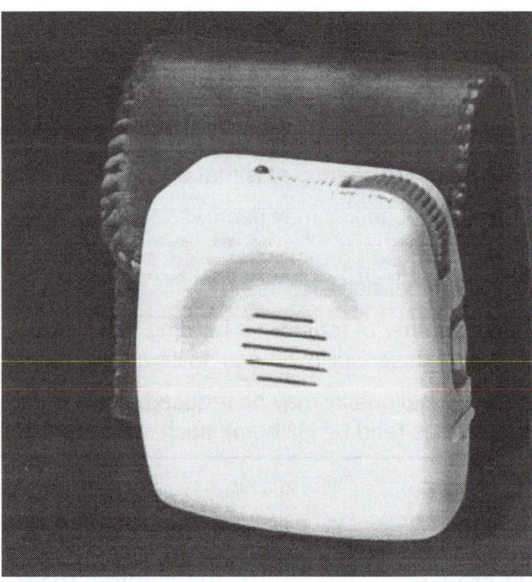

Figure 20–8. An example of a portable telephone amplifier. (Photo courtesy of Ameriphone.)

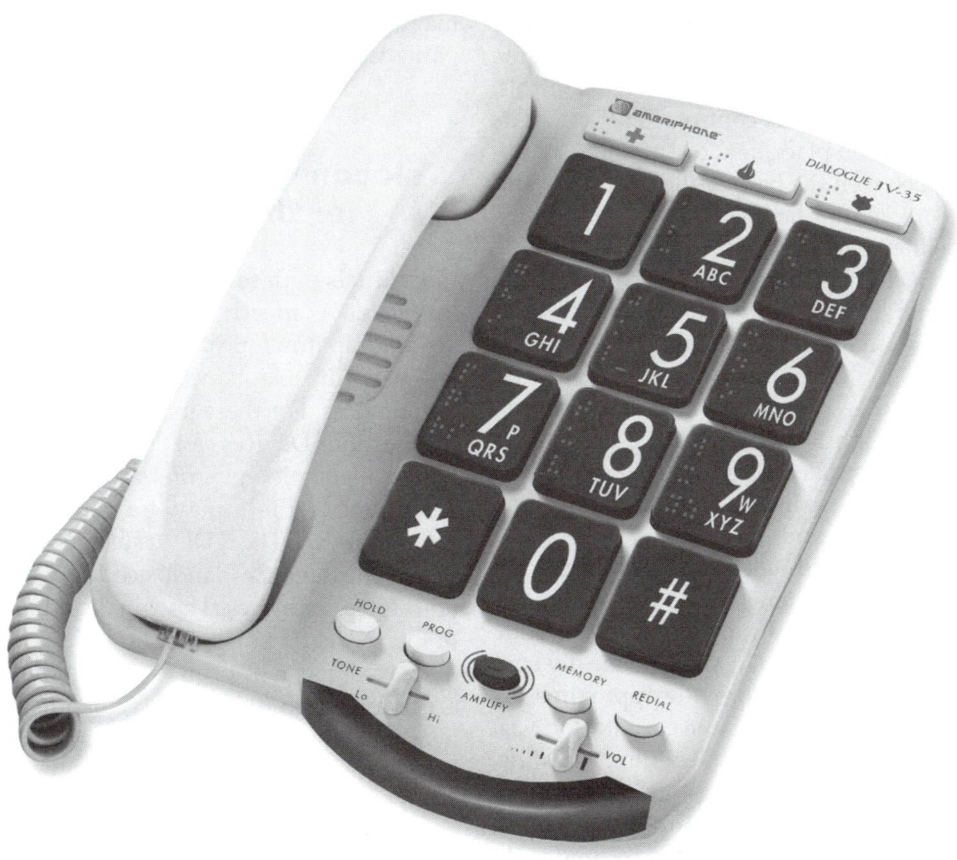

Figure 20–9. Amplified telephone with adjustable volume and tone controls. (Photo courtesy of Ameriphone.)

may also contain low-frequency, high-intensity ringers. Unfortunately, many of the more inexpensive, electronic-based telephones may not provide enough amplification to assist listeners who have more than a mild degree of hearing loss. In addition to amplified telephones, speaker telephones, with adjustable gain characteristics, may also be used by some individuals with hearing loss.

Another form of telephone amplification is amplified replacement handsets. Amplified handsets are generally available with volume control capabilities. In addition, several companies are now dispensing amplified handsets with mute switches, tone controls, and noise cancellation circuitry. Replacement handsets can be attached to most traditional modular telephones. Replacement handsets may not be compatible with many of the newer, more inexpensive, electronic telephone systems. To overcome this problem, amplified replacement handsets may be purchased with their own power supply. It should be noted that when placing a replacement handset on a telephone the impedance characteristics of the replacement handset and telephone must be matched. Otherwise, the gain may not be maximized and the signal distorted. If such handsets are coupled to a hearing aid, it is imperative that the handset is hearing-aid compatible. The Americans with Disabilities Act (ADA, 1990; PL 101-336) requires that all commercially used pay telephones have handsets with adjustable gain controls.

In-line telephone amplifiers are available only with modular telephones. In-line amplifiers come with variable gain controls, frequency response controls, or both. The most common placement of an in-line amplifier is between the base of the telephone and the cord of the handset. In-line amplifiers can either be externally or internally powered. Such amplifiers can also be used with personal rehabilitative technologies. For example, an in-line amplifier can be connected from the telephone base into a FM system. In this case, the individual would receive a high SNR through the FM system and would speak through the handset of the telephone. Most in-line amplifiers are relatively compact and portable.

Portable 20-dB telephone amplifiers, or "strap-on" amplifiers, can be coupled to the telephone acoustically, magnetically, or both. Portable amplifiers that are acoustically coupled to the telephone provide approximately 20 dB of gain and can be used with the vast majority of telephones (cellular, trimline, cordless, and pay phones) on the market today. Portable telephone amplifiers can also be coupled magnetically to the telephone. In this case, the user must switch the hearing aid to the telecoil setting. Magnetic coupling strategies, however, can only be used with hearing-aid-compatible telephones. As of 1991, all telephones manufactured or imported for use in the U.S. were required to be hearing-aid compatible (Public Law 394, The Hearing Aid Compatibility Act, 1988). PL 394 excludes telephones used for the transmission of classified information, public mobile services, private radio services, and residential use if the phone was purchased prior to 1991. Recently, several companies have marketed portable telephone amplifiers that can be coupled either magnetically or acoustically to the telephone. Moreover, there are several acoustic-to-magnetic telephone adapters on the market today. With acoustic-to-magnetic amplifiers, the acoustic signal is received via the telephone handset, amplified, and transduced into an electromagnetic signal. The electromagnetic signal is then picked up via the patients' telecoil.

Telecommunication Devices for the Deaf (TDD)

Individuals with severe to profound hearing losses, poor speech recognition, or severe speech impairments may not be able to effectively use the telephone even with amplification devices. For these individuals, Telecommunication Devices for the Deaf (TDDs) (also called teletypewriters [TTYs] or Text Telephones [TTs]) may be required (see Figure 20–10). The TDD transmits a typed, visual message (in Baudot code) over standard telephone lines. The typed communication appears on either a light-emitting diode display, or it can be printed out. Braille TDDs are available to those with visual as well as hearing difficulties. For a TDD conversation to take place, both the sender and receiver must have TDD instrumentation that is compatible with each other. A TDD system can also be modified to communicate to a computer. To allow this type of communication, an interface option is required to process the slower transmission rate of the Baudot code of the TDD to the faster transmission speed (American Standard Code for Information Interchange — ASCII) of the computer. The ADA mandates that all emergency access services have TDD assessibility.

Telephone relay services (TRS) are available to the TDD user who needs to communicate with a non-TDD user. With the TRS, the individual using the TDD types a message to a state-designated telephone number that is picked up by a normal-hearing operator and transmitted verbally to the non-TDD user. The non-TDD user can then respond to the TDD user by verbally giving the message to the relay operator, who in turn, relays the message via written text to the TDD user. With TRSs, individuals with normal hearing can also telephone persons who use TDDs.

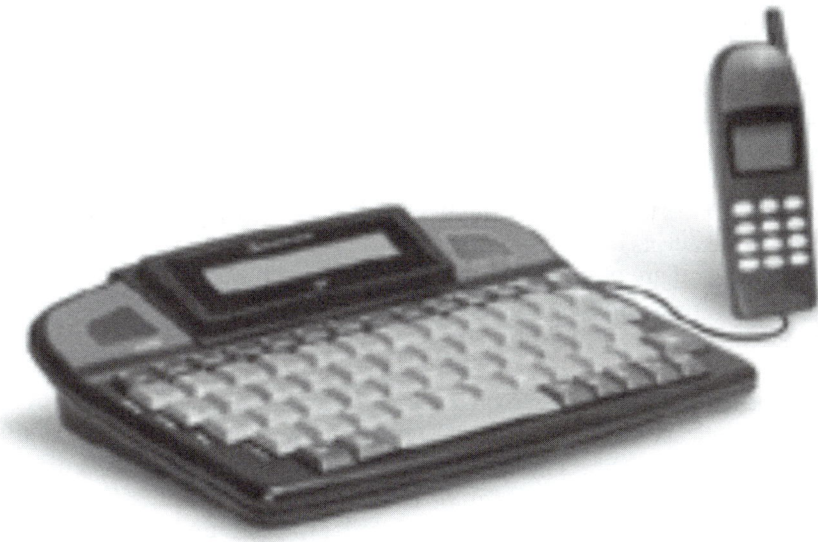

Figure 20–10. A portable Telecommunication Device for the Deaf (TDD). (Photo courtesy of Ameriphone.)

As of 1993, the ADA mandated that all telephone companies provide within- and across-state telephone relay services.

Communication via Computers

In addition to computer-based TDD systems, several teletext computer programs have also become available over the past several years. These personal computer (PC) programs allow the user to communicate to TDD units, computers, or touch-tone telephones via typewritten messages or synthesized voice. In addition, real-time E-mail, "chat room," and video-conferencing technologies offer communicative access for individuals with hearing or speech deficits.

Communication via Facsimile Transmission

An additional form of technology that may communicatively aid the individual with hearing or speech difficulties is facsimile (or fax) machines. With the fax machine, a hard copy message is transmitted over telecommunication lines to another fax machine.

Communication via Video Telephones

Several companies now market video-conferencing technology through either a computer or television. With such systems, a camera-based system is placed on the computer or television. Both audio and video of the person being called are then presented through a standard television or monitor. Systems are now being developed that provide for full-motion video support for sign language. Keyboard-produced text and TDD capabilities are also available options.

IMPROVING RECEPTION OF BROADCAST MEDIA WITH REHABILITATIVE TECHNOLOGIES

Another communicative concern commonly reported by individuals with hearing loss is difficulty hearing and understanding the auditory signal that is broadcast over the television or radio. As was outlined in the first section of the chapter, distance from the sound source, noise, and reverberation can produce a distorted or inaudible signal to the hearing impaired individual. Hearing aids alone often do little to reduce the effects of such environmental disturbances and are often not a solution to improving the recognition (and enjoyment) of broadcast media. Rehabilitative devices such as hard-wired systems, induction loop, FM, and infrared systems can all be used to link the broadcast media to the individual with hearing loss, thus effectively improving the quality of the audio signal received. There are also television-band radios that can be tuned to the channel being watched and placed close to the individual so that the volume can be increased and the effects of distance from the signal reduced. Personal sound-field FM systems are new devices that may be useful as well. The transmitting microphone is placed close to the television or radio speaker, and the receiving speaker amplifier is placed close to the listener. The increased volume and reduction of the effects of room acoustics often significantly improve sound reception.

Closed Captioning

Television viewing can also be enhanced with a running-text subtitle of the audio program in the lower portion of the screen. This running-text subtitling of the broadcast, called closed captioning, is encoded in the television signal and must be decoded to appear on the screen. As a result of the Television Decoder Circuitry Act of 1990 (PL 101-431), all television sets of more than 13 inches must be equipped with a decoder chip so that individuals can have access to closed captioning when available. Most closed captioning is done "off line" and added to the recorded television program before broadcast. Real-time captioning has become available for live broadcasts, such as the news, sporting events, and even meetings. A trained captioner follows the audio signal, and with a delay of 2 to 3 seconds converts it to text that appears on the television screen. Recently voice-to-text technology has become refined enough to use as a real-time captioning device. Using sophisticated voice identification technology, these devices hold promise of directly converting the speech signal into text that can be read by the individual with SNHL.

Two new captioning technologies promise to significantly improve access for people who are deaf or hearing impaired. Discrete personal captioning uses state of the art electronic, optical, and voice recognition technologies to provide text in a "heads-up" display (similar to that found in fighter aircraft) that is built into a pair of glasses. A text readout seems to "float in the air" about 18 inches in front of the wearer. The second technology, called reflective captioning, uses a small handheld LED screen that follows the auditory signal by flashing captions of the signal on the screen. Both technologies are designed to provide equal access to public places by providing an inconspicuous and efficient translation and text display of ongoing auditory signals.

ALERTING SYSTEMS

Alerting devices help alert the individual with SNHL through visual, auditory, olfactory, or vibrotactile outputs (see Table 20–11). Alerting devices can be: (1) hard-wired or wireless and (2) attached to detect one or multiple environmental signals in the home, car, or office. Generally, alerting systems are considered to be beneficial only for individuals with profound degrees of hearing loss. Many alerting devices can also be helpful for individuals with milder degrees of SNHL, however. Persons with high frequency hearing loss, for example, may have difficulties hearing the microwave timer, the doorbell, knocking on the door, or the telephone ringer.

There are three ways that environmental signals can be detected via alerting technology: (1) direct electrical connection; (2) sound

Table 20–11. Sensory modalities used for alerting devices.

Visual
■ Turning on/off lamp
■ Strobe light
■ Bright incandescent light
Auditory
■ Amplified signal
■ Lowered pitch signal
Olfactory
■ Pungent scents
Vibrotactile
■ Pocket pagers
■ Bed shakers
■ Increases in airstream (such as a fan)

activated; and (3) induction based (Larose, Evans, & Larose, 1989). Several examples of alerting devices are found in Figures 20–11, 20–12, and 20–13. Direct electrical connect systems are permanently interfaced with, and directly activated by, the electrical system of the sound-activating device. In this case, the alerting device is directly connected to the telephone, alarm clock, microwave timer, or doorbell. When the device is activated, a visual, auditory, olfactory, or tactile signal is presented to the individual. Direct electrical connected alerting devices, while highly reliable for alerting purposes, are not very portable. Sound-activated systems detect the presence of an environmental sound through the placement of a remote microphone system at or near that device. When the microphone detects the presence of a particular environmental sound,

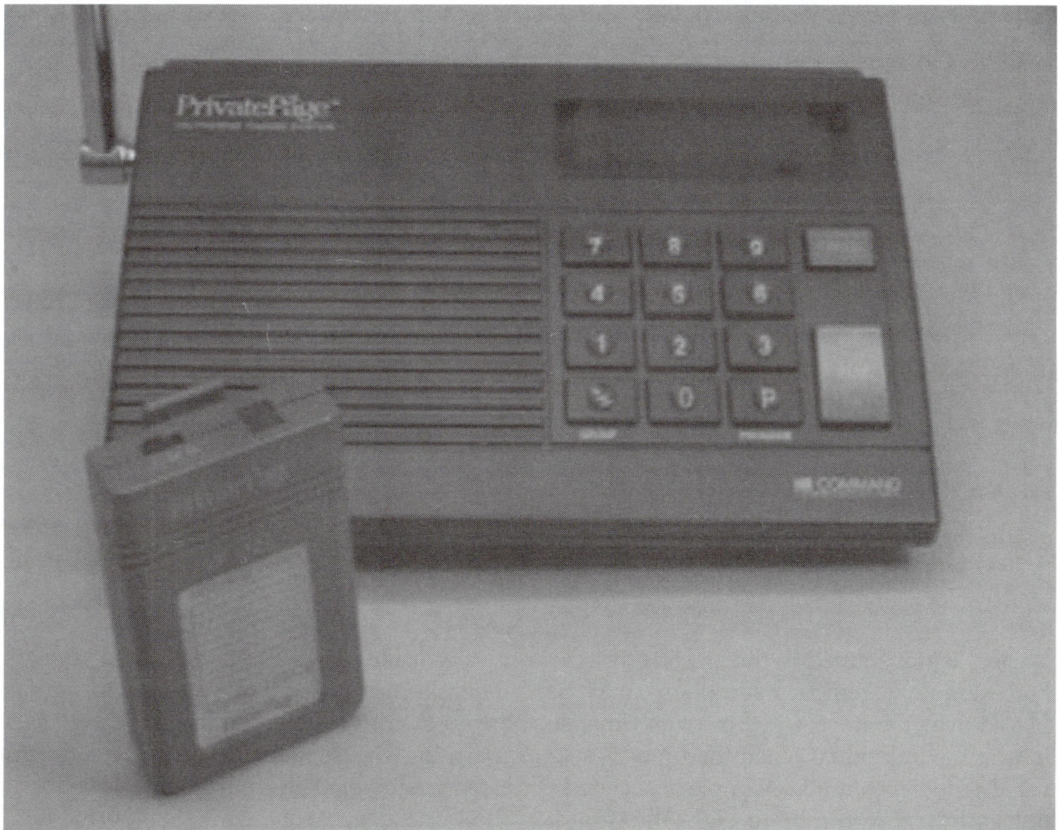

Figure 20–11. An alerting device for various sources with personal pager. (Photo courtesy of Silent Call.)

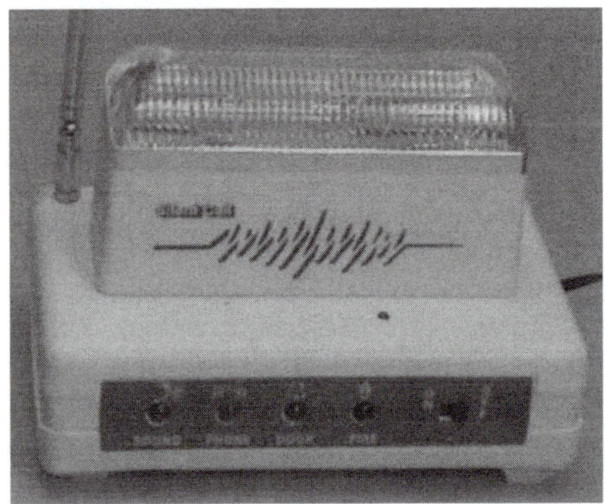

Figure 20–12. An example of an alerting device that uses flashing lights. (Photo courtesy of Silent Call.)

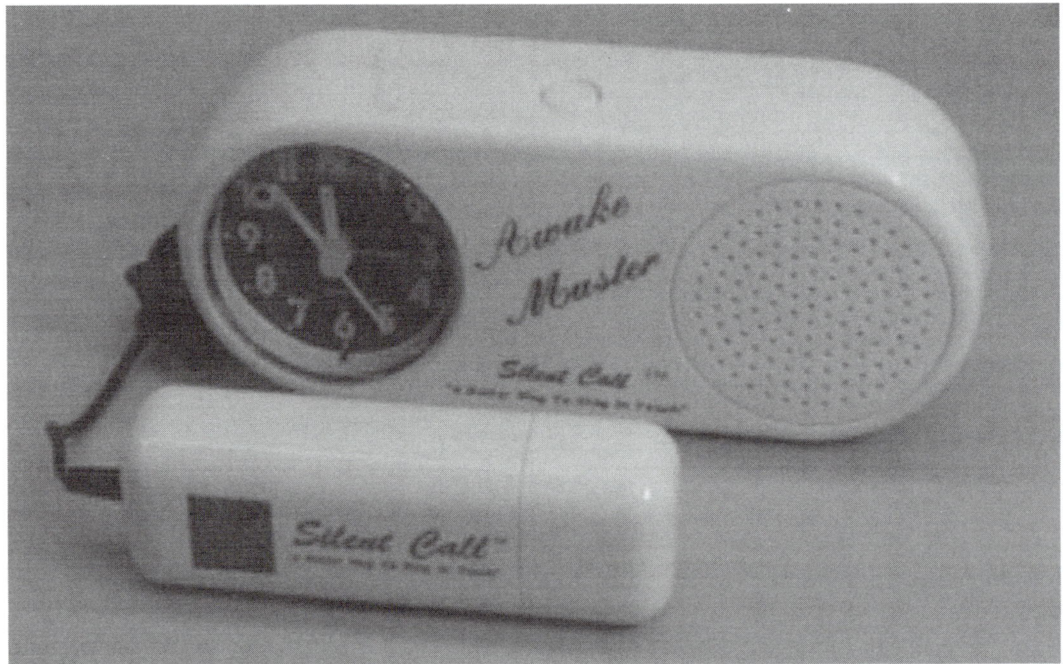

Figure 20–13. An alarm clock alerting device. (Photo courtesy of Silent Call.)

a signal is transmitted to the alerting system. For example, a remote microphone may be placed near the microwave or oven timer to inform the individual when the timer is activated. Another common example of such technology in use would be to place the sound-activated microphone near a baby crib so that the parents can be informed when the child cries or make noises. Sound-activated systems generally have sensitivity settings to reduce the possibility of other environmental sounds activating the system. Recently, sound-activated technologies have been developed that allow the user with hearing impairment to monitor important traffic noises, such as emergency vehicle sirens or car horns. Sound-activated systems are generally portable. Induction-based systems use the electromagnetic field from electrical devices to send a signal to the alerting device. With such systems a suction cup electromagnetic detection device is placed on the desired environmental sound-producing device. When the electromagnetic detection device detects activation of the system, a signal is sent to the alerting system. Although such systems are portable, signal detection may be negatively affected by incorrect placement of the suction cup.

In addition to assistive technologies, dogs can be professionally trained to get the attention of the individual with hearing impairment when particular sounds occur in the environment (door knocking, fire alarm, door bell, telephone ring, and so forth.) and lead them to the source of that sound. In most states, the legislation for hearing dogs is essentially the same as that for seeing eye dogs.

SELECTING REHABILITATIVE TECHNOLOGIES FOR INDIVIDUALS WITH HEARING LOSS AND "NORMAL HEARING"

As previously noted, rehabilitative technologies are designed to minimize the communication deficits caused by a hearing loss. The first step to determine an appropriate rehabilitative device is through a comprehensive evaluation of the audiological dimensions of the hearing loss. In addition to the usual comprehensive evaluative components of thresholds for pure tones and speech, speech recognition in quiet, and immittance measures, the evaluation should include speech-recognition measures in commonly encountered backgrounds of noise. Measures of the central auditory processing (CAP) capabilities of the subject should be conducted as research has demonstrated that some of these individuals do not receive as much benefit from personal hearing aids as persons with intact CAP abilities (Crandell, 1999).

In addition to audiological measures, measures of communication disability and needs are a crucial component of the rehabilitative process. Such forms as the Client Oriented Scale of Improvement (COSI), Hearing Handicap Inventory for the Elderly/Adult (HHIE/HHIA), Abbreviated Profile of Hearing Aid Benefit (APHAB), and the Glascow Scale of Communication function, as well as a detailed case history, have been shown to be useful in assessing such needs and disability. These scales are discussed in greater detail elsewhere in this book. On the basis of the audiological and communication assessments, the audiologist can recommend hearing aids, rehabilitative technologies, communication strategies, and therapies that will minimize the impact of the hearing loss on the client's everyday activities. Unfortunately, too often, the audiologist considers only one of the three important rehabilitative tools: the hearing aid.

Prior to concluding this section, however, it must be noted that evaluating communication needs, and consequently, appropriate rehabilitative technologies, can be a difficult task for a number of reasons (Tye-Murray, 1998). First, communication handicap varies as a function of the communication setting and communication partner. Second, hearing handicap varies with the topic of conversation. Third, handicap does not always happen during conversation; that is, a lack of miscommunication during the assessment process will provide the professional with an inaccurate assessment of the communication handicap the person has under more difficult listening circumstances. Fourth, communication handicap is a construct made up of many dimensions, thus no one assessment measure is likely to capture all of these dimensions. As a result, several assessment measures and a detailed case history should be taken on an individual and interpreted together. Finally, the technology requirements for effective communication for a particular individual will vary depending on location (home, work, travel, and so forth) and on the type of communication (face-to-face, through the media, over the telephone, or as an alerting communication).

Because of the sheer number of possible technologies that should be considered, this decision-making process can be quite complex and confusing. To assist in the selection process, Palmer, Garstecki, and Rauterkus (1990) created a computer software program, the Interactive Product Locator for Assistive Devices, that uses input about the client and the client's communication needs to select from a database of assistive technologies.

As a result of the audiological and communication assessments, recommendations will be made concerning appropriate hearing aids and rehabilitative devices. For these technologies to have a maximum influence on communication handicap, however, individuals must accept that there is a communication problem, be provided with the means to take ownership of their own communication environment, and have the confidence to believe that they have the psychosocial and behavioral tools to minimize miscommunication in everyday listening environments. Singer and Preece (1997) have suggested a three-stage model to assist patient compliance in these areas. The first stage of the model is called "precontemplative." This is the stage where the individual with hearing loss has not accepted that there are problems caused by the hearing loss. The authors suggest that helping the person become aware of the actual problems can be an effective intervention strategy. Hearing handicap scales, such as those previously mentioned, can be used to guide the individual through a discussion of situations that cause listening breakdowns in everyday communication environments. In the second stage, called "contemplation," the individual has become aware of listening problems and is considering ways to solve them. Singer and Preece suggested that the professional can help the individual at this stage by providing accurate information about available technology and rehabilitative options, as well as a realistic assessment of how effective these options might be considering the individual's everyday listening environments. The third stage is referred to as "preparation," wherein the individual with hearing loss is essentially ready to take action to solve listening problems. Having the individual commit to change by signing up for rehabilitation following the fitting of assistive technology often solidifies the readiness of the individual to change. In the fourth or "action" stage, the individual makes tentative decision for change. Singer and Preece suggested that the emphasis should be on the tentative, in that without positive reinforcement for the decisions relating to change (such as the purchase of assistive technology), an individual can revert to an earlier stage in the process that can significantly delay change. The individual might return the assistive technology, for example. In the fifth or "maintenance" stage, the individual truly makes a change, and the benefits to the individual become manifest. During this stage the individual requires support in the use of technology and specific rehabilitative strategy training. In the "termination" stage, the individual has fully accepted the hearing aid and assistive technology, which becomes integrated into his or her everyday listening environment.

In a similar model, Tye-Murray (1998) conceptualized essentially the same process in what she calls communication strategies training. Communication strategies training is composed of three stages. In the formal instruction stage, the client is provided with information about various types of communication strategies and appropriate listening and speaking behaviors. Included here are presentations that describe facilitative and receptive repair strategies and expressive repair strategies; also included are instructions in "clear speech," specific interventions to avoid a miscommunication, and information about how to recover from a miscommunication should one occur. The second stage is called guided learning, wherein the professional creates simulated real-life communication situations where the strategies acquired in the formal instruction stage can be practiced. The audiologist provides feedback and correction to the client as he or she progresses through the simulations. The last stage requires the client to engage in a prescribed real-world listening situation and to answer prepared questions regarding the effective use of information learned in stage one and practiced in stage two.

MEASURING EFFICACY FOR REHABILITATIVE TECHNOLOGIES

Whenever assistive technologies (or hearing aids) are recommended, it is imperative that efficacy be measured. Efficacy is a measure to demonstrate that an intervention was effective or ineffective and that a different intervention may be more appropriate. A number of procedures can be used to quantify the effectiveness of rehabilitative technology on a particular individual (Tye-Murray, 1998). One way of measuring efficacy is through the interview procedure. In this procedure, specific information about the effectiveness of rehabilitative technologies is elicited through the use of informal or formalized questions. One of the problems with the interview procedure, however, is that the patient's responses are hard to quantify. To circumvent these difficulties, forms such as the COSI could be utilized in the interview process. The COSI requires the interviewee to rank in order five handicaps that they perceive are a result of their hearing loss. This initial quantification of the person's problems before intervention can then be used as a measure of whether intervention was effective. A second procedure to measure efficacy is through the questionnaire. As noted above, many hearing-handicap questionnaires have been developed and can be quite useful if the questions match the situation of the individual with hearing loss. If the match is not good, the questionnaire may not provide enough relevant information about communication needs to be useful in the rehabilitative process. A well-matched hearing-handicap scale can provide important information concerning the effectiveness of intervention. If after the intervention there is less hearing handicap, the intervention might be considered effective. One such questionnaire, the Hearing Function Profile (Singer & Preece, 1997) has been developed to determine why an individual is unsuccessful with assistive technology and provides a basis for recommending additional technologies or rehabilitation training. A third procedure to evaluate efficacy is a daily log or diary, wherein the individual with hearing impairment provides qualitative information about communication difficulties with use of the rehabilitative technology over time. These logs provide an ongoing self-report analysis of changes that occur as a result of intervention and can be used to assess the effectiveness of an intervention. Logs can be reactive, however, in that the act of completing the log can affect communication handicap. This is not necessarily bad but lessens the usefulness of the log procedure to gauge the effectiveness of a specific intervention. Group discussion is another possible measure of efficacy. The interactions that occur during a group discussion of persons having hearing loss often forces each individual discussant to introspect and reflect upon their communication problems and rehabilitative technology utilization. Over time, these group interactions can provide important information (and psychosocial support) about technology use. The fifth procedure for measuring efficacy is referred to as structured communication interactions, wherein conversations between the person with hearing loss and the evaluator are simulated to reflect communication situations that are typical for the person. Situations are identified that produce communication handicap under more or less realistic situations. The effectiveness of intervention can be directly assessed by simulating difficult communication situations with and without the assistive technology in use.

INCREASING CONSUMER UTILIZATION OF ASSISTIVE TECHNOLOGIES

Unfortunately, although this chapter has addressed many advantages of having listeners with hearing loss utilize assistive technologies, research suggests that patients are often unaware of assistive technology and that relatively few audiologists are actively dispensing such technologies. It appears that individuals with hearing impairment are unaware of assistive technology due to two factors (Mahon, 1985). First, audiologists have been relatively indifferent to incorporating assistive technologies into their available product line; second, audiologists often have not had an adequate knowledge base to accurately inform their patients about such technologies. McCarthy, Culpepper, and Winstead (1983), for example, showed that a majority of 50 individuals with hearing loss were not familiar with assistive technologies despite the fact that they reported difficulties in most listening situations. Many of the subjects were interested in purchasing assistive technologies when informed about them. Certainly, such data emphasize the need for greater training about assistive technologies for both audiologists and individuals with hearing loss.

It seems reasonable to speculate that, for consumers to accept assistive technologies, audiologists must be convinced first of the value of assistive technologies in the overall rehabilitative plan for an individual. Unfortunately, in audiology training programs, great emphasis has been placed on the proper fitting of hearing aids, but minimal attention has been given to the assistive technology and other rehabilitative needs of the person with hearing impairment (Crandell & Smaldino, 1999a, 1999b). Thus, it appears that the first step in creating consumer acceptance of these technologies is the development of a philosophy of rehabilitation that includes multidimensional assessment of the individuals's auditory and communication capabilities and needs. Within the context of a comprehensive rehabilitative plan the value of assistive technologies will be self-evident because these technologies are not "add ons" but are an integral part of the services provided in the rehabilitative plan for an individual, along with hearing aids and communication strategies training. Ross (1994) eloquently discussed assistive technologies as necessities rather than as a luxury in the rehabilitation process.

In addition to a carefully constructed rehabilitation program, there is a need to engage in activities to enhance consumer acceptance of assistive technology. The same negative stigmas that are attached to hearing loss and hearing aids are attached to assistive devices and even to a greater extent because assistive technologies are typically more noticeable and intimidating than a hearing aid. Sutherland (1995) detailed the following strategies that hearing health care professionals can employ to increase consumer acceptance of assistive technologies: (1) educating consumers about assistive devices including strengths and limitations, (2) training consumers to use technical devices, (3) helping consumers make informed choices, (4) providing consumers with support, (5) encouraging more experienced consumers to help those who are learning about technical devices, (6) empowering consumers by working closely with them as part of a team or partnership, and (7) aligning with consumers to advocate for better laws and services, and for universal accessibility for people with hearing loss.

LEGISLATION FOR ASSISTIVE TECHNOLOGY

There are a number of federal laws that provide for the utilization of assistive technology. Several of these laws have been previously discussed and will not be recapitulated in this section. Beginning in 1975, with the Education of Handicapped Children Act, proceeding through 1997 with amendments to the Individuals with Disabilities Education Act and the Americans with Disabilities Act, and most recently with the amendments to the Individuals with Disabilities Education Act of 1997, there has been a sustained interest in removing barriers for persons with hearing loss and other disabilities. One of the ways that acoustic barriers to communication can be diminished is through the use of assistive listening technology, and these technologies are included as a reasonable accommodation that is required under all of these laws

(Access Board Web site, 1998; Individuals with Disability Education Act Web site, 1998; Individuals with Disabilities Education Act (IDEA) Web site, 1999).

ILLUSTRATIVE CASE STUDIES

The following three cases serve as illustrative examples of the kind of patients that the authors have assisted through the use of rehabilitative technologies. Patients were seen either at the University of Florida Speech and Hearing Clinic or the University of Northern Iowa Audiology Clinic.

Case 1

Case History: Jamie is a college-aged student who was seen in the clinic because of difficulty she was having understanding the professors in class and because she was unable to follow class discussions among other students, especially in large lecture halls. Although she wore hearing aids, she was frustrated because she had been able to get along in high school but now was experiencing great difficulty. The listening difficulties were leaving her fatigued at the end of the day with no energy to properly study or complete assignments. She was thinking of withdrawing from school.

Audiological Assessment: Jamie had moderate SNHL in both ears. Her hearing aids were properly fit and matched NAL targets for the type of aid. Although her aided speech identification was good in quiet, she experienced a loss in ability to hear in noise.

Hearing Aid Assessment: The original dispenser had chosen an ITE model with no telecoil or direct audio input (DAI) options.

Intervention: Although the hearing aids were only 2 years old, they did not have options that would have solved Jamie's main listening problem. New hearing aids were fit incorporating an FM receiver into the hearing aid (assistance for the new aids was obtained through a local vocational rehabilitation office). The use of the transmitting FM microphone nearly eliminated Jamie's trouble hearing in class. In tandem with the new hearing aids, Jamie received communication strategies training to help her cope more successfully in situations where even the new aids are not completely adequate for her listening needs.

Case 2

Case History: Frank is a 42-year-old male with a long history (since childhood) of severe-profound SNHL. The hearing loss was of uncertain etiology, but Frank exhibited a positive family history of hearing loss, thus hereditary hearing loss was suspected. He was seen in the clinic because he noted a change in his hearing. He also noted that he was having increased difficulty in his home environment. Specifically, he complained of not always hearing the telephone, the door bell, the microwave timer, or alarm clock. Frank had been fit with hearing aids at several other clinics but always reported that they offered limited to no benefit. He had returned the hearing aids to the dispenser in each case.

Audiological Assessment: A complete audiological evaluation indicated a bilateral profound SNHL. These results suggested an approximate 10 to 20 dB change in his pure-tone sensitivity over the previous two years. Due to the extent of his hearing loss, speech recognition measures could not be conducted. Speechreading tests indicated that Frank was an excellent speech reader. He was also had extensive sign language abilities. Frank normally uses a TDD at home and at work.

Intervention: Frank was counseled regarding his change in hearing. In addition, the following recommendations were made. First, it was recommended that Frank use alerting devices in his apartment. Specifically, sound activated and electrically activated alerting devices were placed for the following: (1) door knocking, (2) door bell, (3) microwave/oven timer, and (4) telephone ringer. The alerting devices were hooked up to several lamps, which turned on/off in response to a signal and were located in different rooms, and to a personal paging device that vibrated in response to a signal. His alarm clock was hooked up to a bed and pillow vibrator. He reports that these devices help immensely. Second, Frank was recommended for additional auditory rehabilitation at the university and trial utilization of new hearing aids and an FM system. To date, he has not followed up on the hearing aid trial recommendation.

Case 3

Case History: Tommy is an 8-year-old who has a long history of recurrent otitis media. His parents are concerned because he does not pay attention at home, and his teacher believes he is functioning below his capacity. The teacher is also concerned that he has an attention deficit and a developing behavioral problem because he is disruptive in class. While the teacher is aware of his fluctuating hearing loss and has tried preferential seating in the front of the classroom, this has not diminished the problem.

Audiological Assessment: Tommy has had many hearing tests and they often showed a mild conductive hearing loss due to either negative middle-ear pressure, fluid in the middle ear, or both. His medical doctor has treated him with antibiotics and antihistamines when the fluid was present. He never received PE tubes. While his hearing shows a mild conductive loss, there is also a mild sensorineural loss in the higher frequencies. The Listening Inventories for Education (LIFE) (Anderson & Smaldino, 1998) were completed by the teacher, the parents, and Tommy confirming that listening and attention were problems. The Auditory Continuous Performance Test (ACPT) (Keith, 1994) also showed an inability to attend to auditory stimuli.

Intervention: While Tommy's teacher tried preferential seating, it was not successful because the teacher moved around the room during instruction. It was thought that Tommy was exhibiting the "learned" inattentiveness, which often accompanies fluctuating hearing loss with the concomitant inconsistent auditory signal. To provide a consistent signal and to help him focus on important instructional speech, an FM sound-field system was installed in the classroom. The system was designed to enhance the teacher's voice signal about 10 dB consistently throughout the classroom. In addition, Tommy received some listening training to help him "unlearn" the inattentiveness to sound. Almost immediately, the teacher noticed that Tommy was "on task" during classroom instruction and was less of a behavioral problem. A post-test LIFE was administered after a month of classroom amplification and showed improvement in all of the initial areas of concern.

SUMMARY

The deleterious influences of distance, background noise, and reverberation, particularly for listeners with SNHL, are well documented. Unfortunately, hearing aids often offer limited speech-recognition benefit in adverse listening environments. Conversely, many assistive listening technologies such as infrared assistive listening systems, personal FM amplification devices, induction loop, and FM sound- field amplification have been shown to significantly augment speech communication in poor listening environments. Such technologies have also been shown to improve communication of broadcast media and telecommunications. For assistive technology to be accepted and used by an individual with hearing loss, however, the communication needs and proper selection of assistive devices must be conducted within the context of an overall rehabilitative plan. Assistive technology offers the hearing health care professional a challenge, but it also offers an opportunity to maximize communicative abilities for listeners with hearing impairment.

REVIEW QUESTIONS

1. Classroom acoustics are typically characterized in terms of:
a. Standing waves
b. Signal-to-noise ratio
c. Harmonic distortion
d. Transient distortion

2. Assistive listening devices can be grouped as:
a. FM
b. Alerting
c. Inductance loop
d. a, b, and c

3. Assistive listening devices:
a. Should be considered separately from a hearing aid.
b. Should be considered as part of the overall rehabilitation plan
c. Should never be considered with a hearing aid
d. Should be considered after acceptance of a hearing aid.

4. The three stages in communication strategies training are ________, ________ and ________.

5. Closed caption decoders are mandatory on all television sets with screens larger than 13 inches.
a. True
b. False

6. The advantage(s) of the 3D induction loop system as compared to the traditional induction loop system is/are:
a. Easier for the listener to use
b. Spillover is significantly reduced.
c. The signal tends to be more uniform
d. Both b and c
e. All of the above

7. Speech-recognition ability is not significantly reduced in normal-hearing adults until the SNR is reduced to:
a. +5 dB
b. +3 dB
c. 0 dB
d. −2 dB

8. Many electronic-based amplified telephones are advantageous because they are inexpensive and can be used with all degrees of hearing loss.
a. True
b. False

9. When selecting rehabilitative technologies for a particular client, measures of central auditory processing should also be tested.
a. True
b. False

10. According to Singer and Preece's three-stage model of acceptance, "contemplation" is the stage where the individual has not accepted that there are problems caused by the hearing loss.
a. True
b. False

REFERENCES

Access Board Web Site. (1998). http:www.access-board.gov

Americans with Disabilities Act (Public Law 101–336–1990). Web site: http://www.usdoj.gov/crt/ada/adahom1.htm.

American Speech, Language, and Hearing Association. (1995). Guidelines for acoustics in educational environments. *American Speech and Hearing Association, 37*(Suppl. 14), 15–19.

Anderson, K., & Smaldino, J. (1998). *Listening inventories for education*. Tampa, FL: Educational Audiology Association.

Berg, F. (1993). *Acoustics and sound systems in schools*. Boston, MA: College-Hill Press.

Bess, F. (1985). The minimally hearing-impaired child. *Ear and Hearing, 6*, 43–47.

Bess, F., & Tharpe, A. (1986). An introduction to unilateral sensorineural hearing loss in children. *Ear and Hearing, 7*, 3–13.

Bolt, R., & MacDonald, A. (1949). Theory of speech masking by reverberation. *Journal of the Acoustical Society of America, 21*, 577–580.

Boney, S., & Bess, F. (1984, November). *Noise and reverberation effects in minimal bilateral sensorineural hearing loss*. Paper presented at the American

Speech-Language-Hearing Association Convention, San Francisco, CA.

Boothroyd, A. (1991). Speech perception measures and their role in the evaluation of hearing aid performance in a pediatric population. In J. Feigin & P. Stelmachowicz (Eds.), *Pediatric amplification* (pp. 77–91). Omaha, NE: Boys Town National Research Hospital.

Cooper, J., & Cutts, B. (1971). Speech discrimination in noise. *Journal of Speech and Hearing Research, 14,* 332–337.

Crandell, C. (1991a). Individual differences in speech-recognition ability: Implications for hearing aid selection. *Ear and Hearing, 12,* 100–108.

Crandell, C. (1991b). Classroom acoustics for normal-hearing children: Implications for rehabilitation. *Educational Audiology Monographs, 2,* 18–38.

Crandell, C. (1992a). Classroom acoustics for hearing-impaired children. *Journal of the Acoustical Society of America, 92,* 2470.

Crandell, C. (1992b). Speech recognition in the elderly listener: the importance of the acoustical environment. *Texas Journal of Audiology and Speech Pathology, 17,* 25–30.

Crandell, C. (1993). Noise effects on the speech recognition of children with minimal hearing loss. *Ear and Hearing, 7,* 210–217.

Crandell, C. (1998). Hearing aids: Their effects on functional health status. *Hearing Journal, 51,* 22–30.

Crandell, C., & Bess, F. (1986). Speech recognition of children in a "typical" classroom setting. *Asha,* 29, 87.

Crandell, C., Henoch, M., & Dunkerson, K. (1992). A review of speech perception and aging: Some implications for aural rehabilitation. *Journal of the Academy for Rehabilitation Audiology, 24,* 121–132.

Crandell, C., & Smaldino, J. (1992). Sound-field amplification in the classroom. *American Journal of Audiology, 1,* 16–18.

Crandell, C., & Smaldino, J. (1994). The importance of room acoustics. In R. Tyler & D. Schum (Eds.), *Assistive listening devices for the hearing impaired* (pp. 142–164). Baltimore, MD: William and Wilkins.

Crandell C., & Smaldino, J. (1995). An update of classroom acoustics for children with hearing impairment. *Volta Review, 1,* 4–12.

Crandell C., & Smaldino, J. (1996a). The effects of noise on the speech perception of non-native English children. *American Journal of Audiology, 5,* 24–29.

Crandell C., & Smaldino, J. (1996b). Sound field amplification in the classroom: applied and theoretical issues. In F. Bess, J. Gravel, & A. Tharpe (Eds.), *Amplification for children with auditory deficits* (pp. 22–250). Nashville, TN: Bill Wilkerson Center Press.

Crandell C., & Smaldino, J. (1999a). Room acoustics and amplification. In M. Valente, R. Roeser, & H. Hosford-Dunn (Eds.), *Audiology treatment strategies.* New York: Thieme Medical Publishers.

Crandell C., & Smaldino, J. (1999b). Rehabilitative technologies for individuals with hearing loss and "normal hearing." In J. Katz (Ed.), *Handbook of audiology.* New York: Williams and Wilkins.

Crandell C., Smaldino J., & Flexer C. (1995). *Sound field FM amplification: Theory and practical applications.* San Diego, CA: Singular Publishing Group.

Crum, D. (1974). *The effects of noise, reverberation, and speaker-to-listener distance on speech understanding.* Unpublished doctoral dissertation. Northwestern University, Evanston, IL.

Dirks, D., Morgan D., & Dubno J. (1982). A procedure for quantifying the effects of noise on speech recognition. *Journal of Speech and Hearing Disorders, 47,* 114–123.

Duquesnoy, A., & Plomp R. (1983). The effect of a hearing aid on the speech-reception threshold of hearing-impaired listeners in quiet and in noise. *Journal of the Acoustical Society of America, 73,* 2166–2173.

Education of Handicapped Children. Public Law No. 94–142 Regulations. (1977, August, 23). *Federal Register, 42*(163), 42474–42518.

Education of Handicapped Act Amendments of 1986, Public Law No. 99–457 Regulations. (1986, October 8). *United States Statutes at Large, 100,* 1145–1177.

Education of Handicapped Act Amendments of 1990, Public Law No. 101–476 Regulations. (1990, October 30). *United States Statutes at Large, 104,* 1103–1151.

Festen, J., & Plomp, R. (1983). Relations between auditory functions in impaired hearing. *Journal of the Acoustical Society of America, 73,* 652–661.

Finitzo-Hieber, T. (1988). Classroom acoustics. In R. Roeser (Ed.), *Auditory disorders in school children* (2nd ed., pp. 221–233). New York: Thieme-Stratton

Finitzo-Hieber T., & Tillman, T. (1978). Room acoustics effects on monosyllabic word discrimination ability for normal and hearing-impaired children. *Journal of Speech and Hearing Research, 21,* 440–458.

Flexer, C. (1992). Classroom public address systems. In M. Ross (Ed.), *FM auditory training systems: Characteristics, selection & use* (pp. 189–209). Timonium, MD: York Press.

French, N., & Steinberg, J. (1947). Factors governing the intelligibility of speech sounds. *Journal of the Acoustical Society of America, 19,* 90–119.

Gelfand, S., & Silman, S. (1979). Effects of small room reverberation upon the recognition of some consonant features. *Journal of the Acoustical Society of America, 66,* 22–29.

Gengel, R. (1971). Acceptable signal-to-noise ratios for aided speech discrimination by the hearing impaired. *Journal of Audiology Research, 11,* 219–222.

Hawkins, D., & Yacullo, W. (1984). Signal-to-noise ratio advantage of binaural hearing aids and directional microphones under different levels of reverberation. *Journal of Speech and Hearing Disorders, 49,* 278–286.

Hearing Aid Compatibility Act. (1988). Web site: http://www. onclusive.com/pubpol.htm.

Hendricks, P., & Lederman, N. (1991). Development of a three-dimensional induction assistive listening system. *Hearing Instruments, 42,* 37–38.

Houtgast, T. (1981). The effect of ambient noise on speech intelligibility in classrooms. *Applied Acoustics 14,* 15–25.

Humes, L. (1991). Understanding the speech-understanding problems of the hearing impaired. *Journal of the American Academy of Audiology, 2,* 59–69.

Individuals with Disability Education Act Web site. (1998). http://www.edlaw.net/ptabcont.htm

Individuals with Disabilities Education Act (IDEA) Web site. (1999). http://www.ed.gov/offices/OSERS/IDEA/

Keith, R. (1994). *Auditory Continuous Performance Test.* San Antonio, TX: The Psychological Corporation.

Larose, G., Evans, M., & Larose, R. (1989). Alerting devices: Available options. *Seminar on Hearing, 10,* 66–77.

Leavitt, R., & Flexer, C. (1991). Speech degradation as measured by the Rapid Speech Transmission Index (RASTI). *Ear and Hearing, 12,* 115–118.

Lewis, D. (1998). Classroom amplification. In F. Bess (Ed.), *Children with hearing loss: Contemporary trends* (pp. 277–298). Nashville, TN: Vanderbilt Bill Wilkerson Center Press.

Licklider, J., & Miller, G. (1951). The perception of speech. In S. Stevens (Ed.), *Handbook of experimental psychology.* New York: John Wiley.

Lochner, J., & Burger, J. (1964). The influence of reflections in auditorium acoustics. *Journal of Sound Vibrations, 4,* 426–454.

Mahon, W. (1985). Assistive devices and systems. *Hearing Journal, 38,* 7–14.

McCarthy, P., Culpepper, N., & Winstead, T. (1983, November). *Hearing impaired consumers awareness and attitudes regarding auditory assistive devices.* Paper presented at the annual meeting of the American Speech, Language, and Hearing Association Convention, Cincinnati, OH.

Miller, G. (1974). Effects of noise on people. *Journal of the Acoustical Society of America, 56,* 724–764.

Moncur, J., & Dirks, D. (1967). Binaural and monaural speech intelligibility in reverberation. *Journal of Speech and Hearing Research, 10,* 186–195.

Moore, B. (1997). *An introduction to the psychology of hearing.* San Diego, CA: Academic Press.

Nabelek, A. (1982). Temporal distortions and noise considerations. In G. Studebaker & F. Bess (Eds.), *The Vanderbilt hearing aid report: State of the art-research needs.* Upper Darby, PA: Monographs in Contemporary Audiology.

Nabelek, A., & Nabelek, I. (1994). Room acoustics and speech perception. In J. Katz (Ed.), *Handbook of clinical audiology* (4th ed., pp. 624–637). Baltimore, MD: Williams & Wilkins.

Nabelek, A., & Pickett, J. (1974a). Monaural and binaural speech perception through hearing aids under noise and reverberation with normal and hearing-impaired listeners. *Journal of Speech and Hearing Research, 17,* 724–739.

Nabelek, A., & Pickett, J. (1974b). Reception of consonants in a classroom as affected by monaural and binaural listening, noise, reverberation, and hearing aids. *Journal of the Acoustical Society of America, 56,* 628–639.

Needleman, A., & Crandell, C. (1996a). Speech perception in noise by hearing impaired and masked normal hearing listeners. *Journal of the American Academy of Audiology, 2,* 65–72.

Needleman, A., & Crandell, C. (1996b). Simulation of Sensorineural Hearing Loss. In M. Jestadt (Ed.), *Modeling sensorineural hearing loss* (pp. 461–474). Boston, MA: Allyn and Bacon.

Neimoeller, A. (1968). Acoustical design of classrooms for the deaf. *American Annals of Deafness, 113,* 1040–1045.

Olsen, W. (1981). The effects of noise and reverberation on speech intelligibility. In F. Bess, B. Freeman, & J. Sinclair (Eds.), *Amplification in education* (pp. 151–163). Washington, DC: Alexander Graham Bell Association for the Deaf.

Olsen, W. (1988). Classroom acoustics for hearing-impaired children. In F. Bess (Ed.), *Hearing impairment in children* (pp. 266–267). Parkton, MD: York Press.

Palmer, C., Garstecki, D., & Rauterkus, M. (1990, November). *An interactive product locator for the selection of assistive devices.* Paper presented to the Annual Convention of the American Speech-Language-Hearing Association, Seattle, WA.

Plomp, R. (1978). Auditory handicap of hearing impairment and the limited benefit of hearing aids. *Journal of the Acoustical Society of America, 75,* 1253–1258.

Plomp, R. (1986). A signal-to-noise ratio model for the speech reception threshold for the hearing impaired. *Journal of Speech and Hearing Research, 29,* 146–154.

Ross, M. (1978). Classroom acoustics and speech intelligibility. In J. Katz (Ed.), *Handbook of clinical audiology* (pp. 469–478). Baltimore, MD: Williams and Wilkins.

Ross, M. (1994, July). Assistive devices: Luxury or necessity? *The Hearing Review, 13.*

Siebein, G. (1994). *Acoustics in buildings: A tutorial on architectural acoustics.* New York: Acoustical Society of America.

Siebein, G., Crandell, C., & Gold, M. (1997). Principles of classroom acoustics: Reverberation. *Educational Audiology Monographs, 5,* 32–43.

Singer, J., & Preece, J. (1997). Hearing instruments: A psychological behavioral perspective. *Hearing Review, 1,* 23–27.

Suter, A. (1985). Speech recognition in noise by individuals with mild hearing impairments. *Journal of the Acoustical Society of America, 68,* 887–900.

Sutherland, G. (1995). Increasing consumer acceptance of assistive devices. In R. S. Tyler & D. J. Schum (Eds.), *Assistive devices for persons with hearing impairment* (pp. 251–256). Needham Heights, MD: Allyn and Bacon.

Television Decoder Act (PL. 101-431). (1990). Web site: http://www.onclusive.com/pubpol.htm

Tye-Murray, N. (1998). *Foundations of aural rehabilitation.* San Diego, CA: Singular Publishing Group.

Van Tassell, D. (1993). Hearing loss, speech, and hearing aids. *Journal of Speech and Hearing Research, 36,* 228–244.

Wang, M., Reed, C., & Bilger, R. (1978). A comparison of the effects of filtering and sensorineural hearing loss on patterns of consonant confusions. *Journal of Speech and Hearing Research, 24,* 32–43.

Weinstein, B., & Amsel, L. (1986). The relationship between dementia and hearing impairment in the institutionalized elderly. *Clinical Gerontology, 4,* 3–15.

CHAPTER 21

Cochlear Implants

MARY JOE OSBERGER, PH.D.
DAWN BURTON KOCH, PH.D.

CONTENTS

A cochlear implant is a surgically implantable device that provides hearing sensation to individuals with severe-to-profound hearing loss who cannot benefit from hearing aids. By electrically stimulating the auditory nerve directly, a cochlear implant bypasses damaged or undeveloped sensory structures in the cochlea, thereby providing usable information about sound to the central auditory nervous system.

Although it has been known since the late 1700s that electrical stimulation can produce hearing sensations (see Simmons, 1966), it was not until the 1950s that the potential for true speech understanding was demonstrated. In 1957, two French surgeons placed an electrode on the auditory nerve of a deaf man during an operation for facial nerve repair (Djourno & Eyries, 1957). When current was passed through the electrode, the patient could discriminate some sounds and understand a few simple words. Based on that observation, several research groups began exploring the feasibility of an implantable electrical stimulator that could be used on a long-term basis by individuals with hearing impairment

By the 1980s, cochlear implants had become a clinical reality, providing safe and effective speech-perception benefit to adults with profound hearing impairment. Since that time, the devices have become more sophisticated, and the population that can benefit from implants has expanded to include children as well as adults with some residual hearing sensitivity. (For a history of cochlear implant development, see Beiter & Shallop, 1998; Loizou, 1998; Shannon, 1996; Wilson, 1993.)

This chapter describes the basic characteristics of cochlear implant systems, highlights some of the significant differences among the devices available in the United States, and discusses the regulatory issues associated with the distribution of cochlear implants. It then details clinical applications, including evaluation procedures, candidacy criteria, and cochlear implant outcomes in adults and children. Finally, the chapter considers some of the important issues that impact current and future uses of cochlear implant technology.

COMPONENTS OF A COCHLEAR IMPLANT

The function of a cochlear implant is to provide hearing sensation to individuals with severe-to-profound hearing impairment. Typically, people with that level of impairment have absent or malfunctioning sensory cells in the cochlea. In a normal ear, sound energy is converted to mechanical energy by the middle ear, which then is converted to mechanical fluid motion in the cochlea. Within the cochlea, the sensory cells—the inner and outer hair cells—are sensitive transducers that convert that mechanical fluid motion into electrical impulses in the auditory nerve. Cochlear implants are designed to substitute for the function of the middle ear, cochlear mechanical motion, and sensory cells, transforming sound energy into electrical energy that will initiate impulses in the auditory nerve.

Common Components

All cochlear implant systems comprise both internal and external components (Figure 21–1). The external components, which are worn on the head over or next to the ear, include (1) a microphone, which converts sound into an electrical signal; (2) a speech processor, which manipulates and converts the signal into a special code (i.e., speech processing strategy); and (3) a transmitter, which sends the coded electrical signal to the internal components. The internal components are the parts of the system that are surgically implanted under the skin behind the ear. They include (1) a receiver, which decodes the signal from the speech processors, and (2) an electrode array, which stimulates the cochlea with electrical current. The entire system is

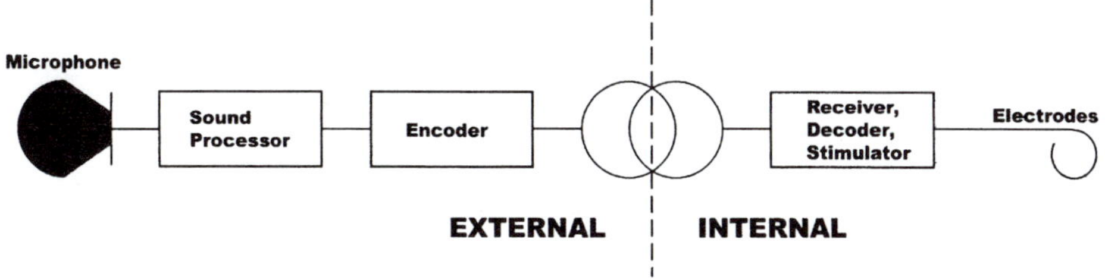

Figure 21–1. External and internal components of a cochlear implant system.

powered by batteries located in the speech processor.

Component Variables

Although all cochlear implant systems have basic features in common, they differ in how those features are implemented. Important differences exist in the transmission link, implanted electronics packaging, electrode design, stimulation waveform and temporal pattern of stimulation, speech coding strategy, and telemetry.

The following discussion compares these features for three cochlear implant systems available in the United States in 1999—the Clarion Multi-Strategy Cochlear Implant (Advanced Bionics, USA; Figure 21–2), the Nucleus CI24M Cochlear Implant (Cochlear, Australia; Figure 21–3), and the Med-El Combi 40+ System (Med-El, Austria; Figure 21–4).

Transmission Link

The transmission link is the manner by which information is sent from the external parts of the implant system to the implanted components. For all current systems, the connection is made through transcutaneous inductive coupling of radio frequency (RF) signals. In this scheme, an RF carrier signal—in which the important code is embedded—is sent across the skin to the receiver. The receiver extracts the embedded code and determines the stimulation pattern for the electrodes. Disadvantages to an RF link are (1) the amount of information that can be transmitted may be limited and (2) a significant amount of power is required.

Some earlier implant systems (e.g., Symbion/Ineraid) used a percutaneous connector that was affixed to the underlying skull and passed through the skin. The connector allowed direct communication to the electrodes, consumed little power, and required no implanted receiver. The disadvantage to this link was that the skin was perforated and susceptible to infection.

Electronics Package

Cochlear implant systems use one of two biocompatible materials to encase the implantable electronics—titanium or ceramic. The Nucleus system uses a titanium case surrounded by a silicone capsule. Titanium is a flexible and very strong metal that allows the casing to be small and thin. In this design, the receiver antenna is placed outside the titanium case.

In contrast, ceramic housings are used in the Med-El and Clarion implants. Although expensive to manufacture, ceramic is becoming increasingly the material of choice in many modern medical and electronic applications. Unlike metallic materials, a ceramic case does not interfere with signal transmission and allows the transmission of a large amount of information with low energy requirements. In addition to favorable electrical characteristics, the ceramic material used in

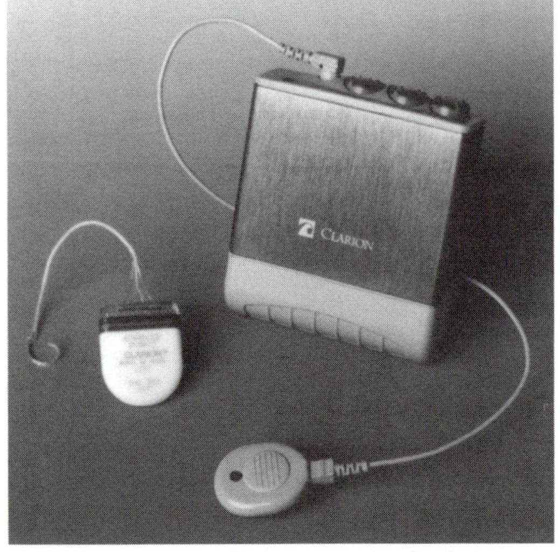

A

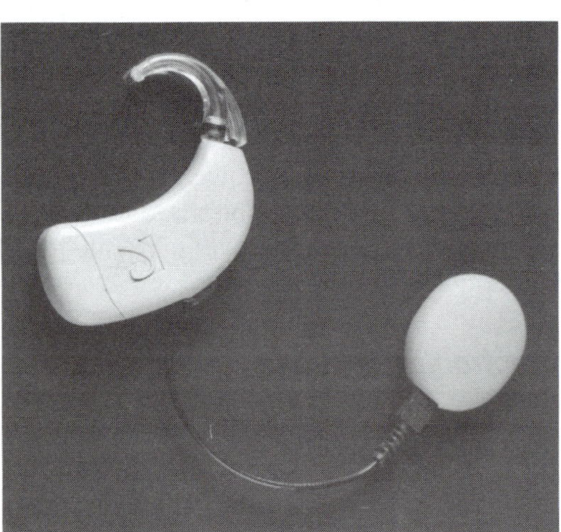

B

Figure 21–2. The CLARION Multi-Strategy Cochlear Implant System. **A.** S-series speech processor and headpiece (right), implantable receiver and electrode array (left). **B.** Behind-the-ear speech processor and headpiece. Photos courtesy of Advanced Bionics Corporation, Sylmar, CA.

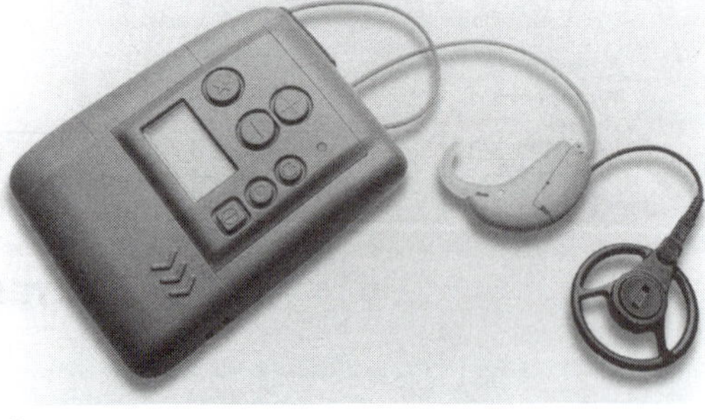

A

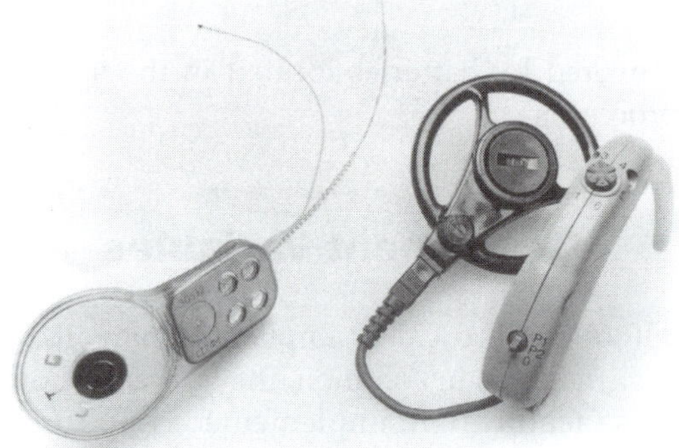

B

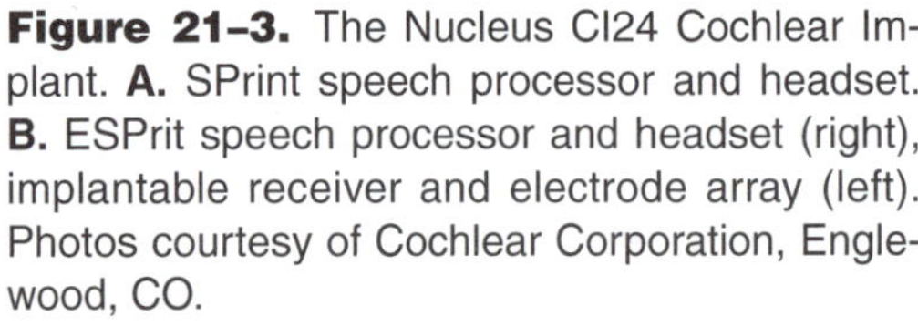

Figure 21–3. The Nucleus CI24 Cochlear Implant. **A.** SPrint speech processor and headset. **B.** ESPrit speech processor and headset (right), implantable receiver and electrode array (left). Photos courtesy of Cochlear Corporation, Englewood, CO.

implants has high mechanical strength and is similar in hardness to the surrounding bone.

Electrode Design

Typically, cochlear implant electrodes are inserted into the scala tympani of the cochlea longitudinally to take potential advantage of the place-to-frequency coding mechanism used by the normal cochlea. Information about low-frequency sound is sent to electrodes at the apical end of the array, whereas information about high-frequency sounds is sent to electrodes nearer the base of the cochlea. The ability to take advantage of the place-frequency code is limited by the number and pattern of surviving auditory neurons in an impaired ear. Unfortunately, attempts to quantify neuronal survival with electrophysiologic or radiographic procedures before implantation have been unsuccessful (Abbas, 1993; Jackler, 1988).

There are two basic types of electrode designs. The Nucleus and Med-El electrode car-

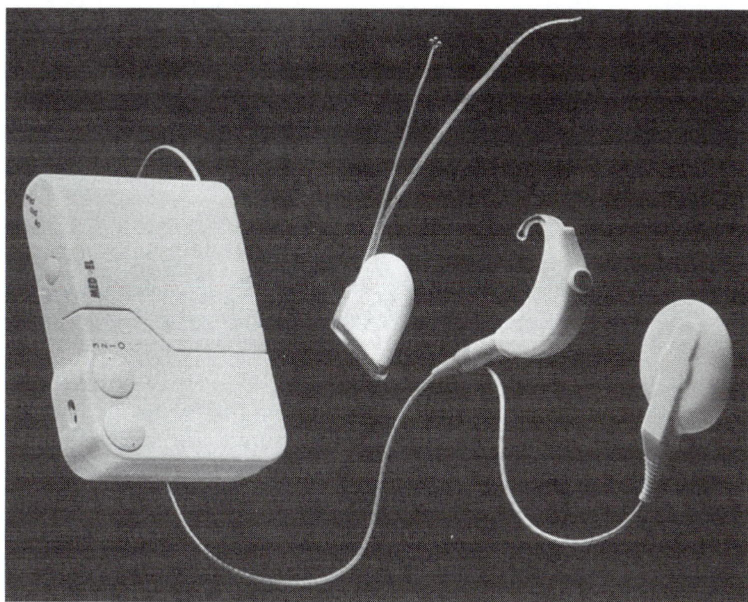

A

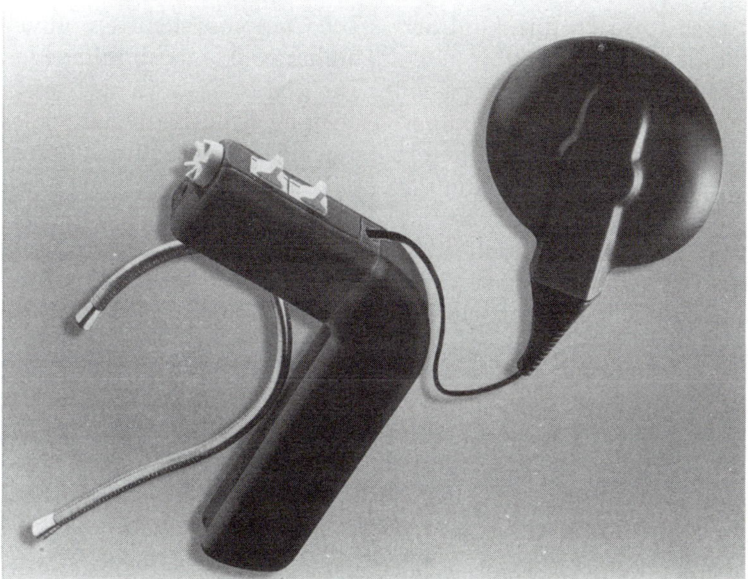

B

Figure 21–4. The COMBI 40+ Cochlear Implant. **A.** CISPRO+ speech processor and implantable components. **B.** TEMPO+ speech processor. Photos courtesy of Med-El Corporation, Research Triangle Park, NC.

riers are straight and thin to minimize occupied space within the scala tympani. The Nucleus array is 25 mm long and has 22 electrode bands arranged longitudinally. The Med-El has 12 dual electrodes (24 contacts) and is 30 mm long.

In contrast, the Clarion electrode carrier is spiral-shaped to follow the curve of the scala tympani so that the contacts will sit close to the target neurons. The precurved Clarion electrode requires a special tool for insertion so that it can be maintained in a straight position during the insertion process and then, as the electrode is released from the tool, it reassumes its spiral shape. The Clarion 25-mm electrode array consists of 16 contacts arranged in 8 medial-lateral pairs. The electrodes are ball-shaped and oriented toward the medial spiral curve of the carrier. In addition, the Clarion system uses an Electrode Positioner (EP), which facilitates consistent placement of the electrode array along the modiolus close to the spiral ganglion cells. The EP is a thin piece of silastic, with its own insertion tool, which is inserted behind the Clarion electrode. By positioning the electrode array closer to the spiral ganglion, the EP should increase spatial selectivity, reduce channel interaction, and reduce the amount of current required to reach threshold and most comfortable listening levels.

For all systems, electrical current is passed between an active electrode and an indifferent electrode. If the active and indifferent electrodes are remote, the stimulation is termed monopolar. When the active and indifferent electrodes are close to each other, the stimulation is referred to as bipolar. Bipolar stimulation focuses the current within a restricted area and presumably stimulates a small localized population of auditory nerve fibers (Merzenich & White, 1977; van den Honert & Stypulkowski, 1987). Monopolar stimulation, on the other hand, spreads current over a wider area and a larger population of neurons. Less current is required to achieve adequate loudness levels with monopolar stimulation, whereas more current is required for bipolar stimulation. The use of monopolar or bipolar stimulation is determined by the speech processing strategy and each individual's response to electrical stimulation.

The Nucleus 24, Clarion, and Med-El cochlear implants all have extracochlear electrodes so that monopolar stimulation can be implemented. The Nucleus 24 and the Clarion also can implement various bipolar stimulation modes.

Stimulation Waveform

Two types of stimulation are currently used in cochlear implants, analog and pulsatile. Analog stimulation consists of electrical current that varies continuously in time. Pulsatile stimulation consists of trains of square-wave biphasic pulses. The pattern of stimulation can be either simultaneous or nonsimultaneous (sequential). With simultaneous stimulation, more than one electrode is stimulated at the same time. With nonsimultaneous stimulation, electrodes are stimulated in a specified sequence, one at a time. Currently, analog stimulation is simultaneous, and pulsatile stimulation is sequential.

The Nucleus and Med-El implant offer only nonsimultaneous pulsatile stimulation. The Clarion system can provide both nonsimultaneous and simultaneous stimulation. The Clarion also has the capability of implementing hybrid strategies that combine analog and pulsatile stimulation and simultaneous and nonsimultaneous stimulation.

Speech Coding Strategy

Coding strategy defines the way the implant system transforms sound into electrical stimulation of the auditory nerve. In particular, coding strategies differ in the way they transform the acoustic speech signal into an electrode stimulation pattern.

A cochlear implant must analyze and encode the frequency, amplitude, and timing parameters in the acoustic speech signal. For example, in the time domain, a basic property of the speech signal is a series of peaks and valleys in the amplitude envelope. These amplitude fluctuations are heard normally as variations in loudness and are closely tied to the syllable-based rhythmic structure of speech. In the frequency domain, speech is characterized by rapidly changing amplitude peaks and valleys across the spectrum. Those fast spectral variations arise from the filter characteristics of the vocal tract, which enhances the energy in certain frequency regions and attenuates the energy in others. Because the vocal tract filter changes constantly in running speech as the tongue and lips move to articulate the various speech sounds, the frequencies of the peaks and valleys in the spectrum change constantly.

Therefore, in order to represent speech faithfully, the coding strategy must reflect three parameters in its electrical stimulation code—frequency, amplitude, and time. Frequency information is conveyed by the site of stimulation, amplitude is encoded by amplitude of the stimulus current, and temporal cues are conveyed by the rate and pattern of stimulation. The speech processing strategies available in the current implant systems are described below.

Simultaneous Strategies

Currently, the Clarion implant is the only device that supports simultaneous stimulation. The simultaneous strategy currently available is the Simultaneous Analog Stimulation (SAS) strategy. The SAS strategy evolved from compressed analog (CA) schemes that used a vocoder approach. In that approach, a bank of filters separated the incoming sound into different frequency bands, and the resulting analog waveforms were compressed and delivered to appropriate electrodes. In the Clarion, a digitized version of the incoming acoustic signal is filtered, compressed, and processed, then transmitted to the implanted electronics. Following digital-to-analog conversion, the analog waveforms are sent simultaneously to all electrodes (Kessler, 1999). One problem encountered with simultaneous stimulation is channel interaction. Channel interaction results from the spread of current from the targeted nerve population to neighboring nerve fibers, thereby degrading channel independence (i.e., frequency selectivity), which, in turn, adversely affects speech understanding (White, Merzenich, & Gardi, 1984). Therefore, a bipolar electrode coupling mode is typically used to limit the area over which the electrical current spreads around each contact (Figure 21–5). Channel interaction is further reduced with use of the Electrode Positioner.

Additional simultaneous strategies are under development or evaluation for the Clarion. The Simultaneous Pulsatile Strategy (SPS)

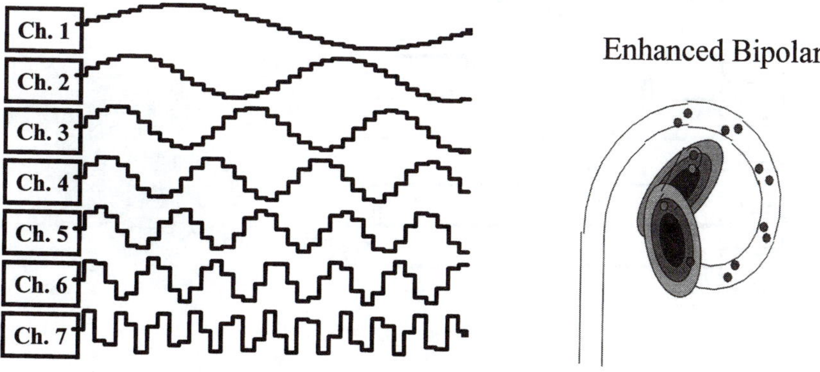

Figure 21–5. Schematic of the Simultaneous Analog Stimulation strategy and enhanced bipolar stimulation mode used in the CLARION cochlear implant.

uses simultaneously presented bipolar pulses rather than analog waveforms. The Paired Pulsatile Sample (PPS) is a partially simultaneous strategy that stimulates two nonadjacent electrodes at the same time with biphasic pulses. The Hybrid Analog Pulsatile (HAP) strategy combines simultaneous analog stimulation of the apical electrodes with nonsimultaneous, pulsatile stimulation of the basal electrodes (Kessler, 1999).

Nonsimultaneous Strategies

These strategies fall into two general categories: continuous interleaved sampling (CIS) and "n of m" strategies. In a CIS strategy, trains of biphasic pulses are delivered to the electrodes in an interleaved or nonoverlapping fashion to minimize electrical field interactions between stimulated electrodes (Wilson et al., 1991). The amplitudes of the pulses delivered to each electrode are derived by modulating them with the envelopes of the corresponding bandpassed waveforms. A CIS strategy uses the full spectrum of the incoming acoustic waveform without compromising temporal information. The rate at which the pulses are delivered to the electrodes is an important variable in the implementation of CIS strategies. High-rate stimulation typically results in better speech understanding than low-rate stimulation (Wilson, 1993). Because only one channel is stimulated at a time, monopolar electrode coupling is typically employed with this type of strategy (Figure 21–6). All three implant systems can implement a CIS strategy, although the number of analysis channels, number of electrodes, and stimulation rates differ among them.

In an "n of m" strategy, a specified **n**umber of electrodes out of the **m**aximum number available are stimulated. The implementation of this type of processing in the Nucleus implant is referred to as the spectral peak extraction (SPEAK) strategy (Skinner, Holden, & Binzer, 1994). SPEAK analyzes the incoming sound to identify the filters that have the greatest amount of energy, selects a subset of filters, and then stimulates corresponding electrodes (always less than the total number of electrodes in the cochlea). The stimuli are pulsatile and nonsimultaneous. With SPEAK, 6 to 10 electrodes are activated sequentially at

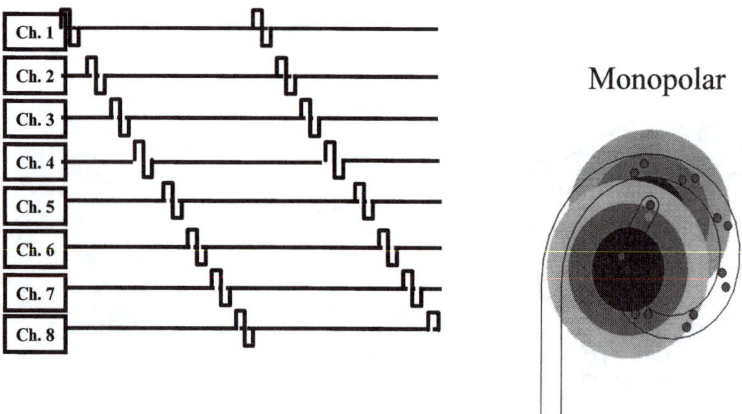

Figure 21–6. Schematic of the Continuous Interleaved Sampler strategy and monopolar stimulation mode used in the CLARION cochlear implant.

a rate that averages approximately 250 pulses per second on each activated electrode. The investigational Advanced Combination Encoder (ACE), offered in the Nucleus CI24M, combines the spectral maxima detection of SPEAK with a higher stimulation rate (Cochlear Corporation, 1999). With ACE, the number of maxima and electrodes used, which will influence the stimulation rate, can be specified for each patient. The Med-El system also offers an "n of m" strategy with a fixed number of channels stimulated at a high rate.

Telemetry

Back telemetry is available in all three U.S. cochlear implant systems. Back telemetry allows the implanted components to send information back to the speech processor, thereby providing data on the function and integrity of the internal electronics and electrode array. The Clarion is the only implant that employs continuous bidirectional telemetry because it has two independent RF carriers, one that transmits data to the internal device and one that sends information from the internal device to the speech processor (Kessler, 1999). The Nucleus CI24M offers Neural Response Telemetry (NRT). NRT allows clinicians to stimulate one electrode within the cochlea while recording the response of the auditory nerve using another electrode. This feature is intended to assist clinicians in programming the implant, especially in young children (Abbas et al., 1999; Brown, Abbas, & Gantz, 1998).[1]

REGULATION OF COCHLEAR IMPLANTS

Unlike hearing aids, cochlear implants are regulated by the U.S. Food and Drug Administration (FDA). Prior to commercial distribution, they must be evaluated for safety and efficacy in clinical trials monitored by the FDA under what is termed an Investigational Device Exemption (IDE). During an IDE study, patients who meet specified criteria can be implanted at a limited number of investigational clinics. These clinics, under supervision from local Institutional Review Boards (IRB), implant patients and collect safety and efficacy data, which then is sent to the implant manufacturer. The manufacturer compiles the data and submits an application for Pre-Market Approval to the FDA. After review, the FDA then may grant the manufacturer a release to distribute the cochlear implant in the United States. Typically, the device is released for a defined population (e.g., profoundly deaf adults), so additional clinical trials must be conducted if other populations (e.g., children) are to receive the device. Moreover, additional clinical trials are required if changes are made to the device itself.

In general, the safety information required by the FDA includes operative and postoperative complications (e.g., infection at the implant site, facial nerve paralysis, device migration) and device reliability and stability (e.g., failure of the internal device requiring explant and re-implant). Efficacy data are collected so that the manufacturer may make statements, or claims, about benefits that may be expected from the implant. Typically, cochlear implant claims revolve around the primary benefit of the device, that is, that patients experience improvements in speech-perception skills with the implant relative to their preoperative abilities with hearing aids. In children, claims about secondary benefits of improved speech production and language skills also may be made.

Although clinical trials are costly in both money and time, they have advanced the development of implant designs, provided longitudinal data on implant benefit, and sparked development of assessment tools

[1]Readers Note: A videotape with an animated display of how a cochlear implant works is available from Advanced Bionics. Readers may request a copy of "Clarion: the Link between Silence and Sound" by calling (800) 678–2575.

that now have become standard in audiologic practice. The results of clinical trials over the years also have led to expanded candidacy criteria. In other words, the improvement in benefit experienced by patients using new technologies has allowed implants to be made available to more individuals, including those who are very young and those who are not profoundly deaf.

COCHLEAR IMPLANT EVALUATION, SURGERY, AND PROGRAMMING

Medical Evaluation

Experience with cochlear implants indicates that individuals with nearly all causes of severe and profound hearing loss may be appropriate candidates for implantation. With few exceptions, stimulable auditory nerve fibers appear to be present even in profound deafness, irrespective of etiology (Hinojosa & Marion, 1983; Otte, Schuknecht, & Kerr, 1978).

Medical and otologic evaluations are required before an individual is considered further as a cochlear implant candidate. The primary care physician's examination ensures that an individual is able to undergo surgery without risks to general health. The otolaryngologist's evaluation ensures that an individual is a suitable implant candidate and that no otologic conditions exist that contraindicate ear surgery. In addition, a radiographic evaluation consisting of high-resolution computed tomography (CT) evaluates the anatomical integrity of the cochlea. Usually, congenital malformations of the inner ear (e.g., Mondini deformity) do not preclude cochlear implantation (Jackler, Luxford, & House, 1987; McElveen, Carrasco, Miyamoto, & Linthicum, 1997). Anatomical contraindications to implantation are Michel deformity (complete absence of the cochlea) (Miyamoto, Robbins, & Osberger, 1993) and small internal auditory canal syndrome in which the VIII-th nerve may be absent (Shelton, Luxford, Tonokawa, Lo, & House, 1989) Chronic otitis media must be resolved before implant surgery can take place.

CT scans also reveal cochlear ossification, a condition that frequently occurs following deafness from meningitis. Cochlear ossification may be partial or complete and may be localized to one or more cochlear turns (Becker, Eisenberg, Luxford, & House, 1984; Swartz et al., 1985). The obstructive intracochlear bone and soft tissue often requires modifications in implant surgical technique and, in some cases, a complete insertion of the electrode array cannot be achieved (Balkany, Gantz, & Nadol, 1988; Bird et al., 1999; Gantz, McCabe, & Tyler, 1988). Nonetheless, if the ossification process is identified in its early stages, a full electrode insertion often can be made, offering the individual the best potential for speech-perception benefit. Current clinical practice suggests that all individuals with profound hearing loss should have high-resolution CT scanning of the cochleae within the first 2 months following the onset of meningitis. If early signs of ossification are detected, and there is no evidence of hearing recovery, implantation is recommended as soon as possible (Novak, Fifer, Barkmeier, & Firszt, 1990).

It is anatomically feasible to implant children as young as 2 years of age and even younger. Although the cochleae are adult sized at birth, there is approximately 2 to 3 cm centimeters of temporal bone growth through adolescence (Jackler & Bates, 1989). All cochlear implants have an expandable lead between the electrode array and the receiver package to accommodate this head growth. Results in children implanted under the age of 2 years have shown no increased risk for extrusion of the electrode due to head growth, occurrence of labyrinthitis, or meningitis due to the higher frequency of otitis media in this age group, or facial nerve damage (Lenarz et al., 1999; Mack, Müller, & Helms, 1997).

Audiologic Evaluation

A comprehensive audiologic evaluation is performed to establish the degree and type of hearing loss, and to assess functional hearing aid benefit. Air and bone conduction thresholds are measured in each ear under earphones. All candidates must demonstrate a severe-to-profound sensorineural hearing loss bilaterally. Impedance testing is conducted to rule out middle ear infections and to demonstrate absent stapedius reflexes. Auditory brainstem response (ABR) testing is performed in young children to verify the presence of a profound hearing loss bilaterally. Routine speech audiometry is conducted under earphones; however, implant candidacy is determined by speech recognition performance with hearing aids rather than on results obtained under earphones.

Evaluating Hearing Aid Benefit in Adults

The audiologist must establish that the individual is using amplification appropriate for the degree and configuration of hearing loss and that the hearing aids meet the specifications of the manufacturer. Skinner, Holden, and Binzer (1994) suggested that patients with severe-to-profound hearing loss should use hearing aids with 50 to 70 dB gain and maximum power output of 120 to 140 dB SPL. Real ear measurements should be interpreted with caution in persons with profound hearing loss and should be used in conjunction with aided soundfield testing. The individual should have at least 1 or 2 months experience with a hearing aid to ensure that a plateau in performance has been reached with acoustic amplification. Exceptions to this guideline are persons with sudden onset of bilateral profound deafness (e.g., due to meningitis) who demonstrate no response to sound at the audiometric limits or responses that are suggestive of vibrotactile rather than auditory sensation, that is, responses only to low-frequency sounds at high intensity levels (Boothroyd & Cawkwell, 1970). In these individuals, a hearing aid trial can be waived if they demonstrate no residual hearing and will derive no benefit from acoustic amplification. If, on the other hand, the audiologist determines that the individual is not using an appropriate hearing aid or the hearing aid has not been set appropriately, then a hearing aid trial of approximately 30 days is recommended.

Functional assessment of hearing aid benefit includes aided soundfield (warble tones) thresholds and speech recognition testing. Speech recognition testing consists of open-set word and sentence tests using recorded materials presented at 70 dB SPL. Typically, sentence tests are administered in the "best-aided condition" to simulate the individual's performance in everyday listening situations. Open-set word tests are administered to each ear monaurally and in the binaural condition to assist in selecting the ear for implantation and to identify the "best-aided" condition for sentence recognition testing.

In 1996, a committee comprised of representatives from the American Academy of Audiology (AAA), the American Academy of Otolaryngology—Head and Neck Surgery (AAO-HNS), and cochlear implant manufacturers convened to identify a set of materials to be used clinically and in research studies to assess the performance of adults with cochlear implants. The Hearing in Noise Test (HINT) (Nilsson, Soli, & Sullivan, 1994) and the Consonant/Nucleus/Consonant (CNC) test (Peterson & Lehiste, 1962) were selected. A CD recording was made of the test materials and is distributed as the Minimum Speech Test Battery for Adult Cochlear Implant Users (Nilsson, McCaw, & Soli, 1996).

The HINT consists of 25 equivalent lists of 10 sentences that have been normed for naturalness, difficulty, and reliability (Nilsson et al., 1994). Although the HINT was designed to be administered adaptively, a fixed presentation level is used when testing adults with cochlear implants. Two lists of 10 sentences are presented, with performance scored as the percentage of words correctly identified. If an individual scores ≥ 20% in quiet, then testing in spectrally matched background noise is conducted at a +10 dB signal-to-noise ratio (SNR). Testing at less favorable SNRs (i.e., +5 dB or 0 dB) can be conducted if a good score is obtained in less difficult noise conditions.

The CNC test consists of 10 lists of 50 monosyllabic words with equal phonemic distribution across lists. Each list has approximately the same phonemic distribution as spoken English, and each word has a frequency of occurrence greater than four per million (Lehiste & Peterson, 1959; Thorndike and Lorge, 1944). Because words from the CNC lists were used to construct the NU-6 lists (Northwestern University Auditory Test No. 6; Tillman & Carhart, 1966), the two tests are considered to yield comparable results.

Although not part of the recommended protocol, the Central Institute for the Deaf (CID) Everyday Sentence test (Davis, 1978) also is used often in a cochlear implant evaluation. The test has been re-recorded by Cochlear Corporation as five lists of 20 sentences, with three practice sentences at the beginning of each 20-sentence list. Performance is scored as the percentage of key words correctly understood in the 20 sentences (i.e., 100 per 20 sentences). Because of improvements in implant technology and expanded candidacy criteria, many individuals score nearly 100% on the CID sentences after relatively limited implant experience (i.e., 1 to 3 months). Therefore, more difficult measures such as the CNC and HINT tests now are used routinely to assess pre- and postimplant speech recognition skills.

Evaluating Hearing Aid Benefit in Children

The appropriateness of the hearing aid fitting also must be assessed in children. It is important to examine the maximum power output setting on the child's hearing aids to ensure that the level is not below the child's behavioral thresholds, a situation that might occur because of concern for overamplification (Seewald, 1991). Typically, a child must use hearing aid amplification for at least 6 months before a plateau in the development of auditory skills can be established or it is determined that progress is substantially slower with hearing aids than that observed in children with cochlear implants. A shorter hearing aid trial may be conducted in young children who demonstrate no functional benefit even with appropriate amplification and intensive auditory rehabilitation.

Functional hearing aid benefit in very young children (i.e., ≤3 years of age) is based on reaching basic auditory milestones. Two measures can be used to assess auditory development in young children, the Meaningful Auditory Integration Scale (MAIS) (Robbins, Renshaw, & Berry, 1991) and the Infant-Toddler Meaningful Auditory Integration Scale (IT-MAIS) (Zimmerman-Phillips, Robbins, & Osberger, 1999). These measures employ a parent interview technique to quantify the frequency of occurrence of target behaviors during everyday situations. During a structured interview, information is obtained from the parent about the frequency with which the child demonstrates 10 different behaviors. A rating is assigned to each target behavior based on the frequency of reported occurrence by the parent, using the following scoring system: 0 = never (i.e., the behavior is never observed); 1 = rarely; 2 = occasionally; 3 = frequently; 4 = always. The MAIS was developed for school-aged children and later modified for infants and toddlers (IT-MAIS) (Table 21–1). Strict scoring criteria have been developed for the two measures to ensure uniformity among examiners in scoring the parents' responses. Inter-rater reliability is high (i.e., 0.90) on the MAIS (Robbins et al., 1991). In addition, postimplant performance on the MAIS is highly correlated (r = 0.70) with performance on the Phonetically-Balanced Kindergarten (PBK) test (Haskins, 1949; Robbins, Svirsky, Osberger & Pisoni, 1998). The MAIS and IT-MAIS have been

Table 21–1. Probes on the Infant-Toddler Meaningful Auditory Scale (IT-MAIS).

Vocalization Behavior

1. Vocal behavior affected while wearing hearing aids?
2. Production of syllables and syllable sequences recognized as speech?

Spontaneous Alerting to Sound

3. Spontaneous alerting to name in quiet with auditory cues only?
4. Spontaneous alerting to name in noise with auditory cues only?
5. Spontaneous alerting to environmental sound with auditory cues only?
6. Spontaneous alerting to sounds in new environments with auditory cues only?

Derives Meaning from Sound

7. Spontaneous recognition of sounds with auditory cues only?
8. Discriminates between two speakers' voices with auditory cues only?
9. Discriminates between speech and nonspeech stimuli with auditory cues only?
10. Response to changes in intonation (motherese) with auditory cues only?

used extensively to examine postimplant performance and to determine candidacy in young children (Osberger, Geier, Zimmerman-Phillips, & Barker, 1997).

In older children, hearing aid benefit is determined using tests of closed- and open-set word recognition. The Early Speech Perception (ESP) test (Moog & Geers, 1990), the Phonetically-Balanced Kindergarten test (Haskins, 1949), the Lexical Neighborhood test (LNT) and Multisyllabic Lexical Neighborhood test (MLNT) (Iler-Kirk, Pisoni, & Osberger, 1995), and the Hearing in Noise Test (HINT-C) for children (Nilsson, Soli, & Gelnett, 1996; Nilsson, Soli, & Sumida, 1995) are used most often. Additional tests that have been employed to assess pre- and postimplant performance are found in Tyler (1993).

The Early Speech Perception (ESP): Monosyllable Word Identification Test (Moog & Geers, 1990) contains three subtests: Pattern Perception, Spondee Word Identification, and Monosyllable Word Identification. The Low Verbal version of the test is administered to young children, and the Standard version is used with older children. Although all three subtests provide useful information, performance on only the most difficult subtest, the Monosyllable Word subtest, is used in an implant evaluation. The Monosyllable Word subtest consists of one-syllable words that differ primarily in the amount of vowel information. The Low Verbal version implements the use of real objects and the response set consists of only four choices. This version presents 12 trials (three repetitions of each item in random order). The child is asked to point to the object representing the word spoken. Chance performance is 25%. The Standard version consists of 12 items presented to the child on a picture plate. It presents 24 trials to the child (two repetitions of each item) in random order. The child is asked to point to the picture representing the word spoken. Ideally, a recorded presentation of the test should be used. Chance performance is 8%.

The PBK test consists of lists of monosyllabic words that are phonetically balanced (Haskins, 1949). Although each list consists of 50 words, typically only half lists (25 words) are used pre- and postimplant. The child is instructed to repeat what he or she hears. Performance is scored by number of phonemes and words correctly understood. A recorded version of the test should be used. Consonant blends are counted as one phoneme, so the child must repeat the entire blend to receive credit for it. Chance performance is 0%.

The Lexical Neighborhood Test (LNT) (Iler-Kirk et al., 1995) was designed to assess speech recognition in children while controlling for lexical properties of the stimulus words. Unlike previous measures of speech recognition (i.e., PBK test), the LNT equates words for the number of phonemes shared by other words and for the frequency of occurrence of the words in spoken English. For example, the word "cat" is considered to have many "lexical neighbors" or words that rhyme (e.g., hat, bat, mat, etc.). It also is a high-frequency word. In contrast, the word "juice" has few lexical neighbors (i.e., few words that rhyme with it) and is a low-frequency word. The LNT consists of monosyllabic words, arranged in lists of "easy" and "hard" words. There are 25 words on each list that are scored for the number of phonemes and words correctly understood.

The Multisyllabic Lexical Neighborhood Test (MLNT) (Iler-Kirk et al., 1995) was developed using the same principles used for the LNT. It consists of multisyllabic rather than monosyllabic words to make the task easier for younger children. It is an open-set test consisting of lists of lexically "easy" and "hard" words. Each list contains 24 words that are scored for the number of phonemes and words correctly understood. Chance performance is 0%.

The Hearing in Noise Test for Children (HINT-C) (Nilsson et al., 1996) is a children's version of the HINT test. It consists of a subset of the sentences used in the adult version that could be repeated by 5- to 6-year-old children with normal hearing. The test consists of 130 sentences sorted into 13 lists of 10 sentences each with approximately equal phonemic content. Two lists of 10 recorded sentences are administered at each evaluation session. Performance is scored as the percentage of key words and sentences correctly repeated. Chance performance is 0%.

Cochlear Implant Referral Guidelines for Adults and Children

Referral guidelines, based on current clinical practice, are listed in Table 21–2 for adults and children. These guidelines are more liberal than current FDA-approved indications for implants because candidacy criteria are constantly changing. In addition, it is important that individuals and their families have access to cochlear implant information as soon as possible, even if candidacy has not been clearly established. It usually takes many months for an individual to reach a decision regarding implantation. Moreover, securing reimbursement for the cochlear implant and associated costs may be a lengthy process.

Cochlear Implant Surgery

Cochlear implant surgery is performed under general anesthesia and ordinarily takes between 1.5 and 3 hours. The procedure can be done in either an inpatient or outpatient setting. Patients usually are able to get out of bed and walk around the day after surgery and generally are discharged from the hospital on the first postoperative day.

The most widely used surgical approach for cochlear implantation is the facial recess approach (Kveton & Balkany, 1991). Skin incisions are designed to provide coverage of the external portion of the implant receiver while preserving the blood supply of the postauricular flap. Following the incision, a complete mastoidectomy is performed, and a bed for the receiver is drilled. The facial recess is opened, and a cochleostomy is performed, followed by insertion of the electrode array into the scala tympani. Fascia is packed around the electrode at the cochleostomy, the receiver is securely affixed to the skull with sutures, and the incision is closed (Balkany, Telischi, & Hodges, 1994; Kveton & Balkany, 1991).

Medical and surgical complications are rare with an incidence, including device failures, of less than 1% (Cohen & Hoffman, 1991; Hoffman & Cohen, 1993). Major complications are those that require additional surgery or hospitalization for treatment or correction (e.g., re-implant following device failure). Facial nerve palsy or paralysis is classified as major complication even though no further surgery is required. Minor complications are those that can be resolved with outpatient treatment.

Table 21–2. Cochlear implant referral guidelines for adults and children.

Audiological Criteria for Adults

- Severe-to-profound bilateral, sensorineural hearing loss (3-frequency pure-tone average ≥70 dB HL)
- Limited benefit from appropriately fitted hearings, defined as a monosyllabic (e.g., CNC, NU6) word recognition score ≤ 30%

Other Considerations for Adults

- Limited interactive telephone conversations, even with amplification devices
- Relies on TDD and other written telecommunication forms
- Relies heavily on speechreaching in face-to-face communication
- Limits his or her social and business life as a result of severe-to-profound hearing loss

Audiological Criteria for Children

- Profound bilateral sensorineural hearing loss (3-frequency pure-tone average ≥90 dB HL)
- Plateau or limited progress in acquisition of auditory skills with appropriate hearing aids and rehabilitation
    - Children <3 years of age
        - Limited hearing aid benefit, defined as failure to acquire basic auditory milestones (e.g., spontaneous response to name and environmental sounds) (i.e., IT-MAIS score ≤2 on 5 or more items) even with appropriated fitted hearing aids and rehabilitation
    - Children 3 to 5 years of age
        - Limited hearing aid benefit, defined as an open-set word recognition score ≤30% (e.g., MLNT test)
    - Children ≥5 years of age
        - Limited hearing aid benefit, defined as an open-set word recognition (e.g., PBK test) or sentence score (e.g., HINT-C) ≤30%

Programming the Cochlear Implant System

Following release from the hospital, individuals return home for a period of 4 to 6 weeks to allow complete healing around the implant site. Following this healing period, the individual returns to the clinic to be fitted with the external components of the system. This first session is often termed the "initial stimulation" session. At that time, electrical threshold and most comfortable listening levels are determined for each electrode, and other psychophysical parameters of the speech processing scheme are programmed into the speech processor. This programming is accomplished using a personal computer, device-specific software, and an interface that allows the computer to communicate with the patient's speech processor. At the end of the first session, a patient goes home with programs downloaded onto the speech processor. Multiple visits to the implant center are necessary during the first months of implant use as the individual grows accustomed to sound and as tolerance for loudness increases. Following the period of initial device adjustment, visits may occur at less frequent intervals (e.g., every 6 months). In addition to making adjustments in threshold and most comfortable listening levels, individuals can be fit with different speech processing strategies at follow-up programming sessions.

In children, programming adjustments may be required more frequently over a longer time period, depending on the reliability of their responses during the programming sessions. The use of objective measures (stapedius reflex thresholds, auditory evoked potentials, and compound action potentials) can be helpful for estimating psychophysical thresholds in young children (Brown et al., 1998; Brown, Abbas, Fryauf-Bertschy, Kelsay, & Gantz, 1994; Brown, Hughes, Lopez, & Abbas, 1999; Firszt, Rotz, Chambers, & Novak, 1999; Hodges, Butts, Dolan-Ash, & Balkany, 1999; Shallop, VanDyke, Goin, & Mischke, 1991). In addition, Kileny (1991) advocated the use of intraoperative electrical auditory brainstem responses (EABR) to assist in the selection of the ear to be implanted.

COCHLEAR IMPLANT BENEFITS

Adults

Speech-Perception Results

Most adults with postlingual onset (i.e., onset ≥6 years of age) of severe or profound hearing loss demonstrate dramatic improvements in speech recognition abilities after relatively limited implant experience. Figure 21–7 shows mean preoperative speech-perception scores obtained with hearing aids compared to 1- and 3-month postoperative performance for adults implanted with the Clarion device plus Electrode Positioner.

Figure 21–8 shows individual word-recognition scores at the 1- and 3-month postoperative intervals. These data illustrate both learning effects and the wide range of individual differences. Performance continues to improve during the first year of implant experience, although in many individuals the most dramatic increases in speech recognition performance occur during the first few months of use. Loeb and Kessler (1996) reported that 59% of the first group of adults to receive the Clarion implant reached a plateau in speech-perception performance after only 3 months of implant experience. In contrast, the other 41% of the adults continued to show improvement at variable rates.

Postimplant speech recognition performance is lower and the rate of learning is slower in adults who have a longer duration of deafness or who are older at time of implant (Geier, Barker, Fisher, & Opie, 1999; Osberger, Fisher, Kalberer, submitted; Rubinstein, Parkinson, Tyler, & Gantz, 1999; Tyler & Summerfield, 1996; Tyler, Parkinson, Woodworth, Lowder, & Gantz, 1997). Figure 21–9 shows mean CNC word scores after 3 months of implant use plotted as a function of duration of

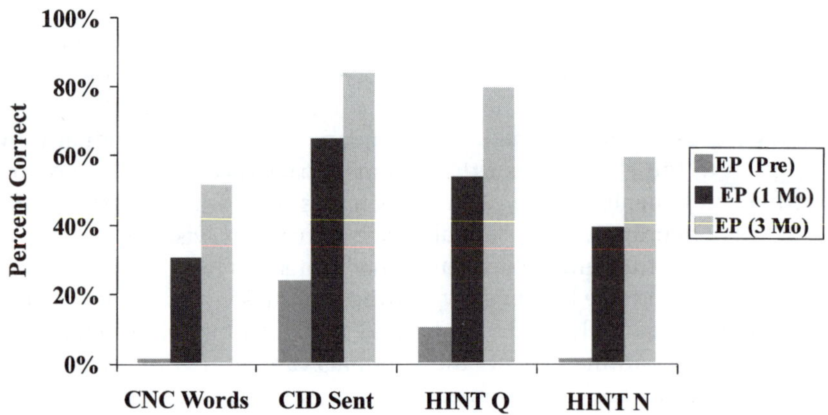

Figure 21–7. Mean pre- and postoperative CNC word, CID sentence, HINT sentence in quiet, and HINT sentence in noise scores for adults using the CLARION device plus Electrode Positioner.

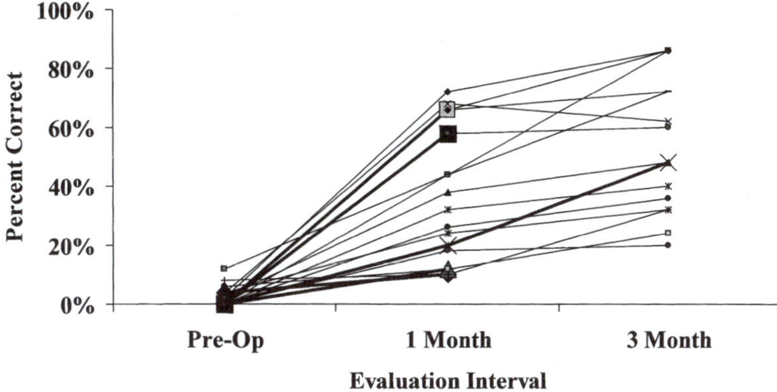

Figure 21–8. Individual postoperative CNC word scores for adults using the CLARION device plus Electrode Positioner.

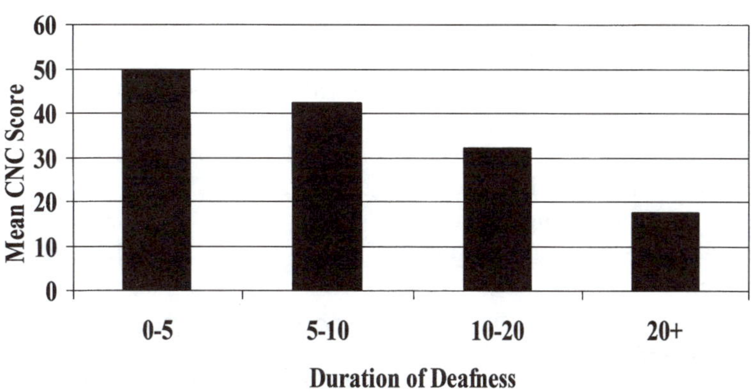

Figure 21–9. Mean CNC word scores as a function of duration of deafness for adults using the CLARION cochlear implant.

deafness in a group of adults who received the Clarion device. In this figure, there is a systematic decrease in performance as duration of deafness increases. *These findings indicate that adult candidates should be implanted as soon as possible to derive the maximum benefit from the device*. Nonetheless, individuals who have long duration of deafness or who are elderly still are considered viable candidates because of the potential benefits they can derive from an implant relative to those derived from acoustic amplification. It is important, however, that these candidates be counseled regarding potential benefits and the relatively long learning period that might be required to achieve optimal performance with a cochlear implant.

Rubinstein et al. (1999) also found that preoperative sentence recognition performance had a significant impact on postimplant word recognition scores. Patients who had better preoperative scores on the CID sentence test achieved higher word recognition scores postimplant. Specifically, Rubinstein and colleagues reported that each additional 2% on the CID test preoperatively resulted in a 1% increase in the postimplant CNC word score. These researchers caution, however, that individuals who show no preoperative speech recognition scores (i.e., score of 0% on sentence tests with hearing aids) also do extremely well postimplant, although even small amounts of residual hearing are associated with a higher average performance and lesser variance. The findings of this study support the current trend to implant adults with more residual hearing.

The number of prelingually deafened adults seeking cochlear implants is increasing as the candidacy criteria are expanded and there is more widespread use of the technology. Research shows that these individuals also derive substantial benefit from cochlear implants, although their performance on speech recognition tests is poorer than adults with postlingual onset of severe or profound hearing loss (Waltzman & Cohen, 1999; Zwolan, Kileny, & Telian, 1996). The ideal candidates with prelingual severe or profound hearing loss are adults with a consistent history of hearing aid use, preferably with some residual hearing, who also use oral communication. Counseling regarding appropriate expectations with an implant is important for these individuals.

Psychosocial Benefits

Research has shown that the use of a multichannel cochlear implant by adults with postlingual onset of hearing loss yields psychological benefits. Knutson et al. (1998) reported significant improvement on measures of loneliness, social anxiety, and distress within 1 year of implant use. Improvement on measures of marital satisfaction and assertiveness became apparent after more long-term implant experience.

Two questionnaires that can be used to assess implant benefits, the Social Benefits Questionnaire and the Self-Reported Benefits Questionnaire, appear in the Appendix. Both questionnaires were developed by personnel at Advanced Bionics to assess perceived benefits in a variety of social and communication situations and to evaluate quality of life. Test-retest reliability is high on both measures (i.e., r = .79 for the Self-Reported Benefits Questionnaire; r = .70 for the Social Benefits Questionnaire). Table 21–3 summarizes results obtained on the Social Benefits Questionnaire, expressed as the percentage of patients who agreed or strongly agreed with each item. The results are based on responses from 36 Clarion users with a mean duration of implant use of 10 months. The findings indicate improvement in a wide range of areas after relatively limited implant experience. For example, although it might be expected that an implant might have a more pronounced effect on job opportunities (item 7), 19 of the 36 patients indicated that the item was not applicable to them for reasons other than hearing (e.g., retirement, other disabilities preventing employment, etc.). Measures such as these provide valuable information that can be used in conjunction with more traditional speech recognition measures to better understand the benefits that individuals derive from a cochlear implant.

Children

Speech Perception Results

In contrast to adults, children with cochlear implants show improvement over a longer time period. Figure 21–10 shows PB-K phoneme scores as a function of time after implantation for 50 children implanted consecutively during the Clarion clinical trial. Mean age at implant for the younger children was 3 years compared to a mean age at implant of 9 years for the older children. All children were prelingually deafened (onset before 2 years of age) and demonstrated profound hearing losses (mean pure tone average = 111 dB HL). The results indicate that, after 2 years, the older children were beginning to plateau on this test, while the younger children were catching up and might overtake the performance of the older children. Other new evidence also suggests

Table 21–3. Percentage of patients who agreed or strongly agreed on the Social Benefits Questionnaire ($n = 36$).

Items	*Percent (%)*
1. My overall quality of life has improved.	58%
2. I am a happier person.	61%
3. I am more comfortable with strangers.	28%
4. I participate in more social activities.	45%
5. I am more relaxed in social situations.	53%
6. I have more confidence.	50%
7. I have increased job opportunities.	19%[a]
8. I depend less on lipreading.	45%
9. I have increased social contacts.	31%
10. I enjoy listening to music.	42%
11. I enjoy going to movies more.	22%[b]
12. The quality of my speech improved.	39%
13. I am better able to control loudness of my voice.	56%
14. I feel safer.	53%
15. I rely less on others.	47%
16. I do things I was uncomfortable doing before.	42%
17. I am more independent.	47%
18. Using the telephone is less frustrating.	36%
19. I enjoy calling family and friends.	44%
20. I feel less isolated.	47%

[a] 19 individuals responded not applicable
[b] 9 individuals responded not applicable

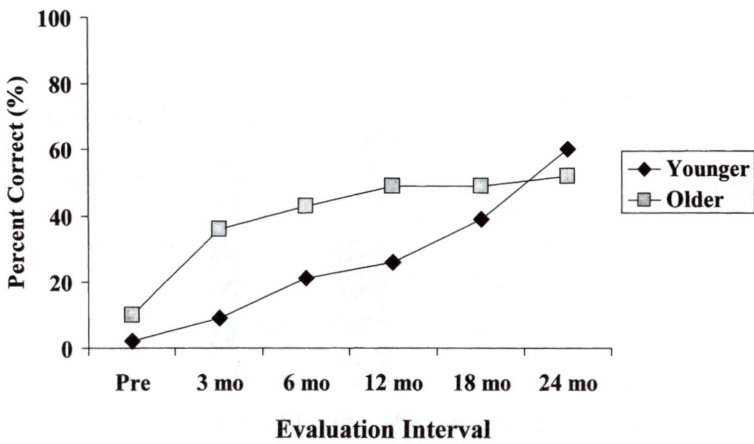

Figure 21–10. Mean pre- and postoperative ESP Word Identification scores for children implanted with the CLARION cochlear implant.

that children implanted at a younger age have the potential to achieve higher speech-perception performance than children who receive implants at an older age (Fryauf-Bertschy, Tyler, Kelsay, Gantz, & Woodworth, 1997; Waltzman & Cohen,1998).

The long time course of learning for younger children may be influenced by the fact that they have limited language and test-taking skills early in the implant process. Consequently, it may take several years for their language skills to catch up and be reflected in a speech-perception test. Nonetheless, on the IT-MAIS, a test that evaluates milestones in speech and auditory perception skills, very young children showed significant improvement even in the first 3 months after implantation, with continued improvement over time (Figure 21–11). The data in Figure 21–11 were obtained from 10 children implanted between the ages of 18 and 23 months with the Clarion implant. Following implantation, the most obvious improvement occurs in vocalization behaviors, followed by spontaneous alerting to sound. More dramatic improvement in deriving meaning from sound occurs after 12 months of implant use

Other factors besides age influence cochlear implant benefit in children. For example, educational method impacts the performance of older children. Children who use primarily oral communication have higher speech-perception scores than children who are educated using a total communication approach (Osberger, Fisher, Zimmerman-Phillips, Geier, & Barker, 1998; Somers, 1991; Staller, Beiter, Brimacombe, Mecklenburg, & Arndt, 1991; Svirsky & Meyer, 1999). Moreover, children who had some preoperative speech-perception skills using hearing aids do better than children who showed no hearing aid benefit (Osberger & Fisher, 1999). Nonetheless, children with no preoperative auditory perceptual skills still show significant speech-perception benefit after implantation.

Language and Speech Production Results

In addition to auditory perceptual benefit, children with cochlear implants show significant improvement in their receptive and expressive language development (Bollard, Chute, Popp, & Parisier, 1999; Dawson, Blamey, Dettman, Barker, & Clark, 1995; Robbins, Bollard, & Green, 1999; Robbins, Green, & Bollard, 1999; Robbins, Svirsky, & Kirk, 1997). During the first 12 months of implant use, a group of 18 Clarion users showed significant language growth on the Reynell Developmental Language Scales,

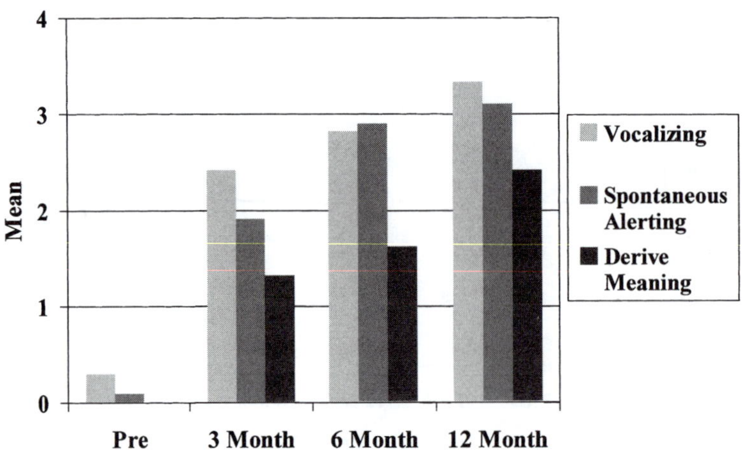

Figure 21–11. Mean pre- and postoperative IT-MAIS scores for very young children implanted with the CLARION cochlear implant.

Revised (RDLS; Reynell & Huntley, 1985). Moreover, the rate of language acquisition exceeded that of normal-hearing children with equivalent language age. That increased rate, especially during the first 6 months after implantation, reflects an acceleration of learning when auditory information became available through the implant. Nonetheless, even with the marked improvement in language development, the implanted children still remain delayed compared to their peers with normal hearing of the same chronologic age. They do not continue to fall farther behind in their language performance, however, as has been reported for their peers with profound hearing impairment who use hearing aids (Moeller, Osberger, & Eccarius, 1986).

Speech production skills also improve after implantation (Osberger, Robbins, Todd, Riley, & Miyamoto, 1994; Robbins, Kirk, Osberger, & Ertmer, 1995; Tobey, Geers, & Brenner, 1994; Tobey & Hasenstab, 1991). Brown and McDowall (1999) evaluated speech production before implantation and 3 and 6 months after implantation in 24 children who received the Clarion device. They used the Identifying Early Phonological Needs in Children with Hearing Impairment (IEPN) assessment procedure (Paden & Brown, 1990), which is designed to measure children's spontaneous use of early developing phonologic patterns in words. The results showed that the greatest improvement in speech production occurred between 3 and 6 months after implantation. The greatest gains were made in the production of nonsegmental features, vowels, and diphthongs, although improvement also was seen in consonant production. These data indicate that speech production improvement occurs after limited implant use even in young children who have little or no auditory experience before implantation.

Educational Benefits

A recent study by Francis, Koch, Wyatt, and Niparko (1999) indicated that the educational cost/benefit ratio for cochlear implants is low. A comparison of 50 implanted children and a similar group of profoundly deaf children with hearing aids showed that the implanted children were mainstreamed at a much higher rate, and that their need for special support services dropped significantly after the first two years. Strikingly, the researchers calculated that the cost savings were between $100,000 and $150,000 each (K–12) for the implanted children compared to profoundly deaf children who do not receive cochlear implants.

FUTURE DIRECTIONS

Cochlear implants have become an accepted medical treatment for severe-to-profound sensorineural hearing loss in children and adults. Candidacy is determined only after comprehensive evaluations by a team of highly skilled professionals. These implantable hearing prostheses provide a range of perception benefits to postlinguistically deafened adults—from awareness of environmental sounds to the ability to converse on the telephone. Moreover, a cochlear implant improves social and communication abilities and quality of life. The level of benefit is dependent on several factors including duration of deafness, age, preimplant speech-perception ability, and severity of hearing loss. Prelinguistically deafened adults also derive benefit from a cochlear implant, but their abilities may be poorer than those adults who have heard before or have some residual hearing.

Children also benefit from cochlear implantation. The outcomes of recent studies of cochlear implantation in children are important for determining implant candidacy in the future and for counseling parents. The results indicate that implanting children as young as possible will give them the most advantageous auditory environment for speech and language learning. Furthermore, providing auditory input early will increase a child's ability to learn in a normal classroom setting and reduce the need for special education services. Older children still can benefit significantly from a cochlear implant, especially if they use oral communication, but their benefit may be limited if they have been deaf for a long time or if they use total communication.

An important aspect of the cochlear implant process is follow-up rehabilitation, a topic beyond the scope of this chapter. Rehabilitation with adults typically focuses on effective use of communication strategies and orientation to listening situations that are now viable with cochlear implant use. A comprehensive rehabilitation guide for adults has been developed by Wayner and Abrahamson (1998). Children with implants continue to require intervention services, as do any children with significant hearing impairment. An overview of available resource information is presented in the *Educator's Guide*, distributed by Advanced Bionics (1999). A videotaped series, demonstrating the principles of cochlear implant rehabilitation with children (Koch, 1999), also is available.

The future of cochlear implants is bright. Technological advances should result in the development of electrode/neural interfaces that better focus electrical stimulation to reduce channel interaction. Speech processing strategies that use a variety of stimulation waveforms and patterns will allow implants to be tailored to each user. New miniaturization processes will result in smaller behind-the-ear processors and, eventually, a completely implantable system. Moreover, technological advances also will result in improved implant reliability and enhanced speech-perception benefit. As the perceptual benefits improve, the candidacy criteria will expand to include other individuals with hearing impairment who do not benefit from acoustic amplification.

REVIEW QUESTIONS

1. Stimulation mode describes
   a. how sound is converted to electrical pulses.
   b. how current flows between active and indifferent electrodes.
   c. the analog signal delivered to the implanted electrodes.
   d. how electrical signals are sent across the skin to the implant.

2. The Nucleus implant system has
   a. 22 intracochlear electrodes.
   b. analog stimulation.
   c. SPEAK speech processing strategy.
   d. both a and c.
   e. both a and b.

3. The Clarion implant system has
   a. simultaneous analog strategy.
   b. continuous interleaved sampler strategy.
   c. SPEAK strategy.
   d. both a and b.
   e. both b and c.

4. Telemetry is
   a. how information is programmed into the speech processor by the audiologist.
   b. how data is sent between the internal and external implant components.
   c. how the speech processor can be connected to a telephone.
   d. how current passes from an active to a ground electrode.

5. An Investigation Device Exemption (IDE) signifies that
   a. a cochlear implant will help all deaf individuals.
   b. a cochlear implant is to be used only in research.
   c. a cochlear implant is undergoing clinical trials.
   d. a cochlear implant can be marketed in the United States.

6. List three criteria for referring an adult for a cochlear implant.

7. Name four tests that can be used with children to assess speech-perception skills.

8. Describe three benefits experienced by children with cochlear implants.

REFERENCES

Abbas, P. (1993). Electrophysiology. In R. S. Tyler (Ed.), *Cochlear implants: Audiologic foundations* (pp. 317–355). San Diego, CA: Singular Publishing Group.

Abbas, P. J., Brown, C. J., Shallop, J. K., Firszt, J. B., Hughes, M. L., Hong, S. H., & Staller, S. J. (1999). Summary of results using the Nucleus CI24M implant to record the electrically evoked compound action potential. *Ear and Hearing, 20*, 45–59.

Advanced Bionics Corporation. (1999). *Educator's guide*. Sylmar, CA: Advanced Bionics Corporation.

Balkany, T., Gantz, B., & Nadol, J. B., Jr. (1988). Multichannel cochlear implants in partially ossified cochleas. *Annals of Otology, Rhinology, and Laryngology, 97*(Suppl. 135), 3–7.

Balkany, T., Telischi, F. F., & Hodges, A. V. (1994). Cochlear implant basics. In R. K. Jackler & D. E. Brackman (Eds.), *Neurotology* (pp. 1361–1377). St. Louis, MO: Mosby-Year Book, Inc.

Becker, T. S., Eisenberg, L. S., Luxford, W. M., & House, W. F. (1984). Labyrinthine ossification secondary to childhood bacterial meningitis: Implications for cochlear implant surgery. *American Journal of Neuroradiology, 5*, 739–741.

Beiter, A. L., & Shallop, J. K. (1998). Cochlear implants: Past, present, and future. In W. Estabrooks (Ed.), *Cochlear implants in kids* (pp. 3–29). Washington, DC: Alexander Graham Bell Association.

Bird, P. A., Balkany, T. J., Hodges, A. V., Butts, S., Gomez, O., & Lee, D. (1999). Using the Clarion cochlear implant in cochlear ossification. *Annals of Otology, Rhinology, and Laryngology, 108*(Suppl. 177), 31–34.

Bollard, P. M., Chute, P. M., Popp, A., & Parisier, S. C. (1999). Specific language growth in young children using the Clarion cochlear implants. *Annals of Otology, Rhinology, and Laryngology, 108*(Suppl. 177), 119–123.

Boothroyd, A., & Cawkwell, S. (1970). Vibrotactile thresholds in pure-tone audiometry. *Acta Otolaryngologica, 69*, 384–387.

Brown, C. J., Abbas, P. J., & Gantz, B. J. (1998). Preliminary experience with neural response telemetry in the Nucleus CI24M cochlear implant. *American Journal of Otology, 19*, 320–327.

Brown, C. J., Abbas, P. J., Frayauf-Bertschy, H., Kelsay, D., & Gantz, B. J. (1994). Intraoperative and postoperative electrically evoked auditory brainstem responses in Nucleus cochlear implant users: Implications for the fitting process. *Ear and Hearing, 15*, 168–176.

Brown, C. J., Hughes, M. L., Lopez, S. M., & Abbas, P. J. (1999). Relationship between EABR thresholds and levels used to program the Clarion speech processor. *Annals of Otology, Rhinology, and Laryngology, 108*(Suppl. 177), 50–57.

Brown, C. J., & McDowall, D. W. (1999). Speech production results in children implanted with the Clarion implant. *Annals of Otology, Rhinology, and Laryngology, 108*(Suppl. 177), 110–112.

Cochlear Corporation. (1999, Spring). *Nucleus news*. MUN 060 (p. 1). Englewood, CO: Cochlear Corporation.

Cohen N. L., & Hoffman, R. A. (1991). Complications of cochlear implant surgery in adults and children. *Annals of Otology, Rhinology, and Laryngology, 100*, 131–136.

Davis, H. (1978). Audiometry: Pure-tone and simple speech tests. In H. Davis & S. R. Silverman (Eds.), *Hearing and deafness* (pp. 183–221). New York: Holt, Rinehart & Winston.

Dawson, P. W., Blamey, P. J., Dettman, S. J., Barker, E. J., & Clark, G. M. (1995). A clinical report on receptive vocabulary skills in cochlear implant users. *Ear and Hearing, 16*, 287–294.

Djourno, A., & Eyries, C. (1957). Prosthese auditive par excitation electrique a distance du nerf sensoriel a l'aide d'un bobinage inclus a demeure. *Presse Med, 35*, 14–17.

Firszt, J. B., Rotz, L. A., Chambers, R. D., & Novak, M. A. (1999). Electrically evoked potentials recorded in adult and pediatric Clarion implant users. *Annals of Otology, Rhinology, and Laryngology, 108*(Suppl. 177), 58–63.

Francis, H. W., Koch, M. E., Wyatt, R., & Niparko, J. K. (1999). Trends in educational placement and cost-benefit considerations in children with cochlear implants. *Archives of Otolaryngology—Head and Neck Surgery, 125*, 499–505.

Fryauf-Berschy, H., Tyler, R., Kelsay, D., Gantz, B. J., & Woodworth, G. G. (1997). Cochlear implant use by prelingually deafened children: The influences of age at implant and length of device use. *Journal of Speech and Hearing Research, 40*, 183–199.

Gantz, B. J., McCabe, B. F., & Tyler, R. S. (1988). Use of multi-channel cochlear implants in obstructed cochleas. *Otolaryngology—Head and Neck Surgery, 98*, 72–81.

Geier, L., Barker, M., Fisher, L., & Opie, J. (1999). The effect of long-term deafness on speech recognition in postlingually deafened adult Clarion cochlear implant users. *Annals of Otology, Rhinology, and Laryngology, 108*(Suppl. 177), 80–83.

Haskins, H. (1949). *A phonetically balanced speech discrimination test for children*. Unpublished master's thesis, Northwestern University, Evanston, IL.

Hinojosa, R., & Marion, M. (1983). Histopathology of profound sensorineural deafness. *Annals of the New York Academy of Science, 405*, 459–484.

Hodges, A. V., Butts, S., Dolan-Ash, S., & Balkany, T. J. (1999). Using electrically evoked auditory reflex thresholds to fit the Clarion cochlear implant. *Annals of Otology, Rhinology, and Laryngology, 108*(Suppl. 177), 64–69.

Hoffman, R. A., & Cohen, N. L. (1993). Surgical pitfalls in cochlear implantation. *Laryngoscope, 103,* 741–744.

Iler-Kirk, K., Pisoni, D. B., & Osberger, M. J. (1995). Lexical effects on spoken word recognition by pediatric cochlear implant users. *Ear and Hearing, 16,* 470–481.

Jackler, R. K. (1988). CT and MRI of the ear and temporal bone: Current state of the art and future prospects. *American Journal of Otology, 9,* 232–239.

Jackler, R. K., & Bates, G. J. (1989). Medial and surgical considerations of cochlear implantation in children. In E. Owens & D. K. Kessler (Eds.), *Cochlear implants in young deaf children* (pp. 153–181). Boston: College-Hill Publications, Little, Brown and Company.

Jackler, R. K., Luxford, W. M., & House, W. F. (1987). Sound detection with the cochlear implant in five ears of four children with congenital malformations of the cochlea. *Laryngoscope, 97*(Suppl. 40), 15–17.

Kessler, D. K. (1999). The Clarion multi-strategy cochlear implant. *Annals of Otology, Rhinology, and Laryngology, 108*(Suppl. 177), 8–16.

Kileny, P. R. (1991). Use of electrophysiological measures in the management of children with cochlear implants: Brainstem, middle latency, and cognitive (P300) responses. *American Journal of Otology, 12*(Suppl. 12), 37–42.

Koch, M. E. (1999). *Bringing sound to life.* Baltimore: York Press.

Knutson, J. F., Murray, K. T., Husarek, S., Westerhouse, K., Woodworth, G., Gantz, B. J., & Tyler, R. S. (1998). Psychological change over 54 months of cochlear implant use. *Ear and Hearing, 19,* 191–201.

Kveton, J., & Balkany, T. J. (1991). Status of cochlear implantation in children. *Journal of Pediatrics, 118,* 1–7.

Lehiste, I., & Peterson, G. E. (1959). Linguistic considerations in the study of speech intelligibility. *Journal of the Acoustical Society of America, 31,* 280–286.

Lenarz, T., Lesinski-Schiedat, A., von der Haar-Heise, S., Illg, A., Bertram, B., & Battmer, R. D. (1999). Cochlear implantation in children under the age of two: The MHH experience with the clarion cochlear implant. *Annals of Otology, Rhinology, and Laryngology, 108*(Suppl. 177), 44–49.

Loeb, G. E., & Kessler, D. K. (1996). Speech recognition performance over time with the Clarion cochlear prosthesis. *Annals of Otology, Rhinology, and Laryngology, 104*(Suppl. 166), 290–292.

Loizou, P. C. (1998, September). Mimicking the human ear. *IEEE Signal Processing Magazine,* pp. 101–130.

Mack, K. F., Müller, J., & Helms, J. (1997). Dimensions of the temporal bone in small children in relation to the cochlear implant—analysis of CT scans. *Advances in Otorhinolaryngology, 52,* 57–59.

McElveen, J. T., Carrasco, V. N., Miyamoto, R. T., & Linthicum, F. H., Jr. (1997). Cochlear implantation in common cavity malformations using a transmastoid labyrinthotomy approach. *Laryngoscope, 107,* 1032–1036.

Merzenich, M. M., & White, M. W. (1977). Cochlear implant—The interface problem. In F. T. Hambrecht & J. B. Reswick (Eds.), *Functional electrical stimulation: Applications in neural prostheses* (pp. 321–340). New York: Marcel Dekker.

Miyamoto, R. T., Robbins, A. M., & Osberger, M. J. (1993). Cochlear implants. In L. A. Harker (Ed.), *Otolaryngology—head and neck surgery* (Vol. 4, 2nd ed., pp. 3142–3151). St. Louis, MO: Mosby-Year Book, Inc.

Moeller, M. P., Osberger, M. J., & Eccarius, M. (1986). Receptive language skills. *ASHA Monographs, 23,* 87–91.

Moog, J. S., & Geers, A. E. (1990). *Early speech-perception test.* St. Louis, MO: Central Institute for the Deaf.

Nilsson, M. J., McCaw, V. M., & Soli, S. (1996). *Minimum speech test battery for adult cochlear implant users.* Los Angeles, CA: House Ear Institute.

Nilsson, M. J., Soli, S., & Gelnett, D. J. (1996). *Development of the hearing in noise test for children (HINT-C).* Los Angeles: House Ear Institute.

Nilsson, M. J., Soli, S., & Sullivan, J. (1994). Development of the Hearing in Noise Test for the measurement of speech reception thresholds in quiet and in noise. *Journal of the Acoustical Society of America, 95,* 1085–1099.

Nilsson, M. J., Soli, S. & Sumida, A. (1995). *Development of norms and percent intelligibility functions for the HINT.* Los Angeles, CA: House Ear Institute.

Novak, M. A., Fifer, R. C., Barkmeier, J. C., & Firszt, J. B. (1990). Labyrinthine ossification after meningitis: Its implications for cochlear implantation. *Otolaryngology—Head and Neck Surgery, 103,* 351–356.

Osberger, M. J., & Fisher, L. (1999). Preoperative predictors of postoperative implant performance in children. *Annals of Otology, Rhinology, and Laryngology.* Manuscript submitted for publication.

Osberger, M. J., Fisher, L., & Kalberer, A. (1999). Speech perception results in children implanted with the CLARION Multi-Strategy cochlear implant. *Advances in Otolaryngology.* Manuscript submitted for publication.

Osberger, M. J., Fisher, L., Zimmerman-Phillips, S., Geier, L., & Barker, M. J. (1998). Speech recognition performance of older children with cochlear implants. *American Journal of Otology, 19,* 152–157.

Osberger, M. J., Geier, L., Zimmerman-Phillips, S., & Barker, M. J. (1997). Use of a parent-report scale to assess benefit in children given the Clarion cochlear implant. *American Journal of Otology, 18*(Suppl.), S79–S80.

Osberger, M. J., Robbins, A. M., Todd, S. L., Riley, A. I., & Miyamoto, R. T. (1994). Speech production skills of children with multichannel cochlear implants. In I. J. Hochmair-Desoyer & E. S. Hochmair (Eds.), *Advances in cochlear implants* (pp. 503–508). Vienna, Austria: Manz Publishing.

Otte, J., Schuknecht, H. E., & Kerr, A. G. (1978). Ganglion cell population in normal and pathological human cochlea: Implications for cochlear implantation. *Laryngoscope, 38,* 1231–1246.

Paden, E. P., & Brown, C. J. (1990). *Identifying early phonological needs in children with hearing impairment.* Washington, DC: Alexander Graham Bell Association.

Peterson, G. E., & Lehiste, I. (1962). Revised CNC lists for auditory tests. *Journal of Speech and Hearing Disorders, 27,* 62–70.

Reynell, J. K., & Huntley, M. (1985). *Reynell developmental language scales* (rev. ed., 2nd ed.). Windsor, England: NFER-Nelson Publishing.

Robbins, A. M., Bollard, P. M., & Green, J. (1999). Language development in children implanted with the Clarion cochlear implant. *Annals of Otology, Rhinology, and Laryngology, 108*(Suppl. 177), 113–118.

Robbins, A. M., Green, J., & Bollard, P. M. (1999). Language development in children following one year of Clarion implant use. *Annals of Otology, Rhinology, and Laryngology.* Manuscript submitted for publication.

Robbins, A. M., Kirk, K. I., Osberger, M. J. & Ertmer, D. (1995). Speech intelligibility of implanted children. *Annals of Otology, Rhinology, and Laryngology, 104*(Suppl. 166) 399–401.

Robbins, A. M., Renshaw J. J., & Berry S. W. (1991). Evaluating meaningful auditory integration in profoundly hearing-impaired children. *American Journal of Otology, 12*(Suppl.), 151–164.

Robbins, A. M., Svirsky, M., & Kirk, K. I. (1997). Children with implants can speak, but can they communicate? *Otolaryngology—Head and Neck Surgery, 117,* 155–160.

Robbins, A. M., Svirsky, M., Osberger, M. J., & Pisoni, D. B. (1998). Beyond the audiogram: The role of functional assessments. In F. H. Bess (Ed.), *Children with hearing impairment* (pp. 105–124). Nashville, TN: Vanderbilt Bill Wilkerson Center Press.

Rubinstein, J. T., Parkinson, W. S., Tyler, R. S., & Gantz, B. J. (1999). Residual speech recognition and cochlear implant performance: Effects of implantation criteria. *American Journal of Otology, 20,* 445–452.

Seewald, R. C. (1991). Hearing aid output limiting considerations for children. In J. A. Feigin & P. G. Stelmachowicz (Eds.), *Pediatric amplification* (pp. 19–36). Omaha, NE: Boys Town National Research Hospital.

Shallop, J. K., Van Dyke, L., Goin, D. W., & Mischke, R. E. (1991). Prediction of behavioral threshold and comfort values for Nucleus 22-channel implant patients from electrical auditory brainstem response test results. *Annals of Otology, Rhinology, and Laryngology, 100,* 896–898.

Shannon, R.V. (1996). Cochlear implants: What have we learned and where are we going? *Seminars in Hearing, 17,* 403–415.

Shelton, W., Luxford, W. M., Tonokawa, L., Lo, W. M., & House, W. F. (1989). The narrow internal auditory canal in children: A contraindication to cochlear implants. *Otolaryngology—Head and Neck Surgery, 100,* 227–231.

Simmons, F. B. (1966). Electrical stimulation of the auditory nerve in man. *Archives of Otolaryngology, 84,* 2–54.

Skinner, M. W., Clark, G. M., Whitford, L. A., Seligman, P. M., Staller, S. J., Shipp, D. B., Shallop, J. K., Everingham, C., Menapace, C. M., Arndt, P. L., Antogenelli, T., Brimacombe, J. A., Pijl, S., Daniels, P., George, C. R., McDermott, H. J., & Beiter, A. L. (1994). Evaluation of a new spectral peak coding strategy for the Nucleus 22-channel cochlear implant system. *American Journal of Otology, 151*(Suppl. 2), 15–27.

Skinner, M. W., Holden, L., & Binzer, S. (1994). Aural rehabilitation for individuals with severe and profound hearing impariment: Hearing aids, cochlear implants, counseling and training. In M. Valente (Ed.), *Strategies for selecting and verifying hearing aid fittings* (pp. 267–299). New York: Thieme Medical Publishers.

Somers, M. (1991). Speech perception abilities in children with cochlear implants or hearing aids. *American Journal of Otology, 12*(Suppl.), 174–178.

Staller, S. J., Beier, A. L., Brimacombe, J. A., Mecklenburg, D. J., & Arndt, P. (1991). Pediatric performance with the Nucleus 22-channel cochlear implant system. *American Journal of Otology, 12*(Suppl.), 137–143.

Svirsky, M., & Meyer, T. A. (1999). Comparison of speech-perception in Clarion cochlear implant and hearing aid users. *Annals of Otology, Rhinology, and Laryngology, 108*(Suppl. 177), 104–109.

Swartz, J. D., Mandell, D. M., Faerber, F. N., Popky, G. I., Ardito, J. M., Steinberg, S. B., & Rojer, C. L. (1985). Labyrinthine ossification: Etiologies and CT findings. *Radiology, 157,* 395–398.

Thorndike, E. L., & Lorge, I. (1944). *The teacher's word book of 30,000 words.* New York: Bureau of Publications, Teachers College, Columbia University.

Tillman, T. W., & Carhart, R. (1966). *An expanded test for speech discrimination utilizing CNC monosyllabic words. Northwestern University Auditory Test No. 6.* (Technical report No. 1 SAM-TR-66–55). USAF School of Aerospace Medicine, Brooks Airforce Base, TX.

Tobey, E. A., Geers, A., & Brenner, C. (1994). Speech production results and speech feature acquisition. *Volta Review, 96,* 109–130.

Tobey, E. A., & Hasenstab, S. (1991). Effects of Nucleus multichannel cochlear implant upon speech production in children. *Ear and Hearing, 12*(Suppl.), 48S–54S.

Tyler, R. S. (1993). Speech perception by children. In R. S. Tyler (Ed.), *Cochlear implants: Audiological foundations* (pp. 191–256). San Diego, CA: Singular Publishing Group.

Tyler, R. S., Parkinson, A. J., Woodworth, G. G., Lowder, M. W., & Gantz, B. J. (1997). Performance over time of adult patients using the Ineraid or Nucleus cochlear implant. *Journal of the Acoustical Society of America, 102*, 508–522.

Tyler, R. S., & Summerfield, A. Q. (1996). Cochlear implantation: Relationships with research on auditory deprivation and acclimatization. *Ear and Hearing, 17*(Suppl. 3), 38–50.

van den Honert, C., & Stypulkowski, P. H. (1987). Single fiber mapping of spatial excitation patterns in the electrically stimulated auditory nerve. *Hearing Research, 29*, 195–206.

Waltzman, S. B., & Cohen, N. L. (1998). Cochlear implantation in children younger than 2 years old. *American Journal of Otology, 19*, 158–162.

Waltzman, S. B., & Cohen, N. L (1999). Implantation of patients with prelingual long-term deafness. *Annals of Otology, Rhinology, and Laryngology, 108*(Suppl. 177), 84–88.

Wayner, D. S., & Abrahamson, J. E. (1998). *Learning to hear again with a cochlear implant*. Dallas, TX: Hear Again.

White, M. W., Merzenich, M. M., & Gardi, J. N. (1987). Multichannel cochlear implants: Channel interactions and processor design. *Archives of Otolaryngology, 110*, 493–501.

Wilson, B. E. (1993). Signal processing. In R. S. Tyler (Ed.), *Cochlear implants: Audiological foundations* (pp. 35–85). San Diego, CA: Singular Publishing Group.

Wilson, B. E., Finley, C. C., Lawson, D. T., Wolford, R. D., Eddington, D. K., & Rabinowitz, W. M. (1991). Better speech recognition with cochlear implants. *Nature, 352*, 236–238.

Zimmerman-Phillips, S., Robbins, A. M., & Osberger, M. J. (1999). Assessing cochlear implant benefit in very young children. *Annals of Otology, Rhinology, and Laryngology*. Manuscript submitted for publication.

Zwolan, T. A., Kileny, P. R., & Telian, S. A. (1996). Self-report of cochlear implant use and satisfaction by prelingually deafened adults. *Ear and Hearing, 17*, 198–210.

APPENDIX 21A

CLARION® MULTI-STRATEGY™ COCHLEAR IMPLANT
Adult Social Benefits Questionnaire

NAME ______________________________ TODAY'S DATE ______________
CLINIC ______________________________ SURGERY DATE ______________

Please indicate the average number of hours that you use your CLARION daily: _________Hours

INSTRUCTIONS:

Please circle the answers that come closest to your feelings. Use the following scale as your guide. You should check *not applicable (NA)* **for a situation only if you do not, or cannot, participate for reasons other than your hearing loss. If, however, your hearing loss is the main reason for not participating, then you should mark one of the other choices.**

0 = Not Applicable

1 = Strongly Disagree

2 = Somewhat Disagree

3 = Disagree

4 = Agree

5 = Somewhat Agree

6 = Strongly Agree

APPENDIX 21B

CLARION® MULTI-STRATEGY™ COCHLEAR IMPLANT
Adult Social Benefits Questionnaire

Post-operative: **Since I have had my Clarion cochlear implant:**	**Not Applicable**	**Strongly Disagree**	**Somewhat Disagree**	**Disagree**	**Agree**	**Somewhat Agree**	**Strongly Agree**
				Circle One			
My overall quality of life has improved.	0	1	2	3	4	5	6
I am a happier person.	0	1	2	3	4	5	6
I am more comfortable in the company of strangers.	0	1	2	3	4	5	6
I participate in more social activities.	0	1	2	3	4	5	6
I am more relaxed in social situations.	0	1	2	3	4	5	6
I have more confidence.	0	1	2	3	4	5	6
I have increased my job opportunities.	0	1	2	3	4	5	6
I depend less on lipreading.	0	1	2	3	4	5	6
I have increased my social contacts.	0	1	2	3	4	5	6
I enjoy listening to music more.	0	1	2	3	4	5	6
I enjoy going to the movie theater more.	0	1	2	3	4	5	6
The quality of my speech has improved.	0	1	2	3	4	5	6
I am better able to modulate the loudness of my voice.	0	1	2	3	4	5	6
I feel safer.	0	1	2	3	4	5	6
I rely less on others.	0	1	2	3	4	5	6
I do things that I was uncomfortable doing before.	0	1	2	3	4	5	6
I am more independent.	0	1	2	3	4	5	6
I find using the telephone a less frustrating experience.	0	1	2	3	4	5	6
I enjoy calling family and friends.	0	1	2	3	4	5	6
I feel less isolated.	0	1	2	3	4	5	6

APPENDIX 21C

CLARION® MULTI-STRATEGY™ COCHLEAR IMPLANT
Adult Self-Reported Benefits Questionnaire

NAME ______________________ TODAY'S DATE ____________
CLINIC ______________________ SURGERY DATE ____________

INSTRUCTIONS:

Please circle the answers that come closest to your "everyday" experiences. Use the following scale as your guide. You should check *not applicable* (NA) for a situation only if you do not, or cannot, participate for reasons other than your hearing loss. If, however, your hearing loss is the main reason for not participating, then you should mark one of the other choices.

0 = Not Applicable	
1 = Never	
2 = Rarely	**(25% of the time)**
3 = Usually	**(at least 50% of the time)**
4 = Frequently	**(at least 75% of the time)**
5 = Always	**(100% of the time)**

APPENDIX 21D

CLARION® MULTI-STRATEGY™ COCHLEAR IMPLANT
Adult Self-Reported Benefits Questionnaire

Pre-operative: When I am wearing my hearing aid. **Post-operative: When I am wearing my Clarion cochlear implant.**	**Not Applicable**	**Never**	**Rarely**	**Usually**	**Frequently**	**Always**
	Circle One					
At the post-operative intervals only: I use a hearing aid in my other ear.	0	1	2	3	4	5
I am able to participate with little difficulty in a conversation with three or four others in a quiet environment.	0	1	2	3	4	5
I am able to participate in conversations with one or two others in a noisy environment such as a crowded restaurant.	0	1	2	3	4	5
I am **unable** to understand what is being said by someone who is speaking to me from across a room.	0	1	2	3	4	5
I am able to follow a lecture or sermon when I am able to see the speaker.	0	1	2	3	4	5
I am able to follow a lecture or sermon when I am **not** able to see the speaker.	0	1	2	3	4	5
I am able to understand the dialogue in a movie or at the theater.	0	1	2	3	4	5
I am able to understand the news on the car radio.	0	1	2	3	4	5
I am able to understand the news on the television without the use of captioning.	0	1	2	3	4	5
I am **unable** to participate in meetings with four or more others.	0	1	2	3	4	5
I am able to enjoy live music performances.	0	1	2	3	4	5
I am able to enjoy recorded music played on a stereo, Walkman or radio.	0	1	2	3	4	5
I am able to enjoy music on the car radio.	0	1	2	3	4	5
I am able to understand when an announcement is made over a public address system.	0	1	2	3	4	5
I am able to converse in an automobile when I am driving.	0	1	2	3	4	5
I am able to converse in an automobile when I am not driving.	0	1	2	3	4	5
I am able to participate in conversations with one or two others in a quiet environment.	0	1	2	3	4	5

Pre-operative: When I am wearing my hearing aid. **Post-operative: When I am wearing my Clarion cochlear implant.**	**Not Applicable**	**Never**	**Rarely**	**Usually**	**Frequently**	**Always**
	Circle One					
I am **unable** to converse over the telephone when I am familiar with the person speaking.	0	1	2	3	4	5
I am comfortable using the telephone.	0	1	2	3	4	5
I am able to converse over the telephone when I do not know the person speaking but know the topic being discussed.	0	1	2	3	4	5
I am **unable** to make appointments and reservations over the telephone.	0	1	2	3	4	5
I am able to converse over the telephone when I do not know the topic being discussed or the person speaking.	0	1	2	3	4	5
I am able to identify who is speaking over the telephone.	0	1	2	3	4	5
I am **unable** to tell the difference between male and female speakers over the telephone.	0	1	2	3	4	5
I am able to hear someone coming up behind me.	0	1	2	3	4	5

CHAPTER 22

Legal and Ethical Considerations in Hearing Instrument Dispensing

MICHAEL J. METZ, PH.D.

OUTLINE

(continued)

One of the most challenging issues of hearing health care concerns legal and ethical issues. Yet many dispensers, audiologists, and physicians—those professionals involved in dispensing of hearing instruments—may not be able to rationally discuss the issues at the base of our continuation in the health care field. Most who read this chapter belong to a professional organization. Yet relatively few have read the Code of Ethics of the organization to which they belong. One Code of Ethics is just like another, right? Furthermore, nobody likes to discuss ethics and morals. It just gets you into trouble because we cannot agree on what is right, wrong, or ethical. The individual can seldom convince his or her colleagues that one method of professional behavior is correct or ethical. Because we cannot legislate ethics or morals, discussing such questions doesn't change anyone's mind. Such attitudes can be dangerous. Frank and open discussions of the issues facing hearing instrument dispensing are essential if continued growth and appropriate professional recognition are to be achieved.

A clear definition and understanding of an ethical stance is necessary, not only to those who belong to a profession, but to those served by the profession—the consumers of products and services. Those both in and out of any professional field must know where the profession stands. This understanding is part of what is involved in belonging to a "profession." Understanding and consensus are necessary so that members of the profession follow the same rules in monitoring their own behavior and that of their colleagues. This chapter outlines the legal requirements and ethical objectives in the field of hearing instrument dispensing. Examples are offered so that those interested in such issues will have a place from which to depart on discussions regarding legal and ethical issues that affect the professional growth of hearing instrument dispensers.

In a litigious society, the issues of what is legal and ethical arise most often in the courts in the form of complaints against professional practices. Although extreme legal consequences do not happen regularly in the field of hearing instrument dispensing, it is unwise to wait until such legal actions occur before we consider, discuss, and arrive at a consensus of what we believe to be solid ethical and legal foundations.

As any profession evolves, ethical issues related to that profession generally tend to solidify. It is important that each member of the professional group understands and follows the rules, allowances, methods, and limitations of that group. In the 1970s and 1980s, many professions, including hearing instrument dispensing, were besieged with issues of state licensing and federal regulation. The resolution of these issues made hearing instrument dispensing more broadly accepted as a professional activity and tended to solidify methods of operation. This was accomplished despite arguments by opposing factions. In the 2000s, the field of hearing instrument dispensing is faced with the possibility of increased government regulation and control, especially in the context of health care changes. The inclusion of a chapter treating legal and ethical issues is a positive indication of increased interest in legal and ethical standards of practice.

DIFFERENTIATING LEGAL AND ETHICAL ISSUES

A discussion of laws and ethics must start at the level of differentiation between the two areas. There is an essential difference between law and ethical principle. For example, traffic laws require that you use an automobile turn signal indicator. If you make a turn without using the correct signal, you have broken the law and are subject to legal penalties. Contrast this illegal offense with the concept of driving courtesy, allowing a driver to merge ahead of you, for example, or changing freeway lanes to allow faster drivers to pass you. Such courtesies are examples of the difference between legal behavior and ethical behavior; they are also examples of socially conscious behavior. One can think of this responsibility to others as an awareness of the correct way to act and a willingness to do so.

Both ethics and the law are founded in public policy. Public ethics are concerned with following a socially accepted code of behavior, as determined by what society considers the right thing to do. Professional ethics are founded in the policy of professional organizations. Members of a professional body are expected to hold to a different level of function than would be seen in the behavior of others not in the professional organization. Professional members must not only function in a socially correct manner, they also are expected to function in a manner consistent with other members of the profession. Adherence to these correct behaviors is an inherent part of belonging to a professional body. Indeed, following professional guidelines of behavior is typically required for membership in the professional organization.

Professional ethics have a direct impact on every member of a given profession. The behavior of each member of any professional group affects all other members of the group. Even the behavior of others doing the same job as members of the professional group will determine what is correct. Individual behavior determines, in large part, the viability and credibility of the profession. Any professional group is composed of its members; the behavior of the members tends to define the group. Insofar as the standard behavior of members in the professional group differs from the expected and socially accepted public behavior, that behavior will define the profession. As a member of that profession, defined by expected behaviors, each member of the professional group will be held to the performance expectations of the others in that profession.

This level of expected professional behavior is a higher level than is generally expected from a social standpoint. Does the public expect a different level of behavior from a professional member, compared to a member of the general public? Yes, they do! The public expects the health care professional to perform his or her services on behalf of the consumer. This expectation of professional behavior extends to the point that those who provide services related to the profession are expected to perform at the same level of consumer awareness. For example, a nurse or other health care person working in the office of a physician and performing services on behalf of the physician is expected to comply to the same extent with the ethical requirements of the medical field.

ETHICAL CONCERNS OF THE HEARING INSTRUMENT DISPENSER

As a hearing instrument dispenser, you will be held to the ethics of your professional affiliation. Increasingly, you may be held to the standards of other organizations if you perform the same duties, imply that you perform the same duties, or have represented yourself in any manner as being associated with any other profession. If one attempts to create the impression that his or her duties are similar to another profession (such as medicine or law), one may be expected to live up to that standard of practice.

Even without formal training, for example, it has become the responsibility of the hearing instrument dispenser to be aware of ear diseases when fitting a hearing instrument. That is, the hearing instrument dispenser (HID) is expected to recognize some medical problems associated with hearing loss, despite the lack of a universal requirement that dispensers know specifically about ear diseases. The ability to determine if an ear is infected, diseased, or otherwise in need of medical treatment is presumed in the "warning signs" that HIDs must evaluate prior to taking an impression or fitting an instrument. It is presumed that awareness of these signs, and the subsequent appropriate referral, is necessary for the protection of the consumer. Protecting the consumer has become a part of the HID's responsibilities, in part because the HID has requested that responsibility. The profession of dispensing has evolved to the point that identifying such problems has become the normal standard of practice. Even though it is clinically impossible for the HID to function on the same educational or clinical plane as a physician, the dispenser may be held to the same standards of practice. Obviously, a provider who makes claims of possessing skills outside his or her scope of practice and training assumes the risk of serious legal consequences. The general term applied here is misrepresentation.

An example of expanding responsibilities involves the prerogative of diagnosis. Audiologists do not hold appropriate professional license, nor can they assume the privilege or responsibility of making a medical diagnosis. Yet if the test procedures that audiologists use involve tests for the presence or absence of an VIIIth nerve tumor, the reporting of tumor-positive results and appropriate follow-up for such a test finding may have legal and ethical consequences. It has become the standard of care that the audiologist report these findings as "indicative" of a serious medical problem. Failure to do so may be viewed as being inconsistent with the generally accepted standard of care rendered by an audiologist. In this situation, the audiologist may face serious legal consequences if appropriate reporting, referral, and follow-up procedures are not performed.

Even though it would be illegal for the audiologist to make a specific diagnosis, he or she must function as though such a diagnosis has been made. Functioning in such a manner has become the standard scope of audiological practice. It is assumed that anyone doing such tests is capable of correctly interpreting the tests and making judgments appropriate to the audiology profession. Therefore, although making a medical diagnosis is illegal, *not* making decisions about test results may not only have legal consequences, but also may be considered unethical.

CONTROL OF PROFESSIONAL DESTINY

Audiologists have learned through past experiences that, as a professonal entity, we should be the ones who determine our own destiny. Recall the past deliberations of the United States Food and Drug Administration (FDA) and United States Federal Trade Commission (FTC) hearings of the 1970s, which instituted mandatory trial periods, instrument guarantees, standard purchase agreements, and so forth. The actions of the FDA and FTC in 1993, which resulted in dictating to hearing aid manufacturers what and how they could advertise, serve as a particularly painful reminder that the government is taking close notice of what we say and do. As members of the profession to which we have elected to belong, we must be involved in the making and changing of the laws that affect our livelihoods. If we make or change laws, we will be codifying our standards of practice (our ethics) and allowing for enforcement of these ethical standards in the legal arena. The establishment of legal standards or laws is often preceded by the embodiment or codifying of standards of ethical practice.

If one conforms to the laws that govern the business aspects of a dispensing practice, the first criterion of professional business is met. Meeting the ethical requirements will serve to "seal" the public confidence in the profession. Differences between legalities and ethical considerations involve thoughts suggesting that:

- Individuals must obey the law; however, legal does not equate to ethical, and illegal does not equate to unethical.
- An individual may violate some ethical principles and still be legal. If specific issues arise and are warranted, one may be judged unethical by a governing professional body, but one cannot be prosecuted for violation of any written law.
- Legal and ethical issues are related. Unfortunately, at times they may be either closely or distantly related.
- Sometimes unethical is illegal, but one can conform to existing laws and still be judged unethical.
- Most of the time, illegal is unethical, because the ethical standards of organizations do not necessarily imply illegalities.
- Ethical behavior is always legal behavior.

Hearing health care professionals should control situations that threaten the ability to govern their own ethical proclamations. We must strive, perhaps, to make our ethics equal to or better than other health care providers. If we assume a professional provider position in the health care system and not one of sellers of prostheses, we cannot operate our practice solely as a sales-oriented entity. We cannot ignore profit, but must place it in a different role secondary to the well-being of the consumers we serve. This level of function is different from the function level of salespeople; it is one of care provider. When we control our own professional and ethical destiny, appropriate laws governing what we do and how we do it will follow.

The principle that "laws-follow-ethics" progression should teach us that while we can't legislate ethics, professional behavior dictated by ethical standards of our professional group can set the stage for the establishment of suitable ethical standards. We can determine the legal posture we will assume as professionals. Establishing a long-term legal position is absolutely necessary if hearing instrument dispensing is to flourish as a full-fledged member of the health care profession. The degree to which one is involved in these types of ethical decisions and the degree to which we all agree on what is the "right thing," will determine the speed at which the field progresses. It determines also the extent to which we will be included in health care plans.

SOME ETHICAL QUESTIONS

If we are concerned only with the technicalities and business aspects of instrument dispensing, legal and ethical behaviors may not take a primary position. We get involved only when a legal or ethical issue threatens our business. Misconceptions concerning ethics may be more easily understood if one considers the following "rules":

Rule 1

Everyone functions in what he/she perceives to be his or her own best interest. This is a basic rule of human behavior.

Rule 2

You don't want someone to tell you when you are illegal and/or unethical. This rule is inherently not true except on the level of personal standards of behavior. That which is legal is determined by law. You establish moral rules of conduct for yourself. All professions must adhere to laws governing their practice. Ethical issues are different. Ethical behavior is not situational, nor is it up to the person to determine. Personal ethics may be called morals. Morals, dependent on the individual, are subject to some degree of personal interpretation and can be influenced greatly by religious and other beliefs. Ethics are always based on what a group decides is right or correct. Sometimes individual interpretations of what the group would likely consider correct are allowed, but generally the members of the group as a whole determine what is correct. It is the responsibility of the group to determine appropriate behavior and to communicate this behavior standard to other members of the group. It is the responsibility of individual members of the group to function in a manner prescribed by the group.

Rule 3

Everyone who fails to act as you do is either illegal, unethical, or both. This rule is obviously not true. There are many things wrong with this rule.

The legal stance of any profession is determined by the educational and licensing requirements of the state in which the provider practices. There is no apparent argument here. Everyone would agree with this statement. The ethical stance of a profession, especially a health care profession, depends on the degree to which the provider of health care places the benefits to the other party ahead of the benefits to him/herself. On the surface, this statement of "patient-before-provider" would appear clear and obvious to most health care providers. Nonetheless, it is in this area that an emerging professional field struggles to rise to a level perceived by the public as acceptable. This raising of ethical standards and the relationship of ethics to legal requirements are best illustrated with examples.

Example 1

A business person is expected to provide adequate information to the customer. The customer may expect this information to be somewhat biased towards a particular product. An additional expectation is that the business person charge a "fair market" price for his or her goods and services. Profit is the motive of business, and the consumer usually realizes that fact. Deliberate ignorance of the truth will not be tolerated, but the salesperson may be expected to proclaim the benefits of the product perhaps to the exclusion of the problems. The consumer usually takes this sales approach with "a grain of salt." The business person is expected to take only a reasonable profit. The ethics of business are determined by the group to which the salesperson belongs—the business community. There is a hierarchy of business practices within the business community. Some business people may take more liberty with the facts than do others. A typical example of these different expectations may be found in the selling of automobiles. What is the typical impression of an automobile salesperson held by the general public? Is this impression different than that held for an insurance representative or a department store manager? Where does the leniency of the sales pitch become "failure to disclose"? Inspection of the generally held values to which we hold these and other members of the business world will reveal that while we expect honesty, we seldom expect such individuals to function in our best interest to the exclusion of their primary motive.

Example 2

Typically, a friend with whom a person does business is expected to act with more integrity, a higher standard, and with unquestioned honesty. That is, when the consumer deals with the business person who is a friend, it is typical that a higher level of disclosure is expected in the transaction. As such, a higher level of honesty is assumed by the buyer. This businessperson/friend is expected to function less in the interest of profit and more in the interest of the friend. When possible, that is why many people seek out a personal friend with whom to do business. The social ethic dictates against telling untruths to friends and tempers the business approach.

Example 3

A physician is expected to function in the best interest of the patient. Profit is still a motive for the physician, as it is for all those required to make a living. Nonetheless, the profit motive is placed in a different perspective in that the public expects the physician to serve the needs of the patient. Patient service takes a primary position in the physician's standards of practice. It is so stated in the physician's code of ethical behavior and historically has been practiced by all members of that profession. The public expects the physician to perform in this more selfless manner. The professional image of the physician requires this level of ethical performance.

PROFESSIONAL CATEGORIZATION

The general public places members of hearing health care professions in the same category as other medical professionals. Generally, health care professionals have made a great effort to place themselves in a position to inspire public trust. The expectations of the public are that, as licensed professionals dealing with health-related issues, we will put the patient's immediate needs ahead of our own.

This higher level of professional function or ethical behavior is what helps to define a profession. Professional behavior in the health care field requires that the person providing service function on behalf of another individual. The level at which the professional functions for the benefit of the other party, as well as the degree of the benefit to the other party, determines the level of ethics to which that professional is held. The converse of this statement is also true: The level of ethics adhered to by the professional field determines the expected altruistic behavior of the person providing the care.

Salesmen, professional carpet layers, or members of any profession that does not act specifically to protect its customers, may belong to a trade group and may even have a Code of Ethics or Behavior. They are not, however, subject to professional standards and ethical levels of function other than those that apply to the correctness of their business practices.

At this point, one should be aware of the evolution of the hearing instrument dispensing field in which the level of provision of goods and services to the public may no longer be sufficient to avoid reprisals on ethical or legal grounds. A higher level of functioning may be necessary not only because of the educational and technical advances, but because of the level of service provided by others who offer similar goods and services. Over the years, hearing instrument dispensing has made significant progress in presenting a professional image to the consuming public. A part of this changing professional image involves a change in ethical behavior. Ethics cannot be taught, but ethics and ethical standards can be explained. Behavior can be changed. The better hearing instrument dispensers understand ethical questions and the more that they function in the best interest of their patients with hearing impairment, the better prepared they will be to meet consumer needs.

LEGAL CONSIDERATIONS

Hearing instrument dispensers make every effort to be legal. Legal behavior consists primarily of two functional areas—advertising and contracts. Other legal considerations may arise from time to time, such as sales approaches, descriptions and predictions of benefits, pricing of the products and accompanying services, disclosures, and required legal statements. Legal issues involving contracts and advertising constitute the baseline, however. To a large extent, contracts and advertising set the tone for the professional dispensing practice.

Defining Legal Contracts

Hearing instrument sales contracts should outline exactly what is expected from each party involved in the contractual agreement. From a legal standpoint, a contract should limit the liability of all parties to the contract and should specify each party's responsibilities. Usually, contracts relating to hearing instrument sales and services involve only the buyer of the instrument and the dispenser of that instrument. There is, however, a large variation in contracts and contract language. Many contracts lack the basic fundamentals of what is legally required.

The minimum legal requirements for the delivery of a hearing instrument may vary slightly by state. Nonetheless, the essential elements of the contract will remain the same.

- In return for the charges relating to the instrument and associated services, the consumer expects to find considerable information specified on the contract. A simple bill of sale is usually not sufficient for such transactions.
- Instrument cost, dispensing services, earmolds, batteries, and all other supplies given to the consumer should be detailed on the contract. This protects not only the consumer, but also the dispenser.
- Terms of the guarantees, if any, should be clearly stated, as should any fees or costs not refundable to the consumer.
- The name of the consumer and the hearing instrument dispenser should appear on the contract. Typically, addresses and telephone numbers of both parties are incorporated into the identifying information.
- It is required that the manufacturer, instrument model number(s), and serial number(s) of the instrument(s) appear on the agreement. These items are basic and should appear on all contracts regardless of the state in which the hearing instrument dispenser practices.
- The return policy as specified by the state in which the transaction is consummated must be outlined on the contract.
- The standard and required length of a trial period is 30 calendar days from the date the contract is signed. This time period may be extended but cannot be shortened. The dispenser expects the instrument to be returned by the end of the trial period if the consumer requests a refund. The dispenser expects the instrument to be returned in normal, working condition. It is generally agreed that if the consumer damages or loses the instrument within the trial period, he/she cannot expect money to be returned. Without specifically stating such on the contract, this return for credit policy may not be enforceable.

The consumer expects the hearing instrument(s) to be delivered in proper working order. The consumer expects that the dispenser will provide all services related to the fitting of the instrument and the earmold. The consumer expects the instrument to be warranted against defects. In brief, the contract should be clear and unambiguous with respect to such items as:

- Make, model, and serial number(s) of the instrument(s) being sold.
- Names and addresses of the buyer and the seller.
- Exact costs (these should be itemized to delineate products from services).
- A statement concerning instrument condition, such as new, reconditioned, as-is, and so forth.
- Current hearing instrument dispenser license and/or certification information.
- Specifics of instrument warranty or guarantee.
- Return policies, specific lengths of time, and exact specification of expiration date(s).
- Fees that are or are not refundable (these should be itemized in exact detail).
- Follow-up services and tangible goods that are included in the agreement.
- The sources of all additional charges made to parties of the contract.

- The date the contract was signed by both parties.
- The signatures of all parties involved in the contract.

Some states may require additional contract information. For example, California *requires t*he Assistive Device Warranty Act (the Song-Beverly Consumer Warranty Act) wording, set in 10-point sized type. Such wording must appear on all sales contracts. Some states may require additional information. Cooling off periods and notification of such time periods may be required on out-of-office sales. Should the instrument be used or reconditioned, or should it be sold with less than the standard warranty, the contract should be clear in defining these limitations.

Contract Modifications

Modifications of contracts, as determined by the dispenser, should be considered carefully. For example, if the dispenser adds that batteries are included with the hearing instrument without specifying how many batteries and for how long, the contract may be interpreted that batteries are included for the length of the warranty. Another additional example concerns the 1-year loss and damage policy provided for most hearing instruments. Most contracts fail to inform the buyer that, if the instrument is replaced during the coverage period for loss and damage, the manufacturer has fulfilled its legal obligation. That is, the manufacturer will not be obligated to replace the instrument if lost a second time. Some dispensers have discovered this the hard way. If the contract does not specifically state the terms of the loss and damage policy, the dispenser, not the manufacturer, is the one to whom the consumer turns for resolution.

Additions to contracts that support or clarify the dispenser's business practices may appear to be appropriate but may lead to future trouble. One should consider the following.

- Does the contract contain promises that cannot, or will not, be realized?
- Do contract modifications imply benefits that are impossible to achieve?
- Do the contract modifications make things more or less clear?

Federal Trade Commission regulations are presented here in a summarized form (courtesy of the Hearing Aid Dispensers Examining Committee, State of California, 1994). These regulations require the following information to appear on any hearing instrument sales contract:

- Warrantor's name and mailing address.
- Who is protected by the warranty, including limitations.
- Precisely what parts, components, or characteristics and properties the warranty covers and what it excludes.
- What items or services the warrantor will pay for, and those, if any, for which the consumer must pay.
- When the warranty term begins (if other than the date of purchase).
- The warranty's duration.
- Whom to contact to obtain warranty service (including names, addresses, and telephone numbers).
- Step-by-step instructions to follow to obtain service.
- Any expenses the consumer may be required to pay.

It is important to have contracts reviewed by an attorney. No one would ask an attorney's advice on how to fit a hearing instrument, but it would seem reasonable to ask an attorney's advice relative to legal contract issues. Although most contract attorneys cannot be legally bound to ensure that your contracts conform to all existing laws, they will find the obvious errors in almost all contracts.

Regarding contracts, a dispenser gets little assistance from most hearing instrument manufacturers. Dispensers presume that providing customers with legal advice involves a more visible legal profile than is necessary for their functioning. The manufacturers hesitate to assume legal responsibility when they do not have to do so. If the manufacturers gave legal advice, their attorneys would probably advise that they charge for it because it increases their legal liability. No one should increase legal exposure without being adequately compensated for such exposure. More importantly, manufacturers may not know much about local or state requirements beyond those that are required in the manufacturing procedures.

There is no such thing as a perfect contract. There are, however, basic documents that will help you to draw up a legally viable agreement. Most libraries have reference books on basic business agreements. These basic forms may need modification, but they provide a reasonable starting point. It may be more cost effective for a dispensing group to produce a standard contract and then share the cost of an attorney's review. If in doubt, the attorney's fee can be significantly less than the cost of being sued by the consumer.

A few thoughts are in order concerning spoken and unspoken agreements. There are other expectations, by the consumer and the dispenser, which do not appear on the contract. These expectations, when inadequately covered in written form on the contract, can be viewed as legally binding on both parties to the contract. For example, most dispensers expect that the consumer will be cooperative. This cooperation is essential to the correct fitting of an instrument, but required cooperation is subjective and typically is not mentioned in the contract. The contract usually does not mention that the consumer will not use the instrument in a damaging manner and will try to the best of his or her ability to use the instrument in a logical and effective manner. If the consumer does not use the instrument correctly or damages the instrument during the course of normal use, there can be no penalties unless stated in the contract. The consumer may have some responsibility for hearing aid misuse, even if it is not stated in the contract. It is difficult to outline such expectations in a contract. When hearing instrument misuse occurs, it is more likely than not that the dispenser will return the instrument and refund money to the consumer. This may be so even though it may be determined that the consumer failed in the proper performance of what the instrument dispenser expected from the user.

Attorneys who have dealt with dispenser-versus-consumer complaints and subsequent legal actions state that many of these actions arise out of issues promised, implied, or otherwise incorrectly alluded to by the dispenser. The consumer-turned-plaintiff alleges that the dispenser-turned-defendant promised that the instruments would eliminate background noise, be invisible in the ear, never need batteries, and so forth. The dispenser replies that these promises were never made and that the consumer-plaintiff did not understand what was truly stated. Too many hearing aid sales have been made with these types of misunderstandings as an implied part of the agreement. The buyer may expect things that are unrealistic, and the dispenser fails to clarify these misconceptions. The question is, "Where is the responsibility?" The answer, of course, has considerable legal precedent in the realm of complete disclosure.

What the dispenser agrees to deliver to the consumer is obvious in the exact terms of the contract. What is actually delivered may not be so obvious. Failure to communicate specific information means that the buyer may assume more than intended or expect less difficulty than is reasonable. The medical profession has learned, via rather large monetary settlements in some cases, the consequences of failure to completely disclose all aspects of surgery, care, or treatment. The hearing health care professional may expect similar, although not so serious, consequences of failure to disclose or failure to adequately explain. These behaviors may be judged illegal. Recall that all illegal actions most likely also will be judged as unethical.

Here is a suggestion to help determine the atmosphere in which consumers are treated in a legal manner. How one deals with a patient/client/customer may help the hearing health care professional make a meaningful differentiation. That is, the way one thinks about patients/clients may help to determine how they are to be treated. Thinking of the consumer as a person needing service, expertise, and sophisticated clinical help may aid in putting the consumer's needs in the appropriate primary position. One should think of the consumer as more of a patient and less of a source of profit. One should establish the boundaries of a dispensing practice according to good business principles: location, advertising and promotion, necessary clinical tools and technical skills, appropriate accounting practices, and reasonable prices. Then, the clinician may proceed with dispensing *clinical* services to individuals with hearing impairment. This approach assures legality and also puts one well on the road to functioning legally and ethically.

Make sure that sales contracts are in order. Make sure that they contain all the required information and protect not only the dispenser, but also the consumer. If the contract does not protect both parties, it generally will be held invalid. Assure that all necessary contracts are in place before proceeding. Sales contracts, rental contracts, contracts for loaner instruments, additional services, insurance, and so forth, are a part of the required paperwork. Be sure that everybody involved in the contract receives a complete copy of the agreement. No-carbon-required (NCR) copies assure that all parties to the contract get identical information. Copies are less expensive than legal expenses.

Specify exactly what is to be delivered for an agreed upon price. Do this not only on sales contracts, but also on any price quotes. Estimates of the cost of goods and services are acceptable if they are specified as estimates. It would be prudent to specify the expiration date of the estimate. One would be hard pressed to honor an estimate for the purchase of a hearing instrument that was 2, 3, or more years old.

Repair Contracts

Hearing instrument repair contracts are another problem source. Repair contracts are simple to devise. What happens when the consumer is quoted the usual price for repair and warranty and the factory cost is twice what was expected? A well-worded repair contract not only limits the dispenser's liability in assuming more of the cost than good accounting practices would dictate as normal, but makes the repair cost understandable to the consumer. A good repair contract will protect both parties and eliminate arguments when higher-than-normal repair charges are received.

Loaner hearing aid contracts are essential if one provides this service to the consumer. Otherwise, one may loan and subsequently lose instruments that are better than those being repaired. How does one enforce the replacement cost of lost loaner instruments? What happens if the consumer causes the loaner instrument to malfunction? All these things must be stated in the loaner hearing aid contract to provide this service in a legal manner. What if the consumer is so pleased with the loaner instrument that he/she does not return it? Without a valid loaner hearing aid contract, one has no legal recourse to be compensated for the "lost" instrument.

Consumer Complaints

Suppose one fails to write all these things down as a standard contract? Where do consumers go when problems arise and specifics are not in writing? If hearing instrument specialists do not satisfy the consumer, the consumer will generally file a complaint with the Better Business Bureau, the State Licensing Board, or local and state professional organizations. The Better Business Bureau will generally call or write asking for the dispenser's understanding of the disagreement. The Bureau generally keeps a list of companies that have complaints lodged against them. The Bureau has no power to enforce but does communicate with law enforcement agencies when situations or circumstances demand some type of action.

Trade, local, or state organizations also have no legal authority but can help solve the consumer's complaint before a government agency intervenes. Generally these organizations conduct a superficial investigation by talking to both parties and attempting to arrive at a compromise at best, and full restitution to either party at worst. A good example of the interceding activities of a typical organization is the "ethics committee" of state or local dispensing organizations.

If the consumer lives in a state with an enforceable licensing law, there is a state licensing board. This board seeks information about the supposed "wrongdoing" and may take one of several courses of action. This board may abandon the complaint due to a misunderstanding by the consumer. If the complaint has merit, the board may issue warnings or impose censure on the dispenser. The board may remand the case to local law enforcement authorities for further investigation, arrest, detainment, or other legal action if the complaints are sufficient in degree or number to warrant such action.

PRODUCT ADVERTISING

It is tempting to manage this topic with only two words of advice—don't advertise. The rationale for this approach involves the widespread aversion to any type of public or media advertising held by many professional people. This professional, no-advertising stance still represents the standard of practice by many clinicians in other professions. It is neither illegal nor unethical to advertise. The law allows truthful advertising as a protection to the consumer. It has been decided in legal proceedings that professional groups and ethical boards of professional organizations cannot prohibit advertising.

The issue of advertising was highlighted by a legal decision in 1978 (National Society of Professional Engineers vs. United States, 1978) involving a professional engineering association that ruled the advertising by one professional engineer violated the Code of Ethics of his profession. The engineer brought legal action against the association and prevailed in the appellate courts. The legal logic was that an organization cannot censure the individual's attempt to place his or her name before the public in the form of advertising. It was ruled that such action constituted a restraint of trade and a violation of an individual's right to free speech. This legal decision has been construed to allow members of all professional organizations to advertise their services. Prior to this decision, all media advertising by members of the medical and dental professions, hospitals, and suppliers of professional goods and services had not been deemed appropriate on ethical grounds.

This legal decision changed the way in which some professional bodies looked at advertising. It has influenced current methods of advertising that many dispensers employ. Prior to this decision, hearing health care professionals commonly advertised price, products, and services. Many dispensers advertise in this manner. The effect of advertising by professional groups is also evident in the deliberations of the Food and Drug Administration and the Federal Trade Commission (FTC) (1993).

Federal government agencies have stated and supported their decisions with definitive actions. Manufacturing claims and those of the dispensing community that cannot be documented by peer-reviewed research will not be tolerated. Claims of noise reduction capabilities of hearing aid circuits based only on anecdotal information, for example, have been disallowed by these government agencies. Following the decision by the FDA and the FTC, considerable discussion occurred regarding questions of what constitutes legitimate advertising and appropriate, substantiating research for claims of instrument performance. It may be some years before these issues are completely resolved.

The issues themselves, however, indicate the gradual change from a strictly business approach in advertising to an approach based on professional practices. That is, it may have been considered borderline to make claims of instrument performance in the past. Now federal and state government agencies, as well as the ethics committees of professional organizations, are monitoring the advertising practices of their constituents.

In a larger sense, it behooves all dispensers to maintain a level of advertising that places an increased emphasis on the professional aspect of the dispensing field. If the profession is to be judged publicly, the appearance of advertising and the gradual movement of the dispensing community into the area of "professionalism" requires this constraint. Although some dispensers adhere to old advertising patterns, over time these methods may be judged unethical.

Unethical advertisement may never be judged illegal. Issues such as these have been ruled on by various courts, including the United States Supreme Court. For specific discussions regarding advertising, the reader is referred to the following cases:

- Medical Association versus Federal Trade Commission, 638 f.2d 433, 449 (2d 1980.
- Arizona versus Maricopa County Medical Society, 457 U.S. 332, 348-49, 1982.
- Brunswick Corporation versus Pueblo Bowl-O-Mat, Inc., 429 U.S. 477, 488, 1977.
- Goldfarb versus Virginia State Par, 421 U.S. 773, 1975.
- National Society of Mechanical Engineers versus United States, op.cit.

In short, these cases made clear that many types of professional regulation or limitation of advertising violate the laws governing restriction of trade. As such, there are no legal limitations on the type, quality, quantity, and direction of advertisement other than what would violate the truth. These violations of truth are typically defined by the Business Codes or the Business and Professions Codes of each state. As disconcerting as this concept may be, there are complex and confusing legal principles involved. The truer course is that the nature and extent of advertising should be determined by a peer group of professional associations affected. Recall that people who perform the same professional duties are essentially members of the same professional group whether they elect to join the group or not.

State and federal business codes prohibit advertisement that is false, misleading, or deceptive. The codes prevent the advertiser from stating claims that are false or misleading. They prevent implying statements that are deceptive. A reasonable model for legal advertising has been determined in California. The following are requirements under California Business and Professions Codes:

> *Price advertising must be exact, without the use of phrases like "as low as," "and up," "lowest prices," or words or phrases of similar import. (Advertising a discount is not illegal unless it is misleading or false.)*
>
> *Any advertisement using words of comparison must be based on verifiable data substantiating the comparison.*
>
> *In price advertising, the price for each product or service must be clearly identifiable.*
>
> *The price advertised for a product must include charges for related professional services, including dispensing and fitting services, unless the advertisement clearly states otherwise.*
>
> *The dispenser may not compensate or give anything of value to a representative of the press, radio, television, or other communication medium for professional publicity unless the fact of compensation is made known in the publicity.*
>
> *Business names should not be so broad as to connote comprehensive and diagnostic hearing services unless the dispenser is also licensed as a physician or audiologist. (For example, it would be considered incorrect to advertise the "XYZ Hearing Aid Center" as the "XYZ Hearing Center.")*
>
> *Dispensers should not advertise "free hearing test" or hearing tests without further*

qualification, because the statement connotes comprehensive, diagnostic testing not within a hearing instrument dispenser's scope of practice. It is acceptable to advertise "free test to determine if you could be helped by a hearing aid" or to use words of similar import to clarify the nature of the testing performed by a hearing instrument dispenser.

Sending consumers preset appointment information as part of a direct mail solicitation is prohibited because it is deceptive and misleading and thus constitutes a violation of the code.

Hearing Instrument dispensers should not utilize anonymous or blind advertising, but should disclose the name of the business or dispenser in each ad. For example, it is incorrect in the context of an ad to state, "If you have a hearing problem, call 123-4567. Instead, it could be stated "For information on how you can be helped by a hearing instrument, call Mr. Dispenser, a licensed hearing instrument dispenser, at the XYZ Hearing Aid Center."

If an ad refers to a dispenser's board certification, the ad should indicate specifics, written in a manner that is easily understood by consumers. Also, the California licensing law provides for licensing dispensers, not specialists.

Correct: John Doe, Hearing Aid Dispenser

Jane Doe, Board Certified Hearing Instrument Specialist

Incorrect: Jack Doe, BC-HIS

Jill Doe, Hearing Aid Specialist

Laws and regulations regarding correct advertising may vary depending on the state in which the dispenser practices, but the rather strict and prohibitive California law represents the direction in which the regulations concerning advertising are moving. It would appear that such movement is necessary to enable consumers to differentiate between more simple business entities and professional entities.

The California regulations may provide a model for any state regulation in that it would generally be considered fairly conservative in scope and yet broad in application. The state licensing board where a dispenser practices should be contacted to procure the specific regulations that apply in that state.

ETHICAL ISSUES

At this juncture, let us discuss when ethical considerations, as they apply to a clinical practice involving hearing instrument dispensing, must be considered. Ethical behavior is that which is considered by the group as the right thing to do. Stated another way, ethics are "a consensus of norms and behaviors" founded in public policy and based on public opinion but applied to a specific group of people. Ethical behavior involves the concept of what would be considered "correct" group behavior.

Ethical professional behavior is defined by comparing individual behavior to that of the average peer member of the group. Until recently, most hearing instruments were dispensed by members of a group that did not have professional licensure. This group was composed of people who managed the retail aspects of hearing aids. In the 1980s and 1990s, however, retail instrument sales changed. Today audiologists or physicians dispense a significant number of the hearing instruments in the United States.

The hearing instrument dispenser of today has more education, more clinical skills, and better access to technology. Because the composition of the peer group has changed, comparisons to the "average" dispenser have changed. It is no longer correct to assume that a hearing aid will be dispensed by a salesperson with little or no health-based training. As more dispensers have training in audiology and medicine, things considered correct, ethical, and legal in the past may not be correct, ethical, or legal today. Additionally, dispensers who behaved in a certain manner in times past may not act similarly now because aspects of that past behavior may be judged unethical or illegal in light of the new make-up of the profession of dispensing.

Correspondingly, the privileges and expanding responsibilities of a dispensing professional may be of more concern to those who have been dispensing for a long time rather than those just entering the field. This expanding professional responsibility is evident in the requirement to refer consumers who demonstrate ear and hearing problems that are beyond the clinical skills of the dispenser. Not meeting this particular responsibility may lead to ethical censure or legal difficulties. This aspect of responsibility for referral without privilege of diagnosis may be difficult for some to accept. An argument that experience in practicing will suffice for academic training is not sufficient for reasons that ought to be obvious to anyone who gives more than cursory thought to the problem. Caring for ill people for any number of years will not teach the caregiver the practice of medicine. Although the dispenser may have a high success rate of fitting hearing aids, the treatment of hearing loss encompasses much more than that. Successful hearing instrument fittings are not the measure of clinical prowess any more than bandaging a wound is the measure of medical expertise.

The professional practice of hearing instrument dispensing, in moving from a retail business to a more science-based discipline, is changing quickly and dramatically. Factors defining ethical behavior are also evolving as the "peer group" is changing and growing. The ethical behavior required by the group is reflective of the time in which the behavior occurs. This does not mean that unethical behavior is situational. It simply means that, when the act or action was committed, the judgment of ethics must take place in that time. Prior to the early 1980s, for example, it was considered unethical for audiologists to dispense hearing instruments. Audiologists who did dispense prior to those years were judged to be unethical by the audiology profession. Audiologists who dispensed hearing instruments before 1979 were considered unethical by the peer group to which those individuals belonged. In the year 2000, the same action could be judged as ethical by the group because attitudes and regulations have changed. Stated another way, ethics change with respect to time, educational degree, who they include, what is good and bad, what actions are accepted, how they used to be, what they may become, and so forth. Professionalism through ethical stance has to do with the relationship the individual has with the group at that time. One cannot persist in methods that were correct in the past without risk of being judged unethical.

Although ethics cannot be legislated in the typical sense, they can be defined and enforced in both the legal and professional arenas. Ethical conduct should be judged by the group to whom such conduct applies. Should the professional group fail to pay close attention to issues that affect the public, there are alternatives that may be set into motion. If ethical matters are not judged closely and in the public interest by the professional group, they may end up before the public courts. When ethical matters are judged by the public or legal interests, the interpretation of an ethical violation may be different than that which the associated group would have interpreted. Consider the following examples.

Examples of Ethical Issues

Example 1

It is generally believed that hearing loss detracts from the pleasures of life determined by adequate communication and that hearing better is a positive contribution to living a better life. Being able to hear and understand more is good. When the FDA ruled on this matter, however, they concluded that equating better hearing with better life could be construed by the consumer differently than what was intended by the manufacturer. Therefore, this statement constituted illegal advertising. Having the FDA judge this matter was not in the best interest of the dispensing profession. How could this situation have been avoided? Who should make the decisions concerning how and what to advertise? What sanctions should be carried out when rules of advertising are violated?

Example 2

In one state, an attorney employed by the state's board of licensing offered a legal opinion: The removal of cerumen by an audiologist constituted "the invasion of a bodily orifice" and thus was not within the audiologist's scope of practice. This ruling, while not constituting a legal interpretation of the licensing law of that state (only the attorney general or the legislature of the state can so bind the interpretation of the law), precluded audiologists from the management of cerumen. (It really does not prevent an audiologist from managing cerumen, it just precludes his or her malpractice insurance from covering problems arising from such management.) It becomes, in a practical sense, "illegal" or ill advised to do such management. This stance makes the management of cerumen removal risky in that state. It may be legal as well as ethical in other states. Clearly, this is an example of someone not well versed in the professional training, abilities, and scope of the profession making a judgment about the legalities and ethical behaviors of that profession. This judgment is not considered to be in the best interest of audiologists or hearing instrument dispensers. It would have been better if the decision about what lies within the scope of professional practice had been left to the professional people affected by such a decision. How does this decision or situation affect the ability of the hearing instrument dispenser to expand the scope of practice? Would the removal of cerumen by an audiologist be considered illegal, unethical, both, or neither?

The first example is illustrative of the fact that actions that seem right may be judged wrong. The second example illustrates that actions may be illegal but may not be unethical. In general, it is generally conceded that most illegal actions are also unethical. Nonetheless, this seemingly obvious statement may not always be held correct.

It is always interesting to present examples of ethical dilemmas. Discussion of, or thought directed to, these examples may help clarify thinking about ethical issues. Recall that ethical decisions cannot be made without judging how the professional group would agree or disagree with the decision. The behavior and the group go together.

Examples of Ethical Dilemmas

Ethical Dilemma No. 1

What happens when what you think is good for your business profits conflicts with what is best for the customer or the patient? (Does your choice of descriptor for the consumer define the situation as primarily being one of a business or of a professional relationship?) The way you think about patient versus customer may determine your answer to this conflict. Individuals trained in the fields of medicine, audiology, and instrument dispensing are obligated to treat the consumer in a professional manner. This obligation should be tantamount to all others. If you hold yourself to be a professional, the public expects a higher standard with respect to the manner in which the consumer is treated. This professional treatment also holds with respect to profits. That is, if you act as a professional, you will be expected to place the benefits to the consumer (patient) in the foremost position. You can be concerned with profits, but only in a secondary manner. This difference may be the most definitive in comparing a professional relationship to a business relationship.

As any observer can verify, the relationship of business to the health care profession became one of the most difficult to define in the closing years of the 20th century. The advent of managed health care and the concomitant application of business principles to patient management have produced quandaries with which state and federal governments have grappled. As the millennium turned, there had yet to be a resolution of the ethical conflicts of business versus health care. This conflict is present in the hearing health care arena as witnessed by the next dilemma.

Ethical Dilemma No. 2

Is it best for your business to maximize profits by charging the most for your products and services? Is this practice ever in conflict with your professional ethics or the professional ethics of persons in the same or similar situations? Of course it conflicts! It usually conflicts when that which is professionally appropriate interferes with the maximum profits generated in the relationship between you and the consumer. If it did not conflict, there would be no dilemma, and everyone would always do the "correct" thing. The resolution of this conflict is the key issue. The manner in which you approach the situation determines whether the resolution is ethical. Unfortunately, some may decide to manage the situation in a manner that significantly differs from the way in which other members of the profession would resolve the problem. If your decision differs from that which would come from the group, your resolution of the situation may be judged as unethical.

Ethical Dilemma No. 3

There is a classic story of a student in a college class of business ethics who told the instructor that he understood the concepts of ethics, but asked the instructor to give examples of what constituted good *business* ethics. The instructor replied that the student really did not understand, and the question he asked was a demonstration of this lack of understanding. Some people don't understand this example. Do you?

There is an adage that states all is fair in love, war, and business. What the professor was trying to get across to the class was that all may not be "fair" in business. There are rules of conduct in the business world that relate to fairness, profit, and general methods of operation. If a person in business acts in a manner that is not "fair" or not "morally correct," it would be consistent that the manner in which that person conducts business corresponded to a given set of *personal* morals. A person who acts "fairly" would be judged as "ethical," no matter if the action is in the personal or the business arena. The professor expected that student to realize that all people have a sense of what is fair and reasonable. To violate that sense just because the arena changes in the business world is inconsistent. The maintenance of profit does not make all business decisions valid.

Ethical Dilemma No. 4

If the consumer can be helped equally well with hearing instruments that are appropriate but less expensive, are you unethical if you recommend the more expensive instruments? (Is an auto salesman unethical by recommending all the options?) What if you believe the more expensive instruments may be better, they just haven't been proven yet? What are your professional responsibilities for knowing what constitutes the newest technologies and applications? What are your professional responsibilities for being well versed in the research and clinical literature related to hearing aid dispensing? Could you ever fit a patient with instruments that have not been verified in terms of demonstrable benefits?

Belonging to a professional group implies that certain minimum behaviors are maintained. Among them are appreciation and protection for the consumer of professional services and professional knowledge. The maintenance of professional knowledge—keeping current with technology and the ability to apply the technology effectively—is so important that most professional organizations require continuing education as a criterion for continued membership. Indeed, this aspect of "professionalism" is so important to the consumer that it has been legislated into many state licensing laws to assure compliance of the members of the profession.

This dilemma poses difficult decisions. Many times, new technology reaches the marketplace quickly without the necessary, objective clinical research to prove its efficacy. Widespread advertising encourages consumers to investigate, and the dispenser is faced with an eager patient/customer and only the anecdotal verifications of the manufacturer or advertisement to support the new technology. As digital signal processors expand the hearing aid marketplace, this dilemma may become more pronounced.

Ethical Dilemma No. 5

It is argued that "I must make a reasonable profit so I can stay in business and my consumer can be given continued (or correct, best, appropriate) services." That profit mandate enables the hearing health care professional to assess a reasonable charge (or more than the guy down the street who doesn't know as much as I do). This could be a "closer call" than the prior example because higher levels of training, more experience, and so forth, ought to be worth more than inexperience or no training. The judgement of ethical versus unethical lies in how the other members of the professional group to which the clinician belongs (or aspires to belong to) would judge this situation. If that professional group thinks those costs are right, then they are right by definition.

The difficulty is that you do not get to belong to two different groups depending on the decision you want at the time. That is, it would be inappropriate to hold the patient's interest in the highest position until such time as it becomes more beneficial to consider profits. A correct professional decision may not be the same as the correct business decision. If the decisions were the same, the answer would be obvious, and no dilemma would exist.

This dilemma is slightly less obvious when one considers the situation in which a dispenser attempts to make the impression that there is more education, more clinical expertise, or more sophistication present than actually exists. Consider, for example, a dispenser in a white laboratory coat, offering information of a diagnostic or therapeutic nature to a consumer sitting in a typical physician's examination chair. Is the consumer's impression in this situation consistent with the education of the professional involved? Would the consumer be more likely to place more confidence in the advice of this person? Why? Is the impression one suggesting that provider of these services appears to be a "doctor"? If the provider is not a physician, under what circumstances would this situation be judged as unethical?

Ethical Dilemma No. 6

For many years, hearing instrument dispensing practices included dispensing offices that sold products from only one manufacturer. Recently, we have seen the advent of large "chains" of offices. What types of situations could occur in these employment settings that would pose an ethical dilemma? The difficulties in what used to be known as a "single-line" office, such as lack of current technology that exists in an instrument from another manufacturer, have been replaced to some degree with similar problems facing a multiple-line office chain.

Consider a situation in which the home office has arranged for exceptionally deep discounts from a certain manufacturer. This arrangement appears in each chain office as an "encouragement" for selling instruments from this manufacturer in preference to other manufacturers. If the sale of instruments is based on financial considerations only and not on clinical appropriateness, would this constitute an ethical dilemma?

Assuming that a sales goal has been met, does it pose a conflict of interest for the dispenser or audiologist? That is, should the dispenser or audiologist be compensated in accordance with the number of sales from the company offering the deepest discount? Does it place the provider of hearing instruments at ethical risk to be considered for retention or promotion based on the quantity of sales?

Is it unrealistic to expect that the managers of the corporation will select provider/employees for other types of rewards (trips, vacations, or other incentives) based on factors other than profit? How does an ethical provider of health services of any kind solve these potentially unethical situations?

Ethical Dilemma No. 7

At the end of the year, having met a sales goal for instruments dispensed, the hearing health care provider is taken on a pleasure trip along with many other providers who have met similar goals. What situations or conditions would change the ethical dilemma? What would you think of a physician who prescribed specific brand medications based on the reward of a "free" trip at the end of the year?

Ethical Dilemma No. 8

In the late 1990s, there appeared on the World Wide Web various sites that permitted a person to purchase hearing aid(s) at considerable discounts from typical retail price. These Web sites and promotional methods caused considerable debate among dispensers. Legal as well as ethical considerations of such practices were questioned.

There are some interesting dilemmas presented in this example. If the actual business location to which the Web site pertains is located in a state that allows mail-order sales of instruments, is the sale of instruments to citizens of those states that do not allow mail-order sales illegal? Consider the dispenser who participates in such sales by providing ear impressions, instrument fitting and setting, follow-up services, and so forth. Is this dispenser acting in a legal and ethical manner? What are this dispenser's obligations if the instruments ordered "independently" were inappropriate for this patient or the hearing loss? If these instruments do not work properly, how much of this responsibility must the local dispenser assume? How much responsibility does the Web site assume? For that matter, is the operator of the Web site acting in an ethical manner?

Sales of hearing instruments costing thousands of dollars will eventually involve different methods to lower retail costs. These methods will no doubt fall outside the limits of what the dispensing field now considers legal and ethical. Incorporation of these methods into the field of hearing instrument dispensing will alter many perceptions.

Ethical Dilemma No. 9

What's wrong with this statement: "An ethical act is any act after which you feel good?" Answer: "Nothing," so long as it applies to a personal ethical system. What does this statement say about everyone establishing his or her own ethical standards? (Recall that professional ethics are the standards of a group.) Could this be stated more appropriately, "A professional ethical act is any act after which the group would feel good"?

It is easier to define legal than it is to define ethical. If it's legal, it's in the book and can be readily referenced. If it's ethical, it's only written down in general terms in a Code of Ethics. Furthermore, the decision of "correct" must always be representative of the consensus thinking of the group at that particular time. As the group opinions of right and wrong change, so does the ethical judgement. That is one reason why ethics (and, on a personal basis, morals) are not legislated in the standard manner. The legislative act would need to be changed too often. This changing concept of correctness makes it harder for us to define ourselves. The extent to which we are professional is determined, to some degree, by the altruistic level of these concepts of the right way to effectively manage our consumers. We define ourselves by our actions. That is why ethics are a more interesting topic and give rise to more arguments. It is these arguments and discussions that help us as a profession to define what we do and the methods of behavior that will become the consensus of the group.

CONCLUSION

The reality that people expect more from doctors, lawyers, and other recognized professionals than they do from most business people has been reviewed in this chapter. When the members of the public believe that they are not being served on a professional level, their emotional responses may be ones of betrayal, disbelief, or skepticism. Why is this true?

Stromberg (1990), in a paper presented to the American Speech-Language Hearing Association, speculated on the skepticism in the minds of both the public and the profession itself.

> One reason (for the skepticism) is that most fields have experienced an erosion of professional sovereignty in the face of demands that professionals be more "accountable" to the public. In past eras, doctors, lawyers, engineers, and other professionals were viewed with awe and treated with deference. This is far less so today. Instead, there is a common perception, as George Bernard Shaw said, "Every profession is a conspiracy against the laity [the public]." The remoteness and paternalism of many professions are no longer acceptable. Consumerism and the proliferation of information have reduced people's willingness to defer to professional's judgements. Today, people want to feel empowered. They demand to know what lies behind the professional's decisions. And when clients or patients second-guess the professionals, they are willing to question not only their competence but also their ethics.

This public skepticism that gives rise to professional accountability is a major driving force in the rising expectations that both professionals and the public place on hearing instrument dispensing. Our field has requested and worked hard for recognition and concomitant responsibility. When the public experiences products, product claims, or services that are less than proclaimed, the skepticism may be warranted. This must not be allowed to happen.

Each of our actions adds, detracts, or maintains our ethical position. If more providers detract from that which is expected, the field of hearing instrument dispensing may not rise to the desired professional level. Stated another way, as the field of hearing instrument dispensing establishes itself as a professional entity, the more the altruistic interests of the patient become the guiding principle. Fixation on the profit motive to the exclusion of the patient's best interests may place professional goals at the level of business-only ethics. The alternative is to resist change and remain only a business, forfeiting the professional status afforded by many states.

Does the current professional position place the hearing instrument dispensing field in a position that requires, demands, or expects more public trust? In the final decades of the 20th century, federal and state regulations changed. As licensing, educational requirements, advertising, fitting appliances, and methods evolved, the field has become more professional, and the public expects more. When one observes government (FDA, FTC) involvement in the hearing aid dispensing field, it is reasonable to expect that the position of this field in the hearing health care arena will be more defined. As a result, the public will continue to demand higher ethical standards in the future.

In a sense, we are asking the public to place more demands on us as we gain increased sophistication and expertise in our field. We ask for an elevated position when we request to become the entry point for hearing health care. We seek this level of responsibility when we expect to bill third-party payers for our products and services. We invite closer public scrutiny of our standards when we license ourselves and move beyond a simple sales-oriented approach to products and services.

The ethical standards to which we must adhere can be summarized simply: Do the right thing as determined by the group. That is the essence of all professional ethics.

Where can hearing health care professionals learn more about the ethical issues we now face and those that will arise in the future? Obtain appropriate references and read the few sources that pertain directly to our field. Become involved in the issues that face the profession. Demand of yourself and of others that everyone "do the right thing" at all times. Why should we be concerned with the ethical behavior of others in our chosen field? If we don't, who will? Perhaps our methods of managing these ethical issues are the indicators or the true measure of our emergence as a genuine consumer-related professional group. We should not tolerate persons who fail to perform at a level directed by professional standards. Our professional standards must evolve not by state or federal mandate, but by members of our profession.

The author realizes that some of the content of this chapter may be offensive. Certainly, it has not been the purpose of this chapter to indict, demean, or question the legal or ethical behavior of a given individual or group. Instead it was intended to comment on changes that have occurred over time. Further, it was the intent of the author to comment on these changes or observed behaviors as they relate to legal or ethical concerns. The dilemmas delineated here were used as an pedagogic method for reviewing that which may reflect current conditions or portend future events.

REVIEW QUESTIONS

1. Ethical considerations are based on mandatory laws defined by state and local officials. (Explain why you agree or disagree with this statement.)

2. Is it possible for the hearing health professional to be legal but unethical? (If so, how can it be evident in clinical practice?)

3. Do you agree that contracts are legal documents? (Explain your answer.)

4. Do you agree that both ethics and law are founded in public policy? (If this statement is true, why is it so?)

5. Although hearing health professionals are not physicians, are they obligated to perform tests that contribute to the physician's understanding of the hearing loss problem? (If true, are they practicing medicine without a license?)

6. Is it unethical to accept a European tour offered by a hearing aid manufacturer, if the hearing health professional qualifies based on total number of sales? (If so, explain your answer.)

7. Are the ethical standards of hearing instrument dispensing above those of automobile salespersons? (If so, how do they differ?)

8. Relative to legal contracts regarding the sale of hearing instruments, what items should be included?

9. What is wrong with the following statement? Product advertising is correct if the patient buys the hearing aid and does not return it.

10. Is it both legal and ethical for hearing health professional to make claims of better hearing with hearing aid X before evaluating the patient?

REFERENCES

American Medical Association v. Federal Trade Commission, 638 f.2d 433, 449 (2d Cir.) (1980).

Arizona v. Maricopa County Medical Society, 457 U.S. 332, 348-49 (1982).

Brunswick Corporation v. Pueblo Bowl-O-Mat, Inc., 429 U.S. 477, 488 (1977).

California Business and Professions Code, Sections 651, 3301, 3401(1), and 3428.

Goldfarb v. Virginia State Bar, 421 U.S. 773 (1975).

National Society of Professional Engineers vs. United States, 435 U.S. 679, 697-98 (1978).

Resnick, D. M. (1993). *Professional ethics for audiologists and speech-language pathologists*. San Diego, CA: Singular Publishing Group.

Stromberg, C. et al. (1988). *The psychologist's legal handbook*. Washington, DC: Council for the National Register.

Stromberg, C. (1990). Key legal issues in professional ethics, in reflection on ethics. In *A compilation of articles inspired by the May 1990 ASHA Ethics Colloquium*. Rockville, MD: American Speech-Language-Hearing Association.

CHAPTER 23

Observations And Future Considerations

ROBERT E. SANDLIN, Ph.D.

OUTLINE

(continued)

In 1988, the first edition of the *Handbook of Hearing Aid Amplification* was published. Since that time, some of the prognostications of future needs have been realized. Today two general areas of concern remain. First, we must create a diagnostic protocol that provides sufficient data about impaired auditory performance to permit the development of hearing aid systems that better meet acoustic needs of our patients. The second area of concern is still one of achieving the maximum processing of information in various environmental backgrounds. It is becoming increasingly evident, however, that advances in diagnostic protocols and achieving better information processing in noise is not enough. Understanding patient motivation related to psychological and emotional states (see Chapter 17), as well as determining patient acceptance of and satisfaction with amplification (see Chapters 16 and 17), are important issues that will require creative thinking to surpass the methods now used to assess these subjective measures.

This revised chapter takes a more broad-based look at what the future portends than did the original chapter. Not only is emphasis placed on advances in hearing aid technology, but a number of other concerns about amplification for individuals with hearing impairment are reviewed as well. In part, observations presented here are based on the author's biases arising from many years of working with persons with hearing loss. This chapter looks at future implications regarding ethics in hearing instrument dispensing. It examines the effect of managed care agencies on dispensing practices, the probability of mandatory hearing aid performance standards, rehabilitation practices, and the psychological and emotional concerns of the patient related to the acceptance or rejection of hearing aid devices.

The hearing health care professional must become more than just a "fitter" of electroacoustic devices. Future developments regarding federal or state regulations, technological advances, and effective management strategies will demand a new breed of professionally trained and dedicated clinicians.

HIGH-FIDELITY SOUND REPRODUCTION

The holy grail of hearing aid development is that of producing an instrument that provides the best possible solution to problems facing individuals with hearing impairment in responding appropriately to information-bearing stimuli in a number of listening environments. Such an instrument would by its nature be one of high-fidelity sound reproduction (see Chapter 5). Although there is no consensus as to a universal definition of high-fidelity sound, it seems logical to suggest that it include a minimum of signal distortion, broad-based frequency amplification, and excellent reproduction of sound quality and audibility of a frequency range sufficient to understand speech. In essence, the ultimate high-fidelity hearing aid amplification presupposes an *acoustic transparency*. Acoustic transparency suggests that the hearing aid user's reception of sound with a high-fidelity hearing aid would not differ significantly from what the hearing impaired person receives when listening directly.

The reproduction of high-fidelity sound has been an ongoing concern since the creation of electric hearing aids more than 70 years ago. Even casual perusal of available literature documents advances made in high-fidelity sound reproduction. Killion (1993, p. 31), however, stated that, ". . . problems of size, response of smoothness, bandwidth limitations, and noise level have now been completely solved." Although there may not be universal agreement with this statement, it is true that significant advance has been made in the reproduction of high-fidelity sound. Much remains to be accomplished in reducing the signal degrading propensity of distortion products produced by the hearing aid, however. Further development in analog and digital signal processing (DSP) technology will provide answers to problems associated with distortion due to hearing aid devices operating in or near saturation.

Relative to the determination of high-fidelity sound reproduction, coherence measures (Preves, 1990) will continue to serve as a means of validating the fidelity of sound reproduction. Nonetheless, current measures offer only a partial solution to the hearing aid saturation problem. Bentler (1994, p. 344) defined coherence as, "that portion of the output signal that is directly related to the input signal. Coherence measures indicate the total distortion and noise measured at the output of a hearing aid (harmonic and intermodulation distortion as well as circuit noise)." Coherence is a measurement of the linearity of the hearing aid. It measures what part of the output signal is due to the input signal. A coherence of 1, for example, would mean that there is a 100% correspondence between the input signal and the amplified output signal. A coherence value of .9 would mean that the output contains a 10% distortion factor. Standardizing the use of a coherence measure would give the hearing health care professional a numerical value to determine, in part, the "quality" of the recommended instrument. The onus, then, is placed directly on those who produce the instrument and those who fit the instrument. As such, there is a measurement device that can be implemented in the selection process. Granted, this is not a panacea, but a significant step forward in assessing hearing aid performance and probable benefit.

Currently, greater coherence can be realized by reducing the gain at high input levels or by increasing the SSPL 90. Technological developments designed to reduce distortion beyond its present level await discovery and resolution. Also, solutions will be forthcoming relative to distortions produced by nonlinearities of amplifier response. It seems improbable that advances in analog technology will contribute greatly to the resolution of these problems. Although one should not overemphasize the contributions of DSP, it appears likely that appropriate algorithms will be developed to offer permanent solutions to problems of distortion and the subsequent degrading of speech signals. There is considerable time and distance to be covered before we have resolved those problems associated with distortion products due to nonlinear performances of the amplifier. Continued developmental efforts contribute to resolution of these problems.

Regarding high-fidelity hearing aids, it is naive to suggest that the end result of technological advance in hearing aids is that of generating high-fidelity response, which offers the greatest potential for signal processing by the users of amplification. Ongoing advances in transducer efficiency, coupled with continuing advances in amplifier technology, will add greatly to achieving high-fidelity response. This chapter, in part, is an overview of probable future advances that will contribute to the development of high-fidelity hearing aids.

LINEAR VERSUS NONLINEAR PERFORMANCE

Certainly, the future of hearing aid performance must transcend reliance on linear amplifiers to meet the complex acoustic needs of individuals with hearing impairment. In this instance, linear amplification is defined as equal changes in output as the input signal is increased or decreased. Somewhat disturbing are consistent reports that in the United States, about 80% of hearing instruments fitted are those with linear amplifiers (Cranmer, 1992). The reliance on linear amplifiers to resolve amplification needs of nonlinear neurosensory systems remains a mystery. Given irrefutable evidence that the human ear is a nonlinear system in its neurophysiologic performance, how does one justify the large number of linear amplifiers used to resolve the electroacoustic needs of those with impaired hearing? With the rather recent introduction of analog nonlinear systems, and especially nonlinear digital signal processing instruments, reliance on linear type amplifiers probably will be reduced greatly as the clinician becomes aware of the many benefits to be derived from new technology. Linear amplifiers are only linear to the point of saturation (e.g., peak clipping), at which time the output is nonlinear with changes in input level. The disastrous consequence of instrument performance in saturation, however, is a highly distorted signal at the output stage. Intermodulation and harmonic distortion products contribute the most to the degradation of the output signal. Linear hearing aids fail to satisfy audibility requirements and at the same time control MCL and UCL requirements. Nonetheless, linearity of response is not all that negative. If speech input is audible over a broad frequency range and below the peak clipping level, speech discrimination (word recognition) is optimized. This is so because the speech envelope, or the dynamic range of the instrument, is not compressed, and as a result, there is no spectral smearing. Spectral smearing can occur with some compression-type hearing aids. Perhaps the best of both worlds is achieved when the linearity of the speech envelope is maintained in an otherwise nonlinear system. There is one manufacturer of digital signal processing hearing aids that uses the principle of maintaining, as much as possible, linearity of the speech envelope by not compressing, or only minimally compressing, the dynamic range within a given frequency band.

Tangentially related to the use of a linear amplifier is the knowledge required of those who dispense hearing aids. This is not an indictment of the hearing health care professional's intelligence or dedication, but rather one of questioning motivations for using linear amplifiers when nonlinear systems may have better served the needs of patients. Perhaps some of the more advanced instrumentation (i.e., nonlinear, multichannel, and digital processing systems) pose a technological threat to those who have failed to keep current with advances. With current emphasis given to such advances in technology and with the level of training provided by several manufacturers and professional bodies, it can be reasonably predicted that the numbers of underinformed hearing health care practitioners will diminish significantly. These statements are not to indict analog linear amplifiers but to suggest that their clinical value is limited and falls to the approximate functional efficiency of most nonlinear systems.

FUTURE IMPLICATIONS OF DIGITAL SIGNAL PROCESSING HEARING INSTRUMENTS

Without question, the future of technological advance is directly coupled to DSP hearing aid systems (see Chapter 8). The major reason for this optimistic projection is based on the following: *Once the analog input signal has been converted (digitized) to a series of numbers (or digits expressed in binary form), there are unlimited ways in which those numbers can be manipulated by the microprocessor to achieve subsequent processing schemes.* That is, digital conversion of the input signal makes it possible to process the signal in ways that are *impossible with analog systems.* There are limits imposed regarding the amount and magnitude of possible changes and the range of the changes that can be accomplished in analog circuitry. Certainly, the sophistication of current and future microprocessors permits the engineer to develop appropriate and sophisticated algorithms to best interface with electroacoustic need. What is currently lacking in DSP is related to our lack of knowledge regarding the functional efficiency of impaired auditory systems and the ways in which acoustic signals should be processed to achieve the greatest correspondence with need. We are at the threshold of utilizing the advantages offered by DSP technology. Once the analog signal is converted to a digital one, it can be manipulated in unlimited ways. As one gains more information about cochlear mechanics and auditory processing of acoustic signals, appropriate algorithms will be developed to create the best interface with amplification needs.

The jury is still out regarding the question of open or closed platforms. An open platform implies that all functions are described in software and that unlimited variations in the response characteristics can be made. A closed platform implies that the DSP system is a dedicated one, that modifications of electroacoustic performance are limited, and that major changes in performance would require a new dedicated system. Currently, there is some question regarding open platform DSP systems. Kuk (1997) examined the issue of closed or open platforms and presented cogent arguments about their present status and utility.

It is quite possible that DSP instruments of the future will have open platforms. The skill level of those fitting and dispensing DSP systems will have to be significantly more advanced to maximize the benefits of open platforms. Perhaps one of the limiting factors for an open platform may be the reluctance of manufacturers to support its introduction. It is conceivable that any technological advance offered by a given manufacturer could be replicated by an open platform system, thus limiting the commercial advantage of innovative design.

One of the current advantages of DSP is that of the physical dimensions of the integrated chip (IC). Hearing aid size no longer is of concern to many individuals with hearing impairment. The IC allows manufacturers to produce an instrument housed in a small physical space without sacrificing electroacoustic performance. This is not to suggest that cosmetic appearance is the only concern of the manufacturer, but rather that there are no longer significant size constraints. Whether rational or not, there will always be persons with hearing impairment whose use of amplification is governed by cosmetic concerns dictating purchase, acceptance, and use of hearing aid devices. Another potential advantage of reducing chip size is that of "stacking" one IC on another. As more processing potential becomes available, new ways in which the input signal can be manipulated can be introduced. By so doing, there will a quantum leap in signal processing potential housed in the same hearing aid casing. One cannot stress too strongly the advantages offered by increasing the capabilities of digital signal processing. As more complex cochlear models are conceived, and as we gain more knowledge of human auditory performance, algorithms will be developed to process the signal in ways consistent with the model. As the IC becomes smaller, the use of multiple chips in the same hearing aid housing probably will become commonplace. What, then, are some of the current and future contributions of DSP technology that portend significant advantages to the individual with hearing impairment?

Parallel Processing

Parallel processing, as an integral part of digital signal processing, allows several processing tasks to be handled simultaneously. Analog hearing aid circuits are able to manipulate only a limited number of electroacoustic parameters. Parallel processing permits a number of parameters to act differentially on the input signal at the same time. Among those areas of concern to improve hearing aid performance, one may consider the following:

Speech Enhancement

Current DSP technology has provided marked improvement in speech enhancement techniques. Through an ongoing statistical analysis of the input signal, it is currently possible to differentiate the modulation rate of speech and noise. As a result, depending on the number of discrete channels in which the analysis is taking place, background noise suppression permits an improved SNR that increases the possibility of signal or word recognition. It has yet to be determined how many independent channels are needed to maximize the speech enhancement process. Continued research will provide rational answers to this question. One of the major problems related to speech enhancement utilizing multiple channels is that imposed by the transducers. It is the receiver that causes the problem. The maximum slope per octave of a given frequency band is dictated by the receiver. Theoretically, it is of little consequence if a DSP system can provide much steeper slopes; it is the receiver that dictates the permissible steepness of the slope before the introduction of distortion. The question is one of how many channels can be utilized in the processing of signals before interchannel distortion degrades word recognition or signal distortion. Future advances may solve the problem of channel interaction, making possible an efficient system with a number of channels to process information with only minimal negative consequences.

Differentiating speech and noise by identifying modulation rates is not the same as separating speech and noise and processing them independently. Future technological advances may make it possible to accomplish this separation. Currently, the consensus is that multiple microphone arrays are necessary to truly process noise and speech as separate acoustic occurrences. We can remain optimistic, however, that differential processing of speech and noise is possible and can be accomplished by advances in processing strategies without excessive current (battery drain) demands.

Other approaches to speech enhancement have been presented by a number of investigators, who have examined unique methods for enhancing the perception and discrimination of speech (Boers, 1980; Bustamante & Braida, 1986, 1987; DeGennaro et al., 1986; Dillon, 1989; Fortune & Preves, 1991; Freyman & Nerbonne, 1989; Plomp, 1998; Tetzeli et al., 1991; Villchur, 1976). Some of the concepts inherent in these reports can be greatly expanded in their utilitarian value with the possible application of DSP technology.

Loudness Mapping

Loudness mapping algorithms have been utilized to control gain requirements for signal audibility and most comfortable listening levels and to avoid uncomfortable listening levels. Future developments will permit DSP instruments to be more interactive. Gain functions will be determined by the environment in which listening takes place. The ability to locate the signal source in a milieu of noise, as well as the ability to program audiometric data into the system to greatly expand its value to the hearing impaired population, will be exhibited in hearing aids of the future. Relative to audiometric data input, future DSP systems will look at more frequency data points instead of octave or half octave values. The greater the analysis of data points, the more sophisticated and efficient the loudness mapping function will be.

Internal Noise Reduction

During the past decade, significant advances have been made to reduce audible internal noise. Transducer technology, especially evident in microphone performance, is such that the noise floor of the hearing aid is now of relatively minor concern to the engineer and clinician. Given a reduced noise floor and algorithms that automatically attenuate internal noise below the point of audibility, the problem has been greatly reduced. In future developments, however, even greater noise reduction will be realized and improved threshhold sensitivity will be achieved utilizing microphone technology or digital signal processing.

In Situ Measurement

One of the more recent developments in DSP function, and one which bodes well for the future, is the application of "in situ" measurement. Although in situ measurement is an integral part of real ear assessment, the magnitude of measurement error is greater than that of in situ measurements in which the test signal is generated by the hearing aid. That is, by having the hearing aid produce its own test signal, measurement error is greatly reduced.

For several decades, hearing health care professionals have relied on threshold-based and suprathreshold-based measurements to set predicted insertion gains to selected target frequencies. (Berger, 1979; Bragg, 1988; Bryne & Dillon, 1986; Cox et al., 1982, 1985; Hawkings, 1992; Libby, 1986; McCandless, 1983; Pascoe, 1976; Seewald, 1992; Shapiro, 1976; Skinner et al., 1982) Several of the currently employed fitting formulae use threshold-based or suprathreshold-based values to establish the electroacoustic performance of the hearing aid. Most fitting formulae were developed to assess gain requirements for those with sensorineural impairments who used linear amplifiers and occluding earmolds.

The application of various formulae presents a problem relative to the variability of threshold values from true organic thresholds. Without knowing the actual sound pressure level at the eardrum or actual sound pressures generated during loudness mapping procedures, preciseness of measurement is in jeopardy. Inaccurate assessment lends itself to a lack of predictability. Therefore, if one bases the electroacoustic performance of the hearing aid on obtained threshold measures using conventional techniques, there is a high probability of error.

Measurement errors involve the audiometer, earphones, and resonance variations in the outer ear, as well as actual impedance of the eardrum. Furthermore, in the fitting process, additional errors may be generated through traditional methods by which hearing aids are fitted. This magnitude of error is related to the hearing aid, earmold acoustics, residual ear volume, and the impedance of the eardrum. Rankovic (1992) found significant variations in sound pressures produced by a standard TDH 39 earphone placed on the ears of different subjects. The earphone voltage of 1 V was held constant throughout the study. The results demonstrated greater variations in sound pressure at the lower and upper end of the frequency range.

Olsson (1985) reported a study in which 17 different subjects were fitted with the same hearing instrument. The purpose of the study was to measure the range of sound pressures generated at the eardrum of the subjects. The electroacoustic response of the hearing aid was held constant. The insertion gain varied considerably and was greater for the frequency range between 2000 and 4000 Hz. Gain variations were due primarily to the effects of the concha and external ear canal impedance. One may argue that the use of insert earphones can reduce measurement error related to threshold or suprathreshold-based assessment. This argument is correct, but measurement errors continue to exist, reducing the precision of threshold assessment (Ludvigsen & Topholm, 1997).

An in situ procedure in which the hearing aid produces its own test signal provides a more efficient resolution to measurement variation because the clinician knows the exact voltage required to produce signal perception by the individual. There is no sound pressure variation produced by the physical geometry of the ear or the impedance of the eardrum that would alter the validity of the obtained response.

Today there are a limited number of manufacturers using in situ procedures. Future generations of DSP instruments probably will incorporate in situ measurements to obtain more precise assessments of threshold. Consider the following: The functional efficiency of various DSP algorithms is based in part on threshold assessment. Therefore, the more accurate the assessment of threshold, the more precisely the algorithm will perform its dedicated signal processing task.

LOUDNESS FUNCTION

Of major concern in the development of hearing aids are changes in loudness growth resulting from sensorineural impairments. Alterations of loudness function result from damage and loss of outer hair cells (Berlin, 1996). When outer hair cell loss is evident, there is recruitment, and recruitment causes changes in loudness growth. There are a number of studies that review loudness functions relating to loudness discomfort levels. (Beattie et al., 1979; Bentler & Pavlovic, 1989; Cox, 1981; Filion, 1992; Fortune & Preves, 1992; Hawkins, 1980, 1992; McCandless, 1973; Sammeth et al., 1989; Stelmchowicz, 1991).

It is generally agreed that the magnitude of loudness growth change is related to the level of hearing impairment. For instance, a mild sensorineural loss affects only sensitivity to soft sounds. As such, little if any gain is needed for normal speech inputs. As the hearing loss becomes greater, loudness function is altered, and different kinds of amplification schemes are needed to compensate for the loss and subsequent loudness growth. Loudness mapping data used to construct appropriate algorithms to manage loudness growth or to develop analog instruments managing loudness functions for sensorineural losses cannot involve simple, linear amplifiers. It is evident that in most sensorinerual losses, the ear functions normally at some point in terms of loudness perception, relative to the level of the input signal.

Manufacturers of DSP hearing instruments have made promising contributions to the management of loudness growth. Future advances will discover new and unique ways to control loudness function, which will permit much more natural sound. Studies relating to hearing loss and loudness growth may well entail individual assessment of loudness growth over a broad frequency range, rather than relying on group data to determine the response of the hearing instrument as a function of hearing loss magnitude.

Current DSP systems employ loudness mapping strategies based on group threshold, MCL, and UCL data for specific frequencies to construct an appropriate algorithm, which is then applied to an individual's acoustic needs. This statement is not an indictment of current mapping strategies. Indeed, such strategies have been advantageous to individuals with hearing impairment. What is intended here is that future developments of hearing aid systems will improve the efficiency with which disproportionate loudness growth can be managed more effectively.

Binaural Hearing Aids and Signal Perception

All clinicians selecting and fitting hearing aids are familiar with the advantages of binaural hearing aids. Among the advantages offered are improved ability to localize the point source of sound, improved discrimination of speech in noise, improved threshold for signal detection, minimization of head shadow for those with high-frequency loss, and summation affects at suprathreshold levels. With DSP applied to binaural hearing aids, it may be possible to reinstate normal, or near normal, head-related transfer functions (HRTF), which enable the user to more effectively perform in a multitude of acoustic environments. To achieve a higher level of performance, the hearing aids will "talk" to each other to provide optimal processing performance in given listening environments. Communication between binaural systems will undoubtedly employ some type of wireless transmission involving sophisticated DSP technology. With the processing advantages offered by DSP technology such binaural interaction is feasible.

DSP applied to hearing aids is only a tool. It is the way in which DSP is utilized that will determine its benefit to the hearing impairment population. Future generations of DSP systems will greatly eclipse the efficiency of those systems that currently exist.

Understanding Speech in Background Noise

Much remains to be done to optimize the speech signal in a milieu of environmental noise. To date, including current developments in analog and DSP instrumentation, impressive gains have yet to be demonstrated in achieving greater word recognition in noise. What has been achieved is that of providing a more comfortable amplified signal that reduces listener fatigue by attenuating the output in those bands where noise is the dominant signal. In the future, with the interaction of directional microphones and the low compression thresholds possible with DSP control, it should be possible to enhance the detection and discrimination of speech in a background of noise by greatly improving signal-to-noise ratios. (Kuk, 1999; Lee et al., 1998; Rickets & Dhar, 1999; Valente et al., 1999).

The ideal goal is that of digitally separating signal and noise. Perhaps this can be realized at some future date, but greater reliance will probably be given to development of multiple microphone arrays that amplify the point source of the desired message and attenuate other sounds outside the point source. Single directional microphones, although offering measurable advantages in noise reduction when compared to omnidirectional microphones, do not approach the potential clinical utility of multiple microphone arrays. Directional microphones (see Chapter 7) have been proven to be of great clinical value in improving signal-to-noise ratios (SNR). This is true for the application of single directional microphones, as used by one manufacturer of DSP hearing aids. It is highly probable, however, that the use of two or more microphones will enhance the discrimination of speech in noise by creating higher SNR values. The use of beam-forming arrays may provide the best solution for improving speech recognition in backgrounds of noise. It is theoretically possible to develop DSP technology to the point where the hearing aid automatically determines the optimal beam formed by the microphones to enhance the speech signal and attenuate competing noise backgrounds. The hearing aid will determine the location of the speech source by detecting modulation rate and the SPL values of other sound in the environment. This will dictate the behavior of a multiple microphone array to enhance the speech signal while attenuating background noise.

MULTIPROGRAMMABLE HEARING AIDS: ANALOG VERSUS DIGITAL

Most analog programmable hearing aids offer the advantage of multiple memories to enhance speech recognition. For example, programs may be set to optimize listening in quiet environments or to improve sound when listening to music. Program settings can also reduce traffic noise and other aversive stimuli. Such technology offers a host of program settings to meet specific situational needs. Multiple memories utilizing analog technology are necessary because a single memory, analog hearing aid cannot alter its acoustic behavior sufficiently well to achieve desired frequency response changes as listening environments change. Even in view of the limitations imposed by analog technology, the contributions of multiprogrammable systems have been numerous. Although effective in helping the hearing impaired population function better in a number of listening environments, analog programmable systems fall short of achieving the potential processing benefits offered by DSP systems.

Continued development of DSP technology may obviate the need for multiple-memory hearing aids because of the ways in which DSP systems can manipulate input signals. Rather than having multiple memories to enhance performance in a number of listening environments, "intelligent" or "smart" hearing aids will automatically manipulate the input signal to provide optimal word-recognition regardless of the environmental conditions.

One must be careful not to overstate current and future uses of DSP technology. Unfortunately, there is a tendency to do just that because there is no evidence to the contrary. Nonetheless, such technology may well be possible. It is not unreasonable to envision DSP systems capable of enhancing speech recognition in a variety of competing backgrounds.

FITTING AND VERIFICATION STRATEGIES IN THE SELECTION AND FITTING OF HEARING AIDS

A discussion of verification of hearing aid performance can be approached from a number of different directions. For example, one can developed strategies and verification procedures for specific hearing-loss types. Independent strategies exist for noise-induced hearing losses (Bilger, 1984; Fabry, 1991; Lee et al., 1993; Moore et al., 1985; Mueller et al., 1991; Murray et al., 1986; Oticon Research Center, 1989; Rankovic, 1989; Skinner, 1980; Van Tassel et al., 1988). Other strategies exist for verifying binaural amplification for asymmetrical hearing loss (Briskey, 1978; Byrne, 1981; Byrne et al., 1987; Causey, 1980; Courtois, 1988; Cox, 1985; Hawkins, 1986; Libby, 1986; Sandlin,1994; Skinner, 1988; Staab, 1985; Studebaker, 1980). The verification of hearing aid value for unilateral hearing loss has been reviewed in the literature (Bess, 1988; Brookhouser, 1991; Fowler, 1960; Harford, 1965; Harford & Musket, 1964; Hodgson, 1986; Jerger, 1981; Kielmovich, 1988; Markides, 1977; Olyler, 1988; Tilman & Kasten, 1963; Valente, 1991). Unique strategies have been developed for symmetrical hearing impairments (Cos et al., 1981; Cox et al., 1984; Danhauer et al., 1991; Grimes & Mueller , 1981; Hawkins & Yacullo, 1992; Helfer, 1992; McCullough, 1992; Mercola & Wenke-Mercola, 1985; Mueller & Grimes, 1981; Pollack, 1988). Verification of maximum power output has been studied by several investigators (Bentler, 1993; Bentler & Pavlovic, 1989; Cox, 1981; Fortune & Preves, 1991; Hawkins, 1980; McCandless, 1973; Morgan & Dirks , 1974; Skinner, 1988; Stelmachowicz, 1991). There is general consensus that the required maximum output is of great importance in the selection, fitting, and successful use of hearing aid amplification. Differences exist as to measurement procedures and about what constitutes a realistic assessment of maximum power output to meet acoustic needs yet control for UCL.

There is no doubt that various strategies exist for determining specific hearing aid performance characteristics in meeting amplification demands of the person with hearing impairment (Bentler & Pavlovic, 1989; Byrne & Dillon, 1986; Cox & Moore, 1988; Dillon, 1993; Gatehouse & Gordon, 1990; Humes, 1993; Kalikow et al., 1984; Killion et al., 1993; Pavlovic, 1985; Pavlovic & Studebaker, 1984; Pratt, 1993; Preves, 1990; Seewald et al., 1992). It is not surprising that verification strategies are modified as more advanced technologies are developed and more hearing aid response parameters become available. The question to be asked, therefore, is what does the future hold for verification strategies? What issues must be addressed to improve the individual's use of amplification?

There is no need to develop new areas of concern but rather to improve upon those that have been of major concern for decades. We still want the fidelity of amplified signals to enhance speech discrimination, for example. We need to achieve audibility of the signal across a wide frequency range when indicated. We need to improve the fidelity of sound reproduction by minimizing or eliminating distortion products, which degrade word recognition. We need to construct an analog or digital hearing aid that functions at a level below output saturation to avoid harmonic and intermodulation distortion. We need to develop a hearing aid that permits optimal word recognition in a noise background.

More efficient strategies will include criteria by which spatial balance, sound quality, localization ability, listening comfort, smoothing of output performance, and manipulating loudness growth are based on the level of hearing loss. We need to determine whether articulation indices offer a better predictor of word recognition compared to actual speech discrimination tests. Similarly, verification strategies related to hearing aid performance will demand a great deal of the researcher's time and effort.

It is obvious even to the casual observer that advances in verification strategies will be tied to future trends in hearing aid technology. As advanced systems are introduced, their clinical utility will be tied to whether verification strategies, when applied to the new technologies, advance one's skills in determining successful use of hearing aid amplification. Not only that, one must determine whether verification strategies assessing instrumental performance are consistent with the patient's assessment of acceptance, benefit, and satisfaction.

In the final analysis, the question is not one of how the electroacoustic characteristics of the hearing aid are to be measured, but rather how to determine the rationale for adopting any specific fitting and verification protocol and whether or not such rationale meets some standard of performance.

DETERMINATION OF HEARING AID REQUIREMENTS: A DILEMMA

For this author, after more than 40 years of attempting to meet the acoustic needs of those with hearing loss, there has been a recurring thought. There has been no consensus of what audiologic measurements are to be employed in determining the amplification needs of the individual with hearing impairment. Furthermore, even if our profession developed a universal measurement protocol, there is no consensus as to how such clinical data are to be used in determining hearing aid selection.

In the absence of such consensus, we have opted for a rather simplistic approach of measuring threshold sensitivity for discrete frequencies, or discrete frequency bandwidths. From these threshold values, MCL and UCL requirements are determined. The assumption is that the values obtained will either achieve normalization of the acoustic response or equalization of the acoustic response. Normalization can be defined as the restoration of normal loudness for impaired auditory systems by assigning the same gain for the same degree of hearing loss. The assumption is that normal loudness is the desired goal of amplification. For flat losses, this normally results in the same gain for the low frequencies as for the higher frequencies. This can result in more amplification for low frequencies and less amplification for high frequencies than would be evident in the equalization approach. The normalization approach is represented by the IHAFF and FIG 6, as well as some other fitting methods.

Equalization can be defined as the attempt to make each frequency region equally loud by providing different gain for the same degree of hearing loss. The purpose of an equalization approach is to have all frequency regions equally loud at MCL. Normally, there would be less required gain in the lower frequency regions. The equalization approach is used by many linear fitting methods such as the NAL, DSL, and POGO.

At some point in time, one should be able to determine which of the two approaches best meets the acoustic needs of a patient. The dilemma is this: Given identical audiograms for two patients with similar histories of hearing loss onset, one clinician will opt for one method of approach to meet amplification needs; and another clinician will select a different electroacoustic means of resolving amplification needs. It can be argued that the amplification needs of the two patients are identical, yet consensus is not forthcoming as to what method is best. Additionally, two manufacturers, given the identical audiometric data, will not recommend the same hearing aid response characteristics. Additionally, given the same audiometric data and patient history, frequently used fitting formulae recommend different insertion gains to meet acoustic needs (see Chapter 11). Certainly, these statements are not an indictment of the normalization or equalization approach, the clinician, or the manufacturer, but are evidence that a need exists to resolve this perplexing problem of determining optimal acoustic needs based on reliable audiometric data.

Tangentially related to resolving the dilemma of hearing instrument selection is whether linear or nonlinear amplifiers, analog or digital signal processing hearing aids are best suited to provide optimal benefit. The trend over the past five to ten years would seem to favor the use of analog, nonlinear amplifiers. Current emphasis is shifting to a more frequent application of DSP systems. Again, we fail to detect any consensus of what is best for the patient. The data from Kranmer (1992), indicated that about 82% of hearing aids dispensed in the United States are linear amplifiers. Another dilemma presents itself: If the human ear behaves in a nonlinear fashion and the nonlinearity is exacerbated by a sensory or neural deficit, what justification is there in using completely linear amplifiers to solve nonlinear problems?

There are several possible answers. It may be that the retail cost of a Class A, linear amplifier is attractive to those having limited financial resources. Although not as beneficial as nonlinear aids, they provide a certain level of benefit. It may be that the clinician feels "comfortable" with selecting and fitting linear systems and is apprehensive about his or her ability to understand and utilize nonlinear hearing aids. In this instance, the motivation of the dispenser is to maintain a livelihood without having to keep current with advances in hearing aid technology, which may have offered greater benefit to patients. Whatever the reason, the future of hearing aid technology lies with digital signal processing hearing aids. This statement is not to overemphasize the value of DSP systems or to denigrate the use of linear amplifiers, but to point out that technological advances should in part, dictate clinical application of that technology. In the future, those who cannot stay current with advances in technology likely will fall by the wayside. Similarly, those manufacturers relying on the production of linear amplifiers will experience a decreasing market share.

There are a number of factors contributing to successful fittings. What is suggested here is that our profession must develop clinical assessment procedures that dictate the most efficient amplification system for restoring normal hearing function as much as possible. Clinical approaches to meet acoustic needs of patients with hearing impairment will change as more information becomes available. Information in this context refers to technological advances, increased understanding of auditory performance, and effective management strategies related to more human concerns regarding the use of amplification.

FUTURE CONSIDERATIONS BEYOND HEARING AID TECHNOLOGY

Satisfaction, Acceptance, and Benefit

The reader may wonder why verification strategies related to satisfaction, acceptance, and benefit concerns are not covered under the section dealing with hearing aid verification. The answer is straightforward. In this instance, we are looking at the electroacoustic response of the hearing aid and whether it meets some acceptable physical standard. In this section, we are concerned with those standards set for hearing aid performance to meet the needs of the patient, based on a number of nonelectroacoustic factors.

During the 1990s, greater emphasis was given to measures of patient satisfaction and benefit from hearing aid amplification (see Chapter 16) (Byrne & Parkinson, 1982; Cox & Alexander, 1992, Cox et al., 1984, 1989, 1992; Gabrielssonn et al., 1988; Lawson, 1982; McDermott, 1968; Montgomery et al., 1982; Punch & Parker, 1981; Purdy, 1978; Speaks et al., 1972; Studebaker, 1988). Impetus was given to the development of various hearing aid user satisfaction scales (see Chapter 15) because it was evident that meeting target gain requirements, dictated by a given fitting formula, did not guarantee hearing aid acceptance or satisfaction. For far too many clinicians, little attention has been given to what the patient wanted from amplification and whether or not their needs were met. More important, there was no urgency to determine whether the patient's needs could be satisfied, given the current status of technological advance. Furthermore, for some patients, minimal effort was made to assess whether the patient's expectations exceeded the contributions of the hearing aid. Although current efforts to assess benefit are encouraging, more work needs to be done to develop an effective patient management strategy that incorporates the attitudes and expectations of the patients with the performance reality of the hearing aid.

Somewhat disturbing is the observation that some of those who select and fit hearing aids do not utilize the various, excellent *satisfaction, acceptance,* and *benefit* scales available. It is an unsupported assumption, but it seems that most dispensers of hearing aids do not routinely use various assessment scales to determine benefit, satisfaction, or acceptance. Apparently, there is some type of illogical mental processing, which suggests that meeting specified target gains is tantamount to fitting success. This is certainly not to indict the use of target gains, but rather to imply that something more may be needed to assess maximum benefit from hearing aid amplification. With the advent of real ear measurement, computer-assisted fitting strategies, and the use of one or more articulation indices to "predict" performance, less attention has been given to functional measurements of actual patient performance or assessment of benefit. In the future, there no doubt will be greater reliance on analyzing the patient's assessment of hearing benefit that will go far beyond the level of asking the patient two questions: *"How does that sound to you?"* and *"How do you like it?"* Although well intended, these questions provide little if any information about what the hearing aid is doing in specific environments to enhance word recognition or to degrade it. They give the clinician little information about what needs to be changed in hearing aid acoustic performance to achieve greater patient acceptance, use, and satisfaction. In the future, more stress will be given to the benefit of amplification using a number of parameters reflecting the environments in which communication takes place. There will always be, in all probability, the need to "fine tune" the response to achieve greater user acceptance of the hearing aid by altering its frequency/gain response.

Part of the problem in determining hearing aid satisfaction and benefit has to do with the time period patients have to make a decision to purchase or return the instrument(s). Typically, 30 days is the standard time frame. If the patient fails to realize benefit, however defined, the instrument is returned. Unfortunately, for some if not most, it may take longer than 30 days for the patient to really gain maximum benefit. The evaluation period could be much longer before the decision to purchase has to be made. There is no absolute time period when a patient adjusts to a new auditory image, but 60 days does not seem to be overextension of the evaluation period. The optimal time frame to gain maximum benefit from amplification is related to the magnitude and type of hearing impairment, as well as that period from hearing loss onset to the use of amplification.

Of course, an extension of the evaluation period is anathema to some clinicians who dispense hearing aids. Some may feel that it places a needless financial burden on them because the manufacturer's policy on return does not permit time extensions. It does not seem unreasonable that some changes in return policies could be made to encourage longer evaluation periods. It just may be that the acceptance of hearing aid use, and subsequent purchase of it, would result from such a policy. At this moment, there are some manufacturers offering extended evaluation periods. As we gain more information about the time needed to gain optimal benefit from amplification, it is likely that there will be an industry-wide acceptance of the necessity of doing this. It is highly probable that if longer evaluation periods were universally offered, greater emphasis would be placed on measures of satisfaction, benefit, and acceptance. Lacking absolute consensus, the generally accepted timeframe for one to adapt to the new acoustic environment created by the hearing aid is about 6 to 8 weeks.

Psychological Management of the Hearing Impaired Patient

Unfortunately, too many hearing health care professionals fail to appreciate the behavioral and emotional changes that some persons with hearing impairment experience (Goetzinger, 1972; Hansen, 1998; Kaplan, 1992; Orlans, 1985; Ramsdell, 1964; Reiter, 1985; Sandlin, 1974; Sweetow, 1999). The issue is not whether amplification is desirable but whether the individual is emotionally prepared to evaluate or determine its contribution to the quality of life. It is a seeming contradiction that most who select and fit hearing aid devices are well aware of the psychological and emotional manifestations of hearing loss but fail to offer management strategies to deal with them. Most are aware that the severity of the psychological or emotion disturbance is related to the initial onset of hearing loss and its severity, as well as the length of time the hearing loss has been present before the use of amplification. Management protocols depend on this awareness and suggest that those with long-standing impairments may require different management and counseling strategies.

There is an urgent need to develop management strategies that address this issue. If emotional preparedness for hearing aid use were not an issue for many patients with hearing loss, how does one explain the high return rate of hearing aids to the manufacturer? One assumes that hearing aids are recommended based on the level of the hearing deficit and assumptions that they can improve word recognition in a number of environments. The return rate would suggest, in part, that the instrument could have been rejected because acceptance of amplification was not forthcoming. A return rate of 20% or more cannot be accounted for by concluding that the hearing aid was rejected for "unspecified reasons." Such vague statements offer little support for the rejection. Was it the electroacoustic response? Was it the cost? Was it the physical size? Was it cosmetic concern? Future concerns and practices may include some formal declaration for the reason for return of the instrument(s). There is a point in time when the practitioner must examine his or her approach to hearing instrument fitting, including those practices that need to be embraced to provide more than just a hearing aid that meets insertion gain requirements.

We need to give as much professional attention to the patient's emotional and psychological needs as we give to determining the correct electroacoustic performance of the recommended hearing aid. Such additional emphasis may demand a greater amount of professional time spent with the patient and significant others, but if greater attention is given to human concerns rather than just the objective analysis of instrument performance resulting in increased sales, then justification is evident. Meeting patient's "readiness" for amplification and giving clinical attention to acceptance, benefit, and satisfaction are rewarding to the user and to the clinician.

It is a given that those in private dispensing practices are concerned about the "bottom line." The bottom line is whether or not a profit is being realized. Sacrificing financial gain to deal with the psychological and emotional states of the patient is not the goal. One should base part of the retail cost of the hearing aid on patient counseling demands, which can result in a more effective and realistic management of the patient. In essentially all cases of hearing impairment sufficient to interfere with communication, the patient is aware of the problem. The dispenser's task, for the most part, is not to inform the patient that he or she has a loss of hearing based on audiologic data, but to assist the patient in realizing the advantages of amplification in resolving social interaction affected by hearing loss. Current and future challenges facing the hearing health care professional are those of managing the patient in such a manner that emotional and psychological barriers are removed.

The hearing aid candidates of today are much more informed about hearing aids than were their counterparts 10 years ago. They seek professional help and guidance from those whom they feel to be technically competent and who understand their reluctance or apprehension associated with hearing aid use. Future successful practices must include organized management strategies as an effective method of amalgamating behavior-related components into the provision of adequate services.

The Implications of Managed Care Affecting Dispensing Practices

With the emergence of health maintenance organizations (HMOs) and their subsequent competition to attract and keep subscribers, benefits have been extended to include the purchase of hearing aids. As a result, many hearing health care professionals have entered into contracts with one or more HMOs to provide hearing aid services consistent with managed care practices. In reality, the position of the HMO is one of establishing allowable financial assistance for hearing aid purchase. In some instances, the HMO plan may underwrite the cost for one instrument only. One of the possible reasons driving the HMO to offer hearing aids to its subscribers is to maintain or increase members. The more patient services managed care providers offer, the more attractive it becomes for current and potential subscribers.

Unfortunately, the number of dollars the HMO allows for the purchase of hearing aids often falls far short of what the normal retail cost of the hearing aid would be for non-members. The clinician is faced with a decision that may greatly affect his or her practice and introduce possible ethical considerations with which one must contend. Does one offer to the HMO member a discounted price, thus taking possible financial advantage of those patients who do not qualify for a discount? Is the clinician forced to offer discounts to the member as well as the nonmember? If discounts are offered to both, does it affect the selection of instruments best meeting the acoustic needs of the patient? In some practices, greater discounts are given for the less expensive instruments than for the high-performance devices. If discounts are offered to all patients because of contracts with HMOs demanding discounted pricing, does it affect in any way the quality of care? Suppose a high-performance hearing aid has a retail cost of X dollars. The retail cost was determined in part by how much it costs to manage the practice, provide adequate professional services, and support a predetermined lifestyle. What happens when many potential customers in the clinician's geographic area belong to an HMO? The dilemma is one of deciding: (1) Should one enter into a contractual agreement with the HMO to provide audiological and hearing aid services and thus increase one's customer base, (2) ignore the influence of HMOs on dispensing practice and increase a promotion and advertising budget to attract those who do not belong to HMOs, or (3) compete by discounting the cost of hearing instruments to everyone?

If the clinician opts to have a contractual agreement with the HMO, offering discounts becomes mandatory. If discounts are offered, can one continue to offer the same quality of care or provide the same level of technology available in the high-performance hearing aid group? If the quality of care is lessened, has one fulfilled his or her ethical obligations to the patient?

On the other hand, let us assume that the clinician decides to remain independent of HMOs and vigorously implements a promotional strategy to attract new clients into the office. By so doing must he or she increase the retail cost of the hearing aid to cover the additional expense incurred by promotion and marketing activities? If the retail cost of hearing aids is increased, does it introduce a significant barrier to potential users seeking the clinician's services? Lastly, if the clinician decides to compete with the HMO and discounts the retail cost of all hearing instruments, the discounted price will still be higher than the discounted price dictated by the HMO. If such is the case, then the problems facing the clinician are not too different than had he or she entered into some formal arrangement with the HMO. That is, does any discounting reflect on the ways services are rendered?

The HMO influence may be more pronounced in large urban areas. Let us assume there are a number of HMOs in a large metropolitan area; the greater the number of managed care facilities, the greater the number of subscribers in that age group having hearing loss. Let us assume further that the plan of each HMO provides for hearing aids. There is one more assumption to make. In this large metropolitan area, there are a large number of dispensing facilities. Given these "assumed" conditions, the HMO enters into contractual agreements with those dispensing facilities offering the greatest discounted prices. The clinician must decide what the consequences are if a contractual arrangement is made with the managed care facility, as well as determining what the consequences are if he or she does not. Either way, it presents an interesting problem.

This is not to suggest that there is some common ground, or agreement, among managed care organizations that dictates the type of contract offered to the dispensing facility. There is none. For example, if there is only one HMO and one dispensing facility in a given area, the type of arrangement would be significantly different. In all probability, the hearing aid dispensing facility would be in a much better position to get a favorable contract.

The issue that must be decided at some point in time is this: What are the professional responsibilities of the dispensing facility and are they compromised in any way by contractual managed care practices? The author believes that decision making regarding the hearing instrument of choice and the level of professional care should be made, or dictated, by the hearing health care professional and not a bureaucratic functionary working for a managed care facility. Managed care agencies are a part of life. Although they may undergo change, they will not disappear from the health management scene. The professional dispenser must deal with their existence by clearly defining what constitutes a reasonable agreement without sacrificing ethical concerns and meeting the amplification needs of the patient.

Meeting Mandatory Hearing Aid Performance Criteria

With the advent of state licensure for those who dispense hearing instruments and the probable influence of managed care facilities, greater demands will be placed on those who dispense to offer objective support of what the hearing aid is providing to the individual with hearing impairment. In the future, there is a distinct possibility that clinicians will be forced (by law) to submit clinical evidence that the hearing instrument is meeting some mandatory standard of performance. At the moment there is no federal, national, or state mandate dictating what the hearing aid must do in order for a sale to be consummated. State hearing aid dispensing regulatory bodies have some form of appeals board for those patients dissatisfied with their hearing aid or with the clinician's level of service. Complaints are resolved by mutual consent between the two parties, or the "ethics committee" will recommend a reasonable settlement of the dispute. There are no laws dictating that the hearing aid provide a certain level of audibility for a given frequency bandwidth, a specific level of word recognition based on some frequency/gain formula, permissible intermodulation, or harmonic or other types of distortion products. There are no federal, national, or state statutes demanding that a standard of user satisfaction be met based on data derived from current or future subjective assessment tools and that a given level of benefit has been achieved.

These projected future demands may not be unrealistic. It is not beyond reasonable projection that institutional demands (e.g., from HMOs) to meet minimal electroacoustic or subjective performance requirements will become standard practice. Professionally, this may be a positive benefit, both to the hearing instrument dispenser and to the patient. It makes little difference if one is "forced" to abide by mandatory standards established by those outside the dispensing profession. It may be of little consequence whether or not minimal performance standards are developed by professional bodies. The appropriate professional body should shoulder the burden of developing standards of aided hearing aid performance, however.

The important issue is whether a guideline will exist for assuring that the selected instrument is providing positive benefit. Another advantage of such standards is that those patients who would reject the hearing aid on frivolous grounds cannot do so if the minimal performance standards are met.

Ethical Considerations: Future Implications

For most in private practice, hearing aid dispensing is their main source of income. Ethical practice involves something more than a casual familiarity with a "code of ethics" defined by a professional body or agency. It reflects the honesty with which clinical decisions are reached and the ways in which patients are managed. Ethical practice, in effect, must always put the patient first in decision making relating to selection, fitting, and follow-up care. To do otherwise would be to abdicate the professional responsibility one accepts when entering institutional or private practice. Future considerations will involve an ethical defense of practices associated with instrument dispensing and patient management strategies.

There is a marked difference between legal requirements and ethical practices (see Chapter 22). Legally, one must adhere to certain standards of performance. Failing to do so could result in official reprimand or loss of licensure. Ethically, one has a choice related to hearing aid selection and the provision of subsequent care. There is no legal restriction placed upon the selection of hearing aids to meet acoustic needs, for example. Ethically, however, the clinician should be bound to select that instrument most suited for the hearing loss. The clinician should be bound to explain the limitations and advantages of the hearing aid(s) selected and to provide rehabilitative care consistent with the needs of the patient, even though there is no legal requirement to do so. The clinician should be ethically bound to understand technological advances in hearing aids and whether such advances contribute to the ability of the patient to perform as well as possible in a host of acoustic environments. The clinician should be ethically bound to understand the relationship between the existing pathologies and the application of amplification devices in meeting individual needs. The clinician should be ethically bound to discuss instrument costs. Should the patient be financially unable to afford the recommended aid, there should be a frank discussion of the consequences of so doing. The discussion should involve a review of the limitations of the less expensive aid and well as its contributions. There are no legal requirements, other than mandatory continuing education, that the clinician be current (e.g., with the pathophysiology of the auditory system or the implications imposed for those with central auditory processing disorders). Ethically, one should be bound to understand various disorders and the subsequent influence each has in hearing aid use and patient management considerations.

Ethical considerations go beyond fitting a hearing aid to an acoustically impaired ear. Ethical considerations involve an approach to patient management, which says in effect every effort is made to find the best solution to amplification needs. The patient will understand the rationale underlying the selection process, rationale for instrument cost, and rationale for rehabilitative practices involving adaptation to amplified sound and dealing with the psychological and emotional consequences often associated with hearing loss. Future programs for training clinicians to select and dispense hearing aids must include discussions of ethical considerations in the decision-making and management processes.

Retail Costs of Hearing Aids: Another Dilemma

The cost of hearing aids is a matter to be resolved by the hearing health care professional. There is one question to address relating to retail costs of hearing aid systems, however: *"Have the retail costs of hearing aids been overinflated by the introduction of DSP technology and other high-performance hearing aids?"* Some, maybe most, would argue that it should be of little if any concern to anyone other than the individual dispenser. The author would beg to differ. It is true that the introduction of digital signal processing hearing aids has contributed to the abilities of the person with hearing impairment to react more favorably to his or her acoustic environment. It is true that current retail costs of high performance hearing aids have prevented many patients with hearing loss from taking advantage of the advances offered by DSP technology and other high-performance hearing instruments. The dilemma is one of having an excellent product, but one which is not within the financial means of a substantial segment of the population. This is not and argument for a cheap, inferior DSP hearing aid. Nonetheless, inflated hearing aid costs restrict the number of individuals who can benefit.

There are two reasonable paths to follow in reducing retail costs without great financial loss to those involved. One is that of having manufacturers reduce the wholesale cost of the instrument to the dispenser. The other is having the professional dispenser reduce the retail cost. By so doing, there are advantages accruing to each party. The manufacturer produces more units because of the reduction in wholesale costs, and the dispenser increases the number of sales because of the lowering of retail costs. Some may argue that this is a simplistic answer and begs the question involving the rights inherent in free enterprise. The issue here has nothing to do with free enterprise or the capitalistic system. Both are to be cherished and defended. The issue is one of answering two questions: (1) "Am I charging too much for my product and by so doing greatly restricting the number of patients who could benefit from technological advances inherent in DSP products?" and (2) "Is there a positive correlation between the cost of the instrument and perceived or measured benefit?" If one looks at the market penetration of DSP products, it is less than 15%. This is a woefully small market share if one is correct in assuming that it reflects, in part, the relatively high cost of the high-performance product.

Pressure probably will be exerted on the manufacturer and the professional dispenser to take some positive action in more effectively managing the cost of high-performance hearing aids. Groups such as the American Association of Retired People (AARP), managed care facilities, and state and federal agencies underwriting hearing aid costs for qualified persons can and will affect current retail costs. Public opinion can exert great influence on the pricing structure for hearing aids. Focus groups have determined that a significant barrier to instrument purchase is the retail cost. Many of those on fixed incomes must budget their monies carefully. Such budgetary concerns determine permissible costs for a number of personal and assistive items.

Manufacturers may one day develop high-performance products at a lesser cost without sacrificing technical performance. Some dispensers may also readjust their retail cost for the same product to gain a greater patient base or market share. When truly advanced hearing aid technology is introduced, there is a tendency for some to exploit the novelty and advantages by setting retail costs at a relatively high level. This is done not because it must be, but because it can be.

If part of our ethical and professional concerns is to provide amplification systems offering improved performance function, are we not bound to establish a retail cost that permits the majority of those with hearing loss to benefit from technological advance? It is not suggested that one must jeopardize their own financial security to meet amplification needs of the patient or that everyone can afford high-performance hearing instruments. In the real world, there are limitations placed on a number of human conditions and needs reflected in one's ability to afford the best of care. As unfortunate as it may seem, it is a reality. It is equally as real to assume that the manufacturer and the professional dispenser have the right (not the obligation) to decide what is best for their own self-interest (the doctrine of enlightened self-interest) and preservation. In defense of readjusting the costs of high-performance hearing aids, there must be a benefit accrued to each party. These benefits are manifest by lower wholesale and retail sales and, as a result, a greater number of persons enjoy the subsequent benefits of advanced amplification devices. Manufacturers must reclaim the research and development costs for high-performance hearing aids; this is an economic necessity. Nonetheless, there must be a point in time when such R&D costs have been reclaimed, and adjustment of production costs can be entertained.

No one knows what the future holds for the reexamination of hearing aid costs and subsequent advantages to the hearing impaired population. It is quite possible, however, that future events will be determined in part by what the consumer is willing to pay for improved hearing performance. If mandatory minimal performance standards become common practice, will the dispenser always be able to defend the selection of more expensive hearing aid instruments? Therefore, this section of the "future" chapter may be only an academic exercise having little relationship to that which will ultimately transpire.

CONCLUSION

We live in exciting times, reflected in the challenges facing those who dispense hearing aids and the successful management of those who use them. The excitement is enhanced when one realizes that there must be a major revolution in the way we think about hearing aid amplification. Current thinking of some clinicians is mired in old, analog technologies. Outdated assessment procedures must give way to more modern approaches in utilizing the impressive new advances in hearing instrument performance. Greater knowledge will be required to carry out future hearing aid evaluation sequences. There will be significant changes in the ways that hearing aids are selected and fitted. Greater emphasis will be placed on validation and verification of hearing aid performance and use. More organized and functionally efficient rehabilitation programs will be developed. Greater emphasis must be given to patient management (counseling) to accelerate satisfaction and acceptance of hearing aids.

As it was yesterday and is today, future concerns must involve ongoing clinical research to assess the utility of innovative concepts applied to amplification systems. The development of effective verification and validation procedures common to all hearing aids needs to become a reality. Fitting strategies and subsequent software to facilitate and simplify the selection and fitting process will be forthcoming. These will become more important as sophisticated hearing aid systems are developed to interface with acoustic needs that are not being satisfied with current technology.

It must be reiterated that meaningful and intelligent counseling strategies need to be advanced so that clinicians of the future can present to the patient a realistic assessment of what can and cannot be expected from hearing aid amplification. In effect, future strategies will stress the involvement of the patient in determining if needs have been met and whether or not benefits of amplification can be expanded over time as one adapts to amplified sound and a new acoustic environment.

In the future, more demands will be placed on educational requirements before one is qualified to select, fit, and evaluate hearing aids. Universities and colleges will need to expand their current hearing aid science curriculum to keep abreast of technological advances and fitting practices. State and national organizations will place greater emphasis on continuing education. There will be a major increase in the number of professional persons utilizing "distance learning" to fulfill educational requirements for advanced degrees or eligibility requirements to maintain certification or licensure. Advances in technology, increases in the clinician's knowledge of auditory behavior, and greater understanding of human behavior demand that change be made to provide adequate care to the patient with hearing impairment. No longer will a high school education or its equivalent, or the passing of an examination where only minimal knowledge is required to become a licensed practitioner, be sufficient to meet the educational and clinical demands associated with the technology and clinical skills of tomorrow.

Finally, the future holds great promise for understanding and accepting the ethical considerations consistent with providing professional care to a population of persons with hearing impairment. Current observation would suggest that some of us who dispense hearing instruments fall short of absolute ethical practice by sins of *omission* rather than *commission*. Stress on ethical practice will emphasize "total care" of the patient. Not only will clinicians assess the magnitude of the hearing loss and select and fit the appropriate hearing aid, but they will also manage the patient over a sufficient period of time to ensure maximum benefit from amplification use. The patient will understand the limitations imposed by the hearing loss, as well as the limitations of existing technology in meeting acoustic needs. Conversely, the patient will know the benefits of amplification, based on knowledge shared by the clinician with the patient's own assessment of improvement in a number of communicative situations.

Indeed, the future portends a number of unique challenges that will test the academic and clinical skills of those who serve persons with hearing loss. Nonetheless, innovations reflected in technologically advanced hearing aids, advanced fitting and verifications strategies, and sensitive and caring counseling approaches will provide a great deal of personal and professional satisfaction in knowing that one has been instrumental in improving the quality of life for the individual with hearing impairment.

REFERENCES

Box, G. (1957). Evolutionary operation: A method for increasing industrial productivity. *Applied Statistics, 26*, 679–685.

Byrne, D., Parkinson, A., & Newall, R. (1991). Modified hearing aid selection procedures for severe/profound hearing losses. In G. Studebaker, F. Bess, & L. Beck (Eds.), *The Vanderbilt Hearing Aid Report II* (pp. 295–300). Parkton, MD: York Press.

Carhart, R. (1946). The selection of hearing aids. *Archives of Otolaryngology, 44*, 1–18.

Cox, R. M., & Alexander, G. C. (1992). Maturation of hearing aid benefit: Objective and subjective benefits. *Ear and Hearing, 143*, 131–141.

Cox, R. M., & McDaniel, D. M. (1984). Intelligibility rating of continuous discourse: Application to hearing aid selection. *Journal of the Acoustical Society of America, 76*, 758–766.

Cox, R. M., & McDaniel, D. M. (1992). Evaluation ratings of the speech intelligibility rating (SIR) test for hearing aid comparison. *Journal of Speech and Hearing Research, 35*, 686–693.

Dillon, H., & Walker, J. (1992). Comparison of stimuli used in sound field audiometric testing. *Journal of the Acoustical Society of America, 71*, 161–172.

Duffy, J. K. (1967). Audio-visuals speech audiometry and a new audio-visual speech perception index. *Maico Audiological Library Services, 5*(9), 1–3.

Duffy, J. (1978). Sound field audiometry and hearing aid advisement. *Hearing Instruments, 29*(2), 6–12.

Duffy, J. (1987). Sound field audiometry and hearing aid selection. In E. Zelnick (Ed.), *Hearing instrument: Selection and evaluation* (pp. 179–215). Livonia, MI: NIHIS.

Durrant, J. D., & Lovrinic, J. H. (1981). *Bases of hearing science* (2nd ed.). Baltimore: Williams and Wilkins.

Fabry, D. A., & Schum, D. J. (1984). The role of subjective measurement techniques in hearing aid fittings. In M. Valente (Ed.), *Strategies for selecting and verifying hearing aid fittings* (pp. 136–155). New York: Thieme Medical Publishers.

Harford, E. (1969). Is a hearing aid ever justified in unilateral hearing loss? In L. Boles (Ed.), Hearing loss—problems in diagnosis and treatment. *Otolaryngologic Clinics of North America*, pp. 153–173.

Hawkins, D., & Mueller, G. (1992). Test protocols for probe-microphone measurements. In G. Mueller, D. Hawkins, & J. Northern (Eds.), *Probe microphone measurements* (pp. 269–278). San Diego: College-Hill Press.

Hodgson, W. R. (1986). Special cases of hearing aid assessment. In W. R. Hodgson (Ed.), *Hearing aid assessment and use in audiologic habilitation* (3rd ed., pp. 191–216). Baltimore: Williams and Wilkins.

Kuk, F. K. (1994). Use of paired comparisons in hearing aid fittings. In M. Valente (Ed.), *Strategies for selecting and verifying hearing aid fittings* (pp. 108–135). New York: Thieme Medical Publishers.

Lawson, G. D., & Chial, M. R. (1982). Magnitude estimation of degraded speech quality by normal and hearing-impaired listeners. *Journal of the Acoustical Society of America, 72*, 1781–1787.

Mueller, H. G., Hawkins, D., & Northern, J. (1992). *Probe microphone measurements: Hearing aid selection and assessment*. San Diego: Singular Publishing Group.

Munson, W. A., & Karlin, J. E. (1962). Isoreference method of evaluating speech transmission circuits. *Journal of the Acoustical Society of America, 34*, 762–774.

Pavlovic, C. (1991). Speech recognition and five articulation indexes. *Hearing Instruments, 42*, 20–24.

Pollack, M. C. (1998). Special applications of amplification. In M. C. Pollack (Ed.), *Amplification for the hearing impaired* (3rd ed., pp. 295–328). New York: Grune and Stratton.

Posner, J., & Ventry, I. (1977). Relationships between comfortable loudness levels for speech and speech discrimination in sensorineural loss. *Journal of Speech and Hearing Disorders, 42*, 370–375.

Preves, D. (1990). Principles of signal processing. In R. E. Sandlin (Ed.), *Handbook of hearing aid amplification* (Vol. 1, pp. 81–120). San Diego: College-Hill Press.

Punch, J. L., & Parker, C. A. (1981). Pairwise listener preferences in hearing aid evaluation. *Journal of Speech and Hearing Research, 24*, 366–374.

Purdy, S. C. (1990). *Reliability, sensitivity, and validity of magnitude estimation, paired comparisons, and category scaling*. Unpublished doctoral dissertation, The University of Iowa, Iowa City.

Ross, M., & Duffy, J. (1961, November). *Report on sound field audiometry*. Paper presented at the American Speech and Hearing Convention, Chicago, IL.

Sandlin, R. E. (1995). Clinical application of soundfield audiometry. In R. E. Sandlin (Ed.), *Handbook of hearing aid amplification* (Vol. II, pp. 257–278). San Diego: College-Hill Press.

Schwartz, D., Lyregaard, R., & Lundh, R. (1988). Hearing aid selection for severe-to-profound hearing loss. *Hearing Journal, 41*, 13–17.

Shore, I., Bilger, R, & Hirsh, I. (1960). Hearing aid evaluation: Reliability of repeated measurements. *Journal of Speech and Hearing Disorders, 25*, 142–170.

Skinner, M. W. (1988). *Hearing aid evaluation* (pp. 212–219). Englewood Cliffs, NJ: Prentice-Hall.

Speaks, C., & Jerger, J. (1965). Method for measurement of speech identification. *Journal of Speech and Hearing Research, 8*, 185–194.

Studebaker, G. A. (1991). Measures of intelligiblity and quality. In G. Studebaker, E. Bess, & L. Beck (Eds.), *The Vanderbilt Hearing-aid Report II* (pp. 185–195). Parkton, MD: York Press.

Studebaker, G. A., & Sherbecole, R. L. (1988). Magnitude estimation of the intelligibility and quality of speech in noise. *Ear and Hearing, 9*, 259–267.

Sweetow, R. (1994). Fitting strategies for noise-induced hearing loss. In M. Valente (Ed.), *Strategies for selecting and verifying hearing aid fittings* (pp. 156–179). New York: Thieme Medical Publishers.

Tecca, J. (1995). Clinical applications of real-ear probe tube measurement. In R. Sandlin (Ed.), *Handbook of hearing aid amplification. Vol. II: Clinical considerations and fitting practices* (pp. 225–255). San Diego: College-Hill Press.

Thornton, A., & Rafin, M. (1978). Speech discrimination scores modeled as a bimodal variable. *Journal of Speech and Hearing Research, 21*, 507–518.

Valente, M., Valente, M., Meister, M., Macauley, K., & Vass, W. (1994). Selecting and verifying hearing aid fittings for unilateral hearing loss. In M. Valente (Ed.), *Strategies for selecting and verifying hearing aid fittings* (pp. 228–248). New York: Thieme Medical Publishers.

Victoreen, J. (1973). *Hearing enhancement*. Springfield, IL: Charles C. Thomas.

Walden, B. E., Schwartz, D. M., & Williams, D. L. (1983). Test of the assumptions underlying comparative hearing aid evaluations. *Journal of Speech and Hearing Disorders, 48*, 264–273.

Walker, G., Dillon, H., & Byrne, D. (1984). The use of loudness discomfort levels for selecting the maximum output of hearing aids. *Australian Journal of Audiology, 6*, 23–32.

Walker, G. (1990). Technical considerations for sound field audiometry. In R. Sandlin (Ed.), *Handbook of hearing aid amplification* (Vol. I, pp. 146–164). San Diego: College-Hill Press.

Woodward, C. M., & Tecca, J. E. (1985). The use of pure tone stimuli in a soundfield. *Hearing Journal, 38*, 21–27.

Zelnick, E. (1982). Selecting frqeuency response. *Hearing Journal, 35*(3), 31.

Index

A

B

C

D

E

F

I

J

K

L

M

N

O

P

Q

R

S

T

U

V

W

X

Y

Z